ALSO BY JOHN W. FARQUHAR, M.D.

*The American Way of Life Need Not Be
Hazardous to Your Health*

THE
LAST
PUFF

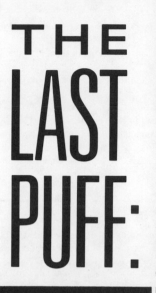

THE LAST PUFF:

EX-SMOKERS SHARE THE SECRETS OF THEIR SUCCESS

JOHN W. FARQUHAR, M.D.
GENE A. SPILLER, PH.D.

W. W. NORTON & COMPANY
NEW YORK LONDON

Copyright © 1990 John W. Farquhar and Gene A. Spiller

All rights reserved.

Printed in the United States of America.

The text of this book is composed in 11/15 Baskerville, with
display type set in Univers 49 and 63. Composition and
manufacturing by The Haddon Craftsmen, Inc.
Book design by Jo Anne Metsch.

First Edition

Library of Congress Cataloging-in-Publication Data

✓Farquhar, John W., 1927—,
The last puff: ex-smokers share the secrets of their success
John W. Farquhar, Gene A. Spiller.—1st ed.
p.   cm.
1. Ex-smokers—Interviews.   2. Cigarette smokers—Psychology—Case
studies.   3. Tobacco habit.   ✓I. Spiller, Gene A.   II. Title.
HV5748.F37 1990
613.85—dc20   89–16182

ISBN 0-393-02789-9

W. W. Norton & Company, Inc., 500 Fifth Avenue, New York, N.Y. 10110
W. W. Norton & Company Ltd., 37 Great Russell Street, London WC1B 3NU

1 2 3 4 5 6 7 8 9 0

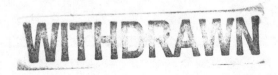

*For C. Everett Koop, who as Surgeon General
of the United States courageously worked for
a smoke-free country.*

*And for the ex-smokers whose stories and ideas
made this book possible.*

CONTENTS

9

CONTENTS

10

AUTHORS' NOTE

The idea for this book came to us when we realized that there was no popular book in which ex-smokers tell their own stories of how they were successful in giving up the habit. We already knew that the great majority of people who have quit—approximately 95 percent, according to recent research—have done so on their own. How did they do it? we wondered. What made them successful—finally? We decided to interview men and women of all ages and many different professions, to try and answer these questions.

The interviews (Chapter 4) are the heart of the book. In the ex-smokers' own words, they reflect their inner feelings and reveal how each person stopped in his or her own way, often inventing a special method. Chapters 1, 2, and 3 set the stage for the stories, and Chapters 5, 6, and 7 discuss some of the highlights of these stories in view of our current knowledge of smoking and addiction.

We want to express our thanks to our many colleagues at the Stanford Center for Research in Disease Prevention, who have contributed so much to our thinking about the issues of smoking and health and whose research is of inestimable help in the battle against nicotine addiction.

A special acknowledgment goes to Christine Farquhar, for her valuable writing and editing skills as *The Last Puff* developed; to Carol Kino, who aided in designing and setting up the early interviews; to Margaret Denny, for her editorial assistance; to Sara Godwin, who carried out some of the interviews and was very valuable in the final stages of manuscript preparation; and to Becki Carr, who transcribed many hours of taped interviews with great professional skill.

A special role was played by Carol Houck Smith of W. W. Norton. From the inception of this work to final edited manuscript, this book would not have been possible without her deep involvement. Her skillful editing and her many suggestions have made this book what it is now. As an ex-smoker as well as an editor, she brought her personal feelings and knowledge to the book in a unique way.

THE
LAST
PUFF

DIFFERENT KEYS,
DIFFERENT LOCKS

What is the pivotal event that makes it possible for someone to quit smoking permanently, often after a long period of excruciating failures? Why do some people decide to give up the habit and never touch another cigarette, while others fail miserably in their repeated attempts to quit smoking?

Consider for example the story of Dick W., a fifty-nine-year-old man. He is a smoker now, but he has tried to quit many times. Once he was successful for fifteen years!

"I had smoked for about eighteen years, from 1948 to 1966, when four of us at work had the urge to quit smoking: We each took $500 and gave it to a fifth person to hold. Anybody who smoked during the course of a year would lose his interest in the pot, and anybody who held out to the end would split the pot.

"Of the three other guys who quit with me, one started to smoke again within two months, another one within six months, so the third guy and I split the $2,000 pot.

"I made it through the next fourteen years without a cigarette, but in 1980 my wife died very, very suddenly. She was only forty-eight and she died in her sleep one night—probably of diabetes.

"I had a cigarette within twenty-four hours after she died. Somebody offered me a cigarette, and I've wanted to cuss him out ever since. I smoked one, and that one led to another, and another led to another. All I had to do was touch one.

"It was the trauma of my wife dying, the sorrow.

"I know I shouldn't be smoking, but I married again at the end of 1982. My new wife is a very heavy smoker, and it's extremely difficult to have just one partner in a marriage give up cigarettes. About a year after we were married we made a pact that we would quit, and we did quit for a month or two. But she was having trouble with her teen-age son and she went back to smoking. That made it very easy for me to go back too. We quit again the first of this year for about a month. I don't know why we started smoking again.

"We keep talking about quitting again. We both want to quit."

While many people will find Dick W.'s story all too familiar, many others have succeeded in conquering their addiction to smoking. It is fascinating to unravel the mysteries of quitting to see how a person evolves from being a smoker to being a non-smoker. The best way to observe the process is to let former smokers tell us why and how they quit.

That is what this book is all about. It's a collection of real, intriguing life stories of people who have successfully quit smoking. You'll meet people from all walks of life, men and women of all ages. You may identify more with some of these people than others, but you should read all the stories. Every one contains fascinating insights into the goals, failures, and ultimate triumph of a former smoker. And each carries the message of hope: You *can* quit smoking. All of these people have done it.

There are about 43 million adult Americans who have given up smoking since 1967. Until now, no one has officially asked them how they did it or gathered their stories in a book. Ninety-five percent or so of those 43 million quit without the help of formal clinics or classes. They quit on their own, by themselves. They did it their own way, every one a different approach, every one a successful solution.

Can the interviews in this book help the 65 million people in the United States who still smoke? Ninety-five percent of those who would like to stop will do it by marshaling their own resources, as most people do. When people see their own experience in someone else's story, they often know better what to do and how to do it and can even gain the courage to do it.

THE FIRST SUCCESS STORY:
SOMETHING CLICKED

Fortunately, ex-smokers are willing to share the secrets of their success. Of course, they deserve to have pride in their accomplishments, but we've also found that people respond in a marvelous way to the idea of helping their fellow humans. That's the spirit you'll find in this book.

For the moment now, John Farquhar is not the physician, the cardiologist involved in preventive medicine who is one of the authors of this book. Instead, John is an ex-smoker, relaxing on his sofa at home and telling his own story. The tape recorder is running. . . .

"When I graduated from high school it was wartime, and I was recruited into a college program called the Army Specialized Training Reserve program. I was seventeen. Toward the end of my first year, I met a girl from California. She was a smoker. We danced to the recordings of the Glenn Miller band and we fell in love. She taught me to smoke. Smoking seemed very sophisticated and very much the right thing to do for a young man in love in wartime. Three months later I was shipped out to basic training. I quit smoking for several months, but the Army's weekly ration of free cigarettes got me started again, and I smoked my way through most of the Occupation.

"In Europe I quit for a while for economic reasons. Our post in Belgium was responsible for shipping the

American troops home. It was standard operating procedure for returning American soldiers to deal in the black market. The opportunity to exchange those free cigarettes for cameras and things of that sort was a very strong motivation to stop smoking. I stayed off cigarettes while I was in Belgium in 1946, and in Germany later on, as well.

"By the time I returned to the United States at age nineteen, I had already started and stopped smoking several times. I started smoking again as an undergraduate at UCLA. I was in a fraternity, and I think the percentage of men who smoked was well over 75 percent. In the immediate postwar era it was standard for men to smoke, particularly those who had been through World War II in any way, shape, or form. I was a confirmed smoker throughout college, four years of medical school, one year of internship, and three and a half years of residency. I was a pack-a-day smoker, as most people were.

"I particularly recall smoking during my internship and residency. There is a certain set formality to making ward rounds in a hospital. It's done in the morning, we were expected to be there fairly early, and we were expected to see every patient. There would be an intern, a medical student, a couple of residents, and perhaps the chief resident, all making the rounds together. We always had an aluminum cart on wheels, about five feet high and three and a half feet wide, which held two rows of patients' charts with aluminum covers on them and a patient's name on each of the slots in front.

"Well, on the top of that chart cart we'd have a couple

of ashtrays. Perhaps one out of four or five of us didn't smoke, but by and large, everyone smoked. We would have our cigarettes in our mouths outside in the hall and we would be smoking and taking a puff and talking about the case and then we would go into the room. If it was a one-bed room or a two-bed room, we would tend to leave our cigarettes burning on the ashtray outside and go in and come out before the cigarette had burned up. But if it was a four-bed room or a six-bed room, we would wheel the cart in and we would go to the bedside. We didn't keep the cigarettes in our mouths while we were listening through the stethoscope—we had enough politeness and wisdom to leave the smoking cigarettes in the ashtray at least—but that's what we did.

"The patients were often very sick, maybe they even had major lung disease, but no one considered whether or not it might be bad for them to have four or five people smoking in their room. It never even occurred to us that it might smell bad, or leave a lingering stale tobacco odor, or offend someone. Why would we consider esthetics when we didn't have the awareness, as physicians, to consider the impact on our patients' health? The whole attitude of society toward smoking was completely different then. We were men; men smoked.

"And there were cigarette machines in the hospital lobby. The patients were smoking, so you would have these hospital rooms full of smoke. That was just the norm.

"There was absolutely no pressure on us in medical school not to smoke. And by this time I had finished my residency and I had finished a year and a half of a post-doctoral fellowship in cardiology, so I was a fully trained physician.

"The only pressure came from my father, who kept after me in a subtle but persistent way. He had been an athlete when he was younger, and he knew instinctively that smoking was bad for the body, but when he would say I should stop he found it difficult to explain why. He just said that it wasn't good for me, and then I'd say, under my breath, 'Well, *I'm* the doctor. What do *you* know?' I dismissed his instinctive knowledge.

"But thinking about the origin of his opposition to smoking, I remember a story he told me about his father, an immigrant from Scotland who lived in Canada. He and his wife raised a large family—there were thirteen children and eight survivors—and his father was a very religious man. Once he caught one of my father's brothers, David, out in the barn smoking. And he said, 'If the good Lord had intended you to smoke, He would have put a smokestack up on the top of your head.' I am guessing that my father may have absorbed a kind of ethos from his father about smoking being wrong.

"In 1958 I had completed my training and was getting ready to move to New York City to work at the Rockefeller Institute for Medical Research. I developed bronchitis. I was coughing, and I knew I had to leave for New York in about a week. It was about eight o'clock at night and I was in a little, damp, musty, windowless San Francisco basement study. I was sitting at my desk and very intense about getting things done that I had to get done.

21

I remember to this day how I felt. I had been sick. I had a bad cold and it had stayed in my lungs; I had bronchitis, and I kept coughing. I was smoking at my desk as usual and I took a deep puff. I inhaled it, blew it out the way you do in ordinary smoking, and as I did, I coughed. I can remember, I had the cigarette in my hand, and I coughed. Suddenly something clicked. I said to myself, 'Hey, this is crazy. Here you are, you've got bronchitis, you breathe in the cigarette smoke, and it makes you cough. That's dumb.' At that moment I quit.

"I had no plans to quit. I had never even thought about quitting before. I hadn't written down a quit date, I hadn't read anything about how you're supposed to do it, and I didn't know anyone who had quit. But from that night on, I have never had a cigarette. After I stopped, I think I probably got a little stubborn about staying off. But there was a weird thing: There were people in my life who were very close to me who knew I smoked. I chose not to announce the fact that I'd quit, and for two weeks no one noticed that I'd stopped smoking. I was upset. Here I'd done something difficult and I was proud of myself and nobody even noticed.

"Did I suffer? I did. I remember being irritable. I remember a good deal of irritability, stress, and discomfort, but I got through by invoking a spirit of stubbornness within. I gave myself a very strong message: 'You are now a non-smoker and you are not going to smoke any more.' Within a few months, I didn't have any desire to smoke.

"Eventually I became the kind of person that a lot of

22

ex-smokers are. You become very, very aware of other people's smoking. I can sniff it out and don't like it at all. Some of my friends tell me that they'll have a nightmare and imagine they are going back, but I don't remember any of that. I don't remember dreams, and I don't remember feeling tempted.

"I've told the medical students in a course I teach in personal health that I wish I'd had teachers who said something about what was good for *our* health. In the first year of medical school there was one doctor who said we ought to have good posture, and he tried to show us what good posture was. Beyond that, it was straight science. We weren't taught how to take care of ourselves; we were taught how to treat various diseases. There was not one whisper about, 'You ought to take care of yourself, you ought to get enough sleep, you ought to eat sensibly, you ought to exercise, you ought to maintain a reasonable weight.' Certainly, no one ever said you shouldn't smoke." The tape recorder is off, John's interview is over.

FORM A BOND WITH SUCCESS

Imagine the interviews in this book as a lock and key. Each lock-and-key combination opens the doors to different houses or cars, but the result is the same: They let you into your own house or car. The diversity in quitting methods is like different keys opening different locks, but the result—quitting—is the same. There is a different lock and a different key for each individual.

What you need to do, then, is find the key among the stories in this book that opens *your* own door to quitting successfully. Look at each key and decide whether it will work for you. The more you see of yourself in the story of someone who used a particular key, the better that key will fit you.

In smoking cessation classes, the participants' smoking histories are revealed and shared by the whole group before they move on to quitting techniques. The problems that each individual encounters on the way toward non-smoking are shared as well. The class develops a group spirit. There is camaraderie, a spirit of helping that extends beyond quitting smoking.

That same spirit of helping and sharing is present in the interviews that follow. If you are a smoker, be inspired, get motivated, learn from these people. They can teach you the tricks of the trade, things that we in medicine don't necessarily have in our bag of tricks. In the interviews you'll hear your own voice coming back to you.

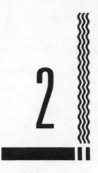

THE LIFE OF A SMOKER:
FROM FIRST TO LAST PUFF

Each smoker's story is different, fascinating, and unique, from the first cigarette to the very last. However, as individual as these stories are, as different as the individual lives may be, they have in common some typical developmental events:

1. The difficult, often nauseating first puff
2. The social pressure to smoke
3. The addiction, physical and psychological
4. A period of heavy smoking with no thought of quitting
5. An incubation period of attempts to quit and relapses
6. A triggering event that leads to quitting (often with a device or personal gimmick)

7. A phase of missing cigarettes and loving secondhand smoke

8. The final phase, when the ex-smoker rejects smoking and typically objects to others who smoke

THE LEARNING PROCESS

The interesting thing about smoking is that it's actually very difficult to get started because the initial experience is usually unpleasant. That first puff can be pretty vile, and many people who never became smokers say it's because they couldn't stand the taste of the first cigarette, so they never had another. One puff is often all it takes to make novice smokers dizzy or nauseated. Inhaling is enough to bring tears to their eyes and make them cough. Lots of first-time smokers feel themselves turning green and end up throwing up. Young people who experiment with smoking sometimes play tough and hide from their friends that they think it's awful. The real wonder is that anybody manages to get through the *first puff* to become addicted to nicotine.

Even though it usually takes a long time before inhaling can be carried off gracefully, new smokers pick up the social aspects of smoking very quickly. We sometimes refer to this as the *acculturation* process. People learn when to light up and when not to. They imitate the style of smokers they admire, in hopes of appearing more mature and in control. By careful observation they learn how to hold the cigarette properly, how to inhale without coughing wildly, and how to affect an appropriately sophisticated expression to go with their newly acquired savoir-faire.

Many people go through the process of learning to smoke secretly and in private, wondering why they are doing it, until the unanticipated moment when the nicotine itself begins to take hold and causes a physical addiction. By then, they may already be psychologically addicted. It takes from six months to a year to get hooked on nicotine.

ADDICTION

Being hooked is another way of saying *addicted.* It's ironic: The smoker who may well have had a tough time getting used to smoking now cannot get through a day without cigarettes. Deprived of the opportunity to smoke for a few hours, the serious smoker will fantasize about smoking, feel desperately uncomfortable, become twitchy and nervous, and go to great lengths to get a cigarette.

Some smokers go out at three in the morning and drive through snow to get a pack of cigarettes. Others pay a small fortune for theater tickets and then run out to the lobby every thirty minutes for a cigarette break, missing a third of the play in the process. This is addiction; this is being hooked on tobacco. Sounds familiar, doesn't it? And yet now people talk about nicotine addiction as if it were a brand-new discovery!

Morphine, cocaine, and nicotine have these features in common:

They are all drugs that act on the brain and the nerves, such as the nerves in the spinal cord.

The spread of dependence is socially mediated and is persistent; relapse is common.

Use persists in the face of serious damage, both individual and social.

These drugs are *psychoactive euphoriants,* two big words that really mean they make you feel happy. Tolerance and physical dependence are produced by repeated drug administration. Tolerance means that after a person has used the drug for a while it takes a bigger dose to produce the same "feel-good" effect. In the case of nicotine, the smoker goes from a couple of cigarettes a day to a pack a day or more.

It is possible, and even likely, that some people are more susceptible to nicotine addiction than others. It is clear that the addiction to nicotine is as strong as the addiction to heroin. The evidence for the powerful hold of nicotine is frightening. If you take people who are smokers and withhold cigarettes from them but give them syringes containing nicotine, they will inject nicotine into their veins, exactly like heroin addicts.

Psychological Addiction

Psychological addiction is closely interwoven with lifestyle. All smokers develop their own habits of smoking: while drinking coffee, talking on the telephone, or driving the car, or after sex. Stress often triggers the urge: having a quarrel, getting caught in traffic, hearing upsetting news. Pleasant situations such as chatting at a party, having a drink with friends, or relaxing after dinner also trigger the desire for a cigarette. Sometimes the trigger is no more than wanting to have something to do with your hands or the familiar ritual of lighting up.

The Russian physiologist Pavlov, in famous experiments with dogs, showed that if a bell was rung whenever the dog was fed, after a few weeks the bell alone would cause the dog to salivate, even if there wasn't any food. Smokers become conditioned in a similar way. They smoke in the context of their daily activities, and after a while certain activities associated with smoking become in themselves a stimulus to smoke.

In the smoking narratives in Chapter 4 you'll read about people who, after stopping smoking, began to play with pens and pencils to keep their hands busy, or ate candy and chewed gum to deal with their desire for oral gratification. They still felt the stimulus to smoke, but they substituted other activities for smoking.

Physical Addiction

Physical addiction is less understood, and much of what is known has been withheld from the American public. This information needs to be made public and emphasized to help young people choose not to smoke.

There are centers in the brain that are crucial in transmitting nervous impulses. These centers use specific chemical substances—*neurotransmitters*—that are synthesized at the end of the nerve, ready to transfer impulses to the next nerve cells. These *nerve endings* become saturated with nicotine, which acts as a substitute neurotransmitter that produces a "jolt" in the brain. The brain records nicotine in these nerve cells as the psychological feelings of tranquility and alertness, and that leads to *dependency* or *physical addiction.*

Research may provide ways to prevent nicotine from affecting the transmission of signals in the brain. For now, the best way to prevent addiction is not to smoke.

The key feature of addiction is that if you do not have the drug, you crave it. And after you take the addicting substance regularly for a long period of time, you become so used to it that you slowly find you need more and more of the substance to get the same effect. This is what happens with nicotine.

Another feature of addiction is that you continue doing it even though it doesn't taste good or feel good and you know it's bad for you. Studies of committed smokers—those famous pack-a-day "average" smokers—have shown that the smoker *wants* only three or four cigarettes a day. The others are smoked to keep the blood level of nicotine up, that is, to satisfy the physical addiction. Watch the faces of addicted smokers having their first puff after not smoking for two or three hours. They will draw the smoke in deeply, hold it a long time, and let it out slowly. A wave of relaxation and pleasure spreads over their faces. That is the nicotine fix.

The most frightening aspect of nicotine addiction is that people will continue their dangerous behavior despite known harm to their health and their bodies, and even when they have personally experienced the consequences they continue to smoke. Some people who have emphysema or who have had a cancerous lung removed continue to smoke in spite of the devastating damage they have suffered. That demonstrates the terrible strength of the addiction to nicotine.

Serious smokers know exactly how many cigarettes to smoke, and when, in order to keep their nicotine level up so they don't start to feel bad. The brain signals, "Okay, it's time," and the smoker starts checking pockets or purse for the pack of cigarettes. Before smokers get on a two-hour flight on an airline where smoking is banned, they are likely to take a few extra-deep puffs because they know the fix has to last. Nicotine produces effects that are considered therapeutic by users; that's part of the euphoriant, "feel-good" effect.

It's important to recognize the connection between nicotine addiction and heroin addiction: The curve of relapse for people who have quit taking heroin and that for people who have stopped smoking are almost identical. In less technical language, nicotine is as addictive as heroin, and the habit is as hard to kick. It is shocking to contemplate that in the United States it is legal to produce, advertise, and sell a drug that is so dangerous to health and so addictive. It seriously threatens the health of the smoker as well as the health of those who merely breathe the cigarette smoke. No government in the world would allow that for heroin!

When cigarette labels were changed a few years ago,

the government did order the cigarette companies to label cigarettes with a variety of warnings about the dangers of low birthweight, heart disease, and various cancers and the fact that nicotine is addictive. The end result was a political compromise. The tobacco industry agreed to include all the health warnings on the warning labels as long as they did not have to state that nicotine is addictive. There is not a cigarette package in the United States that warns smokers that if they use the product exactly as it is intended to be used they will become addicted to a deadly poison—but that is, in fact, the case.

SHARED ADDICTIONS

People who are addicted to one drug often experiment with other drugs, and multiple addictions are not uncommon. Addiction to nicotine, either physical or psychological, is often combined with addiction to other psychoactive drugs, such as alcohol. Studies have shown that the rate of cigarette addiction in adult alcoholics is as high as 90 percent; it is almost universal that people who drink heavily also smoke heavily.

There is more to consider about the mixture of nicotine and alcohol: People who use alcohol increase the number of cigarettes they smoke as they increase the amount of alcohol they drink. In addition, the way they smoke a cigarette changes. Studies show that drinkers inhale more often and more deeply while drinking. Heavy drinkers who smoke inhale the carcinogenic substances of tobacco more deeply than non-drinkers do. This may explain why cancers of the mouth, pharynx, and esophagus are more common in people who drink and smoke: Not only do they tend to smoke more cigarettes, but they inhale more deeply as well.

People hooked on cigarettes to this extent generally do not entertain serious thoughts of quitting.

THE INCUBATION PERIOD:
WEIGHING THE PROS AND CONS

Needless to say, the essential first step in quitting is the decision to stop smoking. Most people consider this step carefully, thinking about it for weeks, months, even years. But they usually don't succeed in their first attempt, which may last only a few hours or days. What's important is that for most people there is an *incubation period,* a time of mulling it over, weighing the pros and cons, that precedes the attempt to quit.

Since 1964, the knowledge of the dangers of cigarettes has made the incubation period more active, because people have become increasingly uncomfortable with smoking. Even when they deny it, they have a nagging suspicion that they shouldn't be smoking. Active incubation includes reading, listening, thinking, analyzing, mulling, denying, questioning, and gathering information. It's one step on the road to motivation.

Failed Attempts and Relapses

As Mark Twain observed, "Quitting smoking is easy; I've done it a thousand times." Many people stop smoking briefly and then suffer a relapse. While Mark Twain's "thousand times" may be an exaggeration for most people—four or five is the norm—a relapse should not send you back to the dungeon. Most people return to the active incubation period, gather more information, marshal more courage and more resolve, and make another serious quitting attempt.

The causes of relapse in smokers have mystified researchers, because after about two weeks all traces of nicotine are gone from the body. Why then is relapse so common?

The two most common reasons are paradoxical: Relapse can occur when the person is in a pleasant, happy situation, or when he is unhappy or under unusual stress. In happy circumstances, such as social situations where alcohol and food are present and other people are smoking, the warm friendliness of the atmosphere sweeps the new ex-smoker back into smoking. That slip of resolve can make the ex-smoker lose faith in her willpower, say "What the hell," and start smoking again. After a week or so, the smoker is not only physically addicted again but disappointed and discouraged about the ability to ever quit once and for all.

The stress factor, our second reason for relapse, is intriguing. Many people who are fired, move from one part of the country to another, go through a divorce, have a serious illness in the family, or experience problems at work start smoking again impulsively. They remember smoking as a stress reliever. There appears to be some sort of residual memory in the nervous system that remains imprinted long after all traces of nicotine have disappeared from the body. What is left that is so indelibly printed on the psychic memory? At this point, science has no answer.

THE TRIGGERING EVENT

After all this incubation, sensitizing, relapsing, something happens—major or minor—that triggers the final attempt at the last puff.

The death of a close friend or member of the family, a personal illness, or some sort of social pressure may make the smoker more sensitive to his smoking habit. These sensitizing episodes can be something major, like a death, or very minor, like being asked to smoke outside a building or not to smoke in somebody's house. Smokers become more acutely aware of a personal habit and are likely to consider the personal and social ramifications every time they light up. Smoking then changes from an unthinking act, an unconscious habit, to a conscious choice each time the smoker takes out a cigarette.

The trigger may be internal or external, in the form of incentives or pressures from without. People are quite ingenious about the incentive, gimmick, or method they use to stop. This rich experience in quitting methods is, perhaps, the heart of this book. Whether it comes from without or within, the trigger is what leads to finally quitting, once and for all.

MISSING CIGARETTES

During the first few weeks, and sometimes for as long as the first few months, ex-smokers have sudden, unexpected urges to smoke. The brain, with all its complex connections and the many chemicals it produces to transmit signals from one nerve cell to another, has become dependent on nicotine. Since nicotine is both a tranquilizer and a stimulant, the brain misses both the calming, relaxing effect and the stimulating effect. When deprived of nicotine, those cells say, "Where is it? Where is it? I want it. I want it." Eventually, as the toxins are diminished in the body, the cells adjust to doing without nicotine, and the craving becomes less frequent and less intense, although sometimes the memory of cigarette smoking as a tranquilizer and stimulant leaves the brain thinking that maybe it ought to go back to it, even after the physiological addiction is gone.

After a few weeks the body is back to normal, however, and is no longer physically dependent upon the effects of nicotine. The return of a normal sense of taste and smell is a pleasure. The improvement in one's skin and general appearance is also a pleasure. The sense of becoming healthier, looking better, smelling nicer, and the pure joy of being able to smell and taste food are all compensation for the occasional urge to smoke.

In people who were heavily addicted, the days of smoking sometimes return in dreams that continue for months. These dreams usually fade with time and eventually cease altogether.

THE FINAL PHASE

The positive results of non-smoking begin to take over after a few weeks or months, depending on the length and intensity of the addiction. Now ex-smokers enter a new phase. Not only do they not crave cigarettes, but they begin to object strongly to cigarette smoke around them. In their place of work, in restaurants, in airplanes, they do not hesitate to make their objection to cigarette smoke known.

The positive effects begin to show. There is an overall sense of greater fitness and health. The shortness of breath disappears, the coughing in the morning is gone, and the aging process that was accelerated by smoking, the "smoker's face," regresses to various extents depending on the age of the ex-smoker and the number of years of smoking. There is a new feeling of health and beauty that had been drowned in a cloud of smoke for many years.

Now food tastes better, and some people do not need to oversalt or overflavor as they used to when their sense of taste was dulled by the smoke and nicotine. The ex-smoker enjoys the fragrance of flowers in blossom in a way that was impossible before. The stale odor of smoke in clothes or old curtains in the house from the smoking days becomes unbearable. It becomes unpleasant if not intolerable to ride in a car where the upholstery smells of smoke. Most ex-smokers cannot go into a hotel room where smokers have been: They are more sensitive to the smell of stale smoke than people who have never smoked. It's interesting that most of these people did not have this sensitivity in their smoking days.

When these positive effects begin, smokers know that their attempts to become ex-smokers have succeeded. They have an inner confidence that their smoking days are gone forever.

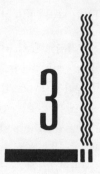

CONCERNS AND QUESTIONS
OF EX-SMOKERS

WHAT ABOUT DEPRESSION AFTER QUITTING?

Some ex-smokers go through a period of anxiety and have some difficulty functioning normally during the first week or two after quitting, but most people don't get depressed. That statement does not alter the fact that nicotine is a stimulant and that the absence of that stimulant may leave some people with a sense of torpor and lethargy, in effect a sense of mild depression. But the lack of a familiar stimulant is significantly different from severe clinical depression requiring professional psychological help or anti-depressant drugs. The lack of this stimulant *can be* a problem for creative people who use the "brain hit" of nicotine to move their brain into high gear. Fortunately this dependency also passes, especially when exercise (an excellent antidote) takes over.

However, given how common depression is in adults, ex–cigarette smokers who later become depressed are susceptible to relapse just as alcoholics are, because depressed people don't care much about anything, including their personal health. That may prompt them to start smoking again. It may help to keep in mind that smoking only makes life more difficult by leaving a person who's already feeling sad and angry to cope with all the hassles of nicotine addiction again. Certainly a feeling of depression in an ex-smoker should be a strong signal to seek professional help and not just "fight it out."

WHAT ABOUT RELAPSE AFTER MANY SMOKE-FREE YEARS?

What leads to relapse after many years without direct exposure to nicotine? It is often the memory of what cigarette smoking did for them when they were sad, tense, or anxious. There is a temptation to fall back on old habits for comfort. Many people feel that since they have conquered their addiction so well, one cigarette won't restart the cycle. This is seldom true: Most of the time that one cigarette means the ex-smoker will soon smoke a pack or two a day. This is true in many other types of addiction as well.

Most people who have stopped smoking and have taken up the habit again will say that they lost their willpower. Some psychologists say there is no such thing as willpower; rather, there are simply certain skills that need to be learned to control behavior. They don't like the word *willpower* because it implies some mystical property that can't be measured. But in practical terms we still need to understand that when people say that they have lost their willpower they mean they've lost a sense of control over their lives. They have been carrying an image of themselves as non-smokers, and if they suffer relapse, they may feel that their life is starting to fall apart. People who lose their self-esteem, confidence, and optimism are more inclined to return to behavior that has comforted them in the past, to go back to an old, familiar habit, even when they know it isn't good for them. They lose their self-respect, and that includes the respect for their bodies.

WHAT ABOUT ALCOHOL?

The combination of alcohol and stress may lead ex-smokers down the path to relapse. Alcohol releases both social and personal inhibitions, which helps undermine the ex-smoker's determination. Though initially a stimulant—alcohol makes people feel reckless and carefree—subsequently it is a depressant, making people feel that it doesn't matter what they do. Neither of those feelings is helpful to ex-smokers, who need to keep their wits about them to resist the temptation to light up "just this once." "Just this once" is the signpost that marks the road back to smoking.

WHAT ABOUT CRAVING SWEETS?

There is another side effect of nicotine addiction: When people stop smoking they develop a passion for sugar. In one study, those who gained weight responded to the increased desire for sugar by eating more sweets without increasing their exercise. Ex-smokers have to be careful about increasing the number of calories they consume from sugar, particularly since many sweets are combined with calorie-laden fats in foods like chocolate, dough-nuts, and ice cream.

It's best to try to satisfy the craving for sweets with the natural sugars found in fresh fruits. Fruit also satisfies the desire for oral gratification and answers the need to find something to do with your hands. Fruits that need peeling—oranges, tangerines, tangelos, and bananas, for example—serve all three purposes. They also in-crease your carbohydrates and fiber, so you can feel dou-bly virtuous. Besides, it's practically impossible to get fat eating fresh fruit. You may even *lose* weight, because the fruit provides enough bulk to satisfy your hunger, so you may not eat as much as you did before you quit smoking.

The other alternative to eating sweets is increasing physical activity. Swimming, cycling, and working out with weights all burn calories and keep your hands busy and your thoughts off smoking. Once again, you get to feel virtuous: You've quit smoking *and* you're getting more fit.

WHAT ABOUT WEIGHT GAIN?

Is it true that people gain weight after they quit smoking? How much? Is it inevitable? Can it be prevented? What is its cause? The increased craving for sweets is one reason some ex-smokers gain weight. Once the craving for sweets comes under control, the weight gain can be reversed.

Animal experiments have shown that animals with free access to food lose weight when they are given nicotine. The higher the dose of nicotine, the more weight they lose. It may be that nicotine reduces their appetite. Studies with humans, however, suggest that appetite does *not* decrease among smokers, and that smokers don't consume fewer calories.

Nicotine and other constituents of cigarette smoke are poisons. They are often called metabolic poisons because they affect the basic mechanism of different cells of the body. The way these poisons work is not completely understood. It could be that the human body does not assimilate the calories from food normally, either in the process of digestion or in the transformation of calories to fat. This means that the body cannot use those calories for energy or energy storage. The net result is that people lose weight.

Even though nicotine has these effects on cells of the body, it is not true, fortunately, that weight gain is the norm. In one research project where large numbers of

43

ex-smokers were tested, two-thirds either stayed at the same weight or lost weight. Only one-third of the ex-smokers gained weight, and the average gain was only a few pounds, although for some there was a larger weight gain.

Our culture places such a premium on slimness that often even normal weight is perceived as fat. Both men and women worry about gaining weight but, because our society places a greater importance on women's appearance than on men's, women worry more. Some women refuse to stop smoking because the fear that they will gain weight is so intense.

Even if ex-smokers gain a moderate amount of weight, the risk to their health is far less than the risks inherent in smoking. Those who lose or do not gain weight after quitting smoking often change other aspects of their lives as well. They take the next step toward better health and fitness by choosing foods more carefully and eating more fresh fruits, vegetables, and whole grains, and less high-fat meats and cheeses; they work toward greater fitness by getting more exercise. It is important to make some changes in the diet at the time of quitting if the ex-smoker wants to prevent weight gain. These changes promote good health in many other ways, and the benefits can be substantial.

WHAT ABOUT DEVICES TO PREVENT RELAPSE?

The stories that follow show that people have been successful using a variety of items that give their hands something to do when they would normally be playing with a cigarette. To satisfy the need to have something in your mouth in place of a cigarette, chewing gum and, in the early stages after quitting, even lollipops and other candies may be justified. You'll find other suggestions in the stories in Chapter 4.

In extreme cases some of the drugs, such as nicotine gum, that are used to help people to stop smoking may be useful in preventing relapse.

A final suggestion: In the early stages after quitting, avoid situations that once triggered cigarette smoking. For example, for a few weeks stay away from social events that may be strongly associated with smoking, such as cocktail parties, and don't visit friends who are heavy smokers.

THE VOICES OF
EXPERIENCE: EX-SMOKERS
TELL THEIR STORIES

These are the stories of people (like you) who smoked—
until one day they found the key that unlocked the door
to freedom from smoking. They are people of all ages
and all professions, males and females. Different as their
stories are, each with its subtext of upbringing, environment, and social attitudes toward smoking, all have the
theme of failure followed by success. See which stories
most closely parallel your own smoking pattern. Perhaps
you will find the key there.

SAMANTHA G.
I Can Quit Anytime I Want

Samantha G., now sixteen, comes from a family with a long history of addiction to cigarettes. Her father, aunt, grandfather, and both grandmothers all smoked heavily at some time in their lives; all have struggled, with varying degrees of success, to quit. Samantha began smoking two years ago at age fourteen, just before she entered ninth grade. She thinks she might give up smoking when it's time for her to start her own family.

While the men and women in all the other stories in this book have successfully quit smoking, Samantha is the exception; as a teen-ager, she thinks she can quit whenever she wants to. All the stories that follow prove that this is not the case: quitting is not easy, and there can be many relapses.

Before I started smoking I was always saying, "You put that cigarette out! Na-na-na-na-na! You're gonna die! Blah-blah-blah-blah-blah." I was totally against it. But here I am, smoking right now. Yeah, I smoke every day. A pack lasts me about three or four days. It's not like I'm going to get cancer next year.

I had my first cigarette at the end of eighth grade. A friend of mine was smoking and we were walking home, and I said, "Well, here, let me try one." And I did! And I liked it. "Give me another one!"

That first time was neat. I don't know if it was the

nicotine, but the first time I smoked it, yeah, it gave me a little head rush. It was like, "Wow!" At first I thought it was a cool thing to do and I'm all, "Hey, give me a smoke." It wasn't like I was smoking constantly. I'd have a few cigarettes, and then maybe two or three weeks would go by and I'd see some friends and they'd have smokes so I'd go, "Can I have a cigarette?" "Well, sure!"

It was fun. Other kids were doing it, and since I was a freshman, I thought, "Well, gee, maybe they'll think more of me if I smoke cigarettes." I thought it was the cool thing to do. (Now it's not cool.)

I never bought a pack of cigarettes until the middle of ninth grade. I'd see friends and I'd say, "Can I have a drag? Give me a drag," but I wouldn't buy a pack 'cause there was no way I was going to smoke the whole thing. I don't do that now. I don't buy a pack, smoke it in two minutes, and go out and buy another pack. A pack'll last me a couple of days—unless I'm at a party and I've given them all out.

My parents won't let me smoke at home. They say the house could go up in flames in a minute, and besides, they're parents, you know. Parents don't want their kids to smoke cigarettes. They say it's bad for you.

It gets on my nerves—my parents telling me not to smoke in the house like that's going to keep me from smoking anywhere else. I just go outside. I can smoke there, but I can't smoke in the house. That makes me mad because my grandmother smoked in the house for years. She owns it.

Smoking relaxes me. I can do my homework easier. I

can sit down calmly and do my homework instead of sitting there looking at my homework thinking, "I don't wanna do this." It's not a hundred percent difference. It just makes me go "Aaahhh." It's like a baby with a bottle. You know, when a baby is crying and it starts sucking a bottle and it shuts up. But since I can't smoke when I do my homework, I don't get my homework done!

A bunch of my friends smoke, but there're some who don't like it. Then there are some who say they've quit and then I'm all, "When did you quit?" "Yesterday." And then they'll ask me for a cigarette. That's a worthless cause. I only do it because it's something to do. But it gives me bad breath so I carry Certs or something with me.

My dad quit smoking. He's straight. He won't touch anything now. He doesn't drink or smoke or anything. He goes to A.A. a lot.

If my parents bought me a car, I would quit in a minute. Nothing like a pair of shoes or something; a pair of shoes is gone in a month, but a car would last me. If they give me a car, I'll quit! And if the car breaks down, I'll get it fixed, because once I quit smoking, I probably wouldn't start again. Hopefully. Knock on wood.

I don't smoke instead of eating. There'll be days when I'll have a couple pieces of fruit, and nothing else, and smoke, but it's not like I'm smoking to become anorexic. But that's not every day. There'll be days when I pork out, you know? Sometimes I get mad and I think, "I know, I'll go eat some food." And then the next day I'll go, "Uuuhh," and then just sit and smoke cigarettes.

If I'm pissed off, I'll smoke a pack, but I'm usually not pissed off 'cause it's summertime right now. I get pissed off when my parents get on my nerves, or if it's a gloomy day, or if it rains. I don't like the rain.

I usually have a cigarette in the morning around nine or something and then about three o'clock. Every day, I have one in the morning, and then at lunch, and then after school, and then the rest of the day I'll have a cigarette here and there. After school I go out with my friends and we'll all be smoking cigarettes. I go to a store to buy them.

When I'm out of school, I can see myself smoking once in a while. But I want to have a family, which means I'm gonna have to stop, because it's very dangerous if you're pregnant and you smoke. There is no way I am going to smoke when I am having kids. I know I'll quit smoking by then. Until then, who knows?

When my grandmother smoked, it didn't upset me except when we'd be eating dinner, and she would be smoking, and she'd have three cigarettes in the fifteen minutes. That was really sick. I don't smoke when I eat a meal. I'll have one afterwards, because okay, you're full, no more. Here, relax. Have a cigarette. But my grandmother did it before, during, and after, and it was so disgusting. She had cartons everywhere.

Older people do it because they're addicted. And they've probably been smoking for a long time. Or their parents did it, or brothers or sisters, or their husbands or wives.

They keep doing it because it is too hard to quit. My

other grandmother quit smoking at sixty-seven. She shouldn't have done it because she's really heavy and she's got bad arthritis, and when she stopped smoking she gained a lot of weight. And it was like, "Well, why are you doing it now?" Not to say, "Why are you doing it now, you're not gonna live much longer," but, "Why are you doing it now, because it won't make much difference."

I think she would be better right now if she was still smoking, because then she wouldn't have gained as much weight as she did. That's not good because she's got bad arthritis, and she's going to have to have surgery on her knees. And it's kind of sad, too. Also, I love her.

But I don't think I'll be smoking then, because, like I said, if I am going to have a family, I don't want to be smoking. I don't want my kids saying, "Mommy, what are you doing? Mommy, stop smoking!" Or if I had a lot of kids: "Mom, gimme a cigarette!"

I wouldn't want to smoke around my kids. Little kids should not be brought up with smoke because they're so alive with energy. And they might start smoking at an earlier age than me.

I don't think I have cancer yet. I mean, I shouldn't— I've only been smoking about a year and a half.

AMANDA M.
Nicotine Slavery

Amanda M., now thirty-seven, studied modern dance in New York and worked for many years as a dancer and choreographer. Later, she pursued her dance career on the West Coast until an injury forced her to retire. She has embarked on a new career in advertising. She used to worry, after seventeen years as a smoker, that she wouldn't be able to dance if she stopped smoking.

When I was smoking and living in New York, I would go out on a Saturday night, come home at two in the morning, and realize I was out of cigarettes. I'd pick butts out of my ashtray or trash can and smoke them. You know, with coffee stains or bits of food or lipstick on them. It was nicotine slavery!

Nobody is born needing to smoke. Nobody starts out needing to be a drug addict. You do it to yourself. I remember in high school thinking, "God, how disgusting! How could anybody ever even want to smoke? And what would that wanting to smoke feel like? I can't imagine such a weird thing." The first cigarette I ever smoked was in my junior year in high school. I smoked one or two, thought it was stupid, and stopped doing it. All the other kids in my school were doing it, so I thought I should try it. It was horrible. It tasted disgusting, and it made me shiver and shudder.

I didn't smoke again until I was in Czechoslovakia on a trip with a group from my prep school. It was a very loosely arranged two-month tour of Europe. My best friend was on the trip with me. She was five-foot-ten, thin and slinky, and very glamorous. And she smoked! I wanted to emulate her.

I would smoke a couple of cigarettes, come home, and lie in front of the TV feeling nauseous. I don't know why I kept doing it. I guess I thought I was being risqué. And, more importantly, I was doing something my parents absolutely forbade.

Nobody in my family smoked. Never. They were always ranting about it. My grandfather died of emphysema from smoking in 1970. And my father is a pathologist. My parents are against it because they're health-conscious people and they know that smoking can kill you. My father had smoked in the forties and fifties and had quit. It wasn't a struggle for him. He just quit.

Neither my brother nor my sister has ever smoked a single cigarette. I'm the oldest. I smoked as an act of rebellion against my family. I was eighteen and getting seriously into adolescent angst and rebellion. I wanted to assert my independence. Still, it wasn't exactly open rebellion: In seventeen years of smoking I never once lit a cigarette in front of my parents.

All my friends smoked in college. We sat around and smoked cigarettes, middle-class girls sitting around being sullen, hating the establishment and objecting to the war in Vietnam. We smoked and talked and stayed up much too late. And we smoked a lot when we studied and stayed up all night for exams. We all knew smoking was bad for us, but it was somehow like thumbing our noses at the rules, particularly since our parents said it was horrible.

We smoked cigarettes, smoked pot, and took Dexedrine so we could stay awake and talk some more. We spent endless hours philosophizing about life. I associated smoking with thinking deeply and being intellectual.

I had an eating disorder where I would get really uptight or mad, or something wouldn't turn out well, and I'd think, "*I* don't care. I'll just eat. I'll be ugly and stupid and eat up all this stuff." I would eat too much, get furious with myself, and then smoke to kill my appetite, so I wouldn't binge any more.

When I graduated I said, "Ah, now I can quit smoking because life is going to be ever so much simpler now that I'm not in school any more. All my troubles are over." Now that seems kind of a funny statement! I moved to New York, and of course, living there was more a panic than anything else I had ever experienced.

I worked in offices during the day. I'd get bored and I'd smoke out of boredom. In the evening I had dance classes at the studio, and all the dancers smoked waiting for class to start and then they'd smoke after class, cooling down. New York is a smoking culture.

Those were the days when some dance teachers smoked while they were teaching. I don't think they are allowed to now. I think all of the ones who did are dead. I do! They don't do that any more.

Dancers smoke partially to not eat, I think. A lot of dancers have poor eating habits, particularly ballet dancers, and smoking has a lot to do with not wanting to eat. And partially it's something to do to kill time at rehearsals while you're waiting for your turn to dance. That was in New York. And if you live in New York City the air is so polluted, you honestly wonder what difference smoking is going to make. In California, hardly anybody in dance smokes. I can't think of anybody who does. Being a dancer is very stressful. You're always exhausted, you're always running around trying to whip together dance concerts, rehearsing, going to class, and working some miserable daytime job as a secretary or waitress so you can pay the rent and buy groceries. I saw myself as a groovy dancer or *artiste*—a New York *artiste*—not as self-destructive but as committed to creating art.

I worked in a publishing house as an editorial assistant five hours a day. I rehearsed in the afternoon, went to class at six o'clock every night, got home about eight-thirty, and had dinner. I usually went out because I was too tired to cook. I would end up eating hamburgers, stay out smoking and talking, talking and partying. And I'd drink, and smoke.

Every time I smoked I'd think, "This is really stupid. Why are you doing this? This could kill you. Why are you doing this? It's gonna make you wrinkled. It'll make you go through early menopause. It will make you old, and stinky, and ugly. Why are you doing this?" But I wasn't ready to stop, I guess. The little voice that tells you to stop hadn't spoken and said, "No! Enough!"

I never took drugs after college, but I smoked when I was bored or nervous or happy or having fun. Or because I was mad. Smoking blocks out emotions. If I got upset about something, I wanted to have a cigarette. It puts a lid on things and takes away the immediacy of what you're feeling.

The first time I tried to quit, I was living in Minneapolis, not New York. I wasn't dancing. I was living in a nicer place, and I wasn't as nervous as I used to be. That's basically what it was. There were still a number of people around who smoked, but there were also women I knew who had smoked about as long as I had who were quitting or who had quit recently. That's what motivated me to think about quitting, but my attempts to quit were half-hearted. I would always cheat.

I said, "This is for the birds," and I signed up for a quit-smoking class, and I went, and I *still* cheated. I never really stopped smoking. I would smoke, maybe, two cigarettes a day. I had all these signs—"Thank you for not smoking"—and brochures about smoking and all sorts of charts, stuff that's part of a packet of non-smoking material they give you when you sign up for the class. I did cut down for a couple of months. Way down. But then I started smoking more, and as soon as I allowed myself to do it once, I did it again. And again. I became lax, and gradually, over a week or two, I was smoking.

I went back to smoking my habitual amount, fifteen to twenty cigarettes a day. I think everybody has a different level of how much they will smoke, given free rein. My limit was about a pack a day. Some people smoke two packs a day, some people smoke three packs a day. It is incomprehensible to me that anybody could stand to smoke that much.

The man I was living with also smoked, but he didn't have any compulsion to smoke, as I did. He smoked mostly to be social. He could go out to a party, smoke a pack, and not smoke again for three days. We had our own apartment, and we both smoked. Then he quit. We went to see his parents and his father is a very heavy smoker. He quit because it made him sick to see his father smoking. Then he would tell me not to smoke in the car when he was in it. I would do what he asked because I knew it was annoying, but I still smoked at home.

Then we moved to California into a group house where they had a rule: no smoking in the house. We did it on purpose. But since I couldn't smoke in the house, I went out in the backyard to smoke instead.

At the same time, I quit drinking coffee, which made it much easier for me not to smoke in the morning. I used to stagger to the coffee pot, smoke while I waited for the coffee to drip, and have a cigarette or two with my coffee.

I smoked at work still. I was a secretary in San Francisco, at two different corporations. And I started dancing again. There were only one or two other people who smoked in the class. It wasn't the same kind of studio atmosphere as in New York, where everybody hangs out in the studio and smokes. In California you go to class, take the class, and go home. I didn't have all my smoking friends here. It wasn't the same at all.

A year before I quit smoking, that guy Latka on "Taxi"

died of lung cancer, but it wasn't from smoking. He was only one year older than I was, and that really gave me the creeps. I was thirty-four—and he died of lung cancer! I thought, "Oh, God, this is horrible. He is only a little bit older than me and he has died of this weird cancer." From that day I made a rule that I could smoke no more than six cigarettes a day.

Then they passed the law in San Francisco that said you couldn't smoke in an office building unless you had a private office with a door. That cut my smoking down even more.

It was hard at first, because it's such a habit. It's like not exercising when you're used to exercise. You feel like, "Eeyuchh!" You want to scream or something. I'd get nervous and irritable, and I'd want to stuff my face. I'd drink diet pop or eat Cheetos. I got used to it, though.

I read a lot of quit-smoking books, and one really got to me. It talked about all of the physiological changes that one cigarette causes in your body. It was amazing. Worse, it said that you can smoke about 100,000 cigarettes and not necessarily cause permanent physical damage, but after that, with each one you smoke, you're playing Russian roulette, because that one could give you cancer or emphysema or heart disease. *That one.* Reading that did it, because I was sure I had probably smoked that many. I was sick of smoking. It was a pain to deal with it any more.

I still had a studio in New York, where I had my things in storage. I decided I wasn't going to live there, so I went back to arrange for everything to be shipped to

California. I was still smoking my six cigarettes or less a day that I started when that guy on "Taxi" died.

At JFK Airport, waiting for my flight back to California, I had one cigarette left in the pack. I smoked it, crumpled up the pack, and said, "That's that!" And that *was* that. I didn't decide ahead of time. The day came when it was time to stop, and I stopped. Perhaps I associated it with closing the chapter on my life in New York, my years of adolescent rebellion, my image of myself as the driven *artiste*. I was leaving all of that stuff behind.

I used the things I learned in the quit-smoking class in Minneapolis—the signs and things they gave me. I put one up on my desk at home, and I put one up at work. They were sort of boosterish messages to myself. They say, "Thank you for not smoking," and I would say to myself, "Thank you for not smoking." Every time I looked at them, I would thank myself.

I didn't get nauseous and throw up, or get constipated, but I was nervous and wanted to eat. Every night I ate a giant bowl of popcorn with no butter, a huge bowl of popcorn. I would sit there and stuff my face with it around nine or ten at night. I did it every night for six months. Then I did it about three nights a week. And then about six months ago, I couldn't stand the sight of popcorn any more.

Now that I've stopped smoking, I feel better. When I drank coffee and smoked I was very sluggish when I got up. Now I just wake up and I'm awake. I can even have a normal conversation within three minutes of getting up.

It's like being a kid. I don't drink any stimulants like coffee or caffeine tea when I get up. I just drink water and leave the house and I'm fine.

I haven't noticed food tasting better or smelling things more, but my clothes smell better, and I smell better. And I have much better color. I used to get really pale, and I think it was from smoking. When I first was in New York, my cheeks would get rosy when I danced, and after seven years of smoking, they didn't. My wind is obviously much better. I used to get winded going up the stairs for a subway, even though I danced hours every week.

I had always been very interested in health and nutrition. I always ate basically healthy food—broiled chicken, steamed broccoli, and baked potatoes. There were things that I ate then that I wouldn't eat now. Candy and cake and coffee, for example.

I didn't drink at all when I first quit because I couldn't separate the two in my mind; they really went together. Now I drink wine, but I don't need to smoke when I do it. I don't even think about it any more. I just don't smoke.

I thought that choreographing without smoking would be a problem, but it wasn't. When I moved out here no smoking was allowed in dance studios, so even though I was still smoking, I couldn't smoke when I was in the studio. I adapted to the situation. I used to worry that I wouldn't be able to dance and choreograph any more, the way writers quit smoking sometimes and think they can't write without a cigarette hanging out of their mouth, but it's not a problem.

I used to think about having a cigarette every day, but

every time I wanted to smoke I'd say to myself, "Just wait it out, it'll pass." And I'd get over it. I'd go for a walk, exercise, or do long stretches and wait until the moment passed. That's how I did it: As the urge came to smoke, I would wait until it passed. They became farther and farther apart, and I thought about smoking less and less. Now, most of the time, I never think about smoking, unless someone is smoking near me, and then I get disgusted. I hate it and I don't let anybody ever smoke in the house where I live. I hate the way it smells, and it makes me feel like I'm choking: It's as simple as that!

I always was a weird smoker. I couldn't be in smoky bars for very long because the smoke hurt my eyes. It was very difficult—my eyes would get red and burn. And if I had gone for twenty-four hours without smoking, the first time I would smoke a cigarette would give me those shudders. I mean it physically affected me in a disgusting way.

When I was smoking six or less a day, every time I smoked I could feel the hit. I could feel my heart rate increase, and I could feel myself getting wired. The physiological things were as plain as day. It's the same thing that coffee does to me.

Smoking always seemed like it wasn't me. As I became an adult, I started associating smoking with people who were uneducated, who didn't know any better, who didn't take responsibility for their health. I felt weird about smoking toward the end. I thought, "This is a creepy thing to be doing." I was embarrassed that I did it. I felt humiliated at myself. I wasn't feeling very good about myself in general, and so these feelings about smoking reinforced my lousy self-image as an inadequate twit. Somebody who wasn't quite with it. Somebody who wasn't successful.

I feel tremendously clean from not smoking. Now I see myself as an energetic person who is bright and fun to be around, somebody who's disciplined and had the strength to quit smoking.

Every once in a while I'll just get this flash: "Gee! I'd like a cigarette." I get them at all different times. I'll be driving down the street and all of a sudden have this feeling of wanting to smoke, or be talking to somebody and want to smoke. I just put it out of my mind.

After I quit, I dreamed about coughing up blood. I was coughing and there was blood on my pillow. I dreamt it twice. I never dreamed about it while I was smoking, but after I quit I did. It gives me the creeps.

My ex-boyfriend started smoking again. He asked me, "Don't you ever sneak a puff or anything?" No. I never do. I never will, because I can't. I was addicted to nicotine. And he is, too.

Sometimes I feel weak when something horrible has happened. I had another boyfriend who turned out to be a terrible jerk. I was really upset, and I talked to a friend of mine and I said, "I feel like having a cigarette." She said, "Don't do it; he's not worth it. Nothing is worth it. Don't do it." Every time I'm really upset about something and I find myself thinking, "I want to smoke," I think instead, "It's not worth it. This piece-of-shit person is not *worth* smoking over. This ridiculous work situation isn't *worth* smoking over. It's no big deal, nobody's going to die—except me, if I start smoking again."

JAMES V.
Pictures of Smokers' Lungs

James V., in his late fifties, has been a truck driver for thirty years, delivering tons of gravel to construction sites. The roads are sometimes steep, the traffic is often heavy, and the trucks are always loaded to their legal limit of 80,000 pounds. As James says, "You don't want to hit anybody because these big trucks kill people real easy." Even the dumping must be done with care and skill to keep the truck from overturning.

I started smoking when I was eighteen years old—just about the time I went into the Navy in 1950. I enlisted to go to Korea and started smoking when I was in training in San Diego.

In the service they used to have a saying, "The smoking lamp is lit," and whenever they told you that, you could stop and smoke. Or if there was a coffee shop nearby, you could have coffee and smoke. All of that kind of goes together. Even if you didn't smoke when you went in, you'd probably start in the service. My brother, who didn't smoke until he was almost twenty-five, started smoking in the service.

In the beginning, smoking would make me dizzy. If I went without smoking for too long, maybe a few hours, and then took a drag on a cigarette, I'd get dizzy. Pretty soon the dizziness was over and I'd feel all numb—almost like taking a drink.

In my smoking days, I remember there were spots along the road, certain places where the truck goes slow, and I'd take out a cigarette and light it and smoke it while I went up the hill. Then thirty or forty minutes later I'd have to have another one. I'd get the craving, and there'd be another spot on the highway for the next smoke. I'd been doing that since I started driving in 1958.

When I first started, I smoked Lucky Strikes with no filter, and then after my grandfather died—he was a heavy smoker—I started smoking filter cigarettes. I started with filters as soon as they came out. Later I switched to True—less nicotine, less tar, and all of that baloney. They're supposed to do you less harm. Well, I talked my wife into smoking them too, but now she smokes more than she did before, because she gets less out of them. I was the same way—you just smoke more cigarettes.

I was raised as a Seventh Day Adventist. I went to religious schools up to high school, and I didn't believe in smoking or drinking or theaters or even hardly holding hands with girls, so I was raised up real strict. But when I thought I was old enough, and I was on my own, I figured I could do what I wanted. Nobody could tell me what to do. I was rebelling against my folks and religion. I quit going to the church, and I started smoking and drinking and chasing girls.

My folks never smoked, either one of them, because of

their religion, and because they didn't think they should. They said smoking was bad even back then, but they didn't tell us why. They just said it was bad. And I figured, well, it's because of their religion—that's why.

I was about eighteen when I started and I was thirty-three when I realized that my relatives were dying because of their smoking habit. None of them were Seventh Day Adventists like my mother and father. My grandfather died and my uncle and another uncle, and they all smoked and smoked and smoked since they were little children. They came from the Midwest, where tobacco was plentiful. They all died young: My grandfather died when he was sixty-four; one uncle died of a stroke when he was around sixty; and another one died from lung cancer around sixty-two. I realized then that, "Hey, something's wrong, something is causing that." So I decided to quit when I was in my early thirties.

I was driving trucks then, too. As I've said, that's quite stressful. I realized how much better I felt the first time I quit. It takes a little while to start feeling better. For a while you still have that great desire, but you have to overpower it mentally, you have to think it away.

Nobody told me I should quit: I decided I had better quit or I would end up like my grandfather and my uncles, and so I did quit—I just made up my mind one day. I had tried to quit quite a few times before that, but after a few days I would sneak a cigarette and think, "It won't hurt me." I would have a drag, start to smoke the cigarette, and it would make me dizzy, so I would put it out, but after a while it breaks your will down. I would say,

"Well, I've already had one, so I might as well try another one," and pretty soon I'd try another one ten hours later, and the next day I'd try another one. Within a day or two I'd buy another pack and put it back in my pocket and I was hooked again. You can't fool yourself, that nicotine makes you want more.

Finally I said, "Well, this is no good." You can't cheat; with smoking, there is no cheating. So I said, "This is it. This is the last one, and no more." After I quit, I would wake up in the morning, and no cigarette, and I would fight all day long with myself mentally.

I did not smoke for nine years. Then my first wife and I split up after nineteen years of marriage. She pulled away, she left me. I was about forty-one. After the divorce, the stress was kind of heavy. I started drinking more, and I was so emotionally upset, I didn't care whether I lived or died. I was really in love with her. After nine years I started smoking again and kept smoking clear up until last year.

The reason I quit this time is that my lungs started hurting me. I was hurting, and I could tell I wasn't normal. I would take a deep breath and I would get dizzy. I went to a lung cancer specialist and had my lungs X-rayed and checked for cancer, and I went to a throat specialist and had my throat checked out for cancer. It all came out negative, but I decided, "Well, that's it. I am not taking no more chances, because I'm no kid no more, and it can catch up with me." So I quit, and I had to fight the desire to smoke again—just like it was the first time I quit.

It took about six months, but the first few days were the worst. And then gradually, the craving gets less and less. Your system gets used to not having the nicotine. Now I hardly crave it at all.

The wife I am married to now smokes a whole bunch. She smokes about two or three packs a day. She is quite a bit younger than I am, but if she is going to smoke, she is going to smoke. I can't stop her. Everybody has to quit themselves, if they want to. I don't nag her. I let her do what she wants to do. I just told her, "I hate to see you kill yourself like that, but it will happen if you keep going. I have seen too much of it." I stick right with her, whether she smokes or not.

Now I snack quite a bit, but I try to snack on health foods, like cereals. Once in a while I get a package of peanuts or sunflower seeds—it gives me something to do with my hands. When I first quit, I started doing that—it gets your mind off cigarettes, because you're sitting there picking shells off sunflower seeds or peanuts.

I used to dream a lot when I first quit. I'd dream I was smoking, and it would scare me when I woke up because I thought I had been smoking, which I hadn't been. You'd wake up and say, "What's happened here?" Then you realize you didn't smoke and you're real glad, real happy.

Another thing that helped me to quit this last time were these colored pictures I saw somewhere of a good, non-smoking lung and of a smoker's lung. The smoker's lung looked like a roast beef compared with the non-smoker's lung. You could hardly tell what it was from the pictures. On the good lung you could see everything very plain, but the smoker's lung looked like it was cooked.

It has been a year this spring since I quit. One of my uncles passed away at that time. Before he passed away, he would come and stay at my house for a few days. When he came back last time he was complaining of hurting and hurting and hurting. He had been a smoker since he was six years old, and he was sixty-five when he died. He only lived with me a few months before he died. He wouldn't talk very much, he would just say, "I'm hurting." He couldn't eat hardly any food. I said, "Well, you got to eat," and I took him to my doctor, who said, "He's got lung cancer," so they gave him cobalt treatments and the cobalt treatments hurt him bad. The day before he died, he wanted a cigarette, so I went and got him some cigarettes. I had quit by then. He helped me make up my mind that I had better stay off cigarettes because I had seen too much of what they can do with him and his brothers and his dad.

My mother passed away last year just after I quit smoking and she was eighty-two. My dad is eighty-four now, and he is still going strong. He's got good lungs and a good mind and he is still all together. He was a nonsmoker. My mother's brothers are the ones who died young, and her father died young, and they were all smokers. My wife's mother has one sister who is a nonsmoker and she is still going good, but she has another sister who is about to die, and she is a smoker. To me, that is proof in my mind as to what smoking will do to you. It is all black and white in my own family—the ones that don't smoke live a long life and the ones that do smoke die young. That tells me a lot.

Something else has helped me to quit. I listen to the radio every day going down the highway from one until two in the afternoon. I listen to this doctor, Dr. Dean Edell, as he talks about the hazards of smoking, and addiction to smoking, and how heavy a drug it is, and how they have come out recently that smoking is just as hard to quit as heroin. They say if you can quit smoking, and if you're a druggie or an alcoholic, you can quit any of them, because smoking is the toughest one to quit. He has helped me; I have listened to him for years. He helped encourage me a little bit, and then my uncle dying, that really encouraged me.

DAVID GOERLITZ
The Winston Man

For six years, David Goerlitz was the Winston Man, the model who represented Winston cigarettes in newspaper and magazine advertising. He was a three-pack-a-day smoker who smoked Winstons and was proud of it. When he gave up smoking, he stopped modeling for Winston—and walked away from $75,000 a year in doing so. Figuring that he persuaded many young people to start smoking in his years as the Winston Man, he is now committed to persuading people to stop. He is thirty-nine years old.

Doesn't it seem odd to you that 95 percent of the people who die of lung cancer are smokers? Or that 78 percent of the people who die of heart disease are smokers? It's a horrible feeling to be aware of what cigarettes do to people's health, knowing that I was the main reason that Winston became the number-two-selling cigarette over a four-year period. I have a very guilty conscience about that.

I loved smoking, loved it. I didn't just light cigarettes; I *smoked* them. I wasn't even out of bed when I had my first cigarette. The first thing I did in the morning was smoke a cigarette; the last thing I did at night was smoke a cigarette. I started when I was fifteen, and I smoked for twenty-four years. I was up to three and a half packs a day when I quit.

There wasn't a day that went by that I didn't smoke. It didn't matter if I had a cold, I smoked. When I was in the hospital with my whole left side paralyzed, I smoked. I was working as Harrison Ford's double in *Witness*, doing stunts, and the last week of the shoot, my left side suddenly became paralyzed. They gave me VIP treatment in the hospital, complete with a private room, and in my room I could do anything I wanted, including smoke. The first thing I did in the morning was smoke a cigarette, and the last thing I did in the evening was smoke a cigarette.

The evidence of addiction became more and more undeniable as I got older. I would not go to sleep if I was down to fewer than ten or twelve cigarettes. I would go out and buy a pack of cigarettes so I'd have them in case I woke up in the night and needed them. That *never* happened, but the fear that it *might* only grew stronger as the years went by. I would literally get out of bed on a cold night, get dressed, shovel the snow off my car, and go out to find a store that was open twenty-four hours a day to buy a pack of cigarettes, to be sure those cigarettes were there, just in case.

I used to hide cigarettes under the seats of my car. If I had a pack of cigarettes in my pocket that only had four or five cigarettes left, I'd take that pack and put it under the seat of the car and put a fresh pack in my pocket. I'd store them up just the way a little chipmunk or pack rat would do. I didn't care if they got stale; it didn't matter.

I would go through ashtrays to find a butt that had maybe as much as an inch of tobacco left in it, and I would save those, too. I hoarded them against an emergency, against the day I might need them. I wish I were as good with my money as I was with my cigarettes. I always knew where my cigarettes went, and I always knew where to find some when I needed them.

For twenty-four years I smoked. For four years the neurosurgeon told me I'd better lay off the cigarettes because of the paralysis I had. That didn't stop me. My son, who's now ten, begged me every year on his birthday to stop smoking as his birthday present. That didn't stop me. My mother sent me pictures of tar-coated lungs in the mail. That didn't stop me. My gums had been bleeding for four years, and everyone in my family complained about the way I smelled from smoking. That didn't stop me either.

What stopped me was seeing kids twelve and thirteen buying cigarettes and lighting up, and the fear that I might have influenced them to smoke. What stopped me was the realization that the tobacco industry commits murder, and I have been an accessory for six years. The tobacco industry is pushing a substance as addictive as cocaine or heroin that kills 400,000 people every year from diseases *directly* related to smoking.

Smoking-related diseases are the biggest public health issue in the United States today. Not AIDS. Not drugs. Not even highway deaths. More people die every year from smoking-related diseases than from any other single cause in this country's history, with the exception of World War II. The Surgeon General has declared that secondhand smoke causes lung cancer, and women who don't smoke but whose husbands do have a 40 percent greater chance of getting lung cancer than women who are married to men who don't smoke.

There are 50 million smokers in the United States. That's 26 percent of the population. Every year it's decreased by 4–5 percent. The 4–5 percent who quit are over forty years of age. Look at the figures. Fifty million smokers spending $2 per day is $100 million per day, $700 million per week. The tobacco industry generates $15 *billion* per year. To maintain those kinds of revenues the tobacco industry needs to recruit 5,000 new smokers every single day to offset those who quit—and those who die. The tobacco industry would rather addict the young. They'll be customers longer. That's why cigarette advertising is aimed at teen-agers.

I also feel guilty about having been an inconsiderate smoker. I honestly felt that non-smokers who asked me not to smoke were infringing on my civil rights. "I can smoke if I want to; it's not illegal!" was my resentful reaction. I didn't care about the non-smoker, second-hand smoke, the offensive smell, or any of that stuff.

Now it seems to me that the tobacco companies use the "right to smoke" issue as a diversionary tactic. If smokers and non-smokers fight with each other, maybe they'll never notice that smokers are paying for the dubious privilege of allowing the tobacco companies to reap huge profits from systematically poisoning their customers. Any other industry that did that would be shut down instantly and ordered to pay heavy damages to those who were sick and to the families of those who died.

I have three children in the public schools. They are exposed every day to secondhand smoke from teachers who smoke. Not one of my children smokes, but all of them are exposed to nicotine addiction from their teachers' smoking. The dangers are all clearly detailed in the Surgeon General's 1986 report *Health Effects of Secondary Smoke.* Not to mention the simple hypocrisy of the teachers coming back from their cigarette break and telling the kids to "just say no." I think the 74 percent of us who don't smoke should protect our children's health by making it illegal to smoke anywhere on school property.

I've had great things happen since I stopped smoking. For one thing, I have much more self-esteem and confidence, and that makes my work better. I lost eleven pounds. And I used to worry that sex wouldn't be the same without a cigarette after. I was right; it's not the same. It's better!

TONY B.
I Quit Cold, and That Was It

Tony B., sixty-six, has recently retired as vice-president of CBS Entertainment Productions at CBS Television. One of the pioneers of early television programs, he started out stage-managing, and eventually directing, such live-performance classics as "Playhouse 90," "Studio One," and "Climax." Many of his shows are now considered among the finest ever produced on television.

My mother had a heart attack on Monday. On Tuesday my older brother had a heart attack. On Wednesday my mother died. I was in Los Angeles working in television, and nobody in the family wanted to upset me, so nobody told me what was going on until they called me to come home for my mother's funeral. After going to the funeral, I went to visit my brother, who was so depressed over his condition that nobody had told *him* our mother had died for fear the shock would kill him, too.

I was scared to death. I knew that smoking was bad for me. I'd been thinking about quitting for a long time, but I hadn't done it. When I got back to Los Angeles, I started having chest pains. I kept telling myself it was psychosomatic, that I was making it up because I was upset about my mother and brother. The pains persisted for a couple of weeks, and finally I went to the doctor. He did an examination, and when he was done he said, "Well, of course you're having chest pain. You've had bronchitis for weeks." I almost died of relief.

I reached into my pocket, pulled out my pack of Marlboros, threw them across the desk, and said, "You can have these. I don't need them any more." He laughed, opened his top desk drawer, put them in it, and said, "They'll be here if you decide you want them." I've never touched another cigarette, and that was more than thirty years ago. I had been smoking three packs of cigarettes a day for more than twenty years.

I was uncomfortable for the first three days, and after that the urge just disappeared. I was psychologically prepared for it. That's the key. A person has to be ready to quit smoking, and they have to really want to give it up or need to give it up. I kept thinking to myself, "This is ridiculous. Why should I keep smoking? It's bad for me, it's scaring the hell out of me, and there's no point." I quit cold, and that was it.

I've never had another drag on anything. I don't want to put anything with smoke in my mouth because I *know* that I was addicted. Even now I'm not sure that if I took even one drag that I wouldn't want more. I have no yearning for it, no craving at all, but I just don't want to take the chance.

I dislike it when other people smoke around me, not because it makes me want a cigarette—it doesn't—but because it smells bad. It gets in my hair and on my clothes, and I don't like it.

The real horror, to me, is that the tobacco industry is well aware of how lethal their product is, yet it keeps saying that it's not lethal, that it's okay to smoke, they're putting in filters and there's nothing to worry about. Driven by greed, they continue to foist poison, *real poison*, on the public *knowingly.* That's the horror to me.

Hollywood has a reputation for being stressful and tension-ridden, especially the movie and television industries. You might assume a lot of people in the industry would smoke, but that's not the case. Very few of the people I worked with at CBS or in the studios smoked. They had either quit or never started. For myself, I knew that smoking doesn't relieve tension. That kind of stuff is all in people's heads. I had to learn how to deal with stress in productive ways, not by killing myself.

I jog regularly, and I play a lot of golf. I'm convinced that if I had not quit when I did I wouldn't be able to do the things that I'm doing today. Every time I hear more evidence about how harmful smoking is to the lungs, the heart, the whole cardiovascular system, I thank God that I quit when I did. I'm sure I couldn't enjoy my life as much as I am now if I hadn't quit.

My wife quit smoking a year after I did, and she just came back from a week of whitewater rafting, and a few days later she went backpacking in the Sierras for another week. You can't do that if you can't breathe, or you're worried about your heart.

My brother was only forty-eight when he had his heart attack, and the first thing the doctors told him was to quit smoking. He couldn't do it. Smoking is an addiction. He lived another fourteen years, babying himself so he wouldn't strain his heart and sneaking off to smoke in the bathroom. What a waste, what a *waste.*

MARION R.
I Was a Closet Smoker

Marion R. was born in Austria during World War II. She spent her childhood in convents and private schools. When she was nineteen, she came to the United States and received her higher education here. She was one of the first female computer systems analysts on the East Coast and worked in the computer industry for eight years. Now married, she has two teen-age children and is writing a novel based on her own life. She realizes now how difficult she made her task by constructing private games about her smoking.

I had gone through two years of trying very, very hard to stop smoking, allowing myself only an occasional cigarette here and there. I didn't smoke in the house, I didn't smoke in front of my husband, I didn't smoke around other people. Life became very difficult with all the restrictions I invented for where and when I could smoke. For two years I played these little games with myself, hoping they would help me cut down on my smoking.

What all this really did was to alienate me from other people. I used to disappear so I could have a cigarette while nobody could see me, but they didn't know where

I'd gone or why. It was like being a closet alcoholic—I was a closet smoker. I was embarrassed because I always made this big deal, "I am going to give up smoking," and then didn't. I didn't want anybody to know that I didn't manage it again.

In the end, I didn't sleep well any more—I woke up every night at two o'clock in the morning berating myself, saying, "You worthless human being, why can't you manage to get a better hold of yourself? You can't let cigarettes control your life."

Every night I would say, "Next morning when I get up I won't have a cigarette," and then someplace along the line, I would have one again. I prepared myself seriously for two years to do it, and I half-heartedly quit a couple of times here and there, but that was different from this last time. I went through the whole thing of getting nicotine gum and various and sundry other things as part of my preparations. A couple of times when I had tried to stop previously I had experienced withdrawal symptoms of chills and shaking and being miserable. I imagine that's how it is for alcoholics who stop drinking. This time I got myself ready in case this happened; I had the nicotine gum and everything. One day I chewed a piece of that gum and it was so vile tasting that I said to myself, "Come on . . . you can do without that, can't you?" I chewed the gum for a little while, but that was it. I didn't need the nicotine.

Psychologically, my failures to quit caused me hell. Finally, it was close to my husband's birthday, and I was thinking, "What can I do that is really special?" Although he knew I was smoking, we never talked about it. I decided, "Well, this is it, for myself, for him, for the whole family, for the peace of everybody, I am going to give it up this time and this is going to be it." And I did. It was very simple; it was the easiest quitting episode I have ever had.

I remember so well how it happened. . . . It was the strangest thing; I woke up and I thought, "This is it." Never once in the back of my mind did I even consider sneaking a puff here or there. Overnight, I had the feeling that I was rid of it. The monkey was off my back, and I was not going to smoke ever again. Now I have absolutely no desire to smoke—no desire.

I was not really worried about my health. It wasn't the fear of lung cancer so much, or heart disease. My main reason for wanting to stop smoking was to be in control of myself; the other reasons were all window dressing.

I had smoked for many years before I quit. I began to smoke at thirteen. I thought smoking was very glamorous. Practically every one of my friends smoked—we shouldn't have, but we were really not told not to. I liked smoking right away. I kept on trying to give it up because I couldn't afford cigarettes. There wasn't a lot of money in Austria after the war, and certainly very little for a girl who ran away from home at fourteen. For financial reasons I had to give it up a few times as a teen-ager.

I gave up smoking voluntarily when I became pregnant with each of my children, although it had not been proven at the time that smoking was dangerous to fetuses. By then I was living in the United States. When I had my first child in 1969—I was thirty at that time—I gave up smoking before I became pregnant and didn't smoke for about two and a half years. I guess I thought it was better for pregnant mothers not to smoke. When my son was about eighteen months old, I started smoking again. I had a house guest for two and a half months. She smoked, and having the smoke around me all the time reminded me that I missed it.

The second time around, I gave up smoking before I became pregnant with my second child, in 1972. I kept it up until she got sick when she was a year old. She had to be hospitalized with a terrible flu. I was at the hospital at two in the morning, found a cigarette, and started smoking again. I was terrified of losing my daughter. I was under a lot of stress.

Ever since then I've tried to give it up. I'd quit for two months, or three months or six months, and then I'd fall on my face.

I have always been very athletic, and I found it a bit obscene to be a tennis player hanging around with a cigarette in her hand. I also ride a great deal, and it's very dangerous to have cigarettes around stable areas. I really didn't want to smoke. It frustrated me to keep losing the battle. I hated not wanting to do something but feeling compelled to smoke, hated being addicted to something that I knew was bad for me.

I've tried to quit ten or twelve times in the last twenty years. And very, very rarely did I give up smoking for only a couple of days—I have always given it up for at least two months, most of the time for six to nine months. Every time I went back to smoking, it was as though I had never stopped smoking. I didn't get dizzy, lightheaded, or anything like that, the way it was when I tried smoking the very first time.

About four years ago I had stopped smoking again. For about seven months I did not smoke. I had taken the children skiing and was driving our station wagon at night when I was hit head-on by a drunk driver in a pickup truck. The car spun around, and my head went through the windshield. (The kids weren't hurt, thank heaven.) I had to go to the hospital to have my head sewn up, and as I was recovering the next morning, I thought, "Why am I worrying about the cancer that might kill me if I smoke? Here is this drunken idiot out there who almost killed me, and I'm putting myself through all this agony to stop smoking?" So I started smoking again.

You may wonder why I am so sure this time that I'll never smoke again. Two things are different now. One is that when I stopped before, I used to smoke in my dreams, and I used to wake up hyperventilating from smoking in those dreams. Even when I quit for two and a half years, I used to smoke in my dreams. I have not dreamed that I was smoking since I gave it up this last time, except once. I woke up one night, and I was so disappointed because I dreamed I'd had one puff of a cigarette. It never happened again because I couldn't stand the sense of disappointment.

Something else is different this time. That's how I know I have finally quit at last. For years I went around saying, "Someday I am going to write a book, a novel, but really the story of my life." About two years ago that "someday" arrived. I started off with an outline, did a lot of soul searching, went through a lot of emotional pain, agony, pleasure, exhilaration, a lifetime-size bundle of emotions. I was forced to look at myself in certain ways and didn't feel very comfortable doing it, but I did it anyway. I was able to forgive myself for some of the things I felt I needed to forgive myself for, pat myself on the shoulder for some of the things that I deserved to be patted for. I made peace with some of the figures in my past, made peace with myself partially, and knew that there was no way I could make peace with myself if I let things I didn't like control me—stupid habits like smoking and drinking and such, like little clowns that had a stranglehold on my life.

When I began to write the book two years ago, I began taking the first serious steps toward quitting smoking. I hadn't seen this correlation before, but now that I think about it, it's true. Now that the book is almost finished, I have stopped smoking. The book is the story of my life. I have rediscovered myself by writing the book. That's why I know I'll never smoke again.

DON C.
I Thought It Was Indigestion

Don C. was vice-president of human resources in a major corporation with more than 600 employees when he had a serious heart attack. He and his wife, Mary Jane, have been married thirty-one years. When Don came home from the hospital, Mary Jane was still smoking.

I remember the last day I smoked all too well. It was Labor Day, 1983. I was at home. It was a warm day, the temperature was in the eighties, and I felt extremely hot and tired. In the morning I had had some chest pains that I thought were indigestion. There was a cord of firewood in the driveway to be stacked, there was some shrubbery to clear away, and I wasn't looking forward to all this physical work because I just didn't feel good.

I did it anyway, but by late afternoon, when I'd nearly finished it, I realized something was seriously wrong. I began to perspire heavily, and the pain became more intense and spread across my shoulders. I knew I needed to cool off fast, so I put the garden hose over my head and yelled to my wife to get me to the doctor immediately. She took me to an emergency medical clinic. It only took about five minutes to get there, but something was telling me that every minute counted.

I wasn't fully aware of everything that was going on. They took an electrocardiogram, listened to my heart, asked me a few questions, and diagnosed it as a heart attack. They gave me some nitroglycerin and called a cardiologist. They transported me to a large hospital and put me in the coronary intensive care unit. They thought my condition had stabilized when I went into ventricular fibrillation [extremely irregular heartbeat]. It's a good thing the cardiologist was there. I feel to this day that he saved my life. They put tubes up my arm directly into my heart and they had got out those special electric paddles used to get your heart going again after it stops . . . which frightened me. When I heard them ask if there was a priest on duty, I think that frightened me more than anything else.

I remember hearing the beeping sound from the electronic equipment that I was hooked up to. It was beeping rather rapidly . . . but I was not aware of any pain or any serious discomfort, and I had the feeling that this couldn't really be happening to me.

At any rate, there was full blockage in one of the arteries in the upper left part of the heart. I was in the hospital ten days. I finally realized the full scope of the damage that had been done. I went home for six weeks and then returned to the hospital for an angiogram, a way to photograph the arteries of the heart. It showed partial blockage in two other arteries. A week later I underwent triple-bypass surgery on my heart.

All this put sufficient fear in me that I realized I had to change my life-style. Various cardiologists, before and after the surgery, told me that the operation would not do me any good in the long run if I went back to smoking and if I wasn't more careful about what I ate. In the three years before my heart attack I had been eating less meat and cutting down on fried food, but I hadn't gone far enough. I needed to get into a regular exercise program.

Before all this happened I had been trying to cut down on my smoking, was doing a little exercise, and experiencing some angina—chest pain—but I always thought it was indigestion. When I had asked a doctor about it, he told me it was probably indigestion. I had just taken a physical exam six weeks before my heart attack, and so I knew what I needed to do: exercise more, watch my weight, watch what I was eating. But as one of the cardiologists told me later, the blockage in those arteries occurred over a period of years—not in the last six months. And he told me that I had a good chance to live to a ripe old age if I would pay more attention to these things. If I went back to smoking and my old eating habits, he couldn't guarantee anything. I felt as if I had been hit by lightning, and I don't need to be hit by lightning twice.

I have not touched a cigarette or a pipe or anything resembling tobacco since my heart attack. My last cigarette was on that Labor Day, 1983.

Once I experienced the nearness to death during my heart attack, there was absolutely no question in my mind that I would never have a cigarette again. When my children and my wife came to see me in the hospital, I knew that I could not and would not have a cigarette or pipe ever again.

When I got home from the hospital my wife was still a smoker, and the cigarette smoke still smelled good to me. I used to tell smokers around me, "It's all right to smoke; in fact, it kind of smells good." I have since come to very intensely dislike people smoking around me. I don't like people to smoke in my home, in my car, and I certainly don't let people smoke in my office. I dislike, very much, being around smokers.

I had many thoughts when I realized what had happened to me, regarding my life and my priorities in life. I felt inadequate, incompetent, as they say in management. I thought, "Why did this happen to me? I know people who are obese, who smoke much more than I do, who get absolutely no exercise. Why did this happen to me?" I was only five to ten pounds overweight, I was a smoker, but not a heavy smoker, and I just couldn't understand it. I had great concern for my longevity and a high interest in what I needed to do to live to a ripe old age. It made me stop and think about my children, the importance to me of work, the importance of my friends, the quality of my life. These are the things I thought about while I was in the hospital, having little else to do other than stare up at the ceiling.

I had smoked for a long time, starting at about sixteen years old. It seemed like very nearly every boy in my high school class was a cigarette smoker. I was smoking unfiltered cigarettes, as was common in those days, about half a pack a day. It was very much the thing to do.

It was difficult to start. I remember it well. My father had a philosophy that if you are determined to smoke, don't sneak around—do it at home.

My father smoked. As I recall, he smoked Lucky Strikes and Chesterfield cigarettes, which were popular brands in those days. I remember I was in my bedroom listening to the radio and reading a magazine and having a cigarette, and I was eating some French bread, and it made me very sick. I had to go to the bathroom and throw up, and my father laughed because he thought that would teach me not to smoke.

The whole thing made me very ill. In fact, I got sick two or three times. But because of peer pressure in high school to smoke and to drink beer—in those days there was no temptation towards marijuana or anything—I kept trying to get used to smoking, and eventually I did. It took me two or three weeks, maybe even two months— not trying it every day, just on occasion—until I got accustomed to smoking.

Later I switched brands to a filtered brand, Kent, after high school when I went in the Navy in the early fifties. I smoked about a pack a day. All of the years that I smoked cigarettes, I found that I could never smoke more than a pack a day. In the late afternoons and evenings they did not taste good. They left a foul taste in my mouth, and anticipating the cigarette was better than the reality.

In the mid-seventies I quit cigarettes, and to this day I don't know why. I just threw a pack away one day and decided I was not going to smoke again. I took up smoking a pipe. I started smoking about three pipes a day. Eventually, I was smoking five or six pipes a day. I had a pipe in my mouth almost constantly, whether it was lit or not. I had some colleagues and friends who also smoked pipes, and it was something to do together.

Some of my friends who smoked pipes later quit smoking the pipes and took to cigarettes. I found that if I was around them and I didn't have my pipe with me, I would borrow one of their cigarettes. I would tell myself, "Well, one cigarette is not going to get me back to smoking cigarettes," but of course, it did!

So from the mid-seventies until 1983, I was smoking

both cigarettes and a pipe. By 1983 I was smoking about a half a pack of Marlboros a day. I wasn't fooling around with low-tar and -nicotine cigarettes, and since I didn't allow smoking in my office, I would take cigarette breaks in other smokers' offices. I smoked in the evening and on my way to work. I smoked half a pack of cigarettes a day, and my pipe about twice a day, until I had my heart attack. In fact, that very day I remember having some cigarettes and thinking they tasted particularly bad. But right up to the day that I had the heart attack, I was a smoker.

After I quit, I wanted to talk to my wife, Mary Jane, about her smoking and her health. She got angry at me and didn't want to talk about it. She already knew that she shouldn't smoke, but the time had to be right for her to quit. She had my sympathy, because she was trying, but she had smoked since she was a teen-ager and smoked heavily—at least two packs of Marlboros a day.

One day, after she attended Smokenders without telling me, I realized that she hadn't had a cigarette all day. She didn't want other people to know because she was afraid of failing, but she was trying to quit. It was hard for her to get through that first week, but now she is very proud of the fact that she hasn't smoked in more than a year.

Before that she had tried hypnosis. She didn't even want me around when she was listening to the audio tapes on how to quit! She had heard a lot of people say, "Well, I quit for six months," and it was discouraging for her. She was afraid that if she quit and then started again she might never be able to quit permanently.

She was also concerned that if she quit smoking she would gain weight—and she did. She now plans to get into a diet program to lose the weight. She had to lick the smoking problem first, and she did. She's sure she will never smoke again.

For me, the temptation to smoke is completely gone. I just don't like the smell of cigarette smoke. It seems like a dirty habit. Occasionally, and this may sound crazy, but occasionally, on a winter evening, I will get the urge to smoke my pipe. A pipe is something of an evening, indoor activity. Or I'll smell pipe smoke, and that will remind me how enjoyable it was. (Actually, though, it smells better than it tastes, as most pipe smokers would agree.) But it isn't a serious urge; it's not going to turn me back into a smoker. I can pass a pipe shop and say, "Gee, it's like cookies baking, but I am not going to have one." It's pure nostalgia.

It took me about one year or, at most, a year and a half to really dislike smoking. Some people have asked me, "Why didn't you quit sooner? The information was out there about how bad it was for your health." Well, tobacco is like a drug. I had started smoking at a time when you went to the movies and you saw Humphrey Bogart smoking, and it was a very manly thing to do—very macho to have a cigarette dangling from your lip. There was a popular fantasy that the girls thought you were that much more masculine if you had a cigarette after sex.

No one ever said how harmful it was the first ten or fifteen years I was smoking. No one except my mother, who would say, "Why are you doing that? It is going to stunt your growth." But I looked around and I didn't see only short people walking around smoking, so I thought that was all a bunch of baloney that mothers would tell their children to scare them.

Years ago, athletes advertised cigarettes and doctors smoked. I collect old *Life* magazines. I have seen ads in some of them that say, "Doctors who smoke recommend Chesterfield cigarettes." How terrible that in the late thirties *doctors* were recommending brands of cigarettes! That just shows how common smoking was. I mention this only because cigarettes really hooked me. My first fifteen years of smoking, the thing to do was to have a good American breakfast of bacon and eggs and white toast with butter and maybe some coffee, and then to finish that off with a couple of cigarettes. You know what? That's the recipe for a heart attack.

JONI L.
An Ad on TV Convinced

Joni L. was in her early twenties when her parents died. Both had been smokers, and both died of cancer. After she went through a sizable inheritance, she had to make drastic changes to put her life in order. For the past twenty years Joni, now in her early fifties, has worked as a legal secretary and a paralegal, specializing in litigation.

Both my father and mother were smokers. My father had always been a smoker, but not my mother. My mother told me that she had smoked as a teen-ager before I was born. When she found out she was pregnant with me, she stopped smoking. She started again when I was in high school. I am afraid that I may have triggered that, because when she found out that I was smoking on the side in high school, she said, "Well, I used to smoke."

"Oh, Mother, you never did."

"Oh, yes, I did."

"Did you inhale?"

"Yes."

"Show me," I said.

And she did. And that triggered her desire to smoke again after all those years. I guess she thought that if I, her child, was smoking, why couldn't she? She smoked from that day on until she died of cancer. I have carried a terrible guilt all these years as I think I may have been responsible for my mother starting to smoke again.

I remember the way I began to think about smoking. I was about five years old and I was riding my tricycle out in front of the house with a neighborhood playmate. We were talking about what grown-ups did: getting married, having children, drinking, and smoking. I remember saying, "Well, I don't want to get married, I don't want to have children, I'll never drink, but I will smoke." I made a conscious decision for what was, to my child's mind, sophistication. Most adults smoked and I figured it must be fun. I followed my father's example.

When I was about eleven, I got into my dad's cigarettes, stole some matches, and, with my little girlfriend, hid in the weeds of a vacant lot not far from my home. We figured if we hunched down we could smoke and nobody would see us. We didn't realize that the smoke was circling over our heads. I didn't like it: It tasted awful.

I didn't smoke again until I was seventeen. I was a senior in high school, and all of my friends were smoking because it proved you were very grown up, very sophisticated, very much accepted by your peers. Peer pressure and the desire for sophistication and social acceptance triggered my smoking. Still, I had known from the time I was five that I would probably smoke someday.

I was never a heavy smoker. In high school it amounted mostly to going out to the cars in the school parking lot at lunchtime. A group of girls would take their lunches, go out to somebody's car, pile in, laugh and giggle and talk about boys, smoke a couple of cigarettes, and then go back to class. I have never smoked more than a pack a day, very often only three-quarters of a pack a day.

I realize now that I never really liked the taste of cigarettes. I couldn't smoke without having just drunk something or eaten something. If I was under stress and wanted a cigarette to relieve the stress, I would very often have to eat something before smoking. Eating and smoking went hand in hand. I was not a person who could smoke alone. I never got up and smoked first thing in the morning, never smoked last thing before I went to bed. I was never a *heavy* smoker, but I was a *chronic* smoker for nearly eighteen years.

The years 1957 and 1958 were extremely stressful for me. My mother passed away of cancer in the latter part of 1957, I divorced my husband, and in the early part of 1958 my father also died of cancer. In less than fourteen months I had three major traumas. It was a very, very difficult time.

In the 1960s, having gone through most of a large inheritance, I ended up having to sell my home in Menlo Park. It was an extremely difficult period because I was not used to being poor, I was trying to break into the business world in Los Angeles, and I had no connections. I was not smoking any more heavily than before, but still I was smoking, and the stress was mounting.

Then I saw an advertisement on television and it was the actor who played the district attorney on the old "Perry Mason" television program, William Talman. I believe he made the commercial for the American Cancer Society. He was dying of cancer, and he made some television advertisements against smoking which showed him as he appeared on the "Perry Mason" show when he was in good health, and then the camera panned back to him as he looked dying of cancer: emaciated and obviously close to death. His message was, "If you don't smoke, don't start, and if you have started, quit."

That actor reminded me very much of my father. I had lost my father from cancer, my mother from cancer, and now here was this actor in my living room on my television screen telling me why I should stop smoking. He reminded me so much of my father: It was the perfect message for me.

I thought about it for a couple of weeks. I could not shake the memory of that man, that wonderful actor. His face was constantly before me, even while I was at work. Finally I reached the decision to quit. I quit cold turkey after eighteen years.

My method was probably unique to me. I had never heard of anything like it before: I call it the sleep method. I decided to take three days off and do nothing but sleep, which for me was sleeping, getting up, eating, going back to bed, and going to sleep again. I repeated this cycle each day. I did nothing else, had no stress; I just rested and slept. On the fourth day I got up and went to work. I must have read somewhere or heard that by the third or fourth day your body is relieved of the physical craving and after that you just had to work on the mental aspect of smoking. I felt that if my body wasn't craving cigarettes, surely I could control my mind. From that day in 1969, I never touched a cigarette again. It is twenty years now since I quit, and I'm very glad I did!

To show the resolve I had in quitting smoking, on the fourth day after I had quit I started a new job as a legal secretary in Beverly Hills. I had to sit next to another secretary who smoked at her desk. I was surrounded by cigarette smoke, but I never wavered, never took another puff from a cigarette.

Now I cannot be around smokers and I cannot be in a

room full of cigarette smoke. I have developed an allergy to it. I can't breathe, and I get very ill. I feel I owe all this to William Talman and the commercial he did against smoking. He was the one who brought the connection between smoking and cancer into sharp focus for me. I thank God for the new laws prohibiting smoking in the workplace because I have not been able to work in some law firms since I refuse to work around smokers now.

PATRICK REYNOLDS
Committed to Help Others

Patrick, thirty-nine, is the grandson of the founder of the R. J. Reynolds Tobacco Company, one of the largest tobacco companies in the world. As a boy, he watched his father, a heavy smoker, die a slow death from emphysema. In spite of that experience, Patrick started smoking himself. It took him ten years to kick the habit successfully. Today he has invested his inheritance from the R. J. Reynolds fortune in a program to help people quit smoking.

My grandfather, R. J. Reynolds, chewed tobacco and died of cancer of the pancreas. My father smoked heavily and he died at fifty-eight after years of suffering from emphysema. My father's sister, Nancy, smoked, and she also died of emphysema. His other sister smoked and died of cancer. One of Nancy's children, my cousin, smoked, and died recently of cancer. My mother smoked, and I believe that smoking contributed to her death as well.

I started smoking at seventeen, sneaking smokes in the basement at Hotchkiss, the prep school where I boarded. I would sneak down to the basement to have one little cigarette once or twice a week from a stale pack of cigarettes. It was very unpleasant initially. Nobody ever inhaled their first few cigarettes without coughing, including me.

I started smoking mostly because it was against the school rules. In fact, smoking was grounds for expulsion. It was an act of pure adolescent defiance. Cigarettes were a way of breaking the rules, and breaking the rules felt great. It was my way of expressing my anger against the school, against authority, against having to take on adult responsibilities. I was really angry about being locked up in boarding school, in classes wearing a coat and tie six days a week.

Occasionally I would smoke in my room. That required elaborate preparations. I put a towel in the crack under the door to keep the smoke from escaping. I would crack the window in such a way that the smoke would flow out the top of the window and the fresh air would flow in the bottom. I'd blow the smoke out the top crack. I had room deodorizer, mouthwash, special soap, cologne to throw around the room and douse my hands in, everything at the ready, in case there was a knock at the door. I thought it all worked because I never got caught, but I found out later that one of the masters at school did see smoke coming out of my room one day and decided not to report me.

As far as I knew, none of my friends smoked because it

wasn't something I did with friends. I did it alone. It was my own personal, private rebellion. I couldn't imagine expressing my anger to adults directly, so I turned the anger inward and did something self-destructive—smoked—instead. All I accomplished was hurting myself. Sixteen or seventeen is a difficult period in life, and that's why so many people are vulnerable to starting smoking at that age.

Once I got to college in California, I was hooked. I smoked a pack a day, and it made me feel older and more confident. It seemed grown-up and sophisticated to smoke. By comparison with all the drugs and craziness that were going on at Berkeley in 1967, smoking was one of the milder forms of rebellion. The peer pressure there was to smoke marijuana.

Cigarettes are a good anxiety-reducer. And once I got accustomed to it, I liked the taste of tobacco. The deep inhaling, deep breathing, is an ancient yoga practice for inducing a calm, meditative state, and smoking helped calm me. Plus, I was a Reynolds; let's not overlook that. The family had helped popularize cigarettes, so there was a certain amount of pride in lighting up a Winston. I always smoked the family products.

I wanted to stop smoking within a year of starting, but I didn't start trying to quit for several years. I tried hypnosis, but I was too uptight to allow myself to let go enough for it to be an effective therapy for me. I really believed that I was so strongly addicted that I couldn't let go of that idea even under hypnosis.

Then I tried Smokenders, which was a system of cutting down on smoking. You start by marking a cigarette to smoke only part of it. I think that takes more willpower and strength than quitting cold turkey. It didn't work because every time you put a cigarette in your mouth you are restimulating the habit and your enjoyment of it. Every time I got to have a cigarette, even when I was down to four or five cigarettes a day, it was very upsetting because I was only going to get that one more cigarette that day, and oh, my *God* . . . So Smokenders didn't work. It might work for someone else, but it didn't work for me.

I tried going cold turkey on my own a few times. I'd make it for a couple of weeks, but it was a very hairy, difficult experience. I was crabby to my friends, I was nervous, I bit my fingernails. The feeling deep inside that I really, really *wanted* a cigarette remained. So that didn't work.

I even tried acupuncture, but I thought the acupuncture was going to make it easy, that it was going to do it for me. It helped a little bit, but it wasn't enough by itself, so I failed. I hadn't really prepared myself to fight the battle of withdrawal. Maybe if I'd tried the acupuncture in conjunction with a strong commitment to being a nonsmoker it would have worked. But I didn't, and it didn't.

The best program I tried was Schick. Of all the methods I tried, it was the most effective one, but in the end, it didn't work either. J. Patrick Frawley was the chairman, and we talked, and he loaded me up with materials about addiction, books to read, videos, everything.

The program takes a week. They give you a mild electroshock every time you take a puff in order to give your-self negative reinforcement to counter the positive rein-forcement you get from the pleasure of smoking. Now if each cigarette takes fifteen puffs, and you smoke twenty cigarettes a day, twenty times fifteen, you get a lot of positive reinforcement for your habit. Multiply that by the number of days or weeks or years you've smoked, and your unconscious mind has hundreds of thousands of positive associations with smoking. You can make a conscious decision to quit smoking, but your conscious mind and unconscious mind don't necessarily work to-gether. All your unconscious mind knows is that smoking feels good. What Schick does is help deprogram the un-conscious mind.

I had such a strong addiction that I went through the program five times. I'd last three or four weeks or three or four months and once I lasted eight months, but then I'd start smoking again. They held follow-up seminars after the program, but they were really boring. I didn't like getting in the car, driving to a meeting, and sitting around listening to people talk about how badly they wanted a cigarette. I knew that already, and I didn't want to burn up two hours of my life sitting around listening to it.

I smoked from 1967 to 1984. That's seventeen years, but I had periods of non-smoking during that time that cut the number of years I actually smoked regularly to more like ten. The thing that would trigger the relapses was always stress, whether it was positive or negative. I'd have an argument with my ex-wife, and I'd take out my anger at her by having a cigarette. Or a lonely moment. Or a sad moment. Positive stress had the same effect. The hardest times for me even now are when I'm relaxed, say, on vacation at a friend's estate. I've had a beautiful meal, we're having an espresso, a friend lights up a cigarette, and I really, *really* want one. It's as though everything is perfect except that one thing is missing: *my* cigarette. Before, I didn't realize that all it takes to get me hooked again is one cigarette. Now I've learned to recognize the danger in these moments, so I'm very wary and careful. I tell myself, "Take it easy, the desire will be gone in five minutes, so just wait it out." I make a conscious decision not to have a cigarette at that tempting moment. I haven't smoked for four years, and now those moments occur much less often.

The thing that finally worked was to quit by myself with an assist from a behavior modification program that I got from a psychologist. When I put together the Reynolds Stop Smoking Program, that was the technique we used. Research done on corporations that support programs to help employees stop smoking finds that smokers do best quitting on their own or with minimal intervention programs, like cassette tapes. They do much better than those in group programs. Only a very small percentage of those in group seminars quit successfully. I invested the money I inherited from my grandfather's fortune into this corporation. I hope I can help undo some of the damage that's been done by tobacco, or at the very least discourage young people from ever starting to smoke.

MICHAEL G.
I Got Tired of the Rigmarole

Michael G. has a Ph.D. in ethnographic history, but has changed careers to become a broker, contracting computer experts to companies. Married for twenty-five years, he is the father of a five-year-old daughter.

I've not smoked for twenty years. I was twenty-five when I quit, and I had smoked for ten or eleven years. I started when I was about fourteen or fifteen, back in prep school in a small town just north of New York City. It started as a game but, sooner or later, everybody got hooked. My father was a very heavy smoker. I ended up smoking Lucky Strike unfiltered cigarettes. I smoked about half a pack a day during high school, close to a pack a day in college and at the Lutheran seminary where I went after college.

After I graduated from the seminary and had already been accepted at graduate school, I worked in a warehouse to earn some money for graduate school and my wedding. There was a lot of dust and gas-driven forklifts, which probably didn't improve the quality of the air (these were pre-EPA days), and I happened to work a forklift a fair amount of the time.

I usually worked lots of overtime because that was the only way you made money in those days. I'd often work over sixty hours a week. I remember this one gray day, the sun was just breaking through the clouds and the breakfast truck had come around for the mid-morning snack, that usual awful sugary kind of food. . . . Anyway, I bought a doughnut and had it with my coffee.

That morning I lit up a cigarette and said, "Hey, I don't like this any more." I put out the cigarette and looked at the cigarette machine: Cigarettes were getting expensive. Now they were forty, maybe forty-five cents a pack, and that had been bothering me. When I was younger I could get cigarettes for as little as twenty-three cents a pack.

Something else was bothering me: Besides carrying around cigarettes in your pocket, you either have to carry enough matches to pass as a pyromaniac, or you carry lighters. And lighters take fluid and flints and you are always diddling around with them.

At least the logistics of smoking cigarettes were not as complicated as the logistics of smoking a pipe, which I had also tried. Smoking a pipe was too much of a pain. I didn't want to carry around a small brain surgery kit just to smoke a pipe for five minutes. I tried cigars and found they didn't taste very good. I even tried a hookah, a bubble pipe, once.

But, back to that morning at the warehouse. . . . I had half a pack of cigarettes with me. That pack stayed in my pocket that whole afternoon. In the evening I threw the pack out on a card table in my bedroom, asked my brother-in-law, "Do you want some cigarettes? Do you want a lighter?" and gave him the cigarettes and the

lighter. About two nights later I had one filter cigarette at a party and it didn't taste very good. I was just
plain getting tired of smoking. That was the last time I
smoked . . . that's about twenty years ago.

You can say that I quit out of sheer laziness. I didn't
want my life to revolve around cigarettes, I didn't want to
have to worry about the change in my pocket, or running
out on holidays, or stuffing a lighter, or carrying all of
this stuff around. Not smoking made life so much simpler! I gained back my shirt pockets, and my pants pockets no longer had long holes torn in them. Suddenly I
didn't have to worry about running out of cigarettes. I
had had this constant worry about supply and logistics. I
came to the conclusion that if I wasn't enjoying it, quit.
The money arguments didn't work, the cancer arguments didn't work, the fitness and health argument
sounded too much like a Southern Baptist summer camp
(they are probably very nice people, but . . .); in the end
smoking was too complicated and too time consuming. I
had to think about too many things to smoke, and I had
plenty of other things I wanted to think about.

This crazy thing of logistics is what really bothered me.
Sometimes you put a pack in your back pocket and sit
down and *crunch*! Or you have tobacco on your lips, and
straight raw tobacco, no matter what the quality, doesn't
taste very good. The nicotine burns. Then there is the
mess, the ashes, what you do with the cigarette if you
want to do something else with your hands. . . .

I still like to play with my hands, but now I do it with
computer keyboards or telephone keyboards, or I'll read

and flip through the pages of computer magazines or journals. There is more than enough to keep one's hands busy; that's never a problem.

CHRIS J.
I Don't Like Feeling Out of Breath

Chris J., thirty-five years old, is a social psychologist evaluating how various groups and organizations promote good health in the community. She was born in England and brought up in the United States. During her childhood her family moved frequently; Chris attended more than twenty schools, most of them in Southern California. Her smoking "career" lasted almost ten years, but it began at age thirteen.

I stopped smoking when I was twenty-two. What happened was that the things you think of as the rewards of smoking when you are young simply aren't there anymore when you become an adult. I mean, you find that smoking is commonplace, and if you are in it for the sophisticated image, that image fades away. And by then, if you're lucky, your sense of self is better developed. Other things are more rewarding as an adult—like your schoolwork, physical activity, and social interactions—so that smoking becomes unimportant to you. Then all you're stuck with at that point is the physiologic component—the addiction—and the smell.

I remember being bothered by having my clothing smell like tobacco, and the fact that people could tell I smoked when I walked into a room even if I wasn't holding a cigarette. In college I supported myself by working in a bank part time. I couldn't smoke on the job. If I wanted to have a cigarette, I had to get up and leave. It got to be a real hassle to have a cigarette.

I started smoking at the end of elementary school, when I was about thirteen. I had a strong interest in horseback riding. A friend and I used to ride horses together after school; we actually trained horses. Her father smoked. He was a farmer from South Dakota, and he smoked unfiltered Camel cigarettes. He also rolled his own cigarettes. She and I used to go home after school and change our clothes and then go out to the stables. Occasionally, she would show up with a pack of cigarettes. I remember walking out to the horses; it was just a ten- or fifteen-minute walk, but it was long enough . . . that is where it all began. She would try smoking—I wouldn't have called it peer pressure then, though I might call it that now. At the time it was just that she was smoking, why wasn't I smoking?

She was my age; we were only two weeks apart. There was something else going on—there was an older girl, probably fifteen or sixteen, who was much more sophisticated than we were, and we looked up to her. She was in high school, and she was someone who did her hair and dressed well, and *she* smoked. She owned one of the horses that we trained, and we wanted very much to be like her. Looking back, I think she was influential in making us want to smoke and be sophisticated in the way that we thought she was.

I remember a few things that I liked about smoking. It was all very image related; one part was the sophistication, and the other was the packaging. I don't know if there is a gender difference here or not, but I think—and this is a terrible stereotype—that women like little things in cute packages. I think this is true for a lot of women, and I remember there was something very attractive about going and buying these little packs of cigarettes. The other thing was the cost—a pack of cigarettes then used to cost around thirty-five or forty cents, which was affordable even for an elementary or high school student. You could get a lot of sophistication and image building for a very small amount of money.

It was easy to buy cigarettes from small liquor stores and gas stations, even though we were obviously too young to buy them legally. It was more difficult and much less likely that we would try to buy them from a large grocery store, like a Safeway.

One day my mother came to me. I can remember the time of day and where I was in the house and all that. It was evident that I had been smoking because I smelled like a cigarette, and she said, "If you do nothing else for me in terms of the way you dress and the way you behave as an adolescent, please don't smoke." She was very sincere, pleading with me not to smoke. I think that probably planted a seed in my mind; it made me think about wanting to quit. I thought, "Boy, she really means this. I probably shouldn't smoke." There was probably a rebellion/defiance component to my smoking, since it was something my parents didn't want me to do.

Neither of my parents ever smoked, and never have. I attribute the ease with which I was able to quit smoking later to that. It seemed natural to me that I shouldn't smoke, and that the whole time I was smoking I probably shouldn't have been smoking.

When I was eighteen I went to England. It was fun to smoke there because English cigarettes are very different—they are smaller and they taste different. American cigarettes are stronger. We used to exchange cigarettes and talk about different brands. At that point, it was still enjoyable to smoke.

Smoking was much more socially acceptable in England than in the United States. Everybody smoked. At that time I smoked about a pack a day, ranging between, say, fifteen cigarettes a day and a pack and a half.

In the beginning, I didn't like smoking: I was trying to start with Camel unfiltered cigarettes, which were just awful. I can't even describe it. To this day, fifteen to twenty years later, I remember how terrible it was. Then, our sophisticated high school friend said, "Well, try these." They were Larks. I don't think Larks are a cigarette anymore, but I remember the purple package with the gold or white labeling. They were very mild cigarettes, but they still weren't mild enough for me. I remember searching for the mildest cigarette I could find. I switched to Tarrytons, which were low tar, low nicotine.

My friend branched off into Marlboros and other very

strong cigarettes. To this day, she still smokes Marlboros. I couldn't go that way; physiologically, I didn't
like it. In the early days, I felt nauseated when I smoked,
light-headed and dizzy. I just did not feel good.

I was a true smoker by the time I was fifteen, and I
smoked all the way through age twenty-one or twenty-
two, so it was six or seven years. I smoked Lark cigarettes
or something equivalent to them in terms of the strength
of the tobacco.

Throughout elementary and high school I was very
athletic—riding horses, playing softball, running, that
sort of thing. I actually ended up buying my own horse in
high school, and I did a lot of riding. But when I moved
to San Diego to go to college I left the horse behind. I
found myself in a new situation—living in the dorms—
and smoking was still very acceptable. That's when you
start drinking if you're inclined, and I did, so there was a
lot of going out to places where smoking and drinking
were important focuses. My exercise and physical activity
sort of fell by the wayside during the first few years in
college.

It was when I began to miss physical activity that I
started on the road towards quitting smoking, because I
thought, "Well, gee, I want to start exercising again." I
could tell I was getting out of shape, and I missed being
in shape. I got a bike for my birthday—actually, I got two
bikes, one from my boyfriend and one from my parents
because they all knew I wanted to get back into physical
activity. That was my twenty-first birthday.

I started cycling again. San Diego is a great place to

cycle. I lived in Point Loma, which is a very hilly area, at the midpoint on a very steep hill. One day I went out on my bike with one of my college roommates and started to head up the hill. I realized that I was having a difficult time breathing, and I didn't attribute it all to the hill: I attributed it to my smoking.

From the time I went to San Diego until getting on this bike, there had been two years that I had been physically inactive and smoking at an increased rate. I attributed feeling out of shape and having a hard time breathing not so much to not exercising but to smoking. I thought, "I don't like feeling like an old person. I don't like feeling out of breath." It was a steep hill, but nevertheless for someone who was twenty-one years old, it was very telling. I remember standing on the top of the hill and looking at my roommate and saying, "It's just not worth it. You know, smoking is a bad thing." And that was it. That was the last time I smoked.

I think there were several things that led up to my quitting, but that was the final thing, the most significant thing. I had tried to stop before that, but I can't remember giving it a really hard try. I'd stop for one week or two weeks, just putting the cigarettes aside, and trying not to pick them up again. When I finally decided that there was a good reason to quit smoking, it seemed easy.

I never thought too much about things like cancer. I was too young at the time I quit to worry about that sort of thing. It was very much oxygen related, something that is important if you exercise a lot. Even now when I am feeling lazy and say, "I don't want to get out on my

109

bike," I think about the air, about how good it feels to get plenty of oxygen into your brain after sitting in an office all day, and that is enough incentive to get me out. I was used to the high that exercise gives, so it's a good incentive for me.

Now looking back, I do remember a pain in my lungs that I had not felt before—a raspy feeling. When I heard friends who coughed a lot in the morning from smoking I thought, "Am I going to be that way in a few years?" I didn't think about cancer or heart disease, I am sure I didn't think about chronic disease, but I did think about clogging up my breathing system and being less physically capable of exercising.

The interesting thing is that I had a roommate who smoked and I had a boyfriend who smoked, and that was a problem with the boyfriend. It began to bother me. I think you have to go one way or another—either other people's smoking bothers you or you start smoking again. It's hard to stay neutral about having close friends who smoke when you don't.

When I go to hotels I always request non-smoking rooms now. In restaurants and on airplanes I request the non-smoking section. If I am in a non-smoking section and someone is smoking, I'll ask them to put their cigarette out. A neighbor came over and wanted to give me some little housewarming gifts, and she asked if she could come in. I said, "Yes, you can, but your cigarette has to stay outside."

I live alone now, but I wouldn't date or get into a relationship with someone who smoked. Wouldn't it be awful to meet a terrific person who smoked? That would be tough.

BOB L.
My Wife and I Quit the Same Day

Bob L., forty-nine, has worked a granite rock quarry for twenty-three years, first as a heavy equipment operator and then as supervisor of rock crushing. Bob and his wife have three grown children, with children of their own. On weekends, he and his wife take off in their motor home. They both enjoy fishing.

About three years ago I quit smoking for the last time, because of my wife. Smoking was starting to bother her health—she was coughing a lot. She said, "Honey, I'm going to stop smoking." And I said, "Well, honey, if you're going to quit, then I'm going to quit, too." She smoked about three packs a day, the same kind of cigarettes I did. I thought, "If she is going to quit, it would be a lot easier for her and me to quit together." We both quit on the same day, the same week.

If it weren't for her health, I probably would still be smoking because it didn't bother my system. I know it really bothers a lot of people. But I have to say honestly that it never bothered me. But it made my wife cough a lot and get real deep chest pains. And, no joking, money was a big factor. We figured it up one time and it cost $1,100 a year for her and me to smoke. That played some part in deciding to quit, but the biggest part was the health factor.

I still craved cigarettes for some time after I quit. I had to have the willpower to say, "No, I am not going to take one." Your body does crave those cigarettes for quite a while—like maybe three, four, or five months. I think the key to quitting smoking is yourself: I don't think anybody can tell somebody to quit; it has to be your own decision. Once you make up your mind, you can quit. I don't think you can go to a hypnotist or to a school. I think it is all up to the individual. A lot of people say they can't quit, but down deep, I don't think they want to quit. They really want to smoke. They say, "How did you do it? I just can't quit smoking." Well, you *can* quit, because the day you say, "That's it. I am not going to smoke," you can flat out quit.

Since I quit, I eat a little more. Food tastes a lot better, and with the food tasting better, instead of grabbing a cigarette, we tend to eat more. My wife has gained weight since we've quit smoking.

I can honestly say that quitting did make me a little bit nervous in the beginning. I got tense because sometimes my subconscious mind was saying, "I want a cigarette," and then my conscious mind would say, "No, you're not going to have a cigarette," so I had a tug-of-war between my subconscious mind and my real mind.

I remember how my dad smoked until he was about forty-five, and one day he quit. He just threw his cigarettes out the window, and that was the last time he smoked. He just flat quit, and that was it.

I started smoking young, probably fourteen years old, about 1952. I think one of the reasons I started is that all the other kids were doing it, so it was something like, "The other kids do it, so why not me?" I think it's the same with drugs and everything else.

In the beginning my body tried to reject the nicotine. But I told myself, "I'm going to make myself smoke," because everybody else was doing it, and I thought it was kind of a smart thing. Pretty soon your body builds up a tolerance to it, and you're hooked. I would say it took my body a couple of months to get hooked on it.

I used to smoke about two, two and a half packs a day. I usually smoked filter cigarettes—Virginia Slims. My wife did, too. We both smoked when we got married; I was nineteen and she was seventeen. I smoked two and a half packs a day for thirty-three years.

I had quit once before, about ten years ago. At that time I decided to quit because it interfered with my work. I was always grabbing a cigarette, trying to smoke it while I was working, and it got in the way. I got mad at myself for smoking and just threw the things away and said I wasn't going to smoke no more. When you're trying to do something and you have a cigarette in your mouth and the smoke is in your eyes and your eyes are watering, you just get mad. I said, "That's it, I am not smoking no more."

I didn't smoke for a year. Then I started again. The reason is that a lot of times you're sitting around with the guys and having a beer or something, and the next thing you know, "Well, I'm going to have me a cigarette." So

I'd have a cigarette, and the first one made me dizzy. It took a little while to get used to it again. That dizzy spell is your body trying to reject the nicotine, but pretty soon I was smoking again anyway.

When other people smoke it doesn't bother me a bit. As a matter of fact, I can smell their smoke, and I don't even crave one. But for the first few weeks, whenever I smelled a cigarette, I had to have some willpower not to ask for one. I really had to watch myself, but once I got over that hump it was fine.

I am happy I have quit, you bet. I'll never, ever start back again. My wife either. We will never, ever go back to smoking again. Now my house is clean. Oh, it used to smell of smoke. We had to wash the walls down. When you're smoking like that you don't know how dirty the house gets from just nicotine and smoke. It's unbelievable.

LOUISE G.
The Change in Public Attitude
Has Helped Me

Louise G., sixty-three, and the mother of five children, practiced law for seventeen years before retiring to devote her considerable energy to tennis, bridge, and Scrabble. She lives in a turn-of-the-century house in a quiet town south of San Francisco. Her smoking led to the trauma of a bad fall.

I had a weight problem when I was young, and smoking changed my metabolism so that I could eat as much as I wanted without gaining weight. I started smoking when I was sixteen. My brother and I would sneak into the bathroom with a pack of Camels and smoke. I enjoyed it right away. I was a senior in high school then, and by the summer between high school and college, I was smoking a pack a day.

I always smoked a pack a day. I smoked all through college. I smoked through my four pregnancies and five children. Nothing could convince me to stop smoking.

Every one of my children objected to my smoking—loudly and often. They left no doubt as to the intensity of their disapproval. Worse, they set me a good example: Not one of them ever smoked. Even worse were my four grandchildren, who begged me to stop smoking practically from the time they could talk. But none of this inspired me to stop. I didn't have a cough. I had no trouble breathing. And I liked smoking.

Two of my daughters are nurses, and they, of course, were the most outspoken of my children about how bad smoking was for my health. They would say, "We'll take you to the hospital and make you look at the emphysema patients. *That* will convince you to quit." The idea that someday I might not be able to breathe was very frightening, but even that didn't work. Nothing worked.

There were some things I just couldn't do without a cigarette. Ironing was one, sewing was another. When I was working with my hands I liked to have a cigarette going at the same time. I would stop smoking when I had a cold. I had one fairly serious illness when I was in my early thirties, and for a long time I couldn't smoke. Well, I could hardly wait until I could start smoking again. I really looked forward to it, as that was the only way I enjoyed doing things like sewing: Sewing and cigarettes always went together for me.

I used smoking as a pleasant way to break up the day. When the mail came, I'd sit down, light a cigarette, and read the mail. Or I'd tell myself, "First I'll have a cigarette, and then I'll do that chore."

There were some problems with smoking. I had an awful tendency to burn holes in my clothes and in the car upholstery. I worried constantly that I'd left a cigarette burning when I left the house, and I'd go back home to reassure myself that I hadn't.

Another problem was that, even when I smoked, I hated the smell of stale cigarette smoke. I remember now how offensive and unpleasant it was to open the door of my car and smell the stale tobacco. I didn't mind having other smokers around me. I played bridge with three other smokers, and the smell was not particularly objectionable. I was so used to the odor of cigarette smoke that I didn't even notice immediately if a smoker had been in my house. I couldn't smell the smoke on clothes either. It was only the smell of stale smoke that was so terribly unpleasant.

Anyway, not even the offensive smell of stale smoke in the car or the holes I routinely burned in my clothes deterred me from smoking until something happened one morning in the fall of 1983. I will never forget the details of that morning as long as I live.

That morning I got up, went to the bathroom, brushed my teeth—I couldn't stand to smoke until I had brushed my teeth—and then I lit a cigarette. That had been my routine for years. I truly enjoyed that first cigarette; it tasted *so* good.

That morning I lit my first cigarette and after a few puffs I felt terribly sick to my stomach and terribly dizzy. I felt sicker and worse than I ever had in my whole life. I was so dizzy that I fell down, cracking my head on the bathroom floor. You know how you feel when you are afraid you are going to die? That's how I felt. It was awful. My kids took me to the hospital and I realized that I should never smoke again. And I haven't.

That was my last puff, that cigarette in the bathroom. Smoking is permanently intertwined in my mind with that awful fall, that terrifying sick and dizzy sensation. I am sure that it was the cigarette that triggered the sickness, that dizziness and weakness and bad fall. I have a very definite connection in my mind between the cigarette and the fall. That's what has kept me away from cigarettes since that day. I haven't touched one since.

I am fairly sure that if I smoked a cigarette now and didn't get sick that I'd probably be hooked again. I've dreamed that I smoked and wakened not quite sure whether it really happened. That's scary, because I don't ever want to smoke again. I've made a bargain with myself about cigarettes exactly like the one I've made about candy: never again, not even one!

Never again? Well, maybe when I'm eighty I'll have another Hershey bar, but I haven't had one in forty-two years. And sometimes I think that if I make it to ninety-five, and there isn't much I can do with myself anyway, maybe I'll try smoking again. . . .

Could I get hooked again if I tried one cigarette? I think so. The only way I've been able to stay away from cigarettes for the last four years is to know that I can never have another cigarette, not one.

Before my collapse I had tried to cut down on smoking with low-tar cigarettes. I ended up smoking three packs a day instead of one, and not enjoying it. In the last few years before I quit, I'd started asking clients if they minded if I smoked while they were in my office. I guess that was my attempt to integrate myself into the new world, the world where smoking was no longer socially acceptable. There were ten lawyers in my law office, and I was the only one who smoked.

The change in attitude toward smoking from the fifties to today helped me make the connection between smoking and my fall. It's interesting to watch movies of the forties, fifties, and sixties—everyone's smoking! If there had not been so much public information about how bad smoking is for your health, I'd probably have started smoking again the minute I recovered from my fall.

My life changed when I stopped smoking. I gained thirty pounds, most of which I've taken off. I can't eat as much as I used to without gaining weight. It wasn't that I ate more when I quit; it's that the same amount I ate then now makes me put on weight, so I have to eat less and play tennis more. I appreciate the fact that my car doesn't smell of stale tobacco any more, and I don't burn holes in my clothes and the car upholstery any more, and I don't worry about burning the house down any more. These are big differences. As far as my general health goes, I don't believe it's made any difference.

It makes me very sad that my fifteen-year-old granddaughter has started smoking. I understand smoking has become epidemic among teen-age girls. When she was eight or nine, she used to beg me to stop: "Don't smoke, Granny. I don't want you to die." Her eight-year-old sister wrote an essay in school that said, "This is a description of a happy day. A happy day is one that my sister would stop smoking so her lungs and teeth would not get black and she would not die. I am worried about her smoking. I want her to live to a hundred and two." That story is pasted on our refrigerator, but I'm afraid the fifteen-year-old doesn't pay much attention to it.

≈≈≈

JUNE H.
Something Is Different . . .

June H., in her mid-thirties, is a vivacious woman who works in the public relations department of a major corporation. As a single parent, she has two daughters. Recently she moved to a quiet suburb outside the city and is looking forward to going back to school. After many efforts to quit, she says she doesn't care about smoking anymore.

119

I was pregnant in 1980 with my second daughter, and during that whole pregnancy my doctor kept saying, "June, the baby is not growing. You have to quit smoking." And the more she told me, the more I smoked. It was weird. Every Monday I would say, "Okay, this is my last cigarette," but I couldn't quit. I would think, "Oh, no. Something is going to be wrong with my baby," but I'd still have the cigarette.

After the baby was born, every Monday for three years I woke up saying, "I'm not going to smoke anymore." I would make it through the day, but then Monday night I would smoke, and I'd say, "Well, I'll quit next week." And I'd try to quit again the next week. This went on for years.

I started smoking when I was fifteen, in the tenth grade. Everyone else did, and we thought it was in. I got pregnant when I was in the eleventh grade. I was sixteen. I couldn't smoke during that pregnancy—it was a difficult pregnancy—but when my daughter was four months old, I started smoking again.

When you have smoked your whole life, it takes time to change. I tried to quit almost from the beginning. One time I went to a hypnotist and quit smoking for about two days—that was it! I was always a nervous kid, and I always thought that I smoked out of nervousness. That was my release. . . . If something was going wrong, smoking was the way I released all of the tension.

After that I tried to quit many times. When I came to work for this corporation in 1979, they offered the employees a Smokenders program. The company paid for part of the program, and if you still weren't smoking in three months you would get half of your money back. After six months, you would get all of your money back. When I went into this program, I quit smoking for three weeks.

In 1985 I quit for one month, then I started again. In 1986 I quit for about two months on my own. See, I always wanted to quit, but something always came up that made me nervous, and I would smoke again. Either something happened in my family or something happened on the job. I was very nervous, unsettled. I am real hyper, so I used that as an excuse.

In March of 1987, my younger daughter's father, who is a smoker, had one lung collapse, and we went to visit him at the hospital. On the way home I lit up a cigarette, and my youngest girl started crying and said, "Mom, if you don't quit smoking, you are going to die like my father." Her father didn't die, but we had just seen him in the hospital, and he had all of these tubes coming out from his body all over the place.

I felt bad. . . . I put down that cigarette and didn't smoke for about eight weeks. Then I started again. It seemed like I could only make it without smoking for about eight weeks.

In 1987 I went through a period when I started getting chest pains. One night I was smoking a cigarette, and when I inhaled, it felt like a hand had just squeezed my heart. I caved over a little bit, and I thought, "My God, I'm not even thirty-five, and I am going to end up having a heart attack."

And what did I do? I went and smoked three cigarettes in a row. I thought, "Oh, no. I might die of a heart attack." Yet, all of this time, I was just puffing one cigarette after another.

Smoking became an obsession, and it wasn't fair to anyone around me. The whole house, everyone, was complaining about my smoking. It got to the point where the only place I could smoke was in the bathroom. I found myself in the bathroom the majority of the time that I was at home because that was the only place they would let me smoke. Smoking wasn't much fun any more.

I felt sorry for my older daughter because I would give her my cigarettes and say, "Give me two a day," but then I would end up asking her for more. One night I woke her up at one in the morning. I said, "Michelle, where did you put my cigarettes?" because she would hide them. I looked in her closet and her drawers. She said, "Mom, I am not giving you one." I said, "Michelle, either you are going to give me a cigarette, or else I am going to get up and go to the store." She got up, threw my cigarettes at me, and said, "Mom, don't bother me with your not smoking any more."

This time something is different. I have not smoked for over five months. It all started last June. Michelle was going to graduate from high school. Just before she graduated, I started getting headaches from smoking. I would cough every morning and cough up phlegm. I would gag when I brushed my teeth in the morning.

After her graduation party I had a couple of cigarettes,

and all my girlfriends told me, "Well, June, you said when Michelle graduated you would quit smoking." And I said, "I am, I will." Michelle said, "Well, Mom, I graduated, so I guess you have to quit smoking." I said, "I guess I have to."

The next day when I woke up I didn't have any more cigarettes in the house, but there was half a butt in the ashtray and I unrolled it, straightened it out, struck a match and inhaled the smoke. I literally choked on the cigarette and I thought, "What am I doing? Here I go, I am going to kill myself again, I am back to the same old thing. . . ." As soon as I lit the cigarette I started getting my headache again, the same headache I had been getting for a couple of weeks, and I thought, "June, you're going to die with a cigarette in your mouth." And so I crushed that cigarette out that Friday morning and I haven't had one since.

I quit cold turkey. Everything seemed to come together all at once. In March 1987, my younger daughter's father's lung collapsed, and he had to have it removed. That same month, my uncle, also a heavy smoker, died of cancer. In June my older daughter graduated, and I'd sworn for years that I'd quit when she graduated. I'd been smoking a pack a day for twenty years, but I quit cold.

It was hard for the first two months. I was very nervous, and my stomach was upset practically all the time. That had always been more than enough to get me back to smoking in the past, but this time I dealt with the issues. I said, "June, having a cigarette isn't going to make you less nervous. It'll make you more nervous because you'll be smoking again and worrying about coughing up phlegm and cancer and heart attacks again." Every time I felt lousy I told myself it was because my body was getting rid of the poison, getting the nicotine out of my system.

There was one time when if it hadn't been for the worst hurricane in history I would have gone out and bought a pack of cigarettes. That was the last day of my vacation in Jamaica, and Hurricane Gilbert was coming. My friend and I were preparing ourselves for the hurricane to hit. Everything was fine. When we went into our hotel room it started to rain, and I felt this tremendous urge to smoke. If I could have gone to the store, I would have bought some cigarettes, and I would have smoked. And the more it stormed, the more the wind howled, the more I wanted a cigarette.

I thought, "If I am going to die, I might as well smoke." I told my friend, "If I could get a cigarette right now, I would be smoking." "June, don't," he said, "because the hurricane is going to be over, we are going to go back home, and then you are going to regret it."

When I got back home, my kids said, "Mom, we can't believe that you didn't smoke while you were there." Out of my whole vacation that was the only time that the urge came. Other than that, I was swimming every day, and I felt great.

I think I have done it this time. I feel so much better now. My headaches aren't as bad. I have not gagged at all since I quit smoking.

Now that I have not smoked for five months many things are changing. I wear contact lenses, and often when I was smoking my eyes were red and sticky. It seemed like I had to rinse out my contacts a couple of times a day. But now I don't. I put in my lenses in the morning, and they last all day.

Under my eyes my skin used to be so tight, but now it isn't. It feels good. Around my cheekbones, it feels good. In fact, my skin feels cleaner, and it looks cleaner, and the dry feeling it used to have is gone. A lot of people recently have said, "June, what are you doing to your face? It looks so clear." One friend said, "June, you look like you've gotten two years younger." But they didn't know I'd quit smoking, because I'm not going around telling everyone I quit. People say, "God, you look so young since the last time I saw you. What have you done?" And I say, "I don't know, but I think it's because I quit smoking."

Food tastes different too; my whole cooking style is different. I don't put a lot of salt or pepper on my food anymore. I used to dump lots of spices into my food just to be able to taste it, and now I don't. I used to have to have a lot of sweets, but now when I eat a candy bar, I don't like it anymore. I used to eat about three candy bars a day. I could always have a doughnut in the morning, but now I don't want all of that sugar. I don't need it like I used to.

To me, tobacco is worse than heroin. I worked at Stanford University at a drug clinic in 1974, and I saw people who were hooked on heroin, and do you know, I always felt like cigarettes were just as bad because there is a terrible withdrawal. You get depressed when you quit, physically you go through a lot, and you are always thinking about cigarettes. It is an obsession.

Now the only time that I think about cigarettes is at the end of a day, when I say to myself, "June, you are doing great." I tell myself that every day. All my friends who have gone through my millions of assertions, "I'm going to quit this week, I'm going to quit this week," say, "June, I never could believe that you would quit smoking." All of them tell me that. Even my daughters. They say, "Mom, I can't believe you haven't had a cigarette." They can't believe it because they heard me tell them a million times before that I was going to quit.

I don't think I'll smoke again this time. Now I don't care about it. I really don't.

LESLIE M.
Things Smell Good Now

Leslie, thirty-one, is a writer and poet. She has spent all of her adult life in the university world: ten years in undergraduate and graduate studies in creative writing and English and four years as a teacher of creative writing at a small women's college. She is certain that her academic background not only allowed but encouraged her smoking habit for a number of years. Leslie's interview is followed by excerpts from letters she wrote to a close friend soon after she had smoked her last cigarette.

I have been a non-smoker for a hundred and twenty days today—but my eleven years as a chain smoker are still as vivid and sweet to me as youth itself. I have not had so much as a puff of a cigarette since I paid $200 to have myself hypnotized one afternoon last May, but I have watched hungrily as other people smoked around me, and hundreds of moments already I have been on the verge of reaching for someone else's cigarette left burning in an ashtray or waving near my face.

Like most young people of my generation, I was certain the world was a dangerous place and would do me in before I could do myself in with something like cigarettes. My first cigarettes were those we snuck down by the ravine in my subdivision. As a daughter of the white upper middle class, I was terribly interested in passive rebellion, and smoking was one of the most available expressions of that. Of course, those first cigarettes tasted vile, and staggering up out of the ravine, a little dizzy from the experience, my girlfriends and I chewed onion grass to hide the smell on our breath. Between the ages of sixteen and nineteen or twenty, I confined my smoking to parties, bars—situations where alcohol was the primary agent of rebellious behavior—but I was still often repelled by people who chain-smoked in the daytime.

Nineteen seventy-four was my first year in college; I don't know if it was indicative of the times or the place or both, but women there seemed to be taking up smoking in great numbers. My favorite professors, sassy, smart, professional women, held court in tiny offices crammed with impressive-looking books and blue clouds of smoke. It was not unusual for them to smoke during class, gesturing with their cigarettes. It was also not unusual then to find classrooms supplied with stacks of ashtrays. No one asked if anyone minded smoking. All the campus radicals I admired most seemed to chain-smoke. I was trying to make myself into a woman writer, a poet: I had a photograph of Edna St. Vincent Millay holding a cigarette and looking pensive; I saw Jane Fonda play Lillian Hellman in the movie *Julia*, chain-smoking and throwing her typewriter dramatically out of the window. I associated smoking with bluestocking women, independent women who turned their intelligent eyes on men who annoyed them and blew smoke in their faces. I found smoking a very useful deterrent to drunk and potentially pawing fraternity boys, a socially acceptable way of surrounding oneself with boundaries.

Then I fell madly in love with a dangerously handsome man who told me right off that he couldn't stand to see attractive women smoking cigarettes, and I didn't much care because I didn't then feel I *needed* to smoke. But when he suddenly disappeared from my life and couldn't be reached even by phone, I decided to mourn his passing with a bottle of scotch and a chain of Salem Light 100s that lasted a few days, at the end of which I realized I had come to like the taste of cigarettes, scotch or no scotch. And in playing out my agony over the loss of my beautiful boyfriend, I had hung over the typewriter pounding out stories and poems of revenge and made the most powerful association of my life: cigarettes with writing.

Four months after having my last cigarette and it is still difficult to be at the typewriter without a cigarette in the ashtray. I still believe that cigarettes actually helped me think, that they helped me focus and make the connections that I need for effective communication. I liked being a smoker for many years. I liked pictures of myself looking writerly in profile with a cigarette in my hand. I liked the fraternal feelings of hanging out in student lounges and dark pubs with other writers who were chain-smoking, and now I am a little unhappy sometimes that I have to avoid such scenes because they make me too nostalgic for my old smoking self.

Quitting smoking was one of the hardest things I have ever done, so hard, so painful that the strongest deterrent to my taking up smoking again is the thought of ever going through withdrawal again. I began to quit in stages: First I bought a new car and decided I was never going to smoke a cigarette in that car, even though I was—and intended to continue being—a chain smoker then. I did not smoke in that car, and I wouldn't let anyone else smoke in it either, which seemed odd to my many smoker friends, but it was the first of a number of inconveniences I tried to cause myself over smoking. The second step was the loss of my cigarette case, a metal case with an enameled design that I had bought the very month I began smoking full time. I loved that cigarette case; it kept my cigs dry and smooth and found its way back to me on numerous occasions when I had left it at parties or bars. But I lost that case one night about a year before I actually quit smoking. I knew where I had lost it, a little jazz club on the edge of town, but I decided not to call about it the next day. I thought if I had to live with no cigarette case, my cigarettes would get wet and smashed and the inconvenience would eventually convince me I didn't need to smoke any more.

Then I tried a trial run: I went to teach creative writing at a summer school/camp for the arts where I have spent a number of happy summers. I knew that the effects of the altitude would make smoking yet more problematic for me when I first went up, and I knew that being out in the woods it would be inconvenient for me to drive into town to buy cigarettes. I also resolved to buy cigarettes I didn't like so that I would only smoke when I was desperate. This way, with sheer willpower, I managed to get myself down from a pack and a half a day to three cigarettes a day. I thought I would leave the mountains a non-smoker, but I then was scheduled to attend a writers' conference and I was terrifically nervous about that because I was to read my poems to an audience of rather important and intimidating people. On the flight to the conference I opted for the non-smoking section, but the man who met my plane was happily smoking away, and when we arrived at the party of writers in progress at the convention center, all happily yakking away in their clouds of smoke, I greedily smoked a whole pack. I was a hacking, wheezing chain smoker once again.

It was another year before I again decided I needed to

quit smoking. But this time I had clear reasons: I had just passed the age of thirty. I began to feel old, a little dried-up looking. I could see the beginnings of "smoker's face" on me: the sallow skin, the bags around my eyes, the dry cross-hatching. I admit I am vain, and my vanity was much more powerful, finally, in persuading me that smoking was detrimental to me than any of the hundreds of pamphlets and articles on the nasty effects of smoking that my mother sent me regularly in the mail. I looked in the mirror and thought that quitting smoking might be like getting oneself a very expensive facial: my color would improve, my hair would be healthier, my eyes brighter.

I called a hypnotist and made an appointment. I called my mother and told her I was quitting smoking for her Mother's Day present so I couldn't back out. I sat on a bench outside the hypnotist's office and had my last cigarette. I said to myself: This is my last cigarette ever. I took every drag deeply. A few men in business suits passed me on my bench and smiled. I wondered if they suspected that I was a woman smoking the last cigarette of her life. I smoked that cigarette right down to the butt, and then I threw the rest of the pack, lighter and all, in the nearest trash can.

The next three days were a nightmare, and the whole first month of withdrawal was a trial I never wish to repeat. During that month I was trying to write a lot of letters to a very close friend of mine, partly because writing letters helps me keep sane and in control of my feelings and partly because I wanted to keep myself comfortable at the typewriter and try to prevent my decision to quit smoking from affecting my writing.

The excerpts from those letters describe some of the things I worked through as I cast off the most powerful habit of my life. . . .

May 8, 1988

Dear Joanne,

I have actually done it—gone to the hypnotist and gotten the stop smoking routine. I became a non-smoker at 3 P.M. on Friday, and now, about noon on Sunday, I am rather a mess about it. I figure that at a pack a day and about ten minutes per cigarette, I was spending somewhere between three and four hours a day with a cigarette in my hand—times twelve years. No wonder I feel fragmented, confused, unfocused. Writing is very difficult; paying attention to anything for very long is difficult. I began a letter to you yesterday, got about a page written, spaced out, and shut off the power to the computer before I had saved the file, so the whole page I'd written was zapped. I'm not sure that the hypnosis is really the miracle cure they claim it to be. I want a cigarette more than ever, but after I paid two hundred bucks to have someone tell me I don't want a cigarette, I think of all the money down the drain if I do smoke a cigarette.

I get absentminded and find myself going to the drawer where I kept my cigarette supply, or digging in my purse while I am on the phone. I tried chewing gum, but that makes my jaws hurt after a while, and so I went to the grocery this morning and bought a box of wooden toothpicks. I have them here by the typewriter and find that they are the best answer to cigarette cravings. I remember that one of my teachers quit a long smoking habit when I was his student, and we all used to think it was pretty funny how he'd sometimes have two toothpicks hanging on his lip—he had a very hard time quitting smoking—he finally managed it. But I am having trouble hanging onto ideas, trouble sitting here at the computer and having the same sort of concentration I used to have when I did smoke. I wonder if smoking really did help me focus and concentrate or if I only believed that it did. I'm sure the latter. Well, this morning when I got up, I reached into the cupboard for some clothes and noticed the smell in there—the general stale smell of cigarettes—my whole closet reeks—and I never noticed it before. My mother always swore that the suitcases I left at home were full of cigarette smell, and I thought she exaggerated. I spent a good portion of my time yesterday cleaning the nicotine stains off the windows, picture glass, walls, and blinds. That's an activity that always grosses me out because the nicotine is so sticky and yellow and nasty—I figured grossing myself out that way would reinforce my resolve. I notice that even after a day and a half, my own sense of smell is improved many times and the inside of my mouth tastes good—sort of fruity and sweet. I never realized how ugly that taste of cigarettes was in my mouth. My friend Janet told me that when she quit smoking, she was sure that her lips got fuller and the bags under her eyes went away.

Probably the most effective motivation for my decision to quit was the face of a woman. . . . She's a great lady, feisty, older, smart—but her face is positively an example of the smoker's face they show you in those scare tactic programs. It's true that smoking ages the skin in a way nothing else does. Women who have smoked for a long time begin to look like ashtrays themselves. This woman is a prime example. Her skin is wrinkled and gray, and her gums and teeth are yellowish like dog teeth. If you look hard, you see that this woman is neither very old nor naturally very ugly. She also has that thinning, limp smoker's hair and yellowish fingers. I was so frightened of becoming like that that I was motivated to quit. So this is all to say that it's vanity that made me quit—and vanity that will probably keep me a non-smoker.

Janet tells me that when she quit, she cried for two weeks and the horror of the whole experience was enough to keep her from ever smoking again. She's been helping me along—telling me things like how her hair got bright and shiny again after she quit, how her skin plumped up and glowed, and her energy level soared, but she told me as well that I would have to remember that I would always be an ex-smoker, that if I ever even took so much as a puff of a cigarette again, I could ruin all my hard work, trigger the addiction anew. It's all an interesting psychological experiment—the gaps in my experience—all my adult life to have been a smoker. I try to remember it all—it was before I became a writer, before I knew anything about anything. The only time I was a non-smoker was when I was a kid—and then I began smoking, though not chain-smoking, when I was sixteen, and I became a smokestack when I was about nineteen and had gotten very fat from endless dorm food and adolescent depression. The smoking had a great many functions in my life then—it helped me thin down; it was a great social control, a way to keep one's physical distance from a man in a bar or at a fraternity party. One thing I am feeling now that Janet said she felt too—was vulnerability. The habit is some sort of wall between you and the world, and really a weapon too. Blowing smoke in someone's face is a good way to get them to leave you alone. But the whole thing also functions as a psychological wall between the self and the world, and I do feel rather exposed right now, as if I am wearing my heart on my sleeve.

I've been riding my bike a lot these last two days, and when I'm out riding, I don't feel as inclined to want a cigarette. Yesterday I rode to the park and the place where the fountain surrounded by magnolia trees is. There weren't many folks out, so I helped myself to one of those basketball-sized magnolia blossoms, put it in my backpack, and rode on home with it; it's so huge it takes up a whole big serving bowl, and the perfume from it is overwhelming—all through the house I can smell it. Amazing. I don't know if the blossom is really unusually powerful or if my non-smoking status renders my nose so much more capable I can smell anything. I know that riding my bike today was more pleasurable than yesterday because I could smell every flower I passed and often identify it—and while the smells are strong enough for even a smoker to detect, the pleasures are much heightened now. I'm wishing I could have that house full of lilacs before me again—now I could appreciate them all the more.

May 13, 1988

Dear Joanne,

Today marks exactly one week without a cigarette, and though it's a lot better than it was the first three days, I am still missing cigs a lot. The first three days were hell. I was feeling crazy, mean, restless, and had terrific nightmares in which I was smoking like crazy. When I woke up, my chest hurt as if I had been chain-smoking; my throat was sore and I felt positively battered. The next few nights, I couldn't sleep at all. I got up and wandered around the house in the dark sucking on toothpicks and wanting a cigarette so badly I thought I'd get dressed and go out to an all-night store. But I held out. I inspect my face every day now to find the changes—the slow but wonderful changes in my skin and hair. My face is getting softer and the bags under my eyes are actually fading. This is not my imagination. There simply seems to be more moisture under my skin. It looks plump. In order to keep myself from wanting cigs, I've taken endless bike rides and am enjoying the way my lungs feel better and cleaner every day. I can't believe how much more breath I have. When I exert myself, I don't feel that pain in my chest—and there seems to be more room in me for air in general. I've been riding first thing in the morning and just before dark at night—mostly on the park bike path, which is probably a four-mile run if I do full circle. It takes about an hour to do the whole thing and back from my front door. Last night I did it all twice, till my legs ached—and last night was the first night that I actually slept soundly and well since I quit smoking. I am growing to love that park and bike path. It's so amazing both morning and night.

Probably my single greatest benefit in quitting smoking is what I can smell now—since I am a person who responds so much to smell. And since I have ridden that path so many times this week, I've gotten to know which spots will smell what way, and I can anticipate each tree and patch of flowers before I get to it. The other great thing to do on the park trail is check out the joggers. They are almost all men and quite an attractive bunch. I can smell them too when I whiz past on my bike as they huff and puff in the Texas heat. They, of course, have no idea how deeply I am breathing in their intimate smells, and I love the secret feeling of stealing those smells from them. And already I am beginning to get a sense of who the regulars are, who does the loop more than once, and how long it takes each one to get around.

God how I miss smoking. I have a toothpick in my mouth at this very minute. I've become as addicted to them as I ever was to cigarettes, and the toothpick is quite an ugly habit. I look like a real hick. If my mother could see me, I'm sure she'd rather have me smoking.

Last night I went to a small party. On the late end of the party there were a number of people smoking—probably everyone in the room except three of us. Of course, they were all writers. At first I loved the smoke and breathed deeply of it, but after about an hour, it started to smell bad and I got a headache. When I came home I noticed the smell of smoke in my hair and clothes and had to take a shower before bed because it bugged me so much. I thought maybe that was some sort of break-through, a sign that I really am changing my mentality from that of a smoker to that of a non-smoker. I did talk to two other folks last night who had quit long-time smoking habits. One woman told me that she slept dif-ferently now, that she dreamed more and slept more soundly since she quit smoking, but also that she went to bed much earlier because there was something about smoking that kept her awake. And it's true I have been dreaming much more and sleeping differently, though at first I had great insomnia, and the dreams are not all that soothing.

Last night I could smell each person I talked to. I could smell the fabric of their clothes and the soap they'd used to shower. If I get close to people's hair, I can smell shampoo and that fur smell that hair has. There's some-thing very sensuous about not smoking. I want to touch everyone, get close, smell skin. I want to put my nose against heads and shoulders and arms. I smell my own skin, my hands and wrists and breasts. It's quite wonder-ful and sexy. I feel sort of sexually charged by it all and wonder if I haven't been missing out on something all these years.

Of course, bad smells now are exaggerated, too. The fruit stand next door has begun to stink. They throw the rotting stuff out back and it continues to rot in the sun. My neighbor and I are worried about it because the smell drifts in our windows when the wind is going a certain direction—and the loose rotting produce has drawn some monster city rats. I haven't seen them, but my neighbor has, and he says they are big as cats. There's a load of rotten watermelons under my window and they smell like vinegar. But mostly things smell good: I stick my nose in my herb box every day. The basil and mint are heavenly. When I run my fingers through them I can smell it on my fingers. Yesterday I did some ironing and I put starch in some cotton shirts and skirts. The smell of the hot starch was so wonderful that I ironed everything in my closet—now all my clothes are stiff and crisp, but they smell fresh and clean too. I love the smell of laundromats in general now, and warm sheets and the smell of leather shoes in the back of my closet. I can hardly wait to get to the mountains and discover all the smells I've missed there the last two summers. Already I imagine how the cabins will smell, the dust and stone and old wood, old curtains and ashes, the horses and the grass and the flowers.

NEIL B.
The Doctor Said to Cut Back . . .

Neil B., with an M.B.A. in labor relations, is personnel director of a large corporation. His wife is an accounts payable supervisor at a bank. Both were heavy smokers, and they gave up smoking on the same day. Both are in their forties.

When we met, my wife had not smoked for five years. About nine months later, she picked up a cigarette again, and within a week she was up to a pack a day. We both smoked and smoked and smoked. I would say I was smoking two and a half packs of Marlboros a day.

139

The last year of my smoking, I got a sore throat on two or three occasions. It was only when I would swallow in certain ways, and it always went away. It would come for a while. Then it would go away.

The day I quit smoking, I went for a walk after lunch, and I coughed. It actually brought tears to my eyes, it hurt so bad. I did an about-face, went in and called my doctor, and asked him to recommend a throat specialist. That afternoon I took off from work and went to see the specialist. I remember on the way there, I thought, "Now he is going to tell me that I should quit smoking. And I am not going to do it." Every doctor says it: "You should quit smoking." And I got tired of that. I'd heard that so many times. They didn't understand my feeling. The thought of quitting caused me sheer panic. The thought of not having a pack of cigarettes in my front pocket just scared me to death. And the thought of never smoking another cigarette was something I couldn't even contemplate, it was so scary.

But when I was walking into his office, going into the examining room, I walked by a sign that said: "If you are contemplating quitting smoking, we have prescription drugs that can help you. Ask us about them." When I got into the examining room the doctor found a lesion on my vocal cord. He said he didn't think it was anything to worry about, it wasn't malignant, but it would probably help if I could cut back on smoking for a while. That was probably the best thing he could have said to me, rather than, "You've got to quit smoking!"

Something snapped inside of me at that moment. It was not fear. I didn't have a fear of this lesion on my vocal cord. But there was something that told me to quit. I said to him, "If you'll give me some drugs, I'll quit."

He said he would give me a prescription for nicotine gum. I didn't even know what it was that one took to quit smoking. My wife had been wanting to quit. She had talked about quitting, but I'd kept telling her, "No, no, I'm really not interested in quitting." So I said to the doctor, "If you give my wife a prescription, she'll probably quit too." Medicine being what it is, he couldn't do that. But he did give me a liberal prescription, and I could do with it as I chose, I guess. I assume this nicotine gum was not something dangerous.

I walked out of the doctor's office, got in my pickup and my cigarettes were on the seat beside me. I actually picked them up, but then I said to myself, "If you're going to quit, you had better not smoke this one." So I didn't.

On the way home I stopped at the drugstore, bought the gum, took it home, and set it on the table—I got home before my wife did that day—and didn't smoke. When she got home, I told her the throat specialist had found a lesion on my vocal cord and he was doing a biopsy to make sure it wasn't cancerous. He didn't think it was anything to be concerned about, but I had decided that I was no longer going to smoke.

I said, "I got you some gum, too." She said, "I'm not ready. This has happened too quickly. I'm not prepared to quit." I said, "I don't care whether you quit or not, I am. I'm done. And I'm never going to smoke another one."

That night, she smoked one more cigarette. I didn't even open up the gum until after we had had dinner. She had that one, last cigarette, and I chewed a piece of the nicotine gum.

When I wanted a cigarette there was a feeling in my chest that was only relieved by smoking. I assume nicotine caused that sensation. Well, when I chewed this gum, that feeling went away, and at that point I knew I had beaten it. For me, there were two parts to this habit. One was this feeling that I had in my chest, which was the need for nicotine. And the other part was, "What do I do with my hands?" I couldn't beat both of them at the same time. I had tried. I had tried quitting two or three times. Couldn't go a week. I was just climbing the walls. But I *could* handle one at a time, and that's what the nicotine gum made possible. It made the feeling in my chest go away.

Well, I chewed two more pieces that night. The next day I chewed the gum almost constantly. I had a burn from the tip of my tongue clear down into my stomach because of nicotine. The instructions said, "Chew it slowly," and I don't chew anything slowly, so I was tenacious even in chewing this gum! But it worked. It helped. I didn't have that physical need to smoke.

When I first quit I'd reach into my coat pocket for my cigarettes every time I reached for the telephone. It was such a habit, but I finally broke it. I was anxious to get rid of the gum because it struck me immediately that I had replaced cigarettes with this gum. I consciously started cutting back on it. My wife did the same thing.

Two months after we started on the gum, we were both taking some vacation time to work on a new house we'd bought. It's an hour and a half away from the city, where the prescription for the gum was. We were down to our last two pieces of gum. We had a decision to make: Were we going to take time out to go get gum? Or were we going to say, "The hell with it, that's it?" We talked about it and said, "That's it." So we quit the gum together, just the way we quit smoking together.

I started smoking when I was twelve or thirteen years old. I remember telling my mother how ridiculous it was that people became hooked on cigarettes and had to rely on these things. Shortly thereafter I became fascinated by cigarettes. I look back in old magazines, and in most of the photographs everybody's got a cigarette in their mouth. According to the ads, more doctors smoked Kents than any other brand when I was growing up. Older people, adults, smoked. There was quite a pressure to smoke, particularly if you wanted to grow up fast, and I did.

I had to put a lot of effort into learning to smoke, because in the beginning it made me sick. I began smoking Marlboros. I think that had as much to do with the Marlboro Man as it did anything else! By the time I graduated from high school, I had the habit.

Shortly after that I went into the Army. The Army at that time was particularly conducive to smoking. People who didn't smoke already started in the Army, because every break was a "smoke break." Army life was surrounded by cigarettes. There was no tax on cigarettes at the PX, so you could get them for practically nothing.

After I got out of the Army I went to college, and at that time cigarettes and coffee were very much in vogue at the student unions, the coffee shops. It seemed as though every university had three or four coffee shops, and the ones I went to were no exception. Adults smoked and adults drank coffee, and suddenly we were adults. You could tell we were adults because we smoked and drank coffee.

My first wife did not smoke. Throughout our marriage she disliked smoking and didn't understand what it's like to be hooked on them. I had absolutely no interest in quitting. In fact, I used to comment to people at that time that if a doctor told me that I had six months to live if I continued smoking, or forever if I quit, I would have been hard pressed to make a decision! That's how much I enjoyed smoking. At times my wife would tell me, "It would really be great if you quit smoking because it smells." I used to tell her that I smoked when we got married, and she was just going to have to accept that. I had no interest in changing.

The medical evidence—I'm amazed that one still hesitates to say "evidence"—but about five years ago I began to recognize that the evidence was overwhelmingly against smoking. At that time, too, the social acceptability of smoking changed considerably. Now it was:

You could smoke in a restaurant, and somebody might ask you not to. Being of the nature I am, I would probably tell them to go to hell. But at least I was becoming conscious that smoke probably did offend some people. The fact that smoking not only *didn't* turn me into the Marlboro Man—even after all those years of brand loyalty—but was, instead, making me offensive to people, began to bother me.

Finally I took a giant step forward and switched from Marlboros to a low tar: Merit. I had tried previously to go to various low-tar, low-nicotine–type cigarettes, but it didn't work. It didn't work at all. But I went to these Merits. After you get used to less hit . . . I don't know how to describe it, particularly for a non-smoker, but there is a feeling you get when you take a huge bunch of smoke into your lungs—there is a physical feeling when you do this. The lighter the cigarette, the lighter the hit. You have to get used to a lighter hit. Once I got used to that, those cigarettes were fine, but I smoked just as many, maybe more.

I certainly don't regret the decision to quit; I am very pleased that I quit. But I am pleased from a health point of view, which may have been what snapped inside of me. I suddenly said, "I've got to quit because of my health." I never had that kind of determination hit me before. Something swept over me that gave me that determination. Without it, I wouldn't have done it. Smoking has such a hold on you. You've got to have that determination. You've really got to believe you're going to do it.

Just no doubt in your mind that you can do it.

Since that time I have not even been tempted to smoke a cigarette. Now, that's not to say I haven't missed them. I missed a cigarette at lunch today. One thing that would make a non-smoker sick—as well as a smoker who still smoked—is that if today they decided that cigarettes weren't bad for you I would go down right now and get a pack of cigarettes, and I would start smoking probably two packs a day. I love to smoke. But I know I cannot smoke one, or I will smoke. So I am not even tempted to smoke. It is something like the alcoholic. One drink puts you back into it. There is no doubt in my mind that one cigarette would put me back into it.

I think one of the significant things is I never remember what day it was. People who quit a lot of times will say, "I have quit now for one year, two months, one week, and three hours," or something like that. But I still don't remember what day it was because that wasn't as significant to me as I was never going to smoke again. It has been over three years now.

Every night when I would go to bed I would cough a real deep cough, once, and then I would go to sleep. This was every single night. Also, if I would sing—you know how your vocal cords, when your volume is up, have a vibration to them? That would cause me to cough. And that's gone away.

Things that have not changed are the things that I was told would change. That things would taste better: I don't notice that at all. I would have more lung capacity:

I haven't noticed that. In fact, I had a doctor tell me, on a lung X-ray taken while I still smoked heavily, that he was amazed that I smoked, because my lungs didn't look as though I did.

The down side of quitting is that I have now, for the first time in my life, a weight problem. I *look* at French fries and I gain weight. Although now that I am understanding nutrition more, that might be a blessing in and of itself. French fries don't rank very high on the good nutrition list, what with all the fat and salt.

My wife is really bothered by being around smokers. She's an accounts payable supervisor. She has asked the people who work for her who smoke not to smoke in her office. The smoke really bothers her, where it doesn't seem to bother me.

I have not become one of those offensive ex-smokers. In fact, I eat lunch quite often in the smoking section. It doesn't bother me. If people want to smoke in my office, I don't care. People who smoke around me don't bother me. Now, at times though, the smell of smoke does, but I don't say anything. I guess my feeling is that if secondhand smoke is that bad for you, living in a city is just as bad, so I don't get enough secondhand smoke to worry about.

LISA M.
I Let Myself Smoke in My Dreams

Lisa, thirty and single, grew up on Long Island, New York, and now lives on the West Coast, where she works as a sales coordinator for a video game manufacturer.

I come from a family of smokers. As long as I can remember both my parents smoked heavily, and so did my aunts, uncles, and cousins. In fact, I don't know how my brother escaped. He is the one person in my family who doesn't smoke, and he absolutely hates to be around people who are smoking.

When I was twelve, I wanted to be cool, so I learned to smoke, to swear, and to do all those things that kids do to be cool. In college I smoked probably a pack a day, but by the time I quit—depending on how late I stayed up at night—I was smoking between a pack and a half and two packs a day. If I was at a party or at a bar drinking and up until two o'clock in the morning, then I would smoke about two packs a day.

I smoked for about eighteen years. I thought about quitting many times and I thought, "Well, when I really want to quit I'll quit." There were all kinds of reasons why I didn't want to quit just then. When I did try to quit, it was very half-hearted. I never really made that commitment, that decision to quit. I would quit for a couple of days or I'd have a cigarette here, a cigarette there.

Last Christmas I went home to New York. My great aunt—I was very attached to her—had just died of emphysema and she was a heavy smoker who refused to quit. She was seventy-five when she died, but for years she suffered and would sit in a chair and huff and puff but she would still keep smoking. And I could never say, *"Why don't you quit?"* because I still smoked.

My dad, who's fifty-eight, is a very heavy smoker too. In spite of the fact that he had a triple bypass a few years ago, in spite of the fact that he has high cholesterol, and in spite of the fact that he is overweight, he is still chain-smoking two packs a day.

While I was home for Christmas, my dad, my mom, and I were on our way out to brunch and my dad was smoking a cigarette while driving the car. He started to cough, that smoker's kind of cough, and got so red in the face he was purple. He couldn't get any air; but as soon as he could get his breath, he finished smoking that cigarette. *"That's it,"* I thought! So I rolled down the window of the car and threw my pack of cigarettes out. My dad said, *"What are you doing?"* and I said, *"I don't want to end up like you when I'm fifty-eight!"* I have not had a cigarette since.

It was frightening to me to see how my father was, and to realize that if I didn't quit I was going to end up just like that, as I know I am very much like him. Now I feel great, I feel I can breathe and smell the fresh air again!

The first week after I quit was easy because I was all fired up and that was it, *I was going to quit.* But after the first week it got a little bit harder, but every time I did feel the urge to smoke I would get this picture in my mind of my aunt, how she looked and how she could hardly breathe before she died and how she was so thin and so ill. Then I would get this mental picture of my father with that red face.

Those images would give me enough reasons why I shouldn't smoke. Then I'd give myself a mental image of my boyfriend and how happy he would be if I wasn't smoking because he cares and worries about me.

My uncle, who quit three years ago, said something to me: "Lisa, when you get a yen for a cigarette, and you really want one, that feeling is going to go away whether you smoke a cigarette or not, so why smoke a cigarette?" And I would think about that every time I got the urge for a cigarette and say to myself: "Okay, this is going to go away."

I still get yens for a cigarette but mostly when I am under a lot of stress. I'll be damned if after all this time I am going to start smoking again and have to go through the effort of quitting again at some later point in my life. This is it for me.

I dream about smoking all of the time. And I let myself smoke in my dreams. That is not going to hurt me. It is funny, because I know I am dreaming and I'm saying to myself: "If this wasn't a dream, I wouldn't be doing this." I know I'm smoking in my dream but that's okay: If that is where I gotta do it to keep off smoking, that's where I'll do it.

ANDY G.
A "Type A" Sort of Person

Andy G., now forty-nine, left an Eastern university to become director of athletics at a major university in California. His jurisdiction includes everything from football games to tennis matches, from physical education instruction to fund raising. It takes $19 million a year and a staff of over 150 people to get it all done. His success depends on the success of a lot of other people, especially athletes. Their attitude about smoking strongly affected him.

When I came to the West Coast I was smoking quite heavily. Smoking is stress related in my life: The harder things were, the more I wanted a cigarette, and the more cigarettes I smoked. Something happened to me when I smoked a cigarette that relieved, or that I thought relieved, my stress. I call it digital satisfaction. I smoked for about twenty years off and on, but when I smoked heavily, I chain-smoked. I was not only a heavy smoker but a heavy drinker as well. I am a risk taker, an entrepreneur, a type A sort of person. People like me operate aggressively; we're not afraid to take chances. We even take chances with our health and our lives.

About three or four years ago I realized I wasn't feeling very well. I was overweight and felt a great deal of personal dissatisfaction with almost everything. I chose to work on some things in my personal life. I quit smoking. I quit cold turkey; I just stopped. Two years later—I remember the exact day, in fact—I had my last drink of alcohol. Giving up these bad habits was an attempt to get some discipline and control in my life. I see smoking and drinking as related activities; I see them both as substance abuse. Nicotine and alcohol were substances I felt I needed, rather than something that I enjoyed.

I quit smoking because I didn't feel very well, and I thought that was unattractive. My wife's father died of lung cancer, and he had been a heavy smoker. My first boss in this business died of emphysema a few years ago, and he was a heavy smoker. I simply realized that it was stupid. I might die early anyway (I may already have smoked too much—I don't know how much damage I did, but so far my chest X-rays are good), but why *create* the reason?

I was also clearly influenced by things I had read, like the Surgeon General's report, the warnings on the cigarette packs, and the research that's reported in the newspapers and on television. It's hard to be ignorant of the dangers of smoking here at this university, with all the research on smoking that is being done here in our medical school, the committees that work on smoking policies in campus buildings, and stuff like that. People in California are very aggressive about not liking smoking. Those that don't like smoking *really* don't like it. They don't want you smoking around them, and they say so. I respect that. I don't like smoking around me now. It bothers me.

I can't think of a single athlete here at the university

that I have seen smoking. They are very aware that it would affect their physical performance. I know for a fact that a great many of them don't respect smokers and don't want people smoking around them. I'm sure their attitude influenced my decision to quit.

I remember the day I quit. I was in my office—I think I had burned a hole in a pair of pants, or knocked over an ashtray, or something—and I said to myself, "Stop. Just stop." I got up, walked out the back door, and threw the cigarettes (I think I had about seventeen cigarettes left in the pack) in a dumpster rather than throw them in the wastebasket in my office, because if I threw them in the wastebasket I could fish them out again. I threw them in a place where I couldn't get them back. That was it. I never smoked again.

I don't recall quitting as being traumatic; it wasn't something I needed to taper off or get counseling or help with. I just stopped. It was pretty easy for me the first few weeks because I had made up my mind that I wanted to give up smoking. Now instead of cigarettes I keep things around my desk that I play with, like Captain Queeg in *The Caine Mutiny*: I have a coin, I have a dish of rubber bands, and I'll just sit here talking with somebody, quietly twisting a rubber band.

I still get the urge to smoke—it comes and goes. I am nervous and intense during games. My job is very stressful because it involves the performance of other people. My success is dependent upon the success of lots of other people, and I find that nerve-racking. During the games, I have a straw or toothpicks or what-have-you, something in my hands that I can fool around with. That need hasn't gone away. I still need to cope with nervousness and stress, I am still a type A, I still take risks, but now I express those characteristics in different ways. That is what I mean by drinking and smoking being substance abuse. It wasn't for pleasure; it was a necessity.

It is incredible how much healthier I feel now that I have stopped smoking. After I stopped drinking, I felt even healthier. Looking back, I associated smoking and drinking. Now I attend a lot of Alcoholics Anonymous meetings. Talk about smoke-filled rooms! I was astounded at how many recovering alcoholics smoke. I am proud of the fact that I quit smoking and drinking.

MIKE B.
His Wife Had a Smart Idea

Mike B. is a successful businessman who was able to retire at fifty-five and to build himself an exceptionally well-equipped studio. He is a serious sculptor, calling on the influences of primitive art. He and his wife travel extensively to study ancient civilizations and primitive cultures.

It was such a trauma that I remember every detail of how I quit. My wife had been bugging me for seven years. She had smoked earlier in her life, and she had quit. One day she said to me, "I know you want a new Mercedes." We were going to drive our son back to college in Ohio.

"Instead of taking the old car, let's get a brand-new Mercedes, *but you can't ever smoke in it.* If you'll agree never to smoke in it, then I'll agree to buying the Mercedes." That was her way of manipulating me, and I agreed to go along with her.

My wife was very devious. She planned a three-week photographic safari through some of the most beautiful parts of Canada and the United States. She plotted a route up the California coast, across British Columbia, through the Canadian Rockies, down into Ohio to Oberlin, and then back to California through some of the great American national parks like the Grand Canyon. I went for it. If she hadn't used these incentives and said, "Let's get a new car," I think I would still be smoking.

Not smoking in the car was terrible. I went cold turkey after thirty years of three packs a day. I was very tense. I had never quit for more than half a day, and the trip took three and a half weeks. I kept my word: I never smoked a cigarette in that car. I screamed for three weeks, I was terribly irritable, but I never smoked cigarettes again.

The trip broke all my associative patterns, all my habits of going to work, smoking with coffee, smoking while making long business phone calls, smoking with drinking (we didn't drink on the trip since we were driving most of the time). We had a wonderful trip photographically, and I never once smoked a cigarette in that car. That car never smelled of tobacco.

We went up to Seattle and through Vancouver. I was cranky and kept getting worse, so I began to eat Life Savers. I consumed about five packs of Life Savers a day, maybe more. It gave me some oral gratification.

By the time we got to Ohio, I was much better; I was calming down. It took two weeks to get to Ohio, and the kid was being a pain, which is what teen-agers do for a living, and between him and me, my wife should be nominated for the Nobel Peace Prize. Anyway, we said goodbye to the kid in Ohio, and then my wife and I were together. It was a very nice time for us. I was a lot better by then, as we headed home. It took us a week. We went the southern route because it was already getting toward the middle of September. We stopped at a couple of the national parks, like the Grand Canyon.

The car was the device, the trigger, and it was a very clever one. We could have afforded the car anyway; that didn't have anything to do with it. It was just a gimmick. My wife is very clever. She knew that once I stopped, I probably would stay that way.

When I got home and was back in my office environment, I found it much easier than I had anticipated. I got a lot of reinforcement from people around me who had stopped smoking, although it was tough to have meetings with my staff if they smoked, but I learned to live with it. It was very hard to break the habit of smoking while I was on the phone. Two key associations I had with cigarettes were with coffee in the morning and when I talked on the telephone. These activities always prompted a cigarette response. Before quitting, I was on the phone all day, so I smoked all day. When I had a drink in the evening, I found that a very nice combination was vodka and a cigarette. That was a great combo and was very hard to give up. I have really missed it.

I dreamed about cigarette smoking for months. It still happens. I just had a dream last week that I was smoking, and I quit fourteen years ago.

I craved tobacco probably for three years after quitting. For a while, if people were smoking around me, I would say to them, "Blow the smoke at me, so I can smell it," because I loved tobacco. I ate two or three packages of mints a day for a few months, until my dentist told me to stop. I gained about five pounds.

I started to smoke in the Army. I was eighteen years old at the end of World War II, which would be 1944–1945. It was the fall of 1944, and they shut down all of the Army college programs and sent me off to basic training. In December of '44 I found myself in Arkansas with a gun in my hand, getting ready to go to the Battle of Bastogne to fill the battle lines.

Everybody was smoking, everybody. It was part of being grown up. It took me a couple of weeks before I was really hooked, and in the interim I got sick. It ruined my appetite and ruined my sense of taste.

Of course, I knew smoking could kill me. I didn't want to die of lung cancer or coronary disease. I have spent almost all of my life in the health industry, so I read all the medical literature. Before 1975 I had tried many times to quit. I quit twenty or thirty times. I tried everything. I tried gums and candies and everything. Nothing worked. I always went back to cigarettes. And I switched to mild cigarettes, but all I did then was smoke four packs a day instead of two. That is when Carltons came out, I think. I smoked Carltons, and they were terrible.

By 1975 I was ready to quit—I was forty-nine years old, I had been smoking thirty years, and my wife kept pestering me to quit. She made a nuisance of herself about how unpleasant it was, how bad I smelled, and how I was hurting my health. Then when the Surgeon General put all that stuff on the cigarette pack, it had quite an impact on me. I became convinced that there was a real problem here. I started to feel physiological changes. In 1970 a friend who smoked four packs of cigarettes a day dropped dead at forty-seven—that scared the hell out of me! I cut back for a while after that, but then I went right back to three packs a day.

I was a very nervous person in my work. I was always pushing very, very hard. I had a lot of feelings of inadequacy and anxiety about my work. In terms of position and responsibility, I was always way above what I felt I was trained to do. That was a pattern I always had. In those days I was vice-president of a major pharmaceutical company. It was a very nerve-racking job, because I was in an area that the rest of the company wasn't very interested in and I was trying to make it successful so I kept pushing, pushing, pushing—all of that created a lot of anxiety. I used cigarettes to help reduce the anxiety. The more anxiety I felt, the more cigarettes I smoked. They gave me a way to pause and think. There were a lot of wonderful aspects to that lousy habit.

In the seventies, after I left my position as vice-president of that pharmaceutical firm, I started a new corporation, which was very successful. Later, I helped a Chicago corporation go public, and that was a huge success; they make intravenous drugs for the hospital market. When I was fifty-five I achieved the financial target I had set for myself and I quit being a businessman to retire and take up sculpting seriously. I quit the boards of all my companies and I sold all my shares of stock.

The one real solid thing in my life was my good marriage. One thing that made me able to quit was the pressure from my wife and her support. My marriage was—and is—the most important thing in my life. For other people, it's their work or some hobby, but for me, it's my marriage.

In the fall of 1975 I quit smoking cigarettes. And I never had another. But ten years after quitting cigarettes, I started smoking cigars. I started in January of '85 and smoked for five months, until May. I was starting to do some excellent work in sculpture. I loved to sit and savor a cigar and sculpt. When I started smoking cigars, I thought I would smoke just one or two a day, but by May, I was up to twelve cigars a day so I quit again. I realized I could never touch tobacco in any form.

CELESTE HOLM
Smoking Was Chic

Celeste Holm's extraordinary acting career began when she created the role of Ado Annie in Oklahoma *and later replaced Gertrude Lawrence as Anna in* The King and I. *She won an Academy*

Award for Gentleman's Agreement, *and was knighted by King Olav of Norway in 1979—her title is Dame Celeste Holm. A public-spirited woman, she personally raised $20,000 for UNICEF (United Nations International Children's Emergency Fund) by selling her autographs for fifty cents—which means 40,000 autographs!*

I started smoking because in 1938 it was *chic.* I was fourteen years old, and I wanted to grow up. I thought smoking was a sign of growing up. It was absolutely idiotic, of course. I didn't know it could kill you. Nobody did. When I look back at it now, my Lord, I was fourteen! I see fourteen-year-olds now, with those eager little eyes, declaring, "I'm grown up!" Well, they push it, and so did I. Some friends and I once decided to give ourselves a challenge: to fill an entire shoebox with cigarette butts. It was ridiculous.

My friends and I didn't inhale when we smoked. The first time I ever inhaled was when someone gave me marijuana. I was seventeen. I was at a party given by musicians, and somebody said, "Hey, I brought back some of those funny cigarettes from Mexico," and everybody said, "Whee!" They handed me one, and I did my usual number, and they said, "No, no, you're not doing it right. You've got to do *this*" [demonstrating inhaling]. It was astonishing. I immediately began hallucinating. I kept seeing clouds. I sat down on the floor, my back leaning against the wall, closed my eyes, and started seeing clouds in pink and blue rushing by at high speed. When I opened my eyes everybody was moving in slow motion. I passed the cigarette on to somebody else; one inhalation was enough.

I started looking for the guy who'd brought me to the party, and he was nowhere in sight. I found him in the bathroom in front of the mirror making faces at himself, like John Barrymore. At least, that's what *he* thought.

I said, "Take me away from here." He said, "Why did you bring me here?" I stared at him. I didn't know any of these people. I hated him. He hated me. Absolute paranoia, both of us.

We went into Walgreen's in the basement of the Times Building in New York. I went up to the pharmacist and said, "Somebody gave us some funny cigarettes, and I can't stand it, and I want to come back." The man behind the counter looked at me and said, "How old are you?" I said, "Seventeen." He gave us big bowls of chili and crackers and milk and we wolfed it all down. I still didn't like the guy I was with. But that's how I started inhaling. I don't think I ever would have inhaled if it hadn't been for that miserable experience.

I never tried marijuana again, but I smoked cigarettes for twenty years after that, inhaling every one. I never thought about it harming my health, or threatening my career, or even being offensive to anyone else. Many of my parts involved singing and dancing as well as acting, but I never considered what smoking might do to my voice or my wind. I don't know whether no one knew then what cigarettes do to your lungs and throat and larynx or whether it was simply that no one talked about it. In either case, I didn't draw any connection between the fact that I sang for a living and the fact that I smoked.

Twenty years later, in 1961, I was singing in Las Vegas. It was summertime, 104°F outside, 64°F inside, and I got what's called Las Vegas throat. It comes from going back and forth between the hot, dry desert air outdoors and the cool, moist, air-conditioned air indoors. The typical symptom is that you lose your voice. Speaking professionally, it means you have no middle register at all. The middle register is where you speak. I could sing high and I could sing low, but there was nothing in the middle. Here I was trying to make a living using my voice, and it wasn't there. I said, "This is dumb." So one day I stopped smoking, and I never did it again.

The first day I quit, I wanted a cigarette, but I said, "This is ridiculous." The second day I kind of wanted a cigarette, but I said, "This is silly." The third day I didn't want it that much, and the fourth day it was over. I stopped entirely. I never took another cigarette. I had no support group for this decision. What for? It was nobody's business but mine. It wasn't so much a health issue as a livelihood issue. I couldn't continue to earn my living as an actress and singer if I smoked. Once I realized that, there was no question in my mind. I had to quit.

I hate it when other people smoke. I'm offended by the smell. Smokers don't seem to realize that the smoke from their cigarette drifts around the room, so I just complain consistently. I move away from people who are smoking. They're affecting my life. I wish they'd go away. When people ask if I mind if they smoke, I say, "Yes."

ALLEN S.
You Can't Do It Until You're Ready

Allen S., forty-six, is president of a multinational corporation that manufactures and sells health products. Gradually he began to feel that it was an intolerable contradiction to be a smoker and part of a major health products manufacturer. He stopped smoking in 1984.

If I were like my wife, I'd still be smoking. She can smoke a cigarette or two a day or none; enjoy them if she has them, and if she doesn't have them, not miss them. She's never bought cigarettes, ever. When I stopped buying cigarettes, she stopped smoking. Where she is a very controlled person, I tend to be compulsive.

The first time I quit was about fifteen years ago, in the early seventies. I was about thirty, and I did it on my own, without getting involved in a group or cigarette substitutes or anything. I quit for one year, and I honestly thought I was over cigarettes and smoking. Then I began to believe that I could indulge myself with an occasional cigar after dinner. I often traveled for business, and I remember waking up in my hotel room and looking at the dresser across from my bed and seeing a large number of empty cigar five-pack boxes. I realized that I was smoking cigars the way I'd smoked cigarettes. I was going through twenty or thirty cigars a day, inhaling them, and using them exactly like cigarettes. I was smoking all the time, but instead of smoking cigarettes, I smoked cigars. It sort of sneaked up on me.

I had never made a conscious decision to start smoking again. I thought, "Well, I can have a cigar after dinner," and then, two cigars after dinner, and then all the usual habit triggers came into play—the phone ringing, or getting in the car. Eventually it came down to waking up in the morning and I'd have to have a cigar. When I saw all those cigar boxes in my hotel room, I said, "The heck with that. I'm going back to my cigarettes." Which I did.

The second time I stopped was in 1981 or 1982, while working for this corporation, before I became president. This is a company involved in manufacturing and selling healthful products, and I was under significant peer pressure to quit. I agreed to join a company-sponsored Smokenders program. I went to the meetings and I did all of the little things you're supposed to do each week to go through a controlled withdrawal. And I did stop smoking for a short period of time—about six months. I became such a miserable person—I was really unhappy. I made myself stop smoking by sheer force of will, but I never stopped wanting to smoke. It was awful. In fact, a group of people put up a petition in the Oakland office where I worked—I had several hundred people working for me—asking me to go back to smoking. Which I did.

There was no question in my mind that it was stupid to smoke. Here I was increasingly responsible for a company whose business is health and taking control of one's life, and I was embarrassed as much as anything. It seemed so completely out of character to be a part of this company, part of its management, and continue to smoke. It was a contradiction of everything the company stood for.

That I *should* quit had certainly been on the top of my mind for at least ten years before I actually did it. I had smoked since I was about thirteen. My father smoked cigarettes, and two of my four sisters did as well. My father quit, but by then I had been smoking for years. He quit long before I did. Most of my life—twenty-eight years of it—I was a steady, two-pack-a-day Marlboro smoker. The last few years I smoked Merits on the theory that they had less nicotine. The only result of switching to Merits was that I went from two packs a day to two and a half packs a day!

As my three daughters got older, the pressure at home to stop smoking became more significant, particularly since none of my kids smoked. They were very vocal about wanting me to quit!

When I quit this last time, more than anything else I felt I had come to the point where I'd had it. I didn't want to smoke any more, which was very different from all of the other times I quit smoking. Every other time I quit, it was because I felt I *should* quit smoking. I think I understand now why people say, "You can't do it until you're really ready." I don't know what you have to do to get really ready, but the biggest difference between the other times I quit and this time was that I *wanted* to quit.

One day about five years ago I told my family that I

would stop smoking when we left on our annual vacation—I always take the last two weeks of December off. I
told them in October that I would have my last cigarette
when that vacation started. I smoked right up through
the day we left. We were driving down to the desert from
San Francisco. As I got on to Highway 5, I still had a
couple of cigarettes left. I smoked down to the end of
that pack and said, "That's it, guys. I quit smoking." And
I did.

It was a good thing that I was going away for two weeks
of vacation. I was away from familiar surroundings, I was
away from the telephone, and I was away from the office.
That helped me get through the early part of it, because I
was in a no-pressure situation. I was away from all the
things that tended to trigger smoking.

I knew that I was never going to smoke again, and I
didn't. It was not that difficult. I never had the miserable
feelings or symptoms that I'd had at previous times.
What I did was gain thirty pounds, which I've had on and
off and on and off, but today I still have that same thirty
pounds on me. I gave up smoking for eating.

I've never had addictions other than food and cigarettes. I'm a compulsive person. I do things compulsively, and I know that. I work compulsively, I eat compulsively, and I used to smoke compulsively. I would
never fool around with anything like drugs that could be
addicting. It scares me, given that I know how compulsive I am.

One other thing happened that made me want to quit:
a friend of mine—a smoker—had a heart attack and

triple-bypass surgery. It happened less than a year before I quit. I remember going to see him at the hospital after he had his bypass. He had been a strong, robust guy, and he looked so weak and frail—and he was a smoker. I don't know if his heart attack had anything to do with the fact that he smoked—he may have had a lot of other things in his life-style or genetic background that caused it—but nonetheless, smoking was the thing he and I had in common.

When I went to see him in the hospital, it was awful. His wife was waiting in the hallway, wringing her hands. He was trying to put up a good front for his kids and me. He hadn't shaved in a while, he didn't have much strength, and he was lying there in a private room in a little hospital. I thought, "My God, this is awful." It was awful for him and it was awful for everybody around him. That really set my resolve to quit.

I always knew it was bad to smoke—you couldn't be a reasonably intelligent person and not know! I had seen the movies, I had seen the photographs, and I have known other people who have had heart attacks and cancer. You don't make it to my age in life without being exposed to that sort of thing, but seeing a close friend in that shape traumatized me in more ways than one.

I made several resolutions that day. The only one I've kept is the one to quit smoking. I also resolved to get back in shape and to quit working as hard. I still work very hard, and I am not in shape, but at least I don't smoke.

Now I hate cigarettes. I don't like being around smoke.

If I'm in a restaurant where someone is smoking, it makes me crazy. My eyes water. It is as though I have a strong, physical, allergic reaction to tobacco smoke. Still I must tell you honestly, I know if I had a cigarette I would be a three-pack-a-day smoker tomorrow. With all the knowledge, with all the resolve, with all the revulsion over cigarettes, I know for a fact that if I had a cigarette, I'd smoke again. I don't know what drug addiction feels like, but I think of the way that I react to cigarettes as an addiction. I know that as much as I hate them, that if I smoked even one, I'd be hooked again.

STEVE G.
Drinking and Smoking Went Together

Steve G. teaches English and history at a private boarding school, where he also coaches the soccer and basketball teams. His avocation is singing with a local opera company. A recovered alcoholic with fifteen years of sobriety, Steve is active in Alcoholics Anonymous. He quit smoking and drinking within a few years of each other. For a time he found A.A. meetings difficult because of "all the smoking."

In junior high school I was contemptuous of smoking and drinking, very puritanical, because I was an athlete. I was on all the all-star teams. But during the summer between the ninth and tenth grade I went through many changes. I lived in Los Angeles in a big house, and it seemed as though every room in the house had little containers of cigarettes. There were cigarettes every-where, like candy in a candy dish; they were so accessible. My mother smoked, and my father smoked sporadically.

Anyway, I remember sitting there with a cigarette, playing with it and lighting it up a few times during that summer. It was something to do that was kind of taboo, since not many kids smoked during that period. There was no cancer scare. Adults said it would stunt your growth or cut down your wind, but I never experienced that.

I was a ninth-grader, at the top of the heap in a three-year junior high school. A three-year junior high allows you to make your mark, as you do in high school, unlike the two-year middle school system we have now. And then when high school started I was back at the bottom of the heap. Suddenly I wasn't the greatest athlete, there were 3,600 kids in the three-year high school to compete with, and the girls that I'd gone out with started going out with the senior boys. I felt rejected. On top of it all, I had to follow my older sister through the process, who was a saint—who *was* and still *is*—and who every teacher revered. I was constantly compared to her. I decided that I would be a rebel because I was not going to be cut from the same cloth as my sister. I started smoking when I entered high school; I was fifteen.

That sense of loss in going from the top of the pecking order to the bottom is why a lot of college freshmen start smoking. How many people never smoke until they are college freshmen? There's a tremendous vulnerability when you've been at the top and you have to start all over again from the bottom. Teaching school, I see it all the time, in seniors. High school seniors are often much more mature in their behavior than college freshmen are.

I continued to play sports and smoke clandestinely, because in those days if you got caught smoking you were off the team. But it didn't seem to affect my wind, so I continued to smoke. A lot of it was social. Everybody smoked Marlboro hard pack, because it was the macho thing to do. Although I think I was getting addicted, I didn't realize it at the time. I never even thought about quitting.

In the first year of college I became a serious smoker, and my drinking intensified. I couldn't imagine drinking without smoking—the two went hand in hand. About that time I began to have problems with alcohol. I was aware of it. I was getting in more and more trouble, but it was hard for me not to drink and smoke. At the end of my freshman year I was tossed out of UCLA for disciplinary reasons.

I went in the Army. Of course, smoking was a way of life in the Army. I smoked Camel non-filters, about a pack a day. It's funny, I never was what one would call a chain smoker. I would never light a cigarette and put it down and light another one. Smoking Camel non-filters, too: They were so strong, I didn't have to smoke that often. Again, it went hand in hand with the drinking.

I was stationed in France. Alcohol was readily available even though we were under age: It was very cheap. We would go to the EM Club every night after work, and we would smoke and drink. I smoked French cigarettes occasionally—they were incredibly strong. We could buy cigarettes in the PX for twelve cents a pack because they were tax-free. They were almost like fringe benefits. You could get a drink for five cents or ten cents during happy hour. If you were a compulsive-obsessive, as I am, it was a dream come true. You could get drunk on a dollar and smoke for practically nothing.

Anyway, smoking and drinking began to affect my health in my twenties. In the Army I began to have stomach problems. I also remember waking up coughing. Sometimes, with the combination of the alcohol, I remember waking up coughing and vomiting. I think one of the blessings in my life is that drugs—I consider nicotine a drug—affected me at an early age. I had very strong reactions.

My father died of cancer of the esophagus when I was about twenty-two. It was probably the most traumatic event of my life, and it accelerated my drinking. Three weeks after he died, I went to my first A.A. meeting, at the age of twenty-three, which was very young at that time. That was 1965. I continued to smoke, because in Alcoholics Anonymous the attitude was, "Well, you don't drink now, so smoking's okay." That was the prevailing attitude in Alcoholics Anonymous until very recently. You felt guilty if you didn't smoke at an A.A. meeting. After about six years of sobriety, by the way, I experimented with social drinking for a couple of years and it was disastrous. But I went to A.A. during that time.

171

I was smoking during that time, too.

I had quit drinking for a number of years, married, had children, graduated with honors, secured a teaching position, and felt comfortably successful, but smoking was still a very active part of my life. I taught in a boarding school. The majority of the people there did not smoke—the kids did, but the faculty did not. I taught English and drama and coached athletics. I probably smoked more at school than anyplace else. I would smoke when I rehearsed; I would smoke sometimes even in the classroom.

This was still prior to the real cancer scare and the real stop-smoking era. It was the late sixties, early seventies, when they were just beginning to make the connection between smoking and cancer. It was rumored that smoking stunted your growth. There were similar scare stories, too, that we whispered to each other when we were younger, something to do with masturbation stunting your growth as well. I always laughed at them. I often wondered how tall I would have been if I hadn't smoked or masturbated.

I still smoked probably a pack a day, but I started trying to quit smoking. I would go awhile without smoking, and then I'd start again. I was influenced by the fact that I was in a very healthy environment. Few adults at the school smoked; I lived out in the country; my wife did not smoke. It is marvelous that she managed to live with a smoker—I am now so intolerant of it myself. The smell, the ashtrays, and everything else.

My first major attempt at quitting was in my late twenties for six months. I ended up getting very heavy. Instead of exercising to compensate for the change in metabolism, I started smoking again. All it took was one drag on a cigarette and that was it, I was off to the races. In view of my experience in Alcoholics Anonymous, where you learn that one drink starts you drinking again, I should have realized that one cigarette would start me smoking again. And it did.

Probably the single most important event was Thanksgiving in 1972. We were invited to a party at this guy's house. He was a doctor. We went in, I lit up a cigarette, and he said, "I'm sorry, but you can't smoke in the house." Nobody had ever told me that before. It was a cold rainy day and everybody was inside; nobody else smoked. I went outside and smoked a cigarette, and I felt so alienated, so anti-social, so *excluded*. I had never been put in that position before. Nowadays it's quite common; lots of people won't let smokers smoke in their house or their office or their car.

This doctor was a cold bastard, very aloof, and I really hated his guts for making me do this. But years later, when I saw the same doctor, I told him how grateful I was because that was the turning point for me in terms of my attitude toward smoking. I had felt that alcohol was not socially acceptable—or more accurately, my *reaction* to alcohol was not socially acceptable—but I'd never felt that way about smoking. Cigarettes were always socially acceptable.

In February of 1973, for some unknown reason, I am not sure why, I just said, "Well, I am going to quit again." There was no preparation for it. I am sure this had weighed on my mind, but I was not aware of it. I did not set a date. I quit, and that was the last time I had a cigarette. I remember because I took a group of school kids on a week-long trip. It was the worst possible time to quit. I gave those poor kids holy hell. I was on edge; my nerves were raw.

I began to gain weight again, and this time I started running. I had gotten some exercise before, coaching the soccer and basketball teams, running up and down the sidelines. I decided to run every day, starting with a quarter of a mile. It was a good, healthy replacement habit. Although I gained weight, the exercise evened it out. I was in the best shape I've ever been in in my life.

I did some other things, too, which other people might find rather absurd. I would go to A.A. meetings and take carrots and celery to munch on. I ate junk food. That's a compulsion I have to this day, an addiction that I haven't quite got rid of, so my weight fluctuates.

And then I did something else. I realized that a lot of the pleasure of smoking was the oral gratification, the sucking. I had an infant at the time, so I took her baby bottle, put orange juice in it, and sucked on her baby bottle when I watched television in the evening. It worked! It had a tremendous pacifying effect.

I would never do this in public, but in my own house, when I'd come home after a hard day, it worked. The end of the day is usually the time I'm looking for some small reward. I couldn't drink. I could eat junk, but even that was hard because we lived out in the country. I'd take the baby's bottle, fill it up with orange juice, and I would sit there and watch TV, sucking on this bottle. It took a long time to drink orange juice this way because the pulp would clog the nipple. When the end of the nipple would get stuck with stuff, I'd clean it out and start over again. And it worked fairly well as oral gratification. I'm pleased to report that I did not become addicted to the baby bottle.

The key this time was not thinking in terms of quitting for the rest of my life; I quit one day at a time. I used the A.A. principles. I could smoke tomorrow without any problem. So rather than swearing off and making the "I'll never smoke again as long as I live" vow, I used the A.A. principles. That is what sustained me through the first year or two. Then, after two years, not smoking became a habit just as smoking had been.

It was very hard to go to A.A. meetings for a long time because of all the smoking. I would go home and I could smell the stale smoke on me. I would breathe it in. Sometimes I'd get headaches. I can see the danger of second-hand smoke. Fortunately, now there is a new consciousness in A.A., so there are lots of smoke-free meetings. I don't have to feel guilty.

My daughter now smokes! I notice teen-agers, particularly girls, smoke now. It's chic. When they quit they gain weight, so a lot of teen-age girls smoke to keep their weight down. It's become part of our cultural obsession with weight control.

My younger sister smoked. She's also in A.A., and she quit smoking and drinking. My mother quit a few years ago because of social pressure in her family. My mother had a tremendous weight gain after she quit smoking, which resulted in her having bad knees. Her knees couldn't support the extra weight. She's had some other health problems, too. It's been a mixed blessing. But she just couldn't stand the social pressure any more. The same with my mother-in-law, with whom I live. I think she quit because of social pressure from the family. It's nice to have her quit smoking because she smoked in the house.

People associate smoking and drinking; they have to do one with the other. A lot of people always have a cigarette with a drink. I come from a family of compulsive-obsessive people. There's a lot of alcoholism in my family and a long history of smoking. My father smoked, and he died of cancer of the esophagus. My mother and sister smoked until very recently. My uncles, my father's brothers, were alcoholic, and they all smoked. They all died of alcoholism.

I've had some wonderful benefits from quitting. I'm a singer. I sing opera. I'm a tenor, but my speaking voice has always been placed low. I also coach athletics after school, which involves a lot of yelling and cheering. I developed a tumor on my larynx, and I went in to have it removed. The first question the doctor asked me was, "Do you smoke or drink?" and fortunately I could say that I had been off both for a long time. He said: "There's no doubt in my mind that if you had smoked and drunk during that time you would have cancer of the throat now. Between the use and abuse of your speaking voice from coaching and yelling without a megaphone or bullhorn, if you'd been smoking and drinking too, you'd have had cancer of the throat." It was one of those grateful moments where I could see that quitting made a difference. The tumor was nonmalignant, it was removed, and since then I have been singing and my voice is as strong as ever. That alone makes it worth it to quit.

BETSEY W.
A Compulsion Lasts about Two Minutes

Betsey W. took her degree in economics at a major university in preparation for the family business, from which she retired as president in 1987. Now she works part time doing public relations and assembling a history of the granite mining industry. She and her husband have been married since 1948. Gradually, she lessened the number of situations in which she smoked.

I always loved mountain hiking, so I decided that after I retired—in January of 1987—I was going to hike the John Muir Trail. It's over 200 miles of rugged mountain terrain in the Sierra Nevada in California. I knew I had to quit smoking in order to have the endurance I'd need.

I smoked my last cigarette the morning of December 31, 1986, and I told myself that I could have a cigarette again when I came down off Mount Whitney, the end of the John Muir Trail and the highest peak in the lower forty-eight states.

I'd smoked for about thirty years. I started when I was close to thirty years old, much older than most people. I had managed to resist smoking all through high school and college, though I tried my first cigarette when I was around fourteen. Four or five girls from my high school went to a friend's house. She had some old cigarettes, and we tried smoking them; they were pretty awful. They were all dried up. At any rate we tried them, and then we got worried that her mother would find out that we had been smoking so we put a lot of toothpaste in our mouths. Of course, we didn't have our own toothbrushes at her house!

But I didn't really smoke until much later. I was president of the family business in the early fifties and we were having a lot of conflict. My mother had been running the company and we asked her to leave. But she was suing us, and it was very difficult having her and her attorney at board meetings. Someone suggested that I smoke during these meetings because it gives you a chance to do something, to think for a minute, because the ritual of pulling a cigarette out of a package and putting a match to it gives you a little time. People will wait for that time, and you can get your thoughts together. So that's what I did. I smoked only at board meetings for a few years, then I started smoking more often.

I also had a housekeeper who smoked, and I admired her a lot. Smoking was something that I could do to be like her. A strange thing, but true.

I found it rather difficult to quit when I tried after a few years—so I must have been addicted. I eventually smoked about a pack a day. I have always been a physically strong person—I have only been in the hospital twice, when I had my two sons—and I thought I was the healthiest smoker in the world!

Sometime in the early seventies I tried to quit smoking. I managed to stay off cigarettes from three to six weeks. That sounds like a short time, but it is not a short time for somebody who is quitting smoking. Once in a while I would try—every New Year's I would think about whether this was the year that I was going to quit smoking. Oh, but I didn't sign up for a course or any of that stuff.

I don't think my husband has ever smoked a cigarette. I don't think he even tried one when he was a teen-ager. He didn't like to see me smoking. But I told him I wished he would stop fussing with me about smoking. I think I was smoking partly in defiance of his wanting me to quit because I am a stubborn, defiant person. "I want to make up my own mind, please!"

In November of 1985, I was thinking more and more about quitting smoking. What I did first was to stop smoking in places or situations where I was used to smoking, and the first one was in the car. Now I admit that I smoked before getting in the car and I would smoke in parking garages when I got *out* of the car if I drove up to San Francisco. I would always light a cigarette the minute I got out of the car, and that went on through all 1986. I was still smoking, but never in the car.

Something else helped. Not many people at the company smoked any more. The few who did went outside the building—their co-workers won't allow them to smoke in the office. My son had stopped smoking in September of 1986. When he told me that, it made me think even harder about quitting.

I disconnected myself from smoking at parties sometime during 1986. Cocktails and smoking were kind of a connection, but I managed to go to parties and not smoke. Some days I didn't smoke at work. I'd say, "Hmm, I went through the whole day without smoking."

The only thing I didn't manage to do in 1986 was to stop smoking when I got home, because my routine was to leave the office and stop by the grocery store every night on the way home. We eat lots of fresh vegetables, and when I shop every day at the same store I get to know the vegetables personally. I really do: I can recognize that they were there yesterday—they look the same, but a little older. Things like eggplant, a store has for days, and the eggplant waves and says, "I saw you before," and I say, "Well, you can stay here. It's nice seeing you again but. . . ." Anyway, when I got home I would put that bag of groceries down, pour myself a glass of wine, and light a cigarette. That is the only smoking I didn't manage to stop before the end of 1986.

I think there were times in 1986 when I got down to half a pack a day, but I was normally a pack-a-day smoker. I wanted to stop smoking and *had* stopped smoking in some situations on a trial basis. I was trying this and trying that in 1986. I knew I was going to retire at the end of 1986, and I wanted to do the John Muir Trail in 1987, but my breathing was not too good when it came to high altitudes. The John Muir Trail is over 200 miles long, all at high altitude!

I knew I had to stop smoking or I would never have the endurance to hike over 200 miles all the way to the top of Mount Whitney. In August of 1986 I had made some friends who were also interested in doing that hike. We started training together, and five of us went on a hike on the back side of the Sierras in August 1986. I had a terrible time. It's an easy hike, from Twin Lakes to Peter Lake, out of Bridgeport, northeast of Yosemite. Well, I didn't even get to Barney Lake, and that's only four or five miles from the trailhead. I began to feel terrible just before the switchbacks where the trail starts to get steep. I gave out before that, feeling awful.

I said, "I don't feel good. I don't think I should go any farther." The rest of them went up to Barney Lake, but I stayed and slept at the bottom of the switchbacks that night. I felt fine the next morning. I suppose it was the smoking and the altitude—about 7,000 feet—that made me feel the way I did the night before.

After that experience I knew that if I wanted to do the 211 miles of the John Muir Trail in one summer I had to stop smoking. One of the things that I hadn't done was the John Muir Trail. I decided that I was going to do the trail that following summer. I had to stop smoking, at least until after the hike. My son was going to meet me at Mount Whitney, and he was going to bring me cigarettes. That cigarette *after* the Mount Whitney climb was my dream.

I had figured that to do 211 miles it would take twenty-one days. But ten miles a day is a long way at a high altitude. You start adding some rest days, and it took us more time: It took us forty-one days. We had good weather. It didn't rain once. It snowed a little, and it hailed a little, but that's all. We washed everything we had when we laid over. We would dry some things, and then we would put on those clothes and wash the others. We'd start after each rest day with ourselves clean and our clothes clean, one way or the other.

We started the John Muir Trail on July 8, from Yosemite Valley. As we passed people on the trail they would ask, "How far are you going?" I'd say, "We're going to Whitney," and the fellow with us who had hiked a lot said, "Don't say that; you might not make it." And the three of us who hadn't done any of this before said, "Oh, of course we will. We won't make it if we *don't* say it. We have to keep that goal out for ourselves." It did seem impossible for the first few days. We reached the top of Whitney on August 17.

Before the trip I would say, "Well, you can't smoke today because you are going to do this hike next summer. You can't have a cigarette today." I knew myself well enough. If I had one I would smoke the whole pack. I mean, what are you going to do with the rest of them? I did say to myself, "I can quit smoking for seven and a half months until I get off Mount Whitney." Now I was up on Mount Whitney, and I never even thought about smoking one way or the other.

When we were coming down Whitney we met a lot of people who were going up, and we asked, "Can we get a cold beer down at the store when we come down off the mountain?" It isn't the beer so much as the coldness and the bubbles because that is different from the stream water. My husband met us at the end of the trail with a watermelon and lots of fresh fruit, and we went through that whole watermelon.

By this time, cigarettes were completely forgotten. Cigarettes were out. I had lost my interest in cigarettes as the hike went along, and I never did have that cigarette when I came down off Whitney. I haven't smoked yet, and I probably won't smoke ever again.

Oh, once in a while I think about smoking. My husband said something to me that was helpful: "You know, I have read somewhere that a compulsion lasts about two minutes." When I think about wanting a cigarette, or when I see a friend smoking, I sometimes think, "Hmm, maybe this cigarette will be what I hope for in cigarettes. Maybe I could ask her for a cigarette. . . ." Then my husband's suggestion runs through my mind. If I can live through one or two minutes, then the feeling goes away. I also pretend to smoke. Pretending smoking to me is deep breathing. So I take a few deep breaths, and I hold a pen as a cigarette and I play with the pen a lot. I wreck more pens because I pull them apart playing with them, and that is one of the things that I do instead of smoking.

Since I stopped smoking I have developed an addiction to corn chips. I used to smoke two or three cigarettes while I was cooking dinner and have a couple of glasses of wine. Now I have to have something with the wine so I eat corn chips. I eat an immense amount of corn chips. But I can get by without corn chips if there aren't any. It's not like cigarettes used to be where I'd have to go out and find some. Still, I do make sure that I have plenty of corn chips at home.

As a non-smoker, one of the things I notice now is that when I pass people in the grocery store I can smell if they're smokers. And it does not smell good to me. Now that I realize how bad people who smoke smell, I don't know how my husband, who never smoked, ever managed to stand me all those years, almost thirty years.

My next ambition is to do the Inca Trail in South America with a Stanford group. I was at Machu Picchu in the Peruvian Andes and I had such terrible altitude sickness—it's over 10,000 feet—that I never saw the ruins, even though I was very interested in them and in the sense of continuity of human beings going back hundreds of years in one place. So I want to go back again to see them.

I'm also going to do a shorter Sierra trip this year, 150 miles. It's twenty-one days, though, half the time of last year's trip.

One of the things I found out since I stopped smoking is that whatever I was looking for in cigarettes had never been there. I don't know how to define it exactly. It was the feeling of emptiness some people feel at times, as I did. But smoking never filled this internal emptiness. I kept hoping that the next cigarette would. But it never did.

JOHN G.
He Wrote Tobacco Advertising

*John G. has been an advertising copywriter for almost forty years,
on Madison Avenue and on the West Coast.*

I quit smoking because it began to nauseate me that I was
a slave to tobacco. My whole life revolved around being
able to smoke. I even resented going to sleep because it
meant I couldn't smoke. Concerts, the theater, movies,
all were damned uncomfortable. I couldn't last longer
than twenty or twenty-five minutes, thirty at the outside,
before I had to run out to the men's room to have a
cigarette. Of course, when I came back I'd have missed
key parts of the movie. Say you have a ninety-minute
show, and three interruptions of about ten minutes each,
that's thirty minutes, or a third of the movie. I used to say
the same thing to every person I ever went to a movie
with. I'd say, "God, that movie didn't make much sense.
It really didn't hang together." I didn't know who had
died, and where the dog went, and why they were now in
Alaska when they had been in Florida. . . .

And I hated the bookkeeping of smoking. When I took
the dogs out for a walk, I had to tap my shirt pocket to
make sure I had cigarettes, and then I had to check to
make sure I had more than six cigarettes left. I had to
check to see if I had my lighter, and be sure that I had

matches with me in case my lighter didn't work. Maybe I'd better look to see if I've filled the lighter and have fresh flints. Heck, maybe I'd better take a fresh pack in case I get into a conversation with somebody.

My wife, now my former wife, was also a heavy smoker. We'd buy cigarettes by the carton, but still sometimes I'd have to go out at three o'clock in the morning, with a foot of snow on the ground, to some all-night diner that had a cigarette machine. Or we'd fish butts out of the wastebasket.

The amount of planning that smoking required was ridiculous. If I was going on a long drive, I'd have to remember to put an extra pack of cigarettes in the glove compartment. It was a constant preoccupation. It was crazy.

It wasn't even that I enjoyed smoking, but I was so damned uncomfortable when I *wasn't* smoking. If I had to go a whole hour without a cigarette I'd get a crawly, itchy feeling. It was terribly distracting. If I was at a lecture or in a meeting where I couldn't get out to have a cigarette, it wasn't long before I couldn't hear what the lecturer was saying. All I could think about was how much longer it would be until I could smoke.

I smelled like an ashtray most of the time, but so did almost everyone else. I started smoking when I was ten years old, sneaking off on Saturday mornings with my friends. We all knew we were going to smoke when we grew up; it was just a matter of when. My father was a physician and my mother was a registered nurse, and they both smoked. All the adults I knew did. There was much more acceptance for smoking then. It would never have occurred to anyone to ask you not to smoke or to tell you that they did not allow smoking in their house. It simply wasn't done.

It was considered bad form to light up during a meal between courses, but if I thought I could get away with it, I did. I always had a cigarette after meals. A cigarette, a cigar, a pipe, I used them all.

I always had a cigarette after lovemaking. That's a particularly agreeable time to have a cigarette. And with a cup of coffee; coffee and cigarettes just seemed to go together. The best cigarette of the day for me was the first one, as soon as I woke up. When you have a cigarette with nothing else in your system, it goes straight to home plate. It was nice. It felt good.

But that's remembering back a long time, because I haven't smoked for twenty-five years. I was a heavy smoker by the time I was sixteen, I smoked until I was thirty-two, quit for seven years, and then deliberately decided to start smoking again. I had put on some weight and I knew I was hitting the sweets pretty hard, and I remembered that smoking had cut my appetite. I thought if I started smoking again it would be easier to control my weight. I started out with two or three cigarettes a day, and within a week I was back to smoking three packs of Camels. I smoked heavily for a year, quit again, and haven't touched a cigarette or wanted one in twenty-five years.

I found a book by the late Herbert Brean, a writer for *Life* magazine, called *How to Stop Smoking*, which was very valuable. It's out of print now. I had tried to stop smoking several times and was unable to. I could make it maybe as much as two days without a cigarette by myself.

The book excited a different feeling about quitting in me; it changed my attitude. It's a funny book. The first chapter is why you *shouldn't* quit smoking. Then, if you read as far as the second chapter, he points out how essentially insane it is to allow your entire life to be dominated by a little white tube of paper with some chopped-up weeds in it. His key tip was that once you quit, pamper yourself in every other way you can think of so you don't feel sorry for yourself. For the first few weeks of quitting he says to take it easy on yourself with everything else— buy yourself some little thing you want, eat a whole bag of cashews, have a dessert with lunch. It's very wise advice because there is a terrible tendency to feel deprived, and if you do, you can't quit. Self-pity will wreck it every time. He made it clear that there are lots of things other than smoking that can make you feel good.

I realized what a grip tobacco had on me the first time I tried to quit. I hadn't had a cigarette for a week, and I went into a restaurant in New York for lunch. The service was typically slow and typically rude, really standard-issue stuff for New York, and I walked out in tears because I was sure they were being mean to me. God! I knew it must have been nicotine withdrawal, because even New York waiters had never reduced me to tears before. I was thirty-two years old.

Brean, in his book, was very cheerful and very optimistic. He said that you could quit if you sincerely wanted to, and he suggested telling everyone you knew that you were quitting. By telling everyone you created your own peer pressure to really quit, and you created a support system for your quitting as well.

He also suggested distracting yourself, so you don't sit around thinking about this great sacrifice that you've made. Go to four movies in a week, take up needlepoint, just don't think about what a poor, unloved child you are because you've quit smoking. And he tells you what a great sense of victory there is when you've finally quit. And it's true.

I've become a trifle fanatical about cigarette smoking, and especially about the calculated promotion thereof by people who ought to know better. The tobacco advertising I wrote in my days on Madison Avenue was tacitly, but clearly, aimed at the young. We knew that habit patterns in smoking tend to be well formed before one achieves maturity. It is a truism that rather few people start smoking after their mid-twenties. Today the ads depict people even younger than the models we used to use, and always with the theme that this is the passport to being "with it."

Promoting tobacco shows an unmistakable contempt for human life. No tobacco company could do well if its customers were moderate users. The five-cigarettes-a-day smoker is never the target market. The *heavy* smoker is the target, and we were never for an instant uncertain or confused about that when we were composing our lyrics.

We are so concerned about whales, sea otters, snail

darters, and the like that it seems just plain crazy for us to make so little protest in behalf of our own kind. If there were a movement to poison deer and peregrine falcons with toxins as potent and damaging as tobacco, a hue and cry would be raised that would jail the promoters of such a scheme overnight.

I don't write tobacco advertising any more; I haven't for many years, and I've become convinced that to do so is criminal. Quitting smoking is the smartest decision I've ever made.

STEVE W.
She Said, "Oh, You Smoke?"

Steve W. is president of a large business that has been family-owned for three generations. At the age of thirty-five, he shares the title of president with his brother. He has a master's degree in psychology and enjoys skiing as a sport. He never thought about quitting until he actually did quit.

I know a lot of smokers who have tried to quit a lot of times and to them "trying" means not buying a pack of cigarettes, and then not having any cigarettes for a whole morning or maybe a whole day. I always said to myself if I ever wanted to quit I would quit and never smoke again. I didn't know if I was fooling myself or not, because I had never tried.

I had a kind of a nagging, half-conscious concern about my health, but never really up front. Besides, it was always easy to find an older person, eighty or ninety, who was smoking, and with that I could justify all the cigarettes I'd ever had, and was going to have.

My mother was a smoker, too. She recently quit smoking, and I think that she is one of those people who have tried to quit, which means that she has set down cigarettes for weeks, even months, over the last ten years, and then has started smoking again.

When I finally quit I had smoked for about twenty years. I would say I probably had my first puff of a cigarette when I was fourteen. Some older kids had cigarettes that they had taken from their parents and would pass them around in a hideaway, dark-alley–type situation. It was exciting to sneak a puff of a cigarette.

I didn't really like it at first, because it burned my throat and made me cough, but I figured it was something to overcome, like other adult tastes. In the very beginning I probably smoked once or twice a month. Then there was a gradual increase up to about a pack and a half, maybe even two packs per day, when I was about seventeen. It took three years to progress—if you can call that progress! I smoked at that level until I quit two years ago. I quit because I'd gotten a date with a very pretty girl.

It happened that I asked this girl, Janet, to go out with me. She was very, very pretty, and I was very much attracted to her. She was quite health conscious—health club every day, health foods, but not overboard. I knew she would have nothing to do with me if I smoked, and so the night I was to take her out I brushed my teeth fifteen times, washed my hair six times, put on a clean set of clothes, and did not have a cigarette on the way to pick her up, did not have one the entire time I was with her that evening.

Janet didn't know I was a smoker. I had cleaned my car very well. She spent the night at my house that evening. We didn't have sex, but we did share my bed because we had had a lot of wine and she didn't want to drive home. It was a very clean first date—no sex. When we got up that Sunday morning, she made some breakfast and we sat out by my swimming pool in the sun, and we were just going to have a relaxing day around the pool. Meanwhile, I hadn't had a cigarette. I had never gone that long without a cigarette since I was around sixteen or seventeen, when I got to the pack-and-a-half deal. And I said to myself, "Well, I like her." It was then about two o'clock in the afternoon, and I still hadn't had a cigarette. I had a cup or two of coffee, and so the need for the other half of that experience—a cigarette—was very much there all morning.

Finally I said, "Oh, hell. Either she likes me for who I am, or she doesn't." I went into the house, got my pack of Camel filter cigarettes, went out by the pool, and said, "Oh, it's about time for a cigarette." And she said, "Oh, you smoke?" And I said, "Oh, occasionally." I didn't want her to know I was a big-time smoker. I lit it up and got about halfway through the cigarette, which is maybe four or five puffs, and I could literally feel the drug of the cigarette taking hold. I could feel my body getting very small shakes.

She didn't say anything, and I didn't say anything to her, except, "This cigarette isn't that great." She didn't know that it was unusual for me to put a cigarette out half-smoked, or to react to it like that.

Tuesday night of the following week, I went to dinner with her again. I still hadn't had a cigarette. I was still sticking to the commitment that I don't need to have that shaky feeling and I don't need all of the other negative things that go along with cigarettes. It wasn't a health decision—it was more cosmetic. Cigarettes make you smell like an old ashtray. They mean your teeth get brown—I have pretty nice teeth. Plus all of the other things that go along with smoking.

That pretty girl that first night was the inspiration. After our second date, she put a pack of candy cigarettes in my mailbox because I told her that, indeed, I was a more-than-occasional smoker. We were having fun with her bringing me candy cigarettes.

The first three weeks of not smoking I was concerned that I wouldn't be able to go through with it, because some of the people in my office who noticed I wasn't smoking—there was no cloud of smoke billowing out of my office door—began to make me think that there were going to be withdrawal symptoms. My secretary was saying, "Boy, you're irritable," and I thought, "Well, hell."

Some of my friends who had paid a lot of money for Smokenders' seminars brought me stacks and stacks of literature about what types of withdrawal symptoms to expect. Irritability is one of the things to watch out for, and some of my co-workers told me that I was a grouch. Either I was having a physical withdrawal to not having a cigarette or it was purely psychological, but at any rate, within two months I was more or less back to my old self.

After reading all the literature on smoking and hearing about everyone else's problems with quitting, I thought, "My God, maybe I do need some props." I went out and bought a whole bunch of Life Savers and gum, and I found myself eating more. I don't know if I really needed to or if it was because of the influence of all the damn literature. I quit and then I started reading the literature and thought, "Well, hell, I had better have some Life Savers in my pocket." Sometimes I feel that I would have been better off without reading all that literature!

I never broke down since that half a cigarette the first day, although I have smoked two cigars without inhaling since then. That was on a weekend in Las Vegas. With lots of cocktails, it seemed like the time to have a very expensive cigar, and I smoked two of them, one each night. That was about a year after I'd quit. I have not smoked since, and I mean no cigars either!

I know that now I have a lot more lung capacity. Skiing is one of my greatest physical exertions every year, and now I can go down hills where I used to have to stop three or four times to catch my breath. I think it is just great—my excitement in skiing is not held back now. I can do more, and that is great.

In the last year and a half I have had three or four dreams about smoking. I have waked up and said to myself, "Crap, I've had a cigarette; in fact, I've had several." And then I tell myself, ";Oh, hell, it was just a dream." But still, I feel really bummed out that I let a small urge to smoke overcome my greater need not to.

An interesting point: Most of the people I know try to quit smoking by eliminating the accessibility of cigarettes. They don't have a pack of cigarettes in their desk drawer, in their car, in their shirt pocket. I have given this kind of quitter many a cigarette! I think that's ridiculous. When I went out with that girl, Janet, the first night, I had a full pack of Camel filters, my favorite brand at the time, in my car. I had that full pack in my kitchen that night, and of course, the next day, that Sunday afternoon, I had a full pack of Camel filters. That same full pack was in my shirt pocket for the next six weeks. I never had that cigarette pack out of my reach. It dwindled because my friends who were continually in and out of my office would bum cigarettes from me. Eventually, the pack was finished, but not by me. It was a nice, secure feeling that if I ever had one of those situations where I *had* to have a cigarette—I could light one up. But when my friends finally bummed all the cigarettes in that pack, I never bought another pack.

My daily routines, such as checking to make sure I had a pen in my top pocket, my wallet in my back pocket, and my comb in my right back pocket, used to include making sure that I had a pack of cigarettes and a pack of matches. Now I've eliminated two items in my life, which is a great freedom. When I "pack up" in the morning, I don't have to look around for cigarettes and matches.

Other habits have changed, too. I drink a lot less coffee now, probably 30 percent of what I drank before. Over the last ten years that I smoked, I was probably drinking eight cups a day—and I am talking mugs, not tea cups. Now, two or three at the most. Interestingly enough, I now get mild headaches from coffee if I drink "too much," which I didn't when I smoked.

Now, after I get home from a nightclub, or a bar with a band for dancing, and I smell my clothes, I think, "My God, I was wearing these? They smell so horrendous from the cigarette smoke."

Why did I quit? My quitting was kind of an accumulation of disliking my clothes and my hands smelling like cigarettes, combined with the probable health consequences of smoking—death. It all just came to a head on that date. People used to tell me that if I didn't smoke I wouldn't be limited as to the type of girl that I could go out with. Well, I found out that was total bullshit because now *I* will not go out with smokers. I'll only go out with girls who don't smoke.

CHRIS S.
For a While I Quit Quitting

Chris S., twenty, is assistant manager at a gourmet coffee and tea shop. He is a college student majoring in business administration. He found out that smoking is less attractive for people in his age group than it used to be.

I knew smoking wasn't very good for me. I knew people died from smoking cigarettes. I just figured I would quit when I wanted to. I would do it for a few years and quit. My father had been telling me for years to quit smoking, but I didn't listen to him. I said I would quit when I was ready. I knew I could quit sometime, but I got pretty nervous for a while when I was smoking two packs a day and found out that it was going to be harder to quit than I thought.

I had tried smoking when I was in third grade with my cousin, trying to be cool, but I hated cigarettes. My parents smoked. My dad quit, but when my parents got divorced he began to smoke again. I lived with my father and stepmother. My father finally quit again about two years before I started high school. I was the one who got him to quit. I kept telling him how bad smoking was and everything.

When I started high school the crowd of people I hung around with all smoked, so I started smoking. That was in Ohio. When I moved to California to go to high school here, I smoked more than ever. I smoked Marlboro Reds. I started to smoke at fourteen and stopped just after I turned twenty—that's about six years of smoking. At the end I was smoking about a pack a day, but when I was working at a gas station, where all I did was sit in a box by myself, I smoked almost two packs of cigarettes a day. Everyone at the gas station smoked cigarettes. I went back to one pack a day when I began to work in this coffee and tea shop.

I had quit before and started again, and quit and started, and then I pretty much quit quitting. It hadn't worked out. I switched cigarettes, went to light cigarettes, smoked only a few a day, and then I just went back to my normal Marlboro Reds, smoking a pack a day. I figured I would quit when I wanted to quit.

And then one day, out of the blue, I decided that when I'd finished the pack I was smoking I wasn't going to have any more. I had one cigarette left though, just in case I needed it, but I've never had another one since then. I kept that one cigarette around for about two weeks and then it disappeared. Someone took it from my room and smoked it or something.

I feel a lot better since I quit. For the first few weeks I almost seemed sicker, I coughed more, but I guess that was my body just getting over it. I think I am still recovering from the years of smoking, but in the next few years I should be a lot healthier.

It was tough at first, but I didn't have many withdrawal symptoms. Wanting to have a cigarette was on my mind constantly. Some of my friends still smoked, and it was hard when I saw them smoking. But gradually I just got over it. Then three or four of my friends quit smoking too. They all quit after me, and none of us have smoked since. We are all about the same age, but I believe they had smoked for a shorter time than I had. They were about a year and a half younger than me, so they hadn't smoked quite as long or quite as much.

I quit on my own. I didn't have any withdrawal that I can think of, except that mentally I wanted to smoke. But I kept saying, "I have gone a day, so I will go another day; I have gone two days, so I will go another day." Now I have gone four or five months, and I don't even think about smoking. I actually view smokers as sort of outcasts. They seem different from everyone else. I see someone smoking, and it just doesn't seem natural or right, whereas before, a cigarette was like part of my body. I had one going all the time. Now I don't like people smoking in my apartment. If people are going to smoke, they have to go outside.

Smoking now seems to be more of a teen-ager–type thing. It is getting less and less popular in my age group—twenty, twenty-one years old—but I still see a lot of high school kids out in front of schools sneaking a smoke.

ELTON W.
He Changed His Attitude about Quitting

Elton W., a magazine editor for many years, is now director of public relations for an advertising firm. In his late forties, he also is a dedicated fly fisherman and photographer, having won numerous awards for his photographs.

I tried to stop smoking any number of times before I finally quit. I would make little deals with myself: "Today I am going to not smoke." That would last until about eleven o'clock in the morning. Or I'd decide I'd only have a cigarette if someone offered me one. In those days, the correct cigarette protocol, if you were going to smoke, was to offer anyone in the immediate vicinity a cigarette, too. Sometimes I'd deliberately not buy cigarettes and just mooch instead. That never lasted very long. Eventually some exasperated colleague would say, "Why don't you buy your own damn cigarettes?" I switched brands. I tried filters. I tried low-tar cigarettes. Those had an interesting effect: I went from one pack a day to three. Just as much tar and nicotine and three times the oral gratification. I tried quitting when I was out of town on assignment in remote locations. All I accomplished was feeling wretched, sleeping badly, and coming back thoroughly miserable. I tried smoking a pipe and once, very briefly, cigars.

I was the classic quitter. I knew everything there was to know about quitting. After all, look at how many times I'd done it. I tried every trick in the book. It's a good thing I never had access to classified information. All they would have had to do to get me to tell them everything would have been to take my cigarettes away. "Here are the atom secrets, just give me a cigarette." I wanted to quit for several years before I actually started trying to quit, and I tried to quit for a couple of years before I accomplished it.

And yet in thirteen years of smoking I never bought more than two packs of cigarettes at a time. A carton was more of a commitment to smoking, more of an admission that I was addicted, than I was willing to make.

I used to say that I belonged to the caffeine-nicotine school of writing. My cup of coffee was on the left, my cigarettes and ashtray on the right, and my typewriter in the middle. When I would try to quit I'd go through all the symptoms of withdrawal—anxiety, irritability, insomnia, hyperactivity, an inability to concentrate—to the point where I couldn't write. I was secretly terrified that I couldn't write without cigarettes. That was very scary since that's how I earned my living!

The discomfiture was extreme for weeks. On a number of occasions the withdrawal symptoms were so disabling that I started smoking again just to be able to function effectively. It wasn't weakness of will; it was simple practicality. I had a family, and I had to be able to earn a living. The discomfiture does fade, but it fades gradually over a period of five to six weeks. It was a couple of months before I felt good about my writing again.

There's a certain amount of evidence that I did not handle my various attempts at quitting with all the charm and savoir-faire with which I ordinarily conduct myself. On one occasion, when I was five days into quitting, my wife went out and bought me a carton of cigarettes. She presented them to me with the announcement that she didn't like my smoking but she'd rather I smoked than continue to behave the way I had for the past few days.

I started smoking when I was thirteen or fourteen because my best friend had started. The crowd we traveled with was bright and precocious, and smoking was one of those sophisticated affectations that made us feel independent and adult. We were in our sophomore year of high school.

Smoking was a difficult habit for me to acquire. It tasted bad, it made me cough, and it burned my throat. That was a bit of an obstacle to overcome, but I persevered in the name of social *panache*, and within a few weeks I was walking around with a pack of cigarettes in my pocket all the time.

Cigarettes were ubiquitous when I was young. In the world I grew up in, the majority of adults smoked, though my father didn't, and my mother smoked only socially. All the actors and actresses in the movies smoked and they looked sophisticated, so I was sure that eventually I would, too. Judging from what we saw on the screen, practically every social situation was enhanced by a cigarette.

I practiced appropriate facial expressions and ways of holding the cigarette to appear properly jaded and elegant. My mother told me plainly I looked foolish, and she was right. My father, a doctor, told me smoking wasn't good for me—cigarettes had been called coffin nails for many years before I started smoking. He also told me I'd probably outgrow it, which, given the fact that I wanted to appear adult and not as though I were going through another adolescent phase, was an excellent strategy.

By the time I graduated from high school, I had the habit. I was smoking a pack or pack and a half a day, and I smoked all through college. I went into journalism, working at one of the largest magazines published in the West. I don't know that the journalism profession is inherently high-stress, but my reaction to it was high-stress. I was very driven, and I worked very hard.

Still, smoking did serve some useful purposes in the thirteen years that I smoked. It gave me something to do with my hands. Now I fiddle with pens or shred Styrofoam coffee cups or play with my glasses. It also allowed me to look thoughtful. When someone would throw me a question for which I didn't have an instant answer, I would take out my pack of cigarettes, carefully select one, tap it to pack the tobacco, fumble around for matches or my lighter, light the cigarette, inhale deeply, and by that time I'd have thought of something to say. And I looked as though I was considering the best approach instead of scrambling madly for a response. Pipes are the best for that purpose. A good pipe smoker can stretch out the ritual for two or three minutes with practice. Properly managed, a pipe can increase perceived I.Q. by twenty-five points.

What finally made me determined to quit was editing a college text called *The Psychophysiology of Respiration and Lung Disease* for a friend. The chapter on emphysema opened with the lines, "No one likes an emphysema patient. Their doctors don't like them, their families don't like them, and they don't like themselves. Their doctors don't like them because they don't get better. Their families don't like them because strong emotion can trigger an emphysema attack, so emphysema patients typically become cold and withdrawn in an attempt to forestall an attack. And they don't like themselves because they don't dare express their strongest feelings." That sounded like a rotten way to spend the last years of life. I smoked steadily the whole time I was editing the book, and when I was done I smoked one last cigarette, and that was it. I had been smoking a pack or pack and a half a day for thirteen years.

At the time, two things conspired to make me successful. I had received a promotion, so I was in the process of winding up my old position without having yet taken on any major projects for my new one. There were no critical deadlines for a couple of weeks.

The key thing was that I changed my attitude toward quitting entirely. In all the previous attempts I acted out of a spirit of self-sacrifice. I was giving up something that I liked and quitting was unpleasant. I felt like a real martyr. I'd go three days without cigarettes and feel as though I deserved the Congressional Medal of Honor *and* the Nobel Peace Prize.

This time I didn't. I had to commute across the bridge every morning, so as soon as I hit the bridge I started saying out loud, to myself, "No, thanks, I don't smoke." I'd imagine myself in all kinds of situations where people might offer me a cigarette, and then I'd say, out loud, "No, thanks, I don't smoke." Not, "I'm trying to quit," but, "No, I don't smoke." I was practicing, trying on, inventing a new identity for myself, as a non-smoker. Not an "ex-smoker" or a "reformed smoker" but a *non-smoker*. I imagined this super-wholesome, super–Boy Scout persona for myself, the sort of person who would *never* smoke. I was a Boy Scout leader at the time, so I pretended that I was the kind of squeaky clean purist who would be shocked and offended by smoking, the sort that people would hardly even think of offering a cigarette to. I imagined this person as a real Goody Two-Shoes, but I don't think I ever took it that far in reality. That was just for the person I was creating in the car on the commute twice a day: "No, thanks, I don't smoke." God knows what the other commuters thought of me smiling and nodding pleasantly and obviously talking to myself every morning and evening.

I also kept a generous supply of carrot sticks and celery sticks around to deal with the oral gratification issue. In the past I'd tried chewing gum, but since I hate chewing gum it didn't work very well.

I haven't smoked in over twenty years. It's not a struggle at all. In fact, I find that now that I no longer smoke

I'm offended by the smell of tobacco on someone's clothes or hands or hair. I've even checked out of hotel rooms rather than stay in one that smelled of tobacco. I guess I just outgrew it, exactly as my father said I would.

ARLENE H.
I Had Lost Control of My Life

On Arlene's twenty-third wedding anniversary, her husband announced that the marriage was over and walked out. The next day a postcard came in the mail from the local hospital announcing an introductory open house for people who were interested in quitting smoking. Arlene had smoked for thirty-two years, but, as she says, "I didn't have any plans for that evening. I didn't have any plans for the rest of my life. So I went."

It was like beating cancer. It was like climbing Mount Everest. It was one of the most incredible experiences of my life. Everyone who knew me well said, "Arlene, I can't believe you did that!" And that made it even better. The last cigarette I had was January 14, 1985. I have never had another puff on a cigarette. I have no desire to smoke. Occasionally, a particular place or particular people will trigger a memory of when it was comfortable for me to smoke, but I don't want to go through all the rigmarole of smoking again. It isn't worth it. I'm more comfortable *not* smoking than I ever was smoking. To this day, my daughter celebrates that anniversary. She sends me a card and takes me to lunch. She's very proud of the fact that I quit.

I started smoking when I was fifteen and a half. My parents had said that I could not smoke until I was sixteen, so the day I turned sixteen, I walked into the house smoking a cigarette. My parents couldn't figure out how I'd learned to smoke so fast. Well, I'd been practicing for six months, that's how.

I wanted to smoke because all my friends smoked. We thought it was really neat. It was adult, sophisticated. The older kids smoked, and we wanted to smoke, too. The athletes smoked. Everybody smoked. But for all my desire to be sophisticated, it was very difficult for me to learn to smoke. I coughed. I got sick. I almost threw up. It was very difficult to inhale. It was awful. Now I realize that I was introducing a foreign substance into my body, and my body didn't like it. It never occurred to me that it was bad for me.

We smoked all the time as kids. When we were studying, walking to school, in the car going to football games, at the movies, everywhere. As I got older, I smoked more. At work, my pack of cigarettes was right there next to my typewriter. I smoked going to work, we always went out for a drink after work and I smoked there, I smoked going home, wherever I was, I smoked. I was smoking a pack and a half a day when I quit—and I'd been smoking for thirty-two years.

I would never leave the house without being sure that I had at least two full packs of cigarettes, just to be sure I didn't run out. I always carried an extra pack or two of cigarettes. I bought cigarettes by the carton. If it was eight o'clock at night and I had only one pack left, I'd go to the store and buy a new carton. It was too frightening to run out of cigarettes. I think I only ran out once, when someone came over and they were smoking my cigarettes. I was being polite, but I kept thinking, "What if we finish this pack? What am I going to do?" I was really angry.

Now lots of stores are open twenty-four hours, but I had been known to drive quite a distance to find a store that was open before that was true. Mostly it was to be sure I'd have cigarettes for the next day, just in case the forty-day flood came or some other calamity occurred. It was so time-consuming to be constantly planning, pre-planning, to have enough cigarettes. I also had cigarettes in three or four different rooms of the house. I had a pack in the bathroom, a pack in the kitchen, a pack in the living room.

Now that I am able to be honest about it, I don't think I ever really enjoyed smoking. I enjoyed the situations in which I smoked, but smoking did not enhance them or make them any better.

I smoked from the moment I got out of bed. I couldn't talk on the phone without a cigarette. I couldn't write a letter without a cigarette. I smoked when I was angry. I smoked when I was happy. Sometimes when I couldn't smoke for one reason or another I'd long for one, but when it was over I'd think, "I feel so good not smoking. What if I didn't smoke?" But then another voice would say, "Aw, c'mon. You deserve it. Be good to yourself," and I'd light up. I think truly the more you smoke, the more you want it.

Other times I'd wake up hating the taste of tobacco in my mouth. I remember not feeling good in the morning. I'd worry about my coughing. I'd think, "It smells so bad, maybe it would be great if I didn't smoke." I'd make myself little promises, like, "Today I'm not going to smoke until five o'clock." Within twenty minutes I'd have a cigarette in my hand. And then, of course, I'd beat myself up for being so weak. I thought about quitting for ten years before I did it.

My family wanted me to quit, too. Neither of my children smoke, and my ex-husband quit a three-pack-a-day habit cold turkey fifteen years before I quit. I tried quitting with him. He smoked cigars, I smoked cigarillos, but then I went back to cigarettes. They all wanted me to quit. My daughter was dating two boys in med school and they would talk to me about it. I kept saying, "Look, I smoke and it doesn't affect me. I don't think you understand. I walk and I run and I play tennis, and smoking doesn't affect me." I was convinced that smoking did not affect me because I was a very strong person and my lungs were extremely strong. My final rationale was that I could be run over by a truck tomorrow, so what difference did it make?

Then my husband announced on our anniversary that our marriage of twenty-three years was over, and the next day I got this little postcard about a behavior modification course to quit smoking. They were having an open house to talk about their method for quitting. I thought, "Well, I don't have anything to do for the rest of my life. I have no plans. I might as well go." I was *so* depressed.

I went down to this portable classroom in the hospital parking lot, and there were 120 people there, all coughing and smoking. It was a wary group. We were all just going to look. The people offering the course never talked about quitting. They talked about smoking and why we smoked, and everyone laughed a lot—and smoked. They talked about getting a flat tire, so you have a cigarette, but when you're done with the cigarette, the tire's still flat. That really hit home. Everyone groaned with recognition.

I signed up. I was willing to give it a shot. It was the only positive thing I could think of that I could do for myself. I had totally lost control of my life. My husband was gone. My children were gone. I was alone for the first time in twenty-three years. I was a lost soul. My friends all thought I was insane to try quitting when I was under so much stress. They thought I should smoke *more,* have another drink, kill this pain. I thought maybe they were right, so the first night I went up to the instructors, poured out the whole story, and asked if they thought this was a good time to try quitting. They said it was a perfect time, because the whole point of the behavior modification is to get you to change your routine. There is no better way to change your routine than to discover quite unexpectedly that you are no longer married after twenty-three years.

It *was* perfect. It distracted me from all the pain because I had to concentrate on not smoking. We had homework assignments every day, like calculating how much we had spent on cigarettes—mine came to *$15,000!*—and how much we were likely to spend over the next five years, ten years, fifteen years. We wrote down when we smoked every single cigarette, and why, for a week. We got buttons that said, "I choose not to smoke." We kept all our cigarette butts in a Mason jar someplace where we'd see it often; mine was on the kitchen sink. On top, I had an appalling picture of a man who'd had radical surgery for throat cancer who was still smoking through a little hole in his neck. It was disgusting.

I had a plumber come in while I was taking the course, and he saw this thing on my sink. He stared at it for a minute, and then he said, "I've been in a lot of houses, and I've seen a lot of things, but could you please tell me what this is?" So I told him and explained about the class. He told me his girlfriend smoked and he really hated it and asked if I could get him a copy of the picture so he could give it to her. So I sent him one when I paid the bill.

At the same time that I was quitting, I lost seventeen pounds. Everyone says when you quit, you get fat as a goose. I didn't. I substituted walking for eating. I was doing a lot of healthy things to take care of myself, and I was feeling good and looking good. It was great.

RAY P.
I Finally Quit on Valentine's Day

Ray, in his early forties, has been a hairstylist for twenty-five years. He now owns his own unisex salon. A single parent for the past five years, he lives with his two children, aged twenty and seventeen. Ray has played on local baseball teams for many years. He also coaches a girls' high school basketball team in his free time. He found his own idiosyncratic motivation to stop.

My smoking had a direct correlation to stress. If there was a lot of stress, there was a lot of smoking. If there was less stress, there was less smoking. I smoked in junior high school, I smoked in Vietnam, and I smoked when I was going through my divorce.

I started playing around with cigarettes in the third grade. I quit in the ninth grade because I was interested in sports. If you were an athlete, you didn't smoke. (There was also an old wives' tale that smoking stunted your growth. I don't know if it really makes you short, but it certainly shortens your life!)

I didn't smoke again until I was in Vietnam, with all its anxiety, boredom, tension, and the military's cheap cigarettes. You could buy cigarettes in the PX for a dime a pack. Time really drags standing watch, and the tendency is to fall asleep, so I smoked to stay awake. I quit again when I was discharged in 1968—the price of cigarettes was so much higher than in the Army.

I started smoking in 1982 when I was going through my divorce. In fact, that was practically the first thing I did. It was a Sunday morning, I got in the truck, went out and bought a pack of cigarettes, and smoked. Smoking has always been a crutch for me in times of stress. I started and quit several times before I finally quit in 1988.

I never smoked in front of the girls on the basketball team I coach. I felt funny about smoking in front of them. They were athletes, and I didn't want to set them a bad example. I made sure I never smoked around them because it made me feel like a hypocrite. As a matter of fact, they never knew I smoked until after they graduated and came back to visit me. Then I would light up, and they would look startled and say, "I didn't know you smoked."

I finally quit on Valentine's Day, 1988. It was very symbolic. There are lots of heart problems in my family. My mother had open-heart surgery, my father had heart trouble, I have three brothers with high blood pressure—all the indicators are there for me to have heart problems, too. I began to think seriously about the health hazards of smoking; I don't want to screw myself up. I want to eliminate one of the risk factors. I've never done drugs in my life, but my eating habits are less than ideal, and I don't exercise much when I'm not coaching. I'm not going to stop abusing my body in those ways, probably, so I thought quitting smoking was the easiest step I could take in the direction of preserving my health.

My girlfriend smokes, so in 1987 we started talking about quitting and the various programs that people join to quit. I'm not much of a joiner and I'm not a very good follower; I like to do things my own way. I find my own idiosyncratic motivations. I understand that it is very *in* for yuppies to join programs and support groups, but I didn't want to be like a yuppie. I run away from anything like that, so I used my *machismo.* I'm Mexican American, so I turned to my Latin heritage and told myself that if I smoked I was less than manly, and that a real man could do it on his own. I didn't want to join a group, like some yuppie; I could do it myself. And I did.

Quitting smoking is exactly like being in an athletic competition. The idea that you can do it starts kicking around in your head. You start telling yourself, "This is bullshit. I don't need this." You start little by little psyching yourself up. Slowly you get your thoughts together until you know what you're going to do. When the right day comes, you wake up one morning and say, "Today is the day." That's what I did on Valentine's Day, 1988. I had smoked over a pack of cigarettes a day off and on for more than thirty years.

I find I eat more now, not because I'm hungry, but for something to do. In the hairstyling business, if you're not busy, you're bored. You sit around a lot. I can do some bookkeeping, but it's still just sitting. I miss having something to do with my hands the way I did when I was smoking.

So far there hasn't been any problem, but the idea

keeps nagging me that I quit for five years once before. I liken myself to an alcoholic: I always have to be aware of the problem.

ERIC W.
An Afternoon in Jail

Eric W., now in his late forties, designs communications systems intended to survive under conditions of extreme stress, such as nuclear attack. He describes his job as "tap-dancing on quicksand." He is a serious photographer as well, with subjects ranging from vintage cars to African wildlife.

Here's the scenario. I'm thirty-five years old, and I've made this deal with myself that if I don't have to spend the night in jail I'll quit smoking. My wife arrives with the bail about ninety seconds before they close down releases for the day. Now I'm honor bound to quit, but I've got to deal with the oral gratification issue, so I fixate on Tootsie-Pops, my favorite childhood lollipop. I buy Tootsie-Pops by the bagful. My briefcase is full of Tootsie-Pops. I've got Tootsie-Pops in both pockets of my suit jacket, and I sit in meetings with the Pentagon's top brass wondering what flavors I've got left.

When I can't stand it any longer, I pull out a Tootsie-Pop, unwrap it, and start sucking. You want to bring a meeting to an abrupt halt? You want to change the subject? You want the top brass to hang on your every word? Whip out a Tootsie-Pop in a high-level Pentagon or CIA meeting. Works every time.

But let's begin at the beginning. I started smoking twice, once when I was in high school and again a few years later. I smoked for about a year and a half before I ran away to see the world with the Navy. There were fewer people in the Navy who smoked than there had been in high school, so I quit. The peer pressure to smoke wasn't there. I'd been selected for some very sophisticated training, which meant I spent a lot of time studying, and I just didn't want to be bothered with smoking.

When I started in high school I did it because my friends smoked and because I thought it was the adult thing to do. My dad smoked Camels, so I smoked Camels. They were just wretched. They made me sick the first few times I tried it. I thought you had to prove you were tough enough to take it. I thought all men had to go through that as a dues-paying exercise.

I started again two or three years later, when I was put in an extremely high-stress position. While I was in the service I was on the Western Pacific Nuclear Emergency Team. If there was a Navy weapon that was having a problem, we went out and fixed it. That was sufficiently stressful—as in life-threatening—that I was driven back to smoking. I smoked for fifteen years, until I was thirty-five and change. I started out smoking half a pack a day and ended up smoking two and a half packs a day.

In March of 1976 the police showed up at my door on a

Sunday afternoon and arrested me for failing to pay one overdue $5 parking ticket. I had just moved and apparently the notice to pay hadn't caught up with my new address. In any case, they threw me in the back of the paddy wagon and hauled me off to jail for the afternoon.

The nicest guy in the communal cell was a Hell's Angel gang leader. The rest of the guys were *really* bad. I had some cigarettes in my pocket, so I was doling out cigarettes as a means of bribery. I told myself that if I got out of there that afternoon and didn't have to spend the night in there with those bozos I would never smoke again. I would mend my ways. The decision was made while I was sitting there looking through the bars. I hadn't even been thinking about quitting before that. There was no health issue, no peer pressure, or anything else. I walked out of there without a single cigarette left, and from that moment to this I've never smoked again.

In the three or four hours that I was in jail, Carolyn, my wife, was running around to five different grocery stores, none of which would cash a check for more than $20, to raise the $100 bail. That was back before automated teller machines. She arrived at the jail seconds before they closed down releases for the day. I was down to my last cigarette.

I had a tough time with the withdrawal. The first week was relatively easy because I was on a motivational roll, but then I started to feel the physical craving for a cigarette. I realized I was going to have to deal with the oral gratification issue. I went through bag after bag of Tootsie-Pops. I ate those things constantly. It was the only thing that kept me going. I would reach into my suit coat pocket and feel five or six Tootsie-Pops and wonder what flavors I had left. I would take one out, carefully unwrap it, and then somebody would ask what I was doing. That went on for the better part of a year. I missed the security and reassurance of a cigarette, especially in situations where I had to think fast. Over the years I've learned to tap-dance on quicksand.

There wasn't a lot of support for quitting. Most people wanted to know why, and I didn't have any compelling reason like my doctor told me I'd die if I didn't. I had never questioned the habit at all. More of the people I knew smoked than didn't, so the pressure was to smoke rather than otherwise. That was the norm. The reaction most people had to the announcement that I'd quit smoking was, "What the hell did you do that for?"

The real crisis was in the 90-day to 120-day period after I quit. The frequency with which I wanted a cigarette began to spread out, but the intensity with which I wanted that cigarette got worse and worse and worse. There were times when I really considered that I wasn't going to make it. But there was no backsliding. At no time during that crunch did I ever pick one up.

I went through years and years of watching somebody else go through the ritual after a meal or a drink and living that ritual vicariously. I came close to slipping a few times, less because I wanted the nicotine than because I missed the ritual.

When the desire was greatest, I told myself that I'd never been able to deny myself anything that gave me pleasure, and this was one time I was going to do it. It was a self-test, a good cause, and a good opportunity to see if I could do it. I didn't want to let myself down.

BECKI C.
I Don't Want to Be an Addict!

Becki C., manager of a word-processing business, transcribed the interviews in this book. As she read the stories, she began to think about her own smoking habit. By the time she had finished twenty of the interviews, she was able to quit.

As I listened to the tapes of these ex-smokers, I was struck by how *addictive* nicotine is. I had smoked for more than twenty-five years and had tried quitting, just like a lot of these people, over and over again. The fact that nicotine is a drug really disturbed me. The realization that *I* was an addict was what did it for me. I had worked for years with the Pathway Drug Abuse Council and had put together drug abuse seminars. It was very upsetting to think of myself as being one of the people that I had been trying to help before. It really bothered me to recognize that I was doing something I had no control over. I don't like being in a situation where I'm not in control of myself.

It wasn't even easy for me to get started smoking. I remember standing in front of the bathroom mirror when I was fifteen or sixteen to see what I looked like smoking and watching myself turn green. I didn't smoke much then—maybe a pack a month, mostly what I could cadge from the people I babysat for. Oddly enough, most of the people for whom I babysat were physicians, and most of them smoked. They usually had cigarettes lying around the house, so after the kids were in bed and my homework was finished, I'd practice smoking.

I had smoked for almost twenty years before I tried to quit for the first time. That was in 1979. My husband at that time—a physician, by the way—was a very heavy smoker. He couldn't sit through a movie without getting up to have a cigarette. He couldn't even sleep through the night without waking up for a smoke. He went to Smokenders and quit, just like that! I figured, "If *he* can do it, I'll have no trouble at all." I went to Smokenders and paid the whole amount the first night, I was so sure I'd quit successfully. I was one of three in a class of more than sixty who didn't quit. The other two had quit by the last follow-up class I went to. Me, the one who came in bursting with confidence, sure it was going to be a snap, I didn't.

I had just bought a new BMW when I started Smokenders, so I made a rule that nobody could smoke in my new car, including me. I stuck to that rule for about four years. That was the beginning of my *selective* non-smoking.

Three years ago I had the entire interior of the house repainted and new drapes hung, so I made a rule of no smoking in the house. That one went by the wayside a little sooner. I started cheating and smoking in the bathroom when winter came, because it got awfully cold and wet going outside to smoke.

Two years ago I tried quitting again. I gained thirty pounds. I went back to smoking but managed to keep it down to a pack a day for the last two years. I wanted very badly to quit, but I was afraid of gaining more weight.

Two months ago I quit again. I'd read all these interviews I was transcribing, and I realized how addictive nicotine is. No wonder it's been hard to quit. I haven't been as tense and crabby this time. As long as I'm busy and there are things to do, it really doesn't bother me. I do have to stay away from alcohol; it lowers my defenses and makes it much harder to resist smoking. I feel I'm doing well. I want this to be the last time I quit. I don't want to be an *addict*.

JOHN A.
I Saw What Could Happen

John A. is a doctoral candidate in clinical psychology and a supervisor at a clinic that specializes in rehabilitating people who have suffered brain injuries. He also does group and individual therapy and psychological testing at a state prison, where he works as an intern. He is twenty-seven years old.

Two things made me decide to quit smoking. One was that I had been experiencing some respiratory congestion and headaches from smoking. I knew smoking was bad for me and I knew I needed to come to terms with the habit. The other, that hit very close to home, is that a good friend, a neighbor who's only sixty-three, is dying of emphysema. He's in a great deal of pain and can only walk a few steps without being out of breath. He was a heavy smoker for fifty years. He talked to me about how wise it is to stop smoking now and not risk what he is suffering in the future.

That had a big impact on me because, like me, he started smoking when he was young. I saw with my own eyes what can happen from prolonged smoking. I know him well, and he's dying slowly in a lot of pain.

I started smoking when I was eleven or twelve, in the sixth grade. It was just something to do with the neighborhood kids, not a habit, but still I smoked five or six cigarettes a week until my last year in high school. Then I quit for a year and started smoking again in college. I smoked anywhere from a couple of packs a week to half a pack a day for more than ten years, and I always smoked strong, unfiltered cigarettes, like Camels.

I'd been having headaches and nasal congestion for two years, and that disturbed me. I've always been very athletic, and I noticed I was losing my wind. It's important to me to be in good shape physically, not necessarily to compete in sports, but just to be generally fit. I knew it was because of smoking, so I decided to improve my health and do away with the silly habit.

I had tried to quit before; most smokers have! I've made many attempts over the years to stop. They all succeeded for a few months. Then I'd start again, because I was feeling stressed, or I was in a bar with a friend who was smoking.

This time I had a kind of internal dialogue with myself. I realized that the time had come to use my willpower, so I said to myself, "That's it. I'm quitting cold turkey." And that's what I did.

The first couple of weeks were very difficult. It's not easy to break a habit of ten years' duration. But once I decided that was what I was going to do, it wasn't so hard. I was in a lot of situations where I was tempted, but I didn't follow through with the temptation.

It would make sense to say that all my training in psychology helped me, but I don't think it did. I wish all that learning and education made a bigger difference, but I honestly think it was my own determination that helped me to quit for good. When I feel confident that I'm making the right decision, I have the willpower to do what I need to do.

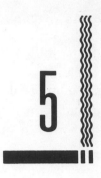

THE LESSONS OF
EXPERIENCE

THE MOMENT OF DECISION

For everyone there seems to be a moment that is right for making a major decision, for making a significant change of behavior. This is true in all kinds of addictions, where several attempts to quit are common before achieving success.

The moment of decision that leads to successful quitting is like the release of a tightly wound spring. Many people remember the day, and even the hour of their decision. Some decisions seem born of the events of a moment, as when Don C. (p. 82), suffering a serious heart attack, heard the hospital staff asking if there was a priest who could administer the last rites, or when Louise G. (p. 114) experienced an ambulance trip after she blacked out, fell, and hit her head.

Some decisions to quit appear impulsive but are, in fact, often preceded by a long period of thought, emotional preparation, and unsuccessful attempts to stop smoking. The moment of decision may come as a shock—for example, the desperation, emptiness, and loneliness felt by Arlene H. (p. 206) in the few days after her husband walked out on their twenty-third wedding anniversary, never to return. Arlene's story demonstrates how extraordinary external stress can lead to the decision to quit smoking. Arlene had thought about quitting for ten years before that moment.

Other people's decisions to quit appear to be purely spur-of-the-moment. Eric W. (p. 215) was anxious not to spend the night in jail with a gang of ugly-tempered cellmates and gave away his cigarettes, one by one, as bribes. Peering through the bars, he promised himself that if he was sprung before lock-down that evening he would quit smoking.

THE POWER OF INCENTIVES

Some quitters came up with incentives for stopping that were more appealing than continuing to smoke.

Our most expensive example occurs in Mike B.'s story (p. 154), when his wife agreed to the purchase of a new Mercedes Benz, *if* he never smoked in the car. Mike took the bait and decided to quit smoking the day they drove off on their three-week cross-country trip surrounded by brand-new upholstery and its "new car smell."

Good incentives can help overcome some of the obstacles to the final decision to quit smoking. There is another new-car story buried in the pre-quitting history of Betsey W. After her husband bought her an expensive new car, to keep it smelling fresh and new, she dissociated her smoking habit from one part of her life: driving her car (p. 177). She did not stop smoking completely for a year, but this was an important part of the incubation process.

The potential health damage of cigarettes is the decisive factor in quitting for many people. Fear is often aroused when something happens to the smoker personally—such as a heart attack or a physical abnormality discovered during a medical examination—or by seeing friends or family suffering from a painful, disabling, smoking-related disease. Sometimes fear for one's health is aroused by news items in newspapers, articles in magazines, or radio and television programs and advertising.

Celeste Holm, the actress and singer, was afraid that she would lose her voice, which was essential to her career, unless she stopped smoking (p. 159). All the symptoms of a small problem that could eventually threaten her livelihood were there in Las Vegas, a place where her nightclub act and her career depended on her singing. Louise G. wanted to avoid fainting and falling again and hurting herself even more seriously than she had the first time. Fear of not being able to be physically active and symptoms such as shortness of breath, developing a cough, or having chest pain when they breathed deeply led several people to quit smoking.

And a healthy vanity played a part in the decision for those who dreaded the smoker's wrinkles, the dry skin, the pallor, the yellowed teeth, the tobacco-stained fingers, and the smell of stale tobacco in their hair and clothes.

Behavior changes can take place when thinking changes, and many people found the courage and strength to stop by associating powerful images, both positive and negative, with smoking.

A good positive image is to imagine yourself as a non-smoker. Visualize yourself with smoother skin, healthier color, and whiter teeth, able to breathe deeply without pain or wake up in the morning without coughing, able to taste and smell again. Think of the smell of flowers, clean mountain or sea air, and the taste of your favorite foods. Imagine yourself achieving new levels of accomplishment for whatever physical activities you do—whether it's walking up stairs without getting winded, hiking farther, running faster, or playing tennis better.

Negative or depressing images are often created by accidental events, but their impact is tremendous on the minds of smokers who have been considering quitting. Joni L. responded to the American Cancer Society television ad in which William Talman, dying of lung cancer, pleaded with the audience not to smoke (p. 90). Talman reminded Joni of her father, who had smoked and died of cancer. Joni said, "I thought about it for a couple of weeks. I could not shake the memory of that man, that wonderful actor. His face was constantly before me, even while I was at work." Joni was haunted by the image of the dying actor, coupled with her fears of the health hazards of smoking after losing both parents to cancer. The combination of the two images helped her quit.

Leslie M.'s experience also bears out the power of negative images as probably the single most effective motivation for her decision to quit was the face of a woman (p. 126). Leslie described the woman, whom she much admired: "Her skin is wrinkled and gray and her gums and teeth are yellowish, like dog's teeth." Leslie, a writer, was surrounded by talented, creative, intellectual women and men who smoked constantly. Leslie saw herself beginning to look like some of her friends and decided to quit smoking.

Amanda M. admired the actor who played Latka on the television series "Taxi," a man only a year older than she was. When she learned that the actor had died of lung cancer, she said: "Oh, God, this is horrible. He is only a little bit older, and he died of this weird cancer" (p. 52). This image was coupled with a statistic she had read that said that there is a certain number of cigarettes that can be smoked before the next one might cause serious disease. Every time she smoked, she coupled the thought of that statistic with the image of Latka, and the combination pushed her toward her decision.

Many images came from something that was read or seen: A picture of a man who had only tubes where his throat had been, still smoking, is known to have influenced many people in the 1970s.

Some images are drawn from experiences closer to home. James V.'s uncle lived in his house for the last few months of his life, and the pain he suffered from lung cancer made James determined to quit smoking (p. 63). A neighbor of whom he was very fond and who was suffering from emphysema warned John A. of the dangers of smoking, and John heeded his warning (p. 221). He could see himself ending up like his sad, shuffling neighbor if he kept smoking. Allen S. described eloquently the devastating impact of visiting a friend who had had a heart attack (p. 163): "It was awful. His wife was waiting in the hallway [of the hospital] wringing her hands. He was trying to put up a good front for his kids and me. He hadn't shaved in a while, he didn't have much strength, and he was lying there in a private room in a little hospital. I thought, 'My God, this is awful.' It was awful for him and it was awful for everybody around him."

Effective negative images need not be so direct. David Goerlitz, the Winston Man, realized that he was helping cigarette companies recruit new young smokers by symbolizing a good-looking, healthy, active young man—the kind of person kids want to be—in Winston's advertising (p. 69). Seeing children twelve to thirteen years of age buying cigarettes triggered the guilt that led to his decision to quit smoking *and* quit modeling for the Winston commercials.

CREATING YOUR OWN POWERFUL IMAGES

Your own personal images will help you quit smoking. And you can create them without having a heart attack, or watching a neighbor die of emphysema, by using a combination of positive and negative images.

As you are working toward the decision to quit and strengthening your motivation, imagine yourself achieving a new level of physical fitness. Visualize how much better your clothes, car, and house would smell if they were free of stale smoke.

Then create negative images, such as a lung full of tar. If a clear image doesn't come to you, hold a sponge in your hand and pour molasses over it. Then squeeze out the sponge, and think of it as your lung with the tars that have accumulated from years of smoking oozing out. This image was used in a public service advertisement in Australia and was extremely effective. It was identified by thousands of people as having a major impact on their decision to quit.

Imagine a person dying of emphysema, gaunt, with a thin, haggard face, a grayish pallor, walking with halting steps and scarcely able to breathe. People with emphysema cannot take a deep breath—every breath is shallow—and doctors can recognize people with early emphysema from twenty feet away by the way they breathe—or, more accurately, don't breathe. Call up that image as part of your decision-making process.

In addition to lung-related problems, cigarettes cause thick, fatty cholesterol deposits to develop in the coronary arteries, the arteries that bring blood to the heart muscle. Most people are more afraid of contracting cancer of the lung than they are of a heart attack, but the fact is, cigarettes cause more heart attacks than they do lung cancer. Smokers are known to have two to four times more coronary attacks than non-smokers.

Imagine the inside of a coronary artery. It is pink and lovely, the red blood cells are floating by, the artery is opening and closing as the blood pulses through it, and it is alive and wonderful. Then imagine what happens as a smoker continues to smoke. Thick, yellowish cholesterol sludge builds up along the sides of the artery over a ten- to twenty-year period until 60 percent of the artery is clogged. The blood has a tough time flowing through it, and a heart attack looms on the horizon.

PERSONAL TRANSFORMATION

Most people in this book, after trying to quit smoking and failing, reported achieving a different state of mind, a different level of conviction, and even a degree of inner tranquility that convinced them that *this* attempt to quit would be the last one.

Marion R. (p. 77) wrote a book about her own life in which she was "able to forgive myself for some of the things I needed to forgive myself for, pat myself on the back for some of the things that I deserved to be patted for. I made peace with some of the figures in my past, made peace with myself partially. I told myself I couldn't make peace with myself totally if I let smoking control me. . . . I woke up one morning and said, 'This is it.' I had the feeling that the monkey was off my back."

Ray P. (p. 212) challenged himself to use his Latin heritage to help him quit smoking. As he put it, it was a "macho" thing to do, because he considered it unmanly to keep smoking when he wanted to quit. It was more macho to quit cold turkey, without the support of a group or seminar, and he reinforced his decision by deciding that this was a macho, not "yuppie," way of doing it.

Elton W. came to look at quitting in a new way (p. 200). "The key thing was that I changed my attitude toward quitting entirely." He had felt like a martyr on all his previous attempts. "I would go three days without cigarettes and feel that I deserved the Congressional Medal of Honor *and* the Nobel Peace Prize." His change of attitude was precipitated by editing a book that in one section discussed why no one likes emphysema patients, including they themselves. The editing job forced him to see the health hazards of smoking in a different light.

Another rather similar personal transformation occurred during the writing of this book. After transcribing twenty interviews, Becki C. (p. 219) convinced herself that nicotine was, in fact, addicting, and she didn't want to see herself as an addict. June H.'s battles with frequent relapses and broken promises to herself ended when she convinced herself that she had to live up to her commitment to her daughter and her daughter's friends that she would quit when her daughter graduated from high school (p. 119). Allen S. made many earlier attempts to quit only "because I felt I should." But his last attempt was different: "This time I really wanted to quit." He made a commitment to his family two months before he quit and used the powerful image of his friend's heart attack and bypass operation to give him the strength to follow through with it.

All of the people above finally took responsibility for their habit. Once that was acknowledged, the personal transformation became possible.

HOW TO ACHIEVE PERSONAL TRANSFORMATION AND SELF-CONFIDENCE

If you're a heavy smoker, how can you achieve personal transformation? Does this sound like an impossible quest? The stories in this book show that each one of these people did it. But you need to surmount the barrier of negative thinking that is inside each person addicted to smoking, a barrier that keeps you from reaching the level of confidence where you can say, "I have stopped. This is the last time."

This confidence gradually comes during the incubation period described on page 33 and easily recognized in many of the stories. Recall how many of the men and women had that inner feeling that "this is the day." With patience and awareness, you can reach the point where there is a level of inner peace and strength that says your chances are good that you can make it.

For some successful quitters that point is achieved during a calm period in their lives—when they are on vacation or when job pressures are less. For others a period of maximum stress is the time to take on the challenge of giving up smoking; quitting then becomes a distraction from the stress. Either way, you must feel certain that you are ready. You must have the confidence you can carry it through.

For some, this confidence comes as the person is solving other health problems. Succeeding at one thing gives the confidence needed to succeed in others. Success is contagious. Lesser behavioral changes can also point the way. Taking small steps, such as improving your nutrition by eating fresh fruit instead of sweets or increasing the amount of your daily exercise by walking briskly for thirty minutes at lunch, can build the confidence you need to take a big step like quitting smoking.

Many of our quitters gained confidence by realizing that they had succeeded, *at least temporarily*, in previous quit attempts. They borrowed various methods that they learned from each quit attempt—such as planning rewards during the first week or two—and then used a number of these techniques to quit once and for all. They also gave up blaming themselves for the failure of previous attempts, concentrating on the aspects that were successful instead of saying, "I'll *never* be able to quit."

WHAT ABOUT FRIENDS AND RELATIVES?

Many non-smoking spouses have waited for years for their partners to quit. Remember Steve G.? He told us: "A fact which I now think is marvelous is that she [his wife] could live with a smoker for four years, because now [as a non-smoker] I am so intolerant of it myself. Just the smell, the ashtrays, and everything else." Steve looked back and realized how much his wife had put up with.

Smokers need to accept the pressure to stop smoking from friends and relatives in the loving spirit with which it is intended—these people want you to live a longer, healthier life. Friends and family should be careful to express their feelings in a gentle and loving way without resorting to nagging. At the same time they should recognize that the response of smokers may well be to reject that advice, sometimes for years, before they're ready to stop smoking.

Bob L.'s story (p. 111) is an interesting reversal, indicating true generosity of spirit. Bob was perfectly content to continue smoking but stopped because his wife wanted to quit, and he realized it would be easier for her if he stopped smoking at the same time. June H. broke innumerable promises to herself to quit smoking, but when she kept her promise to her daughter to quit the day she was graduated from high school she was successful. Commitments can feel stronger if you say them aloud, or better yet write them down and have a friend or relative sign your statement that you intend to quit.

Sometimes, of course, friends can hamper your efforts: When Eric W.'s friends realized that he had quit smoking, they said, "What in the hell did you do that for?" It was up to Eric to rise above their reactions to his new resolve. Social pressure to smoke is still significant. Preparing yourself for possible negative reactions is as important as asking your friends and family to support you in your effort to quit.

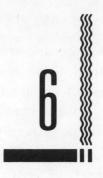

LIFE AFTER SMOKING

THE FIRST WEEK

According to all of our ex-smokers, the first week was the hardest. Eric W. was the sole exception. In Eric's case, he was on a "motivational roll" the first week. His trouble started later, when he felt the need for oral gratification as a delayed reaction. In all the stories there is a common theme of a need to keep hands busy by playing with rubber bands, fiddling with glasses, or shredding paper cups; a need for oral gratification that was satisfied by eating Tootsie-Pops, munching celery or carrot sticks, and even sucking orange juice from a baby bottle. Some people learned to wait out the urge to smoke by taking a brief, brisk walk or closing the eyes and giving a pep talk on how important it is not to have the first cigarette.

Leslie M.'s letters to her friend give a day-to-day history of what happened during the first week. "Today marks exactly one week without a cigarette, and though it's a lot better than it was the first three days, I am still missing cigs a lot. The first three days were hell. I was feeling crazy, mean, restless, and had terrific nightmares in which I was smoking like crazy. When I woke up, my chest hurt as if I had been chain-smoking; my throat was sore and I felt positively battered. The next few nights, I couldn't sleep at all. I got up and wandered around the house in the dark sucking on toothpicks and wanting a cigarette so badly I thought I'd get dressed and go out to an all-night store. But I held out. I inspect my face every day now to find the changes—the slow but wonderful changes in my skin and hair. . . . In order to keep myself from wanting cigs, I've taken endless bike rides and am enjoying the way my lungs feel better and cleaner every day. I can't believe how much more breath I have. . . . Probably my single greatest benefit in quitting smoking is what I can smell now—since I am a person who responds so much to smell. . . . There's something very sensuous about not smoking. I want to touch everyone, get close, smell skin. I want to put my nose against heads and shoulders and arms. I smell my own skin, my hands and wrists and breasts. It's quite wonderful and sexy. I feel sort of sexually charged by it all and wonder if I haven't been missing out on something all of these years."

Leslie gives us a window through which we see some of the suffering of ex-smokers, particularly those who had smoked more than a pack and a half a day. She tells us of the value of distractions—in her case, the extensive cycling and the joy of regaining her sense of smell, which enhanced the sense of her own sexuality. She speaks of the exhilaration of feeling fit and healthy, breathing deeply, and seeing tone and color in her face.

John G., another heavily addicted smoker, reports his feeling of triumph at getting through the first week: "I had a great sense of victory." His advice to smokers is to distract themselves. "Go to four movies a week, take up needlepoint. Just don't think about what a poor, unloved child you are because you've quit smoking." He is right about the self-pity, incidentally, a realization that probably led to his final successful attempt to quit.

Among our stories the choice of distractions is varied. More than one person chose walking; one man has a dish of rubber bands or a coin ready so that when he is in meetings he can act like Captain Queeg in *The Caine Mutiny.* Another tells us about carrot and celery sticks, and still another recommends Tootsie-Pops. Steve G. dealt with oral gratification in the most direct possible way, sucking orange juice from a baby bottle while he watched television for a few weeks after he stopped smoking.

In waiting for the urge to smoke to go away, there are some good tips from Patrick Reynolds (p. 95): "Take it easy, the desire will be gone in five minutes, so just wait it out. I make a conscious decision not to have a cigarette at that tempting moment. I haven't smoked for four years, and now those moments occur much less often." Betsey W. found that after several minutes the urge for a cigarette would go away. Michael G. found that a computer keyboard kept his hands busy when he wanted to reach for a smoke. In a rather unusual method of quelling the urge to smoke, Joni L. allowed herself to sleep for three days. After that the urge to smoke was gone.

Elton W.'s story shows the power of imagining yourself in a new role, or practicing a new role. He found the long trip over the bridge that carries commuters from their hideaways to their workdays in a big city a marvelous opportunity to practice being the non-smoker he wanted to be. He pretended in the car that he was a "squeaky clean purist who would be shocked and offended by smoking." He imagined another person offering a cigarette to him. He would say, over and over again when this person offered a cigarette, "No, thanks, I don't smoke." "God knows what the other commuters thought of me smiling, nodding pleasantly, and obviously talking to myself every morning and evening." In psychologists' jargon this is called *cognitive restructuring*, which is the action of practicing a new behavior. It is a form of playacting in which you take the role of the person you wish to become. Acting and practicing this role makes it easier to do in real life.

Change of environment is another way to deal with the early days after quitting. Mike B. was away from home and work for three weeks, touring the country in a new car. Another of our interviewees did the same, quitting while he was on vacation with his family.

Counteracting some of the physical cravings of the body by using nicotine gum is another way to prevent relapse in the first weeks after quitting. Neil B. (p. 139) found the use of nicotine gum helpful. Usually the gum should be used for a few months, always under a physician's careful supervision, tapering the dose down to zero in the last few weeks. Some people purposely allow themselves a moderate use of alcohol and coffee and eat whatever they want during the first week in order to avoid feeling deprived and sorry for themselves. The Alcoholics Anonymous principle of "one day at a time" can help you to get through the first week. Steve G. says, "I quit one day at a time."

You should expect some discomfort during the first week if you were a heavy smoker. The stories provide graphic descriptions, but fortunately these feelings do not last too long. The time for these feelings to totally disappear varies from person to person. For some people they may last as long as two or three weeks.

Use distractions to allay the discomfort and be ingenious in finding distractions that best suit you. Cultivate activities with your hands; munch on celery, carrots, or fruit; walk, swim, or play tennis. Visualize images of peaceful tranquility and glowing good health. Make changes in your world. Don't try to give up coffee, sugar, and alcohol at the same time you quit smoking. Be gentle with yourself. Don't punish yourself by giving up everything you like just because you're quitting smoking. Not smoking is a step in the direction of a longer, healthier life, not a punishment.

When the urge to smoke strikes, wait it out. After a minute or two the urge goes away. Use your favorite distractions during that time. Keep in mind that each day that passes reduces the amount of nicotine in your body and thus reduces the level of physical dependence as well.

Choose a time to quit when you can make a change in your environment and get away. Even a long weekend away may make it a bit easier to get through the first week of non-smoking. A longer trip is even better. In changing environments, you're probably reducing stress, and that's a bonus in itself.

THE LONG TERM

Some of the methods that are helpful in the first week are good for the long term, too. Although physical addiction to nicotine fades away in a few weeks, people do remain vulnerable to relapse, perhaps for the rest of their lives. The likelihood that relapse will occur diminishes monthly to the point where after a few years it is quite unlikely. There are a few examples of people who went back to smoking after as long as seven years, however, and Dick W. (p. 15) began again after fifteen years. The trick is never to think that one cigarette won't make any difference; it does. Steve G. (p. 168) had been off cigarettes for six months and had gained some weight. This led him to toy with the idea of doing a little bit of smoking. "When I started smoking again I did it by taking just one drag on a cigarette, and that was it—I was off to the races. In view of my experiences in A.A. where one drink

242

starts you drinking again, I should have realized that one cigarette was going to take me back down the same road." Again, as soon as the urge comes, realize that it will go away in a few minutes. If you need help, try visualization techniques. Imagine all the benefits of being a non-smoker in concrete detail.

Don't be deluded, as Mike B. was, by the notion that smoking cigars is not as addictive. Thinking he could smoke just one or two a day, in five months he was up to twelve cigars a day. He realized then that he "couldn't ever touch tobacco in any form."

A good long-term coping skill is to be constantly aware of the kinds of situations that can cause slips or relapses: the stress of divorce, a change of job, unemployment, unexpected stress, and, all too often, too much to drink. Even having one drink cuts down on inhibitions and this—especially in the first few months after quitting— may lead you to think, "Oh, what the hell; just one cigarette won't hurt me." In Alcoholics Anonymous this is what is called "stinkin' thinkin,'" and it's the kind of distorted thinking alcohol causes. Sidestepping a drink is an example of discretion being the better part of valor, at least until you feel completely secure in your status as a non-smoker.

The desire for a cigarette may be especially intense in particular, familiar situations. Even such a strong anti-smoking advocate as Patrick Reynolds occasionally feels the desire for a cigarette after a meal. "The hardest times for me even now are when I am relaxed, say, on vacation at a friend's estate. I have had a beautiful meal, we are having an espresso, a friend lights up a cigarette, and I really, *really* want one. It is as though everything is perfect except that one thing is missing: *my* cigarette."

Make a list of the activities or circumstances you associate with smoking, such as turning on the ignition of your car, having a cup of coffee, or the quiet period after solving a difficult problem. The chance meeting of an old friend who invites you to have a drink and offers you a cigarette may bring back memories of all the times you talked and drank and smoked. Then make a second list of all the positive things about *not* smoking. Make a third list of all the negative aspects of smoking. Carry your lists around with you, and when a tempting situation arises, review your second and third lists to reinforce your determination not to smoke ever again.

MAKING USE OF MENTAL IMAGES

To sidestep the temptation to smoke, use *positive images*: freedom from the foul smell of stale tobacco smoke, freedom from all the paraphernalia of smoking, freedom from the dirty ashtrays filled with cigarette butts, freedom from the coughing and irritated throat of the smoking years, freedom from the headaches, the renewed ability to smell and taste, and your new sense of physical fitness. Visualize your clean, healthy lungs and arteries, and remember that you are now far less likely to suffer the pain and disability of heart and lung disease. Think of yourself as an intelligent person who is no longer addicted to tobacco smoke.

If you need more help to bolster your decision not to smoke, project *negative images.* Think of dying of emphysema or heart disease, or a friend's bypass surgery. Fight the urge to smoke with a mental counterattack. Make it visual. Imagine the face of an emphysema patient with his larynx removed still smoking, and imagine yourself like that.

Reverse imagery works. Remember Leslie M. and her description of a woman smoker's face? "She's a great lady, feisty, older, smart—but her face is positively an example of the smoker's face they show you in those scare tactic programs. It's true that smoking ages the skin in a way nothing else does. Women who have smoked for a long time begin to look like ashtrays themselves. This woman is a prime example. Her skin is wrinkled and gray, and her gums and teeth are yellowish like dog teeth. If you look hard, you see that this woman is neither very old nor naturally very ugly. She also has that thinning, limp smoker's hair and yellowish fingers. I was so frightened of becoming like that that I was motivated to quit."

IF A SLIP OCCURS

All the stories in this book point out that one cigarette, even after years without smoking, can cause a relapse that can lead to a full-fledged habit again. Don't believe that after years of non-smoking you can smoke *just* one cigarette on a special occasion and never touch a cigarette again, or that you can smoke a cigarette once a month and not become addicted again.

If you slip and smoke a cigarette, stop immediately. Do not think that just because you have smoked one you might as well smoke another, or that since one doesn't seem to have caused any terrible harm you can finish the pack and then stop.

While you should try to avoid a slip at any cost, you must also not despair if you slip after not smoking for a while. Don't flog yourself with self-criticism, don't say, "I don't have any willpower. I am no good. What the hell, I might as well smoke again." Be positive. Think, "All that time, and only one cigarette. That's pretty good!" Remember how good and clean it felt when you weren't smoking. Call up the smell of stale smoke on your clothes and car, the awful images of clogged arteries, the gasping breathing of emphysema patients, and the horrors of lung cancer.

And stop right there, with that one cigarette.

ON THE RIGHT PATH

The fact that you are reading this book suggests that you are at least thinking of giving up smoking. If you have already quit, it suggests you want to learn how to avoid starting again. Consider that the reading of this book, even if it was given to you by a friend, is a positive move in the right direction. Use the ideas you find in the stories and picture yourself as a non-smoker, using the methods that work best for you.

Move toward the decision to quit thoughtfully. Let it incubate. Learn more about smoking and what it does. Learn more about quitting and what it can do for you. Read again the interviews that most closely parallel your smoking patterns and habits. Move toward building your confidence, conviction, and commitment to quit.

As noted earlier, there is a right time to quit. It is usually a period of relative tranquility in your life, even if only for a week or two. It could be at the beginning of a vacation or when there are no major changes coming up in your work or personal life.

But the right time could be a stressful time, a time when you might feel that since everything else is going wrong quitting smoking is one good thing you could do for yourself. Pick the time that feels right for you.

ANALYZE YOUR DEGREE OF ADDICTION

It is helpful to know whether or not you are a heavily addicted smoker and whether or not some extra help is needed to quit successfully. Determine your degree of addiction by using this simplified scoring system:

1. **Do you smoke more than:**
   2 packs a day? Give yourself 6 points.
   25 cigarettes a day? Give yourself 4 points.
   Between 10 and 20 cigarettes a day? Give yourself
   1 point.

2. **Do you continue smoking even if you have a cold?**
   If yes, add 4 points.

3. **When do you have your first cigarette of the day?**
   Before breakfast = 4 points.
   After breakfast = 2 points.
   After lunch = 1 point.

Heavily addicted: score greater than 11
Intermediate: 4 to 11
Light: less than 3

If you scored higher than 11 points, you are heavily addicted. It is highly likely that you have inherited a tendency to respond to nicotine differently from those who are able to smoke less than a pack a day. Even though science has not found the answer as to why nicotine affects different people in different ways, we know that quitting is more difficult for people who are heavily addicted. If you are in this category, you might consider using nicotine chewing gum, prescribed by your doctor, when you quit. Use nicotine chewing gum if you have failed once or twice before. Neil B. and his wife used it for two months in their last, and successful, attempt to quit smoking. Heavily addicted smokers must recognize the fact of addiction and be especially kind to themselves when they quit.

Moderate smokers (scores between 4 and 11) need to take their efforts to quit seriously and use whatever techniques will help them stay away from cigarettes. Use the power of mental images (p. 230) in both a positive and a negative way.

Lightly addicted smokers (scores of 3 or less) should be able to quit without drugs like nicotine gum.

FUTURE DEVELOPMENTS:
DRUGS AND PROGRAMS FOR THOSE
WHO WANT TO BREAK THE HABIT

Nicotine gum is an example of a prescription drug that helps not only in quitting but also in preventing relapse in the first few months after quitting. Many people object to replacing the nicotine from cigarettes with nicotine from chewing gum. Yet for a month or two for heavily addicted people, it may be kindest to have something that allows you to decrease the psychological addiction before you go cold turkey on zero nicotine.

New drugs that could help the heavily addicted smoker are currently being tested. These drugs must be used under careful medical supervision. Clonidine, previously used to lower blood pressure, is now under study, in combination with nicotine-containing chewing gum, as an aid to heavily addicted people who have failed many previous quit attempts. Recently, a few anti-depressant drugs have shown some benefit, and nicotine-containing skin patches will soon be available. Any drug has to be used with great caution to avoid substituting one addiction for another.

Scientists and physicians who have worked with these drugs are unanimous in emphasizing that confidence-building and coping skills are the basic foundation of quitting smoking successfully. Intervention with powerful drugs should be undertaken only to decrease initial stress and improve the smoker's chances of staying away from cigarettes. Drugs should be as temporary as crutches for a sprained ankle.

All around the United States people have increased their awareness of the dangers of smoking. Businesses are sponsoring programs that help people to quit. The regulations against secondhand smoke have restricted places where smokers can smoke: Motivation for work sites includes the fact that employee productivity lost to smoking is a serious consideration in the short term, and the cost of medical benefits coverage is a significant capital expenditure in the long term.

Research shows that young people may never start smoking if they are given short courses in how to resist peer pressure. These studies give hope that young people can sidestep smoking in the early teen years, when most people become addicted. Of course, the best way to reduce the appeal smoking has for kids who want to be perceived as grown-up is to make smoking something *real grown-ups don't do.*

HELP OTHERS WHO STILL SMOKE

Giving this book to a friend or relative is a good first step. If you are an ex-smoker who used this book in your decision to quit, your example is a strong statement in itself: Don't underestimate this.

You can do more: Learn how to become a helpful supporter. Nagging doesn't help; quiet encouragement does. Let people know that you will support them if they decide to stop. This is often enough to give smokers who are thinking about quitting the extra motivation they need to do it. You can also become more active (and persistent) if you sense a green light exists.

You can act as a hotline for telephone support or be a jogging or walking partner during the first few weeks of quitting. You can also sign a contract that states your support in a general way.

This book is based on the premise that the inspiration of ex-smokers and their own stories, told in their own way, is the best way to be inspired and to learn how to quit or to stay off if you have already quit. The drama of the life of an ex-smoker is much more intriguing than any scientific lecture.

VIVEKANANDA
His Gospel of Man-making

*"Today man requires one more adjustment on the spiritual plane;
today when material ideas are at the height of their glory and power,
today when man is likely to forget his divine nature,
through his growing dependence on matter,
and is likely to be reduced to a mere money-making machine,
an adjustment is necessary.
The voice has spoken, and the power is coming
to drive away the clouds of gathering materialism.
The power has been set in motion which, at no distant date,
will bring unto mankind once more the memory of its real nature;
and again the place from which this power will start will be Asia."*

– Swami Vivekananda

VIVEKANANDA
His Gospel of Man-making

with A Garland of Tributes
and A Chronicle of His Life and Times
with Pictures

Compiled and Edited by
Swami Jyotirmayananda

Benediction by
Swami Ranganathananda

Foreword by
Swami Tapasyananda

Published by:
© Swami Jyotirmayananda
137, Anna Salai
Chennai-600 002

Email: swamijyoti@hotmail.com
Web site: http://vivekananda-gospel.tripod.com

First Edition – October 1986
Second Reprint – August 1988
Third Edition – December 1992
International Edition – May 1993
Fourth revised and enlarged Edition – August 2000
(*In the context of* "The Millennium World Peace Summit of Religious and Spiritual
Leaders" *organized by the UNO on August 28 to 31, 2000, at New York, U. S. A*)

Library of Congress Catalog Number: 93-900986
International Standard Book Number: 81-85304-66-1

Scanned and DTP-set on 10pt Times New Roman at
'Kwality Xerox', Parsn Commercial Complex, Chennai-600 006.
Printed in India at
Sudarsan Graphics, Chennai-600 017.

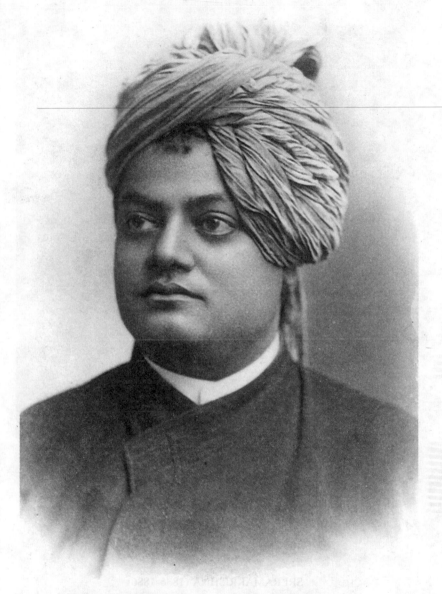

SWAMI VIVEKANANDA (1863-1902)

*"Man-making is my mission in life.... The older I grow the more everything seems
to me to lie in manliness. This is my New Gospel. ....My ideal indeed can be put
into a few words, and that is: to preach unto mankind their divinity, and how
to make it manifest in every movement of life."*

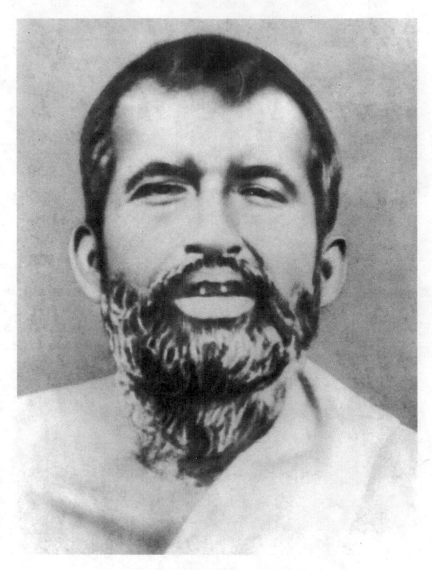

SRI RAMAKRISHNA (1836-1886)

"If there has ever been a word of truth, a word of spirituality, that I have spoken anywhere in the world, I owe it to my Master; only the mistakes are mine."

– Swami Vivekananda

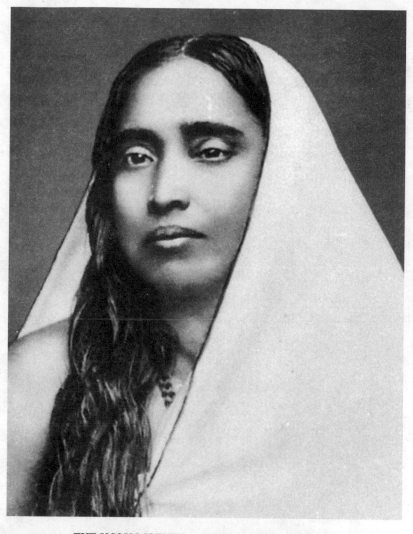

THE HOLY MOTHER, SARADA DEVI (1853-1920)

She gave Swami Vivekananda her blessings, knowing that it was Sri Ramakrishna's wish that he should undertake the journey to America.

SARADA DEVI

RAMAKRISHNA MATH
Ramakrishna Math Marg
Domalguda
Hyderabad-500 029
Ph: 63936 & 63937

Benediction

I have gone through the book by Swami Jyotirmayananda: <u>Vivekananda: His Gospel of Man-making, with a Garland of Tributes, and a Chronicle of His Life and Times, with Pictures</u>. It is a unique book with rich reading material which instructs and inspires the reader. It should find a place in all our libraries of educational institutions and in all our public libraries as well.

Swami Ranganathananda

16 · 11 · 1986

PUBLISHER'S NOTE

The three editions (1986, 1988, 1992) of this book were brought out under the title: *Vivekananda – His Gospel of Man-making, with a Garland of Tributes and a Chronicle of His Life and Times with Pictures.* An International edition (1993) of the same was brought out under the new title: *Vivekananda – A Comprehensive Study*, with an additional part titled: 'Vivekananda – A Voice from Across the Century', in the context of the Centenary of Swami Vivekananda's appearance at the World's Parliament of Religions held at Chicago, on the 11th September, 1893. In this connection, the Compiler-Editor of this volume had an opportunity to attend the 'Global Vision 2000' conference at Washington, and the 'Parliament of Religions' at Chicago, in August-September 1993 (a brief report about which is given at the end of Part Three of this book). The International Edition of this book was introduced in both the above programmes. It was well-received and widely welcomed as a reference work on Swami Vivekananda. There was much appreciation from persons and reviewers.

We are now glad to bring out the revised and enlarged edition of the book in the context of "The Millennium World Peace Summit of Religious and Spiritual Leaders" organized by the United Nations Organization on the August 28-31, 2000, at New York, U. S. A.

The main concern of the world today is peace and harmony. The path that the world has until now traversed in pursuit of technological mastery has imperilled peace. If peace and harmony are to rise and rein in the hearts and minds of all people all over the world, they should have an opportunity to be exposed to the revealing insights of spirituality which Swami Vivekananda has bequeathed to humanity. Hence an earnest and vigorous propagation of his spiritual teachings through books is the most important means of serving that divine mission. The more the life and teachings of the great Swamiji are made known, the more will the spiritual perspective of humanity be widened, thereby paving the way for enduring world peace everyone is hankering for.

Swami Vivekananda is a bridge between the East and the West. He is in fact a dynamic spiritual force to shape the future of humanity. His teachings have set in motion a spiritual force which can eventually bring in the Western civilization the needed qualitative change. Indeed he is the harbinger of peace unto the woebegone humanity.

"The mystics have seen that not till we master the know-how of transforming our human impulses and reactions can we hope to redeem the pitiful state of the world. This pitiful state of our world is but a projection of a dreadful inner disharmony. The new world must come from within and not from without – so the best way is not to be too much preoccupied with the lamentable things that are happening outside, but to grow within so that one may be ready for the new world whatever form it may take."

FOREWORD

The importance of Swami Vivekananda and his message for the revival of India and the welfare of the world at large is now widely recognised. Though the Swami lived only a short life in the latter half of the 19th century, and loomed large in the public eye only for a little less than a decade, the effect of the work he did during that period and the legacy he has left behind will survive through the ages. The chosen instrument that he was of the *yugavatara,* Sri Ramakrishna, his utterances have an unfading freshness and an ever-renewing relevance as of the great scriptures like the Gita and the Upanishads.

We in India look upon him as the patriot-monk, whose clarion call helped our motherland to wake up from her age-long sleep. He was no doubt that, but he was much more. The spiritual regeneration of the whole mankind is the scope of his message. That perhaps is the significance of Providence putting him on the world platforms of New York and London, and making him deliver his message in English, a language which is fast becoming the world language.

Without the acceptance of a spiritual foundation, mankind cannot survive. With the study of Nature alone, eliminating the Spirit that gives value to Nature, man, in spite of the vast powers that the exploitation of Nature gives him, can only be an exalted and extremely skilful animal, endowed also with a degree of cruelty and viciousness to which an animal cannot descend. Such a state of affairs is the direct consequence of the segmented view of man taken by what is called the scientific and modern outlook. A comprehensive philosophy of life should take the whole man into consideration and not merely the development of his body-mind, which is only like the tip of the iceberg in relation to the whole man. The body-mind forms only the evolving medium through which 'the more' in him gets manifestation in slow stages. The non-recognition of this 'more', which Swami Vivekananda, along with all the great teachers of the Vedanta calls the Atman, can produce only the modern elitist philosophy of affluence, which teaches man that to possess and enjoy are the be-all and end-all of life.

Swami Vivekananda stood for an opposite view. The purpose of life is the higher evolution of man and not a stagnation in animality. For, man is essentially Divine. As a spark of a mighty conflagration has all the potentiality of generating an equally big conflagration, the human personality embodies in itself the potentiality of developing into a Divinity. All human institutions, including religion, are valid to the extent they help this process. Affluence which power brings is a curse if it serves only the purpose of possession and enjoyment, and not this higher development of man. The ethical implication of the Vedantic doctrine of the Atman is the development of a polity that helps this process – not for one or a group of elite but for all at different stages of evolution. That is *dharma,* and conceived in this sense, it is an aid to *moksha,* which means the bursting of the shackles of Nature at the maturity of human development. Human development and *moksha* are inseparably related.

Thus Swamiji's message gives mankind a warning against the threat of being devoured by the demon of materialism and an exhortation to listen to the call of Divinity inherent in them. Opposition to materialism does not mean neglecting the improvement of the conditions of man's material life. Such improvement is very necessary for the development of the body-mind of man, which is an essential preparation for spiritual development. But when it is made an end in itself, the consequence is a total denial of man's basic nature and the distortions in individual and social life arising from such a denial.

In the past, religions have been the institutional bottles that preserved spiritual values. But extreme compartmentalisation and alliance with dogmatic and exclusive theologies, together with the firm hold of priesthood with strong vested interest, have politicised these religions and reduced them into cockpits of mutual conflicts and confrontation. Swami Vivekananda's message of the essential Divinity of the human spirit as the main radiating source of all spiritual values, is the one teaching that can purge religions of exclusiveness and fanaticism, and thereby re-fit them to fulfil their spiritual mission. All theologies, rituals and dogmas have nothing sacrosanct in themselves, but are to be valued to the extent they can help man realise and manifest the Divinity latent in him. Harmony and mutual goodwill in the context of religious plurality is possible only in the light of such a universal philosophy that Swami Vivekananda preached.

Dignity of man is the direct consequence of the recognition of the inherent Divinity of the spirit in man. Such a faith in man is the essential pre-requisite of any socio-political gospel which swears by democracy and equality of opportunities for all. A universal spiritual gospel of the kind that Swami Vivekananda preached is a necessity of our times for achieving man's cherished social and political ideals. It is not merely for salvation hereafter, but for salvation here also.

The popularisation of the life and message of such a versatile personality as Swamiji is a necessity of our times. To fulfil this there are already in existence his *Complete Works* in eight volumes and several biographical writings on him by men of great eminence. In the midst of all this what special significance this compilation by Swami Jyotirmayananda has got – is a question that will come to the mind of a reader. It has got a significance which none of the other existing works on the Swami serves. It can be called a comprehensive study of Swami Vivekananda. Not only does it give a brief account of his life and a selected body of his lectures; it gives a variety of essays and utterances by eminent thinkers, a collection of which one can get nowhere except in this book. Besides, it gives also a bird's eye view of the history of the times in which Swamiji spiritual and cultural heritage which show that the melody which Swami Vivekananda sang was not different and he but set the tunes to rhyme with the contemporary conditions. Therein also lay his great genius by which he tried to establish not only the practicality and relevance of our perennial *dharma* in the present-day world but also reiterated the urgent need to follow its tenets for the onward progress of mankind and for the very survival of our planet, the earth.

The first section of the book is a compilation of Vivekananda's thoughts on the art of moulding man, combining scientific temper with a spiritual basis. Man-making was his main pre-occupation, for he believed that in such a free, fearless man of character, enlightenment and love lay the hope of the world. Transformation of man is the only solution for all the ills that are found in the society. Swamiji could cull out from our own philosophy and culture the best of remedies for today's social and global illness.

In the second section we find Swamiji's Man-making ideas springing forth from the fountainhead of his realisation that each soul is potentially divine, getting amplified and reinforced through several scholarly voices. This innate divinity of man was what Swamiji emphasised all the time as he was fully convinced through his own life and of the Great Master that on this foundation alone can be built the beautiful edifice of human life grounded on character, dignity and integrity, not only of the individual but also of the nation.

Through a garland of tributes (section III) the multi-faceted personality of Swami Vivekananda, seen, known, adored and worshipped by many contemporaries, his and ours, gets painted on the canvas of the last one century of Indian cultural history. This section truly reveals the impact he has made on people during his lifetime and thereafter.

Though his voice is without a form today, the vibrations of the same have been caught up in many a heart and have surcharged and transformed them. The third section therefore tries to capture these soul-stirring emotions coming as they are from the best of intellectuals. Therein is revealed the beauty of that wonderful life, nine intense years of which were spent solely in teaching man to see God in himself and in all those around him.

What made Swami Vivekananda stand apart from others is that 'in his life there was made manifest a tremendous force for the moral and spiritual welfare and upliftment of humanity irrespective of caste, creed or nationality'. This power of his is what characterises Swamiji's work even to this day. In the following words his biographer Romain Rolland acclaimed this fact: "I cannot touch these sayings of his, scattered as they are through the pages of books at thirty years' distance without receiving a thrill through my body like an electric shock. And what shocks, what transports must have been produced when in burning words they issued from the lips of the hero."

A rare capacity to stay in the transcendental plane and work in the physical, marked Swami Vivekananda. To religion he gave a scientific basis and to science he added a philosophical background, and, in the truly Indian tradition, transformed every action into worship.

Swamiji equipped Indian Philosophy to face the challenges of today's advanced scientific and psychological discoveries. Having obtained a clear spiritual understanding which revealed to him the universal basic note in all the melody around, the one uniting all the variety of life, Universal Religion, Universal Brotherhood, became naturally the most outstanding feature of Vivekananda's philosophy. A way of life in union with natural laws, rhythms and harmony, in other words, a yogic way of life -- became the culture he propagated.

Today, this culture has a great relevance. At the highest level, among scientists with a real vision, it is this culture that is being discussed and ways and means sought for to actualise it in day-to-day life. The monster of material science is out on a rampage. Our lives, our social relationships, our environment – all are coming under its evil grip. The turning point has to come, very soon indeed. If we are to survive, a new way of life, in consonance with natural laws, in tune with the spirit within, in line with the vision of our ancient seers as endorsed by Sankara, Ramakrishna, Vivekananda and all real visionaries has to emerge before this century bows out. India has all that is needed to give leadership to this new rising culture. In fact, India should shoulder the lion's share of the responsibilities in this cultural transformation, as she is the inheritor of the treasure-chest of spirituality. Swamiji recognised this and hence was his Motherland specially dear to him.

Those who love this Motherland and her wonderful cultural heritage cannot but feel considerable elation and pride recalling what Swamiji did for this country. He, undoubtedly it was, who took India out of her isolation of centuries and exposed her religion and philosophy to the glare of scientific reason and revealed to the world that India's was not a painted veneer which will melt away in light and heat, but her beauty was genuine, a blending of truth, nobility and everlasting splendour based on deep inner fulfilment.

Sardar K. M. Panicker, an architect behind the Indian Union of States, does not exaggerate when he speaks of Swamiji thus: "What gave Indian Nationalism its dynamism and ultimately enabled it to weld at least the major part of India into one State was the creation of a sense of community among the Hindus for which the credit should, to a very large extent, go to Swami Vivekananda. This he could achieve by teaching the universal doctrine of Vedanta as the background of the new Hindu reformation." "No wonder India turned in her sleep at the thunderous reverberations of his words."

Through this commendable work, may many more be attracted to the Vedantic tradition and find in their life a new meaning and fulfilment.

May they come to imbibe the qualities of viveka and vairagya, the hallmark of Swamiji's character as also of our Motherland.

National Youth Day   – Dr. M. LAKSHMI KUMARI
(*Vivekananda Jayanti*)   President
Kanyakumari   Vivekananda Rock Memorial
12th January, 1985   and Vivekananda Kendra

"A BOOK TO BE TREASURED...."*

– M.V. Kamath

There are four important dates in the life of Swami Vivekananda; first, the date of his birth: *Makarasankranti* day, January 12, 1863; second, the year of his first meeting Sri Ramakrishna Paramahamsa (December), 1881; third, the day he addressed the World's Parliament of Religions in Chicago, September 11, 1893; and the last, July 2, 1902, when he attained *mahasamadhi*.

Vivekananda was born in the same year as Henry Ford, Alexander Duff, the Scottish missionary and Thomas Huxley, the British biologist. That was also the year when the famous battle of Gettysberg was fought. Sri Ramakrishna (1836-1886) was then just 27 years old, and had completed the most difficult *Tantrik sadhanas* under the guidance of a sannyasini named Bhairavi Brahmani.

In 1881, Vivekananda (then known as Narendranath Dutta) heard of Sri Ramakrishna for the first time from Prof William Hastie, then principal of the General Assembly's Institution (later to be named Scottish Church College) when he was studying in the F. A. (First Arts) class. Prof. Hastie introduced Sri Ramakrishna by way of an illustration to bring home the concept of a "momentary trance" in Wordsworth's poem 'Excursion'. The professor said: "Such an experience is the result of purity of mind and concentration on some particular object and it is rare indeed.... I have seen only one person who has experienced that blessed state of mind and he is Ramakrishna Paramahamsa of Dakhshineshwar. You can understand if you go there and see for yourself'.

In December 1881, when Ramakrishna Paramahamsa was 45 years old and Vivekananda a fledgling of 18, the two met – and history was made. Narendranath shot his Master one straight question: "Have you seen God?". The reply was instantaneous: "Not only have I seen God, but I can also show Him to you. I see Him more intensely than I see you!".

Narendranath surrendered himself to his Master. In 1886, the Paramahamsa died, aged 50. Narendranath was then a bare 23. But such was his authority that he immediately set about gathering the disciples of the Paramahamsa and to establish a monastery which was, in the years to come, to flower into the Ramakrishna Mission.

In 1893 May, Vivekananda sailed for the United States to attend the World's Parliament of Religions, a stranger to the land. He arrived in Chicago where the Parliament was to be held, alone and penniless. How he was befriended by an American family, and invited to address the Parliament is now history.

During the first day's session, four speakers had addressed the distinguished assembly of over 7,000 people. Vivekananda was then invited

* *Bhavan's Journal*, May 1-15, 1988

to speak. He began with the ringing words. "Sisters and brothers of America". He had hardly uttered those words when the entire audience stood up to give him a prolonged applause. The atmosphere was electric. It was the beginning of Vivekananda's mission. He had gone to Chicago with no one to recommend him. He carried no references. But he had not needed them. Prof. Wright who had introduced him to the audience was to say: "To ask you, Swami, for your credentials, is like asking the sun to state its right to shine!".

The last memorable day is 4 July, 1902. Vivekananda, then, was 39 years, five months and twenty-four days old. He had a premonition of his death. And he told his disciples so.

On that day he was up very early as usual. By 8.30 a.m. he went to the temple to meditate. At 9.30 a.m. he had all doors and windows closed so that he could continue his meditation. He came out at 11.00 a.m. and he was heard to say: "If there were another Vivekananda, he would understand what Vivekananda had done. And yet – how many Vivekanandas shall be born in time?".

He then gave Sanskrit lessons to the assembled *bramacharins*. At 4. p.m. he went for a walk with Premananda and returned at 5.30. p.m. At 7.00 p.m. he went up to his room and asked for a rosary to be sent to him. He went into meditation. At 7.45 p.m. he sent for a *brahmacharin* and asked him to fan him and massage his feet. About 9.00 p.m. he uttered a cry, took a deep breath and his eyes became "fixed in the centre of his eyebrows and his face assumed a divine expression'. All was over. He was gone. His mission, in the circumstances, lasted just about nine years.

Vivekananda was 18 when he lost his Master. His period of preparation to make his debut on the world stage lasted seven years. He was thirty when he addressed the World's Parliament of Religions. And he was thirty-nine when he completed his task.

In 1963, on the centenary of Vivenkananda's birth, the Indologist and historian, Prof A. L. Basham worte: "It is very difficult to evaluate his (Vivekananda's) importance in the scale of world history. It is certainly far greater than any Western historian or most Indian historians would have suggested at the time of his death.... In centuries to come he will be remembered as one of the main moulders of the modern world, especially as far as Asia is concerned, and as one of the most significant figures in the whole history of Indian religion, comparable in importance to such great teachers as Shankara and Ramanuja...."

Basham added: "....He virtually initiated what the late Dr. C. E. M. Joad once called 'the counter-attack from the East'. Since the days of the Indian missionaries who travelled in south-east Asia and China preaching Buddhism and Hinduism more than a thousand years earlier, he was the first Indian religious teacher to make an impression outside India".

There are several excellent to good biographies of Swami Vivekananda. This book is not a biography in the accepted sense of the term. But it places

Vivekananda in the context of his times as no other book has so far done. The book is in four parts. Part I deals with Vivekananda's Gospel of Man-making. If we do not understand that, we understand nothing. Vivekanand said: "Man-making is my mission of life. I am not a politican, nor am I a social reformer. It is my job to fashion man.... I care only for the spirit: when that is right, everything will be righted by itself". On another occasion he said: "First let us be Gods and then help others to be Gods. Be and Make. Let this be our Motto". And on still another occasion he said: "Each soul is potentially Divine. The goal is to manifest this Divinity within by controlling nature, external and internal. Do this either by work or worship or psychic control or philosophy – by one or more or all of these – and be free".

Section (i) of Part I quotes Vivekananda in extenso. Section (ii) gives us Vivekananda's concepts on Education and Religion as interpreted by many of his spiritual followers. Section (iii) consists of tributes to Vivekananda from men and women abroad, from monks, from saints and savants (Sri Aurobindo, Vinoba Bhave, Mahatma Gandhi, Dr. Radhakrishnan, Rabindranath Tagore and statesmen and politicians (Subhas Chandra Bose, K. M. Munshi, Bal Gangadhar Tilak, C. Rajagopalachari et al).

Part II is a Chronicle of important events in the life and times of Swami Vivekananda and tells us a great deal about the events that took place during forty years of the Swami's life. It has been rightly said that the significance of a man's life and activities is best understood in the context of the times in which he lived. The Chronology that Swami Jyotirmayananda has compiled is fascinating on its own.

Part IV provides a portfolio of pictures of Vivekananda from 1881 to the end of his life. Many of them are rare pictures and give us glimpses of a man in his many moods. The book is complete with a general index, a subject index, a bibliography and a list of books by and on Swami Vivekananda. A foreword is provided by Swami Tapasyananda of the Ramakrishna Math, Madras, a Prolegomenon by Dr. M. Lakshmi Kumari, President of the Vivekanand Rock Memorial and Vivekananda Kendra, a Compiler's Note by the compiler himself and a lengthy Introduction.

The Introduction begins with a quote from Christopher Isherwood and it is worth mentioning. Said Isherwood: "The best introduction to Vivekananda is not to read about him but to read him. The Swami's personality, with all its charm and force, its courageousness, its spiritual authority, its fury and its fun, comes through to you very strongly in his writings and recorded words. Reading his printed words, we can catch something of the tone and his voice and even feel some sense of contact with his power.... Vivekananda's English recreates his personality for us even now, three quarters of a century later."

How much powerful must he have sounded when he made his speeches in the United States, in Britain and in Europe! And yet one must remember that while fame came to him, life to him was not all that easy. He often bore the cross of being shunned, laughed at and despised. In the early days of his stay in America he often was refused accommodation in hotels on grounds of colour. Efforts were made by missionaries to discredit him. He was called a fake, a man married to a harem by whom he had "half a regiment" of children! Even an organ of the Brahma Samaj attacked him for his disapproval of Christianity as practised by some. There was jealousy and heart-burning at his success; but Vivekananda endured all the calumny against him serenely. He had conquered his enemies.

What is most fascinating about this book is the Chronology, for it brings to the reader in vivid terms the atmosphere of the tiines in which Vivekananda lived. Newspaper accounts make fascinating reading. And the compiler has provided us long quotes from a variety of sources, both Indian and Foreign. They paint between them such a vivid picture of Vivekananda that he comes through in all his vibrancy. There is something charming in this report, for instance, from The Boston Evening Transcript:

"At the Parliament of Religions, they used to keep Vivekananda until the end of the programme to make people stay until the end of the session. On a warm day when a prosy speaker talked too long and people began going home by the hundreds, the Chairman would get up and announce that Swami Vivekananda would make a short address just before the benediction. Then he would have the peaceable hundred perfectly in tether. The four thousand fanning people in the Hall of Columbus would sit smiling and expectant, waiting for an hour or two of other men's speeches to listen to Vivekananda for 15 minutes. The Chairman knew the old rule of keeping the best until the last."

Annie Besant wrote of him in glowing words, "Monk they called him, not unwarrantably, but warrior monk was he.... Purposeful, virile, strong, he stood out, a man among men, able to hold his own.... On the platform another side came out. The dignity and the inborn sense of worth and power still were there, but all was subdued to the exquisite beauty of the spiritual message which he had brought...."

Will Durant quoted Vivekananda as saying: "It is a man-making religion that we want.... Give up these weakening mysticisms, and be strong.... for the next fifty years.... let all other vain gods disappear from our minds. This is the only God that is awake, our own race, everywhere His hands, everywhere His feet, everywhere His ears. He covers everything. The first of all worship is the worship of those all around us".

Durant's comment on this was "It was but a step from this to Gandhi".

There has never been a book like this before and it is unlikely that there will be another like this again. It brings us Vivekananda in all his magnificence and glory. It recreates for us another time and era. This is a book to be treasured for its own sake and for the sake of Vivekananda.

"A HOMAGE WITH A DIFFERENCE...." *

– Prof. K. R. Srinivasa Iyengar

The serious student of Vivekananda has a generous choice of reading ranging from the *Complete Works* in 8 volumes to the biographical, estimative and interpretative studies by Romain Rolland, Swami Nikhilananda, Sister Nivedita, Swami Avyaktananda, S. N. Dhar, Swami Tapasyananda, R. C. Majumdar and a host of others. Swami Jyotirmayananda's present massive compilation, however, is homage with a difference. While in its weight and varied richness of content it is clearly 'encyclopedic' in scope, it nevertheless avoids uniform alphabetization and is actually a cross between a Vivekananda Handbook and a Chronicle of His Life and Times. The Editor's admirable 17-page introduction sets the tone to the whole endeavour, and is followed by copious extracts judiciously chosen, captioned and arranged – some exhortative, others instructive – from Vivekananda's speeches and writings that cumulatively set forth his 'Gospel of Man-making'. This really means rousing the purblind human race to an awareness of its innate spiritual strength and essential divine nature. Human beings are by no means inheritors of any original 'sin', but truly *'amrtasya putrah'*, children of immortality. Such is Vedanta's Magna Carta for humanity.

In the next section, nearly 40 writers (many of them monks of the Ramakrishna Order, and Arnold Toynbee and R. K. Dasgupta among the others) assess the general thrust of Vivekananda's views on Education and Religion. At a time when there is so much promiscuous talk on "value-based" education, there is much to learn from the critiques here included on moral, ethical, religious and spiritual values in Education.

In Section III, the spotlight is on the Swamiji himself, and nearly 150 tributes to 'Vivekananda: the Man and His Mission'– from fellow monks, prophets, statesmen, thinkers, savants, men of letters and politicians – are assembled together. He is hailed or lauded variously, poetically or picturesquely, and always aptly: "a versatile personality" (Tapasyananda), "Multi-faceted" "multiple personality", "resplendent torchlight", "the morning bird of Indian cultural and spiritual renaissance" (M. Bhaktavatsalam), "a soul of puissance" (Sri Aurobindo), "archetype of the sannyasin" (Justice Chagla), "not a man, (but) a god" (Thomas Allan). Prof. Zaehner thinks that Vivekananda breathed "life into the purely static monism of Sankara", and A. L. Basham believes that the Swamiji virtually initiated "the counter-attack from the East". Writing of Vivekananda's Chicago presence in 1893, Annie Besant wrote: "a lion-head, piercing eyes, mobile lips....warrior monk.... purposeful, virile, strong". For Amaury de Riencourt, Vivekananda is the Eagle pairing with Ramakrishna the Swan,

* *The Hindu,* June 23, 1987.

the Paramahamsa. And Rajaji, recalling his memories of Vivekananda in 1897 in Castle Kernan on the Madras Beach, says succinctly that the Swamiji "saved Hinduism and saved India".

In part II of the volume, 'The Chronicle', spread over 300 pages, Vivekananda's 40-year life-span (1863-1902) is chronologically unfolded in its historical background. The filiations between the Swamiji's life and ministry and the events and personalities of the contemporary world, however obscure, were doubtless there, and the perceptive reader can draw his own inferences about the interpenetrative mystery of our 'bootstrap' universe. Naren was born in the year of the Battle of Gettysburg and the birth of Henry Ford. In mid-August 1886, Sri Ramakrishna communicated his spiritual force and bequeathed his spiritual mission to Naren ("I have given you my all"). Naren became Vivekananda, made history at the Parliament of Religions, and on his return early in 1897 (i.e. 90 years ago) spoke at Colombo on "India, my *punyabhoomi*". Soon after, on 1 May, he launched the Ramakrishna Mission at Calcutta. The Disciple of 1886 returned as the Apostle, and engineered the Man-moulding Mission as his legacy to the world. And when he left his body on 4 July, 1902, *The Hindu* editorially paid a tribute to "all those lessons of nobility, self-sacrifice and enthusiastic patriotism" which the great Swamiji had embodied so splendorously in his all too brief life.

The volume also includes a selection of 80 photographs projecting tapestry-like a visual review of the evolution of Naren into Vivekananda the Prophet of Prabuddha Bharata, of man's awakening into his true self, and of the efflorescence of the Divine in everyday human life.

The Gargantuan editorial work has doubtless been a labour of love and devotion, of total commitment too. This is a book for all libraries, personal and public alike.

COMPILER'S NOTE

"Yes! The older I grow, the more everything seems to me to lie in manliness. This is my new gospel", declared Swami Vivekananda – the great teacher, philosopher, and mystic whose mission was to rouse, in all people, the awareness of the everpresent focus of human dignity, namely the Atman, the Divine Spark, and to help them to manifest that glory in every movement of their life." Never was this gospel of Swamiji more urgently needed than it is now. In the face of the grim challenges confronting us today, we have only one way to deliverance before us, and that is through the realisation and manifestation of the Divine within. Only by doing so can we be true men. We have to wake up from our torpor and move on forward till our goal is reached. This is the essence of Swamiji's great message and it is to be found enshrined in the core of this anthology.

Of the three sections in Part I, the first one, VIVEKANANDA – HIS GOSPEL OF MAN-MAKING, is a bouquet of sublime and soul-stirring thoughts of the Swamiji. It contains significant selection from his highly inspiring speeches and writings, focussing attention on his 'Man-making Gospel' which indeed constitutes the purport and aim of all his utterances. 'Man-making' meant for Vivekananda rousing man to an awareness of his essential divine nature, making him rely always on his innate spiritual strength. "Let man remember his true nature – Divinity. Let it become a living realisation and everything else will follow – power, strength, manhood. He will again become a Man." The first section of the book thus brings together the seminal ideas of Swami Vivekananda on the potential divinity of man and the need for its manifestation in one's own life. It also includes some other fundamental ideas that the Swamiji gave to the world. The passages gleaned and presented herein have been suitably grouped and captioned so as to reveal the main current of thought passing through them. Some twenty-five captions are exhortative and the rest, instructive. Of course, it must be admitted that the compilation is by no means exhaustive.

A miscellany of thought-provoking and enlightening writings of several eminent authors included in the second section, VIVEKANANDA ON EDUCATION AND RELIGION – INTERPRETATION AND ALLIED THOUGHTS, serves to elucidate the ideas of Swamiji contained in the preceding section. As in the earlier case, here too the gleanings have been suitably captioned.

Third section, VIVEKANANDA – THE MAN AND HIS MISSION: TRIBUTES, consisting of glowing tributes paid to the hallowed memory of the great Swami by a galaxy of about two hundred eminent persons from all walks of life, times and climes, reveals the different phases of Vivekananda's multi-faceted genius. Indeed it gives a peep into the charismatic personality of the Swamiji and the grandeur of his life and mission, and enables the reader to ascertain how far the influence of his teachings and personality has permeated the minds of the people at home and abroad. In short, the reader will get a glimpse of the divine personality of Swamiji through these tributes which have been broadly classified, viz a) From Abroad, b) From Monks, c) From Savants and Saints, and d) From the Statesmen and Politicians.

The compiler has spared no pains to make this collection of Tributes as representative and comprehensive as possible within the limitations of space. Inadvertent omissions noticed by readers may kindly be brought to his attention so that he can incorporate them in a succeeding edition.

Part II, A CHRONICLE OF IMPORTANT EVENTS IN THE LIFE AND TIMES OF VIVEKANANDA (1863-1902), aims at presenting Swamiji's historic image in the context of contemporary movements – political, social, cultural etc. This is useful for a proper understanding of Swamiji's mission in world perspective. Besides the principal events in the life of the Swamiji, the Chronicle thus covers significant landmarks in various spheres of human activity in India and abroad during the years 1863-1902. For a clear description of the Chronicle, reference may be made to the detailed account of it under the heading 'A Word about the Chronicle' in the second part.

Part III, VIVEKANANDA – A VOICE FROM ACROSS THE CENTURY: In the context of the centenary of Swamiji's appearance in the World's Parliament of Religions held at Chicago on September 11, 1893, this part highlights his visit to and the impact on the West, and his historic Chicago address. Portraying him as a bridge between the East and the West, it shows how Vivekananda is a dynamic spritual force to shape the future of humanity.

Part IV, VIVEKANANDA IN PICTURES, enables the readers to see Swamiji visually through illustrations. After reading his Gospel, and its elucidations, and hearing what others spoke about him, and perusing the Chronicle of his life and times, it is but natural that the readers should be eager to see Swamiji visually in pictures. The third part consisting of about eighty pictures serves this purpose.

A detailed introduction to the first part highlights the real spirit and purpose of Swamiji's mission. The second part commences with a brief life-sketch of Swamiji and some of his inspiring epigrams under the caption 'Viveka Sutras'. And at the end of the volume, an exhaustive list of books by and on Swamiji is provided, besides a Bibliography of the books consulted in the preparation of the Chronicle.

The compiler need hardly say that between the preparatory processes and the final accomplishment of this venture, he availed himself of the active assistance and willing co-operation of quite a few good friends. He owes them a deep debt of gratitude. He must make special mention of

Swami Vimalanandaji Maharaj (1903-1985), a senior monk of the Ramakrishna Order, who had evinced keen interest in this compilation, and provided encouragement and inspiration. Swami Tapasyanandaji Maharaj, Vice-President, Ramakrishna Math and Mission, graciously offered to commend the book to the public in a Foreword. Thanks are also due to Dr. M. Lakshmi Kumari and Prof. K. N. Vaswani, of Vivekananda Rock Memorial and Vivekananda Kendra, Kanyakumari, for their valuable commendations of this humble venture.

The compiler is very much indebted to the persons who cheerfully undertook the colossal task of typing this large compilation. In the work of reading and correcting proofs and making suggestions for improvement, elaboration and expansion of the reading material, he has received unstinted co-operation from persons too numerous to be individually named. To them also his heartfelt thanks are due.

Prof. C. S. Ramakrishnan, Joint Editor, *Vedanta Kesari,* Sri Ramakrishna Math, Madras, has among other areas of co-operation, rendered a very valuable help by suggesting placement and captions for the collection of illustrations in Part III of the book. The compiler is deeply indebted to him for all his service to this venture.

It is a happy coincidence that this compilation was completed in the International Youth Year (1985) when the Government of India thoughtfully declared the birthday of Swami Vivekananda as the 'National Youth Day', recognizing the fact that 'his philosophy and the ideals for which he lived and worked could be an abiding source of inspiration for the youth.'

The worth and merit of this book are certainly due to the galvanising and lofty utterances of Swamiji incorporated therein, and the learned and insightful writings of the contributors. Defects, if any, are solely due to the compiler, for which he begs the reader to pardon him. He seeks critical comments and useful suggestions from all the enlightened readers to overcome the defects and to enhance the worth of this book in a succeeding edition.

The compiler will feel amply rewarded if this volume would impel some of the readers to a more thorough and intimate study of the inspiring life and message of Swami Vivekananda. "The more the life and teachings of the Swami are made known, the more will the spiritual perspective of humanity be widened", thereby paving the way for world peace.

Namah sriyatiraajaaya Vivekaanandasooraye /
Sachchitsukhaswaroopaya swaamine taapahaarine //

'Salutations to that king of renouncers and controller of passions, the sage, Vivekananda, who is Sachidananda (Existence-Knowledge-Bliss Absolute) Itself, the spiritual preceptor, the remover of distress'.

CONTENTS

CONTENTS

INTRODUCTION

"Surely, Vivekananda's words do not need introduction from anybody; they make their own irresistible appeal."

– Mahatma Gandhi

"The best introduction to Vivekananda is not to read about him but to read him. The Swami's personality, with all its charm and force, its courageousness, its spiritual authority, its fury and its fun, comes through to you very strongly in his writings and recorded words.... Reading his printed words, we can catch something of the tone of his voice and even feel some sense of contact with his power.... Vivekananda's English recreates his personality for us even now, three quarters of a century later."

– Christopher Isherwood

I

Thinking men all over the world feel that the brighter future of the world depends on the understanding by the whole human race of the true nature of man and his potentialities.

Man suffers under the crushing weight of his own self-image. He could not but create such an image as a result of his upbringing in a particular family and environment. He is caught, as it were, in the cocoon of his own limited ideas and attitudes. Nevertheless, he can come out of this narrow and trivial existence, if he holds on to his real nature which is Divine.

Here comes the relevance of Vedanta and the teachings of Swami Vivekananda, the prophet of strength and spirituality and an abiding source of inspiration. His speeches and writings still throb with a rare spiritual power. His message imparts dignity and respect to man however degraded and downtrodden he might be. It gives him immense faith and courage.

The inspirational quality of his teachings can never fade with time as it has a touch of the Eternal.

Divinity of the soul and faith in oneself, unity of existence and universality of outlook, harmony of religions, brotherhood of man and service of God in man – these are some of the fundamental ideas on which Swami Vivekananda structured a philosophy to live by.

In the light of the truths embedded in his teachings, Swamiji wanted young men and women to bring about a regeneration in India, and a silent spiritual revolution in the world at large.

Youth is restless today. Though they have glorious ends to achieve, they feel frustrated for want of dependable guidance. But they can, however, find an unfailing mentor in Vivekananda. He is physically no more. But he lives in his words, whose great power can be felt tangibly as one listens to them. The younger generation will do well to drink at his pure, undefiled well of wisdom and create a brave new world.

II

The greatest benefactor of humanity is the man of pure heart. The moral purity of character qualifies him for an exalted spiritual life which culminates in spiritual enlightenment. The veil of ignorance covering his heart and obstructing his spiritual vision is then torn asunder, and he discovers in his own heart the great effulgent light that is God. He now knows that God, as the One Divine Principle, dwells in the hearts of all and that he has manifested as the whole universe. Seeing the same divinity in all others he dedicates himself to their service. "He who has realised God knows that God Himself has become the world and all living beings. Knowing this he devotes his life to the service of others. He serves all beings, knowing that God resides in everybody's heart." In other words, the enlightened one knows that the same divinity is in all beings, and so none is an alien to him; all are dear to him because he has found that at the source of all these diversities there is the one Divine common to all. So his humanism is based on this spiritual perception which is so vivid and real to him.

"He who has realised the Atman becomes a storehouse of great power. Making him the centre and within certain radius a circle is formed and whoever comes within the circle becomes animated with the ideas of the saint, i.e. they are overwhelmed by his ideas. Thus without much religious striving, they inherit the results of his wonderful spirituality." A living example of realisation of divinity, he inspires others and assists them towards realisation. His life and words now radiate divine wisdom. 'God as One Impersonal Principle is indwelling the heart of every human being', he reminds and goes on to exhort, 'Realise Him through contemplation, backed by universal love and service. Derive courage and inspiration from Him. He is the mine of strength and vitality. Be aware of this spiritual resource and draw it out in your day-to-day life. Then all the divine virtues naturally and spontaneously blossom in you.' 'Let man remember his true nature – divinity. Let it become a living realization and everything else will follow – power, strength, manhood. He will again become a Man.'

According to the enlightened one, only spiritually free and strong men and women taking their stand on the self – the Atman – can truly deify this world, can truly serve it and work in it tirelessly, without desire, motivated by love alone. And only such men and women can meet the unprecedentedly terrible challenge of this age. "Those who give themselves up to the Lord do more for the world than all the so-called workers. One man who has purified himself thoroughly accomplishes more than a regiment of preachers. Out of purity and silence comes the word of power."

In the wake of spiritual knowledge man attains abiding beatitude and perfection. Freed from all worldly shackles, he is ever contented. The divine touch has made him not only dauntless but also gentle and kind in his social dealings. The spiritual experience has mellowed him and rendered him egoless. He knows that he is a mere instrument employed by the Divine

Will and Power. As a divine instrument, while striving to mitigate human sufferings, he also initiates others into a life of dedication and service through the force of his character and austere living. As a wholetime servant of God, he involves himself in the divine dispensation. Ever resigned, he accepts all changes of time and place as determined by Him for the fulfilment of His plan and purpose. He finds that any condition in which he lives is absolutely for his good. He has not the least occasion to get disturbed within and feel sorry or disappointed over anything. Unruffled in weal and woe, he lives a life of perfect unity and harmony with one and all. Perennial joy fills his heart.

The enlightened one unreservedly shares his blessedness with everyone. Through his sayings and doings he executes the Divine Will faithfully, till his last breath. And above all, by his exemplary life and social conduct he not only endears himself to all, but also makes them emulate him, so that they may also rise to the divine heights attained by him. Thus through his noble life and invigorating message, such a one is a great boon to faltering humanity. He is indeed a visible God on earth. His grace descends upon all. His heart goes out to meet everybody. Like a honeycomb he effuses the honey of loving kindness even to the worst 'enemy' or 'sinner.'

To the illumined one, life is no more a woeful prison-house but a 'mansion of mirth', and he really enjoys it at every moment of his earthly sojourn. He witnesses life as a jovial Divine drama in which he actively participates and meticulously performs his part to the best of his ability, but with true discrimination and perfect detachment. While he disseminates Divine Wisdom, his very presence radiates Divine Bliss. His is indeed a beatific life, a life of 'universal love and service.' He does really serve mankind in all possible ways – by his noble thoughts, ambrosial and soothing words and selfless deeds, thereby also elevating everyone and redeeming them from spiritual ignorance. But, all this he does without the least trace of ego which has vanished from him with the dawn of spiritual knowledge. He now lives only to help the world, desiring nothing for himself. His life is a veritable sacrificial offering at the altar of humanity. Verily he is the salt of the earth.

III

The best way, then, to serve society is to purify and ennoble oneself. The ethically and morally perfect prove a boon to the society through their ethical and moral eminence. A rare few who reach spiritual ripeness shower peace and benediction on tormented humanity. "We should never try to be guardians of mankind, or to stand on a pedestal, as saints reforming sinners. Let us purify ourselves and the result must be that in doing so, we shall help others.... The world can be good and pure only if our lives are good and pure. It is an effect and we are the means. Therefore, let us purify ourselves, let us make ourselves perfect."

The society will change when the individuals who constitute it get transformed. When the individual is good, the society becomes good. When the society becomes good, the nation becomes good. And when the nations become good, the world becomes good. "Change the subject, and the object is bound to change; purify yourself and the whole world is bound to be purified. This is the one thing that is required to be taught now more than ever before. We are becoming more and more busy about our neighbours and less and less about ourselves. The world will change if we change. If we are pure, the world will become pure". The world and society can change only when there is a fundamental revolution in the depths of man's mind and heart. A fundamental transformation of human nature alone can bring about a fundamental change in human institutions.

The irony is that everyone thinks of changing the world, but no one thinks of changing himself. Everyone is eager to reform the world without realising that the world is not different from oneself. We experience the world according to our own nature. Hence, reform to be effective must start with the individual. What is therefore necessary today is 'self-reform' – a 'moral and spiritual revolution' in man. "Political revolution must be a futile and disastrous experiment unless there is first a moral and spiritual revolution changing human nature and creating spontaneous love for a just social order." "Self-reform automatically brings about social reformation. Confine yourself to self-reformation. Social-reform will take care of itself." The real beginning of reform lies in the individual, since society is made up of individuals and the aggregate of individuals' homes.

The individual being raised, the society is bound to rise. When all inldividuals live an ideal life, or even if a choice few sincerely strive to inculcate moral and spiritual values in their lives, society will get transformed of itself. The enlightened ones have also testified to this effect. Their considered views are as follows:-

> We cannot transform the world; we can transform ourselves. Society improves, nations attain to a higher scale of civilisation, to the extent individuals better their lives. A saint lives his silent life and his influence becomes tremendous over the whole humanity.

> If there be righteousness in the heart, there will be beauty in the character. If there be beauty in the character, there will be harmony in the home. If there be harmony at home, there will be order in the nation. If there be order in the nation, there will be peace in the world.

> By changing the mind man can be changed and not by reforming the external environment. Change should come from within. Change the man and everything becomes changed.

The erring race of human beings dreams always of perfecting their environment by the machinery of Government and society. But it is only by the perfecting of the soul within, that the outer environment can be perfected. What thou art within, that outside thee thou shalt enjoy; no machinery can rescue thee from the law of thy being.

They have found out that no amount of political or social manipulation of human conditions can cure the evils of life. It is a change of the soul itself for the better, that alone will cure the evils of life. No amount of force of Government, or legislative cruelty will change the conditions of a race. But it is spiritual culture and ethical culture alone that can change wrong racial tendencies for the better.

The basis of all systems, social or political rests upon the goodness of man. No nation is great or good because Parliament enacts this or that, but because its men are great and good.

Great indeed are the manifestations of muscular power, and marvellous the manifestations of intellect expressing themselves through machines by the appliances of science, yet none of these are more potent than the influence which spirit exerts upon the world.

Neither science nor politics can give man peace or happiness, joy or fulfilment. It is spiritual awareness alone that generates real peace and happiness, love and unity in the world.

The deplorable failure of many outward and isolated reforms is traceable to the fact that their devotees pursue them as an end in themselves, failing to see that they are merely steps towards the ultimate, individual perfection.

All true reforms must come from within, in a changed heart and mind. It is good, therefore, to cleanse the heart, to correct the mind and to develop the understanding, for we know that the one thing needed is a regenerate heart.

Reforms are not material things. It is a matter for the inner self. One cannot reform through legislature. What we need is knowledge, what we need is the flowering of the self.

Unless man's psyche changes, society cannot be deeply and permanently changed. After all, our society is an exact replica of ourselves.... The various social, political and economic problems in the world are only the outward symptoms of an inner psychological malaise.

The crisis that the world faces is not so much a crisis of material wants as one of character. Human miseries cannot be removed until man's nature or character changes. The solution lies in his attainment of knowledge and purity. Let men have light, let them be pure and spiritually strong and educated; then alone will misery cease in the world, not before.

Our economic and social crises come from the withering away of spiritual values and the consequent moral vacuum in public life.

Frequently the man of passion is most eager to put others right; but the man of wisdom puts himself right. If one is anxious to reform the world, let him begin by reforming himself.

Seek not to transform the world before you have wrought the needed change in yourself.

Reform yourself before reforming others.

Be busy in making thyself good. Thine example would talk a million times louder than words.... Reform thyself; and watching thine example, let others be inspired to reform themselves. That is what is wanted and needed in this world.... Be attentive to thine own mental house-cleaning, and perchance others will be encouraged to get busy doing the same for themselves.

Before we think of changing others we have to change ourselves. I cannot continue to remain what I am and insist on everybody or everything else, be it my neighbour, my Government or my environment, changing. I may not have the power to change others, but I have always within me the power to change myself if I will.

In a world that is becoming utterly chaotic, there must be a human transformation, a great, deep psychological revolution. Man has experimented centuries upon centuries with revolutions of the bloody kind; he has tried to change the environment through bloodshed and violence of every kind, and apparently he has not succeeded at all. He has brought about certain destructive changes in the environment, but not a deep and radical psychological transformation in man.

In the long and chequered course of the earth's history and human history, various attempts have been made to change outer nature, the structure of society, and the ways of the individual and collective man. But only the spiritual revolution can really touch the heart of the problem.

It is a spiritual, an inner freedom that can alone create a perfect human order. It is a spiritual, a greater than the rational

enlightenment that can alone illumine the vital nature of man
and impose harmony on its self-seekings, antagonisms and
discords.... only a spiritual change, an evolution of his
being from the superficial mental towards the deeper spiritual
consciousness, can make a real and effective difference.... It
means that no machinery invented by the reason can perfect
either the individual or the collective man; an inner change is
needed in human nature.... If this is not the solution, then
there is no solution; if this is not the way there is no other
way for the humankind.

The solution of the problem which spirituality offers is
not a solution by external means, though these also have
to be used, but by an inner change, a transformation of the
consciousness and nature.... Spirituality cannot be called upon
to deal with life by a non-spiritual method or to attempt to
cure its ills by other panaceas, the political, social or other
mechanical remedies which the mind is constantly attempting and
which have always failed.

This is the first necessity that the individual, each individual,
shall discover the spirit, the divine reality within him and express
that in all his being and living. A divine life must be first and
foremost an inner life; for since the outward must be the
expression of what is within, there can be no divinity in the outer
existence if there is not the divinization of the inner being.

The manifestation of the divine in himself and the realisation of
God within and without are the highest and most legitimate aims
possible to man upon earth.

Man, thou art of one nature and substance with God, one soul
with thy fellowmen. Awake and progress then to thy utter
divinity, live for God in thyself and in others.

Recover the source of all strength in yourselves and all else will
be added to you, social soundness, intellectual pre-eminence,
political freedom, the mastery of human thought, the hegemony
of the world.

Teach yourselves, teach everyone his real nature, call upon
the sleeping soul and see how it awakes. Power will come, glory
will come, goodness will come, purity will come, everything
that is excellent will come when the sleeping soul is roused
to self-conscious activity.

The foregoing thoughts culled from the writings of several saints and
savants of India and the world stress, again and again, one point:

what is truly needed is an 'inner transformation of man' – a 'spiritual revolution' in him. All reforms must come from within. Superimposition can have no lasting influence. It is always a change within that leads to change outside – it is out of inner victory that there comes the outer conquest. Hence, the 'inner man' is to be set right first, and the externals will take care of themselves. When a man has succeeded in governing the within, he is best equipped to govern the without.

The need of the hour therefore is 'moulding of man, instilling in him the strength to overcome human frailties and stand up as a shining symbol of manhood embodying within himself the virtues of love, self-restraint, sacrifice, service and character'. In short, what is needed is self-development and self-transformation – a qualitative improvement of man, of oneself. If we do not attend to this, our problems cannot help mounting; we cannot help becoming problems to ourselves. Let us therefore reform our lives in such a manner as to become a shining example in character and spiritual strength believing in the dictum 'service to humanity is the best worship of God'.

IV

Life is a bounteous gift of nature; but noble living is a rare gift of wisdom. In the company of the enlightened ones we derive the light of wisdom. A spiritually enlightened man is a veritable mine of spiritual wisdom. He is a repository of all divine virtues. In his life there is a peculiar power. In his company our hearts get purified, we get inner strength. He gives us right understanding which is the greatest need on the spiritual path and the path of life. He helps us to steer clear through the riddles of life.

We should try to follow in his footsteps. Our inner life is to be cultivated along the path laid down by him.We should make ourselves adherents of the pattern of divine life which he has worked out and try to emulate his example and carry out his teachings with sincerity. This emulation will be the greatest tribute we can pay him.

Even after his exit from the world, the saint inspires and guides the aspirants for an enlightened life and leads them towards the *summum bonum*. His exemplary life and invigorating message act as a beacon light in the midst of the encircling gloom. It is he who holds the key to an ideal life. Blessed are those who avail of it and unlock the mysteries of life.

Such a key to an ideal life can be found with the great Vedantic monk, Swami Vivekananda, whose one major task in life was to elevate man from the sensate level to sublimity. "To be satisfied with life in the senses is the way of the beast and base man. Seeking life at the intellectual level is the way of the ordinary man. It is the superman that seeks to live at the ethical and spiritual level. The superman invariably lives an exalted spiritual life for the commonweal and not for his petty, selfish ends. To make human life sublime and abundantly fruitful was the mission of Swami Vivekananda."

In order to accomplish his mission effectively and thoroughly, Swamiji found it imperative to awaken the latent spiritual powers of man – to enkindle the dormant divine consciousness in him, thus revitalizing him and reviving his divine glory. "The light Divine is obscured in most people. It is like a lamp in a cask of iron; no gleam of light can shine through it; gradually by purity and unselfishness, we can make the obscuring medium less and less dense, until at last it becomes as transparent as glass."

Swamiji was never tired of reminding man of his essential divine nature. He in fact dinned the message of 'spiritual dimension of human personality' into the ears of everyone. He repeatedly pointed out that man is not a conglomeration of body and mind – a mere psycho-physical organism. He is not a helpless, limited being as he deems himself to be, but birthless, deathless, glorious child of Immortal Bliss. Swamiji taught that man is ever the Pure One, that he is wholly divine, that he is replete with the qualities of divinity, and that he can boldly assert this truth. "Fill the mind with it day and night" he cried. "You are not this body and must always have the realisation that you are the Atman."

Man is a veritable dynamo of enormous spiritual power; every man has in him immense potentialities and that to realise this is to be possessed of joy, strength and blessedness. "In every man there is the eternal Atman. The Self, the beginningless and endless light without a shadow – the source of all strength and courage, purity and holiness and wisdom – is fraught with immense possibilities for the future." Every man is born to rediscover his divine nature. But alas! oblivious of his glorious divine heritage, he thinks he is a pauper. "None is poor. Everyone has got rubies in his bundle. But how to open the knot, he does not know. And therefore he is a pauper." "Each one of us is a spark from the Divine Fire. Everyone of us has the potentiality to become a blazing radiance. But the spark in us is mostly covered over with ashes. So the latent divinity is not an experienced reality with us. Because of this want of realization we suffer. Not knowing our real nature, which is perfection, we chase imperfections and waste our substance. If our actions are imperfect and entail infinite sorrow, it is because we crave for the insubstantial, unaware of our inner plenitude."

Swamiji, therefore, made up his mind and girded his loins to awaken man from his deep slumber of spiritual ignorance. Like a mighty lion he rose and roared and roused the dozing souls. Diving deep in the Ocean Immortal, he came up again to guide the mortals. And all his sayings and doings were mainly aimed at dispelling the sombre cloud of ignorance which was an obstacle to the unfoldment of the Divine within us. As he observed, we are like men walking over a gold mine, thinking we are poor. We are like the lion cub in the story which thought it was a sheep. When the wolf came, it bleated with fear, quite unaware of its true nature. Then one day a lion came, and seeing it bleating among the sheep called out 'you are not a sheep, you are a lion. You have no fear.' The lion cub at once became conscious of its nature, and let out a mighty roar.

When man is roused to an awareness of his Divine nature, all glory and goodness naturally blossom forth in its wake; all blessed qualities emerge in consequence, nay, man becomes a repository of all divine virtues. He becomes unselfish and loving to others.

When spiritually awakened, man is capable of solving for himself his problems. He not only attains a spiritual outlook on life, but also a sterling character, graceful manners, a virile mind and a humane spirit. It is only then that he becomes a Man, an embodiment of manliness, piety and wisdom. Swami Vivekananda expected everyone to be a Man in this sense. And therefore everywhere he taught man to realise his Divine heritage. The innate Divinity of man was the constant theme of all his teachings. His Gospel cuts across all divisions based on political or religious affiliations. Its assimilation by man will make for character at once deep and broad. The more spiritual a man, the more universal he is. Hence "the more the life and teachings of the Swami are made known, the more will the spiritual perspective of humanity be widened."

Swami Vivekananda expects man to lead his life in such a way that he attains his spiritual realisation, freed from all bonds. Not only that, he must also be able to promote the welfare of others. The idea is, in the inmost core of his being, man has to realise the Godhead; again, he has to experience Him as manifest in all. Thus, just as man tries to be free, he should also try to help others to be free.

In order to aid the manifestation of Divinity in man, Swamiji advocated the synthesis of the fourfold paths of yoga, allowing fuller expression to a particular path according to the temperament of the aspirant. Each soul is potentially divine, he reminds us and goes on to point out that the purpose of life is to make this potential Divinity kinetic by conquering nature external and internal. This can be done through reasoning, devotion, meditation and disinterested action. These constitute the four yogas of jnana , bhakti, dhyana and karma.They can be practised singly or in suitable combinations according to the capacities and tendencies of the aspirant. "Man is constituted of the will, emotion, and cognition. These faculties can be harnessed and sublimated to the Divine level. Karmayoga and rajayoga are the paths both to vitalize and spiritualize the will in man. Bhaktiyoga purifies and divinizes emotion and raises man to Godhead. Jnanayoga sharpens the intellect and transforms it into intuition. These paths are not exclusive of one another but they blend into a wholesome self-culture. The message of Swami Vivekananda is to evolve superman by inculcating the practice of these time-honoured yogas."

Swami Vivekananda stood for the integration of human personality. He advocated a harmonious development of every aspect of the individual: body of perfect health and strength, mind with all clarity and control, intellect as sharp as razor, will of steel, heart full of love and sympathy, a life dedicated to the commonweal, and realisation of the true Self.

Swamiji decried a lopsided growth. "Would to God that all men were so constituted" said he, "that in their minds all these elements of philosophy, mysticism, emotion and work were equally present in full! That is my ideal of a perfect man. Everyone who has only one or two of these elements of character I consider one-sided and this world is almost full of such one-sided men with knowledge of that one road only in which they move, and everything else is dangerous and horrible to them. To become harmoniously balanced in all these four directions is my ideal."

"Swamiji feels that by the combination of the fourfold paths of yoga, it is possible to produce a balanced character free from the possible defects of each of these exclusive paths – the heartlessness of the intellectual, the aloofness of the meditative and the arrogance of the active."

Thus in order to develop a well-balanced spiritual character, Swamiji required the aspirants to harmonise the intellect, intuition, emotion and action. In other words, he laid equal emphasis on the culture of the head, heart and hand. For, "mere work uninspired by religion and unaccompanied by meditation, discrimination and other spiritual exercises, degenerates into a kind of mere social service activity. Such mechanical work, when not attuned to a higher conception of life, piles bondage upon bondage. Hands can work for the desired end when the vision is clarified and the heart finds facilities for its full expression. Again, simple discrimination or study of scriptures ends in mere intellectual gymnastics, dry and insipid, if it does not express its conclusions in terms of the actualities of life. Similarly devotion degenerates into meaningless and often dangerous sentimentalism if it disassociates itself from discrimination and work. To know the Truth, to feel its presence in the innermost recesses of one's heart and to realise its expression all round – these are but three aspects of the same highest Divine Realisation". Hence Swamiji laid stress on the cultivation of an integrated life in which the pursuit of knowledge, devotional absorption, mystic communion and selfless work find their proper place.

Swami Vivekananda has thus provided man with the quintessence of a comprehensive philosophy of life. The humblest and the highest can put into practice and in the process grow in all dimensions, physical, mental and spiritual. The secular and the sacred blend in this process, providing man with a practical design for a peaceful as also a useful earthly career. And in today's murky atmosphere of character crisis due to the erosion of moral values all around, the gospel of Vivekananda gains in relevance and importance.

V

It is indeed seldom that such an eminent personage of light and leading as Swami Vivekananda appears amongst mankind. His was a multi-faceted personality whose emotions, words and deeds exhibited a profound harmony. Endowed with a sharp intellect, noble heart, and a powerful mind, his whole being was ever engaged in the amelioration of suffering humanity. "His compassion for the poor and downtrodden, the defeated, was a passion. One did not need to be told, but seeing him one knew that he would willingly have offered his flesh for food and his blood for drink to the hungry". Immaculate purity, voluntary poverty, self-abnegation, deep devotion to his Master and disinterested love for humanity were the major characteristics of this great servant of God. He exemplified the ideal of the four-fold yogas. He was indeed the living example of Vedanta.

Sri Ramakrishna Paramahamsa was undoubtedly the source and support of his intellectual and spiritual effulgence. It was Paramahamsa's divine touch that awakened all the latent powers in Swami Vivekananda and charged him with the mission of rediscovering for India its soul and quickening a mighty renaissance in every field of creative work. Swami Vivekananda was thus Sri Ramakrishna's gift not merely to India but to the whole humanity.

The initial stage of Swamiji's life was characterised by a passionate search for God. And that spiritual hunger brought him, ultimately, to the feet of the God-intoxicated saint, Sri Ramakrishna, in whom he found a seer of the highest order. In the holy company of t'.is great saint of Dakshineswar, Vivekananda underwent a course of self-culture for nearly half a decade. Sri Ramakrishna revealed to Vivekananda his true spiritual stature, and not only led him on to the spiritual realm but also transmitted to him all his accumulated spiritual powers, thus equipping him well for the future role he was to play as the world awakener and teacher. 'Self-dedication to all life' – was the great ideal Ramakrishna placed before Vivekananda. And he realized, more and more, that as one moves on the path of selfless service one experiences, more and more, union with the world spirit. So does true 'service' become 'sacrifice.' Thus the contact with Sri Ramakrishna, the Great Master, conferred on Swamiji God-realisation, which, in turn, led him to a state of exalted self-dedication to the commonweal.

In fulfilment of his spiritual mission, Vivekananda attended the World's Parliament of Religions held at Chicago, U. S. A. He was indeed India's, spiritual ambassador to the West, where he delivered the message of Vedanta as lived and exemplified by his Great Master Sri Ramakrishna. It was the message of India's Eternal Wisdom, a message of harmony and goodwill, of strength and fearlessness, of unity of existence, of universal love and service. While Vivekananda delivered his message eloquently, forcefully and logically, he carried out his mission with sincerity, statesmanship and with deep respect for other faiths. His message of Vedanta had a tonic effect on the materially advanced but spiritually impoverished life of the Occident.

Truly, he dazzled the West by dint of his fascinating personality, scintillating intellect and powerful oratory. And the newspaper columns testified to that effect: "The most impressive figure of the Parliament was Swami Vivekananda. He was an orator by divine right and his strong, intelligent face in its picturesque setting of yellow and orange was hardly less interesting than his earnest words, and the rich rhythmical utterance he gave them.... Those who heard him once were so impressed by the magnetism of his fine presence, the charm and power of his eloquence, his perfect command of the English language and the deep interest in what he had to say, that they desired all the more to hear him again." "He is undoubtedly the greatest figure in the Parliament of Religions. After hearing him we feel how foolish it is to send missionaries to his learned nation". This is typical of the comments made by contemporary American newspapers and periodicals.

After being successful in planting the seeds of India's spiritual wisdom in the very heart of the English speaking world – in New York and London, Swami Vivekananda came home to be welcomed as a conquering hero by his proud and grateful countrymen. His achievements abroad created in the average Indian mind a pride in the past and a confidence in the future. It looked as though a miracle had happened and the country appeared to be waiting for his message. And the Swamiji set about his task with systematic thoroughness. He felt the pulse of India and found out what she wanted. Through his soul-stirring outpourings he roused the slumbering spirit of his countrymen and galvanised it into dynamic activity. He sought to draw out the spiritual resources of the people. He endeavoured to enkindle the fire of manliness and vigour in them. He emphasised the greatness of the spiritual ideas enunciated in the Vedanta, the important role it was destined to play in elevating the whole of mankind. But he said, this great mission of India would remain unfulfilled as long as India continued in her present state of abject poverty and squalor. The material greatness of India was, therefore, indissolubly bound up with the spiritual regeneration of India and mankind.

Swami Vivekananda's public life covered a period of about ten years from 1893, when he appeared at the Parliament of Religions in Chicago, to 1902, when he gave up his body. These were years of great physical and mental strain as a result of extensive travels, adaptation to new environments, opposition from detractors both in his native land and abroad, incessant public lectures and private instructions, a heavy correspondence and the organising of the Ramakrishna Order in India. Hard work and ascetic practices undermined his health. Nevertheless he kept himself engaged in some work or other. "When death is inevitable, let the body fall in serving a noble cause". "Let this body, since perish it must, wear out in action and not rust in inaction" – that was his firm determination till the last. "Let this body which is here be put to the use of others. The highest truth is this: There is no other God to seek. He alone serves God who serves all beings"– that was his sublime realisation. "Have immense faith in yourself. That faith calls out the Divinity within" – these were his watchwords. Time and again he exhorted everyone to be strong, fearless, cheerful and charitable. He insisted on everyone living up to the teachings of Vedanta, as that was what the world needed. He regularly imparted his instruction in this regard and also set himself to mould the character of his followers, until the fourth of July 1902, when he shed his body, as a true yogi and liberated himself from all bonds, by entering into the state of superconsciousness, from which he never returned, thus fulfilling the prediction of his Master, that when he would accomplish his divinely ordained mission on earth, he would get back at the time of giving up the body the treasure of spiritual realisation. "Having given his ideal a firm practical shape, having inspired millions of people with the noble ideals of 'Renunciation and Service', having made India conscious of her glorious past and having awakened her to future tasks, Vivekananda wound up his earthly career at the age of thirty-nine years, five months and twenty-four days, thus fulfilling his own prophecy: 'I will not live to be forty years old.' "

Only one person was able to gauge the potential of the phenomenon known to the world as Swami Vivekananda and that person was his own Master Sri Ramakrishna, to whom he was totally dedicated and in whose hands he became a humble instrument. His gurubhakti was unique. Whatever he could achieve, in thought, word and deed, during his brief earthly sojourn, he offered it all at the holy feet of his guru. He owed everything to him. In fact, Vivekananda considered himself as the most obedient servant of his Great Master. He said that he had not one word of his own to utter, nor one infinitesimal thought of his own to unfold; everything, all that he was himself, all that he could be to others, all that he might be to the world, came from that single source, Sri Ramakrishna. "All that I am, all that the world would someday be, is owing to my Master, Ramakrishna. If there has been anything achieved by my thoughts or words, or if from my lips has ever fallen one word that has helped anyone in the world, I lay no claim to it; it was all His. All that has been weak has been mine, and all that has been life-giving, strengthening, pure and holy, has been His inspiration, His word – and He Himself. I am an instrument and He is the operator. Through this instrument He is rousing the religious instincts in thousands.... 'He makes the dumb eloquent and makes the lame cross mountains'. I am amazed at His grace.... They call me the 'cyclonic Hindu'. Remember, it is His will – I am a voice without a form." "My supreme good fortune is that I am his servant through life after life.... O, I am the servant of the servants of his servants.... If there has been a word of truth, a word of spirituality that I have spoken in this world, I owe it to my Master. Only the mistakes are mine."

In the words of Sister Nivedita, "The shastras, the guru and the Motherland – are the three notes that mingle themselves to form the music of the works of Vivekananda.... These are the three lights burning within that single lamp which India by his hand lighted and set up for the guidance of her own children and the world."

VI

Whether we regard Swami Vivekananda as a teacher, patriot or saint and whether we accept his teachings only partially or in their entirety, no one can deny that in his life there was made manifest a tremendous force for the moral and spiritual welfare and upliftment of humanity, irrespective of caste, creed, nationality or time.

There was indeed an air of divinity about him. Everyone who saw him felt it. No one near him could avoid feeling the force of his divine power almost like shock-wave.... He was a veritable thunderbolt of Shakti, a human dynamo of energy. He lived like a lion, he died like a lion. And even after his death, his bones continue to work wonders. And Vivekananda is today a voice without form. His invisible evangelic personality works as a dynamic spiritual force. It permeates the re-awakening India. It re-vitalizes man. It infuses new life and strength. Acquaintance with him opens a new portal to life. Accepting his message and applying it in full makes one's life exalted.

A prophet of strength and spirituality, Vivekananda impressed on the human mind the importance of courage and manliness. "He wished to build up men and women of strength on every level of human activity and in every social stratum and condition of life. He also wished to infuse India's oldest, highest, and broadest truths back into the very blood of the people." "Manliness in his view, emanated from the Atman, permeating the whole empirical man – body, senses, mind, heart, and will. To have the quality of manliness was to be established in the Self, to rejoice in the Self, to want nothing, to fear nothing, to dislike nothing, to serve all." Swamiji gave the message of action, of dynamic and dedicated life. He made it clear that he was not a politician, nor a social reformer. His job, he said, was to transform man. 'Man-making' as he called it, formed the central task of his life on earth.

"Man-making is my mission of life", declared Swamiji, "You try to translate this mission of mine into action and reality." He also said: "The older I grow the more everything seems to me to lie in manliness. This is my new gospel." And in consonance with his 'new gospel' he wanted to make man his own master, to give him self-confidence and to show him how to draw forth, from within himself, by himself, the infinite power of spirit. Swamiji, therefore, declared that his ideal was to rouse in all people the awareness of the everpresent focus of human dignity and glory, namely the Atman, the Divine Spark in all men and women, and to help them to manifest that glory in every movement of their life. He pointed out that enormous potential is within us, if only we would assiduously actualize it. When we realize the profundity of our spiritual life, our external life becomes smoother, tension-free and radiant. Thus, his one dominant theme was 'the innate spiritual nature of man and the need to discover it and express it in life and action'. In fact that was the keynote of his teachings. 'Throughout his mission this ideal – to preach unto mankind their divinity – was central to Swamiji's teaching. It was indeed more than central; it was the ground in which all else was rooted and the light towards which all else aspired'.

"I am born to proclaim to them that fearless message – 'Arise! Awake!' " he declared, and urged his disciples: "Be you my helpers in this work. Go over from village to village, from one portion of the country to another, and preach this message of fearlessness to all, from brahmana to the chandala. Tell each and all that infinite power resides within them, that they are sharers of immortal bliss. Thus rouse up the rajas within them. First make people of the country stand on their own feet by rousing their inner power.... in everything the austere spirit of heroic manhood is to be revived."

"Everyone should start with the highest of truth, 'I am the Self, the Omniscient One', making this bedrock fact the foundation of his total mental outlook.... my mission is to bring manhood to my people.... We must teach them, we must help them to rouse up their infinite nature. This is what I feel to be absolutely necessary all over the world.... Let the world resound with this idea and let the superstition vanish. Tell it to men who are weak and persist in telling it: 'You are the Pure One.' "

"There is no sin in thee", asserted Vivekananda, "There is no misery in thee, thou art the reservoir of omnipotent power.... All power is within you, you can do anything and everything. Believe in that, do not believe that you are weak.... You can do anything and everything without even the guidance of anyone. All power is there.... Arise, awake, and manifest the divinity within you and everything will be harmoniously arranged around you." And again he exhorts: "Awake from this hypnotism of weakness. None is really weak; the soul is infinite, omnipotent and omniscient. Stand up, assert yourself, proclaim the God within you.... Teach yourselves, teach everyone his real nature, call upon the sleeping soul and see how it awakes. Power will come, glory will come, goodness will come, purity will come and everything that is excellent will come, when the sleeping soul is roused to self-conscious activity."

Reiterating that infinite power and indomitable energy lie hidden in every man, Swamiji points out: "This infinite power of the spirit brought to bear upon matter, evolves, material development, made to act upon thought, evolves intellectuality and made to act upon itself, makes man a God. First let us be Gods and then help others to be Gods. 'Be and Make'. Let this be our motto. Say not, man is a sinner. Tell him that he is God.... Say that to the world, say it to yourselves and see what a practical result comes, see how with an electric flash everything is manifested, how everything is changed.

Tell that to mankind and show them their power. Then we shall learn how to apply it in our daily lives."

As has rightly been pointed out, the social service, as envisaged by Swami Vivekananda, does not stop with the establishment of general material well-being or the diffusion of intellectual enlightenment. It aims at liberating the strength of man, born of his intrinsic divinity so that he may creatively shape his own divine destiny. The dire sin of weakness has to be eradicated. Man, as the divine spirit, has to be awakened to self-consciousness. Towards that consummation Swami Vivekananda laboured, even as he asserted: "Let everyone be taught that divine is within and everyone will work out his own salvation."

The greatest of all benefactions, according to Swami Vivekananda, is the act of rousing man to the glory of the divinity within.The a wakened man solves for himself all his problems, secular and sacred. "The solution to all human problems is in man's becoming Man in all his dimensions, by manifesting his divinity. Problems are understandably many. But the solution is one – to become the new kind of man, who being simultaneously scientific and spiritual, eventually becomes free. It is this new man, pure in heart, clear in brain, unselfish in motivation, who works in a balanced manner with his head, heart and hand, who has shed all his smallness and illusions, who has experienced unity of existence in his expanded consciousness – this selfless, spotless and fearless man of character, enlightenment and love, is the hope of the world. The more we can produce such men, the greater is the hope of the world. Hope is not in more machinery, wealth, politics of cleverness and power. The world is looking forward to the coming of this new man – who is aware of his own divinity and is always anxious to discover and worship the same divinity in all others – in ever increasing numbers."

PART ONE

Section I

VIVEKANANDA
–HIS GOSPEL OF MAN-MAKING

"Man-making is my mission of life....
The older I grow, the more everything
seems to me to lie in manliness.
This is my new gospel."

---

*This Section quotes generously from the writings and speeches of Swami
Vivekananda. It speaks for Vivekananda more than an orthodox biography would
have done. As Gandhi said of himself, the Swami's life was his message. Anyone
who wants to know Vivekananda could do no better than read this Section most
carefully.*

– M.V. Kamath

CONTENTS:

VIVEKANANDA
– HIS GOSPEL OF MAN-MAKING

Man-making is my Mission

I have a message to give; let me give it to the people who appreciate it and who will work it out. What care I who takes it? 'He who doth the will of my Father' is my own.

I know my mission in life, and no chauvinism about me; I belong as much to India as to the world.... I hate cowardice; I will have nothing to do with cowards or political nonsense. I do not believe in any politics. God and truth are the only politics in the world, everything else is trash. Let no political significance be ever attached falsely to any of my writings or sayings.

I am not a politician, nor am I a social reformer. It is my job to fashion man.... I care only for the spirit – when that is right, everything will be righted by itself.

Man-making is my mission of life. You try to translate this mission of mine into action and reality.

Yes, the older I grow, the more everything seems to me to lie in manliness. This is my new gospel.

I never make plans. Plans grow and work themselves. I only say 'Awake, awake'.

I direct my attention to the individual, to make him strong, to teach him that he himself is divine, and I call upon men to make themselves conscious of this divinity within.

My ideal indeed can be put into a few words, and that is: to preach unto mankind their divinity, and how to make it manifest in every movement of life.

Let man remember his true nature – divinity. Let it become a living realisation and everything else will follow – power, strength, manhood. He will again become a Man.

My sons, all of you be men. That is what I want! If you are even a little successful, I shall feel my life has been meaningful.

Today man requires one more adjustment on the spiritual plane; today when material ideas are at the height of their glory and power, today when man is likely to forget his divine nature, through his growing dependence on matter, and is likely to be reduced to a mere money-making machine, an adjustment is necessary. The voice has spoken, and the power is coming to drive away the clouds of gathering materialism. The power has been set in motion which, at no distant date, will bring unto mankind once more the memory of its real nature; and again the place from which this power will start will be Asia.

Yield not to Unmanliness

As I always preach that you should not decry a man by calling him a sinner but that you should draw his attention to the omnipotent power that is in him, in the same way does the Bhagavan speak to Arjuna. 'It doth not befit thee!' 'Thou art Atman imperishable, beyond all evil. Having forgotten thy real nature, thou hast, by thinking thyself a sinner, as one afflicted with bodily evils and mental grief, thou hast made thyself so – this does not befit thee!'– so says the Bhagavan! 'Yield not to unmanliness, O Son of Pritha.'

If you, my son, can proclaim this message to the world, then all this disease, grief, sin, and sorrow will vanish off from the face of the earth in three days. All these ideas of weakness will be nowhere. Now it is everywhere – this current of the vibration of fear. Reverse the current; bring in the opposite vibration and behold the magic transformation!.... Proclaim to the whole world with trumpet voice, 'There is no sin in thee, there is no misery in thee; thou art the rerservoir of omnipotent power. Arise, awake and manifest the Divinity within....'

The Hindu believes that he is a spirit. Him the sword cannot pierce, him the fire cannot burn, him the water cannot wet, him the air cannot dry. The Hindu believes that every soul is a circle whose circumference is nowhere, but whose centre is located in the body, and that death means the change of this centre from body to body. Nor is the soul bound by the conditions of matter. In its very essence it is free, unbound, holy, pure and perfect. But somehow or other, it finds itself tied down to matter, and thinks of itself as matter.

De-hypnotise Yourself

I will tell you a story. A lioness in search of prey came upon a flock of sheep, and as she jumped at one of them she gave birth to a cub and died on the spot. The young lion was brought up in the flock, ate grass, and bleated like a sheep. It never knew that it was a lion. One day, a lion came across this flock and was astonished to see in it a huge lion eating grass and bleating like a sheep. At his sight the flock fled and the lion-sheep with them.

But the lion watched his opportunity and one day found the lion-sheep asleep. He woke him up and said: "You are a lion."

The other said, 'No' and began to bleat like a sheep.

But the stranger lion took him to a lake and asked him to look in the water at his own image and see if he did not resemble him, the stranger lion. He looked and acknowledged that he did. Then the stranger lion began to roar and asked him to do the same. The lion-sheep tried his voice and was soon roaring as grandly as the other. And he was a sheep no longer.

My friends, I would like to tell you that you are mighty as lions.

Allow me to call you brethren, by that sweet name – heirs of immortal bliss – yea, the Hindu refuses to call you sinners. Ye are the children of God, the sharers of immortal bliss, holy and perfect beings. Ye divinities on earth – sinners! It is a sin to call a man so; it is a standing libel on human nature. Come up, O lions, and shake off the delusion that you are sheep. You are souls immortal, spirits free, blest and eternal. You are no matter, you are not bodies; matter is your servant, not you the servant of matter.

Aye, let every man, woman and child, without respect to caste or birth, weakness or strength, hear and learn that behind the strong and the weak, behind the high and the low, behind everyone there is that Infinite Soul, ensuring the infinite possibility and the infinite capacity of all to become great and good. Let us proclaim to every soul – Arise, awake and stop not till the goal is reached. Arise, awake! Awake from this hypnotism of weakness. None is really weak, the soul is infinite, omnipotent, and omniscient. Stand up, assert yourself, proclaim the God within you, do not deny Him!... dehypnotise yourselves.... Teach yourselves, teach everyone his real nature, call upon the sleeping soul and see how it awakes. Power will come, glory will come, goodness will come, purity will come, and everything that is excellent will come when the sleeping soul is roused to self-conscious activity.

Awake and Arise

You are the pure one; awake and arise, O mighty one, this sleep does not become you. Awake and arise, it does not befit you. Think not that you are weak and miserable. Almighty, arise and awake and manifest your own nature. It is not fitting that you think yourself a sinner. It is not fitting that you think yourself weak. Say that to the world, say it to yourselves and see what a practical result comes, see how with an electric flash everything is manifested, how everything is changed. Tell that to mankind and show them their power. Then we shall learn how to apply it in our daily lives.

Let us take our stand on the central truth of our religion – the spirit of man – the Atman of man – the immortal, birthless, all-pervading, eternal soul of man whose glories the Vedas cannot themselves express, before whose majesty the universe with its galaxy upon galaxy of sun and stars and nebulae is a drop. Every man or woman, nay, from the highest devas to the worm that crawls under our feet, is such a spirit evoluted or involuted. The difference is not in kind but in degree.

The Infinite Being is also the same finite soul. The Infinite is caught, as it were, in the meshes of the intellect and apparently manifests as finite being; but the reality remains unchanged. This is, therefore, true knowledge: that the Soul of our souls, the Reality that is within us, is That which is unchangeable, eternal, ever-blessed, ever-free.... Therefore, there is hope for all. None can die, none can be degraded for ever. Life is but a playground, however gross the play may be. However we may receive blows, and however knocked about we may be, the Soul is there and is never injured. We are that Infinite.... Be not afraid. Think not how many times you fail. Never mind. Time is infinite. Go forward; assert yourself again and again, and light must come.... Get hold of the Self, then. Stand up. Don't be afraid. In the midst of all miseries and all weaknesses, let the Self come out, faint and imperceptible though it be at first. You will gain courage, and at last like a lion you will roar out, 'I am He! I am He!'

All Power is Within You

Do you know how much energy, how many powers, how many forces, are still lurking behind that frame of yours? What scientist has known all that is in man? Millions of years have passed since man came here and yet but one infinitesimal part of his powers has been manifested. Therefore you must not say that you are weak. How do you know what possibilities lie behind that degradation on the surface? You know but little of that which is within you, for behind you is the ocean of infinite power and blessedness.

Never think there is anything impossible for the soul. It is the greatest heresy to think so. If there is any sin, this is the only sin, to say that you are weak.

Never forget that all your strength is within yourselves.

All power is within you, you can do anything and everything. Believe in that. Do not believe that you are weak.... You can do anything and everything, without even the guidance of anyone. All power is there. Stand up and express the divinity within you.

Arise, awake, sleep no more. Within each of you there is the power to remove all wants and all miseries. Believe in this, and that power will be manifested.

If you can think that infinite power, infinite knowledge and indomitable energy lie within you, and if you can bring out that power, you can also become like me.

Remember Your True Nature

'I have neither death nor fear, I have neither caste nor creed, I have neither father nor mother nor brother, neither friend nor foe, for I am Existence, Knowledge, and Bliss Absolute; I am the Blissful one. I am not bound either by virtue or vice, by happiness or misery. Pilgrimages and books and ceremonials can never bind me. I have neither hunger nor thirst, the body is not mine, nor am I subject to the superstitions and decay that come to the body, I am Existence, Knowledge, and Bliss Absolute; I am the Blissful one, I am the Blissful one.'

This, says the Vedanta, is the only prayer that we should have. This is the only way to reach the Goal, to tell ourselves, and to tell everybody else, that we are divine; and as we go on repeating this, strength comes. He who falters at first will get stronger and stronger, and the voice will increase in volume until the truth takes possession of our hearts, and courses through our veins, and permeates our bodies. Delusion will vanish as the light becomes more and more effulgent, load after load of ignorance will vanish, and then will come a time, when all else has disappeared and the Sun alone shines.

Rise, thou effulgent one, rise thou who art always pure, rise thou birthless and deathless, rise almighty and manifest thy true nature.... This is the one prayer, to remember our true nature, the God who is always within us, thinking of it always as infinite, almighty, ever good, ever beneficent, selfless, bereft of all limitations.... Our only work is to arouse this knowledge in our fellow-beings. We see that they too are the same pure self. Only they do not know it; we must help them to rouse up their infinite nature. This is what I feel to be absolutely necessary all over the world. These doctrines are old, older than many mountains possibly. All truth is eternal. Truth is nobody's property; no race, no individual can lay any exclusive claim to it. Truth is the nature of all souls. Who can lay any special claim to it. But it has to be made practical, to be made simple (for the highest truths are always simple) so that it may penetrate every pore of human society, and become the property of the highest intellect and the commonest minds, of the man, woman and child at the same time. All these ratiocinations of logic, all these bundles of metaphysics, all these ideologies and ceremonies, may have been good in their own time, but let us try to make things simpler and bring about the golden days when every man will be a worshipper and the Reality in every man will be the object of worship.

Manifest Your Innate Divinity

Manifest the divinity within you, and everything will be harmoniously arranged around you. Bring forth the power of the spirit, and pour it over the length and breadth of India; and all that is necessary will come by itself.

Infinite power is within you....

This infinite power of the spirit, brought to bear upon matter, evolves material development; made to act upon thought, evolves intellectuality, and made to act upon itself makes man a God.

First, let us be gods, and then help others to be gods. 'Be and Make.' Let this be our motto. Say not man is a sinner. Tell him that he is God.

Have Faith in Yourself

Have faith in yourself.... I see it clear as daylight that you all have infinite power in you. Rouse that up; arise, – apply yourselves heart and soul, gird up your loins. What will you do with wealth and fame that are so transitory. Do you know what I think – I don't care for mukti and all that. My mission is to arouse within you all such ideas. I am ready to undergo a hundred thousand rebirths to train up a single man.

The history of the world is the history of a few men who had faith in themselves. That faith calls out the divinity within. You can do anything. You fail only when you do not strive sufficiently to manifest infinite power. As soon as a man or a nation loses faith, death comes.

If you have faith in all three hundred and thirty millions of your mythological gods, and in all the gods which foreigners have now and again introduced into your midst, and still have no faith in yourselves, there is no salvation for you.... Why is it that we three hundred and thirty millions of people have been ruled for the last one thousand years by any and every handful of foreigners who chose to walk over our prostrate bodies? Because they had faith in themselves and we had not.

Faith, faith, faith in ourselves, faith, faith in God, this is the secret of greatness.

Whatever you think, that you will be. If you think yourself weak, weak you will be; if you think yourselves strong, strong you will be.

Let people say whatever they like, stick to your own convictions, and rest assured, the world will be at your feet. They say, 'Have faith in this fellow or that fellow', but I say, 'Have faith in yourself first', that is the way. Have faith in yourself – all power is in you – be conscious and bring it out.

The Vedanta teaches men to have faith in themselves first. As certain religions of the world say that a man who does not believe in a personal God outside of himself is an atheist, so the Vedanta says, a man who does not believe in himself is an atheist. Not believing in the glory of our own soul is what the Vedanta calls atheism. To many this is, no doubt, a terrible idea; and most of us think that this ideal can never be reached; but the Vedanta insists that it can be realised by everyone. There is neither man nor woman nor child, nor difference of race or sex, nor anything, that stands as a bar to the realization of the ideal.

All the powers in the universe are already ours. It is we who have put our hands before our eyes and cry that it is dark. Know that there is no darkness around us. Take the hands away and there is the light which was from the beginning. Darkness never existed. Weakness never existed. We who are fools cry that we are weak; we who are fools cry that we are impure.... As soon as you say, 'I am a little mortal being', you are saying something which is not true, you are giving the lie to yourselves, you are hypnotizing yourselves into something vile and weak and wretched.

The greatest error, says the Vedanta, is to say that you are weak, that you are a sinner, a miserable creature, and that you have no power and you cannot do this and that. Every time you think in that way, you, as it were, rivet one more link in the chain that binds you down, and add one more layer of hypnotism on to your own soul. Therefore, whosoever thinks he is weak is wrong, whosoever thinks he is impure is wrong, and is throwing a bad thought into the world.... This false life must go, and the real life, which is always existing must manifest itself, must shine out. No man becomes purer and purer, it is a matter of greater manifestation. The veil drops away, and the native purity of the soul begins to manifest itself. Everything is ours already – infinite purity, freedom, love and power.... The actual should be reconciled with the ideal, the present life should be made to coincide with life eternal....

These are the principles of ethics, but we shall now come down lower and work out the details. We shall see how this Vedanta can be carried into our everyday life, the city life, the country life, the national life, and the home life of every nation....

The ideal of faith in ourselves is of the greatest help to us. If faith in ourselves had been more extensively taught and practised, I am sure a very large portion of the evils and miseries that we have would have vanished. Throughout the history of mankind, if any motive power has been more potent than another in the lives of all great men and women, it is that of faith in themselves. Born with the consciousness that they were to be great, they became great. Let a man go down as low as possible; there must come a time when out of sheer desperation he will take an upward curve and will learn to have faith in himself. But it is better for us that we should know it from the very first. Why should we have all these bitter experiences in order to gain faith in ourselves? We can see that all the difference between man and man is owing to the existence or non-existence of faith in himself. Faith in ourselves will do everything. I have experienced it in my own life, and am still doing so; and as I grow older that faith is becoming stronger and stronger. He is an atheist who does not believe in himself. The old religions said that he was an atheist who did not believe in God. The new religion says that he is the atheist who does not believe in himself. But it is not selfish faith, because the Vedanta, again, is the doctrine of oneness. It means faith in all, because you are all. Love for yourselves means love for all, love for animals, love for everything, for you are all one. It is this great faith which will make the world better.

If a man, day and night, thinks he is miserable, low and nothing, nothing he becomes. We are the children of the Almighty, we are sparks of the infinite, divine fire. How can we be nothings? We are everything, ready to do everything, we can do everything, and man must do everything. This faith in themselves was in the hearts of our ancestors, this faith in themselves was the motive power that pushed them forward and forward in the march of civilisation; and if there has been degeneration, if there has been defect, mark my words, you will find that degradation to have started on the day our people lost this faith in themselves. Losing faith in one's self means losing faith in God. Do you believe in that infinite, good

Providence working in and through you? If you believe that this Omnipresent One, the *Antaryamin,* is present in every atom, is through and through, *ota-prota,* as the Sanskrit word goes, penetrating your body, mind and soul, how can you lose heart?

For centuries people have been taught theories of degradation. They have been told that they are nothing. The masses have been told all over the world that they are not human beings. They have been so frightened for centuries, till they have nearly become animals. Never were they allowed to hear of the Atman. Let them hear the Atman – that even the lowest of the low have the Atman within, which never dies and never is born.... Let them have faith in themselves.... You have been told and taught that you can do nothing and non-entities you are becoming everyday. What we want is strength, so believe in yourselves.

The idea of true *shraddha* must be brought back once more to us. The faith in our own selves must be reawakened and then only all the problems which face our country will gradually be solved by ourselves. What we want is this *shraddha.* What makes the difference between man and man is the difference in the *shraddha* and nothing else. What makes one man great and another weak and low is this *shraddha.* My Master used to say: He who thinks himself weak will become weak; and that is true. This *shraddha* must enter into you. Whatever of material power you see manifested by the western races is the outcome of this *shraddha,* because they believe in their muscles; and if you believe in the spirit how much more will it work.

I beg you to understand this one fact, no good comes out of the man who day and night thinks he is nobody....

To preach the doctrine of *shraddha* or genuine faith is the mission of my life. Let me repeat to you that this faith is one of the most potent factors of humanity. First have faith in yourselves. Know that though one may be a little bubble and another may be a mountain-high wave, yet behind both the bubble and the wave there is the infinite ocean. The infinite ocean is the background of me as well as you. Mine also is that infinite ocean of life, of power, of spirituality as well as yours. Therefore, my brethren, teach this life-saving, great, ennobling, grand doctrine to your children even from their very birth.

Be Strong and Fearless

Be strong! Be brave! Strength is the one thing needful. Strength is life! Weakness is death! Stand up! Be bold! Be strong! India calls for heroes! Be heroic! Stand firm like a rock! India calls for infinite energy, infinite zeal, infinite courage. Let our youths be strong, – strong first. Religion will grow out of strength!

What makes a man stand up and work? Strength. Strength is goodness, weakness is sin. If there is one word that is coming out of the Upanishads like a bombshell upon masses of ignorance, it is the word fearlessness. And the only religion that ought to be taught is the religion of fearlessness. Either in this world or in the world of religion, it is true that fear is the sure cause of degradation and sin. It is fear that brings misery, fear that brings death, fear that breeds evil. And what causes fear? Ignorance of our own nature.

The best guide in life is strength. In religion, as in all other matters, discard everything that weakens you, have nothing to do with it.

Being reminded of weakness does not help much; give strength, and strength does not come by thinking of weakness all the time. The remedy for weakness is not brooding over weakness, but thinking of strength. Teach men of the strength that is already within them. Instead of telling them they are sinners, the Vedanta takes the opposite position, and says, "You are pure and perfect, and what you call sin does not belong to you."

You have been told and taught that you can do nothing, and non-entities you are becoming everyday. What we want is strength, so believe in your- selves. We have become weak, and that is why occultism and mysticim come to us – these creepy things; there may be great truths in them, but they have nearly destroyed us. Make your nerves strong. What we want is muscles of iron and nerves of steel, inside which dwells a mind of the same material as that of which the thunderbolt is made. Strength, manhood, *kshatra-virya* plus *Brahma-teja.*

We have wept long enough. No more weeping, but stand on your feet and be men. It is man-making religion that we want. It is man-making theories that we want. It is man-making education all round that we want. And here is the test of truth – anything that makes you weak physically, intellectually and spiritually, reject as poison; there is no life in it, it cannot be true. Truth is strengthening. Truth is purity, truth is all knowledge; truth must be strengthening, must be enlightening, must be invigorating. Repeat and pray day and night: 'O Thou Mother of the Universe, vouchsafe manliness unto me! O Thou Mother of Strength, take away my weakness, take away my unmanliness, and make me a Man.'

Strength, strength is what the Upanishads speak to me from every page. This is the one great thing to remember, it has been the one great lesson I have been taught in my life; strength, it says, strength, O man, be not weak.... Aye, it is the only literature in the world where you find the word *abhih*, "fearless", used again and again; in no other scripture in the world is this adjective applied either to God or to man. *Abhih;* fearless! And in my mind rises from the past the vision of the great Emperor of the West, Alexander the Great, and I see, as it were in a picture, the great monarchstanding on the bank of Indus, talking to one of our sannyasins in the forest; the old man he was talking to, perhaps naked, stark naked, sitting upon a block of stone, and the Emperor, astonished at his wisdom, tempting him with gold and honour to come over to Greece. And this man smiles at his gold, and smiles at his temptations, and refuses; and then the Emperor standing on his authority as an Emperor, says, "I will kill you if you do not come", and the man bursts into a laugh and says, "You never told such falsehood in your life, as you tell just now. Who can kill me? Me you kill, Emperor of the material world! Never! For I am Spirit unborn and undecaying: never was I born and never do I die; I am the Infinite, the Omnipresent, the Omniscient; and you kill me, child that you are". That is strength!... Therefore, my friends, as one of your blood, as one that lives and dies with you, let me tell you that we want strength, strength, and every time strength. And the Upanishads are the great mine of strength. Therein lies strength enough to invigorate the whole world; the whole world can be vivified, made strong, energised through them. They will call with trumpet voice upon the weak, the miserable and the downtrodden of all races, all creeds and all sects to stand on their feet and be free. Freedom, physical freedom, mental freedom and spiritual freedom are the watchwords of the Upanishads.

A religion that does not infuse strength into its believers is no religion to me.... Strength is religion and religion is strength.... Be not afraid of anything. You will do marvellous work. The moment you fear, you are nobody. It is fear that is the great cause of misery in the world. It is fear that is the greatest of superstitions. It is fear that is the cause of our woes. And it is fearlessness that brings heaven in a moment....

Be strong and stand up and seek the God of Love. This is the highest strength. What power is higher than the power of purity? Love and purity govern the world. This God of love cannot be reached by the weak; therefore be not weak, either physically, mentally, morally or spiritually. There must be no fear, no begging, but demanding – demanding the highest. The true devotees of God are as hard as adamant and as fearless as lions.... Make God listen to you. None of that cringing to God. Remember. God is all-powerful. He can make heroes out of clay.

Read what your Scriptures say of the Lord, – calling Him *abhaya*, fearless! Dare to be *abhaya*, fearless, and you will be truly free!

One must admit that law, government, politics are phases and are not final in any way. There is a goal beyond them where law is not needed. Christ saw that the basis is not law, that morality and purity are the only strength. You have the saying that man cannot be made virtuous by an act of Parliament. And that is why religion is of deeper importance than politics since it goes to the root and deals with essentials of conduct.

Practise Spiritual Boldness

"....The sun cannot dry, fire cannot burn, sword cannot kill, for I am the birthless, the deathless, the ever living, Omnipotent, Omnipresent Spirit." This is spiritual boldness.... Stand up, men and women, in this spirit, dare to believe in the Truth, dare to practise the Truth! The world requires a few hundred bold men and women. Practise that boldness which dares know the Truth, which dares show the Truth in life, which does not quake before death, nay, welcomes death, makes man know that he is the Spirit; that in the whole universe, nothing can kill him. Then you will be free. Then you will know your real soul.... Talk not about impurity, but say that we are pure. We have hypnotised ourselves into this thought that we are little, that we are born, and that we are going to die, and into a constant state of fear.... You are lions, you are souls, pure, infinite and perfect. The might of the universe is within you. 'Why weepest thou, my friend? There is neither birth nor death for thee. Why weepest thou? There is no disease nor misery for thee, but thou art like the infinite sky; clouds of various colours come over it, play for a moment, then vanish. But the sky is ever the same eternal blue.'

Be Kind and Benevolent

Our duty to others means helping others; doing good to the world. Why should we do good to the world? Apparently, to help the world, but really to help ourselves. We should always try to help the world, that should be the highest motive in us, but if we consider well, we find that the world does not require our help at all. This world was not made that you or I should come and help it. I once read a sermon in which it was said: 'All this beautiful world is very good, because it gives us time and opportunity to help others'. Apparently, this is a very beautiful sentiment, but is it not a blasphemy to say that the world needs our help? We cannot deny that there is much misery in it; to go out and help others is, therefore, the best thing we can do, although in the long run, we shall find that helping others is only helping ourselves.... The only help is that we get moral exercise. This world is neither good nor evil, each man manufactures a world for himself. If a blind man begins to think of the world, it is either as soft or hard, or as cold or hot. We are a mass of happiness or misery; we have seen that hundreds of times in our lives. As a rule, the young are optimistic and the old pessimistic. The young have life before them; the old complain their day is gone; hundreds of desires, which they cannot fulfil, struggle in their hearts. Both are foolish nevertheless. Life is good or evil according to the state of mind in which we look at it; it is neither by itself. Fire, by itself, is neither good nor evil. When it keeps us warm we say, 'How beautiful is fire!' When it burns our fingers, we blame it. Still, in itself, it is neither good nor bad. According as we use it, it produces in us the feeling of good or bad; so also is this world. It is perfect. By perfection is meant that it is perfectly fitted to meet its ends. We may all be perfectly sure that it will go on beautifully well without us, and we need not bother our heads wishing to help it.

Yet we must do good. The desire to do good is the highest motive power we have, if we know all the time that it is a privilege to help others. Do not stand on a high pedestal and take five cents in your hand and say: 'Here, my poor man', but be grateful that the poor man is there, so that by making a gift to him you are able to help yourself. It is not the receiver that is blessed, but it is the giver. Be thankful that you are allowed to exercise your power of benevolence and mercy in the world, and thus become pure and perfect.

The great secret of true success, of true happiness, then, is this: The man who asks for no return, the perfectly unselfish man, is the most successful. It seems to be a paradox. Do we not know that every man who is unselfish in life gets cheated, gets hurt? Apparently yes. 'Christ was unselfish, and yet he was crucified'. True, but we know that this unselfishness is the reason, the cause, of a great victory – the crowning of millions upon millions of lives with the blessings of true success.

Ask nothing, want nothing in return. Give what you have to give; it will come back to you – but do not think of that now. It will come back multiplied a thousandfold – but the attention must not be on that. You have the power to give, give, and there it ends. Learn that the whole of life is giving, that nature will force you to give. So, give willingly, sooner or later you will have to give up.... It is because we dare not give, because we are not resigned enough to accede to this grand demand of nature, that we are miserable. The forest is gone, but we get heat in return. The sun is taking up water from the ocean, to return it in showers. You are a machine for taking and giving, you take, in order to give.

Ask, therefore, nothing in return; but the more you give, the more will come to you. The quicker you can empty the air out of this room, the quicker it will be filled up by the external air; and if you close all the doors and every aperture, that which is within will remain, but that which is outside will never come in, and that which is within will stagnate, degenerate, and become poisoned. A river is continually emptying itself into the ocean and is continually filling up again. Bar not the exit into the ocean. The moment you do that, death seizes you.

Be Strictly Moral

Be moral, be brave, be a heart-whole man – strictly moral, brave unto desperation. Don't bother your head with religious theories. Cowards only sin, brave men never; no, not even in mind. Try to love anybody and everybody. Be a man and try to make those immediately under your care.... brave, moral and sympathising.... No religion for you, my children, but morality and bravery. No cowardice, no sin, no crime, no weakness – the rest will come of itself.

Perfect morality is the all in all of complete control over mind. The man who is perfectly moral has nothing more to do; he is free. The man who is perfectly moral cannot possibly hurt anything or anybody. Non-injuring has to be attained by him who would be free. No one is more powerful than he who has attained perfect non-injuring. No one could fight, no one could quarrel in his presence. Yes, his very presence, and nothing else, means peace, means love, wherever he may be, nobody could be angry or fight in his presence. Even the animals, ferocious animals, would be peaceful before him.

Truth, purity, and unselfishness – wherever these are present, there is no power below or above the sun to crush the possessor thereof. Equipped with these, one individual is able to face the whole universe in opposition.

I have experienced even in my insignificant life that good motives, sincerity and infinite love can conquer the world. One single soul possessed of these virtues can destroy the dark designs of millions of hypocrites and brutes.

That soul has not been awakened that never feels weakness, never feels misery. That is a callous state. We do not want that. At the same time, we do not only want this mighty power of love, this mighty power of attachment, the power of throwing our whole soul upon a single object, losing ourselves and letting ourselves be annihilated, as it were, for other souls – which is the power of the gods – but we want to be higher even than gods. The perfect man puts his whole soul upon one point of love, yet he is unattached.

Who will give the world light? Sacrifice in the past has been the law, it will be, alas, for ages to come. The earth's bravest and best will have to sacrifice themselves for the good of many, for the welfare of all. Buddhas by the hundred are necessary with eternal love and pity.

Build up Your Character

Build up your character and manifest your real nature, the Effulgent, the Resplendent, the Ever Pure and call it up in everyone you see.

Religions of the world have become lifeless mockeries. What the world wants is character. The world is in need of those whose life is one burning love, selfless. That love will make every word tell like a thunderbolt.

The first great thing to accomplish is to establish a character, to obtain, as we say, the *pratishtita prajna* (established wisdom). This applies equally to individuals and to organised bodies of individuals....

Neither money pays, nor name, nor fame, nor learning; it is character that can cleave through adamantine walls of difficulties. Bear this in mind.

The character of any man is but the aggregate of his tendencies, the sum total of the bent of his mind.

This is really what is meant by character; each man's character is determined by the sum total of these impressions. If good impressionsprevail, the character becomes good; if bad, it becomes bad. If a man continuously hears bad words, thinks bad thoughts, does bad actions, his mind will be full of bad impressions; and they will influence his thought and work without his being conscious of the fact. In fact, these bad impressions are always working, and their resultant must be evil, and that man will be a bad man, he cannot help it. The sum total of these impressions in him will create the strong motive power for doing bad actions. He will be like a machine in the hands of his impressions, and they will force him to do evil. Similarly, if a man thinks good thoughts and does good works, the sum total of these impressions will be good, and they, in a similar manner, will force him to do good even in spite of himself. When a man has done so much good work and thought so many good thoughts that there is an irresistible tendency in him to do good, in spite of himself and even if he wishes to do evil, his mind, as the sum total of his tendencies, will not allow him to do so, the tendencies will turn him back; he is completely under the influence of the good tendencies. When such is the case, a man's good character is said to be established.

It is said, 'Habit is second nature', it is first nature also, and the whole nature of man, everything that we are, is the result of habit. That gives us consolation, because, if it is only habit, we can make and unmake it at any time. The *samskaras* are left by these vibrations passing over our mind, each one of them leaving its result. Our character is the sum total of these marks, and according as some particular wave prevails, one takes that tone. If good prevails, one becomes good; if wickedness, one becomes wicked; if joyfulness, one becomes happy. The only remedy for bad habits is counter-habits; all the bad habits that have left their impressions are to be controlled by good habits. Go on doing good, thinking holy thoughts continuously, that is the only way to suppress base impressions. Never say any man is hopeless, because he only represents a character, a bundle of habits which can be checked by new and better ones. Character is repeated habits, and repeated habits alone can reform character.

If you really want to judge the character of a man, look not at his great performances. Every fool may become a hero at one time or another. Watch a man do his most common actions; those are indeed the things which will tell you the real character of a great man. Great occasions rouse even the lowest of human beings to some kind of greatness, but he alone is the really great man whose character is great always, the same wherever he be.

Entertain Positive Thoughts

We see the world as we are.... Do not talk of the wickedness of the world and all its sins. Weep that you are bound to see sin everywhere, and if you want to help the world, do not condemn it. Do not weaken it more. For what is sin and what is misery, and what are all these, but the results of weakness? The world is made weaker and weaker everyday by suchteachings. Men are taught from childhood that they are weak and sinners. Teach them that they are all glorious children of immortality, even those who are the weakest in manifestation. Let positive, strong, helpful thoughts enter into their brains from very childhood. Lay yourselves open to these thoughts, and not to weakening and paralysing ones. Say to your own minds, "I am He, I am He" (pure, free, immortal spirit). Let it ring day and night in your minds, like a song, and at the point of death declare: "I am He". That is the Truth; the infinite strength of the world is yours. Drive out the superstition that has covered your minds. Let us be brave. Know the Truth and practise the Truth. The goal may be distant, but awake, arise, and stop not till the goal is reached.

Think, all of you, that you are the infinitely powerful Atman, and see what strength comes out.... Self-deprecating; what is it for? I am the child of the infinite, the all powerful Divine Mother. What means disease or fear or want, to me? Stamp out the negative spirit as if it were a pestilence and it will conduce to your welfare in every way. No negative; all positive, affirmative. I am, God is, everything is in me. I will manifest health, purity, knowledge, whatever I want.... 'Thou art Energy, impart energy unto me. Thou art strength, impart strength unto me. Thou art Spirituality, impart spirituality unto me. Thou art Fortitude, impart fortitude unto me.'

One must think of oneself as strong and invulnerable.

'This Atman is first to be heard of.' Hear day and night that you are that Soul. Repeat it to yourselves day and night till it enters into your very veins, till it tingles in every drop of blood, till it is in your flesh and bone. Let the whole body be full of that one ideal: 'I am the birthless, the deathless, the blissful, the omniscient, the omnipotent, ever-glorious soul'. Think on it day and night; think on it till it becomes part and parcel of your life. Meditate upon it and out of that will come work.

Doing is very good, but that comes from thinking. Fill the brain, therefore, with high thoughts, highest ideals; place them day and night before you; and out of that will come great work.

It is thought which is the propelling force in us. Fill the mind with the highest thoughts, hear them day after day, think of them month after month. Never mind failures; they are quite natural, they are the beauty of life, these failures. What would be life without them? It would not be worth having if it were not for struggle. Where would be the poetry of life? Never mind the struggle, the mistakes. I never heard a cow telling a lie, but it is only a cow never a man. So never mind these failures, these little backslidings; hold the ideal a thousand times, and if you fail a thousand times, make the attempt once more.

'Out of the fullness of the heart the mouth speaketh', and out of the fullness of the heart the hand worketh also. Action will come. Fill yourselves with the ideal; whatever you do, think well on it. All your actions will be magnified, transformed, deified, by the very power of the thought. If matter is powerful, thought is omnipotent. Bring this thought to bear upon your life, fill yourselves with the thought of your almightiness, your majesty and your glory.

Make Your Own Future

Know that you are t`he creator of your destiny.

Every thought that we think, every deed that we do, after a certain time becomes fine, goes into seed form, so to speak, and lives in the subtle body in a potential form, and after a time it emerges again and bears its results. These results condition the life of man. Thus the human being moulds his own life. Man is not bound by any other laws excepting those which he makes for himself.

Once we set in motion a certain power, we have to take the full consequence. That is the law of karma.

We are responsible for what we are; and whatever we wish ourselves to be, we have the power to make ourselves. If what we are now has been the result of our own past actions, it certainly follows that whatever we wish to be in future, can be produced by our present actions; so we have to know how to act.

Men in general lay all the blame of life on their fellow-men, or failing that, on God, or they conjure up a ghost, and say it is fate. Where is fate, and who is fate? We reap what we sow. We are the makers of our own fate. None else has the blame, none has the praise. The wind is blowing, those vessels whose sails are unfurled catch it, and go forward on their way, but those which have their sails furled do not catch the wind. Is that the fault of the wind? Is it the fault of the merciful Father, whose wind of mercy is blowing without ceasing, day and night, whose mercy knows no decay, is it His fault that some of us are happy and some unhappy. We make our own destiny.... His infinite mercy is open to everyone, at all times, in all places, under all conditions, unfailing, unswerving. Upon us depends how we must use it. Upon us depends how we utilise it. Blame neither man, nor God, nor anyone in the world. When you find yourselves suffering, blame yourselves, and try to do better.... Therefore, stand up, be bold, be strong. Take the whole responsibility on your own shoulders, and know that you are the creator of your own destiny and all the strength and succour you want is within yourself. Therefore, make your own future. 'Let the dead past bury its dead.' The infinite future is before you, and you must always remember that each word, thought, and deed, lays up a store for you, and that as the bad thoughts and bad deeds are ready to spring upon you like tigers so also there is the inspiring hope that the good thoughts and good deeds are ready with the power of a hundred thousand angels to defend you always and for ever.

So if the responsibility is thrown upon our own shoulders, we shall be at our highest and best. When we have nobody to grope towards, no devilto lay our blame upon, no personal God to carry our burden, when we are alone responsible, then we shall rise to our highest and best. I am responsible for my fate. I am the bringer of good unto myself, I am the bringer of evil. I am the pure and Blessed one. We must reject all thoughts that assert the contrary.

That is what the Vedanta teaches. It does not propose any slipshod remedy by covering wounds with gold leaf and the more the wound festers, putting on more gold leaf. This life is a hard fact; work your way through it boldly, though it may be adamantine; no matter, the soul is stronger. It lays no responsibility on little gods; for you are the makers of your own fortunes. You make yourselves suffer, you make good and evil, and it is you who put your hands away and see the light; you are effulgent, you are perfect already, from the very beginning.

Love all Beings as Yourself

In every nation the truth has been preached from the most ancient times – love your fellow-beings as yourselves, I mean, love human beings as your selves. In India, it has been preached, love all beings as yourselves; we make no distinction between men and animals. But no reason was forthcoming, no one knows why it would be good to love other beings as ourselves. And the reason why, is there in the idea of the impersonal God; you understand it when you learn that the whole world is one – the oneness of the universe, the solidarity of all life – that in hurting anyone I am hurting myself, in loving anyone I am loving myself. Hence, we understand why it is that we ought not to hurt others.

In the lowest worm, as well as in the highest human being, the same divine nature is present. The worm form is the lower form in which the divinity has been more overshadowed by *maya;* man is the highest form in which it has been least overshadowed. Behind everything the same divinity is existing, and out of this comes the basis of morality. Do not injure another. Love everyone as your own self, because the whole universe is one. In injuring another, I am injuring myself; in loving another, I am loving myself. From this also springs that principle of Advaita morality which has been summed up in one word – Self-abnegation. The Advaitist says: This little personalised self is the cause of all my misery. This individual self, which makes me different from all other beings, brings hatred and jealousy and misery, struggle and all other evils. And when this idea has been got rid of, all struggle will cease, all misery vanish. So this is to be given up. We must always hold ourselves ready, even to give up our lives for the lowest beings. When a man becomes ready even to give up his life for a little insect, he has reached perfection.

Do you feel for others? If you do, you are growing in oneness. If you do not feel for others, you may be the most intellectual giant ever born, but you will be nothing; you are but dry intellect, and you will remain so.And if you feel, even if you cannot read any book and do not know any language, you are in the right way.... Feel like Christ and you will be a Christ; feel like Buddha and you will be a Buddha. It is feeling that is the life, the strength.

All expansion is life, all contraction is death. All love is expansion, all selfishness is contraction. Love is therefore the only law of life. He who loves lives, he who is selfish is dying. Therefore love for love's sake, because it is the only law of life, just as you breathe to live.

Love binds, love makes for that oneness, you become one, the mother with the child, families with the city, the whole world becomes one with the animals. For love is existence, God Himself; and all this is the manifestation of that one love. The difference is only in degree, but it is the manifestation of that one love – throughout.

Nothing else is necessary but these – love, sincerity, and patience. What is life, but growth i.e. expansion, i.e. love? Therefore, all love is life. It is the only law of life; all selfishness is death, and this is true here or hereafter. It is life to do good; it is death not to do good to others.... Feel, my children, feel; feel for the poor, the ignorant, the downtrodden; feel till the heart stops and the brain reels and you think you will go mad; then pour the soul out at the feet of the Lord, and then will come power, help, and indomitable energy. Struggle, struggle, was my motto for the last ten years. Struggle, still say I. When it was all dark, I used to say, struggle; when light is breaking in, I still say, struggle. Be not afraid, my children.

You are Everywhere

We have always heard it preached, 'Love one another.' What for? That doctrine was preached, but the explanation is here. Why should I love everyone? Because they and I are one. Why should I love my brother? Because he and I are one. There is this oneness, this solidarity of the whole universe. From the lowest worm that crawls under our feet to the highest beings that ever lived, all have various bodies, but are the one Soul. Through all mouths you eat; through all hands you work; through all eyes you see. You enjoy health in millions of bodies, you are suffering from disease in millions of bodies. When this idea comes and we realize it, see it, then will misery cease, and fear with it. How can I die? There is nothing beyond me. Fear ceases, and then alone come perfect happiness and perfect love. That universal sympathy, universal love, universal bliss, that never changes raises man above everything.

The infinite oneness of the Soul is the eternal sanction of all morality, that you and I are not only brothers – every literature voicing man's struggle towards freedom has preached that for you – but that you and I are really one. This is the dictate of Indian philosophy. This oneness is the rationale of all ethics and spirituality.

To every man, this is taught: Thou art one with this universal Being, and as such, every soul that exists is your soul; and every body that exists is your body and in hurting anyone, you hurt yourself, in loving any one you love yourself. As soon as a current of hatred is thrown outside, whomsoever else it hurts, it also hurts yourself; and if love comes out from you, it is bound to come back to you. For I am the universe; this universe is my body. I am the Infinite, only I am not conscious of it now; but I am struggling to get this consciousness of the Infinite, and perfection will be reached when full consciousness of this Infinite comes.

Vedanta formulates not universal brotherhood, but universal oneness. I am the same as any other man, as any animal – good, bad, anything. It is one body, one mind, one soul throughout. Spirit never dies. How can even the body die? One leaf may fall – does the tree die? The universe is my body. See how it continues. All minds are mine; with all feet I walk; through all mouths I speak. In everybody I reside.

There is one Self, not many. That one Self shines in various forms. Man is man's brother, because all men are one. A man is not only my brother, says the Vedanta, he is myself. Hurting any part of the universe, I only hurt myself. I am the universe. It is a delusion that I think I am Mr. so-and-so – that is the delusion.

The soul of man is part of the cosmic energy that exists, which is God.... It is beyond life and death. You were never born, and you will never die. What is this birth and death that we see around us? This belongs to the body only, because the soul is omnipresent.... You are everywhere in the universe. How is that then I am born and I am going to die, and all that? That is the talk of ignorance, hallucination of the brain. You were neither born, nor will you die. You have had neither birth, nor will you have a re-birth, nor life, nor incarnation, nor anything. What do you mean by coming and going! All shallow nonsense. You are everywhere. Then what is this coming and going? It is the hallucination produced by the change of this fine body, which you call the mind. That is going on.... In reality you are neither going nor coming, you are not being born, nor going to be born, you are infinite, ever present beyond all causation, and ever free. Such a question is out of place, it is arrant nonsense. How could there be mortality when there was no birth?

....If we are beyond all law, we must be omniscient, ever blessed, all knowledge must be in us, and all power and blessedness. Certainly, you are the omniscient, omnipresent being of the universe. But of such beings can there be many? Can there be a hundred thousand millions of omnipresent beings? Certainly not. Then what becomes of us all? You are only one; there is only one such self, and that one self is you. Standing behind this little nature is what we call the soul. There is only one Being. One Existence, the Ever-blessed, the Omnipresent, the Omniscient, the birthless, the deathless.... 'He is the Reality in nature, He is the soul of your soul, nay, more, you are He, you are one with Him'. Wherever there are two there is fear, there is danger, there is conflict, there is strife. When it is all one, who is there to hate, who is there to struggle with? When it is all He, with whom can you fight? This explains the true nature of life, this explains the true nature of being. This is perfection, and this is God. As long as you see the many you are under delusion. 'In this world of many, he who sees the One, in this ever changing world, he who sees Him who never changes, as the soul of his own soul, as his own self, he is free, he is blessed, he has reached the goal'. Therefore know that thou art He, thou art the God of this universe, *tat tvam asi*. All these various ideas that I am a man or a woman, or sick, or healthy, or strong, or weak, or that I hate, or I love, or have a little power, are but hallucinations. Away with them! What makes you weak? What makes you fear? You are the One being in the universe. What frightens you? Stand up then and be free. Know that every thought and word that weakens you in this world, is the only evil that exists. Whatever makes man weak and fear is the only evil that should be shunned. What can frighten you? If the sun comes down, and the moons crumble into dust and systems after systems are hurled into annihilation, what is that to you? Stand as a rock; you are indestructible. You are the self, the God of the universe. Say – "I am Existence Absolute, Bliss Absolute, Knowledge Absolute, I am He", and like a lion breaking its cage, break your chain and be free for ever. What frightens you; what holds you down? Only ignorance and delusion; nothing else can bind you. You are the pure one, the ever-blessed.

Silly fools tell you that you are sinners, and you sit down in a corner and weep. It is foolishness, wickedness, downright rascality to say that you are sinners! You are all God. See you not God and call Him man? Therefore, if you dare, stand on that, – mould your whole life on that. If a man cuts your throat, do not say no, for you are cutting your own throat. When you help a poor man, do not feel the least pride. That is worship for you and not the cause of pride. Is not the whole universe you? Where is there any one that is not you? You are the soul of this universe. You are the sun, moon, the stars, it is you that are shining everywhere. The whole universe is you. Whom are you going to hate, or to fight? Know then, that thou art He, and model your whole life accordingly, and he who knows this and models his life accordingly, will no more grovel in darkness.

Give up this mad Pursuit

It is better that we know we are God and give up this fool's search after Him; and knowing that we are God, become happy and contented. Give up all these mad pursuits, and then play your part in the universe, as an actor on the stage.

The whole vision is changed, and instead of an eternal prison, this world has become a playground; instead of a land of competition it is aland of bliss, where there is perpetual spring, where flowers bloom and butterflies flit about. This very world becomes heaven, which formerly was hell. To the eyes of the bound it is a tremendous place of torment, but to the eyes of the free it is quite otherwise. This one life is the universal life, heaven and all those places are here.... When we have become free, we need not go mad and throw off society and rush to die in the forest or the cave; we shall remain where we were, only we shall understand the whole thing. The same phenomena will remain but with a new meaning. We do not know the world yet; it is only through freedom that we see what it is, and understand its nature.... Through delusion we have been trying to forget our nature, and yet we could not; it was always calling upon us, and all our search after God or gods, or external freedom, was a search after our real nature.... In one word, the ideal of Vedanta is to know man as he really is.

Seek God Within

....No perfection is going to be attained. You are already free and perfect. What are these ideas of religion and God and searching for the hereafter? Why does man look for a God? Why does man, in every nation, in every state of society, want a perfect ideal somewhere, either in man, in God, or elsewhere? Because that idea is within you. It was your own heartbeating and you did not know, you were mistaking it for something external. It is the God within your own self that is propelling you to seek for Him, to realise Him. After long searches here and there, in temples and churches, in earths and in heavens, at last you come back, completing the circle from where you started, to your own soul and find that He, for whom you have been seeking all over the world, for whom you have been weeping and praying in churches and temples, on whom you were looking as the mystery of all mysteries shrouded in the clouds, is nearest of the near, is your own Self; the reality of your life, body and soul. That is your own nature. Assert it, manifest it. Not to become pure, you are pure already. You are not to be perfect, you are that already. Nature is like that screen which is hiding the reality beyond. Every good thought that you think or act upon, is simply tearing the veil, as it were, and the purity, the Infinity, the God behind, manifests Itself more and more. This is the whole history of man. Finer and finer becomes the veil, more and more of the light behind shines forth, for it is its nature to shine.

The more you approach your real Self, the more this delusion vanishes. The more all difference and divisions disappear the more you realise all as the one divinity. God exists, but he is not the man sitting upon a cloud. He is pure Spirit. Where does He reside? Nearer to you than your very self. He is the soul. How can you perceive God as separate and different from your self? When you think of Him as someone separate from yourself, you do not know Him. He is yourself.

Adore the Living God

Look upon every man, woman and everyone as God. You cannot help anyone; you can only serve; serve the children of the Lord, serve the Lord Himself, if you have the privilege. If the Lord grants that you can help any one of his children, blessed you are; do not think too much of yourselves. Blessed you are that that privilege was given to you, when others had it not. Do it only as a worship.

You may invent an image through which to worship God, but a better image already exists, the living man. You may build a temple in which to worship God, and that may be good, but a better one, a much higher one, already exists, the human body.

We have to cover everything with the Lord Himself, not by blinding our eyes to the evil, but by really seeing God in everything. Thus we have to give up the world, and when the world is given up, what remains? God. What is meant? You can have your wife; it does not mean that you are to abandon her, but you are to see God in the wife. Give up your children; what does that mean? To turn them out of doors, as some human brutes do in every country? Certainly not. That is diabolism; it is not religion. But see God in your children, so in everything. In life and in death, in happiness and in misery, the Lord is equally present. The whole world is full of the Lord. Open your eyes and see Him. This is what Vedanta teaches.

So work, says Vedanta, putting God in everything, and knowing Him to be everything. Work incessantly, holding life as something deified, as God Himself, and knowing that this is all we have to do, this is all we should ask for. God is in everything, where else shall we go to find Him? He is already in every work, every thought, in every feeling. Thus knowing, we must work – this is the only way, there is no other.

After so much austerity, I have understood this as the real truth – God is present in every *jiva;* there is no other God besides that. 'Who serves *jiva,* serves God indeed'.

I have understood that the ideal of Vedanta lived by the recluse outside the pale of society can be practised even at home and applied to all aspects of daily life. Whatever a man's vocation, let him understand and realize that it is God alone who has manifested Himself as the world and created beings. He is both immanent and transcendent. It is He who has become all the diverse beings, objects of our love, respect or compassion, and yet He is beyond all these. Such a realization of the Divinity in humanity leaves no room for arrogance. By realizing it, a man cannot be jealous of, or have pity for, any other being. Serving man, knowing him to be the manifestation of God, purifies the heart; and in a short time the aspirant who does this realizes that he is a part of God – Existence-Knowledge-Bliss Absolute.

Seek your own Self in every being that breathes, and in every atom of the universe. When you realize this, you cannot live in this world without treating everyone with exceeding love and compassion. This is indeed practical Vedanta.

This is the gist of all worship – to be pure and to do good to others. He who sees Shiva in the poor, in the weak, and in the diseased, really worships Shiva; and if he sees Shiva only in the image, his worship is but preliminary.

We want to worship a living God. I have seen nothing but God all my life, nor have you. To see this chair you first see God, and then the chair, in and through Him. He is everywhere, saying "I am." The moment you feel "I am", you are conscious of Existence. Where shall we go to find God if we cannot see Him in our own hearts, and in every living being? "Thou art the man, Thou art the woman, Thou art the girl, and Thou art the boy. Thou art the old man tottering with a stick. Thou art the young man walking in the pride of his strength." Thou art all that exists, a wonderful living God who is the only fact in the universe.

....The Vedanta says, there is nothing that is not God. It may frighten many of you, but you will understand it by degrees. The living God is within you, and yet you are building churches and temples and believing all sorts of imaginary nonsense. The only God to worship is the human soul, in the human body. Of course, all animals are temples too, but man is the highest, the Taj Mahal of temples. If I cannot worship in that, no other temple will be of any advantage. The moment I have realised God sitting in the temple of every human body, the moment I stand in reverence before every human being and see God in Him, – that moment I am free from bondage; everything that binds vanishes and I am free. This is the most practical of all worship.

No books, no scriptures, no science, can ever imagine the glory of the Self that appears as man, the most glorious God that ever was, the only God that ever existed, exists and ever will exist.

The God in you is the God in all. If you have not known this, you have known nothing. How can there be difference? It is all one. Every being is the temple of the Most High; if you can see that, good; if not, spirituality has not yet come to you.

> From the highest Brahman to the yonder worm,
> And to the minutest atom,
> Everywhere is the same God, the All-Love;
> Friend, offer mind, soul, body, at their feet,
> These are His manifold forms before thee,
> Rejecting them, where seekest thou for God?
> Who loves all beings, without distinction,
> He indeed is worshipping best his God.

Seek for the Highest

Do not go for glass beads leaving the mine of diamonds! This life is a great chance. What, seekest thou the pleasures of the world! – He (God) is the fountain of all bliss. Seek for the highest, aim at the highest and you shall reach the highest.

This world is nothing. It is at best only a hideous caricature, a shadow of the Reality. We must go to the Reality. Renunciation will take us to it. Renunciation is the very basis of our true life, every moment of goodness and real life that we enjoy is when we do not think of ourselves. This little separate self must die. Then we shall find that we are in the Real, and that Reality is God, and He is our own true nature, and He is always in us and with us. Let us live in Him and stand in Him. It is the only joyful state of existence. Life on the plane of the Spirit is the only life, and let us all try to attain to this realization.

There is a joy which is absolute, which never changes. That joy cannot be the joys and pleasures we have in this life, and yet Vedanta shows that everything that is joyful in this life is but a particle of that real joy, because that is the only joy there is. Every moment really we are enjoying the absolute bliss, though covered up, misunderstood, and caricatured.... But to understand that, we have to go through the negation, and then the positive side will begin. We have to give up ignorance and all that is false, and then truth will begin to reveal itself to us. When we have grasped the truth, things which we gave up at first will take new shape and form, will appear to us in a new light, and become deified. They will have become sublimated and then we shall understand them in their true light. But to understand them we have first to get a glimpse of the truth; we must give them up at first, and then we get them back again deified. We have to give up all our miseries and sorrows, all our little joys.

Those who give themselves up to the Lord do more for the world than all the so-called workers. One man who has purified himself thoroughly, accomplishes more than a regiment of preachers. Out of purity and silence comes the word of power.

If a man plunges headlong into foolish luxuries of the world without knowing the truth, he has missed his footing; he cannot reach the goal. And if a man curses the world, goes into a forest, mortifies his flesh, and kills himself little by little, by starvation, makes his heart a barren waste, kills out all feeling and becomes harsh, stern, and dried up, that man also has missed the way.

Regain Your Lost Empire

....You cannot get anything which is not yours already. You are indebted to nobody in this universe. You claim your own birth-right, as it has been most poetically expressed by a great Vedantin philosopher, in the title of one of his books – *The Attainment of Our Own Empire*. That empire is ours; we have lost it and we have to regain it. The *mayavadin,* however, says that this losing of the empire was a hallucination; you never lost it. This is the only difference.

....But the latest and the greatest counsel is, you need not weep at all. You need not go through all these ceremonies, and need not take any notice of how to regain your empire, because you never lost it. Why should you go to seek for what you never lost? You are pure already, you are free already. If you think you are free, free you are this moment, and if you think you are bound, bound you will be. This is a very bold statement, and as I told you at the beginning of this course, I shall have to speak to you very boldly. It may frighten you now, but when you think over it, and realise it in your own life, then you will come to know that what I say is true.

Teach Yourself First

Each one of us is naturally growing and developing according to his own nature; each will in time come to know the highest truth, for after all, men must teach themselves. What can you and I do? Do you think you can teach even a child? You cannot. The child teaches himself. Your duty is to afford opportunities and to remove obstacles.... None can teach you; none can make a spiritual man of you; you have to teach yourself; your growth must come from inside. What can an external teacher do? He can remove the obstruction a little, and there his duty ends. Therefore help, if you can; but do not destroy. Give up all ideas that you can make man spiritual. It is impossible. There is no other teacher to you than your own soul. Recognize this.

Carry the Light of Knowledge

Advaitism – the fairest flower of philosophy and religion that any country in any age has produced, where human thought attains its highest expression and even goes beyond the mystery which seems to be impenetrable.

....Raise once more that mighty banner of Advaita, for on no other ground can you have that wonderful love, until you see that same Lord is present everywhere. Unfurl the banner of love! Arise, awake, and stop not till the goal is reached.

In one word, the ideal of Vedanta is to know man as he really is, and this is its message, that if you cannot worship your brother man, the manifested God, how can you worship a God who is unmanifested?

Vedanta lays down that each man should be treated not as what he manifests, but as what he stands for. Each human being stands for the divine, and, therefore, every teacher should be helpful, not by condemning man, but by helping him to call forth the divinity that is within him.

We shall see how the Vedanta can be carried into our everyday life, the city life, the country life, the national life, and the home life of every nation. For, if a religion cannot help man wherever he may be, wherever he stands, it is not of much use; it will remain only a theory for the chosen few. Religion, to help mankind, must be ready and able to help him in whatever condition he is, in servitude or in freedom, in the depths of degradation or on the heights of purity; everywhere, equally, it should be able to come to his aid. The principles of Vedanta, or the ideal of religion, or whatever we may call it, will be fulfilled by its capacity for performing this great function.

Carry the light and the life of Vedanta to every door, and rouse up the divinity that is hidden within every soul. Then, whatever may be the measure of your success, you will have the satisfaction that you have lived, worked and died for a great cause. In the success of this cause, however brought about, is centred the salvation of humanity here and hereafter.

....I do not believe at all that Monistic ideas preached to the world would produce immorality and weakness. On the contrary, I have reason to believe that it is the only remedy there is. If this be the truth, why let people drink ditch water when the stream of life is flowing by? If this be the truth, that they are all pure, why not at this moment teach it to the whole world? Why not teach it with the voice of thunder to every man that is born, to saints and sinners, men, women and children, to the man on the throne and to the man sweeping the streets?

I only ask you to work to realise more and more the Vedantic ideal of the solidarity of man and his inborn divine nature.

These conceptions of the Vedanta must come out, must remain not only in the forest, not only in the cave, but they must come out to work at the Bar and the Benches, in the pulpit and in the cottage of the poor man, with the fishermen that are catching fish and with students that are studying.

If the fisherman thinks that he is the spirit, he will be a better fisherman. If the student thinks that he is the spirit, he will be a better student. If the lawyer thinks that he is the spirit, he will be a better lawyer.... and so on. If you teach Vedanta to the fisherman, he will say, 'I am as good a man as you. I am a fisherman as you are a philosopher, but I have the same God in me, as you have in you'. And that is what we want, no privilege for anyone, equal chances for all; let everyone be taught that the Divine is within him, and everyone will work out his own salvation.

It may take ages for all minds to receive Monism, but why not begin now? If we have told it to twenty persons in our lives, we have done a great work.

My hope and faith rests in men like you. Understand my words in their true spirit and apply yourselves to work in their light.... I have given you advice enough, now put at least something in practice. Let the world see that your listening to me has been a success.

Be Living Sermons

Men and women of today! If there be among you any pure, fresh flower, let it be laid on the altar of God. If there are among you any who, being young, do not desire to return into the world, let them give up! Let them renounce! This is the one secret of spirituality, renunciation. Dare to do this. Be brave enough to do it. Such great sacrifices are necessary.

Can you not see the tide of death and materialism that is rolling over these Western lands? Can you not see the power of lust and unholiness, that is eating into the very vitals of society? Believe me, you will not arrest these things by talk, or by movements of agitation for reform; but by renunciation, by standing up, in the midst of decay and death, as mountains of righteousness. Talk not, but let the power of purity, the power of chastity, the power of renunciation, emanate from every pore of your body. Let it strike those who are struggling day and night for gold, that even in the midst of such a state of things, there can be one to whom wealth counts for nothing. Put away lust and wealth. Sacrifice yourselves.

But who is it that will do this? Not the worn-out or the old, bruised and battered by society, but the Earth's freshest and best, the strong, the young, the beautiful. Lay down your lives. Make yourselves servants of humanity. Be living sermons. This, and not talk, is renunciation.

Do not criticize others, for all doctrines and all dogmas are good; but show them by your lives that religion is no matter of books and beliefs, but of spiritual realisation. Only those who have seen it will understand this; but such spirituality can be given to others, even though they be unconscious of the gift. Only those who have attained to this power are amongst the great teachers of mankind. They are the powers of light.

The more of such men any country produces, the higher is that country raised. That land where no such men exist, is doomed. Nothing can save it. Therefore my master's message to the world is, "Be ye all spiritual! Get ye first realization!".

You have talked of the love of man, till the thing is in danger of becoming words alone. The time has come to act. The call now is, Do! Leap into the breach, and save the world!

Spiritual Knowledge – The Greatest of all Benefactions

Helping others physically, by removing their physical needs, is, indeed, great, but the help is greater according as the need is greater and according as the help is far-reaching. If a man's wants can be removed for an hour, it is helping him indeed, if his wants can be removed for a year, it will be more help to him; but if his wants can be removed forever, it is surely the greatest help that can be given to him.

Spiritual knowledge is the only thing that can destroy our miseries for ever; any other knowledge satisfies wants only for a time. It is only with the knowledge of the spirit that the faculty of want is annihilated forever, so helping man spiritually is the highest help that can be given to him. He who gives man spiritual knowledge is the greatest benefactor of mankind and as such we always find that those were the most powerful of men who helped man in his spiritual needs because spirituality is the true basis of all our activities in life. A spiritually strong and sound man will be strong in every other respect, if he so wishes. Until there is spiritual strength in men, even physical needs cannot be well satisfied.

Next to spiritual comes intellectual help. The gift of knowledge is a far higher gift than that of food and clothes, it is even higher than giving life to a man, because the real life of man consists of knowledge. Ignorance is death, knowledge is life. Life is of very little value, if it is a life in the dark, groping through ignorance and misery. Next in order comes, of course, helping a man physically.

Therefore, in considering the question of helping others, we must always strive not to commit the mistake of thinking that physical help is the only help that can be given. It is not only the last but the least, because it cannot bring about permanent satisfaction. The misery that I feel when I am hungry is satisfied by eating, but hunger returns; my misery can cease only when I am satisfied beyond all want. Then hunger will not make me miserable; no distress, no sorrow will be able to move me. So, that help which tends to make us strong spiritually is the highest, next to it comes intellectual help, and, after that, physical help.

The miseries of the world cannot be cured by physical help only. Until man's nature changes, these physical needs will always arise, and miseries will always be felt, and no amount of physical help will cure them completely. The only solution of this problem is to make mankind pure. Ignorance is the mother of all the evil and all the misery we see. Let men have light, let them be pure and spiritually strong and educated, then alone will misery cease in the world, not before. We may convert every house in the country into a charity asylum, we may fill the land with hospitals, but the misery of man will still continue to exist until man's character changes.

Spiritual Knowledge – The Highest Utility

Happiness, we see, is what everyone is seeking for, but the majority seek it in things which are evanescent, and not real. No happiness was ever found in the senses. There never was a person who found happiness in the senses, or enjoyment of the senses. Happiness is found only in the Spirit. Therefore the highest utility for mankind is to find this happiness in the Spirit. The next point is, that ignorance is the great mother of all misery, and the fundamental ignorance is to think that the infinite weeps and cries, that He is finite. This is the basis of all ignorance, that we, the immortal, the ever pure, the perfect Spirit, think that we are little minds, that we are little bodies; it is the mother of all selfishness. As soon as I think that I am a little body, I want to preserve it, to protect it, to keep it nice, at the expense of other bodies; then you and I become separate. As soon as this idea of separation comes, it opens the door to all mischief and leads to all misery. This is the utility, that if a very small fractional part of human beings livingtoday can put aside the idea of selfishness, narrowness, and littleness, this earth will become a paradise tomorrow; but with machines and improvements of material knowledge only, it will never be. These only increase misery, as oil poured on fire increases the flame all the more. Without the knowledge of the Spirit, all material knowledge is only adding fuel to fire, only giving into the hands of selfish man one more instrument to take what belongs to others, to live upon the life of others, instead of giving up his life for them.

Spirituality can he Communicated

My master taught me this lesson hundreds of times, yet I often forget it. Few understand the power of thought. If a man goes into a cave, shuts himself in, and thinks one really great thought and dies, that thought will penetrate the walls of the cave, vibrate through space and at last permeate the whole human race. Such is the power of thought; be in no hurry therefore to give your thoughts to others. First have something to give. He alone teaches who has something to give, for teaching is not talking. Teaching is not imparting doctrines, it is communicating. Spirituality can be communicated just as really as I can give you a flower. This is true in the most literal sense.

....Spirituality has nothing to do with the display of psychical powers, which, when analysed, show that the man who occupies himself with them is a slave of desire and a most egotistical person. Spirituality involves the acquisition of that true power which is character. It is the vanquishing of passion and the rooting out of desire. All this chasing after physical illusions, which means nothing in the solution of the great problems of our life, is a terrible waste of energy, the most intense form of selfishness, and leads to degeneracy of mind. It is this nonsense which is demoralising our nation. What we need is strong common sense, a public spirit, and a philosophy and religion which will make us men.

India – The Land of Wisdom

This is the motherland of philosophy, of spirituality and of ethics, of sweetness, gentleness and love. These still exist, and my experience of the world leads me to stand on firm ground and make the bold statement that India is still the first and foremost of all the nations of the world in these respects.

One thing we may note that whereas you will find that good and great men of other countries take pride in tracing back their descent to some robber-baron who lived in a mountain fortress and emerged from time to time to plunder passing wayfarers, we Hindus, on the other hand, take pride in being the descendants of rishis and sages who lived on roots and fruits in mountains and caves, meditating on the Supreme.

Did you ever hear of a country where the greatest kings tried to trace their descent not to kings, not to robber-barons living in old castles who plundered poor travellers, but to semi-naked sages who lived in the forest? Did you ever hear of such a land? This is the land. In other countries great priests try to trace their descent to some king, but here the greatest kings would trace their descent to some ancient priest. Therefore, whether you believe in spirituality or not, for the sake of the national life, you have to get a hold on spirituality and keep to it.

The idea of God was nowhere else ever so fully developed as in this motherland of ours, for the same idea of God never existed anywhere else. Perhaps you are astonished at my assertion; but show me any idea of God from any other scripture equal to ours; they have only clan-Gods, the God of the Jews, the God of the Arabs, and of such and such a race, and their God is fighting the Gods of the other races. But the idea of that beneficent, most merciful God, our father, our mother, our friend, the friend of our friends, the soul of our souls, is here and here alone.

This is the ancient land where wisdom made its home before it went into any other country, the same India whose influx of spirituality is represented, as it were, on the material plane, by rolling rivers like oceans, where the eternal Himalayas, rising tier above tier with their snow-caps, look as it were into the very mysteries of heaven. Here is the same India whose soil has been trodden by the feet of the greatest sages that ever lived. Here first sprang up inquiries into the nature of man and into the internal world. Here first arose the doctrines of the immortality of the soul, the existence of a supervising God, an immanent God in nature and in man, and here the highest ideals of religion and philosophy have attained their culminating points. This is the land from whence, like the tidal waves, spirituality and philosophy have again and again rushed out and deluged the world, and this is the land from whence once more such tides must proceed in order to bring life and vigour into the decaying races of mankind. It is the same India which has withstood the shocks of centuries, of hundreds of foreign invasions, of hundreds of upheavals of manners and customs. It is the same land which stands firmer than any rock in the world, with its undying vigour, indestructible life. Its life is of the same nature as the soul, without beginning and without end, immortal; and we are the children of such a country.

India – The Land of Religious Tolerance

We not only tolerate, but we Hindus accept every religion, praying in the mosque of Mohammedans, worshipping before the fire of Zoroastrians, and kneeling before the cross of the Christians, knowing that all the religions, from the lowest fetishism, mean so many attempts of the human soul to grasp and realise the infinite, each determined by the conditions of its birth and association, and each of them making a stage of progress. We gather all these flowers and bind them with the twine of love, making a wonderful bouquet of worship.

India is the only country where there never has been religious persecution, where never was any man disturbed for his religious faith. Theists or atheists, monists, dualists, monotheists are there and always lived unmolested.

I am proud to belong to a religion which has taught the world both toleration and universal acceptance. We believe not only in universal tolerance, but we accept all religions as true. I am proud to belong to a nation which has sheltered the persecuted and the refugees of all religions and all nations of the earth. I am proud to tell you that we have gathered in our bosom the purest remnant of the Israelites who came to Southern India and took refuge with us in the very year in which their holy temple was shattered to pieces by Roman tyranny. I am proud to belong to the religion which has sheltered and is still fostering the remnant of the grand Zoroastrian nation.

In India there never was any religious persecution by the Hindus, but only that wonderful reverence, which they have for all the religions of the world. They sheltered a portion of the Hebrews when they were driven out of their own country; and the Malabar Jews remain as a result. They received at another time the remnant of the Persians, when they were almost annihilated; and they remain to this day, as a part of us and loved by us, as the modern Parsees of Bombay. There were Christians who claimed to have come with St. Thomas, the disciple of Jesus Christ, and they were allowed to settle in India and hold their own opinions, and a colony of them is even now in existence in India. And this spirit of toleration has not died out. It will not and cannot die there.

In (Hindu) religion, we find atheists, materialists and Buddhists, creeds, opinions and speculations of every phase and variety, some of a most startling character, living side by side. Preachers of all sects go about teaching and getting adherents, and at the very gates of the temples of gods, the Brahmins – to their credit said – allow even the materialists to stand and give forth their opinions.

Thus, India has always had this magnificent idea of religious freedom, and you must remember that freedom is the first condition of growth.

It is here that Indians build temples for Mohammedans and Christians; nowhere else. If you go to other countries and ask Mohammedans or people of other religions to build a temple for you, see how they will help. They will instead try to break down your temple and you too if they can.

Mind you, we have no quarrel with any religion in the world. We have each our *Ishta*. But when we see a man coming and saying, "This is the only way", and trying to force it on us in India, we have a word to say; we laugh at him. For such people who want to destroy their brothers because they seem to follow a different path towards God – for them to talk of love is absurd. Their love does not count for much. How can they preach of love who cannot bear another man to follow a different path from their own? If that is love, what is hatred?

India alone was to be, of all lands, the land of toleration and spirituality.... For one of the greatest sages that was ever born found out here in India, even at that distant time, which history cannot reach, and into whose gloom even tradition itself dares not peep – in that distant time the sage rose and declared: *ekam sat viprah bahudha vadanti* – "He who

exists is One; the sages call Him variously". This is one of the most
memorable sentences that was ever uttered, one of the grandest truths that
was ever discovered. And for us Hindus this truth has been the very
backbone of our national existence. For throughout the vistas of the
centuries of our national life, this one idea – *ekam sat viprah bahudha
vadanti* – comes down, gaining in volume and in fullness till it has
permeated the whole of our national existence, till it has mingled in our
blood, and has become one with us. We live that grand truth in every vein,
and our country has become the glorious land of religious tolerance. It is
here and here alone that they build temples and churches for the religions
which have come with the object of condemning our own religion.

If I ask myself what has been the cause of India's greatness, I answer,
because we have never conquered. That is our glory. You are hearing
everyday, and sometimes, I am sorry to say, from men who ought to know
better, denunciations of our religion, because it is not at all a conquering
religion. To my mind that is the argument why our religion is truer than
any other religion, because it never conquered, because it never shed blood,
because its mouth always shed on all, words of blessings, of peace, words
of love and sympathy. It is here and here alone that the ideals of toleration
were first preached. And it is here and here alone that toleration and
sympathy have become practical; it is theoretical in every other country; it
is here and here alone that the Hindu builds mosques for the Mohammedans
and churches for the Christians.

It has been proved to the world that holiness, purity and charity are
not the exclusive possessions of any church in the world and that every
system has provided men and women of the most exalted character. In the
face of this evidence, if anybody dreams of the exclusive survival of
his own religion and the destruction of the others, I pity him from the
bottom of my heart, and point out to him that upon the banner of every
religion will soon be written, in spite of resistance: "Help and not Fight",
"Assimilation and not Destruction", "Harmony and Peace and not
Dissension."

Spirituality – The Backbone of India

In religion lies the vitality of India, and so long as the Hindu race does
not forget the great inheritance of their forefathers, there is no power on
earth to destroy them.

I have been in the countries of the West, have travelled through many
lands of many races; and each race and each nation appears to me to have
a particular ideal – a prominent ideal running through its whole life; and
this ideal is the backbone of the national life. Not politics nor military power,
not commercial supremacy nor mechanical genius furnishes India with that
backbone, but religion; and religion alone is all that we have and mean to
have. Spirituality has been always in India.

Let others talk of politics, of the glory of acquisition of immense wealth poured in by trade, of the power and spread of commercialism, of the glorious fountain of physical liberty; but these the Hindu mind does not understand and does not want to understand. Touch him on spirituality, on religion, on God, and I assure you, the lowest peasant in India is better informed on these subjects than many a so-called philosopher in other lands.

Here we are, the Hindu race, whose vitality, whose life-principle, whose very soul, as it were, is in religion. I have seen a little of the world, travelling among nations one great ideal which forms the backbone, so to speak, of that race. With some it is politics, with others it is social culture; others again may have intellectual culture and so on for their national background. But this, our motherland has religion and religion alone for its basis, for its backbone, for the bedrock upon which the whole building of its life has been based.

Each nation has its own peculiar method of work. Some work through politics, some through social reforms, some through other things. With us, religion is the main activity along which we can move. The highest ideal in our Scriptures is the Impersonal, and would to God every one of us here were high enough to realise that Impersonal ideal: but as that cannot be, it is absolutely necessary for the vast majority of human beings to have a Personal ideal; and no nation can rise, can become great, can work at all, without enthusiastically coming under the banner of one of these great ideals in life. Political ideas, personages presenting political ideals, even social or commercial ideals would have no power in India. We want spiritual ideals before us, we want enthusiastically to gather round grand spiritual names. Our heroes must be spiritual.

Before flooding India with socialistic and political ideas, first deluge the land with spiritual ideas....

Renunciation and spirituality are the two great ideas of India and it is because India clings to these ideas that all her mistakes count for so little.

But mark you if you give up that spirituality, leaving it aside to go after the materialising civilisation of the West, the result will be that in three generations you will be an extinct race; because the backbone of the nation will be broken, the foundation upon which the national edifice has been built will be undermined and the result will be annihilation all round.

India is immortal if she persists in her search for God. But if she takes to politics and social conflict, she will die.

The main spring of the strength of every race lies in its spirituality, and the death of that race begins the day that spirituality wanes and materialism gains ground.

We Hindus have now been placed, under God's providence, in a very critical and responsible position. The nations of the West are coming to us for spiritual help. A great moral obligation rests on the sons of India to fully equip themselves for the work of enlightening the world on the problems of human existence.

India must Conquer the World with Spirituality

I am an imaginative man, and my idea, is the conquest of the whole world by the Hindu race. There have been great conquering races in the world. We also have been great conquerors. The story of our conquest has been described by that noble Emperor of India, Ashoka, as the conquest of religion and spirituality. Once more the world must be conquered by India. This is the dream of my life.... This is the great ideal before us, and everyone must be ready for it – the conquest of the whole world by India – nothing less than that, and we must all get ready for it, strain every nerve for it.... At the same time we must not forget that what I mean by the conquest of the world by spiritual thought is the sending out of the life-giving principles....

Gift of political knowledge can be made with the blast of trumpets and the march of cohorts. Gifts of secular knowledge and social knowledge can be made with fire or sword. But spiritual knowledge can only be given in silence like the dew that falls unseen and unheard, yet bringing into bloom masses of roses. This has been the gift of India to the world again and again.

We have to conquer the world. That we have to. India must conquer the world, and nothing less than that is my ideal. It may be very big, it may astonish many of you, but it is so. We must conquer the world or die. There is no other alternative. The sign of life is expansion; we must go out, expand, show life, or degrade, fester and die. There is no other alternative. Take either of these, either live or die....

Therefore we must go out, and the secret of life is to give and take. Are we to take always, to sit at the feet of the Westerners to learn everything, even religon? We can learn mechanism from them. We can learn many more things. But we have to teach them something, and that is our religion, that is our spirituality. For a complete civilisation, the world is waiting, waiting for the treasures to come out of India, waiting for the marvellous spiritual inheritance of our race, which through decades of degradation and misery, the nation has still clutched to her breast. Little do you know how much of hunger and thirst there is outside of India for these wonderful treasures of our forefathers. We talk here, we quarrel with each other, we laugh at and we ridicule everything sacred, till it has become almost a national vice to ridicule everything holy. Little do we understand the heart-pangs of millions waiting outside the walls, stretching forth their hands for a little sip of that nectar which our forefathers have preserved in this land of India. Therefore, we must go out, exchange our spirituality for anything they have to give us. For the marvels of the region of matter, we should give marvels of the spirit. We will not be students always but teachers also. There cannot be friendship without equality and there cannot be equality when one party is always the teacher and the other party sits always at his feet. If you want to become equal with the Englishman or the American, you will have plenty yet to teach to the world for centuries to come.

The whole world requires light. It is expectant! India alone has the light, not in magic, mummeries, and charlatanism, but in the teaching of the glories of the spirit of real religion – of the highest spiritual truth. That is why the Lord has preserved the race through all its vicissitudes unto the present-day. Now the time has come.

Up India, and conquer the world with your spirituality.

And I challenge anybody to show one single period of her national history when India was lacking in spiritual giants capable of moving the world. But her work is spiritual, and that cannot be done with blasts of war-trumpets or the march of cohorts. Her influence has always fallen upon the world like that of the gentle dew, unheard and scarcely marked, yet bringing into bloom the fairest flowers of the earth. This influence, being in its nature gentle, would have to wait for a fortunate combination of circumstances, to go out of the country into other lands, though it never ceased to work within the limits of its native land. As such, every educated person knows that whenever the empire-building Tartar or Persian or Greek or Arab brought this land in contact with the outside world, a mass of spiritual influence immediately flooded the world from here.

Political greatness or military power is never the mision of our race; it never was, and, mark my words, it never will be. But there has been the other mission given to us, which is to conserve, to preserve, to accumulate, as it were, into a dynamo, all the spiritual energy of the race, and that concentrated energy is to pour forth in a deluge on the world whenever circumstances are propitious. Let the Persian or the Greek, the Roman, the Arab, or the Englishman march his battalions, conquer the world, and link the different nations together, and the philosophy and spirituality of India is ever ready to flow along the new-made channels into the veins of the nations of the world. The Hindu's calm brain must pour out its own quota to give to the sum total of human progress. India's gift to the world is the light spiritual.

We never preached our thoughts with fire and sword.

Religion is Spiritual Realization

Religion is not talk or doctrines or theories, nor is it sectarianism. Religion cannot live in sects and societies. It is the relation between the soul and God; how can it be made into a society? It would then degenerateinto business, and where there are business and business principles in religion, spirituality dies. Religion does not consist in erecting temples or building churches or attending public worship. It is not to be found in books or in words or in lectures or in organisations. Religion consists in realization.

Religion is realisation, not talk, nor doctrine, nor theories, however beautiful they may be. It is being and becoming, not hearing or acknowledging. It is the whole soul's becoming changed into what it believes. That is religion.

Do not care for dogmas, or sects, or churches or temples; they count for little compared with the essence of existence in each man, which is spirituality, and the more this is developed in a man the more powerful is he for good. Earn that first, acquire that, and criticise no one. Show by your lives that religion does not mean words, or names, or sects, but that it means spiritual realization.

Temples and churches, books and forms, are simply the kindergarten of religion, to make the spiritual child strong enough to take the higher step. Religion is not in the doctrines or dogmas, nor in intellectual argumentation.

Religion is the manifestation of the Divinity already in man.

....It is realization in the heart of our hearts; it is touching God; it is feeling, realising that I am a spirit in relation with the universal Spirit and all its great manifestations.

Man must realize God, feel God, see God, talk to God. That is religion.

The first idea in this attempt to realize religion is that of renunciation. As far as we can, we must give up. Darkness and light, enjoyment of the world and enjoyment of God, will never go together. 'Ye cannot serve God and mammon'. Let people try if they will, and I have seen millions in every country who have tried; but after all it comes to nothing. If one word remains true in the saying, it is: give up everything for the sake of the Lord. This is a hard and long task, but you can begin here and now. Bit by bit we must go towards it.

It is only when the desire to prevent all such bondage to the senses arises that religion dawns in the heart of man. Thus we see that the whole scope of religion is to prevent man from falling into the bondage of the senses and to help him to assert his freedom.

The mind is not to be ruffled by vain arguments, because argument will not help us to know God. It is a question of fact, and not of argument.... Religion is a question of fact, not of talk. We have to analyse our own souls and to find what is there. That is religion. No amount of talk will make religion. So the question of whether there is God or not can never be proved by argument, for the arguments are as much on one side as on the other. But if there is a God, He is in our own hearts. Have you ever seen Him?

This is one great idea to learn and to hold on to, this idea of realisation. This turmoil and fight and difference in religions will only cease when we understand that religion is not in books, and temples. It is an actual perception. Only the man who has actually perceived God and soul, has religion.... Mere intellectual assent does not make us religious.... We often consider a man religious who can talk well. But this is not religion....

Religion comes when that actual realisation in our own soul begins. That will be the dawn of religion.

The end of all religions is the realisation of God....

There may be a thousand different points. There may be a thousand different radii, but they all converge at the one centre, and that is the realisation of God. Something behind this world of sense, world of eternal eating and drinking and talking nonsense, this world of false shadows and selfishness, there is that beyond all books, beyond all creeds, beyond the vanities of this world – and that is the realisation of God within oneself. A man may believe in all the churches in the world; he may carry in his head all the sacred books ever written, he may baptise himself in all the rivers of the earth – still if he has no perception of God, I would class him with the rankest atheist. And a man may have never entered a church or a mosque, nor performed any ceremony; but if he realizes God within himself, and is thereby lifted above the vanities of the world, that man is a holy man, a saint, call him what you will.... I will add that it is good to be born in a church, but it is bad to die there. It is good to be born a child, but bad to remain a child. Churches, ceremonies, symbols, are good for children; but when the child is grown-up, he must burst, either the church or himself.

This is the watchword of Vedanta – realise religion, no talking will do.

Man is to become divine by realising the divine. Idols or temples or churches or books are only the support, the helps of his spiritual childhood: but on and on he must progress.

Cleanse the mind, this is all of religion.

Religion to Suit the Multitude

There are thousands and thousands of varieties of minds and inclinations. A thorough generalisation of them is impossible, but for our practical purposes it is sufficient to have them characterised into four classes.

First there is the active man, the worker; he wants to work, and there is tremendous energy in his muscles and his nerves. His aim is to work; to build hospitals, do charitable deeds, make streets, to plan and to organise. Then there is the emotional man, who loves the sublime and the beautiful to an excessive degree. He loves to think of the beautiful, to enjoy the aesthetic side of nature, and adore Love and the God of Love. He loves with his whole heart the great souls of all times, the prophets of religions, and the Incarnations of God on earth. Then there is the mystic, whose mind wants to analyse its own self, to understand the workings of the human mind, what the forces are that are working inside, and how to know, manipulate, and obtain control over them. This is the mystical mind. Then there is the philosopher, who wants to weigh everything and use his intellect even beyond the possibilities of all human philosophy.

Now a religion, to satisfy the largest proportion of mankind, must be able to supply food for all these various types of minds; and where this capability is wanting, the existing sects all become one-sided.

What I want to propagate is a religion that will be equally acceptable to all minds; it must be equally philosophic, equally emotional, equally mystic, and equally conducive to action.... And this combination will be the ideal, the nearest approach to a universal religion. Would to God that all men were so constituted that in their minds all these elements of philosophy, mysticism, emotion and work were equally present in full. That is the ideal, my ideal of a perfect man. Everyone who has only one or two of these elements of character, I consider "one-sided"; and this world is almost full of such one-sided men with knowledge of that one road only in which they move; and everything else is dangerous and horrible to them. To become harmoniously balanced in all these four directions is my ideal of religion.

If there is ever to be a universal religion, it must be one which will have no location in place or time, which will be infinite like the God it will preach...., which in its catholicity will embrace in its infinite arms and find a place for every human being from the lowest grovelling savage not far removed from the brute to the highest man towering by the virtues of his head and heart almost above humanity, making society stand in awe of him and doubt his human nature...., which will have no place for persecution or intolerance in its polity, which will recognise divinity in every man and woman, and whose whole scope, whose whole force will be centred in aiding humanity to realise its own true, divine nature.

Fourfold Methods of Spiritual Realization

Our main problem is to be free. It is evident then that until we realise ourselves as the Absolute, we cannot attain to deliverance. Yet there are various ways of attaining to this realization. These methods have the generic name of 'yoga' (to join, to join ourselves to Reality). These yogas, though divided into various groups, can principally be classified into four, and as each is only a method leading to the realization of the Absolute, they are suited to different temperaments. Now it must be remembered that it is not that the assumed man becomes the real man or Absolute. There is no becoming with the Absolute. It is ever free, ever perfect; but the ignorance that has covered its nature for a time is to be removed. Therefore, the whole scope of all yogas is to clear this ignorance – and to allow the Atman to manifest its own nature.

We classify them in the following way, under four heads:

1) Karmayoga : The manner in which a man realizes his own divinity through work and duty.

2) Bhaktiyoga : The realization of the divinity through devotion to and love of a Personal God.

3) Rajayoga : The realization of the divinity through the control of mind.

4) Jnanayoga : The realization of man's own divinity through knowledge.

No one of these yogas gives up reason; no one of them asks you to be hoodwinked or to deliver your reason into the hands of priests of any type whatsoever. Not one of them asks that you should give your allegiance to any super-human messenger. Each one of them tells you to cling to your reason, to hold fast to it.

It is imperative that all these various yogas should be carried out in practice; mere theories about them will not do any good. First we have to hear about them; then we have to think about them. We have to reason the thoughts out, impress them on our minds, and meditate on them, realize them, until at last they become our whole life. No longer will religion remain a bundle of ideas or the theories, or an intellectual assent; it will enter into our very self.

Spiritual Science to Bring out the Perfect Man

What you call personal magnetism of the man, that is what goes out and impresses you.... It is the real man, the personality of the man, that runs through us. Our actions are but effects. Actions must come when the man is there; the effect is bound to follow the cause. The ideal of all education, all training, should be this man-making.... The end and aim of training is to make the man grow. The man who influences, who throws his magic, as it were, upon his fellow beings is a dynamo of power, and when that man is ready, he can do anything and everything he likes; that personality put upon anything will make it work.... The science of yoga claims that it has discovered the laws which develop this personality, and by proper attention to those law and methods, each one can grow and strengthen his personality.

The utility of this science is to bring out the perfect man and not let him wait for ages, just a plaything in the hands of the physical world, like a log of drift-wood carried from wave to wave and tossing about in the ocean. This science wants you to be strong, to take the work in your own hands, instead of leaving it in the hands of nature, and get beyond this little life. That is the great idea.

Intense Activity With Eternal Calmness

A man used to solitude, if brought in contact with surging whirlpool of the world, will be crushed by it; just as the fish that lives in the deep sea water, as soon as it is brought to the surface, breaks into pieces, deprived of the weight of water on it that had kept it together. Can a man who has been used to the turmoil and the rush of life live at ease if he comes to a quiet place? He suffers and perchance may lose his mind. The ideal man is he who, in the midst of greatest silence and solitude, finds the intensest activity, and in the midst of the intensest activity finds the silence and solitude of the desert. He has learnt the secret of restraint, he has controlled himself. He goes through the streets of a big city with all its traffic, and his mind is as calm as if he were in a cave, where not a sound could reach him; and he is intensely working all the time.

The doctrine which stands out luminously in every page of the *Gita* (the best commentary we have on the Vedanta philosophy) is intense activity, but in the midst of it, eternal calmness. This is the secret of work, to attain which is the goal of the Vedanta. Inactivity, as we understand it in the sense of passivity, certainly cannot be the goal. Were it so, then the walls around us would be the most intelligent; they are inactive. Clods of earth, stumps of trees, would be the greatest sages in the world; they are inactive. Nor does inactivity become activity when it is combined with passion. Real activity which is the goal of Vedanta, is combined with eternal calmness, the calmness which cannot be ruffled, the balance of the mind which is never disturbed, whatever happens. And we all know from our experience in life that that is the best attitude for work.

Self-abnegation – The Centre of Morality

What is the watchword of all ethical codes? "Not I, but thou".

The happiest moments we ever know are when we entirely forget our selves.

Here are two Sanskrit words. The one *pravrtti* which means revolving towards, and the other is *nivrtti,* which means revolving away. The 'revolving towards' is what we call the world, the 'I and mine', it includes all those things which are always enriching that 'me' by wealth and money and power, and name and fame, and which are of a grasping nature, always tending to accumulate everything in one centre, that centre being 'myself. That is the *pravrtti,* the natural tendency of every human being; taking everything from everywhere and heaping it around one centre, that centre being man's own sweet self. When this tendency begins to break, then it is *nivrtti* or 'going away from', then begin morality and religion. Both *pravrtti* and *nivrtti* are of the nature of work; the former is evil work and the latter is good work. The *nivrtti* is the fundamental basis of all morality and all religion, and the very perfection of it is entire self-abnegation, readiness to sacrifice mind and body and everything for another being.... This is the highest result of good works. Although a man has not studied a single system of philosophy, although he does not believe in any God and never has believed, although he has not prayed even once in his whole life, if the simple power of good actions has brought him to that state where he is ready to give up his life and all else for others, he has arrived at the same point to which the religious man will come through his prayers and the philosopher through his knowledge. Here it is not at all any question of creed or doctrine – even men, who are very much opposed to all religious ideas, when they see one of these acts of complete self-sacrifice, feel that they must revere it. One idea stands out as the centre of all ethical systems, expressed in various forms, namely doing good to others. The guiding motive of mankind should be charity towards men, charity towards all animals. But these are all various expressions of that eternal truth that 'I am the universe; this universe is one'. Or else, where is the reason? Why should I do good to my fellowmen? Why should I do good to others? What compels me? It is sympathy, the feeling of sameness everywhere. The hardest hearts feel sympathy for other beings sometimes. Even the man who gets frightened if he is told that this assumed individuality is really a delusion, that it is ignoble to try to cling to this apparent individuality, that very man will tell you that extreme self-abnegation is the centre of morality. And what is perfect self-abnegation? It means the abnegation of this apparent self, the abnegation of all selfishness. This idea of 'me' and 'mine' – *ahamkara* and *mamata* – is the result of past superstition, and the more this present self passes away, the more the real Self becomes manifest. This is true self-abnegation, the centre, the basis, the gist of all moral teaching; and whether man knows it or not, the whole world is slowly going towards it, practising it more or less. Only, the vast majority of mankind are doing it unconsciously. Let them do it consciously. Let them make the sacrifice, knowing that this 'me' and 'mine' is not the real Self, but only a limitation.

Man is not what He Appears to be

The Real Man is one and infinite, the Omnipresent Spirit. And the apparent man is only a limitation of that Real Man. The apparent man, however great he may be, is only a dim reflection of the Real Man, who is beyond. The Real Man, the spirit, being beyond cause and effect, not bound by time and space, must therefore be free. He was never bound, and could never be bound. The apparent man, the reflection, is limited by time, space, and causation, and is therefore bound. He appears to be bound, but really not. This is the reality in our souls, this omnipresence, this spiritual nature, this infinity. Every soul is infinite, therefore there is no question of birth and death.... The body is not the Real Man, neither is the mind, for the mind waxes and wanes. It is the Spirit beyond, which alone can live for ever.... So this infinite, unchangeable, immovable, absolute is the Real Man. Our reality, therefore, consists in the universal, and not in the limited. These are old delusions, however comfortable they are, to think that we are limited beings, constantly changing. People are frightened when they are told that they are Universal Being, everywhere present. Through everything you work, through every foot you move, through every lip you talk, through every heart you feel.... They will again and again ask you if they are not going to keep their individuality. What is individuality

I should like to see.... There is no individuality except in the Infinite; that is the only condition which does not change. Everything else is in a constant state of flux.... We are not individuals yet. We are struggling towards individuality and that is the Infinite; that is, the real nature of man. He alone lives whose life is in the whole universe, and the more we concentrate our lives on limited things, the faster we go towards death. Those moments alone we live, when our lives are in the universe, in others; and living this little life is death, simply death, and that is why the fear of death comes. The fear of death can only be conquered when man realises that so long there is one life in this universe, he is living. When he can say, "I am in everything, in everybody, I am in all lives, I am the universe", then alone comes the state of fearlessness.... It is only the Spirit that is the Individual; because it is infinite; no infinity can be divided, infinity cannot be broken into pieces. It is the same one, undivided unit forever, and this is the individual man, the Real Man. The apparent man is merely a struggle to express, to manifest, this individuality which is beyond, and evolution is not in the Spirit.... One glimpse of that infinite reality which is behind, but one spark of that infinite fire that is All, represents the present man; the Infinite is his true nature.

The Innate Divinity is Imperishable

The more I live, the more I become convinced everyday that every human being is divine. In no man or woman, however vile, does that divinity die. Only he or she does not know how to reach it, and is waiting for the Truth. ....Man is divine, that divinity is our nature. Whatever else comes is a mere super-imposition, as the Vedanta calls it. Something has been superimposed, but that divine nature never dies. In the most degraded, as well as in the most saintly, it is ever present. It has to be called out, and it will work itself out. We have to ask and it will manifest itself. The people of old knew that fire lived in the flint and in dry wood but friction was necessary to call it out. So this fire of freedom and purity is the nature of every soul, and not a quality, because qualities can be acquired and therefore lost. The soul is one with Freedom, and the soul is one with Existence, and the soul is one with Knowledge. The *Sat-Chit-Ananda* – Existence-Knowledge-Bliss Absolute – is the nature, the birthright of the soul, and all manifestations that we see are Its expressions, dimly or brightly manifesting Itself. Even death is but a manifestation of that Real Existence. Birth and death, life and decay, degeneration and regeneration, are all manifestations of that Oneness. So, knowledge, however it manifests itself, either as ignorance or as learning, is but the manifestation of that same *Chit*, the essence of knowledge; the difference is only in degree, and not in kind. The difference in knowledge between the lowest worm that crawls under our feet and the highest genius that the world may produce, is only of degree, and not of kind. The Vedantin thinker boldly says that the enjoyments in this life, even the most degraded joys, are but manifestations of that One Divine Bliss, the Essence of the Soul.

God – The One Impersonal Principle

Today God is being abandoned by world because He does not seem to be doing enough for the world. So they say: Of what good is He? Should we look upon God as a mere municipal authority?

(In the Upanishads) the personality of God vanishes, the impersonality comes. God is no more a person, no more a human being, however magnified and exaggerated, who rules this universe, but He has become an embodied principle in every being, immanent in the whole universe. It would be illogical to go from the Personal God to the Impersonal, and at the same time to leave man as a person. So the personal man is broken down and man as a principle is built up. The person is only a phenomenon, the principle is behind it. Thus from both sides, simultaneously, we find breaking down of personalities and the approach towards principles, the Personal God approaching the Impersonal, the personal man approaching the Impersonal Man. Then come the succeeding stages, of the gradual convergence of the two advancing lines of the impersonal God and Impersonal Man. And the Upanishads embody the stages through which these two lines at last become one, and the last word of each Upanishad is, "Thou art that". There is but One Eternally Blissful Principle, and that One is manifesting Itself as all this variety.

....Taking for granted that there is but One Impersonal Principle which is manifesting Itself in all these manifold forms, how is it that the One becomes many?.... How is it that this One Principle becomes manifold? And the answer, as we have seen, the best answer that India has produced, is the theory of *maya* which says that it really has not become manifold, that it really has not lost any of its real nature. Manifoldness is only apparent. Man is only apparently a person, but in reality he is the impersonal Being. God is a person only apparently, but really He is the Impersonal Being.

An Integrated Personality

We want harmony, not one-sided development. And it is possible to have the intellect of a Shankara with the heart of Buddha. I hope we shall all struggle to attain to that blessed combination.

What we want is to see the man who is harmoniously developed.... Great in heart, great in mind (great in deed).... We want the man whose heart feels intensely the miseries and sorrows of the world.... And (we want) the man who not only can feel but can find the meaning of things, who delves deeply into the heart of nature and understanding. (We want) the man who will not even stop there; (but) who wants to work out (the feeling and the meaning by actual deeds). Such a combination of head, heart and hand is what we want. There are many teachers in this world, but you will find that most of them are one-sided. (One) sees the glorious mid-day sun of the intellect (and) sees nothing else. Another hears the beautiful music of love and can hear nothing else. Another is (immersed) in activity and has neither time to feel, nor time to think. Why not (have) the giant who is equally active, equally knowing and equally loving? Is it impossible? Certainly not. This is the man of the future, of whom there are (only a) few at present. (The number of such will increase) until the whole world is humanized.

My Master's message to mankind is, 'Be spiritual and realize the truth for yourself....' His principle was: first form character, first earn spirituality, and results will come of themselves....

A man may be intellectual or devotional or mystic or active; the various religions represent one or the other of these types. Yet it is possible to combine all the four in one man, and this is what future humanity is going to do. That was his idea....

The old teachers were rather one-sided, while the teaching of this new teacher is that the best of yoga, devotion, knowledge and work must be combined now so as to form a new society.... The older ones were no doubt good, but this is the new religion of this age – the synthesis of yoga, knowledge, devotion and work – the propagation of knowledge and devotion to all, down to the very lowest, without distinction of age or sex.

Such a unique personality, such a synthesis of the utmost of jnana, yoga, bhakti and karma, has never before appeared among mankind. The life of Sri Ramakrishna proves that the greatest breadth, the highest catholicity and the utmost integrity can exist side by side in the same individual, and that society also can be constituted like that; for society is nothing but an aggregate of individuals.

He is the true disciple and follower of Sri Ramakrishna whose character is perfect and all-sided like this. The formation of such a perfect character is the ideal of this age, and everyone should strive for that alone.

God, though everywhere, can be known to us in and through human character. No character was ever so perfect as Ramakrishna, and that should be the centre around which we ought to rally.... My supreme good fortune is that I am his servant through life after life. A single word of his is to me far weightier than the Vedas and the Vedanta. Oh, I am the servant of the servants of his servants.

Today the name of Sri Ramakrishna Paramahamsa is known all over India by its millions of people. Nay, the power of that man has spread beyond India, and if there has been a word of truth, a word of spirituality, that I have spoken anywhere in this world, I owe it to my Master; only the mistakes are mine.

The Ideal of Education

Education is the manifestation of the perfection already in man.

The ideal of all education, all training, should be this man-making. But, instead of that, we are always trying to polish up the outside. What use in polishing up the outside when there is no inside? The end and aim of all training is to make the man grow. The man who influences, who throws his magic, as it were, upon his fellow beings, is a dynamo of power, and when that man is ready, he can do anything and everything he likes; that personality put upon anything will make it work.

Knowledge is inherent in man, no knowledge comes from outside; it is all inside. What we say a man 'knows', should in strict psychological language, be what he 'discovers', or 'unveils'. What a man 'learns' is really what he 'discovers' by taking the cover off his own soul, which is a mine of infinite knowledge. We say Newton discovered gravitation. Was it sitting anywhere in a corner waiting for him? It was in his own mind; the time came and he found it out. All knowledge that the world has ever received comes from the mind; the infinite library of the universe is in your own mind. The external world is only the suggestion, the occasion, which sets you to study your own mind. The falling of an apple gave the suggestion to Newton, and he studied his own mind. He rearranged all his previous links of thought in his mind and discovered a new link among them, which we call the law of gravitation. It was not in the apple nor in anything in the centre of the earth.

All knowledge therefore, secular or spiritual, is in the human mind. In many cases it is not discovered, but remains covered, and when the covering is being slowly taken off, we say 'we are learning', and the advance of knowledge is made by this process of uncovering. The man from whom this veil is being lifted is the more knowing man and the man upon whom it lies thick is ignorant; the man from whom it has entirely gone is all-knowing, omniscient. Like fire in a piece of flint, knowledge exists in the mind; suggestion is the friction which brings it out. All knowledge and all power are within. What we call powers, secrets of Nature, and force are all within. All knowledge comes from the human soul. Man manifests knowledge, discovers it within himself, which is pre-existing, through eternity.

No one was ever really taught by another. Each of us has to teach himself. The external teacher offers only the suggestion which rouses the internal teacher to work, to understand things. Then things will be made clearer to us by our own power of perception and thought, and we shall realize them in our own souls. The whole of the big banyan tree which covers acres of ground was in the little seed which was perhaps no bigger than one-eighth of a mustard seed. All that mass of energy was there confined. The gigantic intellect, we know, lies coiled up in the protoplasmic cell. It may seem like a paradox but it is true. Each one of us has come out of one protoplasmic cell and all the powers we possess were coiled up there. You cannot say they came from food, for if you heap up food mountains high, what power comes out of it? The energy was there potentially no doubt, but still there. So is infinite power in the soul of man whether he knows it or not. Its manifestation is only a question of being conscious of it.

The light Divine within is obscured in most people. It is like a lamp in a cask of iron; no gleam of light can shine through. Gradually, by purity and unselfishness, we can make the obscuring medium less and less dense, until at last it becomes as transparent as glass. Sri Ramakrishna was like the iron cask transformed into a glass cask, through which can be seen the inner light as it is.

You cannot teach a child any more than you can grow a plant. The plant develops its own nature. The child also teaches itself. But you can help it to go forward in its own way. What you can do is not of a positive nature but negative. You can take away the obstacles, and knowledge comes out of its own nature. Loosen the soil a little, so that it may come out easily. Put a hedge round it; see that it is not killed by anything. You can supply the growing seed with the materials for the making up of its body, bringing to it the earth, the water, the air that it wants. And there your work stops. It will take all that it wants by its own nature. So with the education of the child. A child educates itself. The teacher spoils everything by thinking that he is teaching. Within man is all knowledge, and it requires only an awakening, and that much is the work of the teacher. We have only to do so much for the boys that they may learn to apply their own intellect to the proper use of their hands, legs, ears and eyes.

That system which aims at educating our boys in the same manner as that of the man who battered his ass, being advised that it could thereby be turned into a horse, should be abolished. Owing to undue domination exercised by the parents, our boys do not get free scope for growth. In every one there are infinite tendencies which require proper scope for satisfaction. Violent attempts at reform always end by retarding reform. If you do not allow one to become a lion, one will become a fox.

We should give positive ideas. Negative thoughts only weaken men. Do you not find that where parents are constantly taxing their sons to read and write, telling them that they will never learn anything and calling them fools and so forth, the latter do actually turn out to be so in many cases? If you speak kind words to them, and encourage them, they are bound to improve in time. If you can give them positive ideas, people will grow up to be men and learn to stand on their own legs. In language and literature, in poetry and arts, in everything we must point out not the mistakes that people are making in their thoughts and actions, but the way in which they will be able to do these things better. The teaching must be modified according to the needs of the taught. Past lives have moulded our tendencies, and so give to the pupil according to his tendencies. Take everyone where he standsand push him forward. We have seen how Sri Ramakrishna would encourage even those whom we considered worthless and change the very course of their lives thereby! He never destroyed a single man's special inclinations. He gave words of hope and encouragement even to the most degraded of persons and lifted them up.

Education is not the amount of information that is put into your brain and runs riot there, undigested all your life. We must have life-building, man-making, character-making assimilation of ideas. If you have assimilated five ideas and made them your life and character, you have more education than any man who got by heart a whole library. If education were identical with information, the libraries would be the greatest sages in the world and encyclopaedias the rishis.

Getting by heart the thoughts of others in a foreign language and stuffing your brain with them and taking some university degrees, you consider your- self educated. Is this education? What is the goal of your education? Either a clerkship, or being a lawyer, or at the most a Deputy Magistrate, which is another form of clerkship – isn't that all? What good will it do you or the country at large? Open your eyes and see what a piteous cry for food is rising in the land of Bharata proverbial for its food. Will your education fulfil this want? You consider a man educated if only he can pass examinations and deliver good lectures. The education that does not help the common mass of people to equip themselves for the struggle for life, which does not bring out strength of character, a spirit of philanthropy and the courage of a lion – is it worth the name? Real education is that which enables one to stand on his own legs. The education that you are receiving now in schools and colleges is only making you a race of dyspeptics. You are working like machines only, and living a jellyfish existence.

We want that education by which character is formed, strength of mind is increased, the intellect is expanded and by which one can stand on one's own feet. What we need is to study, independent of foreign control, different branches of the knowledge that is our own; and with it the English language and Western science: we need technical education and all else that will develop industries, so that men instead of seeking for service may earn enough to provide for themselves and save against a rainy day.

The end of all education, all training, should be man-making. The end and aim of all training is to make the man grow. The training by which the current and expression of will are brought under control and become fruitful, is called education. What our country now wants are muscles of iron and nerves of steel, gigantic wills which nothing can resist, which can penetrate into the mysteries and secrets of the universe and will accomplish their purpose in any fashion, even if it meant going down to the bottom of the ocean, meeting death face to face. It is man-making religion that we want. It is man-making theories that we want. It is man-making education all round that we want.

The old institutions of living with the guru and such like systems of imparting education are needed. What we want are Western science coupled with Vedanta, *brahmacharya* as the guiding motto, and also *shraddha* and faith in one's own self.

My idea of education is personal contact with the teacher – *gurugrhavasa;* without the personal life of the teacher, there would be no education. One should live from his very boyhood with one whose character is a blazing fire and should have before him a living example of the highest teaching.

There is only one method by which to attain knowledge, that which is called concentration. The very essence of education is concentration of mind. From the lowest man to the highest yogi, all have to use the same method to attain knowledge. The chemist who works in his laboratory concentrates all the powers of his mind, brings them into one focus, and throws them on the elements; the elements stand analysed, and thus his knowledge comes. The astronomer concentrates the powers of his mind and brings them into one focus; and he throws them on to objects through his telescope, and stars and systems roll forward and give up their secrets to him. So it is in every case: with the professor in his chair, the student with his book, with every man who is working to know.

The more the power of concentration, the greater the knowledge that is acquired. Even the lowest shoeblack, if he gives more concentration, will black shoes better. The cook with concentration will cook a meal all the better. In making money, or in worshipping God, or in doing anything, the stronger the power of concentration, the better will that thing be done. This is the one call, the one knock, which opens the gates of Nature, and lets in floods of light.

Ninety per cent of thought-force is wasted by the ordinary human being and therefore he is constantly committing blunders. The trained man or mind never makes a mistake. The main difference between men and the animals is the difference in their power of concentration. An animal has very little power of concentration. Those who have trained animals find much difficulty in the fact that the animal is constantly forgetting what is told him. He cannot concentrate his mind upon anything for a long time. Herein is the difference between man and the animals. This difference in their power of concentration also constitutes the difference between man and man. Compare the lowest with the highest man. The difference is in the degree of concentration. All success in any line of work is the result of this power. High achievements, in arts, music, etc., are the result of concentration. When the mind is concentrated and turned back on itself, all within us will be servants not our masters. The Greeks applied their concentration to the external world and the result was perfection in art, literature etc. The Hindu concentrated on the internal world, upon theunseen realms in the self and developed the science of yoga. The world is ready to give up its secrets if we only know how to knock, how to give the necessary blow. The strength and force of the blow comes through concentration.

The power of concentration is the only key to the treasure-house of knowledge. In the present state of our body we are much distracted, and the mind is frittering away its energies upon a hundred things. As soon as I try to calm my thoughts and concentrate my mind upon any one object of knowledge, thousands of undesired impulses rush into the brain, thousands of thoughts rush into the mind and disturb it. How to check it and bring the mind under control is the whole subject of study in rajayoga. The practice of meditation leads to mental concentration.

To me the very essence of education is concentration of mind, not the collection of facts. If I have to do my education once again, I would not study facts at all. I would develop the power of concentration and detachment, and then with perfect instrument collect facts at will.

How has all the knowledge in the world been gained but by the concentration of the powers of the mind? The world is ready to give up its secrets if we only know how to knock, how to give it the necessary blow. The strength and force of the blow come through concentration. There is no limit to the power of the human mind. The more concentrated it is, the more power is brought to bear on one point; that is the secret.

Power comes to him who observes unbroken *brahmacharya* for a period of twelve years.

Complete continence gives great intellectual power. Controlled desire leads to the highest results. Transform the sexual energy into spiritual energy. The stronger this force, the more can be done with it. Only powerful current of water can do hydraulic mining. It is owing to want of continence that everything is on the brink of ruin in our country. By observance of strict *brahmacharya* all learning can be mastered in a very short time: one acquires an unfailing memory of what one hears or knows but once. The chaste brain has tremendous energy and gigantic will power. Without chastity there can be no spiritual strength. Continence gives wonderful control over mankind. The spiritual leaders of men have been very continent and this is what gave them power.

Every boy should be trained to practise absolute *brahmacharya* and then, and then alone faith and *shraddha* will come. Chastity in thought, word and deed always and in all conditions is what is called *brahmacharya*. Unchaste imagination is as bad as unchaste action. The *brahmacharin* must be pure in thought, word and deed.

Universal Religion

At the beginning of this century (the nineteenth century) it was almost feared that religion was at an end. Under the tremendous sledge-hammer blows of scientific research old superstitions were crumbling away like masses of porcelain. Those to whom religion meant only a bundle of creeds and meaningless ceremonials were at their wits' end. For a time it seemed inevitable that the surging tide of agnosticism and materialism would sweep all before it. Many thought the case hopeless and the cause of religion lost once and for ever.

But the tide has turned and to the rescue has come what? The study of comparative religions. By the study of different religions we find that in essence they are one.

The proof of one religion depends on the proof of all the rest. For instance, if I have six fingers, and no one else has, you may well say that it is abnormal. The same reasoning may be applied to the arguments that only one religion is true and others are false. One religion only, like one set of six fingers in the world, would be unnatural. We see, therefore, that if one religion is true, all others must be true. There are differences in non-essentials, but in essentials they are all one. If my five fingers are true, they prove that your five fingers are true too.

I find in the study of the various religions of the world that there are three different stages of ideas with regard to the soul or God. In the first place, all religions admit that, apart from the body which perishes, there is a certain part of something which does not change like the body, a part that is immutable, eternal, and never dies. We – the essential part of us – never had a beginning and will never have an end. And above us all, above this eternal nature, there is another eternal Being without end – God. People talk about the beginning of the world, the beginning of man. The word 'beginning' simply means the beginning of the cycle. That which has a beginning must have an end. Wherever the beginning of creation is mentioned, it means the beginning of a cycle. Your body will meet with death, but your soul, never.

Along with the ideas of the soul we find another group of ideas in regard to perfection. The soul in itself is perfection. The New Testament admits man as perfect at the beginning. Man made himself impure by his own actions. But he is to regain his old nature, his pure nature. Some speak of these things in allegories, fables, and symbols. But when we begin to analyse these statements we find that they all teach that the human soul is in its very nature perfect, and that man is to regain that original purity. How? By knowing God.

We find that all the religions teach the eternity of the soul, as well as that its lustre has been dimmed, but that its primitive purity is to be regained by the knowledge of God. What is the idea of God in these different religions? The primary idea of God was very vague. The most ancient nations had different deities – sun, earth, fire, water. Among the ancient Jews we find a number of these gods ferociously fighting with each other. Then we find Elohim whom the Jews and the Babylonians worshipped. We next find one God standing supreme. But the idea differed according to different tribes. They each asserted that their God was the greatest. These races tried to prove it by fighting. The one that could do the best fighting proved thereby that its God was the greatest. These races were more or less savage. But gradually better and better ideas took the place of the old ones. All those old ideas are gone or going into the lumber room. All those religions were the outgrowth of centuries, not one fell from the skies. Each had to be worked out bit by bit.

Next came the monotheistic ideas; belief in one God who is omnipotent and omniscient, the one God of the universe. This one God is extra-cosmic; he lives in the heavens. He is invested with the gross conceptions of his originators: he had a right side and a left side, and a bird in his hand, and so on and so forth. But one thing we find, that the tribal gods have disappeared for ever and the one God of the universe has taken their place – the God of gods. Still he is only an extra cosmic God. He is unapproachable; nothing can come near him. In the new Testament it is taught, 'Our Father who art in heaven' – God in the heavens separated from man. We are living on earth, and he is living in heaven.

Farther on we find the teaching that he is a God immanent in nature; He is not only God in heaven, but on earth, too. He is the God in us.

In the Hindu philosophy we find a stage of the same proximity of God to us. But we do not stop there. There is the non-dualistic stage, in which man realizes that the God he has been worshipping is not only the Father in heaven and on earth but that 'I and my Father are one'. He realizes in his soul that he is God himself, only a lower expression of Him. All that is real in me is He; all that is real in Him is I. The gulf between God and man is thus bridged. Thus we find how, by knowing God, we find the kingdom of heaven within us.

In the first, or dualistic stage, man knows he is a little personal soul – John, James, or Tom – and he says, "I will be John, James, or Tom to all eternity and never anything else". As well might the murderer come along and say, "I will remain a murderer forever." But as time goes on Tom vanishes and goes back to the original pure Adam.

The different stages of growth are absolutely necessary to the attainment of purity and perfection. The varying systems of religion are at bottom founded on the same ideas. Jesus says the kingdom of heaven is within you. Again he says, 'Our Father who art in heaven'. How do you reconcile the two sayings? In this way. He was talking to the uneducated masses when he said the latter, the masses who were uneducated in religion. It was necessary to speak to them in their own language. The masses want concrete ideas, something the senses can grasp. A man may be the greatest philosopher in the world but a child in religion. When a man has developed a high state of spirituality, he can understand that the kingdom of heaven is within him.

Thus we see that the apparent contradictions and perplexities in every religion mark but different stages of growth. And as such we have no right to blame anyone for his religion. There are stages of growth in which forms and symbols are necessary; they are the language that the souls in the stage can understand.

The next idea that I want to bring to you is that religion does not consist in doctrines or dogmas. It is not what you read or what dogmas you believe that is of importance, but what you realise. 'Blessed are the pure in spirit, for they shall see God,' yes, in this life. And that is salvation. There are those who teach that this can be gained by the mumbling of words. But no great Master ever taught that external forms were necessary for salvation. The power of attaining it is within ourselves. We live and move in God. Creeds and sects have their parts to play but they are for children, they last but temporarily. Books never make religions, but religions make books. We must not forget that. No book ever created a soul. We must never forget that. The end of all religions is the realizing of God in the soul. That is the one universal religion.

If there is one universal truth in all religions, I place it here, in realising God. Ideals and methods may differ, but that is the central point.

As soon as a man stands up and says he is right or his church is right and all others are wrong, he is himself all wrong. He does not know that upon the proof of all the others depends the proof of his own.

So far as they are not exclusive, I see that the sects and creeds are all mine, they are all grand. They are all helping man towards the one real religion. I do not deprecate the existence of sects in the world. Would to God there were twenty million more, for the more there are, the greater field there will be for selection. What I do object to is trying to fit one religion to every case. Though all religions are essentially the same, they must have the varieties of form produced by dissimilar circumstances among different nations. We must each have our own individual religion – individual as far as the externals go.

What then do I mean by the ideal of a universal religion? I do not mean any one universal philosophy, or any universal mythology, or any one universal ritual, held alike by all; for I know that this world must go on working wheel within wheel, this intricate mass of machinery, most complex, most wonderful.

What can we do then? We can make it run smoothly, we can lessen the friction, we can grease the wheels, as it were. How? By recognizing the natural necessity of variation. Just as we have recognised unity by our very nature, so must we also recognise variation. We must learn that truth may be expressed in a hundred thousand ways, and that each of these ways is true as far as it goes.

We must learn that the same thing can be viewed from a hundred different standpoints, and yet be the same thing. Take, for instance, the sun. Suppose a man standing on the earth looks at the sun when it rises in the morning, it is a big ball. Suppose, he starts on a journey towards the sun and takes a camera with him, taking photographs at every stage of his journey, until he reaches the sun. The photographs of each stage will seem to be different from those of the other stages: in fact when he gets back, he brings with him so many different suns, as it would appear; and yet we know that the same sun, was photographed by the man at the different stages of his progress.

Even so it is with the Lord. Through high philosophy or law, through the most refined ritualism or errant fetishism, every sect, every soul, every nation, every religion, consciously or unconsciously, is struggling upward, towards God; every vision of truth that man has, is a vision of Him and of none else. Suppose we all go with vessels in our hands to fetch water from a lake. One has a cup, another a jar, another a bucket and so forth, and we all fill our vessels. The water in each case takes the form of vessel carried by each of us. He who brought the cup, has the water in the form of a cup; he who brought the jar – his water is in the shape of a jar, and so forth, but in every case, water and nothing but water, is in the vessel.

So it is in the case of religion; our minds are like these vessels, and each one of us is trying to arrive at the realization of God. God is like that water filling these different vessels, and in each vessel, the vision of God comes in the form of the vessel. Yet, He is One. He is God in every case. This is the only recognition of universality that we can get.

Socialism with a Spiritual Basis

Each individual has to work out his own solution; there is no other way, and so also with nations. Again, the great institutions of every nation are the conditions of its very existence and cannot be transformed by the mould of any other race. Until higher institutions have been evolved, any attempt to break the old ones will be disastrous. Growth is always gradual.

Everything goes to show that Socialism or some form of rule by the people, call it what you will, is coming on the boards. The people will certainly want the satisfaction of their material needs, less work, no oppression, no war, more food. What guarantee have we that this, or any civilization, will last unless it is based on religion, on the goodness of man? Depend on it. Religion goes to the root of the matter. If it is right, all is right.

Human society is in turn governed by the four castes – the priests, the soldiers, the traders, and the labourers.... Last will come the labourer (shudra) rule.

All the members of society ought to have the same opportunity for obtaining wealth, education or knowledge.... Freedom in all matters, i.e., advance towards *mukti*, is the worthiest gain of man.... Those social rules which stand in the way of the unfoldment of the freedom are injurious;

and steps should be taken to destroy them speedily. Those institutions should be encouraged by which men advance in the path of freedom.

Remember that the nation lives in the cottage. The peasant, the shoemaker, the sweeper, and such other lower classes of India have much greater capacity for work and self-reliance than you. They have been silently working through long ages, and producing the entire wealth of the land, without a word of complaint. Very soon they will get above you in position. Gradually capital is drifting into their hands, and they are not so much troubled with wants as you are. Modern education has changed your fashion, but new avenues of wealth lie yet undiscovered for want of the inventive genius. You have so long oppressed these forbearing masses; now is the time for their retribution. And you will become extinct in your vain search for employment, making it the be-all and end-all of your life!

If the labourers stop work, your supply of food and clothes also stops. And you regard them as low-class people and flaunt about your own culture! Engrossed in the struggle for existence, they had not the opportunity for awakening of knowledge. They have worked so long uniformly like machines guided by human intelligence, and the clever educated sections have taken the substantial part of the fruit of their labour. In every country this has been the case. But times have changed. The lower classes are generally awakening to this fact and making a united front against this, determined to exact their legitimate dues.... The upper classes will no longer be able to repress the lower, try they ever so much. The well-being of the higher classes now lies in helping the lower to get their legitimate rights.

When the masses will wake up, they will come to understand your oppression on them, and by a puff of their mouth you will be entirely blown off! It is they who have introduced civilisation amongst you; and it is they who will then pull it down. Think how at the hands of the Gauls the mighty ancient Roman civilization crumbled into dust! Therefore I say, try to rouse these lower classes from slumber by imparting learning and culture to them. When they will awaken – and awaken one day they must – they also will not forget your good services to them and will remain grateful to you.

Hear me, my friend, I have discovered the secret through the grace of the Lord. Religion is not at fault. On the other hand your religion teaches you that every being is only your own self multiplied. But it was the want of practical application, the want of sympathy – the want of heart. This state of things must be removed, not by destroying religion but by following the great teachings of the Hindu faith.

A hundred thousand men and women fired with the zeal of holiness, fortified with eternal faith in the Lord, and nerved to lion's courage by their sympathy for the poor and the fallen and the down-trodden, will go over the length and breadth of the land, preaching the gospel of salvation, the gospel of help, the gospel of social raising up – the gospel of equality.

Before flooding India with socialistic or political ideas, first deluge the land with spiritual ideas. The first work that demands our attention is, that the most wonderful truths confined in our Upanishads, in our scriptures, in our Puranas – must be brought out from the books: brought out from the monasteries, brought out from forests, brought out from the possession of selected bodies of people, and scattered broadcast all over the land.

Your duty at present is to go from village to village, and make the people understand that mere sitting about idly won't do any more. Make them understand their real condition and say, "O ye brothers all Arise!! Awake! How much longer would you remain asleep?"

Initiate all, even down to the chandalas, in these fiery mantras. Also instruct them, in simple words about the necessities of life, and in trade, commerce, agriculture, etc.

We have to give them secular education. We have to follow the plans laid down by our ancestors, that is, to bring all the ideals slowly down among the masses. Raise them slowly up, raise them to equality. Impart even secular knowledge through religion.

The fate of the nation depends upon the conditions of the masses. Can you raise them? Can you give them back their lost individuality without making them lose their innate spiritual nature? Can you become an Occidental of occidentals in your spirit of equality, freedom, working energy, and at the same time a Hindu to the very backbone in religious culture and instincts? This is to be done and we will do it.

PART ONE

Section II

VIVEKANANDA ON EDUCATION AND RELIGION – INTERPRETATIONS AND ALLIED THOUGHTS

"Education is the manifestation of the perfection already in man....
We want that education by which character is formed,
strength of mind is increased, the intellect is expanded
and by which one can stand on one's own feet."

"Religion is the manifestation of the Divinity already in man....
Man must realize God, feel God, see God, talk to God.
That is religion....
Cleanse the mind, that is all of religion."

"This Section consists of comments by various spiritual leaders and few laymen interpreting Vivekananda on Education and Religion. It is useful and relevant supplement to Section One where we have the Swami speaking directly to us. It is not that the Swami wants an interpreter of his thoughts. In fact his message comes through as clearly as a bell and in the same resonant tones. But it is also true that the same simple message may be received differently by different people. An that is worthy of being recorded."

– M. V. Kamath

CONTENTS:

VIVEKANANDA ON EDUCATION AND RELIGION – INTERPRETATIONS AND ALLIED THOUGHTS

The True Aim of Education
– Swami Vireswarananda

Education is not merely imparting knowledge to children about the three 'R's, nor even the imparting of knowledge about any particular subject. But helping the children to get over ignorance and imperfections and becoming mature according to the ideals of the society in which they are born. When we say that the child becomes mature, we mean thereby that it manifests certain inherent qualities or something indicating potential perfection. Our personality is of a two-fold nature – the real and the apparent. The latter is the subject of all empirical sciences and can be studied, while the former eludes such study as it is beyond the senses. This real man within, called variously – the Self, Atman, God etc., is perfect. The more one communes with this inner-self, the more mature or perfect one becomes. That is why Swamiji defines education as "the manifestation of the perfection already in man". So when we are able to manifest in our lives the perfection which is the very nature of the inner man, the Self or Atman, we reach the goal of education. From this point of view we find that Sri Ramakrishna was perfectly educated though illiterate, while we are uneducated though literate. We cannot say that we, with all our imperfections, which form the cause of all our strife and suffering in this world, are educated. It was to impress this point about our present system of education that Sri Ramakrishna refused to get himself educated in the modern sense of the term.

The defect of the present-day education is that it has no definite goal. A painter has a clear idea of the picture he wants to draw, a sculptor has similarly a clear idea of the image he wants to cut out of the marble block, but a present-day teacher has no clear idea of the goal, or rather he has no goal to attain, while he is training the child. We find in the Press discussions about our educational system and various committees are appointed now and then to reorganize the system. But all that centres on the curriculum, and no one discusses the fundamental defect in the system. They stress only secular knowledge or *apara vidya;* they are not at all interested in *para vidya;* they do not think it is necessary. The aim becomes limited to training a child for a career to earn a livelihood. Without *para vidya* nobody can be said to be truly educated.

Even in the *apara vidya* we are after specialization. The child is asked to decide from class IX by what method or profession he is going to earn a livelihood, and when that is selected, all knowledge that refers to this particular subject becomes the main ingredient of his intellectual food and everything else is eschewed. Our present-day education makes a child a specialist in one particular field but gives him no liberal education which would help him to be a human being, an inheritor of the cultural heritage of the past. Imagine an Indian educated as a specialist in one field of technology but who has had no opportunity or time to go through the *Ramayana*, the *Mahabharata* or through some works of Kalidasa or other literary men of the past or present – can such a person be a true Indian?

Another defect in our modern system of education is the want of proper care and training of the instrument, the mind, through which knowledge is acquired. In ancient Indian educational system special attention was paid to the culture of the mind, to control and train it through meditation and concentration and practice of ethical purity, to make it a fit instrument for acquiring knowledge. The seats of learning then were far away from human habitation and were congenial for such culture of the mind. It goes without question that for a sound intellectual life, solitude and deep contemplation are quite essential.

A child imbibes its habits and character from the environment in which it is placed. So if you expect a child to grow up in a certain way, the environment at home and the school should be such as would be helpful to such growth. If you expect a sapling to grow into a beautiful tree and yield beautiful flowers and delicious fruits, you must help its growth with proper manure, water and climatic conditions suitable for its growth as a healthy tree. Similar is the case with respect to a child's growth. So a great responsibility devolves on the parents and the teachers to live the life which they expect the child to manifest when it grows up. In the ancient seats of learning, the *acharyas* were men of exalted character and students under them were inspired by their conduct and life. The modern system is no doubt defective, but the teachers can supplement what is wanting by extra-curricular activities of a cultural and spiritual nature to help the students to imbibe our national ideals along with our modern education. The teacher should convert his home into an Ashram and lead a life like that of the ancient rishis, so that the people of the village or township could go to him for advice and solace and the students could look on him as their friend, philosopher and guide in all their difficulties.

Indian Ideal of Education
– Dr. M. Lakshmi Kumari

In the eradication of *avidya* and the establishment of *vidya* in our lives, lies the essence of true Indian education.

Through his definition of education as 'the manifestation of the perfection already in man', Swami Vivekananda has conveyed all that is to be conveyed about the Indian ideal of education. He draws our attention first to the Indian concept of 'Perfection' which, though beyond the realm of sensory knowledge and intellectual convictions, yet lies within therealizing capacity of man! The real aim of education is to search for this perfection within man, removing all the obstacles on the way to reaching it and having realised it, to manifest it outside in one's own life and activities in a way to benefit humanity.

This perfection is to be understood as the spark of the Infinite Power which resides in everything and everywhere – Sat-Chit-Ananda. To realise this is the ultimate goal of life. True education should, therefore, teach one how to achieve this goal of life through training, pursuit of knowledge and above all through relentless self-effort. An education divorced from this has really no meaning or purpose. On the contrary, if it is clubbed to this central theme, be it art, architecture, music, medicine, science or literature it will blossom in a most unique way, taking one through these very same avenues to the pinnacle of perfection and realization. Only in India can we get such an abiding concept of education covering the entire range of human potentialities.

After understanding the essential nature of this 'perfection', one should identify it with his own self within. For achieving this, ego, ignorance and other false identification which stand in its way should be systematically eliminated. That is, to establish vidya, all avidya should be eradicated. With the acquisition of this true vidya or education, one realises his Self within as the Self everywhere and the absolute oneness and the essential unity of the entire phenomenal world become clear to him. As one draws nearer and nearer to this perfect understanding, farther and farther he moves away from the confusing and confounding world of 'non-self' and ignorance or avidya.

Education in the true sense should help us to universalise our self and link it to the eternal. Only then can it lift us above the narrow grooves of bigotry, crookedness, hypocrisy, fanaticism and selfishness. A fanatic has no claim to be called, 'educated'. A bigoted man, however qualified he may be, for all practical purposes remains 'uneducated'. One who acquires true education simultaneously also acquires qualities of pure love, courage, sense of duty, balance of mind, devotion, faith, discrimination, tolerance, dispassion and above all, knowledge of Self in a most natural way.

True education should aim at giving this 'universal vision' to man. Showing such a universal vision to Arjuna, Lord Krishna lifted him out of the narrow confines of his self and gave him a deep understanding of the entire life. Curiously, knowingly or unknowingly this is what secular education also tries to achieve when Material Science probes to discover that ultimate unit of matter from which all forms must have emerged or that law of nature knowing which all laws can be comprehended or when biology tries to link man with the fundamental unit of structure in the living world and re-creates his family tree to show him his inter-relationship with all that is living!

Just as a true physicist or chemist looking at the world of energy and matter can visualise that they are nothing but manifestations of one and the same energy vibration, so should a man of 'true education', looking around him realise that the so-called phenomenal world of names and forms is nothing but the varying expressions of the one Infinite Self. The gross is only an appearance. Truth is subtle and lies hidden beyond the gross.

When one learns to go beyond the gross appearance to the subtler and subtler realms – barriers break down whether they be in the world of science or spirit. Truth becomes synonymous with perfection. All the rest are appearances. Ultimate in education is the realization of this truth.

Education should also be aimed at maintaining the cultural values of the land, vibrant and ever fresh from generation to generation. Culture of India has its roots in her spiritual values. Unless these values, implicit and explicit in Indian culture, somehow find their way into the thoughts and lives of students, education in India will lose its significance.

Recognition of the time-tested cultural values should therefore become part of the education, not just for the sake of any selfish clannish interest but for the continued maintenance of this perennial supply of spiritual values to the world culture for all times to come. What India can give, no other country can. An Indian, bereft of this pride in his motherland's role in the World Assembly is no Indian at all. Through this knowledge alone can a justifiable pride be generated in our youth and their appreciation of values channelised into true patriotic fervour. Ignorance of this makes our youth look elsewhere for inspiration and guidance, depriving them of the strength and vigour that one gets through one's well-nurtured roots.

Education also means imparting ethical idealism. Each country has its own ethics, almost at par with *swadharma*. Swami Vivekananda refers to religion and spirituality as the very soul of India. Everything that is truly Indian should revolve round this point – the unique spiritual truths which India has propounded from time immemorial and which are truly eternal, catholic and universal. In these eternal, undeniable values lie the everlasting strength and everfresh aroma of Indian culture. It is adherence to these values that has made the country renowned for her capacity for tolerance and universal acceptance. Aggression and domination are unknown to her. India believed and continues to believe that there are as many paths to the top of a mountain as there are climbers wending their way up there.

Inculcating this ethical idealism in our youth is of paramount importance to keep the Indian society from going astray in the way of many others in other parts of the world. This responsibility lies with the educationists, the teachers and the taught.

All efforts at development of one's personality which is one of the purposes of education or any training should aim at this, to make man understand what he really is and having understood that 'perfection' within, strive in every way to manifest it in the outer world. When at least a semblance of this is achieved by a system of education then only can we claim to have really knocked at the doors of Knowledge. Manifestation of this Knowledge, expression of this Oneness in the day-to-day life and transactions must naturally follow, because that is what truly distinguishes a man of worth. How the inner strength and knowledge accumulated through correct understanding are put to use to the advantage of those around – therein lies the real test of education. That is the meaning of 'manifestation'. Swamiji's whole philosophy of karmayoga – combining knowledge with action – has this as the corner stone.

Even a basic understanding of this philosophy is lacking in India today. The vast amount from the exchequer spent on the education of youth is virtually squandered away by the youth themselves, by the politicians who use them and also by the parents who count on education only in terms of their market value. That after acquiring an education at the expense of the tax payer's money, at least a portion has to be returned for their service, is a necessity which we are totally oblivious of. Lord Krishna, in the *Gita*, calls a person, who eats and enjoys at the expense of the society without giving anything in return a 'thief'.

In most exquisite words have our ancient seers sung of the glory of 'education':

> *Asato maa sadgamaya,*
> *Tamaso maa jyotir gamaya,*
> *Mrutyor maa amrutam gamaya,*
> *Om Shantih, Shantih, Shantih!*

Lead me from unreal to the real – remove my attachment to that which has no real existence and attach me to that which is Real....

Lead me from darkness to light – remove from me thoughts, emotions, imaginations and identifications which cloud and darken my mind and lead me towards the light of wisdom, knowledge and true awareness....

Lead me from death to immortality – sever my foolish attachments to things which are impermanent and ephemeral and yoke me on to that which is Permanent, Everlasting and Eternal....

Education in Tune With Religion and Culture
– Swami Harshananda

After independence, tremendous efforts have been made by our governments, by our leaders, to raise the country. But all along somehow or other, raising the country meant to our leaders, raising only the economic standards of our people. The core, the central factor, for raising the country, viz. raising the man himself, who is the basic factor in the national life, seems to have failed to receive much attention. In fact, we are very fond of nationalizing. We have nationalised the banks, we have nationalized industries, we have nationalized the transport system and probably many more ventures will be nationalized in future. But I personally feel, and feel very sore at that, we have failed to nationalize the nation itself. Somehow or other, this has escaped the attention of the great leaders of this country.

It is a very tragic state of affairs. The national consciousness that we are one nation with a great cultural heritage, has not been ingrained in the life of our people. And in our mad rush for building the nation, only looking to the side of economics, we have forgotten our cultural side.

We are blindly imitating the West in toto. The West may be great in science and technology. But why should we imitate in every aspect? In fact, on the other hand, people in the West are fed up with the material life. They are looking towards India for spiritual life, for its spiritual values, for Vedanta and Yoga. So let us not forget that we have to build our nation on our own ideal, and this ideal has been kept before us by Swami Vivekananda. Man-making, character-building, is the primary need of the hour.

The education we impart to our children and youth should be based on moral, ethical and spiritual ideals contained in our religion and culture.

Man is not just the body or even a combination of the body and the mind. He is essentially the spirit encased in the flesh. The aim of education should be to help manifest this spirit in every thought, word and action. So it should aim at a full and harmonious development of the body and the intellect and tune it to the spirit within. In other words, it should help build up an integrated personality, a perfect character.

Though provision is being made in the educational policies of the Government for a harmonious development of the body and intellect, nothing has been done so far for imparting moral, ethical and spiritual training or a character-building education. It is really unfortunate that such valuable reports as those of the Radhakrishnan Commission on University Education which contains an excellent section on religious education, or that of Sri Prakasa Committee which had submitted recommendations on religious and moral instruction have not been implemented. Even the latest Education Commission (The Kothari Commission) emphasizes the importance of moral and spiritual training once again. Religious education is compulsorily imparted in most of the foreign countries. We do not understand why it is not being done even after 35 years of independence, though the above-mentioned Commissions have definitely given us practical suggestions.

Imparting of moral and spiritual teachings through stories and biographies in the lower classes, a regular study of the major religions and religious philosophies of the world in the higher classes, also group prayers and meditation – this is the suggested pattern. We would like to add one more item to this list: The ancient ideal of *brahmacharya*, purity in personal life, and dedication to learning, must be greatly stressed.

Just as social service camps or N. C. C. camps are held, in the same way intensive spiritual retreats of short duration like two weeks may also be seriously thought of and they must be made annual features. Of course, this means that there must be proper teachers specially trained for such purposes. It is then worthwhile seriously considering the starting of special training institutions for such teachers.

What is the fundamental solution to the problems that confront youth? A little reflection will convince us that something more basic in human nature has to be tackled and tackled effectively. It is man that tells lies, steals, robs, commits adultery or murder. All this is done by him in order to get 'happiness' or 'peace' or 'freedom'. But he has taken to the wrong means of achieving them. He commits these crimes, since his mind is not in order! If the mind can be purified and attitudes set in the right direction, the direction of the greatest good of the greatest number, *bahujana sukhaya, bahujana hitaya,* everything is done. Or, to put it in one word, it is 'character' that should be inculcated first and foremost, in the youth. This again becomes possible only when the system of training the youth starting from the home itself, is reoriented to building up a strong moral character. Since it is a burning candle that can light up another candle, a much higher quality of life and conduct is expected of the parents, teachers and leaders of the society, from whom the youth can draw inspiration.

It is here that religion – not in the denominational sense but in the true sense of 'the manifestation of the divinity already in man' as Vivekananda puts it – can play a significant role in the life of the youth, nay, of the whole society.

II

There is a general feeling that the present pattern of education in our country is incomplete and is not capable of improving the code of conduct of the student. Even the best of curriculum will not be conducive to the development of the human personality. Hence many educationists and thinkers have been fervently pleading for the inclusion of moral education as a part of regular study in schools and colleges.

– Dr. H. Narasimhaiah

III

The education we are getting in our schools and colleges is very defective as it has no religious background.

It is a great pity that the education which the Hindu children are getting now has no reference to the Hindu view of life or Hindu ideals. That is why it is so barren of results.

The results of a complete system of education are a spiritual outlook on life, a sterling character, graceful manners, a virile mind and a humane spirit – all these, of course, having their basis in a sound and vigorous body. Mere intellectual education cannot give you all these. So I have always held that the education that is given in our schools and colleges should be supplemented by some kind of moral and religious instructions at home.

– Prof. D. S. Sarma

IV

An academic sell-out in the Indian Universities has been going on with the academicians imitating Western cultural values following Western text-books, authors, systems and structures. If you examine the syllabi of the Indian Universities over the years, fewer and fewer courses are given in Indian culture and it is a pity. There is also no awareness in the Government about the importance of building contemporary ideas and institutions based on India's culture and so the programmes are failing one after another.

– Dr. John W. Spellman

V

Material and psychological conditions of the modern society have created an unhealthy climate for the care and education of the young. The emphasis on commercial and utilitarian ideals has reduced integral education to an absurd irrelevancy. Consequently the new generation is not aware that cultivation of higher values is more important than acquisition of wealth or pursuit of its own good-pleasure. The absence of integral education leads to various disorders, such as neurosis, feeble-mindedness, incapacity for creative effort and moral corruption. The aim of integral education is to prevent the individual from joining the animal kingdom by the manifestation of spiritual values which alone can bring light and joy.

– Swami Adidevananda

Character and Culture – The Prime Requisites
– Swami Vireswarananda

All over the country since Independence there has been a great deal of enthusiasm amongst the people, particularly among our young men, to rebuild our nation. It is very commendable. But then, before one takes up this work one must have a clear idea of India that is to be. A painter paints a picture on the canvas only after he has a clear image, as it were, in his mind of what he wants to paint. Similarly an engineer before he begins the construction of any building, first gets complete information as to what purpose the building will be used – school, hospital, public office, or residence. After that, he draws the plan and then constructs the building accordingly. So we too must have a clear picture of the future India and then begin building the nation. Are we going to make India a great military nation? I am sure we are not, for no military power has lived long. Just see the fate of Hitler and Mussolini.

We are poor nation and we want wealth to be able to feed our masses. But will mere bread and butter solve our problem? Have people of America and other advanced nations peace of mind and true happiness in spite of their wealth? They do not seem to have. Look at the young people of some of these countries, children of affluence, boys and girls, who feel frustration with nothing to achieve in life, wandering about. Some of them are very very rich, but often they feel a sort of terrible purposelessness having no goal in life. We want military strength to protect our freedom and not to rob our neighbours, we want wealth to feed our masses who are poor, but this cannot be the ideal of the nation. Something more is required besides these two. What is that which will bring peace to us along with wealth and power?

It is advisable for us to go through our ancient history and see how great India was in power, wealth, and happiness during the time of Ashoka, Chandragupta, Kanishka, and others. During the Vedic period and during the Buddhistic period evidently we had great ideals that could make India so great in the past. But then how has this degeneration come about? We have to find out the causes that led to our downfall. So in constructing future India we must accept the ideals that made us great, reject what caused degeneration, and supply newly what were not there, at that time, viz. science and technology.

We nowadays swear by science. We say something is not scientific, it is superstitious. But is it scientific to ignore altogether our past, not caring to know what good it contained and what has sustained us as a nation for the last three thousand years, and to run after Western ideas which have not stood the test of time, which are at best two hundred years old and some of even more recent times? Have these ideals solved the problem of the Western nations? Are they happy and at peace? They do not seem to be. So why go after those ideals?

We are human beings. God has given us reason to be used, and not to allow ourselves to be driven like cattle by anyone and everyone who comes and tells us something vehemently. So, I feel that we should gather all materials, all information about our past and present, think well, and plan the future. We should not be led by emotion.

First of all the most necessary thing is character. Without character nothing great can be achieved. Look at Mahatmaji. See how by his character he swayed the nation and forced England to quit India. He did not use guns, atom-bombs, etc. So if we want to make India great, we must build our character first, and then use our reason and find out what sort of India we want to build and then begin to work for it, even if it means sacrificing our lives for it. For this kind of study, Swami Vivekananda's works will be a guide book to us to introduce us to the greatness of Indian culture and ideals.

* * *

India is – our constitution says – a secular State. What do we mean by 'secular State'? You see, that is a negative way of looking at things. We ought to have said that we accept all religions, just as Emperor Ashoka did. Even though he was a Buddhist, he accepted Jainism and Hinduism.

He built monasteries and temples for various sects though he himself was a Buddhist. There was no state religion. Ashoka accepted all the religions. But today we say ours is a secular State, and this has come to mean that we have no religion. We cannot teach any religion to our boys and girls in the schools, for that will not be in tune with the constitution, with our concept of a secular State. Probably nowadays they are just finding it out that this is a rather peculiar situation, and they are now allowing probably religious education in the schools and colleges. But the term 'secular State' represents a negative attitude. We must have it put this way: We accept all religions as true, and therefore we shall not make any distinction between man and man because of his religion. That would have been a very correct statement.

By religion, however, is not meant the common idea about it, that is, a set of beliefs, dogmas or even superstitions sanctified by priesthood or popular customs. Religion is realization of the ultimate Truth. Swamiji says, "Each soul is potentially divine. The goal is to manifest this divine within by controlling nature external and internal. Do this either by work, or worship, or psychic-control, or philosophy, by one, or more, or all of these and be free. This is the whole of religion".

According to Sri Ramakrishna different religions are but different paths to God realization; and he had realized this truth through direct experience. Even intellectually, if we scrutinize the various religions, we find that each of them prescribes only these four yogas, with perhaps stress on one or other. So conversion from one religion to another is to be discouraged, and each person is to rise higher and higher in spirituality by following his own religion and thus realize God.

Religion has to permeate all fields of national life – education, politics, economics, social life, and so on. Education should impart the culture of the land to the younger generation and make them true representatives of the nation; all secular knowledge that is consonant with it should be welcome. Without this, education will be a failure.

II

Swami Vivekananda had tremendous faith in the young people of our country. He considered them as the greatest asset and wealth of India. He believed that they were full of energy, idealism, enthusiasm, hope, optimism and an adventurous spirit and they were the backbone of India. He used to say that if our country has to win back its ancient glory, power and prosperity, it is in the hands of the youth. He felt they would be able to build a New India with their enormous energy and enthusiasm. At present, India is weak, full of poverty, destitution, ignorance, superstition, and disease. What the youth are in need of is inspiration, the right type of education and character. They should be trained to utilize their God-given gifts, their resources, their talents, and faculties for building up their own lives and careers and for uplifting the poor and the down-trodden.

In rebuilding India, we have to take advantage of the modern period. We have to assimilate modern ideals which are healthy and strong. But we need proper guidance in rebuilding India. It is in this context that we have to understand the significance of Sri Ramakrishna and Swami Vivekananda. How many great thinkers, statesmen, writers, philosophers, both Indian and foreign, have paid rich tributes to Sri Ramakrishna and Swami Vivekananda! Not only India, but the whole of modern civilization, has much to gain from the ideas and ideals preached by Sri Ramakrishna and Swami Vivekananda.

Indian young men and women are one of the best amongst the boys and girls of the world. They stand on an equal footing with the young men and women of advanced countries like America, Germany, Japan or Russia in intelligence, brilliance and aptitude in any field of knowledge or adventure. They have made history wherever they have gone by their accomplishments and achievements.

Teachers impart knowledge to the students. The parents impart advice to their children. But what the youngsters need most is inspiration. Nobody – neither the teacher, nor the parents, nor the social and the national leaders – have been giving them inspiration. This does not mean that our young men and women are to remain without inspiration. Swami Vivekananda is a perennial source of inspiration for people of all ages, especially for young men and women.

But we have to remember that today our country is in the midst of distractions, poverty, ill-health and ignorance. What is the duty of every young man and woman today in these conditions? With all the education which you have had in colleges and universities, you are feeling helpless. But if you study the lives and teachings of Sri Ramakrishna and Swami Vivekananda you will get tremendous inspiration and courage, unbounded love and compassion for the poor and the downtrodden; you will be filled with the spirit of service, dedication and patriotism, necessary for serving and saving our country. It is during your young age that you should inspire yourself with these national and human ideas and ideals. The inspiring message of Swami Vivekananda will awaken the tremendous energy and resources lying latent within you. This is what is called character-building. The whole world is in need of your resources of energy and character. With your enormous energy and sterling character, you will re-build a strong, healthy and prosperous India and the world.

Whether you are going to be scientists, doctors, engineers, politicians, journalists, administrators, lecturers or businessmen, you can work for rebuilding India if you imbibe the necessary impulse and inspiration from Sri Ramakrishna and Swami Vivekananda.

We always talk of our troubles, dismal conditions around us, our poverty, our ignorance etc. What are these problems due to? Do we lack man-power? Do we lack resources? Do we lack brains? No. What we lack is character, the spirit of patriotism and service, the will to do hard work, the feeling for the poor and the down-trodden. That is why national problems are multiplying.

Swami Vivekananda says, "Stand on your own feet and be true men and women". If we want to save ourselves, if we want to save our Nation, we must discipline our energies, mobilize them and utilize them for the big task of rebuilding India. We should not waste our energies. This is what we learn from Sri Ramakrishna and Swami Vivekananda.

Strength is life; weakness is death. Accept not what makes you weak physically and mentally. If any food makes you weak, reject it as poison. If any literature spoils your mind and weakens you mentally, reject that literature as poison. If a company of certain people distracts and weakens your mind, reject it as poison. If the cinema makes you weak in body and mind, reject it as poison.

If you want to be good, it is in your hands. Nobody can make you good by force. Likewise, nobody can make you bad against your will. If you are good, the c redit goes to you. If you are bad, you yourself are to be blamed. You are the creators of your destiny. Make your nerves strong. What we want is muscles of iron and nerves of steel. It is man-making education all round that we want.

Be patriots. But who are real patriots? Those who feel for the poor and the downtrodden from their hearts are real patriots. Do you feel for the millions of people who are starving, who are daily sinking more and more in poverty, ignorance, ill-health and destitution before your very eyes? Then you are real patriots.

Do you love your religion and culture? Do you feel proud of them? Do you feel proud of the great men and women of your country? Do you feel respect and reverence for them? Are you prepared to do your best for the upliftment of your country? Then you are patriots. Every educated man and woman should do his or her mite for the welfare of the country.

Once some students asked Swami Vivekananda for a message. Swami Vivekananda told them: "Live and die like heroes for a great cause. Heroes die only once. Cowards die several times".

Today there is an awakening in the students all over the world. They have become conscious of their rights and strength. They want to play a significant role in the affairs of education, of administration and of Government. The Governments of the world can no longer ignore them. They will have to take students into confidence. It is the duty of the Government and educational authorities and parents to understand the genuine problems and aspirations of the students. The students do have the right to express their grievance. Even when they express their genuine greivances, they should do so in a respectful and dignified way. If students do not show respect to authority, how can they expect it for themselves when they themselves one day assume authority?

The students have become very dynamic as a result of their awakening. This dynamism is good. But the question is whether the students are going to direct their awakening and dynamism towards improving the quality of their life and character and their educational excellence, towards improving the prospects of their country or for creating chaos everywhere. Are they going to harness their God-given gifts of youth, energy and vitality for the reconstruction of our society and for the rebuilding of our nation or for the destruction of whatever is good and great and beautiful in our country, in our culture and religion?

How I wish that every boy and girl will promise to himself or herself that from this day he or she will strive his or her best for creating an atmosphere congenial for the development of his or her character, for improving the prospects of their careers, and for the upliftment of our country! How I wish that the Government and the educational authorities try to understand the genuine problems and aspirations of students and establish a rapport with them: The staff members and students should remember that education is a joint venture and so it requires for its success mutual love, understanding and rapport of minds and hearts.

Many of the ailments of our present-day educational systems and many of the maladies affecting students and teachers stem from the narrow educational objectives viz. examinations and jobs. Of course examinations cannot be easily dispensed with and jobs and careers are essential for every student. But students and teachers should not be under the impression that education is merely a system of passing examinations and securing jobs. It is much more than that. Swami Vivekananda says that education is a process of life-building, man-making, character-making assimilation of ideas.

Sri Ramakrishna used to say "As long as I live, so long do I learn". Education is lifelong process. It may begin in schools and colleges, but it does not end there. It is an incessant search for Truth, knowledge, wisdom, experience and faith. A real student is he who goes on assimilating knowledge, experience and wisdom throughout his life and goes on building up his life and chracter. We have to learn not only from books and laboratories but also from our life – its success and failures, ups and downs, joys and sorrows, prospects and problems. It demands the greatest aspiration, dedication, continuous self-effort and industriousness from students.

Service of the country is the prime duty of students. All of us should remember that our mission in life is service of our fellow-men. But in the name of politics, students should not neglect their studies. The greate teachers of mankind are great because of the service they have rendered to mankind.

The principals and professors cannot give students chracter from the pages of books. Character-building comes from their very lives. Students imbibe more from teachers' own lives than they do from the books or lectures. So teachers must have good character.

You are all fortunate to have been born as the sons and daughters of this country which has an ancient heritage and a great history. Our country and countrymen expect you to fuflfil your great destiny and mission i.e., to stirve.to create a glorious and happy future for yourself, for your country and countrymen, with inspiration drawn from the life and messsage of Sri Ramakrishna and Swami Vivekananda.

— Swami Vijananda

Education for Character and Moral and Spiritual Values
— Swami Siddhinathananda

The search for values is purely a human concern. The quality of value will depend upon the worth accorded to man. In common with subhuman creatures, he has a life on the physical level. Food for the preservation of the body and mate for the reproduction of the species are the main objects of search at that level. There man is only a biped, a candidate for manhood. In the animal, the head and the stomach are on the same level. Man is the only animal that walks upright with the head held aloft. In the head he has all the senses meant for gathering external data, and inside his head he has the most wonderful contrivance devised by God and nature which makes him a unique creature – a being who can know himself. That knowledge is the full and final value of man.

Spiritual value means the awareness and attainment of this basic dimension of man, that essentially he is Spirit pure and simple. Man is Spirit caught in the coils of ignorance, impounded in a carnal cage. All his trials and tribulations are a protest against this incarceration and an unconscious struggle to effect a breakthrough. The thirst for freedom is inherent in all creatures; only, at the subhuman level, it is dormant and is expressed as instinct. But man being endowed with a developed brain, he can devise ways and means of attaining his innate, pristine freedom. Man has been described as a teachable animal. Education is the art that transforms the animal-man into human and spiritual-man. Education involves at least two parties, the teacher and the taught. The former must be wise and worthy, and the latter receptive and competent. Proper education must equip the pupil for a full and fruitful life. Life becomes fruitful only when he attains to his spiritual stature. The Spirit is perfect and Swami Vivekananda defines education as the manifestation of perfection already in man. Perfection is inherent in us; imperfection or limitation is accidental. We cannot attain what is not truly ours. What is the meaning of saying that we have to attain what is already ours? We have forgotten our true measure and that has to be brought back to our awareness. If limitation or misery were our true nature, we can never hope to become free. So freedom means the riddance of a non-existent limitation and the recognition of our ever existent – essential nature. An education that enables us to achieve that end alone is real education.

That is the goal. Once the goal is fixed, we have to make the means conducive and commensurate to achieve that end. We have to begin with the grossest in man, namely the body. Man being a social being, he has to learn to live amicably with others. Every creature is selfish. Man is no exception to this. Only he, being intelligent, can be inhumanly selfish. But that will boomerang in the long run. Selfishness is suicidal. So, man evolves social codes of conduct. They are only mutual adjustments of each man's selfish interests. Fear of consequence is what makes such a man submit to social rules and restraints. The biological and economic man may conduct himself in a socially acceptable way. But his correct conduct need not be an expression of a proper character. One may burn inside with envy and anger and at the same time conduct oneself with restraint. But a man of character will be cool within and calm without. Spontaneous noble attitude is what constitutes good character, and good conduct, its natural result. That requires a deeper evaluation of man.

The type of education obtained in schools and colleges nowadays does not make for the cultivation of character. Arts and Sciences are the two main disciplines that are encouraged in the academies. Of them, Science is amoral and studies man mostly at the physical level. Too much science is making man a clever and cruel animal. As for arts, it could, if properly planned, be made to impart instruction which might pave the way for character-building. For that, care must be taken in selecting the teachers and also the contents of the course of study. But unfortunately for us the authorities that direct and control common education plan for only man's stomach and family. They neglect his heart and head. Often, the educational policies are determined, not by educationists, but by politicians. Politicians are after power and their eyes are set on the votes. They do not care much for the real good of man. They cater to the clamouring crowd. They will enlist even God, if possible, for election propaganda. So they plan for an education that will equip man to attain economic security in order that he might indulge in unbridled biological satisfactions. And what is the result? Modern man is restless, inconsiderate to others and unhappy. Peaceful sleep has become a luxury to him. He is an addict to sedatives and narcotics. He has become a nervous wreck. He is a burden and a problem to himself and to the society. All due to wrong values and improper education. And what is the remedy?

The system of education obtained in ancient India was meant for the whole man. It trained the body, the mind and the character. It was a preparation for life and not an indexing of information. It was a total scheme. It viewed man as potential God and valued him as such. Such a view made men value all. Same-sightedness, seeing the self-same Soul in all, was the ideal. And character is the test of realization, said Swami Vivekananda. It is only then that one can love one's neighbour as oneself. When love rules the relation between the members of the human family, noble sentiments towards one another arise spontaneously. That is the sign of noble character. Formation of noble character is possible only when man is appraised as spirit.

Character has to be cultivated slowly and steadily. Proper education is the training ground for it. Man learns both by precept and example, more by example than by precept. The ancient system was *gurukulavasa*, the pupil staying in the preceptor's house serving him and learning from him. The teacher provided the theory and practice and the student learnt noble principles and was given guidance for the cultivation of a proper conduct. The noble character of the teacher keeps the taught on the right path. *brahmacharya* is the ancient term for studentship. *'Brahman'* means the Supreme Truth and also the revelations of the same, namely the Vedas, and *'charya'* means conduct. So a student is one who learns noble lessons and leads his life accordingly. The minimum period of study was twelve years. Repeated habits of good conduct for so long a period guarantees the acquisition of noble character. "Character is repeated habits and repeated habits alone can reform character", says Swami Vivekananda. Rome was not built in a day, nor a noble character. *'abhyasa,'* repeated habit, is the only way for the formation of proper character. Habits, good or bad, are irremovable. All impressions are stored up in the brain, none can be erased. If proper electric impulses are applied to the limbo wherein they are filed, they will come up again. The only way to be rid of evil impressions is to pile up good ones and leave the former alone.

Discipline is the key to success in any walk of life. No education is possible without discipline. Simplicity, humility and service of the teacher are the essential prerequisites for a smooth and successful course of education. Love of luxury and excellence in learning do not go together. Knowledge cannot be bought. It has to be acquired through the favour of the teacher. Humility is the key that will open the heart of the preceptor. Loving service is the fee that the student has to pay. Humility is the root and fruit of education. At the start, it is restraint of the ego, at the end, it is the eradication of the ego which is the same as awareness of the Soul.

The student returns home after acquiring both secular and spiritual knowledge. One requires a minimum of twelve years for the study of the preliminary secular subjects such as semantics, grammar, poetics etc. and at least one Veda. That is sufficiently long a period to lay the foundations of a good character. After returning from the teacher's house, the student takes up the responsibilities of a citizen. He gets married, performs his duties to the family and to the society. That is the period meant for the performance of duties and the discharge of debts. That is the time when his character is put to the test. The education and character that he has acquired earlier stands him in good stead and enables him to carry the burdens of social responsibilities efficiently and honestly. When he reaches middle age and finds the messengers of the final end making their presence felt in the form of wrinkles and grey hairs, he retires from all social responsibilities after entrusting them to his son and goes to the woods, there to devote his wholetime on the ultimate values of life. He lives a strict and disciplined spiritual life, meditates on God and in due time calmly and peacefully gets released from the corporeal prison.

This was the scheme and scope of the ancient system of education. It was a total, life-long scheme. It was a preparation for life as well as for death. Life begins in birth and ends in death. Both these mysteries have to be envisaged in any purposeful education. Only a total view will make us aware of the Spiritual dimension of life. Spiritual and moral values acquire meaning and relevance only when man is viewed as God in disguise. When one discovers the God within, one sees the same God in all creatures. He then treats them as manifestations of divinity. Any lesser view of man will be a devaluation of man. The spiritual relation expresses itself as noble character. And character is the test of realization.

This scheme may sound idealistic and otherworldly. This was the preserve of a handful at the top level of Society. Such criticisms and charges might be levelled against it. Herein we are discussing a scheme for an ideal education. This was the ideal scheme the ancients had evolved. In spite of its social restrictiveness and loftiness of ideal, this has been seriously and sincerely followed with admirable results. Its survival for centuries is proof enough of its validity and vitality. India's heritage in the spiritual, religious, philosophical and moral fields is the golden fruits of such a system of education.

May be the times have changed and much of it is impracticable. We have to adapt to modern conditions. The core of the old scheme is sound and it must be preserved in any reform of the educational system. We have to combine the Indian spiritual wisdom with the modern scientific spirit. That will pave the way for a total education for life which will ensure a noble moral character.

Moral and Religious Education
– Swami Swahananda

The essence of moral education is to present in the form of stories and anecdotes, moral ideas that will become real and part of child's nature through personal experience. Man lives in society. His interests sometimes come to clash with others. There is also moral struggle between self-interest and duty. The existence of the evil of selfishness is a reality. It must be counteracted by training and education. Hence there is the necessity of moral training. Nowadays it is specially proposed as a remedy for certain tendencies that undermine the social morale and cultural standard, and are giving a destructive turn to the youthful energies of boys and girls. Not only the domestic and social authority is threatened by this lack of integration, even the governmental authority is in difficulty. The help of moral education is sought to bring about peace more naturally through education than through force.

True morality is natural, not forced. It is the external manifestation of the inner goodness of man. Efficiency in work comes through moral ideals, through a feeling of equality and not through fear and want, as some people think. Through religious and ethical training only, willing co-operation and responsible work without supervision are possible, for the drive is internal and not external.

India for centuries was guided by a religious pursuit; politics and administration were looked upon as mere auxiliaries. The making of manhood, the development of character was its goal.... The contemporary unrest is a part of the social upheaval due to a change in the pattern of life because of industrialization and technological development.

Not only India but the whole world is passing through moral confusion. Higher ideals are being thrown to the winds, ignoring the fundamental principles of civilization, and the lower conceptions of life are being preached vigorously. The result is tragic. Thinkers with the future welfare of man at heart are trying to find a solution. Religions down the ages were training man in the higher virtues. Their hold being slackened, a substitute in moral education is being sought.

An important factor of the modern civilized societies is the importance gained by education. As long as it was limited to the classes, the spiritual value of education was predominant. But with masses coming in, the increased value of the educated in the labour market became more important. This commercialized view of education coupled with the self-conscious labour brought forth political theories believing in force and violence. This perverted conception of education is the root cause of restlessness in society, specially among the youth. A little moral education for youth or labour is only a symptomatic treatment of the disease without going to its root cause. The essential spirituality of man must be recognised and theories of progress and order must be correlated to it. Man is not a mere living machine: he is spirit with a body and mind and not a mere tool to produce wealth in a capitalistic or communistic pattern or socialistic and economic society.

Proper education presupposes the conception of personality. Our conception is, each soul is potentially divine and perfect. The goal is to manifest that perfection and divinity lying hidden in us. A child is a self-conscious soul with a body, sense organs and a mind which can be trained. So true education will mean the development of his physical, intellectual, moral and spiritual potentialities. Proper control of sense-impulses and instincts, sublimation and proper direction of feelings and sentiments and development of the will and the sense of duty must be learnt by the student. For inculcating higher virtues it is necessary to stimulate the very soul of the child. The greatest incentive to moral life is to be aware of one's pure nature and connection with the Ultimate Reality.

This is the age-old view of man and his place in society. The materialistic view makes man an aggregate of organs and functions. It does not recognise the spirituality of man and believes that his higher nature is determined by his education and environment. Much literature has been produced on this. The Indian idea is to recognise man's nature as spiritual; education is to remove the ignorance that hides his pure, perfect nature. As the goal of life was something non-material, to the old Indian the satisfaction of material wants and sense-enjoyment had only a secondary importance. As he loved peace and was satisfied with the minimum, he did not want conflict or disorder in the outer world too. But now times are changing. The theories of enjoyment are vigorously being preached in every country. But there too competition is inevitable. As a result, the revolutionary theories developed, stressing unrest, conflict and hatred. Boys and girls are naturally affected by these. To counteract this an orientation in Western education is being tried blending technical and moral education. Industrial and technical education will teach people how to earn and live above want, and moral education will teach them the qualities of thrift, temperance, and purity and how to live with other people and the government. By such education, educationists hope that there will be a reign of contentment and happiness, law and order.

In India the situation is a little more peculiar. Here we had a developed social and moral order but a new type of civilization has been thrust on us, bringing in its trail unfamiliar types of social evils. Conflicts of ideals and civilizations, manners and habits are the order of the day. Some of the bad habits are weedy growths, depending on the fashion. If they are to be counteracted, this idea itself must be resisted. Simplicity of life is losing its ground and multiplying things is considered a matter of prestige. So respect for the good traditions also must be kept up, at least for children. Disregard of everything old generates undesirable tendencies in children. This however is being corrected by some leaders nowadays.

A peaceful society requires devotion to one's allotted duty. In Indian tradition a duty is an obligatory action. Every act has two aspects, that of purification of the mind and yielding merits or fruits. The former leads to knowledge, the latter gives enjoyments and is destructible. One is subjective and the other objective. Practical morality requires a certain measure of definiteness. To define a duty with reference to its objective character is to keep its real nature in the dark.... Whatever purifies our mind, elevates our thinking, widens our sympathies, ennobles our feelings and makes us more spiritual is a duty, an obligatory act. Devotion to duty presupposes love. To bring it to children without touching religion will be impossible. For children, love will mean not the mere sentimental attachment but the idea of self-sacrifice and service. The question will arise in their mind why they should love others. The ultimate answer lies in religion only, in the idea that God dwells in every man, that all are His children. Of course, the social reason that by helping others we help ourselves too, though indirectly, is also to be pointed out. The idea of *ahimsa*, of not injuring others is a negative definition. Love is its positive aspect. But love and non-injury are possible only through self-culture. This is then a duty. Duties are directed towards others, so they make us unselfish. This love or non-injury speaks of one's own conduct and will appeal easily to children. Hence both the individual and social ethics commingle. This is the beginning of moral life in man.

Education to Inculcate Moral and Ethical Values
– Swami Vimalananda

Whether judged by ancient standards or modern, absolute chastity of life and purity of thought alone can give happiness to man. The question of health and physical soundness is supremely important for the individual and the nation. A reformed rake does not make a good husband and a woman has every right to except the same purity of life which the man whom she marries demands of her. The consequence of "sowing wild oats" which husbands had in their youth have brought sufferings to many children and wives. The children's inheritance comes from both the parents, and both have to accept the responsibility for what blights the helpless little ones whom they send into the world burdened with physical handicaps from which they can never escape. The consequences of sexual immorality are patent to all, but few take the courage to stem the tide by taking steps to prevent the causative factors. In order to raise the instinct to perpetuate the life of the race to a subline level and to immunize the life of the growing generation against the moral decomposition, a deeper awareness is necessary. The ideal has to be presented every now and then in better light, and competent workers will have to strive with enlightened sympathy. Unless all agencies to educate the rising generation and public opinion come to excercise right influence on the thoughts of the youths and the country in general, this is beyond achievement. And for this obstacles are many.

First of all, our educational institutions usually do not give any clear conception of the ethical ideal or the meaning of human life. Often their environment, and the atmosphere prevailing in them blunt the moral sense of the youngsters that pass through them. Most of the youths do not think that they have to do anything beyond passing some examinations and finding a lucrative profession for earning as much money as they can for increasing their enjoyments or pushing up the social standards which have, generally speaking, only a value of display. Thirst for lust and luxury has been flamed up by ubiquitous cinema houses as well as superficial and fickle political leadership. A wide area of affective literature has been poisoned by commercial writers, and as a consequence, moral and spiritual conceptions preserved in old writings, tested by generations and found useful for human guidance, have been swamped or made suspect in the minds of youths. Widespread propaganda about conception-control in all details, with audio-visual aids and unrestrained display of advertisements, has banished from the minds of young people even a sense of the possibility or need of sexual reticence. The spirit of levity, or *ashraddha*, which openly ridicules and makes light of matters that are to be treated seriously and with reverence, resulting from commercialized education, lack of home care and school discipline, contaminated recreation, and demoralizing amusements, has become the bane of modern society. The unhampered publication of pornographic literature, either in the blessed name of art of masqueraded as 'scientific' literature, has only added fuel to the fire. This has in no small degree contributed to a dislike for established methods, to taking pleasure in lethargy, and to an unwillingness to persevere for any end that does not yield immediate pleasure or money to purchase it. The modern teaching that asceticism, even the mildest form of it, is anti-social and that it is an imperfect, perverse, and erroneous ideal of life, by persons who are incompetent by outlook, training, and individual taste – though they may be applauded as experts in some particular branch of knowledge – also has done great harm. These are signs of a social distemper. It is the bounden duty of all who are interested in the moral and spiritual welfare of the country to protest against the canker that is eating into the nation and to reinforce healthy ideas constantly. The literature of strength, of individual and national purity, and of moral courage alone can do this. It will be a pity if India that boasts of leading mankind to peace and light, at times even causing offence to others, failed to set up a standard of incorruptible purity to herself.

Some Hints on Moral and Spiritual Education
– Swami Gabhirananda

The following is a resume of a detailed discussion which a monk once had with a devotee, in connection with the moral and spiritual education of our countrymen. If the government authorities in-charge of education can implement these ideas, the spiritual, moral and cultural calibre of the nation will certainly improve:

1. Both at the school and college levels, the 'Spiritual and Cultural Heritage of man' should be made compulsory subject of study. The medium of instruction may be English or any other Indian language. But the text books must be the same. Books like *The Cultural Heritage of India*, published by the Ramakrishna Misson Institute of Culture, Calcutta, *The Treasury of Traditional Wisdom*, published by George Allen and Unwin, London, may be used for the preparation of the text books.

2. A condensed and representative selection from the *Complete Works of Swami Vivekananda* (9 volumes) published by the

Advaita Ashram, Calcutta, containing the more fundamental lectures of Swami Vivekananda may be made available to the Higher Secondary and College students at a cheap price (the publication has to be subsidised by the Government of India) in English and other Indian languages. The translation should be done by very able persons who are well grounded in spiritual ideals, so that the spirit of Swami Vivekananada will be conveyed wholly to the readers.

3. The mass media of propaganda like the TV, Broadcasting units, Newspapers etc. should be utilised for the spread of positive and life-giving ideas, which are necessary for social reconstruction. The society has to be educated on the need for an austere and a selfless outlook on life, to help society to separate the grain from the chaff, and to live a life dedicated to the practice of the higher values of life. The parents should inspire their children by their exemplary lives

4. Swami Vivekananda speaks of our national ideals thus: "Renunciation and service are the twin ideals of India. Intensify her in those channels and the rest will take care of itself." A proper study of our history corroborates this view. So this is our national ideal: Renunciation and Service, eschewing selfishness and serving others whole-heartedly. These again are the basic tenets of the religion and culture of India. It goes without saying that our children and youths should be educated and trained on these national ideals.

5. The Government should take immediate steps to put a stop to all kinds of weakening and obscene literature in the country. This will go a long way in educating society to live without the provocative auxiliaries of life. They will not waste their time in reading worthless magazines and novels and lead the children to ruination. Religious classics like the *Ramayana, Mahabharata* etc. must become more and more popular and available for reading. Not only that, the authors of the books and articles and the publishers concerned who cater to the baser instincts of man should be considered as enemies of mankind and are to be prevented from such enterprises by statutory measures. They should not be allowed to talk the nonsense of 'fundamental rights' and eternally demoralize society. This is an imperative duty of the Government which is committed to the welfare of man. This is essential for the survival of the human race itself. The world has been, and is being, fed with weakening and demoralizing ideas since centuries and it is a wonder that no one, with all the boast of culture and education and welfare societies, has done anything to ward off the fast

approaching catastrophe of the world. Rightly has the *Bhagavata* said: "Man is ignorant of his own good and he follows the sensuous pleasure. He foolishly searches for happiness at the very source of misery."

Religious Education – An Indispensable Uplifting Measure

The following are the excerpts from the Memorandum which the General Secretary of the Ramakrishna Mission, submitted to the Universities Commission in 1949:

Our leader, Swami Vivekananda held that humanity would be marching surely towards its doom if modern civilization could not be readjusted on a firm spiritual basis; he would have us believe that India has the Mission of playing an important role in bringing about such a readjustment. In recent years, by pitting the power of the Atman (soul-force) successfully against material power, Mahatma Gandhi demonstrated how the spiritual ideas and ideals that India had been holding aloft through scores of centuries might contribute towards world peace.

We, therefore, feel duty-bound to draw your particular attention to the point that although a considerable leeway has to be made up for ensuring the requisite material prosperity of this land, she cannot and should not, lose her grip on her spiritual heritage. She cannot, because that will go against the grain of her people; she should not, because that may spell extinction of her people by wiping out their individuality as a distinct unit of the human race. She has to advance, as much as she can, on both the fronts – the secular and the spiritual.

Hence, the entire educational programme of this country should be so planned as to enable its people to remain loyal to their spiritual ideals and at the same time to master all that is necessary for making them as intensely practical in secular affairs as any other nation. The objective particularly of University education should be to equip Indian youths for the dual task of ensuring the material progress of this country as also of demonstrating effectively before the world the supreme worth of their spiritual heritage in securing worldwide peace and harmony.

Education should be essentially man-making, character-building assimilation of ideas, as Swami Vivekananda put it. The best elements of Eastern and Western culture should be combined to build up our nation's character. The dynamism and scientific attitude of the West have to be combined with the self-poise and spiritual idealism of the East in order to develop a new type of manhood. University education in this country we humbly suggest, should aim at fostering our national character on this line.

For achieving this end, the Indian Universities have to provide for spiritual education no less than for secular education. In every major religion, beneath the trappings of rituals, mythology and communal custom are found some spiritual truths which are eternal in value and universal in character. They do not belong to any particular age or clime. Like the findings of Science they belong to the whole world. Wherever and whenever put into practice, these are sure to vitalize and ennoble man. If, for instance, University education can invigorate the alumni's faith in the Divinity of man, in the infinite potentialities of the human soul, in the outstanding fact of unity in diversity in the scheme of Nature, in the supreme efficacy of purity (i.e. non-attachment) in attaining perfection, this process is sure to help them become vigorous yet calm, mighty yet tolerant and sympathetic, idealist yet practical, and also to help them extend their love and goodwill beyond communal, national and racial frontiers.

Hence religious education with special emphasis on the fundamental spiritual truth should be treated as an indispensable uplifting measure. Of course, it should be seen that each communal group may develop reverence for all religions as so many approaches to the identical goal of Perfection. It has been illustrated in our age by the life of Sri Ramakrishna that one may be intensely religious and yet behave like an embodied antithesis of all forms of narrowness – sectarian, communal, national or racial. We are firmly convinced that religion really is not to be blamed for the orgies perpetrated in its name anywhere on earth at any time, just as science is not to be blamed for the destructive use of its discoveries. It is only their abuse by man that should be held responsible for such anti-social misdeeds.

The remedy of communal fanaticism and hatred lies obviously not in banning religion from the sphere of education, but in enlightening our people about the correct import of the fundamentals of their religions as also in teaching them to develop a catholic outlook on all the different approaches towards Perfection. This, we believe, will foster natural growth of their personalities and at the same time ensure harmony among all sections of our people.

We, therefore, humbly suggest that in India, the birthplace of spiritual giants, with her memories of Taxila, Nalanda and Vikramshila not to speak of the ancient *gurukulas,* the Universities should provide for a healthy and liberal type of religious education, so that they may turn out saints and philosophers as well as scientists and technicians, statesman and economists and pitch our national character in tune with the comprehensive type of personality advocated by Swami Vivekananda.

The Relevance of Swami Vivekananda's Message
to The Teachers and The Students
– R. N. Haldipur

The present education which is being imparted is not adequate to meet the challenges of the times. It does not try to promote the sharpness and refinement of the mind and arouse intellectual curiosity. It is based upon a banking system, as it were, where information is deposited in the minds of the children without arousing in them the spirit of curiosity which should be the basis for acquisition of purposeful knowledge.

The root of the word "education" means to draw out, to bring out or to develop something latent or potential. It is not putting something in but drawing out what is already within. Education is not stuffing information into the brains of the young ones. It should aim at bringing out their innate excellences in day-to-day life. It should essentially be "character-building" and "man-making" as Swami Vivekananda repeatedly points out. He says, "We want that education by which character is formed, the strength of mind is increased, intellect is expanded and by which one can stand on his own feet". Thus the end and aim of all education ought to be "character-building" and "man-making", according to Swamiji.

In Macaulay's system of education (of which most of us who studied in the early part of the 20th century are the products) the emphasis was on the three "Rs" (reading, writing and arithmetic). But Swami Vivekananda's concept of education lays stress on the rounded perfection of the child's personality. Education should not only stress the child's progress but has to see that it reconciles the child to the home atmosphere, to the society in which it lives and to Nature and environment. A system which ignores this vital aspect, tends to produce educated, but half-baked individuals.

We should adopt the "*gurukula* system" of education with suitable modifications which will stimulate in the student an abiding interest in the world at large. It also should create higher aspirations in the student. In the age-old "*gurukula* system" the students were taught during an intimate and free discussion between the teachers and the taught.There was so much freedom allowed to disciples – to ask openly, contradict and argue with their teachers. As in the *Bhagavad Gita*, where Arjuna and Krishna had a dialogue, and Arjuna could ask question without any mental reservation and Krishna provided the answers most willingly, our teachers and students in the system now envisaged should be partners in the acquisition of knowledge. It could be like the Socratic dialogues recorded by Plato in his famous book "*Republic.*"

Education stands for the blossomming forth of the potentialities already in the student, and in doing this the guru or the teacher should activate and inspire him to think out for himself on various issues and understand the significance of the answer which the teacher provides. This is brought out clearly in the enlightening dictum of Swami Vivekananda: "Education is the manifestation of perfection already in man." If such a systen of education is introduced, the full potentiality of the student is released and he is enabled to think for himself. The role of the teacher and the students undergoes a radical change where they are abled to transform themselves – the teacher instilling the enriching values of life in the student, helping them understand the significance of their inner life, and the students imbibing this precious knowledge vital to their growth in consciousness. Thus the students will be in a position to add to their moral and spiritual stature.

Everything in life finds a place in this scheme of education. Youths will be enabled to bring about intellectual, moral and emotional integration and well-being of the society. The school becomes the cultural centre of the village or the town, the students taking active part in the developmental activites. Such participation will make for national integration and social harmony in the long run.

In any school, involvement of the parents is important. Periodical parent-teacher meetings – involving the parents in various school activities – like collecting materials for building or entertainment with folk music, folk dance, mimicry, puppetry on the Annual Day function – is important from the point of view of establishing a good rapport.

There are a number of schools with a new outlook – some of them are experimental: 1) J. Krishnamurthy's Rishi Valley near Madanapalli in Andhra Pradesh, and Rajghat School in Uttar Pradesh, 2) Warana Nagar experiment in Maharastra, 3) Netherhat Public School in Bihar, 4) Ramakrishna Mission Schools, 5) Vivekananda Kendra Vidyalayas in the North East, 6) Rag Pickers' School in Old Delhi, – each dealing with different problems of different sections. They could well provide us with initiative and enterprise.

Life and Religion
– Swami Swahananda

How far does religion influence our lives? Often is this question asked. With the increase of secularistic ideas, religion is on the defensive. It is of course natural that an older idea is attacked by a newer one and it must support its standpoint. Secularistic people are mainly of two types: egoistical and socialistic. The first group is satisfied with following their individual likes and dislikes, personal enjoyment and happiness. They do not care what happens to the other man. They however are denounced by the religious as well as the socialistic people. The second group thinks more in terms of society. They are not particular about the quality of their individual lives. But they are interested in social growth. This growth however must be tangible and material only. It is this group that can actually question the usefulness of religious pursuits, though while attacking the utility of religion or its metaphysical basis, it makes common cause with the first group.

Generally, the egotistic, individualistic or selfish secular people are not taken into consideration. They are self-condemned. But the vast majority of the secularists belong to this class. They want to be free from all restraints, all considerations for higher ideals or other people. But society cannot progress with such people. So they are to be trained in the tenets of citizenship and a police force also will have to be kept ready for the incorrigibles. This type of selfish nature will be seen among the followers of religion too. And often people ask: What then is the use of religion? What effect has it on the life of the commom poeple? As for the secularistic selfish people this question is not asked. It is taken as a normal thing that man will be selfish. The theories of the socialistic outlook, as well as secularism and materialism are not asked to explain why people are so. For have they not accepted man as an animal or almost a material thing? So there ends their responsibility. If religion speaks of higher values and higher virtues, it must show these virtues manifesting in society. That is the line of argument. If you say non-violence is the ideal, you will be shown immediately half a dozen failures of this principle. If you point out that violence is also untenable as a guide, it becomes only a negative answer!

What then is the balanced view? The point is to be thrust home that the more plausible theory is the correct theory at least for the present, as we accept in the case of scientific truths. Religion as a theory and a way of life will be true and covetable, if compared to other theories and other ways of life, it can solve the problems of life better, and can influence life more deeply.

Following this line of argument, we can easily see that wherever religion fails to influence life, it is not so much its fault as the fault of the 'normal' nature of man as described by the secularists themselves. Looked at from this angle, religion is freed from many of their charges. But still some substance remains in the argument that religion is not so useful unless it brings about a change in the 'normal' life of man. Religious virtues must be manifested in their life. That is also the behest of all religious teachers. 'Religion is realization' said Swami Vivekananda. Unless religious virtues are made practical in the life of the votaries, they remain mere theories, only for arguing and talking. As theories they may stand on equal grounds with other theories, but to be a thing intimately related to life, practice and experience are essential.

It is of course recognized that men with a religious outlook develop the qualities of honesty and dutifulness, qualities that are essential for running the administration as well as the day-to-day affairs. Interpersonal relations require much patience, consideration and love. These qualities are generallyimbibed by such people. Wherever there is a lack of these qualities, we must admit that religion has not penetrated beyond the surface life. There may be still some necessity for it, but the social benefit is little. And people who judge any institution or outlook only from the standpoint of utility will naturally be dissatisfied.

India is often said to be the land of religion. Then why is it that so much of corruption and other evils are seen in this country, is the question often asked. It is a pertinent question too. In the pristine days of India when religion was a reality in the life of the people a very high standard of higher virtues was visible in the society. This becomes clear when we study accounts of Indian society left by Megasthenes and others. We cannot say we maintain the same level even now. After the Independence the sacrificing quality seems to be lessened. The horizontal aspect of religion is surely less, though we still have the vertical one in the lives of rare individuals. If religion is less in the society, it is because we lack the conviction of the ancients. This may be because of the ideological conflict between materialism and spirituality, and the modern emphasis on enjoyment at any cost here and now. It is materialism that fixes man's attention on this life and on pleasure and as a result boosts up self-aggrandizement and other social evils. The way out is not to banish religion, or to declare oneself to be non-religious but to try to be genuinely religious.... By too much criticism more people will be scared to be called religious, and thereby the standard of selflessness will go down even more. Already the rituals of religious life are being given up; criticism will push them out completely. But then religion will lose its power of growth, if completely dissociated from the external, like rice removed of the husk. For a full growth both are necessary.

Let us not banish religion and along with that the basis of unselfishness and higher virtues through our unkind criticism.

Moreover, it is the so-called externals on which depend the peculiarities of a culture. It is often said that a new world order is coming. As a result of the growth of communication and mutual contact between nations, habits, dresses etc. will be standardized and local peculiarities will be obliterated. What then will remain of the culture of a particular country? No nation we think will give way easily. In India we are not very particular about retaining our national characteristics, but dress etc. of other newly freed nations of Burma, Ghana and the like, will show how sensitive they are. Externals are the avenues through which culture expresses itself. With our anxiety for the results we forget that the means are also equally important. To get the kernel of the fruit the skin is also equally important. So devotion to externals, to dresses, habits, language and rituals is essential. It takes generations for an idea to take root in a society and often it is mixed up with many non-essentials. In common man you cannot expect an idea materialized in all its pristine glory. In the so-called enlightened, to whom everything has been relativized, you cannot often get an idea suffusing his life, for he loses the capacity of taking anything as an article of faith.

Improvement of habits, manners and customs, if improvement at all you call it, must be done not by lowering the standard but by pointing out the higher ideal, the better method, and stressing the essential. Then the transition will be less painful and more smooth. And in the process, the fundamental, useful moorings will not be lost. It is because of this, Swami Vivekananda repeatedly warned that while educating the backward, the religious outlook should not be disturbed, for nothing constructive can be implanted in society in one generation. He said:

'We have to give them secular education. We have to follow the plan laid down by our ancestors, that is, to bring all the ideals slowly down among the masses. Raise them slowly up, raise them to equality. Impart even secular knowledge through religion.'

'The fate of a nation depends upon the condition of the masses. Can you raise them? Can you give them back their lost individuality without making them lose their innate spiritual nature? Can you become an Occidental of occidentals in your spirit of equality, freedom, working energy, and at the same time a Hindu to the very backbone in religious culture and instincts? This is to be done and we will do it.'

When we plead for retaining or going slow in changing the age-old customs and habits, we do not say that these externals are inviolables. They can be changed and they are changed. That was how the new *smritis* giving new rules of conduct were promulgated. In this age of easy communication and huddling of men in industrial areas, many of the old habits will have to be changed. Let us not lose the higher moorings embedded in them but adjust them to the new surroundings, by new interpretations and by evolving new habits. Otherwise the vacuum will be filled up by things that degrade men and society,

Religion – The Key-note of Indian Life
– Swami Harshananda

If it is true that in all countries and in all ages, irreligion – or to be more correct, materialism – has held its sway over a section of the people, it is even more true that religion has influenced a much greater number of people and to a much greater extent.

Man being 'cast in the mould of God' cannot easily deny Him. Even great scientists like Newton and Einstein have believed in the existence of God as an intelligent power regulating and guiding the destinies of the Universe.

In the words of Swami Vivekananda, 'Religion is realization'. It is a 'manifestation of the divinity already in man'. And whatever helps in unfolding this divinity inherent in man, is religion. It is not just a dogma or a creed or a set of observances. It is leading the life in such a way that we help manifest our higher nature, truth, goodness and beauty, in every thought, word and deed.

As the saying goes, 'man shall not live by bread alone.' He needs something more, some high ideal to live for. And this ideal is provided by religion, any religion, when understood properly.

It is true that much blood has been shed in the name of religion. World history is replete with crusades and *jihads*. But this is not the fault of religion as such, but due to a misunderstanding of the spirit of religion. No religion ever says that man should shed the blood of man or be cruel to another. It is actually the opposite, the spirit of 'Love thy neighbour as thyself' that has been propagated by religion. And whenever man had heeded this advice, there had been a golden era in history.

And religion has especially been the strong point of India. For centuries India has been producing great personalities who were deeply religious and
who have influenced the national life profoundly. From Rama, Krishna and Buddha in the ancient times up to Ramakrishna, Vivekananda, Ramana, and Aurobindo in the modern times there has been a long procession of these great religious personalities. It is the bounden duty of our students to make a reverent study of the religions of India and draw inspiration from them....

Swami Vivekananda was fond of saying often that each nation has its special characteristic and for India it is religion. Here is a passage from one of his lectures delivered in Madras: "I see that each nation, like each individual, has one theme in this life, which is its centre, the principal note round which every other note comes to form the harmony. In one nation political power is its vitality as in England, artistic life in another and so on. In India religious life forms the centre, the keynote of the whole music of national life; and if any nation attempts to throw off its national vitality, the direction which has become its own through transmission for centuries, that nation dies, if it succeeds in the attempt."

He warned the nation of the disastrous consequences of giving up religion and substituting it with other things, thus: "And, therefore, if you succeed in the attempt to throw off religion and take up either politics or society or any other thing as your centre, as the vitality of your national life, the result will be, that you will become extinct. To prevent this, you must make all and everything work through that vitality of religion." Let us remember that these are the words of a great saint and a modern prophet who provided the inspiration for many of our national leaders in the early part of this century.

II

A reader of Swami Vivekananda's lectures on Indian nationalism will feel a little embarrassed by his uncompromising insistence that religion should form the basis of Indian national reconstruction. For, ever since Independence, our leaders have repeated that India is a secular State and religion should be relegated as a matter of private life. Several sections of people who think that way are motivated only by indifference and insensitiveness to spiritual values. Affluence, which means possession and enjoyment, is the only value to be pursued according to them. There are many others who feel that spiritual values are essential, but they do not think that there is any necessary connection between religion and spirituality. Therefore, according to them, religions should be excluded from the educational system and from the purview of the State's activities in all fields, but spirituality should be encouraged. This denigration of religion in a total or in a partial way has been going on in this country for the past three decades. The cumulative effect of the practice of secularism has only been the growth of corruption and the degeneration of moral standards on all sides.

It is therefore worthwhile to consider whether there is any intimate connection between religion and spirituality. A close scrutiny will show that there is between them an intimate connection, as between a container and the contained. To negate the importance of religion in this respect will be like saying that it is the wine that is important and not the container. In human history religion has always been the container of spiritual values. It has provided through the ages the forms and symbols, the concepts and imageries in which spiritual values have been presented, preserved and transmitted in all societies.

It is also true that religions, as practised in most societies, have included in their scope many anti-spiritual values also. Religion has often provided a favourite rallying ground for bigots and unscrupulous politicians, with the inevitable consequence that religion has been politicised and converted into a mainstream for conveying much of the dirty effluents of human relations. As a consequence religion has got a bad name among a large body of politically minded and patriotic people, and that is why its replacement by secularism has come to be considered as a panacea for all the evils that beset our body politic.

In this predicament it is worthwhile to consider how religion can be freed from the political and social abuses that have brought it bad name. Some of the following steps can help in achieving this:

Religion should become more a matter of realisation than dogmatism. Fundamentalism in religion should be discouraged and the individual must be free to interpret and follow his religion without any external or organisational compulsion.

Religion should not be allowed to obstruct the evolution of a common civil law.

No kind of social institution that goes against human dignity and welfare should be allowed to exist and justify itself in the name of religion.

Religious conversion must be banned by law, as these conversions are effected mainly from political motives and financial inducements, and ultimately go against national integration. This does not however mean the denial of freedom for spiritual conversion, which does not require a change of one's original social and cultural affiliations – not even of one's religious nomenclature.

Religious freedom should mean only freedom to practise a religion and preach it among its own followers for their improvement and not to take any aggressive stance against those who practise other religions or to criticise and caricature their beliefs and practices.

A study of comparative religion should become an important subject in the curriculum adopted in schools and colleges. In a multi-religious country like India textbooks suitable for students of different standards must be pre-pared, not by fundamentalists of different religions but by enlightened people who accept the validity of all religions. These text books must give the principal teachings of all religions in such a way that the students learn to respect all religions.

If the leaders of our country consider spiritual values as essential for the welfare of the people, the State should not harp on secularism and adopt an indifferent attitude towards religion. The State has to play an active part in regulating this all important aspect of human life.

– Swami Tapasyananda

III

Swami Vivekananda warned us against the disastrous consequence of making politics a means of our national salvation. What is happening in our political life at the moment is indeed a tragic fulfilment of his fiery jeremiad against politics as a pursuit of power and his prophetic eyes foresaw that this pursuit of state power would in time become a pursuit of personal power, which ambitious politicians would place above the nation. Today we are facing a dire fate because we did not listen to the great voice warning us against a political approach to our national problems. If today we are unhappy about the vulgarity and shallowness which have entered into our public life, where a public cause is essentially a matter of private ambition, and if we must now deplore a state of affairs in which politics is corrupting our society at all levels, we must blame ourselves for disregarding Vivekananda's view of the dangers of politics.

If we must now endeavour to understand the essence of Vivekananda's message for us and for the world and even in these latter days think of giving a new direction to our thought and action towards a reconstruction of our society, we must first realize that we are today what he wanted us not to be – a nation led by a pack of politicians who can play with the destiny of a whole people for money and for power.

Convinced of the futility of politics in the West, Vivekananda reflected on the genius of the Indian civilization and discovered that in that civilization politics was not in the least an active factor. The average Indian was not a political man and the greatest Indian minds were not political minds. To him the Indian civilization was essentially a non-political civilization and he distinguished it from the Graeco-Roman civilization: In one of his notes of class Talks and Lectures he draws a distinction between the Hindu and the Greek civilization and says that 'the Greek sought political liberty'. 'The Hindu has always sought spiritual liberty'. He does not add that the Hindu is superior to the Greek because he never cared for political liberty. But he draws the distinction and affirms: 'To care only for spiritual liberty and not for social liberty is a defect, but the opposite is a still greater defect'.

Vivekananda was opposed to political revolution because he was opposed to a political approach to human problems. 'If you succeed in the attempt' he says, 'to throw off your religion and take up either politics, or society, or any other thing as your centre, as the vitality of your national life, the result will be that you will become extinct'. 'Before flooding India with socialistic or political ideas' he adds, 'first deluge the land with spiritual ideas'. And he believed that politics was foreign to the genius of the Indian people and in an address he even affirmed: 'The voice of Asia has been the voice of religion. The voice of Europe is the voice of politics'. In his address, *My Master* he says: 'If you come and teach politics to the Hindus, they do not understand; but if you come to preach religion, however curious it may be, you will have hundreds and thousands of followers in no time.... In an interview in England in 1896 he said that 'religion is of deeper importance than politics'.

Vivekananda preached at a time when the Western world itself was raising serious question about the adequacy of politics as an instrument of human good. What made him turn away from politics is the fact that he viewed the contemporary human society as a burning example of the failure of politics. In his own country he saw the grim spectacle of imperial politics.

Vivekananda warned us against the calamitous consequences of an exclusively political approach to our national problems. The voice of warning came from one who had the courage to set himself against the forces of European history and contemplate a society and programme of social action without politics. He conceived a human society free from the evil of State power and he rejected politics because politics is the art of seizing that power for an individual or a party. Neither an individual nor a party can pursue power and at the same time care for principles. If war is the greatest menace to the modern man, you cannot prevent it unless you shun politics, which even in times of peace is essentially an art of conflict. All politics is desire for power and all desire for power is violence even when it is not supported by an army.

Vivekananda fixed his gaze at the primal splendour of his nation's spiritual history and without being guilty of any form of spiritual chauvinism he believed that this was the primal splendour of the entire humanity's spiritual history. That splendour is Vedantic monism. What makes him the greatest of revolutionaries in the world's religious history, a unique example of a renovator of human life as a whole, is that his revolutionary ideal and revolutionary programme are sustained by a philosophy of the Vedanta.

No revolution, political or religious, in the history of the world was so rooted in such a comprehensive philosophy.

A spiritual and moral revolution – a fundamental transformation of human nature alone can bring about a fundamental change in human institutions. Swami Vivekananda was an apostle of such a spiritual and moral revolution. Political revolution must be a futile and disastrous experiment unless there was first a moral and spiritual revolution changing human nature and creating spontaneous love for a just social order.

To Vivekananda, man's liberation must be a Vedantic liberation, the attainment of freedom in a free universe, which is a unity. The revolutionary endeavour is then not an adventitious exercise, something external to what is really the ground of all action and all thought, the Ultimate Reality, which is one and indivisible and in which all things work and move. It is the grand enterprise of man's higher self working towards some cosmic fulfilment.

Vivekananda did not learn his Vedanta from the Vedantic canon alone; he found in his Master, Ramakrishna Paramahamsa, a living embodiment of the finer essence of that philosophy. From his Great Master he received the truth of the Upanishadic doctrine, *tat tvam asi* (That thou art), and he made it a part of his being. That gave him his strength, his hope, his belief in the unity of all thought and all action, his belief in one Supreme Reality.

What is truly revolutionary in Vivekananda's idea of a spiritual and moral revolution is this Vedantic approach to history and man's creative role in it. From this is derived the ethics of man's action in society. When we talk about his revolutionary ideas, it is not enough that we mention his progressive ideas on our social problems, caste, superstition, ignorance, position of women etc. We must first go to the very roots of his gospel of action, his philosophy of revolution. Our radicalism has so far failed us because we have not been radical enough. We have not gone to the roots of things, to the spiritual ground of all work and all thought.

He did not think of building a new society on the quicksands of some imported platitudes, on some progressive ideas that were in the air in his times. He wanted to build on the solid rock of a world-view, a philosophy of action, and he found that rock in the Vedanta as he interpreted it.

Vivekananda's prophetic eyes foresaw how we would make virtues of our vices and how we would abuse our highest ideals for the sake of power and position. He therefore called us into a new understanding of the whole meaning of life, a new perspective of human destiny in a monistic universe where kindness is not a concession to the poor but a means of self-fulfilment, where equality is not a levelling down of all into uniformity but is rooted in a sense of the unity of all life, and where social justice is not guaranteed by a civil code but is ensured by the very spirit of love which must pulsate in a universe which has been realised as a manifestation of Divine Spirit. What a law gives today another law can take away tomorrow. But what flows from love remains and ever increases. And Vivekananda thought that the strength man needed to bring about such a revolutionary change in society could come only from a Vedantic-monistic conception of the universe.

Let us not imagine that this Vedantic-monistic approach to life obliges us to wind up our household and live in the forest for our salvation. What makes Vivekananda a revolutionary in this interpretation of the Vedanta is that he shows its relevance to the life as we live it or wish to live it in our familiar surroundings.... But what he insisted on was character because leadership demanded character. I think he put before the nation the most vital question regarding the instrument of social change, the question of leadership. 'The kings are gone', he said and asked: 'Where is the new sanction, the new power of the people?' He saw the danger of the power going to a small elite of resourceful men who were capable of assuming the authority which once belonged to kings. 'The tyranny of a minority', he said, 'is the worst tyranny that the world ever sees'. Vivekananda therefore put his faith in the congregated strength of a spiritually and morally awakened people and he called his nation and the world to work for that awakening.

His Vedantic monism gives him his conviction that when a nation is regenerated it works for the regeneration of the world. A Vedantist nationalist is necessarily an internationalist. And if Vivekananda was a revolutionary in his idea of nationalism, he was no less a revolutionary as an internationalist. He believed in Vedantism as an agent of a spiritual and moral revolution in the world as a whole and he thought that in a spiritually awakened world there can be no political tyranny or economic injustice. In this faith alone can the world work for its salvation.

– Prof. R. K. Das Gupta

What is Religion?

– Swami Vidyatmananda

Today, as always, man seeks God – and often without knowing he is doing so. All human activity – good, bad, or indifferent – is actually the misapplied search for God,

The fact is that man in his true nature is already divine; but this divinity is covered. Life's one purpose is the realisation of divinity.

Realization of divinity is religion. At base, all religions teach this same truth although accretions often obscure it. Vedanta emphasises the one objective of realization but accepts diverse methods of reaching it.

Realization may be gained by the practice of the yoga of knowledge, or of control of mind, or of selfless work, or of love of God – or by a combination of yogas.

The great prophets of the world afford living examples of the realization of divinity. As models they inspire man, and as dispensers of grace they assist him towards realization.

II

There are many methods by which perfection in God may be reached. Different ways suit different temperaments. In the religious literature of the Hindus, four main paths to the attainment of union with God (known as yogas) are generally recognized.

In karmayoga, the path of selfless work, every action is offered as a sacrament. By dedicating the fruits of one's work to God, one gradually achieves non-attachment and eventually goes beyond both action and inaction – at the same time remaining active.

Jnanayoga is the path of discrimination. By analysing and then rejecting all transitory phenomena, the Reality or Godhead in its impersonal aspect is finally perceived. It is a difficult path, not suited for the majority of spiritual aspirants.

Bhaktiyoga is the path of devotion. By cultivating intense love for God as a personal Being, the worshipper merges his own ego in his Ideal. In this path, God is often worshipped as a divine incarnation – a Christ, or Buddha, or Krishna. Most believers in the world's religions are bhaktiyogis.

Rajayoga is the path of formal meditation. It is the method of concentrating the mind one-pointedly on the Reality until complete absorption is achieved. This path may be followed exclusively, often by those who lead predominantly contemplative lives. But, in a sense, rajayoga may be said to combine the other three paths, since meditation is involved in God-dedicated action, worship, discrimination, and concentration on the chosen ideal of God. Although a balanced spiritual life demands a harmonious combination of all four yogas, one or the other usually predominates, depending on the temperament of the spiritual aspirant. All four paths lead to the same transcendental experience of union with God.

– Swami Prabhavananda

III

Swami Vivekananda summed up the whole of religion in three statements:
1. Each soul is potentially divine.
2. The goal is to manifest this divinity within, by controlling nature – external and internal.
3. Do this either by work, or worship, or psychic control, or philosophy, by one, or more, or all of these – and be free.

"This is the whole of religion," added Swami Vivekananda. "Doctrines, or dogmas, or rituals, or books, or temples, or forms, are but secondary details."

Let us consider these statements as three propositions:

Proposition 1:
Each soul is potentially divine.

What is meant by the term, "divinity"? Most people have a very vague notion about this. Divinity is an existence which is infinite, immortal, imperishable, absolute, all-knowing, all-powerful, and ever-blissful. The word, divinity, therefore, implies the state of (1) absolute existence, (2) unlimited power, (3) infinite knowledge, and (4) eternal bliss. Any conception of Divinity, of God or of an Ultimate State or Being, must include these attributes. Such a Divinity, God, Ultimate State or Being must be perfect, and in order to be perfect it must be of the nature we have just described. Divine perfection is uncaused, unlimited and un-conditioned by time, space, or causation.

In relation to man what do I mean by divinity? I mean that highest ideal of perfection which we all want to attain in the course of our lives. I mean the unfoldment of that state of consciousness in which we will have no defect, misery, suffering, or limitation of any kind. Spontaneously, knowingly or unknowingly, we all respond to an urge for that. What are we all working for? What is our highest goal in life? In short, we are all working for the attainment of the ideal state of perfection, for the attainment of limitless existence, absolute knowledge, and infinite happiness.

We want to live. And we want to live in such a way that there will not be any suffering, disease, death, or an imperfection of any kind disturbing our existence.

We want to know. We spontaneously feel that we have a right to attain a state where there will not be anything in this universe unknown to us. We are all looking for that state of realization. Our discoveries, inventions, and all the advancement of intellectual thought and scientific progress have been possible owing to that inner urge of man. We spontaneously feel that we have a right to be happy. Of course, the philosophy underlying the ideal and the method for the attainment of that state of bliss might be different with different individuals. But, so far as the fundamental urge is concerned, it is one and the same for everyone.

The motive force behind every living being is a similar fundamental urge for the unfoldment of the state of perfect existence, knowledge, and bliss. We do not have to be taught about this state of divinity, for it is not without; it is always within.

Can you find any living being who does not like to live? Can you find a man who has honestly become reconciled to disease and death? Where is the person who is satisfied with the state of imperfection? Can we become reconciled to ignorance? Why this insatiable yearning for more and more knowledge? There is no human being who does not feel a deep sense of protest against the state of ignorance. Tell a human being that he has no right to know, and see how insulted he feels. Why such sensitiveness?

What about happiness? There are people who have been suffering all their lives. But were they reconciled to their state of misery? Were they not always looking for that "silver lining" to the dark cloud of their suffering, either in this life or in a life hereafter? This shows that in man's inner nature there is a firm conviction that he has the right to be happy.

Man's instinctive protest against imperfection of any kind against death, ignorance, suffering, and so on – presupposes that he is born with the unshakeable convicion that infinite perfection is his birthright. That man is divine is shown by his response to this conviction and his resentment towards the contrary, spontaneously and intuitively.

The subjective ideal of perfection, of divinity, has been concretized and objectified in the form of a personal conception of divinity, or God. If you speak to people about God being possessed of these divine attributes – absolute existence, knowledge, and bliss – they will agree. But when you speak of their inner divinity they often seem shocked. Analyse your conception of God and you will find that it is nothing but the concretized picture of the fulfilment of absolute existence, knowledge, and bliss. God does not become old or sick; he does not die. He knows everything; there is no limitation to his knowledge. God has the capacity for the enjoyment of infinite bliss. Nothing can make him sad or depressed. These are the three basic subjective ideals that have been concretized, objectified, and developed into the conception of an objective deity.

Why is that most of you are ready to agree that these ideals describe God, or an Ultimate Being or State, but are not so ready to agree that these may be ascribed to the nature of man also? Why do you hesitate to believe that man is potentially divine? First of all let me ask you that if divinity is infinite, which it must be, will it not pervade everything? Will there be any place where it is not? Could there be anything else besides divinity? No. Because if there were, the infinite would not be infinite. Infinite implies the existence of one only. The existence of anything else would limit it and it would lose its infinite nature.

Proposition 2:
The goal is to manifest this divinity within, by controlling nature, external and internal.

We are divine, but why do we not know it? Why do we feel so powerless to manifest it? Because there are certain obstacles in the way of its manifestation. These obstacles in the way of the manifestation of the Divinity within have to be removed. This is done by "controlling nature, external and internal." Life means the struggle of the soul to assert its own right. The purpose of life is to overcome the obstacles that prevent manifestation of the soul's real nature, which is divine perfection. What are these obstacles? They are: (1) not-knowledge; (2) agitation of the mind-stuff; (3) false self-consciousness; and (4) desire for possessions and attachment to them.

Not-knowledge means indiscrimination and illusion. In Sanskrit this is called *avidya,* this is, not-knowledge or ignorance as to the true nature, the divine nature, of man.

....Divinity is within us, yet all the time we are bewailing its loss. We have been carrying this perfection within us all the time, but because of our misconception of it we do not recognize it. What is actually needed is 'disillusionment.' We have to rouse ourselves out of the state of misconception. We have to wake up from our delusion. When the awakening comes, we realise our mistake. We find that through all our process of searching, we had been carrying within us the very thing we were searching for. We did not have the correct knowledge of the true nature of our Self. This is called *avidya*. Correct knowledge is *vidya*.

The agitation of the mind-stuff is called *chitta-vrtti* in Sanskrit *(chitta,* consciousness, and *vrtti,* ripples or waves). The agitation of the rnind-stuff obstructs the manifestation of divinity. (Actually, nothing can obstruct divinity; it is our understanding of it, our vision, that is obstructed.)

....If you would keep your consciousness transparent and unagitated you would realize the Divinity there. It is external stimuli, worldly thoughts and contacts, and the internal stimuli of desires, hopes, plans, memories, and so on, that keep our consciousness in a state of storm and tempest. How are we to attain that state of quietude? The method is simple enough to state: learn the art of keeping your mind calrn and transparent. There is a special method by which this may be achieved.

False self-consciousness is another obstacle. In Sanskrit this self is called *ahamkara,* or the individualised ego-consciousness. So long as we associate ourselves with the little individualised ego, we cannot realise the Divinity. We have to give up this false self-consciousness.

....Divinities we are, but we have hypnotized ourselves into thinking we are weak mortal beings. We have to rid ourselves of this false self-consciousness. We have to know that we are one with Him.

The desire for possessions, to keep and to add to one's possessions, is called *vasana*. We become attached to possessions, to the transitory things of life, and from this attachment a chain of causation is set in motion in which we become deeply enmeshed. It often becomes so complicated that we completely lose our way in the labyrinth of action. We cannot know our real nature until we rise above all action and attachment to action, and realize our Self as being above these.

These, then, are the four basic obstacles to the manifestation, to the realization, of the Divine within. Now we come to the third proposition. How do we overcome the obstacles to the manifestation of the Divine within?

Proposition 3:
    Do this either by work, or worship, or psychic control, or philosophy, by one, or more, or all of these – and he free.

Humanity may be classified under three broad groups: the awakened, the ready-to-be-awakened, and those who are asleep. The awakened are those who are aware of their divine nature. They may not be completely aware of it, but they are awakened enough. Naturally, they are in the minority. Those who are "asleep" are quite happy with their lives as they are. They do not think beyond this little world of sense objects. They constitute the great majority of mankind. The ready-to-be-awakened are the aspirants in spiritual life.

Again spiritual aspirants are classified under four psychological types, their general characteristics and sources of inspiration being: (1) the discriminating, reasoning type. A philosophical mind responds quickly to this process; (2) the psychic type, which responds more to mental stimuli than to sense stimuli; (3) the devotional, loving type which has a great capacity for feeling; and (4) the active type. Here the appeal is to man's energetic, outgoing propensities.

All these four types are equally important. The principle of the one cannot be applied to another. The systematic method of practice which each type follows for the achievement of the highest goal is called yoga. The word, yoga, is derived from the Sanskrit root, *yuj*, one meaning of which is to join, to unite, to yoke. Hence, the primary meaning of the word is the process by which an aspirant is joined, united, or yoked to his highest Ideal. It means the union of the imperfect self with the divine Self. Each of the yogas can lead an aspirant to the goal, independent of any of the other yogas. Technically, yoga is a special science which enables a seeker of truth to realize the goal. The discriminative type follows the path of jnanayoga. For the psychic type, rajayoga is prescribed. Bhaktiyoga is suitable for the devotional type, and karmayoga is recommended for the active type. However, a general study and practice of the principles of all the yogas is recommended.

Know that all the yogas lead to the same goal. Do not feel too inclined towards only one of them and underestimate the others. Any yoga followed to its logical conclusion, will lead you to the highest goal.

Hindu philosophy is unique in that it has different methods of experimentation. It may, therefore, be called scientific. One who cares to practise conscientiously can learn for himself and judge by his own results.

*   *   *

Let us now review the aims of the four yogas. According to jnanayoga, phenomena are only an appearance; the self is nothing but Brahman, the only Reality. The method of this path is to remove *maya*, the veil of ignorance, by discrimination, and thereby be free and illumined. It is the "royal road of reason."

Rajayoga states that individual consciousness is nothing but Pure Consciousness. Due to agitation within individual consciousness, it appears separate and limited. The method is discipline, concentration, and meditation to calm these agitations which distort consciousness and prevent perfection from manifesting itself.

Bhaktiyoga holds that it is the apparent separation of the individual self, or soul, from its divine source that causes its present imperfection. Union with the divine source is attained by purifying the ego and directing our emotions solely to God.

Karmayoga states that man's perfection is disturbed by his desires, by the setting in motion of the wheel of causation. Neutralisation of karma is the method. When the thread of causality is burnt, perfection manifests itself.

Any one of these yogas prescribed for the different human psychological types, if followed to its logical conclusion, will lead to the highest spiritual realisation. We rarely find, however, a person who is a pure type. The fact is that aspirants lean more towards one of the yogas than others, due to certain natural, inborn tendencies, or *samskaras*. And today, life is so complex that specialization in just one of the yogas is neither practical nor possible. For instance, where is the man who can be a real jnani? Where is he who can honestly say: "I will sit here and deny the existence of everything!"? Today, it is necessary to combine the yogas. The teachings of the yogas should be harmoniously blended in order to develop in us a well-balanced spiritual character.

Swami Vivekananda said: "I want to preach a man-making religion." And he compared the yogas to a bird. "Three things," be said, "are necessary for a bird to fly – the two wings and the tail as a rudder for steering. *Jnana* (knowledge) is the one wing, bhakti (love) is the other, and (raja) yoga is the tail that keeps up the balance."

My criticism of the four yogas, if they stand alone, is this: intellect alone is *stony;* psychic phenomena alone are *spooky*; emotion alone is *sticky;* action alone is *shaky.* We must beware of these four "S's"! We must harmonise our intellect, intuition, emotion, and action.

Now how are we to combine the yogas? Begin the day with rajayoga. Prayer and meditation will give you an undercurrent of poise like the lingering sound of a bell. Strike the "bell" again throughout the day as often as possible, even at work. Whenever you have time to yourself, be a rajayogi. The disciplines of rajayoga develop tenacity and strengthen the will; and they gradually bring consciousness to a state of tranquillity. Close the day, again with rajayoga, with concentration and meditation, eradicating all undesirable concepts that have clung to your consciousness during the day's activities.

Be a bhakta in your contact with others. See God in everything and offer worship to him. You can worship God with flowers or with a broomstick. Establish Him in your home, in your life. Make Him your constant companion. Know that life is the expression of that Divinity. It is He who makes it lovable, makes it livable. With every breath feel that it is He. Nurture and cultivate bhakti in secret, in your heart.... Do not make a display of your devotion; that is cheap sentimentalism. Discipline in bhakti is very necessary.

In the field of action be a karmayogi. Work for the sake of work. let your work be your worship. Always remain unattached to your work and do not let any desire creep in. "Throw self overboard" is the slogan of karmayoga. Be ready to attach and equally to detach your mind from your actions.

A karmayogi knows the skill of adjusting his work and expressions according to the time, place, and environment. Always consider your attitude in all your activities. Be perfect in both the subjective and the objective aspects of activity.

Last but not least, let your life be balanced and controlled by the intellect. Knowledge of fundamental principles gives you latitude and the power of adjustment. It synthesises everything in life; it destroys any superiority complex. Jnanayoga develops discrimination and reasoning. The other yogas are held in form by it. It is the sustainer of the other yogas. Let your entire day nay, your entire life, be controlled and guided by a disciplined and discriminative intellect, which to your life is like the rudder to a boat. ....Sustain all your activities with the knowledge of the fundamental principles of jnana. With that as the basis of your thinking you will not make any mistakes.

By following the principles of the four yogas in your daily life, you will always be in touch with the divine force, at work or at play. You need never be very far from your Ideal.

All the yogas aim at one thing: the attainment of perfection. And we find that the root cause of all the obstacles to the attainment of this perfection in yoga is the misconception we have of our ego-consciousness. From the viewpoint of jnana, the "I-consciousness" has to be understood as an illusion, or a superimposed structure on the Self, and it must be eliminated through discrimination. When "I-consciousness" is eliminated, with it disappears the world. What remains is the Reality – Brahman.

In rajayoga, the strongest and most basic agitation of consciousness is the sense of "I-ness." When that has been subdued, divine Consciousness manifests itself.

In bhaktiyoga the individual ego has to be purified and minimized until it exists no more as such, but loses itself, melts into, as it were, the Divine Consciousness conceived of as the Chosen Ideal.

In karmayoga, "I and mine" consciousness, which leads to desire and attachment, has to be relinquished. The "little I" as the doer of action has to be wiped out, and the "big I", the eternal Witness of all action, has to be realized as one's own Self. in all cases it is ego-consciousness with its various modifications that obstructs us from realizing our spiritual Ideal.

....The practices in yoga are intended to control consciousness at the point where it first becomes individualized, for it is the "I-am" consciousness that is the cause of man's obstacles to the realization of his real nature.... However, although yoga attempts to control and efface the individualized ego, this ego is very, very difficult to get rid of. It comes back, even after realization. So long as we are in a body we will have an ego-consciousness. Sri Ramakrishna often told his disciples: "Let the 'rascal' ego remain, but as the servant, the devotee of God." We must cultivate the ego of devotion, the witness ego, or the ego of knowledge. Establish a definite relationship of your "I-am" consciousness with your ideal.... Depend on God. Then your life will be freed from attachment, freed from fear and from all other things that make you feel small, miserable, and insecure.

All the yogas have been dealt with in a masterly manner by Swami Vivekananda. If you are interested in going more deeply into the study of the yogas there is ample opportunity. But take the study in real earnest, with the intention of putting these grand principles into practice.... There must follow some practices to unfold the inner reality. Live it and feel it at every step of your life. Discover the path that suits you best and follow it.

The practices and disciplines of the yogas are intended to bring the mind of the aspirant to a state of poise and steadiness. Under their influence, the obstacles to the unfoldment of inner perfection will be minimized. Without having attained that state of mental steadiness and calm, the student will find it difficult to follow any of the practices of yoga, much less to concentrate his mind or to meditate. An unsteady and uncontrolled mind is a liability, never an asset. It is of the utmost importance for the spiritual aspirant to attain a refined and calm state of mind.

Give up vain and unnecessary argumentation. Half the literature of philosophy has suffered refutation by others. Don't get yourself involved in such a futile pastime.

Rituals, dogmas, statistics, and logic-splitting philosophy are all primary stage in religion. Real religion begins with being and becoming.

What all the yogas teach is this: know God, realize Brahman. Know that whatever is done through the machinery of your body and mind is because of the omnipotence of God. No matter what your conception of God may be, it is that God, that Infinite Power, which is expressing itself through your "container". Do not pay much attention to the containers. Realise the Substance within, and you are free now.

We have heard enough talk. We have studied enough writings. Now let us be up and doing, for the doing is something that must be done!

– Swami Gnaneswarananda

Four Yogas as Expounded by Swami Vivekananda
– Prof. S. S. Raghavachar

Knowing the Supreme through personal experience is the central substance of religion. This is not something that happens by itself. The seeker should strive and work for this consummation. The ways of realizing are enumerated comprehensively as jnana, yoga, karma and bhakti. Each of them is held to be sufficient by itself. But it so happens that they get mingled and may actually lead to a final synthesis. Swami Vivekananda in his memorable lectures presents these pathways. His manner is systematic and the ancient material, often disorderly, is worked up to an ordered progression.

Jnana Yoga is elucidated in his lectures so named, and we have therein Vedanta marshalled into a profound presentation of Advaita Vedanta.

Bhakti Yoga takes full account of the *Bhagavata* wisdom and combines it with the philosophies of love such as that of Ramanuja and Chaitanya Mahaprabhu, along with a great deal of floating love-mysticism and builds up an impressive ladder of love towards realization. We have a marvellous systematization of highly emotion-ridden material. Each yoga is presented thoroughly as if it were the only way to the Divinity.

Karma Yoga is a striking reshaping of the cardinal teaching of the Gita, convincingly modernised and brought to apply to the ethical needs of contemporary India with tremendous enthusiasm super-added. No wonder Romain Rolland regards it as "most-moving".

Raja Yoga is the exposition of the contemplative technique, formalized by Patanjali, with a great deal of supplementation by other texts. It is mingled with Kundaliniyoga of Tantra and is crowned with a Vedantic orientation. This is a systematic and practical presentation of directions for the practice of spiritual life.

In all this the ancient precepts concerning the pathways to God are rationalized, systematised and brought to focus on the methods of realization. The individual submitting to them either separately or together, marches to the supreme goal. In reality, he is remade, as it were, and attains authentic fulfilment.

It is to be seen that these yogas are individualistic in that through them the individual attains his destiny. Swami Vivekananda fully realized the value of religious institutions, but thought of them as leading to spiritual individualism.

Swami Vivekananda by this grandly conceived yogas worked out the transcendence of the group-bound religiosity and lifted the pilgrim to the plane of universality.

II

According to Swami Vivekananda, yoga is the science of religion. "As every science has its methods, so has every religion. The methods of attaining the end of religion are called yoga (union) by us, and the different forms of yoga that we teach are adapted to the different natures and temperaments of men.... To the worker, it is union between men and the whole humanity; to the mystic, between his lower and higher Self; to the lover, union between himself and the God of love; and to the philosopher, it is the union of all existence. This is what is meant by yoga. This is a Sanskrit term, and these four divisions of yoga have, in Sanskrit, different names. The man who seeks after this kind of union is called a yogi. The worker is called a karmayogi. He who seeks the union through love is called the bhaktiyogi. He who seeks it through mysticism is called the rajayogi. And he who seeks it through philosophy is called the jnanayogi. So this word yogi comprises them all.'

Jnana Yoga (by Swami Vivekananda) based upon the teachings of the Upanishads, which form the philosophical section of the Hindu scriptures, the Vedas, show the way to realize the oneness of the individual soul and the Supreme Soul, through the discipline of discrimination between the real and the unreal. The contents of this book, originally delivered as lectures in America and England, are based upon the Swami's direct experience of Truth. Therein lie their vividness and irresistible appeal. Free from dogmas demanding unquestioning belief for acceptance, *Jnana Yoga* teaches the divinity of the soul, the non-duality of the Godhead, the harmony of religions, and the unity of all existence.

Karma Yoga, perhaps the outstanding book among the works of Swami Vivekananda, shows the way to perfection for the active man of the world, who may be sceptical about the God of the theologians or the various untested dogmas of religion. The Swami contends that a man may, through the right performance of work, reach the same exalted state of consciousness that a genuine Buddhist obtains largely through meditation, and a Christian devotee through prayer. But the performance of work is often irksorne. It seldom leaves time for the other pursuits of life. One activity leads to another. Furthermore, success in work is often accompanied by a desire for power and name; and failure, by frustration and gloom. Yet the life of an active recluse is neither possible nor desirable for all. The Swami asks the active man, conscious of his social duties and responsibilities, to plunge into the world and learn the secret of work; and that is the way of karmayoga. Man need not fly from the wheels of the world-machine, but may stand inside it and learn work's secret. Work properly performed within the machine opens the way out. The secret is non-attachment. Even when the body and sense-organs are intensely active, one can enjoy serenity of soul through non-attachment and realize "non-activity in activity."

Bhakti Yoga teaches man how to train emotions in order to attain his spiritual end; untrained emotion creates a terrible bondage and brings endless miseries. The first part of *Bhakti Yoga* deals with the preliminaries, such as the definition of God, the qualifications of teacher and disciple, the meaning of symbols, the characteristics of Divine Incarnations and the Chosen Ideal, and the details of concrete worship. Next the aspirant is asked to practise the higher discipline described in the second part which is pure love of God, free from dogmas, rituals, and symbols. This is love for love's sake, devoid of fear or punishment or expectation of reward. Through such love the devotee attains the highest intensive knowledge and realises the oneness of the lover, love and the beloved God.

Raja Yoga consisting of the yoga aphorisms of Patanjali with Swami Vivekananda's masterly introduction and penetrating commentary, is perhaps the most widely read of his books in Europe and America. A standard treatise on Hindu psychology, *Raja Yoga* deals with various disciplines for the practice of self-control, concentration, and meditation, by means of which the truths of religion are directly experienced. It was written during the last decade of the nineteenth century, when the physical sciences emphasised the mechanistic interpretation of life and the universe, defining truth as a logical proposition supported by reason based upon sense-experience, and condemning religion as mere speculation incapable of verification by the well-established scientific method of experimentation. The Swami accepted the challenge of science and demonstrated, through *Raja Yoga,* that religion could stand the test of reason and was valid, besides, on the higher basis of man's inner experience, a support that the physical sciences lacked. He showed, further, that the mind possesses unlimited power, which, when properly exercised, enables a man to realize in the end the isolation of the Spirit from the body, this constituting his Highest Good.

Thus the four yogas explained by Swami Vivekananda serve a very useful purpose for the spiritual development of the four types of men: the intellectual, the active, the emotional, and the psychic or introspective. They also help the individual to integrate his diverse faculties and thus endow his action with grace and meaning.

– Swami Nikhilananda

The Source of All Strength
– Swami Pavitrananda

The man who wants to make himself better finds a strong opposing force against him. Why should that be the case? So he begins to search within until he finds that he is much greater than the vagaries of the mind. He discovers that the man only wrongly thinks that he is surrounded by the limitations of nature. Man is much greater than that! All his hankering for more and more in his life indicates that man is much greater than any finite thing in the world. Man is infinite; man is not matter; man is Spirit; man is the Self. Because he does not know this, he suffers. And as long as he does not know that he is the Self, he has to suffer in one form or another. It is man's one problem.

Fortunately for humanity there have been born on earth persons who have come to this plane of human existence to demonstrate that man is the Self. It was not a philosophical speculation with them; it was not theory with them. The Seers of the Upanishads have said: 'I have known that Supreme Being', meaning the Self, 'by knowing which, man attains immortality, man attains bliss – Infinite Bliss.' Now in every individual life also – to the extent this can be realized – man finds himself stronger and happier. For the illumined Soul it was realization, it was a direct experience, it was a fact. And it is a fact also in everyman's life, only he does not know it!

So against all weaknesses, against all handicaps, man has to assert that he is not a bundle of flesh and bones, but that he is the Self. And the more he can assert that, the stronger and happier he will be. There is no other remedy; no other way. Gradually, asserting that, man will one day find himself face to face with the truth that he is the Self, that he is not matter. The only way to attain strength is to assert this fact. Man must find within himself that he is an image of the Self, not flesh and bone. Flesh is weak, but man is Spirit! He is not matter. Matter is an illusion. It is a mistake on man's part that he thinks he is material. It is the fact that he is Spirit, and it is the realization of saints and prophets.

We find it difficult to assert that we are the Self, against so many weaknesses. But we can do the same thing in another way; we can pray to God – for strength and courage, but it is not a God that lives somewhere high above in heaven, who administers justice with a measuring rod – a God who measures merits and judges sins and good acts. But the same Self which is within all. That Self seen through human emotion and human feeling is God.

Our emotions find an outlet when we pray to realize God. Because we go with our emotions, with our feelings to Him, we offer our weakness and strength. Many persons will find it much easier to pray – even monists sometimes pray to God. When man realizes God, he becomes strong and he loses all the limitations of matter. He will undoubtedly connect with the fountain of all wisdom, all power, all bliss, all joy.

We know that we are the inheritors of all these things which we attribute to God. It is said it is our birthright. We are children of God. We need not fear that we are weak. It is a paradox to pray, think and talk of God and at the same time to feel that we are weak. It is a gross paradox to feel that way. One cannot go with the other. Once you feel it is true, once you feel you are a child of God, do not think you are a sinner. You must not think you are weak. That one thinks one is weak is a mistake, an illusion. It is not a fact! Look at the saints, how strong one becomes when one believes in God – when one has come face to face with God.

If we know we are never alone – if we really know that – we become adamant. No weakness, no human misery can touch us when we know that God is always with us.

When we can realize that we are the children of God, we defy all the handicaps by which we are surrounded. We transcend them and we transcend all our limitations and finiteness. That is the only way to get strong.

All things betray us because we deny God – because we do not assert that we are the children of God. That is the only cause and the only remedy.

Then we are to find the method by which we can realize God. For, we can realise God, and we can realise Him as an experience.

What separates man from God? Every saint, every religion, says that God is all-pervading. But where is God? We do not see or know Him. What separates us from God, although God is all-pervading? If there is no spot where God is not, God is closer to us than mind or thought. Where is God then? What separates us?

It is our ego, our I-ness, which is constantly asserting our 'I'-ness and 'my'-ness. Even in a higher level of spiritual life there is that constant struggle. There must be a constant effort to assert that I-ness for good so that the individual may develop spiritually. So long as there is I-ness, I must assert it for my spiritual good so that I can make my life better. But in a high level of spiritual life even that I-ness, if it is there, is a bondage – a hindrance. It must be effaced. When in spiritual life, struggling and struggling so that my strength is almost exhausted, I find nothing else – when this egoness is gone – then I will find there is no difference between myself and God. Through that struggle man finds he himself is God.

When we find our ego is completely gone, we find there is no difference between 'me' and God. It is the same thing! Man finds he is the Self. Here man finds that 'I am one with God.' There is no difference between man and God.

And there is another way – Self-surrender. One sincerely leaves everything to God. It is not a confession of weakness when, through inertia, you say, 'I will leave everything to God.' When man does not struggle and, just to save his face, he says everything is in the hands of God, he is not honest or sincere but when one struggles, it is strength, not weakness.

One should make a conscious effort to kill the ego first. Then he has the right to say, 'I do nothing. Everything is the will of God.' The ego has no real existence, yet constantly we think we are the doers, we are the agents. The whole of our life is centred on this I-consciousness. We know 'I-ness' is a mistaken idea, but still we go after it. This I-ness can be asserted in either of two ways. Always one has to asssert, 'I am not the body or the mind. I am the Self.' If one cannot do that, one should always repeat to oneself, 'Let the will of God be done. Let me surrender everything to the Lord.' By constantly doing either of these two things, one will be able to efface one's ego completely and come face to face with Truth.

So man is weak, man finds himself weak. But one window of his heart is always open to the Infinite. If he can see through that, he will find that weakness is an illusion, bondage is a mirage, that he is one with the Self, and as such, strong as strength itself.

What You Want is – Shakti

– Swami Ramdass

Know that an omnipotent Power which can grant you independent happiness, strength and peace ever seeks revealment in you. Throw open the doors of your soul so that this power may flood your being with pure ecstasy – may permeate your intellect, mind, senses and body with an inexplicable joy. Permit this divine power within you to entirely transform your life to one of light, power and bliss. Remove the restrictions; break down the barriers: root out the impediments that prevent you from having recourse to this great source of your existence. By perfect self-control conserve the energies of your intellect, will and body and focus them all to the one supreme task and aim viz. to realize your Divine existence and nature. Do not fritter away your powers in pursuit of the transient satisfaction and joys of mere external life. Illumine the intellect, develop the will and purify the heart and body, and you will gain immense strength, for the true understanding and perfect enjoyment of an eternal life.

Man unknowingly dissipates his energies in various ways and so concentration on the supreme purpose becomes difficult for him. The result is an unenlightened understanding, an unsteady initiative and a confused activity. So if you would attain to real knowledge, indomitable strength and blissful action, adopt a life of strict discipline in all that you think, feel and act.

Usually man hangs on outside objects for his happiness and he is a slave: but when he has found eternal joy within himself, and does not depend upon external contacts, he is truly a master. Be therefore the master. Be ever in tune with your all-pervading immortal Atman and by handing yourself entirely to the all-inclusive Godhead be a power for righteousness in His omnipotent hands.

You are born to attain the great Truth and to do great things. To lift yourself to this high state is in your making. Waste not your energies in idle hankerings, uncurbed griefs and inharmonious actions. Don't feel dejection or despair under failure and disappointment. For, every attack of anxiety or sorrow dries up in you a great deal of your power – mental and physical. Don't jump into hasty conclusions and judgements: don't be susceptible to the momentary touches of evanescent emotions: don't rush into uncalled for actions with an egoistic impulse.

This life is a rare opportunity for attaining true, real and ever existent bliss and peace. Therefore, go within yourself in a resolute spirit of adventure and discover the immortal source of your being. Then come out with a new vision and become a great force for the uplift of humanity around you. Set fire to the camphor of your soul and convert your life into a flame of Divine effulgence, of offering and sacrifice – in the end to sublimate into your eternal essence.

Be the votary of the almighty Mother of the worlds and achieve this blessedness and liberation – this power and glory – this immortality and bliss. It is Shakti that you want – a Shakti that would lead you upward, that would effect your freedom from the clutches of the mind and the body. The Mother is all mercy to those who believe in Her and give themselves over to Her. Submit to Her will and dispensations and thereby be Her invincible hero, ever eager to obey Her unerring commands. You are not a weak, you are not a puny, you are not a faulty creature, but you are the radiant child of a resplendent Mother whose song of power and victory resounds through worlds and space. Eternal glory be ever yours, O, child of the Mother!

True Prayer
– Swami Abhedananda

O Lord, Thou art the embodiment of infinite energy; fill us with energy.
Thou art the enbodiment of infinite virility; endow us with virility.
Thou art the embodiment of infinite strength; bestow on us strength.
Thou art the embodiment of infinite power; grant us power.
Thou art the embodiment of infinite courage; inspire us with courage.
Thou art the embodiment of infinite fortitude; steel us with fortitude.

May our bodies become pure;
May we be free from impurity and sin;
May we realize ourselves as Light Divine.
May our minds become pure;
May we be free from impurity and sin;
May we realize ourselves as the Light Divine.
May our souls become pure;
May we be free from impurity and sin;
May we realize ourselves as the Light Divine.

O Lord, lead us from the unreal to the Real;
Lead us from darkness to Light;
And lead us from death to Immortality.

Remove all obstacles that prevent the manifestation of Thy Divine power
And do not let us forget that our true nature is one with Thee for ever and ever.

True prayer is the mental and verbal expression of the highest spiritual ideal. It consists not in trying to get anything from outside, but in unfolding the higher powers that are slumbering within the soul. It is the expression of that determination of the individual soul for reaching the highest goal of life; it is the constant desire, or constant aim, or constant thought of attaining to the highest Spiritual Realization.

True prayer is said to be heard by the Supreme Being when we remember our spiritual nature. When an earnest soul longs for spiritual illumination

RELIGION AND EDUCATION   129

and prays for the manifestation of higher powers that are latent, then the Divine Spirit, which is the Soul of our souls, is said to hear that prayer from within and not from outside, and then it manifests its nature.

A true prayer is the expression of that attitude of the human mind which arouses the Divine nature in man and makes it govern the lower, selfish or animal nature by which we are directed in our ordinary life to perform selfish acts. According to Vedanta lip-prayer is no prayer at all. True prayer is always mental. It is the earnest longing of the heart.

Whenever we think of anything, we think in words; and when we mentally repeat the name of the ideal concentrating our mind on it, that prayer is the true prayer. It is another form of meditation. And when such a meditation or true prayer leads to the realization of the Divine Spirit, then it is said, that prayer is heard. True prayer is like a ladder by which the individual soul ascends to the domain of transcendental Reality.

What is Vedanta?
– Swami Bhavyananda

The philosophy of Vedanta has been evolved from the Upanishads which occur at the end of the Vedas. Its key-note is strength, and unity in variety its immortal theme. It demonstrates the essential unity of all religions, recognizing them all as so many paths of the same Truth. It accepts all the great prophets, teachers, and sons of God, for it holds that all are manifestations of the one Godhead; and accepting all, it does not attempt to make converts. It does not inculcate dogmas but offers a rational basis for the principles and practices common to religions everywhere. Therefore its teachings appeal to men and women irrespective of race, nationality and religious persuasion. In the light of its teachings the followers of different religions have a better understanding of their respective religions, and of other religions as well.

Although it possesses the most ancient scriptures now known to the world, Vedanta is yet in harmony with the highest flights of modern science. Its basic theorem is: Atman, the Ultimate Reality underlying man's consciousness, is not essentially different from Brahman, the Ultimate Reality underlying the whole universe. It then asserts that, man's real nature being divine, the aim of human life is to unfold and manifest this divine nature. It also follows that truth is universal, and not the exclusive possession of any one creed, race, or epoch.

The practice of Vedanta is usually called yoga, a general name for the practical techniques by which the theoretical knowledge of the philosophy is realised. It is a much more comprehensive scheme of life than the posture and breathing exercises which sometimes pass for yoga. It is concerned not so much with the subnormal and the abnormal, as with the normal and its evolution into the supernormal.

There are four types of yoga, suited to men of different tastes and temperaments. By jnanayoga the intellect is refined through the practice of discriminating the Real from the unreal, until it becomes capable of clearly revealing Truth. By bhaktiyoga the heart is purified, its powerful emotions redirected to a personal God, through the aid of symbols, rituals, music and prayer. Karmayoga asks the aspirant to purify his active nature by consecrating his energies to selfless service in a spirit of detachment. Rajayoga is the science of psychic and psychological control; through concentration, the transforming of conduct and character leads to a transformation of consciousness.

Finally, the ethics of Vedanta is unshakeably founded on the unity of all existence, which alone provides a rationale for ethics the world over. If I injure anyone, I injure myself, if I help any one, I help myself.

Thus it may be said that Vedanta is philosophy, religion, psychology and ethics in one, integrated in a metaphysics which fulfils reason, and the truth of which man can realize intuitively by undergoing the necessary disciplines.

Vedanta makes itself felt on both levels of human existence. In the personal life of the individual seeker, it provides a solution to the problem of life and death, that is more satisfying than those he had previously been offered. The consequence is a gradual change of heart which in its turn affects the other levels of human existence. In the social life Vedanta affects the individual seeker as a member of the family and the community by reorienting the multifarious strands of life around a super-social ideal, thus knitting them into an organic harmony.

Vedanta has a fascination all its own. For sheer intellectual beauty it is without parallel. But if there were only this to recommend it, mathematics might do as well. Happily, it has nourishment for the other side of man's nature, for it acts 'like the gentle dew which falls unseen and unheard at night but brings into blossom the fairest of flowers at dawn.'

Throughout the centuries Vedanta has produced many great saints and illumined teachers. The latest and in some respects the greatest of these was Sri Ramakrishna (1836-86). Because he had direct experience of the one truth behind India's many sects and went on to find truth behind other religions of the world as well, his life expresses to a greater degree than that of any other teacher the Vedantic idea of religious universality.

Sri Ramakrishna spent most of his adult life near Calcutta, living in the grounds of a temple by the Ganges. Max Muller, Romain Rolland and Christopher Isherwood have written biographies of Sri Ramakrishna with fine understanding. The Advaita Ashrama at Mayavati in the Himalayas and the Ramakrishna Math at Mylapore, Madras, have also brought out valuable books on Sri Ramakrishna. Posterity is especially fortunate in that many of his teachings have been recorded verbatim in *The Gospel of Sri Ramakrishna.*

Several scholars, for instance Max Muller and Paul Deussen, have done most valuable service by disseminating the teachings of Vedanta. The efforts of Swami Vivekananda to make known the teachings were crowned with success, and of all those who laboured in the field it was he alone who founded the first Vedanta Centre in the West, the first being started in the U. S. A., in 1894. The seeds of work in England were sown by him in the following year. Subsequently the Swamis of the Ramakrishna Order quietly consolidated and extended his great work in the West.

II

Vedanta teaches three fundamental truths:

1. That man's real nature is divine.

If, in this universe, there is any underlying Reality, a Godhead, then the Godhead must be omnipresent. If the Godhead is omnipresent, it must be within each one of us and within every creature and object. Therefore man, in his true nature, is God.

2. That it is the aim of man's life on earth to unfold and manifest his Godhead, which is eternally existent within him, but hidden.

The difference between man and man is only a difference in the degree to which the Godhead is manifest.

All ethics are merely a means to the end of this divine unfoldment. "Right" action is action which assists the unfoldment of the Godhead within us; "Wrong" action is action which hinders that unfoldment. "Good" and "evil" are, therefore, only relative values and must not be used as an absolute standard by which we judge others.

Each individual has an individual problem and an individual path of development. But the goal is the same to all.

Because man is divine, he has infinite strength and infinite wisdom at his command, if he will use them to uncover his true nature. This nature can be gradually uncovered and known and entered into by means of prayer, meditation and the living of a disciplined life – that is to say, a life which seeks to remove all obstacles to the divine unfoldment. Such obstacles are desire, fear, hatred, possessiveness, vanity and pride. The Vedantist prefers the word "obstacle" to the word "sin" because, if we think of ourselves as sinners and miserable, we forget the Godhead within us and lapse into that mood of doubt, despondency, and weakness which is the greatest obstacle of all.

Because the Godhead is within each one of us, Vedanta teaches not merely the brotherhood, but the identity of man with man. It says, *"Thou art That"*. Every soul is your own soul. Every creature is yourself. If you harm anyone, you harm yourself. If you help anyone, you help yourself.

Therefore, all feelings of separateness, exclusiveness, intolerance, and hatred are not only "wrong"; they are the blackest ignorance, because they deny the existence of the omnipresent Godhead, which is One.

3. That truth is universal.

Vedanta accepts all the religions of the world, because it recognises the same divine inspiration in all. Different religions suit different races, cultures, temperaments. Every religion, like every individual, is involved in a certain measure of ignorance. But Vedanta does not concern itself with that ignorance. It insists on the underlying truth.

Vedanta is impersonal, but it accepts all the great prophets, teachers and sons of God, and all those personal aspects of the Godhead who are worshipped by different religions. It cannot do otherwise, because it believes that all are manifestation of the one Godhead. Accepting all, it does not attempt to make converts.

It only seeks to clarify our thoughts, and thus help us to a truer appreciation of our own religion and ultimate aim.

– Swami Bhashyananda

Fundamental Truths of Vedanta According to Swami Vivekananda
– Swami Ranganathananda

1. The inherent Divinity of man.

2. The non-duality of the Ultimate Reality, of Brahman or Atman.

3. The Ultimate Reality as Brahman or the Absolute of Philosophy, is also the Intimate Reality as Ishvara or God, of religion.

4. The Ultimate Reality as the Atman becomes capable, of not just a belief in Him, but of the realization or experience or *anubhava* of Him, by man.

5. Such *anubhava,* and the struggle towards it, constitutes dynamic spirituality, and the true meaning of religion, and not just a belief in His existence and a static piety based on it.

6. Such dynamic spirituality means the steady spiritual growth of man, or his growth in his spiritual dimension, by developing increasing awareness by him of his inborn divine nature.

7. Such spiritual growth is to be achieved by man in the context of his life and work by the comprehensive spiritual technique of yoga as taught in the *Bhagavad Gita*, which bridges the gulf between the secular and the sacred, between life and religion.

8. Such spiritual growth through yoga is the prerogative and privilege of every human being, as are the other two prerogatives and privileges of every human being, namely, physical growth, with the help of the science of nutrition and physical exercise, and mental growth, through the science of secular education understood as the training of the mind and not as the stuffing of the brain.

9. Such spiritual growth is achieved, externally, by doing all work in a spirit of service and, internally, by meditation.

10. As a by-product of such spiritual growth, man achieves moral strength, fearlessness, ethical awareness, human concern and aesthetic sensitiveness.

11. Such spiritual growth as upheld in Vedanta is what twentieth-century Biology calls psycho-social evolution, in which the organic evolution, relevant to the pre-human phase, rises to the spiritual dimension, at the human level, in view of nature's giving him the most efficient and versatile organ, namely, the cerebral system which, when released from its thraldom to his organic system and to his ego centred in that system, enables him to expand his psyche in sympathy, understanding, love, dedication and service, and thus manifest his inborn divine nature, his true Self.

12. The technique for achieving this manifestation of innate divinity consists also of the two broad paths of jnana or *neti neti,* 'not this' 'not this', or the path negative, and bhakti or *iti iti,* 'this' 'this', or the path positive, with jnana and karma forming an integral part, of the latter, and, dhyana or meditation forming an integral part of both.

13. Different religions are but different paths, suited to different temperaments and tastes, and designed to help man to manifest his inborn divinity.

14. There is vital need, therefore, to establish harmony between religions, and a spirit of fellowship as between persons wending their way to the same spiritual goal.

The Neo-Vedanta of Swami Vivekananda
– Prof. C. S. Ramakrishnan

Vedanta is not something new, it is as old as the hills. The novelty lies in the thrilling way in which Swami Vivekananda takes us by the hand and leads us step by step steadily to the spiritual summit. The fresh trail he has blazed to the Everest of the soul, he calls practical Vedanta. "Knowledge of Vedanta," he points out, "has been hidden too long in caves and forests. It has been given to me to rescue it from its seclusion and to carry it to the midst of family and social life.... the drum of Advaita shall be sounded at all places – in the bazaar, from the hilltops and the planes". To make the sublime but abstruse philosophy concrete and living in everyday life was his bold mission. Vedanta must come out to work at the bar and the bench, in the pulpit and in the cottage of the poor man, with the fishermen who catch fish and with the students who study.

Standing four square on the *sruti* he does not have to resort to text-torturing, unlike conventional commentators. He insists that religion is realization, that the proof of the pudding is in the eating. For him the different *sruti* passages are not mutually contradictory, but are signposts on different routes to the goal supreme. All paths sincerely pursued lead to the same pinnacle, as his great master has brilliantly demonstrated by his very life. Harmony among faiths, full acceptance and not mere toleration, is the keynote of his famous Chicago address.

The Swamiji has democratized Vedanta. But in presenting it as the universal religion he is far from approving religious conversions. On the contrary, he stresses that understanding Vedanta will make a Christian a better Christian, a Muslim a better Muslim. For, the bedrock of Vedanta is the potential divinity of every soul. Spiritual endeavour consists in striving to manifest this divinity. This can be done by the practice of the four yogas singly or in combination. While the traditional Advaitin will assert that the *jnanamarga* is the panacea, the dualists will swear by the *bhaktimarga*. The Swamiji smiles and says you are free to choose the path to freedom according to your aptitude. And a harmonious blend of all the four yogas is the best.

Renunciation and service are our national ideals, says the Swamiji. This is a bombshell. Renunciation, we can readily understand. The self-abnegating sannyasin has always been held in great reverence. But to expect the world-renouncers to descend and serve the masses! The concept sounded preposterous to the traditional sannyasin. But today, the Ramakrishna Mission has become a byword for selfless service to the ailing and the afflicted, the lowly and the lost. Note, however, that what Vivekananda has introduced is not the run-of-the-mill social service but, solemn and joyous worship of God in man. To the Upanishadic exhortation to serve parents and guests he had added *"daridra devo bhava, murkha devo bhava"* – serve the poor as your chosen deity, serve the illiterate as gods in human form.

Serve Man as God
– Swami Swahananda

Search for unity has been the one passion of all mankind. This is more true of the Indian people. The Vedanta philosophy pointed out that unity of existence is a logical necessity and the saints and the Upanishads asserted that it is a reality. The visible universe, the individual and the ultimate reality are one and the same.... The realization of the eternal self is the goal of all activities of man. Whatever takes man towards that realization is spiritually beneficial. Vedanta is man-centred but man is nothing but the embodied Soul.

The whole point hinges upon our conception of man. In trying to define the real man, rationalism and science find it to be beyond their grasp. Vedanta, too, faced the problem and gave the unique conception of the Atman, the ultimate reality in man. Vedanta analysed a visible man. What is he? Is he the body or the mind or something still finer? Real nature, according to philosophy, means that which does not change. A really real thing must have been in the past, is now in the present and will continue to be in the future too. Is there anything in man that is constant? The body, we know, changes all the time and will not be mine after a certain period of time. It is transitory. So it is not the reality. What about the mind? It, too, goes on changing. And even according to the Hindu philosophy which accords some permanence to it continuing from birth to birth, it dies in final realization or in absorption. Is there anything real at all then in man? The materialists said, 'No'. They were assailed by the argument that a man is a self-evident fact and even if you cannot locate his fundamental reality he still exists and it is an axiom that nothing comes out of nothing. Thus concerned, they said, 'we do not know its nature.' Now this is agnosticism. And, of course, 'we don't know' is a very safe position. Then the retort came, 'Do you know?' Vedanta said, 'Yes; we know it not through reason or physical analysis as such but through intuition, through spiritual absorption.' Sages down the ages have experienced it, and this experience is part of human heritage. And what is it? It is the Atman, the Self, the Spirit, the inmost spiritual core in man, which is his unchanging, real nature. The apparent man is the manifested real man, who is one with Absolute, the Unity of Existence. So service of man is really service to God. Hence it follows that, for Self-realization, disinterested service of man is necessary and perfect men must serve either to set an example or out of sympathy or for both.

....Swami Vivekananda speaks about manifesting the glory of the Atman and that precisely, according to him, is the purpose of life. Service of man helps in the manifestation.

'Ethics is unity', said the Swami, and he often pointed out 'that knowledge was the finding of unity in diversity, and that the highest point in every service was reached when it formed the one unity underlying all variety, and this was as true in physical science as in the spiritual.' Thus, according to him the whole field of moral science was based on the unity of existence and all types of service had this idea of unity as their philosophical basis.

The same idea has been expressed by all religions, though sometimes more pointedly by some. The dictum, 'Love thy neighbour as thyself' or 'Do as thou would be done by' is the the common advice of every faith .

By service, Swami Vivekananda meant not only ameliorative service, but also all types of social welfare. Social reform and social work are all included in his doctrine of service. The major point in this doctrine is that we are to worship God in man by rendering service to the latter. In an inspiring poem he wrote:

> From highest Brahman to the yonder worm,
> And to the very minutest atom,
> Everywhere is the same God, the All-Love;
> Friend, offer mind, soul, body, at their feet.
> These are His manifold forms before thee,
> Rejecting them where seekest thou for God?
> Who loves all beings, without distinction,
> He indeed is worshipping best his God.

Swamiji coined the word *'Daridranarayana'*, God in the form of poor, and asked us to serve him. 'Where should you go to seek God, – are not all the poor, the miserable, the weak, Gods? Why not worship them first?' He believed this type of service is doubly beneficial. If we forget God in the temple the whole service is practically a loss, whereas in this kind of worship at least the sufferings will be physically mitigated. Thus it is more useful type of worship, suitable to the modern temper too.

Manifest The Divinity Within
– Dr. M. Lakshmi Kumari

"Each soul is potentially divine, the goal is to manifest the divinity within," declared Swami Vivekananda.

Purity and goodness are inherent characteristics of the soul and morality is nothing but the assertion of this true nature. In one of his famous lectures on the real nature of the soul Swamiji said: "That is your own nature. Assert it, manifest it. Not to become pure, you are that already. Nature is like that screen which is hiding the reality beyond. Every good thought you think or act upon is simply tearing the veil, as it were, and the purity, infinity, the God behind, manifests itself more and more."

What is the original nature of man that is good? The Upanishadic sages carried out the investigation. They found that the mind consists of subtle matter or energy, is constantly changing and is subjected to various forces, internal and external. Hence it cannot be the eternal, pure, real nature of man. They discovered that beyond the ordinary mind there is the self-luminous, eternal, untainted, immortal Spirit, the true Self, Atman; this alone is the real nature of man.

Why should a man be moral? Because purity is man's true nature which is the Atman. Why should a man do good? Because this Atman is one and indwells all beings. When a person does something immoral or selfish he ceases to be himself, he lowers his own dignity, he loses the glory of his own self. Morality is not a matter of fear, of compulsion, or subservience to an external force. It is simply a matter of being what one really is, simply radiating the true light of one's own soul all around, under all circumstances, at all times.

The doctrine of the eternal, pure, self-luminous and infinite Atman was developed in no other culture in the world; it is India's priceless gift to mankind. But even in India this doctrine had never been made the basis of a universally a pplicable code of ethics until Swami Vivekananda imposed upon himself that task. One of the great contributions of Swami Vivekananda to world culture is to free morality from fear of all kinds and to lay the foundation for a new theory of ethics based entirely on the potential divinity of the soul which will make morality a source of strength, joy and a means of realising all the possibilities of the human soul.

– Prabuddha Bharata, Jan. 1985

II

The foundation of the unique social philosophy of Swami Vivekananda is laid on the fundamental and most universal principle of Advaita, that the individual soul is identical with the Supreme Spirit. On this basic note, which he expressed in his own inimitable way as 'Each soul is potentially divine', has been built up all his other ideas and thought-currents. To understand Swamiji, therefore, it is very essential to absorb the full import and implication of this statement.

The innate divinity of man is what Swamiji stressed all the time and he was fully convinced through his own life and of his Great Master's that from this faith alone can be built up the beautiful edifice of human life founded on character, dignity, integrity, not only of the individual but also of the nation. Whatever may be one's chosen path in life the prime effort of the individual should be to discover within him this essence of Life Eternal and then channelize all his energies for the manifestation of this divinity in the world outside 'through work or worship, psychic control or philosophy, through one or all of them.' All impulses, thoughts and actions that lead one towards this goal are naturally ennobling, harmonizing, fulfilling, positive forces and are ethical and moral in the truest sense, as they take man towards realization of the Ultimate Unity in the Universe and of his own part in it as a viable fraction of that Whole. Everything contrary to this is negative, not congenial for the growth of the individual nor of the society. Only through this understanding can we truly grasp the real significance of observing a code of conduct, obeying a set of moral and ethical principles in life for one's ultimate good. Such an understanding can hasten man's march or evolution towards his divine Super Self as it will give him the power to discriminate between *shreyas* and *preyas* – the temporal and real gains in life.

'What is the purpose of life?' is one question that arises as a corollary of self scrutiny and a correct understanding of the answer is important before elucidating the essential characteristics of morality and ethics. In Swamiji's words, man is like an infinite spring coiled up in a small box. All the time that spring is trying to unfold itself and all the social phenomena that we witness outside are the efforts of this unfolding. Just as a river rushes towards the ocean so does the human soul incessantly struggle to gain its real nature, that of its oneness with the Infinite Universal Self. The realization of this is true happiness. This is true bliss. When one is at peace, or is happy and exalted, he is getting but a momentary taste of this Bliss. These are the rare occasions when he is established in his true self. This identification with the Supreme and consequent feeling of Oneness with all in the Universe is what one should work for, live and die for. *'tat tvam asi'* – that is the truth. Man's struggles to recognise and realize this truth or freedom form the basis of all morality and ethics.

From atom to man, from insentient lifeless particle of matter to the highest existence on earth, the human soul – everything is struggling towards freedom. How to achieve this freedom? How to release the human personality from the shackles of his self, from the limited circle of me and mine? Only absolute selflessness can take man to this freedom. A free man ceases to be Mr. so and so. He acquires an infinite expansion, a universal dimension. This infinite expansion to the level of the Universal Self – One without a Second – Advaita – is indeed the goal of all religions and of all moral and philosophical teachings. Each unselfish action takes us towards that goal. Each selfish action takes us away from that goal. Therefore it follows "That which is selfish is immoral and that which is unselfish is moral." Yoga is one way that makes man realize this innate divinity, through which he enjoys the real freedom within. Then everything else gives way for that. Renunciation takes one through selflessness to freedom and thence to perfect love.

According to Swami Vivekananda, the watchword of all ethical codes which has a direct bearing on the above truth is the concept 'not I, but thou.' The little I, the self which is an expression of the Infinite Self manifested through 'me', must retreat and join the Infinite Self – its true nature. When- ever we truly feel and say 'not I but Thou' we are renouncing the small self and moving towards the real Self. On the other hand whenever we say 'I not Thou' we are taking a false step and slipping down. Renunciation of the small self and replacing it with the greater Self – This is the most important lesson to learn in life.

For that we should learn to withdraw from the world of senses where the 'I' in us usually revels. How? By reversing the process by which we got in. That is where morality and charity begin. Renouncing the interests of the small self is the starting point of a moral behaviour.

There are two powerful forces operative in our lives. One is of unselfishness and the other of selfishness. One has the force of renunciation and the other, the force of acquisition. One gives, the other takes. These forces operate all the time – unifying and differentiating, in various forms, in various names, in different places and in different times. One makes for classes and privileges, the other breaks them down. In metaphysical terms, the 'selfish' in us keeps us at the temporal or phenomenal level, the other elevates us to the spiritual. One urges us to see unity and the other diversity.

Our great seers who recognised the unity behind the diversity concentrated on that Unity, the Self while the West, drawn by the glamour of the diversity in the phenomenal, centred their attention on the non-self. Recognizing the One in the many, Swamiji emphasises, 'ethics is unity, its basis is love'. When one learns to totally renounce the small self and its pre-occupations what remains in the Self is the very fountain of pure love.

The object of all ethics therefore should be to point out this unity or divinity within. Out of this awareness will come the recognition that Infinite strength and power are the property of every one in spite of all apparent weakness. It brings in the realization of the eternal, infinite, essential purity of the human soul in spite of everything to the contrary that appears on the surface.

Today's man with his scientific temper does not want to accept an ethical code as from the mere sanction of a personage. It is neither satisfying nor appealing. He wants to know the rationale behind his philosophy and ethics. What is the eternal truth, principle and sanction behind it all?

According to Swami Vivekananda, "without the supernatural sanction or the perception of the Superconscious there can be no ethics." Only that system which struggles to reach the Infinite alone can give an ideal explanation for ethics. All other systems which bind man primarily to the ephemeral and keep him limited to the scope of his small life or society cannot offer an explanation for the absolute ethical laws of mankind. It is the impersonal idea of God alone that can provide a satisfying explanation for the dictum 'love your fellow-beings like yourself.' Such a belief presupposes that the whole world is one. (Oneness of the universe – solidarity of all life forms the basis of this love. It naturally follows that when I love another I love myself and if I hurt another it is me who gets really hurt!).

"The Infinite oneness of the soul is thus the eternal sanction of all morality – that you and I are not only brothers but we are really one" ....This is the rationale behind all ethics and spirituality. Recognition of this truth – the quintessence of ethics, foundation of all morality – is what all the prophets have preached at all times. This feeling of oneness is the basic note of all ethical codes. That involves a derecognition of 'myself' as the supreme individual in my world. In other words, it recognizes our non-individuality to such an extent that you become part of me and I of you. It brings home the fact that in hurting you I hurt myself, also in helping you I help myself. In being helpful and loving lies my ultimate good. There is no death for me as long as you live, nay as long as any life is there, even be it a worm, because the very life in me pulsates in consonance with that in the worm. By being good, honest, sincere, loving and sympathetic I am only being true to my essential inner nature.

When this truth is understood there is no fear of death and one discovers joy in living, sharing, and in loving. The real taste of life comes from those true moments of life when we live as part of the universal self in others. On the contrary when we live for oneself alone it is truly death. Hence Swamiji declares, "They alone live who live for others, rest are more dead than alive."

What keeps man away from this truth? It is ignorance or in other words the veil of *maya*. How to tear off this veil? It is very simple. Swamiji assssures: Every good thought you act upon is simply tearing the veil, as it were, and the purity, Infinity, the God behind the veil manifests itself more and more.

Further extension of this awareness of his own innate divinity and the external manifestation of it in greater and greater measure is what we see in Swamiji's social ideas as well. Standing on the platform of World Parliament of Religions in Chicago when he thrilled the entire audience with his opening words 'Sisters and Brothers of America', it was this Universal Self in him who spoke creating an instant sympathetic echo of that Oneness in all those who heard him.

A feeling of oneness and fearless rejection of customs based on false notions formed the foundation of Swamiji's social ideas. Differences due to caste, creed, religion, sex etc. held no social meaning for him. Even his childhood prank of smoking the hookah kept for low class people in his father's drawing room is a typical example of this universal trait in his character. Later as a *parivrajaka* going round the country – mingling with people of all types – he learned to see God in a different way. He found Shiva manifested in an infinite variety of *jivas* and became more fully convinced of the essential purity of human soul and the inherent goodness and strength that lie in every human heart ready to be evoked.

His strong conviction in this regard was again and again brought to the forefront in his social behaviour in the West. This was very evident in his treatment of woman. Swamiji did not always observe the conventions of the Western code of behaviour. To quote Sister Christine, "All fine men reverence womanhood. But here was one who gave no heed to the little attentions which ordinary men paid us.... When he sensed our feeling he answered our unspoken thought, 'if you were old or weak or helpless, I should help you.... You are as able as I am. Why should I help you? Because you are a woman? That is chivalry, and don't you see that chivalry is only sex? Don't you see what is behind all these attentions from men to women?' Strange as it may seem, with these words came a new idea of what true reverence for womanhood means. And yet, he it was, who wishing to get the blessing of the one who is called the Holy Mother, the wife and disciple of Sri Ramakrishna, sprinkled Ganga water all the way so that he might be purified when he appeared in her presence!" This truly sums up Swamiji's social ideas.

Manifesting the divinity within him in his behaviour he inspired others to do the same and thus set a unique seal on all his actions. Did he not see this divinity in the nautch-girl of Khetri, whereupon she, sensing his realization of her true nature, gave up her profession, lived a life of holiness, and herself came into the Great Realization? Thus his social ideas belonged to a different realm altogether, often transcending the understanding of our coarse intellects. *"Soham, Soham,"* was the eternal melody to which his being was attuned and this realization permeated all his actions. To understand Swamiji therefore we have to get into the spirit of this universal truth and learn to manifest it in our own lives.

'Be and Make'

– Swami Budhananda

Along with what we are to do in our daily life, we need attend to what is conducive to self-development and self-transformation.

Here is the key idea: qualitative improvement and transformation of man, of oneself. If we do not attend to this, our problems cannot help mounting, we cannot help becoming problems to ourselves.

Unless we daily quietly attend to these requirements of self-development we cannot understand Swami Vivekananda and his message, much less put into practice. And yet in his message there is the solvent of our problems, of mankind.

Those who aspire to follow Swamiji must be ready to mould their lives according to the ideals preached by him.

The first and the most important materials for fashioning life in Swamiji's mould is truth. Those who seek to do so, truth must be the very breath of their life. They must take all their stands in truth, and never forsake truth through fear or temptation. They must be prepared to suffer for holding on to truth under all circumstances of life.... Those who will endure everything for the sake of truth, within them will go open a great power with which they will be able to accomplish much noble things which others will not be able to do.

Truth is the foundation of all strength. Falsehood is the root of all weakness. Those who seek to mould life according to Swamiji's ideal must cultivate strength. In Swamiji's language we need 'muscles of iron and nerves of steel', and also an invincible will power.... The physical strength should be guided and controlled by the mental strength; mental strength should be guided and controlled by the spiritual strength.

It will be soon discovered that neither truth nor strength can be cultivated without moral purity of character.

Along with truth, strength and moral purity, the aspirant who desires to follow Swamiji must cultivate fearlessness. In fact to such as these who cultivate truth, strength and moral purity, fearlessness comes along as a matter of course. They alone – the truthful, strong and pure-hearted – can be fearless under all circumstances of life and also when facing death.

The person endowed with *shraddha* attains knowledge. He who has acquired knowledge develops power to discriminate between the right and the wrong on the one hand and on the other hand a scientific approach to life and affairs of man. Such a person can easily keep himself free from superstition, ancient and also modern, and also cultivate a proper sense of values. One who has developed *shraddha*, power of discrimination and right sense of values on the inner foundation of truthfulness, strength, moral purity and fearlessness, will, spontaneously, develop the most important thing for building life according to Swamiji's ideal: will-power.

This attained will-power will enable one to have three-fold creative faith: Faith in himself, Faith in God and Faith in man.

Swamiji taught: 'Be and Make.' Let this be your motto. To 'be' in the meaning of Swamiji's teaching is to build one's character in the manner we have attempted to narrate. This 'being' has to become one stream with 'making' which is the practice of reverential service to fellow human beings.

That kind of good-doing which has not become my spiritual *sadhana,* out of that not much basic doing-good can accrue to society. This is why Swamiji taught service as worship.

The solution of all the problems of man is becoming better men, greater men, truer men, purer human beings.

If you look around, you will see what an amount of Self-desecration is being practised by human beings who, no doubt, want to improve their lot. One who in his own place, under the given situation, does not do his work properly and wholeheartedly, desecrates himself. Until and unless this self-desecration stops, the man cannot be helped either by the Government or society. Man must take substantial part of his responsibility on himself. This is 'to be', according to Swamiji. Only by 'being' you can 'make' in a manner helpful to all concerned.

Those who have not cared to build their own characters but rush to 'make' others can only ruin the foolish people who follow their leadership.

If we can become such men in whom all the physical, mental and spiritual powers have been developed in a harmonious and integrated manner and these powers have been directed towards the supreme goal of life, then by being such men among the people of the land, we have done something, the value of which cannot be judged by the common standards of profit and loss.

Whatever sociological, political and economic systems we may adopt, they cannot help giving rise to new problems every day. It really does not matter – rather it may help – if we are surrounded by hundreds and thousands of problems.

There is no cause of fear, if only man is man.

If there is darkness around man, he himself has to become the flaming torch. He himself must become light. ....man must become emancipated from the shackles of his own making. It is perfectly open to him to so become.

Let us not suffer from any numerical anxiety. In the dark night, you can see a long distance with the light of a single torch. And around us there are so many human beings ready to blaze forth.

Live a Purposeful Life
– Eknath Ranade

In Swami Vivekananda's words, the goal or purpose of life is to realize the eternity or divinity which is within every individual. It has to be realized only by oneself. Different avenues for the achievement of that goal have also been clearly indicated by Swamiji. It is left to us as to which avenue one should follow to reach the goal. This goal cannot be achieved in one life. The journey is too long, but one has to perform it. If we come across anybody achieving this eternity in this very life, it means that he must have lived thousands and millions of lives before: he must have striven very hard before and this was his last halt to reach the destination. As Tukaram, the celebrated Marathi saint, has affirmed – "In this very body and with these very eyes, I shall enjoy the great festival of final liberation." It is the birthright of every individual to enjoy this. This life must pave a way for the next higher life. But this life is also very short. One has to utilise it in the best possible way, with powers granted to him by God, within the short period at one's disposal. One has to march on the life's way towards the end with the help of five sense organs and five organs of action. Life is a gymnasium where you have to display the best that you possess within the short time allotted to you. You have to be extremely careful to see that the time and the energy are not wasted and that the way for the next higher life is paved by you.

Human life is a combination of time and energy. The five sense organs and the five organs of action consume and utilize energy for their respective functioning. Thus, the organs of understanding and organs of action, are but instruments. There is also the eleventh organ, mind. But all these organs are time-bound. There is a limited time for them and they have to do their best in the allotted span of life. They have to pave the way for the next life and build one's future. The goal is not to be reached in one life, so one must move from target to target and therefore a master plan for this life is most essential. We should live for a specific purpose, lead a purposeful life. Are we living a purposeful life or a moment-to-moment life? A dog's life is a moment-to-moment life. It is propelled by desires and has no purpose in life. The instinct which is predominant for the moment is satisfied by a dog. It feels hungry, it goes in search of food, finds it somehow, somewhere and the hunger is appeased; it has nothing to do thereafter. It feels sleepy; it sleeps; it feels like enjoying; it enjoys; thus, the desire for the moment is sought to be satisfied. There is no purpose or goal of life for which a dog strives and lives. Thus, the four natural instincts or hungers are satisfied by a dog. "Am I to lead a dog's life? What should I do? I am a human being and I must know how to live for a purpose. Why do I live?" These are the questions that every youth must ask himself.

If you ask any Indian youth today why he lives, the reply will be "because he does not die." One must have something to live for and to die for. The pursuit to achieve the goal will not be lost even if one dies. This is the differences between the two types of lives referred to above. A purposeful life is a planned life and there is no importance to personal instincts. Man should not be a product of atmosphere. He should not be at the mercy of circumstances. If the river flows from east to west and if one has to go to the east, he must go against the current. One's life should not be like that of the stray cattle in the cities, moving here and there and finding a way to escape from being impounded in the cattle-pound. It has no goal. It has an instinct only of self-preservation. Many young men are creatures of circumstances. They try to make their way where circumstances are favourable. They aspire to go to medical faculty; if that is not possible, try for engineering side, if not, then be a B. Com., if that is not favourable, then try something else. If the road to one aspiration is blocked, leave it and try another like the cattle and dog which go by the way they find easy. You must always remember that you are a man, a rational animal and you must pave your way for liberation. Strive hard, build up your future and reach the final goal. You have the power and faculties to live a purposeful life. Think always how you can contribute to the betterment of the world. What account of your life are you going to render?

You must refuse to be a slave of circumstances. You must create circumstances. Time at your disposal is very short. There are hundreds of Arts and Sciences; we cannot even think of them, leave alone the idea of even knowing them and much less the idea of mastering them. Life is short and knowledge is vast. So, we must choose the proper mission and utilise the whole life for it. "One life, One mission" should be the ideal. There are, number of attractive things in life, but if they do not fit in with the master-plan that we prepare for the accomplishment of the mission, we must refuse them, however good they may be. Thus, we must possess the discrimination of selection and election in life. There are many people who have not decided about their goal even at the age of sixty, when it is the evening of life and death is just knocking at their doors. Life should not he like a person who goes to a huge library, sees so many books, reads none and gathers no knowledge. "A rolling stone gathers no moss", they say. Only fortunate people decide their goal at the dawn of their life. They have the satisfaction in the evening of life, that, they had not lived vaguely and wasted time in searching for the goal.

Life should be like an arrow hitting the target directly and not going off the mark. Life is like the game of *kabadi*. One can show his skill and play a fruitful game only as long as the breath lasts. Otherwise, one moves about here and there, shouts, dances and returns empty handed. Futile is his play. One must have the full satisfaction of having accomplished one's goal when one breathes one's last. Otherwise, embittered by frustration, one will exclaim, "Life's morning and noon have already gone, the evening has crept in and now the sun is about to set. What have I gained?"

Swamiji understood the goal of life at the feet of his guru. There are hard days and easy days too. But it is time that will decide the exact mission of one's life. There is no compromise and no concession in that. Life is full of obstacles and difficulties. It is like the river which has to reach its destination, the ocean. It is not an air-flight. So, Swamiji also doubted and doubted and ultimately at the southernmost end of our country, at Kanyakumari, he discovered his mission. As a matter of fact, the mission dawned upon him. When such a mission is fixed for anybody, there is only one road to reach it. All other roads are blocked for him. Like a Commander, decide the mission to be fulfilled and then plan the strategy, taking into consideration the power, the potentialities and the limitations. Think of the best manner in which the goal is to be achieved. 'Ifs' and 'buts' have no place in this. After a stern determination, not only the goal and the mission are fixed, but a master-plan will have to be prepared and all the strategy to accomplish it must be settled. Then and then alone something noble can be achieved.

Go Back to Religion
– Swami Vireswarananda

Now we have been an independent nation for the last thirty-six years, but unfortunately, though in certain respects conditions have improved, yet in many other directions the situation has rather worsened. In every part of the country, in fact in every society, we find the conditions are very low from the standpoint of morals and ethics. I need not describe them in detail; you all know very well. For any honest and upright man it has become very difficult to live in such an environment. The present conditions seem to be unavoidable, for when degeneration and disintegration set in a civilization, they run their course to the extreme before they come to a halt and we are able to turn the tide. This is the condition not only in India, but all over the world today. It is the result of neglecting religion and following materialism which has become the goal of life in the West and has through it spread all over the world, India not excluded.

If India gives up religion, she will be extinct in no time, for religion has been the main backbone of her cultural life for centuries. It is, therefore, not possible now to change the ideal, nor is it necessary. We often hear that our present decadence is due to our religion, but Swami Vivekananda says quite the opposite. He says our decadence is because of our not following religion in its true sense.

To set things right again, we have to go back to religion in its true sense, and not merely follow some superstitions. We must know exactly what religion means. To bring us back to true religion from which we had drifted away, two great spiritual personalities, Sri Ramakrishna and Swami Vivekananda, were born in this country in the last century. Sri Ramakrishna preached that the aim of life was to realize God. He firmly declared to a doubting humanity influenced by modern scientific thought that God was a reality and he had realized Him, and that anyone could realize Him by following the right method. This removed all the doubts and objections of the scientific world about the existence of God. According to Sri Ramakrishna religion meant realization or direct experience of the Ultimate

Truth. He pointed out the true meaning of scriptural texts which were forgotten or were wrongly interpreted. He further stated that all religions led to God-realization, and that too through direct experience, which is the only proof that can be convincing to the modern scientific mind. By the extreme spirit of renunciation,which made Sri Ramakrishna to look upon gold and clay alike, he showed to the present acquisitive society that all this accumulation of wealth and grabbing of others' lands was 'vanity of vanities.' He also found that the same Atman existed in all, irrespective of their caste, creed or colour. The same Atman existed behind the rich and the poor, the high and the low, the ignorant and the educated, and behind every man and woman to whatever race he or she belonged.

These differences are imaginary, man made. They are like the waves on the surface of the ocean; down below it is all water. Similarly here, these differences are merely superficial; behind all is the same Atman. From this angle of vision, all humanity is one and there need not be any strife between nations or between races or between classes, which we see today all over the world. As a corollary to this teachirvg, he said 'serve *jiva* as *Shiva'*, and that service to *jiva* with this idea would lead to realization. Thus he harmonized the centuries-old contradiction between work and worship; work can become worship, if it is done in the proper spirit.

The universal message of Sri Ramakrishna is meant not only for India, but for the whole world. We must share it with the outside world, because that is the only way by which we can also help ourselves, for 'expansion is life add contraction is death.' 'We have done this several times before, and we have to do it once more in this age', said Swamiji. That the world is waiting for Sri Ramakrishna's message can be seen from the fact that wherever his message has reached, it has been received with great eagerness.

Swami Vivekananda emphasized one particular teaching of Sri Ramakrishna, namely 'serve *jiva* as Shiva' and placed before the Math and Mission he organized the ideal of *Atmano mokshartham jagaddhitaya cha* – 'For the liberation of the Self and the good of the world'– as it was very essential in this age to establish peace in the world. He had wanted the Advaita Vedanta which was till then confined to the forest retreats and monasteries to be brought to the everyday life of the people. To bring this about, he got the keynote in Sri Ramakrishna's teaching, 'serve *jiva* as Shiva.'

Swamiji found that with this ideal he could bring all people to work for the regeneration of the country without disturbing the national ideal of *moksa*. To him the first step in this direction was to educate the masses and the women. In fact, he used to say that the neglect of the masses and women were the two main causes of India's downfall: 'I consider that the great national sin is the neglect of the masses, and that is one of the causes of her downfall. No amount of politics would be of any avail until the masses in India are once more well-educated, well-fed and well-cared for.... If we want to regenerate India, we must work for them'. We have to raise the backward people culturally and not think that it is 'pollution to touch them or sit with them.' This is not the teaching of the Vedanta of which we are so proud. As a result, we have failed to give practical demonstration of our spiritual ideal, and this has ruined the nation. The higher castes and the richer classes have to undo the mischief they have done, the atrocities they have perpetrated on these backward and poor people and make *prayaschitta* for their sins by serving them, which alone will help us to reconstruct the country. We must give them education and culture, spread our spiritual truths among them, and raise their economic standard by introducing modern methods of agriculture, cottage industries etc. Considering the modern conditions in India, it is everyone's duty to spread Sri Ramakrishna's universal message to all parts of the country, to all strata of society and to work for the uplift of he less fortunate backward and tribal people, to raise them both culturally and economically, and to bring back into society the moral and ethical principles in life to remove the extreme kind of selfishness which prevails today in the country, especially amongst the few, to the detriment of the whole nation.

Women also should be well educated, so that they may solve their problems themselves without the interference of men. Since independence, we find, some progress has been made in this direction, but more needs to be done. Swamiji said, 'Without Shakti there is no regeneration for the world.'

....Mother (Sarada Devi) has been born to revive that wonderful *shakti* in India, and making her the nucleus, once more will Gargis and Maitreyis be born into the world. Swamiji wanted a few educated women to take to the life of sannyasa and take control of the education of girls, so that they might be trained up as ideal women. He wanted the sannyasinis to carry on this kind of work from village to village, so that the whole country, specially the backward people, might be benefited. You all know that such an organization as desired by Swamiji has already come into existence and is working independently for the uplift of women in different parts of India.

I would like to mention that India will progress only according to her national genius which she has cultivated for centuries. Nothing will thrive in India unless it has a religious basis. In religion also, anything that goes against the universal ideal of India would be jarring and not acceptable to the country.

Ramakrishna Lived Religion

– Arnold Toynbee

....Religion is the most important concern of every human being who passes through this world.... Religion knows no barriers of nationality. It may speak through a Hindu mouth or through a Christian one or through a

Muslim one; but if the message does truly come from the source of truth, it speaks to each one of us direct.... This (latter point) is the special insight of Hinduism, and the special gift that Indian religion has to give to the world.

Some of the religions that have arisen to the west of India are inclined to say, "We have the truth." Hinduism would not dispute this, but it would go on to say: "Yes, you have the truth; we have it too, but neither of us has the whole truth or the same piece of it. No human being ever can have the whole truth, because truth has an infinite number of sides to it. One human being will get one glimpse of the truth, another will get a different glimpse. The two glimpses are different, but both are illuminating. Also, two glimpses are more than twice illuminating as one glimpse. Truth is one, but there are many approaches to it. These different views do not conflict; they supplement each other."

This recognition of the many-sidedness of religious insight and experience was part of Sri Ramakrishna's message. It was also part of his life, because – if I am right – his life and his message cannot be distinguished from each other. He gave his message by living as he did.

The goal of Sri Ramakrishna's life was union with God. Having been born in India as a Hindu, he approached this goal first along the Hindu road. Later, he approached it along the Muslim road and then along the Christian road as well. But all the time he was also a Hindu.

A Muslim or a Christian might say: "You cannot do that; you can't take our road unless you give up all others, because ours is the only right one." A Hindu will say: "I can take all these roads and many more, because they are not mutually exclusive."

On this point, I myself believe that Hinduism has seen further into the truth than the Western religions have. I also believe that this Indian understanding of the truth is of supreme significance and value for the human race today.

Of course, it always has been, and always will be, right and good that we should appreciate and value other people's glimpses of truth as well as our own; but this is particularly important today, when the peoples of the world are facing each other at close quarters, armed with fearful weapons. In this situation, the exclusive minded, intolerant temper is not more wrong than it has been in the past; it has always been as wrong as it could be, but today it is more dangerous than it has ever been. The Hindu attitude is the opposite of exclusive mindedness; and this is India's contribution to world harmony.

Sri Ramakrishna was in this world for half a century: 1836-1886. Look up one of the conventional histories of India dealing with those years. You. may not find the name of Sri Ramakrishna in the index. You will find a lot about war and politics; the establishment of British rule over India; the Indian Mutiny. You will find something about economics; the digging of irrigation canals; the building of roads and railways.

Now open a life of Sri Ramakrishna. Fortunately he had a disciple who did for him what Boswell did for Dr. Johnson. This book is a very full record of his conversations, with a great deal too about his religious experiences, recorded at first-hand by an eye-witness. You will find that this book – it is called *The Gospel of Sri Ramakrishna* – mentions none of the things that fill the conventional history books about India in those same fifty years.

Sri Ramakrishna was born and brought up in a village in Bengal. He spent most of his life in a temple on the bank of the Ganges, only a few miles away from Calcutta. Outwardly, his life might seem uneventful. Yet in its own field – the field of religion – his life was more active, and more effective, than the lives of his contemporaries – Indian and English – who were building the framework of modern India in Sri Ramakrishna's lifetime. Perhaps Sri Ramakrishna's life was even more modern than theirs, in the sense that his work may have a still greater future than their work may be going to have.

Sri Ramakrishna's action was communion with God. It drew to him people of all ages, and a group of his younger disciples, headed by Swami Vivekananda, became the first members of the religious Order.... If I am right, Sri Ramakrishna himself did not found his Order in any formal way. You might say that it founded itself after his death through the continuing effect of his life on disciples who had lived with him during his later years.

There can be few people alive today who are old enough to have known Sri Ramakrishna personally. Most of us today can know him only at second hand, in the way we know, say, Socrates or the Buddha or Christ or Mohammed. But we can measure his spiritual power, like theirs, indirectly by seeking the force and impetus of the religious movement which he set in motion.

In history books written fifty years or a hundred years from now, I do not think Sri Ramakrishna's name will be missing (not that it very much matters what does and what does not get a mention). Future histories of India and of the world will, I am sure, have much to say about the practical achievements of modern India. I am thinking particularly of the community development work. This is helping the peasants, in the hundreds of thousands of Indian villages, to realize that they can do something, by their own efforts, to make their lives better. Making them better means making them better materially as a means to making them better spiritually – and this brings us back to religion and to Sri Ramakrishna.

One last word: Indian ideals and Western Ideals are not mutually exclusive. There is room for them both, and need for them both. Put them together, and they will be able, between them, to do great things for humanity.

II

Sri Ramakrishna renounced everything for God and God was everything for him. Those fortunate contemporaries who were attracted to Dakshineswar witnessed his countenance radiating divine love for all, his divine smile, his eyes sparkling with divine joy and listened to a ceaseless flow of words soaked in wisdom. Now he was transfixed in divine vision, now he was singing songs that transported him and those who were present to regions beyond the senses. Every act of his has a stamp of excellence.

Though Sri Ramakrishna's physical appearance was withdrawn from human sight, he was soon transformed into a divine symbol cherished in the hearts of innumerable devotees. As a divine personality he came to exert a more pervasive influence with the passage of time.

Sri Ramakrishna as a divine symbol has grown in stature and has become a cosmic personality today. Through his chosen instrument, Swami Vivek- ananda, unlike many other divine personalities he has created an Order which like his shadow is constantly growing. His influence has overflown the boundaries of India. The Ramakrishna Order has about a dozen centres in America which attract many aspiring souls to his divine personality. Scores of books are published in European countries containing reference to Sri Ramakrishna, his teachings and his influence. Some of these books have their source in academic and intellectual circles. All these circumstances present us evidence to think of Sri Ramakrishna as a growing personality.

In Sri Ramakrishna we have a personality to contemplate, an exemplary life to imitate and teachings of wisdom to inspire.

Sri Ramakrishna has imparted a new vitality to the scriptures by his life in which he has implemented divine wisdom which the scriptures teach.

Today we require equal stress upon purified emotions and uncorrupted ethical will. In Sri Ramakrishna we find an unparalleled combination of the two.

The early life of Sri Ramakrishna is a saga of tremendous spiritual effort for religious realizations resulting in the purification of his emotions to unattainable levels. The middle part of his life was an example of unusual realizations in several religious channels which enabled him to be a genuine teacher of mankind without posing himself as one. In the last period of his life, to quote his own illustration of the flower, he became a fully blossomed lotus attracting innumerable honey-bees to share all that he had to give. Again it is this emotional purification and strength that helped him to see God in everything and to experience directly that all religions are true and lead to the same goal through different paths.

What is the special message Sri Ramakrishna's life holds for us? Swami Vivekananda said that Sri Ramakrishna was not a pure soul but he was purity itself. It is his superhuman purity and God-centered humility that we should specially take note of. To get out of the present-day vicious circle we have to accept the message of religion, the great sympathy, tenderness and unflinching moral purity which Sri Ramakrishna symbolised.

His teachings were simple. He accepted good and evil but he always pointed out to man his spiritual goal. In the pages of the *Gospel of Sri Ramakrishna* are scattered many illustrations of his pure life.

Today we are making frantic efforts to build a better order of society. We have plunged into a vicious circle. Our economic expansion is often at the cost of moral degradation. The medium of communication, the press and radio, are not particularly wedded to truth. Tolerance to truth is dangerously narrowed down in our social transactions. Medium of recreation and enjoyment are fatally contaminated by shocking changes in the values that are created in art. It is at this juncture India and the world need more than ever the example and message of Sri Ramakrishna to draw us out of the morass by his divine sympathy and spiritual guidance.

– Swami Vimalananda

The Wheel of Dharma

– Dr. M. Lakshimi Kumari

Makarasankranti – the auspicious day when the all-illuminating Sun in utmost obedience to the Universal Law of celestial movements, true to his inherent rhythm and *dharma,* retraces his steps from the southern solstice and starts his journey northward. For Indians, it denotes the holy half of the year, a time for celebrations, a time for doing auspicious things and the time to die too. For India, the Holy Day in 1863, was marked by a special event. It saw the birth of her brilliant son Narendranath Datta whose eventful life was to open a new chapter in her history by once again setting ablaze her centuries' old hopes and aspirations. It was to mark India's re-emergence from a period of darkness to light. Presently, 120 years after, how do we recapture the glory of his life and inherit the kingdom he has left behind? Today, what remain with us are the powerful vibrations of his thought-currents and the vibrant, energizing, inspiring, transforming words he spoke with the authority of a realized soul, resplendent with his enduring faith in the values and traditions of his country's philosophy and culture and imbued with his burning passion for the redemption of his Motherland and his suffering brethren. Unfortunately, the fire in his words lies today covered with ashes – of our ignorance, neglect and deliberate indifference. The only way to blow off those ashes and bring back the lustre is to again relive the strength and power inherent in his words by making them part of our *dharma,* the law of being! For this, the *dharmachakra pravartana* which he envisaged should become once again operative in all of us and should also form the ideal of the Nation.

What is the *dharmachakra pravartana* – the wheel of *dharma* that Swami Vivekananda wanted to set in motion?

We Indians can wax eloquent on *dharma* which is explained in great depth in our scriptures where it remains safe beyond the comprehension of the common man, far removed from his day to day life, occasionally to be aired in religious conventions and national seminars.

We also have the *chakra* as an emblem adorning our National flag which we religiously hoist on our national days and which also flies aloft on our government buildings. As a matter of general knowledge, we know that the *chakra* there on was originally part of the great Asoka *chakra,* beyond that we are not worried about its import or importance.

So also we have *pravartana* of various kinds, activities for national reconstruction, social development and for the upliftment of the poor and downtrodden, each set along its planned course, giving an apparent sense of movement and progress, but in truth never reaching anywhere! Why this stagnation, this frustration?

Onward progress is possible only when the wheels move in unison, in harmony, purposefully, co-ordinatedly. Just as the mighty celestial bodies in the cosmic space, by their movement mark Universal Time, as the tiny wheels in the smallest of watches rotating in perfect co-ordination, obeying their law of movement denote the passage of time in our daily lives, so does a man's life evolve and progress when all his movements big and small are harmonized through the law of *dharma. Dharma* divorced from life or *pravartana* is only book knowledge, best left in libraries fit only for scholastic discussions. That is, wisdom or knowledge of *dharma,* if not reflected is one's actions, is not worth its name. Vain indeed is such a knowledge. Similarly, also a man of dynamic action, full of power, energy and strength, but without the backing of a proper philosophy of action, ignorant of his *dharma,* lives like a moth fluttering for a while and then gone forever, leaving nothing positive behind. On the contrary, if action and knowledge be combined through wheel of *dharma,* whose spokes are intellectual conviction, dedication to the ideal, integrity of character, honesty and selflessness in action, attitude of service and surrender – then life acquires a special *dharmic* glow and each of its movement marks an onward thrust towards self-unfoldment and fulfilment. This is *dharmachakra pravartana* that Swamiji envisaged when he used the expressive term of Buddha to emphasize the meaning and purpose of human life. How to combine *dharma* with *pravartana* – adhrence to eternal truth and everlasting values with day to day working systems – therein lies man's genius and ingenuity. The first step is to convince oneself of the power and potency that lie behind the great life principle, the divinity within one and all. This awareness should energise one's life-currents and inspire him to work out his ideals through the multifarious activities of his life. That was what *Sanatana Dharma* was, a unique way of life in consonance with the *dharma,* rhythm of life, in harmony with universal laws, before it got dubbed into an 'ism' and a religion. Unfortunately, when that happened, *dharma* got delinked from *pravartana* and disappeared from our lives. Today, the *dharmachakra* is found fluttering in flags on roof-tops only!

Swamiji asks us to correct this grave mistake first in our own individual lives and then in National life. He proclaimed in no uncertain terms the universal relevance and eternal validity of the *dharmic* principles and gave his call to one and all, irrespective of caste, creed or religion, to acquire the strength and dynamism that such a life can offer so that the *dharmachakra pravartana* would again manifest itself in Nation's life and guide her towards her rightful destiny.

From being just a religion satisfying a few, the eternal principles of *Sanatana Dharma* should again become a universal way of life. Adopting the Universal Principles as one's life principles would mean elevating and merging this small self into the Universal Self. *Dharma* and *pravartana* exist harmoniously synthesised in such a life – knowledge and action become united. Conflicts disappear. Harmony and peace prevail. When the *dharmachakra pravartana* starts operating, the unique Indian national character would be re-established. When, with the knowledge of life's true values, work gets transformed into worship, when renunciation and service become a way of life, man would discover his innate divinity and the Nation would regain her lost identity. This was the man-making, nation-building programme Swami Vivekananda inaugurated before he was snatched away at the young age of 39. The seeds he sowed are today sprouting up in thousands of places in different parts of the world. To inherit the great legacy that Swamiji has left behind, each one of us must make ourselves mini-centres of *dharmachakra pravartana*. Millions of small wheels working in unison would soon create the momentum necessary to move the giant wheel of our *Sanatana Dharma,* to make this *punyabhoomi* into a *karmabhoomi,* a *tyagabhoomi* and, above all, a *dharmabhoomi* where not only Indians but the whole world discover their heaven of Peace and Salvation.

Consequences of Giving up Religion

According to Swami Vivekananda the national union of India must be a gathering up of its scattered spiritual forces. A nation in India must be a union of those whose hearts beat to the same spiritual tune. And Swamiji was fond of saying often that each nation has its special characteristics and for India it is religion: "I see that each nation, like each individual, has one theme in this life, which is its centre, the principal note round which every other note comes to form the harmony. In one nation political power is its vitality as in England, artistic life in another and so on. In India, religious life forms the centre, the keynote of the whole music of national life; and if any nation attempts to throw off its national vitality, the direction which has become its own through transmission of centuries, that nation dies, if it succeeds in the attempt."

So, religion has especially been the strong point of India. For centuries India has been producing great personalities who were deeply religious and who have influenced the national life profoundly. From Rama, Krishna and Buddha in the ancient times upto Ramakrishna, Vivekananda, Ramana, and Aurobindo in modern times there has been a long procession of these great religious personalities.

Swami Vivekananda warned us of the disastrous consequence of giving up religion and making politics as a means of our national salvation: "And, therefore, if you succeed in the attempt to throw off religion and take up either politics or society or any other thing as your centre, as the vitality of your national life, the result will be that you will become extinct. To prevent this, you must make all and everything work through that vitality of religion." Let us remember that these are the words of a great saint and a modern prophet who provided the inspiration for many of our national leaders in the early part of this century.

What is happening in our political life at the moment is indeed a tragic fulfilment of his fiery jeremiad against politics as a pursuit of power and his prophetic eyes foresaw that this pursuit of state power would in time become a pursuit of personal power which ambitious politicians would place above the nation. Today we are facing a dire fate because we did not listen to the great voice warning us against a political approach to our national problems. If today we are unhappy about the vulgarity and shallowness which have entered into our public life, where a public cause is essentially a matter of private ambition, and if we must now deplore a state of affairs in which politics is corrupting our society at all levels, we must blame ourselves for disregarding Vivekananda's views of the dangers of politics.

A reader of Swami Vivekananda's lectures on Indian nationalism will feel a little embarrassed by his uncompromising insistence that religion should form the basis of Indian reconstruction. For, ever since Independence, our leaders have repeated that India is a secular State and religion should be relegated as a matter of private life. Several sections of people who think that way are motivated only by indifference and insensitiveness to spiritual values. Affluence, which means possession and enjoyment, is the only value to be pursued according to them and hence religion should be excluded from the educational system and from the purview of the State's activities in all fields. This denigration of religion in a total or in a partial way has been going on in this country for the past four decades. The cumulative practice of secularism has only been the growth of corruption and degradation of moral standards on all sides.

If the leaders of our country consider spiritual values as essential for the welfare of the people, the State should not harp on secularism and adopt an indifferent attitude towards religion. The state has to play an active part in regulating this all important aspect of human life.

If we must now endeavour to understand the essence of Vivekananda's message for us and to the world and even in these latter days think of giving a new direction to our thought and action towards a reconstruction of our society, we must first realize that we are today what he wanted us not to be – a nation led by a pack of politicians who can play with the destiny of a whole people for money and for power.

Convinced of the futility of politics in the West, Vivekananda reflected on the genius of the Indian civilization and discovered that in that civilization politics was not in the least an active factor. The average Indian was not a political man and the greatest Indian minds were not political minds. To him the Indian civilization was essentially a non-political civilization.

Vivekananda was opposed to political revolution because he was opposed to a political approach to human problems. "Before flooding India with socialistic or political ideas," he said, "first deluge the land with spiritual ideas". And he believed that politics was foreign to the genius of the Indian people: "The voice of Asia has been the voice of religion. The voice of Europe is the voice of politics." "If you come and teach politics to the Hindus, they do not understand, but if you come to preach religion, however curious it may be, you will have hundreds and thousands of followers in no time...." Elsewhere he said that "religion is of deeper importance than politics".

Vivekananda preached at a time when the Western world itself was raising serious questions about the adequacy of politics as an instrument of human good. What made him turn away from politics is the fact that he viewed the contemporary human society as a burning example of the failure of politics.

Vivekananda warned us against the calamitous consequences of an exclusively political approach to our national problems. The voice of warning came from one who had the courage to set himself against the forces of European history and contemplate a society and programme of social action without politics. He conceived of a human society free from the evil of State power and he rejected politics because politics is the art of seizing that power for an individual or a party. Neither an individual nor a party can pursue power and at the same time care for principles. All politics is desire for power and all desire for power is violence.

Vivekananda fixed his gaze at the primal splendour of his nation's spiritual history and without being guilty of any form of spiritual chauvinism he believed that this was the primal splendour of the entire humanity's spiritual history. That splendour is Vedanta. What makes him the greatest of revolutionaries in the world's religious history, a unique example of a renovator of human life as a whole, is that his revolutionary ideal and revolutionary programme are sustained by a philosophy of the Vedanta. No revolution, political of religious, in the history of the world was so rooted in such a comprehensive philosophy.

A spiritual and a moral revolution – a fundamental transformation of human nature alone can bring about a fundamental change in human institutions. Swami Vivekananda was an apostle of such a spiritual and moral revolution. Political revolution must be a futile and disastrous experiment unless there was first a moral and spiritual revolution changing human nature and creating spontaneous love for a just social order.

What makes Vivekananda a revolutionary in the interpretation of the Vedanta is that he shows its relevance to the life as we live it or wish to live it in our familiar surroundings. But what he insisted on was character, because leadership demanded character. He put before the nation the most vital question regarding the instrument of social change, the question of leadership. "The kings are gone", he said and asked: "Where is the new sanction, the new power of the people?" He saw the danger of power going to a small elite of resourceful men who were capable of assuming the authority which once belonged to kings. "The tyranny of a minority", he said "is the worst tyranny that the world ever sees". Vivekananda therefore put his faith in the congregated strength of spiritually and morally awakened people and he called his nation and the world to work for that awakening

He believed in Vedanta as an agent of a spiritual and moral revolution in the world as a whole and he thought that in a spiritually awakened world there can be no political tyranny or economic injustice. In this faith alone can the world work for its salvation.

The greatest of all benefactions, according to Swami Vivekananda, is the act of rousing man to the glory of the divinity within. The awakened man solves for himself all his problems, secular and sacred. The solution to all human problems is in man's becoming Man in all his dimensions, by manifesting his divinity. Problems are understandably many. But the solution is one – to become the new kind of man, who being simultaneously scientific and spiritual, eventually becomes free. It is this new man, pure in heart, clear in brain, unselfish in motivation, who works in a balanced manner with his head, heart and hand, who has shed all his smallness and illusions, who has experienced unity of existence in his expanded consciousness – this selfless, spotless and fearless man of character, enlightenment and love, is the hope of the world. Hope is not in more machinery, wealth, politics of cleverness and power. The world is looking forward to the coming of this new man – who is aware of his own divinity and is always anxious to discover and worship the same divinity in all others – in ever increasing numbers.

Swamiji's art of moulding man combines scientific temper with a spiritual basis. Man-making was his main pre-occupation, for he believed that in such a free, fearless man of character, enlightenment and love lay the hope of the world. Transformation of man is the only solution for all the ills that are found in the society. Swamiji could cull out from our own philosophy and culture the best of remedies for today's social and global illness.

Swamiji's man-making ideas spring forth from the fountainhead of his realization that each soul is potentially divine. The innate divinity of man was what Swamiji emphasized all the time as he was fully convinced through his own life and of his Great Master that on this foundation alone can be built the beautiful edifice of human life grounded on character, dignity and integrity, not only of the individual but also of the nation.

VIVEKANANDA THE MAN AND HIS MISSION - TRIBUTES

Why is it that men of such diverse views and temperaments living in any part of the globe, found in Swami Vivekananda an object of admiration?

Why is it that poets like Tagore, philosophers like Radhakrishnan, men of action like Gandhiji, statesmen like Rajaji, seers like Aurobindo, Marxist ideologists like Rybakov, scholars like Will Durant, and politicians like Jawaharlal Nehru, found in the great Swami a greatness worthy of equal adoration?

What was that spark in Swami Vivekananda, that elicited the spontaneous admiration, bordering on veneration, of these and others, who are by no means men of ordinary stature?

One most dominating factor for this is that the Swamiji was the very epitome of India, of her entire past, present and future, and the very soul of her aspirations.

This Section is one of the most revealing of all. Here we have tributes to Vivekananda from a cross-section of people, foreign, Indian, lay-men, scholars, savants and saints. Suddenly, as it were, Vivekananda comes out alive and aflame. Even at this distance in time, one is amazed at how Vivekananda came across to his contemporaries.

– M.V. Kamath

CONTENTS:

FROM SAVANTS AND SAINTS: 250 - 347

Aiyar, Dr. Sir C. P. Ramaswami: *He united the East and the West* – 250

Apte, Baba Saheb: *His writings are our newest Scriptures* – 250

Asan, Mahakavi Kumaran: *A rare genius* – 252

Aurobindo, Sri: *His influence still working gigantically* – 252

Avinashilingam, T. S.: *His message continues to inspire us* – 253

Bharati, Mahakavi Subramanya: *A unique personality* – 254

Bhave, Vinoba: *He roused us* – 255

C. C. M.: *He went and saw and conquered all* – 255

Chagla, M. C.: *He preached a Universal Religion* – 256

Chatterji, Suniti Kumar: *A divinely inspired and God-appointed Leader* – 257

Chatterji, Dr. U. N.: *One of the rare geniuses* – 260

Dharmapala, M.: *He made an indelible impression* – 262

Dhar, Prof. S. N.: *A Mahayogi* – 264

Dutta, Dr. Tapash Sankar: *He was a prophet in the real sense of the term* – 264

Editor: *Prince of Monks* – 265

Gandhi, Mahatma: *His influence on me* – 266

Ghosh, Hemachandra: *Man-making was his mission* – 267

Golwalkar, Guruji: *Strength and service were the keynotes of his life* – 267

Gore, Dr. M. S.: *His great contribution* – 271

Gupta, Nagendra Nath: *Harbinger of the glorious hour* – 273

Gurudas, Brahmachari: *A lion amongst men* – 274

Iyer, K. Sundararama: *An immortal spiritual personage* – 275

Jagtiani, G. M.: *He created a charter of Hindu Faith* – 276

Katju, Dr. K. N.: *He was proud of being a Hindu* – 277

Lakshmi Kumari, Dr. M.: *He occupies a unique place* – 279

Leelamma, K. P.: *He breathed a new life into India* – 281

Majumdar, Dr. R. C.: *A great saint and fervid nationalist* – 282

Menon, A. Sridhara: *A forceful and dynamic personality* – 285

Mother, The: *His great help* – 286

Nair, V. K. Sukumaran: He *changed the direction of Indian nationalism* – 286

Namboodidpad, Ottoor Subrahmanya: *The universally adored one* – 288

Narang, Dr. Gokul Chand: *Most impressive personality* – 292

Pandit, M. P.: *A multiple personality with multiple vision* – 293

Panikkar, K M: *Unifier of Hindu ideology* – 295

Parameswaran, P.: *His impact and influence still live dynamically* – 295

Pillai, K. Raghavan: He initiated a new movement of humanitarinism – 297

Pillai, Dr. P. K Narayana: *The foremost leader of mankind* – 299

Pradhan, R. G.: *Father of modern India nationalism* – 301

FROM STATESMEN AND POLITICIANS: 348 - 365

VIVEKANANDA
THE MAN AND HIS MISSION
– TRIBUTES

A world embracing personality that Swami Vivekananda was, it is but natural that the whole world should rise as one man to render reverential homage to his hallowed memory. People all over the world have payed glowing tributes to the eminent Swami for his Himalayan attainments in the realm of spirituality, for his enlightening contributions of permanent value to philosophy, for his monumental success in upgrading and enriching the religious consciousness of the world and for his supreme achievement of founding a world-wide Order of monks with 'liberation of self' as its intent and 'service or God in man' as its patent.

What made Swami Vivekananda stand apart from others is that in his life there was made manifest a tremendous force for the moral and spiritual welfare and upliftment of humanity irrespective of caste, creed or nationality. This power of his is what characterizes Swamiji's work even to this day. Though his voice is without a form today, the vibrations of the same have been caught up in many a heart and have surcharged and transformed them. This section tries to capture these soulstirring emotions coming as they are from the best of intellectuals. Therein is revealed the beauty of that wonderful life, nine intense years of which were spent solely in teaching man to see God in himself and in all those around him.

This section comprises not only the importance of Swamiji's life and teachings but also the impact it has produced on world citizens from various walks of life. Starting from those of his contemporaries and friends the expansive list also provides glimpes of what the present-day scholars, philosophers and ordinary men and women from different walks of life feel, how Swami Vivekananda has inspired them, transformed them and elevated them.

The compiler has spared no pains to make the collection of tributes as representative and comprehensive as possible within the limitation of space. He has tried to gather tributes of not merely savants but also all shades of leaders including political leaders because they represent a significant section of Indian society. Many political leaders of India have publicaly acknowledged their indebtedness to Swami Vivekananda. When such a wide cross-section of leaders of all political parties paid glowing tributes to Swami Vivekananda, it not only shows his universal appeal but also brings him out as a focal point of national unity. It also goes to show that all Indians are one in non-political cultural matters and where the Vedantic content of Swamiji's message is concerned. In other words, it testifies to the fact that while political ideologies and politicians divide people, spirituality and spiritual leaders like Swami Vivekananda act as a cementing factor – and effect a union of hearts and minds of people. It is spiritual leaders and saints who alone can truly bring about the national integration (nay, international integration) in the real sense of the term. The spiritual leaders are the salt of the earth and in their exalted life and inspiring teachings do we find a solvent for all our problems, individual, social and national. They are verily the harbingers of much needed peace and harmony on the earth.

TRIBUTES FROM ABROAD

One single man changed the thought-current of half the globe
– Christina Albers

About the spiritual impact of Swami Vivekananda on the West, Christina Albers reminisced:

"I met Swami Vivekananda in San Francisco in California. It was at a lecture in the year 1900....

"He began to speak, and there was a transformation. The soul-force of the great man became visible. I felt the tremendous force of his speech – words that were felt more than they were heard. I was drawn into a sea of being, of feelings of a higher existence, from which it seemed almost like pain to emerge when the lecture was finished. And then 'those eyes, how wonderful! They were like shooting stars – light shooting forth from them in constant flashes. Over thirty years have elapsed since the day, but the memory of it is ever green in my heart and will remain so. His years on earth were not many. But what are years when the value of a life is weighed. Unknown and ignored, he entered the lecture hall of the great metropolis of Chicago in 1983. He left that hall an adored hero. He spoke. It was enough. The depth of his great soul had sounded forth, and the world felt the vibration. One single man changed the current of thought of half the globe – that was his work.

"'The body is subject to decay. The great strain put upon him, weighed on the physical – his work was done. Scarcely forty years of life on earth, but they were forty years that outweighed centuries. He was sent from higher regions to fulfil a great mission, and that mission being fulfilled he returned to his seat among the gods, whence he had come."

He is not a man, he is a god
– Thomas Allan

Having heard of Swami Vivekananda and what a wonderful man he was and what a stir he made at the Parliament of Religions in Chicago in 1893, also having read his book *Raja Yoga,* it was with great joy that I learned of his coming from Los Angeles to this section of the State. He came to San Francisco in February, 1900, and his second public lecture in Oakland was given on 28th February, 1900, in the Unitarian Church, Oakland.... I was at that lecture, and the impression he made on me was: "Here is a man who KNOWS what he is talking about. He is not repeating what other persons told him. He is not relating what he thinks, he is telling what he knows." Going home from the lecture I was walking on air. When I got home I was still acting like a crazy man. When I was asked what sort of man he was, I replied, "He is not a man, he is a god." I can never forget the impression he produced on me. To me he was a wonder, and I followed him to any of the Bay cities where he spoke.

He gave a new ideology
– F. R. Allchin

If in the mature Vivekananda we find less vehemence and a greater insight into the traditional positions of Indian religion and thought, it is because of the influence of his guru, Ramakrishna Paramahamsa, who transformed his ideas and led him to seek an understanding of the past. But, although it was from the wonderful spiritual power of Ramakrishna that he took his inspiration, it was left to Vivekananda himself to remould that power in visible, practical form. This he did mainly in two ways. First, by his years of work in America and Europe, following upon the astonishing success of his participation in the Parliament of Religions in Chicago in 1893, he drew attention outside India to her civilization and to that theme of religion which was its special glory. This in turn changed the relations of Indians to the rest of the world and gave them fresh grounds for self-confidence and self-reliance. The second great step was in the organization of the Ramakrishna Mission, and of the many social works which it undertook. It is clear that Swamiji saw these two as related, as part of the same great task which he had to accomplish, and the order of his undertaking them is significant of their relationship. In general terms, it was only after he had spent his years of travel and teaching in the West that his thoughts turned once more to his own country and to the work which awaited him there. And it was at this moment that his deeply patriotic nature was most strongly influenced by the vision of the poverty and suffering of his fellow-countrymen. In fact it is this love for his native land which forms the cornerstone for all his thinking upon its social problems.

I do not think that it is too much to claim that Swami Vivekananda, more than any other Indian of his time, gave to his countrymen a new ideology. The ideology was a synthesis of many threads: on the Indian side there was the teaching of his guru Ramakrishna, with its devotional and its universalist aspects, and there was the wide philosophical knowledge, particularly centred in the Advaita Vedanta; on the Western side there were

13

the European liberal influences which came to him first through the Brahmo
Samaj, and later from his own wide reading of Western writings and his
own experiences in the West.

Swami Vivekananda took the Vedanta philosophy, one of the greatest
intellectual systems of mankind, and interpreted it in terms understandable
both to the West and to the India of his own times. By so doing he showed
that India had within herself the intellectual means to her own emancipation.

I suppose it is inevitable that one should think of the comparison of
Swami Vivekananda with Sri Shankaracharya, the great exponent of the
Advaita Vedanta, who lived a thousand years before him. Like Shankara,
Vivekananda was a man of incredible energy, who burnt himself up in the
service of his fellow-men within scarcely half the normally allotted span of
life. Like Shankara, Vivekananda has left us two distinct memorials to himself:
a remarkable and great body of writings and an Order of dedicated disciples
to perpetuate his teachings in living form.

A great exponent of religion
– George A. Applegarth

He was so outstanding in the portrayal of his religion that none of the
other speakers could compare with him. They would have made a very poor
showing if they had been called upon to speak after the Swami. The other
addresses had all been more or less complex and obscure. The Swami on
the other hand, presented a philosophy that was so simple and was
presented from such a beautiful viewpoint that people everywhere were
eager to hear more. He had a remarkable command of English and his
lectures were full of colourful metaphors. I was present after some of the
lectures when others spoke to him. He was very approachable.... I talked
to many of the people who had attended his lectures. All were deeply
impressed by the simplicity of his philosophy and by the richness and
beauty of his English.

His noble character and influence
– John J. Bagley

I am glad of an opportunity to express my admiration of his character.... He is a
strong, noble human being, one who walks with God. He is as simple and
trustful as a child.

All who have been brought in contact with him day by day, speak
enthusiastically of his sterling qualities of character and men in Detroit who
judge most critically, and who are unsparing, admire and respect him.... He
has been a guest in my house more than three weeks, and my sons as well
as my son-in-law and my entire family found Swami Vivekananda a
gentleman always, most courteous and polite, a charming companion and
ever welcome guest.

He has been a revelation to Christians.... he has made possible for us
all, a diviner and more nobler practical life. As a religious teacher and an

example to all I do not know of his equal.... He has given us in America higher ideas of life than we have ever had before.

Whenever he spoke, people listened gladly and said, "I never heard man speak like that." He does not antagonize, but lifts people up to a higher level – they see something beyond man-made creeds and denominational names, and they feel one with him in their religious belief.

Every human being would be made better by knowing him and living in the same house with him.... I want everyone in America to know Vivekananda, and if India has more such let her send them to us....

A man of strong personality
– Prof. A. L. Basham

The most important of Ramakrishna's followers was Narendranath Dutta, a well-educated young Bengali who, on the Master's death, became a san- nyasi and devoted himself to the propagation of Ramakrishna's teachings, taking the religious name of Vivekananda. Vivekananda was a man of strong personality and great moral earnestness, and was a very forceful speaker and writer with a good command of English. In 1893 he visited the United States to attend a Parliament of Religions at Chicago. America, always ready to accept new ideas and prepared for Hinduism by the sympathetic interest of a number of her literary men, took Vivekananda to her heart. Wherever he lectured he made a very great impression on a large audience, and several Vedanta societies were founded in the larger cities to continue his work. On his return to India, after a similar lecture tour in Great Britain, he established the Ramakrishna Mission. Organizations for social work had already been founded by Hindus, and the Brahma Samaj had something in the way of famine relief, but the new society while by no means neglecting propaganda, made relief of suffering, its main duty. It marks an important stage in the growth of the Hindu social conscience. Moreover Vivekananda's success in the West further raised the morale of Hinduism. After being subjected to the propaganda of missionaries, whether Muslim or Christian, for seven hundred years, the ancient religion of India was now at last conducting counter-propaganda on the territory of its opponents. At last a Hindu had arisen who could hold his own with the theologians and apologists of other faiths and even gain converts from them.

....Vivekananda restored the educated Hindu's faith as the earlier reformers had not succeeded in doing. When he died in 1902, the new life stirring in Hinduism was quite evident. Vivekananda was a Vedantist of the school of Sankara, in theory completely orthodox. He taught that all institutions and practices of Hinduism were essentially good, though some had become corrupted or were misunderstood. He declared that Hinduism was the oldest and purest of the world's religions and India the most spiritual nation of the world. All that was best in the religions of the ancient

world had come from India. Now India had been outstripped by the West
with its practical and materialistic bent. It was the duty of Indians to absorb
from the West all that was good and useful in science and technology, and
then once more teach the world how to live the life of the spirit in a society
ordered with the furtherance of the life of the spirit as its main aim.... The
old eclecticism of the Brahmo Samaj is no longer a force; the neo-Hinduism
of Vivekananda, in its many developments, is the most potent religious
influence in modern India, and adopted by the genius of Mahatma Gandhi,
has provided the ideology of the Indian Independence Movement.

From the first visit of Vivekananda to America, neo-Hinduism has been
slowly making converts outside India. The Los Angeles branch of the
Vedanta Society counts such well-known literary men as Aldous Huxley
and Christopher Isherwood among its members. In many cities, of Europe
and America, similar societies exist, and teachers of yoga are also to be
found. Through her philosophy Hinduism has long exerted a subtle but
very real influence on the West....

Even now (1963) a hundred years after the birth of Narendranath Dutta,
who later became Swami Vivekananda, it is very difficult to evaluate his
importance in the scale of world history. It is certainly far greater than any
Western historian or most Indian historians would have suggested at the
time of his death. The passing of the years and the many stupendous and
unexpected events which have occurred since then suggest that in centuries
to come he will be remembered as one of the main moulders of the modern
world, especially as far as Asia is concerned, and as one of the most
significant figures in the whole history of Indian religion, comparable in
importance to such great teachers as Shankara and Ramanuja, and definitely
more important than the saints of local or regional significance such as
Kabir, Chaitanya, and the many Nayanmars and Alwars of South India.

I believe also that Vivekananda will always be remembered in the world's
history because he virtually initiated what the late Dr. C. E. M. Joad once
called 'the counter-attack from the East'. Since the days of the Indian
missionaries who travelled in South-East Asia and China preaching
Buddhism and Hinduism more than a thousand years earlier, he was the
first Indian religious teacher to make an impression outside India.

A striking figure
– Annie Besant

A striking figure, clad in yellow and orange, shining like the sun of India
in the midst of the heavy atmosphere of Chicago, a lion head, piercing eyes,
mobile lips, movements swift and fast – such was my first impression of
Swami Vivekananda, as I met him in one of the rooms set apart for the use
of the delegates to the Parliament of Religions. Monk, they called him, not
unwarrantably, but warrior-monk was he, and the first impression was the
warrior rather than of the monk, for he was off the platform, and his figure

was instinct with pride of country, pride of race – the representative of the oldest of living religions, surrounded by curious gazers of nearly the youngest, and by no means inclined to give step, as though the hoary faith he embodied was in aught inferior to the noblest there. India was not to be shamed before the hurrying arrogant West by this her envoy and her son. He brought her message, he spoke in her name, and the herald remembered the dignity of the royal land whence he came. Purposeful, virile, strong, he stood out, a man among men, able to hold his own.

On the platform another side came out. The dignity and the inborn sense of worth and power still were there, but all was subdued to the exquisite beauty of the spiritual message which he had brought, to the sublimity of the matchless evangel of East which is the heart, the life of India, the wondrous teaching of the Self. Enraptured, the huge multitude hung upon his words; not a syllable must be lost, not a cadence missed! 'That man a heathen!' said one, as he came out of the great hall, 'and we send missionaries to his people! It would be more fitting that they should send missionaries to us,'

Indeed a God
.– S. K. Blodgett

I was at the Parliament of Religions in Chicago in 1893, when that young man got up and said 'Sisters and Brothers of America', seven thousand people rose to their feet as a tribute to something they knew not what. When it was over, I saw scores of women walking over the benches to get near him; and I said to myself, 'Well, my lad, if you can resist the onslaught, you are indeed a God'.

A great Hindu Missionary
– Brooklyn Ethical Association

We wish to testify to our high appreciation of the value of the work of Swami Vivekananda in this country. His lectures before the Brooklyn Ethical Association opened up a new world of thought to many of his hearers and renewed the interest of others in the comparative study of religions and philosophy system, which gives breadth to the mind and an uplifted stimulus to the moral nature. We can heartily endorse the words of the Venerable Dean of the Harward Divinity school: "Swami Vivekananda.... has been, in fact, a missionary from India to America. Everywhere he has made warm personal friends and his expositions of Hindu Philosophy have been listened to with delight.... Vivekananda has created a high degree of interest in himself and his work."

We thank you for sending him to us. We wish him Godspeed in his educational work in his own country. We hope he may return to us again, with new lessons of wisdom resulting from added thought and experience. And we earnestly hope that the new avenues of sympathy opened by the presence of himself and his brother sannyasins will result in mutual benefits, and a profound sense of the solidarity and brotherhood of the race.

He added meaning and value to our lives
– Marie Louise Burke

A reversal is taking place in the West, where the people cloyed with material surfeit, are searching for the inner being. The 'spiritual' jolt which Vivekananda gave to the West early in the century is now proving its impact.

Vivekananda understood us; so we are able to understand him. He spoke our language and was thoroughly conversant with our way of life. He added meaning and value to our lives. I am sure that a time would come when the West will discover him as its own hero.

There are already many in the West who are steeped in Vedanta philosophy. These 'unsungdevotees' find in Vivekananda and Ramakrishna's teachings the ways of 'total sacrifice.' Although Vivekananda's teachings are not to be found yet in the mainstream of Western thought and culture, the Christian Church in the West, both Protestant and Roman Catholic, are taking deep interest in Eastern thoughts. Without quite knowing the source, the Americans are influenced by Vivekananda in their 'search for a life within.' The West horrified by the destructive powers of the nuclear forces, is really corroborating the teachings of Vivekananda that a "man with excess of knowledge and power without holiness is a devil."

His heart ached for human misery and degradation on every level – physical, mental, emotional, intellectual, political, and, of course, spiritual. He cried for the hungry, for the ignorant, for the bereaved, for the suppressed, for the miserable of all nations and creeds. Never could he look upon the suffering of men as unreal. Though he saw – truly perceived – man as divine, never did he fail in intense compassion for him. Though he knew that the man who wept in ignorance was here and now God Himself, needing no help at all, yet he wept with him, and he helped him. This blessed contradiction of knowledge and compassion seems to lie at the very heart of prophethood, and nowhere, I think, does one see it more fully manifested than in Swami Vivekananda.

"Man-making"! This.... Swamiji, was to speak as his "new Gospel", applying it not only to sannyasins, not only to Indians, but in its most profound sense, to men and women everywhere. Indeed, to make men and to teach the highest truth constituted in Swamiji's language one and the same mission – and this mission, to his mind, formed the central task of his life on earth.

In consonance with his "new Gospel" he wanted to make man his own master, to teach him to be in full control of his body and mind, to give him self-confidence, to show him how to draw forth from within himself, by himself, all powers of earth and heaven and, step by step, to realize ultimately his identity with the infinite Spirit – Brahman.

Manliness! Swamiji meant a great deal by that term. Manliness, in his view, emanated from the Atman, permeating the whole empirical man – body, senses, mind, heart and will. To have the quality of manliness was to be established in the Self, to rejoice in the Self, to want nothing, to fear nothing, to dislike nothing, to serve all.

Yes, Vivekananda wanted man to be spiritually free for his own sake.... only spiritually free and strong men and women, taking their stand on the Self – the Atman – can truly deify this world, can truly revere it and work in it tirelessly, without desire or fear, motivated by love alone. And only such men and women can meet the unprecedentedly terrible challenge of this age.

He walked with God
– Madame Emma Calve

It has been my good fortune and my joy to know a man who truly "walked with God", a noble being, a saint, a philosopher, and a true friend. His influence upon my spiritual life was profound. He opened up new horizons before me, enlarging and unifying my religious ideas and ideals; teaching me a broader understanding of truth. My soul will bear him eternal gratitude.

He loved the Chinese labouring people
– Huang Xin Chuan

Vivekananda stands out as the most renowned philosopher and social figure of India in modern China. His philosophical and social thought and epic patriotism not only inspired the growth of nationalist movement in India, but also made a great impact abroad. In 1893, Vivekananda visited Canton and its neighbourhood. He noted his impresions of the visit in a letter addressed to the citizens of Madras. He had some knowledge and understanding of Chinese history and culture. He often cited and spoke highly of China in his writings and speeches. He made a prophecy that the Chinese culture will surely be resurrected one day like the 'Phoenix'and undertake the responsibility of the great mission of integrating the Western and the Oriental cultures. His biographer Romain Rolland has narrated the evolution of Vivekananda's idea on this aspect. When Vivekananda went to America for the first time, he hoped that country would achieve this mission. But during his second visit abroad, he realised that he was deceived by dollar imperialism. He, therefore, came to the conclusion that America could not be an instrument to accomplish this task, but it was China which could do it.

Vivekananda had infinite sympathy for the Chinese people living under the oppression of feudalism and imperialism: and he pinned much hope on them. After his visit to China, he made a very interesting comment. He said: 'The Chinese child is quite a philosopher and calmly goes to work at an age when your Indian boy can hardly crawl on all fours. He has learnt the philosophy of necessity too well'. This shows Vivekananda's enormous sympathy towards the miseries of the children of China in the old society.

While explaining his visionary socialism Vivekananda made an interesting 'gospel.' He said that the future society would be ruled by the labouring people and that this would first take place in China. In *Modern India*' he said: 'But there is hope. In the mighty course of time, the brahmin and the other higher castes too are being brought down to the lower status of the shudras and the shudras are being raised to higher ranks.... Even before our eyes, powerful China with fast strides, is going down to shudrahood, ...yet, a time will come when there will be the rising of the shudra class, with their shudrahood, ...a time will come when the shudras of every country.... will gain absolute supremacy in every society.... Socialism, Anarchism, Nihilism, and other like sects are the vanguard of the social revolution that is to follow.'

From the material cited above and his life and works, we can see at least that Vivekananda showed very much concern for, and sympathised with, the people of China who were living under the rule of feudalism and imperialism and placed great hopes on them. But we do not agree with B. N. Datta that the success of the Chinese and the Russian revolutions coming into being at concrete historical moments should be credited to the 'gospel' of Vivekananda. This would make him a divine mystique personality. We have seen that Vivekananda's approach to the laws of social developments was unscientific. However, it is not possible for any advanced thinker to make a correct prediction of the phases and events of the progress of history in every minute details. We should, therefore, appraise Vivekananda in the light of seeking truth from facts.

In conclusion, Vivekananda was the most eminent figure among the democratic patriots in India. He paid high tributes to our glorious ancient culture and loved the Chinese labouring people.

We pay homage to him.

His lofty ideas of humanism
– E. P. Chelishev

Reading and re-reading the works of Vivekananda each time I find in them something new that helps deeper to understand India, its philosophy, the way of the life and customs of the people in the past and the present, their dreams of the future.... I think that Vivekananda's greatest service is the development in his teaching of the lofty ideals of humanism which incorporate the finest features of Indian culture....

In my studies of contemporary Indian literature I have more than once had the opportunity to see what great influence the humanistic ideals of Vivekananda have exercised on the works of many writers.... In my opinion Vivekananda's humanism has nothing in common with the Christian ideology which dooms man to passivity and to begging God for favours.

He tried to place religious ideology at the service of the country's national interests, the emancipation of his enslaved compatriots. Vivekananda wrote that the colonialists were building one church after another in India, while the Eastern countries needed bread and not religion. He would sooner see all the men turn into confirmed atheists than into superstitious simpletons. To elevate man Vivekananda identifies him with God....

Though we do not agree with the idealistic basis of Vivekananda's humanism, we recognize that it possesses many features of active humanism manifested above all in a fervent desire to elevate man, to instill in him a sense of his own dignity, sense of responsibility for his own destiny and the destiny of all people, to make him strive for the ideals of good, truth and justice, to foster in man abhorrence for suffering. The humanistic ideal of Vivekananda is to a certain degree identical with Gorky's Man with a capital letter.

Such a humanistic interpretation of the essence of man largely determines the democratic nature of Vivekananda's world outlook....

Many years will pass, many generations will come and go, Vivekananda and his time will become the distant past, but never will there fade the memory of the man who all his life dreamed of a better future for his people, who did so much to awaken his compatriots and move India forward, to defend his much-suffering people from injustice and brutality. Like a rocky cliff protecting a coastal valley from storm and bad weather, from the blows of ill winds and waves, Vivekananda fought courageously and selflessly against the enemies of his motherland.

Together with the Indian people, Soviet people who already know some of the works of Vivekananda published in the USSR, highly revere the memory of the great Indian patriot, humanist and democrat, impassioned fighter for a better future for his people and all mankind.

A unique preceptor
– Sister Christine

To those who have heard much of the personal appearance of Swami Vivekananda, it may seem strange that it was not this which made the first outstanding impression. The forceful, virile figure which stepped upon the platform was unlike the emaciated, ascetic type which is generally associated with spirituality in the West. A sickly saint every one understands, but whoever heard of a powerful saint? The power that emanated from this mysterious being was so great that one all but shrank from it. It was overwhelming. It threatened to sweep everything before it. This one sensed even in those first unforgettable moments.

Later we were to see this power at work. It was the mind that made the first great appeal, that amazing mind! What can one say that will give even a faint idea of its majesty, its glory, its splendour? It was a mind so far transcending other minds, even of those who rank as geniuses, that it seemed different in its very nature. His ideas were so clear, so powerful, so transcendental that it seemed incredible that they could have emanated from the intellect of a limited human being. Yet marvellous as the ideas were and wonderful as was that intangible something that flowed out from the mind, it was strangely familiar. I found myself saying, "I have known that mind before."

Vivekananda burst upon us in a blaze of reddish gold, which seemed to have caught and concentrated the Sun's rays. He was barely thirty, this preacher from far away India. Young with an ageless youth and yet withal old with the wisdom of ancient times. For the first time we heard the age-old message of India, teaching of the Atman, the true self.

The theme was always the same – man's real nature. Not what we seem to be but what we are....

Vivekananda stood on the platform of the Unitarian Church pouring forth glorious truths in a voice unlike any voice one had ever heard before, a voice full of cadences, expressing every emotion, now with a pathos that stirred hitherto unknown deeps of tragedy, and then just as the pain was becoming unbearable, that same voice would move one to mirth only to check it in mid-course with the thunder of an earnestness so intense that it left one awed, a trumpet call to awake. One felt that one never knew what music was until one heard that marvellous voice.

He had a power of attraction so great that those who came near him, men and women alike, even children, fell under the magic spell he cast.... I had come to one in whom I had seen such spirituality as I had never even dreamed of. From his lips I heard truths unthought of before. He knew the way to attainment. He would show me the way....

He refused to solve our problem for us. Principles he laid down, but we ourselves must find the application. He encouraged no spineless dependence upon him in any form, no bid for sympathy. "Stand upon your own feet. You have the power within you!" he thundered. His whole purpose was not to make things easy for us, but to teach us how to develop our innate strength. "Strength! Strength!" he cried, "I preach nothing but strength...." From men he demanded manliness and from women the corresponding quality for which there is no word. Whatever it is, it is the opposite of self-pity, the enemy of weakness and indulgence. This attitude had the effect of a tonic. Something long dormant was aroused and with it came strength of freedom.... We were taught to think things through, to reject the false and hold to the true fearlessly, no matter what cost. In this process much that had seemed worthwhile and of value was cast aside. Perhaps our purposes and aims had been small and scattered. In time we learnt to lift them into a higher purer region, and to unite all little aims into the one great aim, the goal which is the real purpose of life, for which we come to this earth again an again. We learnt not to search for it in deserts, nor yet on mountain tops, but in our own hearts. By all these means the process of evolution was accelerated, and the whole nature was transmuted.

Blessed is the country in which he was born, blessed are they who lived on this earth at the same time and blessed, thrice blessed, are the few who sat at his feet.

At last, an Indian had shaken the West
– Amaury De Riencourt

Vivekananda sprang from a noble kshatriya family and was every inch a bold warrior. He was essentially a man of action, a master of karmayoga by instinct.

Vivekananda's philosophy of life began to develop gradually as he travelled all over India as a wandering sannyasin, keeping in touch with Ramakrishna's other disciples, watching, learning, meditating. Everywhere he went, he became increasingly conscious of the need for modernization, for breaking with the past and for awakening the dormant potentialities rather than destroying them. He was haunted by the ever-present need for synthesis without sacrificing any of the elements that had made and still make the greatness of Hinduism. Inevitably, something new dawned on him, a crying need for a new dimension of human understanding that had always been sorely lacking in Indian consciousness: historical consciousness, the bold facing of historical reality – not just the prophetic instinct of Muslim culture but the detached, objective and scientific precision with which Western culture was in the process of rescuing mankind's past from oblivion. He longed to see the creation of a school of Indian historians who would bring to life India's past and then awaken a true national spirit in India.

More than anything else, it was human misery that shook him to his depth, the misery of India's mute masses. But what could he do to alleviate the burden crushing India's millions? Social indifference was supreme in the land. And, inevitably, his thoughts began to turn to the West, to the dawning civilization that had been largely responsible for awakening all those thoughts in him.

His thundering success in Chicago electrified the entire Western world and brought India, so to speak, into the consciousness of most thoughtful Westerners – no longer the India of the Theosophists, nor the cold, unrepresentative India of the Brahmo Samaj, but living, dynamic India that was at last awakening. In the words of the *New York Herald,* Vivekananda was "undoubtedly the greatest figure in the Parliament of Religions. After hearing him we feel how foolish it is to send missionaries to this learned nation." But just as promptly quarrels, jealousy, misunderstanding began to mar his great success. Just as he was attacked with unfair violence by a number of clergymen, he was stabbed in the back by all his jealous rivals: members of the Brahmo Samaj, the theosophists, and others who slandered him mercilessly. But a towering giant of Vivekananda's stature could afford to shrug off these frontal and flanking attacks, and he did so with commendable vigour. In addition, the United States, more than any other country of the West, seemed to be ripe for his message. Like Rome in Classical days, the United States was more fundamentally and vitally concerned with religion and religious matters than lands of old culture such as ancient Greece and modern Europe. Prepared by Emerson, Thoreau, Walt Whitman and William James, receptive to new religious ideas and sensitive to great religious personalities, America was less corroded by religious scepticism than Europe on the threshold of its historic decline.

Vivekananda's personality was acute and, although ever ready to flay the West – Christian's hypocrisy, he was evermore ready to humiliate India under the crushing evidence of the West's highly developed sense of social solidarity. Journey to Europe enabled Vivekananda to discriminate between America and the old continent, between the modern Rome and the modern Greece – Europe with its old culture, its higher intellect, its more mature outlook on life, its great Orientalists whom he met and especially England. But he never lost sight of his true mission: welding the immense power of the West and the deep spirituality welling up from the depths of an awakening Hinduism. He felt more at home in Europe than America and, intellectually, more at home with some of the great German minds than with the more pragmatic British. His historic meeting with Max Muller, the greatest Orientalist of the time, elicited enthusiastic comments. He travelled through Germany, saw Paul Deussen at Kiel and talked to members of Schopenhauer Society, and never was more touched than he was by the great German Orientalists

The news of Vivekananda's triumph in Europe and America electrified India. His great success was taken in India as a national triumph, his landing in Colombo in January, 1897, might have resembled the landing of Gautama Buddha himself, such was the size of the shouting multitudes, the singing of religious hymns, the immense processions that greeted him. At last, an Indian had shaken the West and had been able to convey to the Westerners the idea that India had something to offer that the West did not possess.

In a famous message to India, he sounded the call of awakening, in which he summed up his world-view with great forcefulness: "Each nation, like each individual, has one theme in this life, which is its centre, the principal note round which every other note comes to form the harmony.... If any one nation attempts to throw off its national vitality, the direction which has become its own through the transmission of centuries, that nation dies.... In one nation political power is its vitality, as in England. Artistic life in another and so on. In India religious life forms the centre, the keynote of the whole music of national life." And he went on to explain that India would die if its religion were to be discarded, that inevitably social and political reform had to be undertaken by channelling the religious vitality rather than by choking it off. But, he went on, "It is a man-making religion that we want.... And here is the test of truth – anything that makes you weak physically, intellectually and spiritually, reject it as poison, there is no life in it, it cannot be true." But more startling, because it was no longer in the Hindu tradition, he added this warning: "Give up these weakening mysticisms, and become strong". And glancing back at the past, he exclaimed: "Buddha ruined us as Christ ruined the Romans", claiming as a true kshatriya come to life in the modern setting that India's decadence was due to its giving up the heroic virtues of its culture's springtime.

The crowd hailed Vivekananda all over India and howled "Shiva! Shiva!" But there was more smoke than fire at the time. The awakening was slow, gradual, and Vivekananda, although by far the most dramatic of all the awakeners, was only one among many. And the awakening itself did not take place quite the way he would have wished, spilling almost immediately after his death into violent politics. What was enduring in his work, what still endures to this day, is the concrete materialization of his devotion to service: the Ramakrishna Mission, which was founded in 1897 to spread the Master's gospel and to serve in almost all branches of human endeavour except the political; it was divided into an Indian branch with its monasteries (*maths*) and convents, for retreats (*ashrams*), and foreign missions established abroad. To public service was added teaching the Vedanta doctrine.

Thoroughly impressed and silenced, his critics went to work: relief centres for famines, orphanages, training centres, clinics, educational institutions sprouted all over India, caring for all regardless of caste. The most remarkable aspect of Vivekananda's fantastic activity was his ability to attract flocks of Western disciples who went to work in India with the greatest self-abnegation. One would think that with all this, Vivekananda would have become sufficiently Westernized actually to discard most of Hinduism except the vaguest form of Vedantism that could satisfy men of all creeds. But that was not at all the case: as time went on, his personal devotion turned increasingly towards polytheism (with the Advaita's absolute monism in the background): his personal adoration of Kali and Shiva amazed many Westerners who had known him well, but the atavistic call of Mother India was stronger than any foreign influence. Spiritual emotion was welling up in his heart and he could no longer repress it; but he also went on working like a demon and never once forgot service, devotion to his fellow-human beings.

His influence persisted long after his death and inevitably overflowed into politics. The greatest leaders of the early twentieth century, whatever their walk of life – Rabindranath Tagore, the prince of Poets, Aurobindo Ghosh, the greatest mystic-philosopher; Mahatma Gandhi, who eventually shook the Anglo-Indian Empire to destruction – all acknowledged their overriding debt to both the Swan and the Eagle, to Ramakrishna who stirred the heart of India, and to Vivekananda who awakened its soul .

A tremendous force
– The Eastern and Western Disciples

To introduce the life of Swami Vivekananda is to introduce the subject of the spiritual life itself. All of the intellectual struggle, all the doubts, all of the burning faith, all of the unfolding process of the spiritual illumination were revealed in him. As a man and as a Vedantist he manifested the manliness which was sanctity, and the sanctity which was manliness; he manifested the patriotism which came from the vision of the dharma; and he manifested the life of intense activity as well as of supreme Realization, as the fruit of the true Insight of Divine Wisdom. His life revealed throughout the glory of the Supersensuous Life.

It matters not in what light the present generation....may regard the Swami, be it as a teacher, patriot, prophet or saint; it matters not whether they accept his teachings and his ideas only partially or in their entirety; but all will have to admit that in his life there was made manifest a tremendous force for the moral and spiritual welfare and uplifting of humanity, irrespective of caste, creed, nationality or time. The more the life and teachings of Swami are made known, the more will the spiritual perspective of humanity be widened.

He preached a virile creed
– Will Durant

....The most vivid of the followers (of Ramakrishna) was a proud young kshatriya, Narendranath Dutta, who, full of Spencer and Darwin, first presented himself to Ramakrishna as an atheist unhappy in his atheism, but scornful of the myths and superstitions with which he identified religion. Conquered by Ramakrishna's patient kindness, "Naren" became the young Master's most ardent disciple; he redefined God as "the totality of all souls", and called upon his fellowmen to practise religion not through vain asceticism and meditation, but through absolute devotion to men. "Leave to the next life the reading of the Vedanta, and the practice of meditation. Let this body which is here be put at the service of others!.... The highest truth is this: God is present in all beings. They are His multiple forms. There is no other God to seek. He alone serves God who serves all other beings!"

Changing his name to Vivekananda, he left India to seek funds abroad for the Ramakrishna Mission. In 1893 he found himself lost and penniless in Chicago. A day later he appeared in the Parliament of Religions at the World's Fair, addressed the meeting as a representative of Hinduism, and captured everyone by his magnificent presence, his gospel of the unity of all religions, and his simple ethics of human service as the best worship of God; atheism became a noble religion under the inspiration of his eloquence, and orthodox clergymen found themselves honouring a "heathen" who said there was no other God than the souls of living things. Returning to India, he preached to his countrymen a more virile creed than any Hindu had offered them since Vedic days. 'It is a man-making religion that we want.... Give up these weakening mysticisms, and be strong.... For the next fifty years....let all other vain gods disappear from our minds. This is the only God that is awake, our own race, everywhere His hands, everywhere His feet, everywhere His ears; He covers everything.... The first of all worship is the worship of those all around us.... These are all our gods – men and animals; and the first gods we have to worship are our own countrymen.'

It was but a step from this to Gandhi.

He made a great impression
– J. N. Farquhar

After Ramakrishna's death, his chief disciples decided that they must devote their lives to the spread of his teachings. So a group of them renounced the world and became sannyasins. Amongst those by far the most prominent has been Narendra Nath Datta, who took the name of Vivekananda, when he became a sannyasin.

He received a good English education, taking his degree from a Mission college in Calcutta, and distinguishing himself in philosophy. As a student, he came a good deal under the influence of the Brahma Samaj. He had a fine voice, and wherever he went was in great request for the singing of Bengali hymns. After taking his degree, he began the study of law; but, early in 1882, an uncle took him to see Ramakrishna; and that moment became the turning-point in his life.

From the first Ramakrishna singled him out as one destined to do great things for God, and gave him a great deal of attention. On his master's death he became a sannyasin, as we have said, and then spent some six years in retirement in the Himalayas, doubtless studying and thinking about many things. In 1892 he emerged from his retirement, and toured all down the western coast of India, going as far south as Trivandrum (Kanyakumari) whence he turned north again and went to Madras. Preparations were being made at that time for holding the Parliament of Religions in Chicago. Some friends in Madras proposed that Vivekananda should be sent to the Parliament to represent Hinduism. Funds were collected, and he travelled to America by way of Japan. The gathering was held in September, 1893; and Vivekananda made a great impression, partly by his eloquence, partly by his striking figure and picturesque dress; but mainly by his new, unheard-of presentation of Hinduism. The following quotations from American papers show how far those who were most deeply influenced by the Swami went:

"He is an orator by divine right, and his strong, intelligent face in its picturesque setting of yellow and orange was hardly less interesting than those earnest words, and the rich, rythmical utterance he gave them."

"Vivekananda is undoubtedly the greatest figure in the Parliament of Religions. After hearing him we feel how foolish it is to send missionaries to his learned nation."

He stayed some time in America, lecturing and founding Vedanta Societies in several places.

Vivekananda's influence still lives in America. There are societies that teach Hinduism in various ways in New York, Boston, Washington, Pittsburg and San Francisco. His influence seems to be far stronger in San Francisco than anywhere else. There is a picturesque Hindu temple there, in which classes are held and addresses given, and the literature of the mission sold.

Vivekananda started several magazines, which are still published in India. Books written by Vivekananda during his lifetime, and a few others, published by other members of the mission since then, are sold in the various centres.

Vivekananda wished to combine Western and Hindu Education.

He exercised a fine influence on young India in one direction. He summoned his fellow-countrymen to stand on their own feet, to trust themselves and to play the man, and his words were not without fruit.

He summoned his countrymen to practical service, to self-sacrificing work for India.

It is striking to note the harvest that appeared in Vivekananda from the seed sown by his master Ramakrishna.

The work of the Ramakrishna Mission has grown slowly since Vivekananda's death.

His infinite patience
– Mary C. Funke

There were twelve (at the Thousand Island Park, U. S. A.) of us and it seemed as if the pentecostal fire descended and touched the Master Swami Vivekananda. One afternoon, when he had been telling us of the glory of renunciation, of the joy and freedom of those of the ochre robe, he suddenly left us, and in a short time he had written his *Song of the Sannyasin,* a very passion of sacrifice and renunciation. I think the thing which impressed me most in those days was his infinite patience and gentleness – as a father with his children, though most of us, were several years older than he.

His mission was spiritual
– Christopher Isherwood

Vivekananda was profoundly moved by the realization of India's poverty and the state of her oppression under the British colonial rule. And he proposed a revolution. The spirit of this revolution enormously influenced Gandhi and influences Indian political thought to this day.

Vivekananda in this sense is a great figure in Indian history, one of the very greatest historical figures that India has ever produced. But it must always be noted that Vivekananda's revolution, Vivekananda's nationalism, were not like the kind of revolution, the kind of nationalism, which we associate with other great leaders, admirable and noble as they may be. Vivekananda was far greater than that. In fact, when one sees the full range of his mind, one is astounded. Vivekananda looked towards the West, not simply as a mass of tyrants exploiting various parts of Asia, and other undeveloped areas, but as future partners, people who had very, very much to offer. At the same time, without any false humility, he faced the West and said, "we have fully as much and more to offer you. We offer you this great tradition of spirituality, which can produce, even now, today, a supremely great figure such as Ramakrishna. You can offer us medical services, trains that run on time, hygiene, irrigation, electric light. These are very important, we want them, and we admire some of your qualities immensely."

One of the most enchanting things about Vivekananda is the way he was eternally changing sides when he was speaking to different people; he could denounce the British in words of fire, but again he would turn on the Indians and say, "You cannot manufacture one pin, and you dare to criticize the British!" And then he would speak of the awful materialism of the United States, and on the other hand, he would say that no women in the world were greater, and that the treatment of women in India was absolutely disgraceful. And so in every way, he was integrating, he was seeing the force of good, the constructive forces, in the different countries, and saying "why don't we exchange?" So Vivekananda's revolution was a revolution for everybody, a revolution which would, in the long run, be of just as much use to the British as to India. Vivekananda's nationalism, the call to India to recognize herself – this again was not nationalism in the smaller sense, it was a kind of super-nationalism, a kind of internationalism sublimated. You all know the story that Vivekananda was so fond of, about the lion that was brought up with a lot of sheep. Now another lion comes out of the forest and the sheep all run away, and the little lion that had been brought up thinks it's a sheep and runs away too, and how the pursuing lion grabs it, takes it over to a pool of water and says, "Look at yourself, you're a lion". This is what Vivekananda was doing to the Indian people. He remarks in one of his letters, that the marvellous thing about all of the Western nations is that they know that they are nations. He said jealousy is a curse of India. Indians cannot learn to co-operate with each other. Why can't they learn from the co-operation of Western nations with each other?

I am quoting all this because considering all these different attitudes that Vivekananda took, one sees the immense scope and integrity of his goodwill. He was really on everybody's side, on the side of the West, and on the side of India, and he saw far, far into the future; his political prophecies are extremely interesting, and he said repeatedly, that the great force, which would finally have to be reckoned with was China. He also remarked on visiting Europe for the last time in 1900 that he smelled war everywhere, which was more than most professional statesmen did, at that time.

*   *   *   *

Vivekananda taught that God is within each one of us, and that each one of us was born to rediscover his own God-nature.... He was the prophet of self-reliance, of individual search and effort.

Vivekananda was a very great devotee; but he did not proclaim his devotion to all corners. His refusal to do so was a considered decision. Speaking of his work in America after returning to India, he said: 'If I had preached the personality of Ramakrishna, I might have converted half the world; but that kind of conversion is short-lived. So instead I preached Ramakrishna's principles. If people accept the principles, they will eventually accept the personality.'

Vivekananda was the last person in the world to worry about formal consistency. He almost always spoke extempore, fired by the circumstances of the moment, addressing himself to the condition of a particular group of hearers, reacting to the intent of a certain question. That was his nature – and he was supremely indifferent if his words of today seemed to contradict those of yesterday. As a man of enlightenment, he knew that the truth is never contained in arrangements of sentences. It is within the speaker himself. If what he is, is true, then words are unimportant. In this sense, Vivekananda is incapable of self-contradiction.

Vivekananda was not only a great teacher with an international message; he was also a very great Indian, a patriot and an inspirer of his countrymen down to the present generation. But it is a mistake to think of him as a political figure, even in the best meaning of the word. First and last, he was the boy who dedicated his life to Ramakrishna. His mission was spiritual, not political or even social, in the last analysis.

The policy of the Ramakrishna Order has always been faithful to Vivekananda's intention. In the early twenties, when India's struggle with England had become intense and bitter, the Order was harshly criticised for refusing to allow its members to take part in Gandhi's Non-co-operative Movement. But Gandhi himself never joined in this criticism. He understood perfectly that a religious body which supports a political cause – no matter how noble and just – can only compromise itself spiritually and thereby lose that very authority which is its justification for existence within human society. In 1921 Gandhi came to the Belur Math on the anniversary of Vivekananda's birthday and paid a moving tribute to him. The Swami's writings, Gandhi said, had taught him to love India even more. He reverently visited the room overlooking the Ganges in which Vivekananda spent the last months of his life.

You can visit that room today; it is still kept exactly as Vivekananda left it. But it does not seem museum-like or even unoccupied. Right next to it is the room which is used by the President of the Ramakrishna Order. There they are, dwelling side by side, the visible human authority and the invisible inspiring presence. In the life of the Belur Math, Vivekananda still lives and is as much a participant in its daily activities as any of its monks.

Paragon of Vedantist missionaries
– William James

The paragon of all monistic systems is the Vedanta philosophy of Hindustan, and the paragon of Vedantist missionaries was the late Swami Vivekananda who visited our land some years ago....

I have just been reading some of Vivekananda's addresses in England, which I had not seen. The man is simply a wonder for oratorical power.... the Swami is an honour to humanity in any case.

His Divine presence
– Dr. M. H. Logan

His Divine presence spread peace and tranquillity wherever he went; the tumult of uncertainty departed from my soul at the sound of his magic voice. His very form and every mood were those of tender compassion and sympathy. None knew him but to love him; those of us who have had the royal good fortune to meet him in the flesh will some day realize that we have met the true incarnation of the divine One.

To me he is the Christ, than whom a greater one has never come; his great and liberal soul outshines all other things; his mighty spirit is as free and liberal as the great sun, or the air of heaven.

No being lived so mean or low, be he a man or a beast, that he would not salute. His was not only an appeal to the poor and lowly but also to kings and princes and mighty rulers of the earth, to grand masters of learning, of finances, of arts and of sciences, to leaders of thought and of creeds, to mighty intellects, philosophers and poets. Vivekananda shook the world of thought in all its higher lines. Great teachers bowed reverently at his feet, the humble followed reverently to kiss the hem of his garments; no other single human being was revered more during his life than was Vivekananda.

In the few short weeks that I was with him a few could know him better than I. At first I attended him through a severe spell of sickness, then he sat with me partly through a paralytic stroke; he would charm me to sleep and enchant me awake. So passed the sublimest part of my life, and now that sweet memory lingers and sustains me ever and always.

His amazing size
– Josephine Macleod

The thing that held me in Swamiji was his unlimitedness. I never could touch the bottom – or top – or sides. The amazing size of him!.... Oh, such natures make one so free. It's the reaction on oneself that matters really, isn't it? ....It is the Truth I saw in Swamiji that has set me free! It was to set me free that Swamiji came, that was as much part of his mission as it was to give renunciation to Nivedita, or unity to Mrs. S.

Alter ego of Ramakrishna
– E. R. Marozzi

In comparing Swami Vivekananda with other spiritual luminaries of his time Ramakrishna said of him: that if Keshab Chandra Sen had one power which made him famous, Vivekananda had eighteen such powers in the fullest measure; that though the hearts of Keshab and Vijaya Krishna Goswami were brightened by light of knowledge like the flame of a lamp, the very sun of knowledge had risen in the heart of Swamiji and removed from there even the slightest trace of *maya* and delusion; that in taking stock of his special devotees, the *Ishvarakotis* (those who are born with the mission of a Divine Incarnation and have spiritual knowledge from birth), some were like lotuses of ten petals, some like lotuses of sixteen petals and some of the hundred petals – but among lotuses the Swami was a thousand-petalled one; that though the other devotees may be like pots and pitchers, the Swami was a huge reservoir: that though the others were like minnows, smelts, or sardines, Vivekananda was like a huge red-eyed carp. When we remember that those with whom the Swami is thus compared were outstanding spiritual men of India and some of them leaders of the spiritual movements of the time, these are indeed remarkable statements. Nor should we take them to be only glorification and praise from one who loved him much, but rather as proper evaluations from one who could not deviate from truth and who had the insight to understand him thoroughly as none other but the *sadguru* (true spiritual teacher) could. Further, what the Swami became in the end was largely due to what Ramakrishna made him – and we say that Swami Vivekananda the man, as the world knew him, was the spiritual power, Ramakrishna, in another form.

Sarada Devi, the spiritual consort of Ramakrishna, said about the Swami: "Naren is an instrument of Thakur (Master) who makes him write these words for inspiring his children and devotees for doing his work, for doing good to all the world. What Naren writes is true and must be fulfilled hereafter." A few years after the *mahasamadhi* of Ramakrishna, Sarada Devi had a vision in which Ramakrishna was seen going to the Ganges and his body dissolving in the waters. Then Narendra appeared and, crying "Glory to Ramakrishna!", took the water in his hands and began to sprinkle it upon many men and women who had gathered there, who immediately attained illumination. It was a symbolic expression of Swamiji's teaching work and that the being, power, and substance of it were Ramakrishna.

The Swami himself said about it: "All that I am, all that the world will some day be, is owing to my Master, Ramakrishna. If there has been anything achieved by me, by my thoughts or words, or deeds, if from my lips has ever fallen one word that has helped anyone in the world, I lay no claim to it; it was all His. All that has been weak has been mine, and all that has been life-giving, strengthening, pure and holy, has been His inspiration, His word – and He Himself." In a letter from America to a friend in India in 1894 he wrote, "I am an instrument and He is the operator. Through this instrument He is rousing the religious instinct in thousands in this far-off country. Thousands of men and women here love and revere me – 'He makes the dumb eloquent and makes the lame cross mountains.' I am amazed at His grace. Whatever town I visit, it is in an uproar. They call me the 'cyclonic Hindu.' Remember, it is His will – I am a voice without a form."

A remarkable event marked the meeting of these two great souls on spiritual plane and also heralded the coming of Swamiji into the advent of Ramakrishna. The Master narrated it thus: "One day I saw that, through *samadhi*, my mind was going up a luminous path, going beyond the subtle world of ideas. The more it began to ascend to higher and higher strata of that realm the more did I see beautiful ideal forms of *devas* and *devis* existing on both sides of the path. It came gradually to the last extremity of the region. I saw that a fence made of light was there separating the realm of the divisible from that of the indivisible. Leaping over that fence, the mind entered by degrees the realm of the indivisible. I saw there was no more any person or thing there having a form. As if, afraid to enter there, even the *devas* and *devis* possessing heavenly bodies exercised their authority over realms far below. But the next moment I saw seven wise *rishis* having bodies consisting of light only, seated there in *samadhi*. I felt that in virtue and knowledge, love and renunciation they had excelled even the *devas* and *devis*, not to speak of human beings. Astonished, I was pondering over their greatness when I saw before me that a part of the homogeneous mass of light of the 'Abode' of the indivisible, devoid of the slightest tinge of difference, became solidified and converted into the form of a divine Child. Coming down to one of those *rishis*, and throwing Its soft and delicate arms round his neck, it embraced him and afterwards, calling him with Its ambrosial words, sweeter than the music of the *veena*, made great efforts to wake him up from *samadhi*. The *rishi* woke from *samadhi* at the delicate and loving touch and looked at that wonderful Child with half-shut eyes, free from winking. Seeing the state of his bright face, full of delight, I thought that the Child was the treasure of his heart – their familiarity was of eternity. The extraordinary divine Child then expressed infinite joy and said to him, 'I am going, you must come with me.' The *rishi* said nothing at that request, but his loving eyes expressed his hearty assent. Afterwards, looking on the Child with loving eyes for some time, he entered again into *samadhi*. Astonished, I then saw that converted into the form of a bright light, a part of the mind and body of that *rishi* came down to earth along the reverse path. Hardly had I seen Narendra for the first time when I knew that he was that *rishi.*" Later when the Master was asked about the divine Child he said that he himself had assumed the form of that Child. This then is the spiritual event in which Swamiji was called by his Master to accompany Him to earth to carry out His mission.

A monk of commanding presence
– Sir Hiram Stevens Maxim

A few years ago there was a Congress of Religions at Chicago. Many said that such a thing would be impossible. How could any understanding be arrived at where each particular party was absolutely right and all the others were completely in the wrong? Still the Congress saved the American people more than a million dollars a year, not to mention many lives abroad. And this was all brought about by one brave and honest man. When it was announced....that there was to be a Congress of Religions at Chicago, some of the rich merchants took the Americans at their word, and sent them a....monk, Vivekananda, from the oldest monastery in the world. This monk was of commanding presence and vast learning, speaking English like a Webster. The American Protestants, who vastly outnumbered all others, imagined that they would have an easy task, and commenced proceedings with the greatest confidence, and with the air of "Just see me wipe you out." However, what they had to say was the old commonplace twaddle that had been mouthed over and over again in every little hamlet from Nova Scotia to California. It interested no one, and no one noticed it.

When, however, Vivekananda spoke, they saw that they had a Napoleon to deal with. His first speech was no less than a revelation. Every word was eagerly taken down by the reporters, and telegraphed all over the country, when it appeared in thousands of papers. Vivekananda became the lion of the day. He soon had an immense following. No hall could hold the people who flocked to hear him lecture. They had been sending silly girls and half-educated simpletons of men, and millions of dollars, to Asia for years to convert the poor benighted heathen and save his alleged soul; and here was a specimen of the unsaved who knew more of philosophy and religion than all the persons and missionaries in the whole country. Religion was presented in an agreeable light for the first time to them. There was more in it than they had ever dreamed; argument was impossible. He played with the persons as a cat plays with a mouse. They were in a state of consternation. What could they do? What did they do? What they always do – they denounced him as an agent of the devil. But the deed was done: he had sown the seed, and the Americans commenced to think. They said to themselves: "Shall we waste our money in sending missionaries who know nothing of religion, as compared with this man, to teach such men as he? No!" And the missionary income fell off more than a million dollars a year in consequence.

A dominant, majestic personality
– Harriet Monroe

Swami Vivekananda, the magnificent, stole the whole show and captured the town.... the handsome monk in the orange robe gave us in perfect English a masterpiece. His personality, dominant, majestic, his voice, rich as a bronze bell, the controlled fervour of his feeling, the beauty of his message to the Western world he was facing for the first time – these combined to give us a rare and perfect moment of supreme emotion. It was human eloquence of highest pitch.

A luminous personality
– Lillian Montgomery

It was in June 1900 I came in touch with Swami Vivekananda.

Little did I dream I was to see a personality that would be revelation – one that embodied a light I had never seen – nor have I ever seen that light manifest to such a degree of pure glow in any other form.

He rose to speak – phrases flowed forth – without effort – but, every word was moulded round a light that brought new significance to its meaning – he was living the very thought he was expressing.

There seemed an absence of the sense of ego.

As if the outer form were absorbing a light of intelligence pouring from an infinite source!

He was revealing a realm of consciousness unknown to me. I saw as it were a lake of consciousness that filled space back of him, and somehow focussed and was pouring through his words.

Veil after veil was failing from my mind's eye – a new universe was being revealed – the possibility of personality – relationship of the individual soul with divine.

He quoted, "Blessed are the pure in heart for they shall see God."

Words I had learned all my life, but now it was as if the purity of the heart of the speaker was reflecting Divinity at this moment – a new conception of the quotation.

The conviction came then, and has never changed, that he had, within, the 'Pearl of Great Price'– that for which we all longed, and that culture, not possession, was the thing most desired.

There was a brilliance of mind, clothed in the warmth of the heart, and an impressive calmness as he spoke words of wisdom that were leading you into a realm of higher truth unknown.

Being in his presence brought knowledge not to be obtained in book, because you saw he had within himself a Reality that outvalued all the wealth in the world.

I aways left his presence treading air – he had made so clear that life was such a wonderful thing....

Was he so aware of the inner Perfection that he could draw into manifestation for others to witness?....

....Is it strange that to me at that time the luminous flood of consciousness was so apparent?

Or that the voice that flowed from that crystal pure reality should have the ring of Truth, and a sonority of unusual quality and beauty?

And, is it difficult to understand, why, for fifty-four years, Swami Vivekananda has been to me like beacon light "beckoning a distant Goal!"

Archetype of the sannyasin
– Sister Nivedita

There was one thing, however, deep in the master's nature, that he never knew how to adjust. This was his love of his country and his resentment of her suffering. Throughout those years in which 1 saw him almost daily, the thought of India was to him like the air he breathed. True, he was a worker at foundations. He neither used the word "nationality", nor proclaimed an era of "nation-making". "Man-making", he said was his own task. But he was born a lover, and the queen of his adoration was his motherland. Like some delicately poised bell, thrilled and vibrated by every sound that falls upon it, was his heart to all that concerned her. Not a sob was heard within her shores that did not find in him a responsive echo. There was no cry of fear, no tremor of weakness, no shrinking from mortification that he had not known and understood. He was hard on her sins, unsparing of her want of worldly wisdom, but only because he felt these faults to be his own. And none, on the contrary, was ever so possessed by the vision of her greatness.

What was it that the West heard in him, leading so many to hail and cherish his name as that of one of the greatest religious teachers of the world? He made no personal claim. He told no personal story.... He made no attempt to popularize with strangers any single form or creed, whether of God or guru. Rather, through him the mighty torrent of Hinduism poured forth its cooling waters upon the intellectual and spiritual worlds, fresh from its secret sources in Himalayan snows. A witness to the vast religious culture of Indian homes and holy men he could never cease to be. Yet he quoted nothing but the Upanishads. He taught nothing but the Vedanta. And men trembled, for they heard the voice for the first time of the religious teacher who feared not truth.

Man-making was his own stern brief summary of the work that was worth doing. And laboriously, unflaggingly, day after day, he set himself to man-making, playing the part of guru, of father, even of school master, by turns....

He passed, when the laurels of his first achievements were yet green. He passed, when new and greater calls were ringing in his ears....

To his disciples, Vivekananda will ever remain the archetype of the sannyasin. Burning renunciation was chief of all the inspirations that spoke to us through him. "Let me die a true sannyasin as my Master did", he exclaimed once, passionately, "heedless of money, of woman, and fame! And of these the most insidious is the love of fame!"

A teacher of the highest order
– Rhodehamel

It is now more than ten years since Swami Vivekananda lectured to California audiences; it seems but yesterday. It was here as elsewhere; the audiences were his from the outset and remained his to the end. They were swept along on the current of his thought without resistance. Many there were who did not want to resist, whose pleasure and novelty it was to have light thrown into the hidden recesses of their minds by the proximity of a luminous personality. There were a few who would have resisted if they could, but whose powers of resistance were neutralized by the irresistible logic, acumen, and childlike simplicity of the Great Teacher. Indeed, there were a few who arose to differ, but who resumed their seats either in smiling acquiescence or in bewildered impotency.

The Swami's personality impressed itself on the mind with visual intensity. The speaking eyes, the wealth of facial expression, and gesticulation, the wondrous Sanskrit chanting, sonorous and melodious, impressing one with the sense of mystic potency, the translations following in smiling confidence – all these, set off by the spectacular appeal of the Hindu sannyasin – who can forget them?

As a lecturer he was unique; never referring to notes, as most lecturers do; and though he repeated many discourses on request, they were never repetitions. He seemed to be giving something of himself, to be speaking from a super-experience. The most abstruse points of the Vedanta were retrieved from the domain of mere speculation by a vital something which seemed to emanate from him. His utterances were dynamic and constructive, arousing thought and directing it into a synthetic process. Thus he was not only a lecturer but a Teacher of the highest order as well.

Quick, and when necessary, sharp at repartee, he met all opposition with the utmost good nature and even enjoyment. His business was to make his hearers understand, and he succeeded as, perhaps, no other lecturer on abstruse subjects ever did. To popularise abstractions, to place them within the mental grasp of even very ordinary intellects, was his achievement. He reached them all. 'In India', he said, 'they tell me that I ought not to teach Advaita Vedanta to the people at large. But I say that I can make even a child understand it. You cannot begin too early to teach the highest spiritual truths'.

He held purity to be needed for the householder as well as for the monk, and laid great stress on that point. 'The other day, a young Hindu came to see me', he said, 'He has been living in this country for about two years, and suffering from ill-health for some time. In the course of our talk, he said that the theory of chastity must be all wrong because the doctors in this country have advised him against it. They told him that it was against law of Nature. I asked him to go back to India, where he belonged, and to listen to the teachings of his ancestors, who had practised chastity for thousands of years?' Then turning a face puckered into an expression of unutterable disgust, he thundered: 'You doctors in this country, who hold that chastity is against the law of Nature, you don't know what you are talking about. You don't know the meaning of the word purity. You are beasts, beasts, I say, with the morals of a tom-cat, if that is the best you have to say on that subject!' Here he glanced defiantly over the audience, challenging opposition by his very glance. No voice was raised, though there were several physicians present.

Bombs were thrown in all his lectures. Audiences were jolted out of hereditary ruts, and the New Thought students, so-called, were subjected to scathing though constructive criticisms without mercy. Similarly, he would announce the most stupendous Vedantic conceptions so opposed to Christian theological dogmas; then pause an instant – how many, many times, and with such winsome effect! – with his teeth pressed on his lower lip as though with bated breath observing the result; Imagine, if you can, greater violence done to the traditional teachings of Christendom than by his fiery injunction. 'Don't repent! Don't repent!.... Spit, if you must, but go on! Don't hold yourselves down by repenting! Throw off the load of sin, if there is such a thing, by knowing your true selves – the pure! the Ever Free!.... That man is blasphemous who tells you that you are sinners.... And again, 'This world is a superstition. We are hypnotized into believing it real. The process of salvation is the process of de-hypnotization.... This universe is just the play of the Lord – that is all. It is all just for fun. There can be no reason for His doing anything. Know the Lord if you would understand His play. Be His playfellows, and He will tell you all.... And to you, who are philosophers, I say that to ask for a reason for the existence of the universe is illogical, because it implies limitation in God, which you do not admit.' Then he entered into one of his wonderful expositions of the salient features of the Advaita Vedanta.

Energy personified
– Romain Rolland

He (Vivekananda) was energy personified, and action was his message to men. For him, as for Beethoven, it was root of all the virtues.... He had a pair of magnificent eyes, large, dark, and rather prominent with heavy lids whose shape recalled classic comparison to a lotus petal. Nothing escaped the magic of his glance.

His pre-eminent characteristic was kingliness. He was a born king and nobody ever came near him either in India or America without paying homage to his majesty.

When this quite unknown young man of thirty appeared in Chicago at the inaugural meeting of the Parliament of Religions, opened in September 1893, by Cardinal Gibbons, all his fellow-members were forgotten in his commanding presence. His strength and beauty, the grace and dignity of his bearing, the dark light of his eyes, his imposing appearance, and from the moment he began to speak, the splendid music of his rich deep voice enthralled the vast audience of American Anglo-Saxons, previously prejudiced against him on account of his colour. The thought of this warrior prophet of India left a deep mark upon the United States.

It was impossible to imagine him in the second place. Wherever he went he was the first.... Everybody recognised, in him at sight the leader, the anointed of God, the man marked with the stamp of the power to command. A traveller who crossed his path in the Himalayas without knowing who he was, stopped in amazement, and cried, "Shiva!...."

It was as if his chosen God had imprinted His name upon his forehead....

His super-powerful body and too vast brain were the predestined battle-field for all the shocks of his storm-tossed soul. The present and the past, the East and the West, dream and action, struggled for supremacy. He knew and could achieve too much to be able to establish harmony by renouncing one part of his nature or one part of the truth. The synthesis of his great opposing forces took years of struggle, consuming his courage and his very life. Battle and life for him were synonymous. And his days were numbered. Sixteen years passed between Ramakrishna's death and that of his great disciple.... years of conflagration....

He was less than forty years of age when the athlete lay stretched upon the pyre....

But the flame of that pyre is still alight today. From his ashes, like those of the phoenix of old, has sprung anew the conscience of India – the magic bird – faith in her unity and in the Great Message, brooded over from Vedic times by the dreaming spirit of his ancient race – the message for which it must render account to the rest of mankind.

His words are great music, phrases in the style of Beethoven, stirring rhythms like the march of Handel choruses. I cannot touch these sayings of his, scattered as they are through the pages of books at thirty years' distance, without receiving a thrill through my body like an electric shock. And what shocks, what transports must have been produced when in burning words they issued from the lips of the hero!

India was hauled out of the shifting sands of barren speculation wherein she had been engulfed for centuries, by the hand of one of her own sannyasins; and the result was that the whole reservoir of mysticism, sleeping beneath, broke its bounds and spread by a series of great ripples into action. The West ought to be aware of the tremendous energies liberated by these means.

He is dear to the people of the USSR

– R. Ryabakov

The people of the Soviet Union observed the 120th anniversary of the birth of the great Indian thinker and public figure Swami Vivekananda, whose fame has twice outlived his short and dramatic life, entirely devoted to the noble cause of awakening India....

I have recently been to .... Yasnaya Polyana, the house of Leo Tolstoy – the great writer, whose name is equally dear to the peoples of the USSR and India. I saw a group of visitors encircling a large dinner table and my mind conjured up grey-bearded Tolstoy, reading British newspapers out loud in the light of a kerosene lamp. The British Press was full of reports about Vivekananda's brilliant lectures. Sometimes, there was a little truth in them, yet the powerful voice of the Calcutta sannyasi did reach the writer's mind through the filter of the British newspapers. It stirred the writer profoundly and for a while he could not continue reading. He went to the bedroom and read Vivekananda's books all through the night. He marked in his diary: "I was reading Vivekananda again. How much there is in common between the thoughts of his and mine."

That epoch has long since gone. The people who come to the Tolstoy museum and listen to the guide's story were born in the age of space flights, cinema and television and they do not know what colonialism is. The material culture of that time has disappeared and so have clothes and objects of everyday life. But the spiritual culture which unites all nations is alive and continues to exert powerful influence on our contemporaries.

Vivekananda's ideas were dear not only to Tolstoy. They are just as dear to the Soviet people today, primarily, because his life was filled with ardent love for India. Vivekananda had always desired to change the situation in India – the powerful and yet dependent country, fettered by the will of British colonialists, hard vestiges of the centuries-old history and rigid caste conventions and also disintegrated, oppressed and not yet strong to rebel. He had not spared efforts to awaken his countrymen's feeling of national identity, the wish to work for the national benefit and the faith in India's bright future. Neither had he spared sarcasm to stir up the Indians' feeling of shame for their dependent and oppressed position, the shame, which to quote Marx's apt remark, "is already revolution of a kind. Shame is a kind of anger which is turned inward. And if a whole nation really experienced a sense of shame, it would be like a lion, crouching ready to spring." However reluctant, Vivekananda was to get involved in politics, his entire activities were aimed against imperialism and colonialism and he had played an important role in India's becoming an independent state and a leading power.

The essence of Vivekananda's religion is the service to people. "I do not believe in God or religion which cannot wipe the widow's tears or bring a piece of bread to the orphan's mouth", he said. His doctrine was focussed on man. Everything for the good of man – how consonant his idea is with Maxim Gorky's words spoken at about the same time: "The name of Man rings proud." Centering his attention on the Indian reality, Vivekananda explained the national degradation by the indifference of the propertied classes to the people's needs and by the poverty and ignorance of the population. "Contempt for the masses is a grave national sin", he said.

Vivekananda had uncovered yet another cause of India's decline, namely, the country's isolated status. It is only natural that the voice of the man who asserted the idea of equality of all religions and the international fraternity of liberated peoples deeply moved the delegates of the world religious council in Chicago. He was not afraid of reason and relied on it.

"It is better that mankind should become atheist through following reason, than, blindly believe in 200 million gods on the authority of anybody." The supernatural and miracles did not bother him and he refused to accept miracles ascribed to his teacher Ramakrishna. Isn't it a miracle, however, that he had heard the roaring of the coming social and political events of the 20th century in the slow and serene life of 19th century Europe and had aptly foreseen that the liberation would come from Russia.

That epoch is unreachably far away. Kings and kingdoms have disappeared and practically the entire colonial system has collapsed. They say there are old gramophone records of Vivekananda's ardent voice still to be found in India. His voice was admired by Ramakrishna and it produced a tremendous impression on the Chicago religious congress. Those records have been played for a long time already, for there are no gramophones to play them on.

Still, Vivekananda's voice keeps ringing. Celebrating the 120th anniversary of his birth, we recall Rabindranath Tagore's words: "If you want to know India, read Vivekananda."

He interpreted Hinduism to the West
– Prof. Ninian Smart

....The universalist message of Swami Vivekananda, and of his Master, Ramakrishna, genuinely represents a new departure in world religions – the attempt to make the highest form of Hinduism a world faith. In so doing, the Vedanta would cease to be the highest form of Hinduism as such; but it would become the highest form of religion in general. Whether or not this faith will emerge as the unifying factor in the global manifestation of religion is something which will be settled by a process of social dialogue. But it must expect to have rivals from the less synthetically-minded faiths, and probably most of all from Christianity, which combines a strong measure of exclusiveness, characterises the other semetic religions, Judaism and Islam, with a degree of self-criticism and openness to scientific enquiry which is largely lacking in these other faiths.

It may be remarked in the passing that a related challenge faces Christian doctrine. The Theory of Evolution already casts doubt on the doctrine of the special creation of man. Nor is it attractive to postulate the continuous intervention of a supernatural being in grafting souls upon human embryos. Swami Vivekananda was indeed rather scathing about such a doctrine. From the Christian point of view, and bearing in mind the above considerations, it is clear that after all Swami Vivekananda was far nearer the truth than some traditional Christian theology when he wrote: "God being the universal and common cause of all phenomena, the question was to find natural causes of certain phenomena in the human soul, and the *Deus ex machina* theory is, therefore, quite irrelevant." If reincarnation is not accepted, it implies that mental properties have emerged from a material background in the process of evolution, and that this is part of God's continuous creative activity in sustaining and evolving the material world.

....There are many in the West who though superficially indifferent to traditional religious values, still nourish a desire for faith. It is important for them to understand the main issues of religious thinking; in this respect, Swami Vivekananda, by giving such an incisive expression to a revitalized Hinduism ready to break beyond the bounds of India, can clarify men's insights into the choice before them.... Some of the problems tackled by Swami Vivekananda, and his solutions thereto remain, despite changes in the intellectual and scientific climate since he wrote, highly relevant to the contemporary situation. It must be recalled too that not only did he interpret Hinduism to the West so eloquently, but he also interpreted it to India itself.

A shrinking world will surely recognize how much it owes to him, the first man really to bring home to the consciousness of the Western world at large the deeper significance of the *Sanatana Dharma*.

Typical representative of Hinduism
– Merwin Marie Snell

By far the most important and typical representative of Hinduism was Swami Vivekananda, who, in fact, was beyond question the most popular and influential man in the Parliament.... and on all occasions he was received with greater enthusiasm than any other speaker – Christian or Pagan. The people thronged about him wherever he went and hung with eagerness on his every word.... The most rigid of orthodox Christians say of him, 'He is indeed a prince among men.'

A champion of religious unity
– Rev. Sidney Spencer

The thing for which Vivekananda is most widely known is the work which he did on behalf of religious unity. At the Parliament of Religions held at Chicago in 1893 he made in impassioned plea for the recognition of this principle, and it forms the keynote of his teaching. Religious unity was for him at once an ideal and an existing fact. "In essence", he said, "all religions are one."

"There is a tremendous life-power", Vivekananda said, "in all the great religions of the world", and this statement has been abundantly confirmed by subsequent experience. It is Vivekananda's contention that this "life-power" is itself a witness to the fact that all religions have elements of truth and value that all have their own contribution to make to the enrichment of the spiritual life of the world. He is surely right. No religion could maintain itself through the centuries, as all the great religions have done, unless in some degree it met human need, and human need could not be met year by year and age by age by any body of thought and experience which contained no element of enduring validity. "All religions", Vivekananda declared, "are different forces in the economy of God working for the good of mankind."

The problem of religious unity is not to be solved by the victory of any one religion over the others. Such a thing is not within the bounds of practical possibility, neither is it in itself the true direction of advance. Unity, in other words, is not to be identified with uniformity. There is no real incompatibility between unity and diversity. "Unity in variety is the plan of the universe." Human nature is one in essentials, yet it finds an infinite variety of expression. It is, indeed, the very existence of differentiation which makes us what we are. "Variety is the first principle of life."

Vivekananda was the champion of religious unity. But he was not for that reason opposed to diversity of religious thought or of religious organization. He did not depreciate the existence of multifarious sects. "I am a great believer in sects", he said. "I want sects to multiply in every country, that more people may have a chance to be spiritual." He saw that among human beings there are many different types or grades of mind and temperament, and the important thing for him was that men should have the opportunity of satisfying their various needs in the sphere of religion. The greater the variety of religious bodies, the wider the field of selection which is open to us. His attitude affords in this respect the greatest possible contrast to the attitude which is characteristic today of the ecumenical movement in the Christian Church. He laid no stress on unity of organization. That does not mean that he would have favoured the multiplication of sects so far as it arises from differences in small points of doctrine or organization, or from conflicting claims to the possession of a monopoly of saving truth. Sects are valuable, he held, so far as they widen the field of choice for the religious man – so far as they open out the possibility of his finding the form of religious life suited to his particular type of mentality. "So far as they are not exclusive", he said, "I see that the sects and creeds are all mine." He could identify himself with all modes of religious thought and aspiration, without abandoning his own distinctive outlook – except in so far as their attitude was exclusive. "As soon as a man stands up and says he is right, or his church is right, and all others are wrong, he is himself all wrong.... Love and charity for the whole human race, that is the test of true religiousness."

The main fact, however, from Vivekananda's standpoint is not the attitude of Christian Churches to one another, but their attitude to other religions, and here there can be no essential change until there is change of outlook regarding the nature of Christianity. As long as Christianity is regarded as a unique and final revelation of truth, it is impossible for Vivekananda's vision of religious unity to prevail. He saw that in modern times there had been a certain widening of thought among Christian teachers. "They allow that in the older religions, the different types of worship were foreshadowings of Christianity." "This", he said, "is a great advance." Today there are some Christian thinkers who acknowledge, not only that there are elements of truth and value in other religions, but that, wherever such elements are found, they spring from the inspiring activity of God.

For Vivekananda Christianity is a particular expression of divine truth; and if it is to be rightly understood, it must be set side by side with other forms of faith and worship as a manifestation of the one universal religion which underlies them all.

Religious unity is for Vivekananda not merely an ideal for the future; it is a present fact. What we have to do, if we are to realize the ideal, is first of all to discover the essential nature of this fact. "There is only one infinite religion", he says. "This religion expresses itself in various ways in different countries but "the same God is the inspirer of all."

Vivekananda saw religion in all its phases, developed or undeveloped, as man's endeavour to reach out beyond the limits of the physical life and the material world, and to apprehend a deeper and greater Reality. "Every religion", he says, "consciously or unconsciously, is struggling upward toward God.... This is the only recognition of universality that we can get." Again, he says (in a paper on Hinduism read at the Parliament of Religions) "All the religions of the world mean so many attempts of the human soul to grasp and realize the Infinite."

For Vivekananda the mystical experience is the culmination of religion, and it is therefore the clue to its deeper meaning. The end and the inmost meaning of religion is the realization of God in the soul, whereby man is lifted into oneness with God. Everywhere in religion he sees the same moving force, the same inner tendency – the tendency on the part of man to pass beyond the limitations of the senses through contact with the Transcendent. For all the differences which divide them, in this inner tendency, which is their essence, religions are one. However great they may appear, the differences are inessential. The unity of religion reveals itself, not in any common stock of beliefs, but in certain principles which are common to the higher religions of the world.

All religions play their part, for Vivekananda, in helping men to attain their goal. Behind every religion there is a "Soul" "a particular excellence", which marks it out from the rest. The "soul" of Islam is its affirmation of the practical brotherhood and equality of all believers, irrespective of the divisions of race or class. In its emphasis on this truth Islam has a vital contribution to make. It is significant, particularly in view of the history of India since his time, that Vivekananda declared that the hope for India lay in the union of Hinduism with Islam. The "soul" of Hinduism he found in spirituality, grounded in the sense of the immediate presence of God and the possibility of seeing and knowing Him. At its highest level it calls for concentration on that endeavour and so (Vivekananda believed) for renunciation of the world. The Hindu seeks perfection through the merging of his life in the infinite and universal life of God. Hinduism stands thus in principle for universal charity and tolerance. It has its faults, but intolerance is not among them. "If the Hindu fanatic burns himself on the pyre, he never lights the fire of Inquisition."

Vivekananda's watchword is "acceptance, and not exclusion". The religion of the future, he saw, will be one which arises, not from any single stream of tradition; it will be one which finds a place for the vision of all inspired prophets and seers, past, present and to come. Its whole force, as he said in his memorable address to the Parliament of Religions, will be "centred in aiding humanity to realize its own true, divine nature." So far as the spirit of that ideal religion prevails, it gives us the insight to participate in every form of spiritual worship. "I shall go", Vivekananda says, "to the mosque of the Mohammedan; I shall enter the Christian's church and kneel
before his crucifix; I shall enter the Buddhist temple, where I shall take refuge in Buddha and in his law. I shall go into the forest and sit down in meditation with the Hindu, who is trying to see the light which enlightens the heart of everyone."

It is that spirit, which identifies itself with all true worship, because it penetrates beneath the form to the inner substance of faith and devotion, out of which alone a universal religion can emerge. Religion everywhere is one in essence and it is through the sense of that unity, and so through the growth of "fellow-feeling between the different types of religion", that a larger and more comprehensive religion must arise. There is no call for the conversion of believers in one form of religion to another. "The Christian is not to become a Hindu or a Buddhist, nor a Hindu or a Buddhist to become a Christian." What is necessary is that while each preserves his own individuality, he shall at the same time "assimilate the spirit of the others"; he shall enlarge his vision to include the essential truth by which they live, so that he may prepare the way for the universal religion which alone can provide an enduring basis for the unity of mankind.

Confluence of mysticism and the new physics
– Michael Talbot

There are many parallel concepts between the ancient philosophies of the East and the emerging philosophies of the West. Certain concepts are so similar that it becomes impossible to discern whether some statements were made by the mystic or the physicist. Esalen Institute Psychologist Lawrence Leshan gives an example of such an indistinguishable statement: "The absolute (is)....everything that exists....this absolute has become the universe.... (as we perceive it) by coming through time, space and causation. This is the central idea of (Minkowski) (Advaita).... Time, space and causation are like the glass through which the absolute is seen and when it is seen....it appears as the universe. Now we at once gather from this that in the universe there is neither time, space nor causation.... what we may call causation begins, after, if we may be permitted to say so, the degeneration of the absolute into the phenomenal and not before."

The remark was originally made by mystic Swami Vivekananda in *Jnana Yoga*, but the fact that the names of the mathematician who first theorized that space and time are a continuum, Hermann Minkowski, and the great philosopher of Advaita, are interchangeable, demonstrates once again the confluence of mysticism and the new physics.

Vivekananda further expresses a view that has become the backbone of quantum theory: There is no such thing as strict causality. As he states, "A stone falls and we ask why. This question is possible only on the supposition that nothing happens without a cause. I request you to make this very clear in your minds, for whenever we ask why anything happens, we are taking for granted that everything that happened must have a why, that is to say, it must have been preceded by something else which acted as the cause. This precedence in succession is what we call the law of causation."

He radiated divine power
– Robert P. Utter

There was indeed an air of divinity about him. Everyone who saw him felt it. No one near him could avoid feeling the force of his divine power almost like a shock-wave. Yet through all this extraordinary nimbus of vibrant power that seemed to envelop him in a cloud of fire, there hovered an infinite gentleness too, like the sleeping sea, like the sunlight, like moonlight on snowy peaks. He was a poised thunder-bolt forever humming an immortal song like a murmuring stream. He radiated this singing power as the sun shines. It made his abstract, intellectual teachings visible, almost palpable.

A well-known figure
– S. E. Waldo

At a critical juncture in his spiritual life he came under the influence of the great Indian saint Sri Ramakrishna Paramahamsa, whose influence over the young man was immediate and lasting. For the first time he had come in contact with a man to whom God was a living everpresent reality, and who possessed the ability to impart his wisdom to those who were really seeking truth. It must have been a wonderfully powerful character, a holiness and purity beyond all possibility of cavil that was able to impress the young agnostic at the very time in his life when a youth feels his own knowledge and importance to be far in advance of all others.

The high spirited, impetuous boy was no easy conquest, but the love and patience of the Master were boundless, and the force and beauty of his unselfish, utterly unworldly life were so great as to entirely vanquish all opportunities of the wilful disciple, and Sri Ramakrishna's victory was complete. The young man gave up his worldly ambitions, renounced the pleasures that so naturally attract youth, and consecrated himself, body and soul, to his Master's work. His place in the busy world knew him no more, his name was dropped and he became a sannyasin, a pure soul, for whom all earthly allurements were non-existent. Not for him were home and wife and children, not for him were name and wealth and professional success. All these were cast aside as of no value, and in their place he chose yellow robe, the staff and begging bowl of the Hindu monk. Little did he dream that name and fame would ever be his, that he would become far greater than if he had followed the ordinary course of life.

Swami Vivekananda was a well-known figure in England and America, as well as in his native India. He was a man who would shine in any environment, by virtue of his splendid presence, his brilliant conversational powers, his magnetic eloquence and above all by his unworldly simplicity and purity of character.

Under his clear eyes, shams and frauds were quickly unveiled, and for religious hypocrisy he hid nothing but contempt. He demanded truth and sincerity before all else, and became greatly discouraged in his search, by meeting on all sides with shallow pretence and outward show, in place of the earnest sincerity that he was seeking.

Ever enthusiastic in all he undertook, Vivekananda threw his whole heart into his chosen vocation. He travelled on foot all over India, walking barefooted thousands of miles, during many years, teaching and helping the people. In the snowy Himalayas, in the marshy plains of Bengal, amidst pestilence and famine, undergoing privation of every kind, he persevered in his loving ministry, bringing hope and comfort to thousands of disconsolate hearts.

....The Hindu monk was sent across the wide ocean to Vancouver and thence found his way to Chicago in May 1893.... He was alone in a strange land, but fortunately he had a perfect command of the language. He was a dreamy meditative Hindu, suddenly dropped into the whirl and distractions of the busiest city of the Western States of America. It was a trying moment for the young foreigner, then just thirty years of age, but a child in the ways of the world. He said to himself, "If I am really here on God's work, He will take care of me." He gave himself no more concern over a situation that would have seemed desperate to most men in like case. His trust was justified, for friends came forward, people who had never before known of him, but who were instantly attracted to the gifted stranger. He was taken into the family and cherished as a son, and to the end of his life he retained the affectionate regard of these early friends. To know Vivekananda was to like him and to know him well was to revere him.

The instant and overwhelming success of the young Hindu monk in the Parliament of Religions is too well-known. Thousands were thrilled by his eloquence and hung upon his word.

A series of lectures before the Brooklyn Ethical Association, brought him in contact with more earnest people, and early in 1895 his New York work began to take definite shape.

Among the many who came to hear him, some few were found who became his disciples. A dozen of these accompanied him to Thousand Island Park, where during seven weeks he gave them daily instructions, and above all they enjoyed the inestimable advantage of sharing his daily life and seeing the beauty and simplicity of his character.

Vivekananda's success in England was as immediate as it had been in America and he addressed large audiences, besides holding classes for more definite instruction. All his work, both in America and England was done gratuitously, the Swami accepting merely the means to provide for his support and refusing all remuneration for his services, save on the few occasions when he lectured on secular subjects. The Hindu feels that religion cannot be sold.

....He strove to make men understand that all the different religions of the world are but different paths to the one Supreme Being, are but different aspects of one Religion Eternal which is the property of no race or nation, which knows neither beginning nor end, but is the inevitable expression of man's sense of the Divine.

India's spiritual ambassador to the West
– Kenneth Walker

I owe so much gratitude to India and indirectly to India's spiritual Ambassador to the West, Swami Vivekananda. I have never met him but I have been grateful to him..

There is indeed a need for a broader outlook on religion and for a wider recognition of the fact that all the great World Faiths rest on the same, or on very similar, basic truths. All that really differs is the mode of expression of these truths. I am an enthusiastic advocate of a close collaboration between the great World Faiths. I do feel that the time has come for us all to think in terms of World Unity. The speed of modern travel and intercommunication has converted the world into a single whole. Yet we still continue to think of it in old terms of East and West, of Communism and Democracy, of Catholicism and Protestantism, of Moslem and Christian. Let us get rid of these old parish-pump outlooks and let us start to think of humanity as a single whole. Let religious people of all the different faiths set the world a good example by stressing the sameness rather than the differences between the various World Faiths.

It has of course to be admitted that materialism continues to increase in the West and that religion exerts less and less influence over our Western thinking. Many years ago Vivekananda wrote: "Materialism prevails in Europe today. The salvation of Europe depends on a rationalistic religion, and Advaita, the non-duality, the oneness, the idea of impersonal God is the only religion that can have any hold on intellectual people. It comes whenever religion seems to disappear and irreligion seems to prevail, and that is why it has taken ground in Europe and in America." Materialism has an even stronger hold on us now than at the time at which Vivekananda wrote these words, but I am not a pessimist on this subject. I look and hope for a change in outlook.

He spoke up and acted
– Sir John Woodroffe

The qualities I most admire in Vivekananda are his activity, manliness and courage. There are still Indians – though fortunately not so numerous as there were when I first came to India – who seem to be ashamed of and would apologise for Hindu life, Hindu art and philosophy and religion. Vivekananda was not of this sort. His was the attitude of a man. He spoke up and acted. For this, all must honour him, who, whatever be their own religious beliefs, value sincerity, truth and courage, which are the badges of every noble character.

A bright pearl of the Orient sea
– Dr. John C. Wyman

Brother Swami Vivekananda,
Bright pearl of the Orient sea,
Came here with his soul all illumined
By light, love, and liberty.

He came here with greetings fraternal
From the mystical East to our West;
And from those wise Vedas inspired
He taught us the purest and best.

He brought us a message most gracious
From the long past ages of time;
He came as the Priest and the Prophet,
Enthused with a faith all sublime.

Right soon to our hearts he found entrance,
So lovable, so gentle was he, –
And as teacher or friend was so winning,
None could other than love be.

He proclaimed ancient truths with wisdom,
And his eloquence quickly did win
Many earnest and faithful disciples,
Whom he taught of their God-powers within.

God bless our dear brother Swami,
May his path grow ever more bright;
And when his earthly journey is finished
He be clothed in God's garments of light.

He performed an extraordinary feat
– Prof. R. C. Zaehner

Vivekananda performed the extraordinary feat of breathing life into the purely static monism of Sankara. In Europe and America he proclaimed from the house-tops the absolute divinity of man and the sinfulness of the Christian preoccupation with sin. In this obsession with sin and its corollary, the helplessness of man and his absolute dependence on the grace of God, he, like Nietzsche, saw something debilitating and degrading. Man is by nature free (*mukta*), his liberation is permanently with him, and it is he, no other, who binds himself in illusion: he has within himself the power to cast off his chains, and it is only his attachment to his miserable, unreal ego that prevents him from doing so.

TRIBUTES FROM MONKS

A living example of Vedanta
– Swami Abhedananda

Swami Vivekananda is regarded as a patriot-saint of modern India. No country has ever produced such a many-sided character harmoniously combined in one form as we have seen in him. A great yogi, a spiritual teacher, a religious leader, a writer, an orator and, above all, the most disinterested worker for humanity – that was Swami Vivekananda.

I must tell you that I had the honour of living with this great Swami in India, in England, and in this country (America). I lived and travelled with this great spiritual brother of mine, saw him day after day and night after night and watched his character for nearly twenty years, and I stand here to assure you that I have not found another like him in these three continents, and that no one can take the place of this wonderful personage. As a man, his character was pure and spotless; as a philosopher, he was the greatest of all Eastern and Western philosophers. In him I found the ideal of karmayoga, bhaktiyoga, rajayoga and jnanayoga; he was like the living example of Vedanta in all its different branches.

Those who have met him and heard him speak, will remember his fascinating personality, his fine intelligent face beaming with celestial radiance mingled with the innocent smile of a child, his deep musical voice, his uncommon eloquence, and above all, his wonderful oratorical powers which drew from the hearts of his appreciative listeners the exclamation that he was an 'orator by divine right.'

I have met many people in this country (U. S. A.) who regard *Raja Yoga* in the same light as the most devout Christian regards his own Scriptures. It has been a revelation to many agnostic and sceptical minds; it has transformed the characters of many. Every passage of this wonderful book is charged, as it were, with the soul-stirring spiritual power generated by the gigantic battery of the pure soul of our great yogi. This wonderful book, which had been translated into several languages and published in three different countries, has commanded respect among the intelligent, educated classes and the sincere seekers of truth in the three continents – America, Europe and Asia.

After receiving the highest honours from three great nations, Swami Vivekananda's mind was neither elated with pride nor self-conceit; nor was his head turned for half a second from the blessed feet of his beloved, Master. With the same childlike simplicity, with the same humility of character, which he had possessed before he came to America, and keeping the same fire of renunciation alive in his soul he realized the transitoriness of all the triumphal honours which were showered upon him.

Did he belong to any caste? No, Swami Vivekananda had no caste; He had no earthly parents, but he was the child of Ramakrishna. He renounced everything, severed his family relations and was born again of his spiritual father. He never claimed for himself any caste distinction. It was his blessed Master who by the magic of his divine touch brought into play the latent greatness of his soul. Being the most worthy disciple of his Master, he followed the footsteps of Sri Ramakrishna, holding in his heart that he was low, lower even than a *pariah,* so far as caste distinction and social position were concerned. He lived an unmarried life as simple and pure as that of a child; always regarding women as the representatives of the Divine Mother; poverty, self-abnegation, self-renunciation and disinterested love for humanity were the ornaments of this exemplary character.

Man-making was his one great ideal for which he dedicated himself heart and soul. With a heart weeping at the sight of the suffering and degradation of the illiterate masses of India, with a soul glowing with the fire of disinterested love for humanity and true patriotism Swami Vivekananda solved the problems concerning the future of his Motherland by holding before the nation's eyes the ideal of character-building through the light and spirit of Vedanta.

His humility
– Swami Ambananda

It was on the 6th of February, 1897, that Swami Vivekananda, the world renowned Hindu monk, arrived at Madras after a sojourn in the West in fulfilment of his mission. On his arrival he was accorded a grand reception by the citizens of Madras.

Along with a friend of mine, I had gone to see the colourful procession in honour of the great Swami, starting from Egmore Railway Station and proceeding towards the Ice House (now popularly known as '*Vivekanandar Illam*' or Vivekananda's House) at Triplicane beach. We climbed up a roadside tree, to have a glance at the Swami seated in a horse carriage, along with Swamis Niranjanananda, Sivananda, Saradananda and Sri J. J. Goodwin – Swamiji's stenographer. The carriage was being drawn manually in the place of horses.

There was a unique charm in Swamiji's countenance. We were amazed to behold a halo of golden hue shining around Swami's divine face. This scene I could never forget in my life.

When the procession reached the destination viz. the Ice House, a huge public meeting was held there in a specially erected *pandal* in front of the House. I took a convenient position of leaning against a pole near the platform. On that occasion, when Swamiji wanted the audience to ask him questions regarding religious matters, a chemistry professor by name Laxmi Narasu put forth a question. Instead of answering, Swamiji asked him in turn, "Are you an agnostic?" Laxmi Narasu answered in the affirmative. Again when Swamiji asked him the same question in a different way, Laxmi Narasu answered in the negative. On hearing this the whole audience laughed loudly at the professor's folly. Thereafter none dared to ask any philosophical question to Swamiji.

The same day afternoon, Swamiji spoke in another public meeting held at the Victoria Hall. I attended that meeting also and a class talk in the next morning at the Ice House.

I also had the rare good fortune of talking a few words to Swamiji while he was walking along the Marina Beach, conversing with one Sri M. A. Parthasarathy Iyengar, M. A., M. L. On seeing Swamiji, at a distance, three of us walked briskly and approached him from behind. As we were talking aloud, Swamiji turned back and noticed us. We reverentially saluted him. He asked us: "Why are you following me, boys?" I said in reply: "Nothing particular, Swamiji." Then Swamiji said: "We have some important matter to discuss privately. That is why we two came this way. So I am sorry that it is not convenient for me to talk to you now. We shall meet and talk later on, if possible. Aren't you students? It is going dark. So go and study your lessons." We saluted Swamiji and returned to our hostel.

What impressed me most was Swamiji's humility and sense of equality. He never posed himself as a great person. He was very outspoken and hit hard on casteism and superiority complex in his speeches.

His potent influence
– Swami Ananyananda

From about middle of the last century and until almost today, it happened to be a formative period for the expression of our national spirit. The wheel was set in motion by Raja Ram Mohan Roy, and a series of successors followed him strengthening and spreading the movement until, at last, it became a nation-wide movement under the dynamic leadership of Mahatma Gandhi, in our own times.

In this process of awakening India and inspiring her people into a life of thought and action, the influence that Swami Vivekananda, that patriot-prophet of modern India exercised, was one of the most outstanding. He was, as Pandit Nehru beautifully characterizes, "one of the great founders – if you like, you may use any other word – of the national, modern movement of India and a great number of people who took more or less an active part in that movement at a later date drew their inspiration from Swami Vivekananda. Directly or indirectly, he has powerfully influenced the India of today." For the first time in that formative period, he raised his powerful voice 'in defence of India and her people.' His resounding success of the great Parliament of Religions, held in Chicago, in 1893, where he expounded the lofty universal principles of Hinduism as the sole representative of the oldest of living religions, brought India, her people and her thought more prominently before the world than ever before.

India re-discovered herself once again; a certain pride in her own inheritance was instilled in her heart thence forward. That event also marked the beginning of India's influence on Western nations. Since then the process has gone on paving the way for a respectful understanding of the all-comprehensive spiritual and cultural ideas and ideals for which India stands.

Now India is her own master and can shape her affairs without any outside influence or interference, according to her own tradition and genius. For the future of India, Swamiji has given to the nation enough work for centuries to come, as he himself says: "I have done enough for fifteen

hundred years." It is for us, his countrymen, to take up the scheme and
work on for the future glory of India, which, he believed would be far greater
and more glorious than her past.

He promulgated a grand message
– Swami Bhashyananda

Swami Vivekananda was born with a mission. He was not an ordinary
saint who inspires a few people belonging to one part of the country and
who attains his own salvation through spiritual discipline. Sri Ramakrishna
saw him to be one of the universal sages born for the good of the whole
world. Sri Ramakrishna is revered as an incarnation born to fulfil a cosmic
necessity. To free religion of the crust of superstition, Swami Vivekananda
was interpreter of such a religion and gave his interpretation to the whole
world.

As St. Paul was to Christ, Ananda was to Buddha, Swami Vivekananda
was to Sri Ramakrishna. Sri Ramakrishna was a prophet too spiritual to face
the rough and tumble of life. He required therefore a sturdy instrument to
propagate his message to the whole world. Swami Vivekananda gave that
message in 1893 in the World's Parliament of Religions at Chicago where
had gathered the flower of thinking human beings. The nineteenth century
is characterized by a profound change in human thinking. Naturally the
very important department of human activity called religion was also equally
affected. A great reaction against religion was created by science and
technology. The pre-scientific age was the age of faith. God was considered
an extra-cosmic reality. Religion consisted of dogmas and creeds laid down
in the scriptures. There was no place for reason except within the framework
of revelations. Salvation was only for the believers. People were satisfied
for 1,500 years with creeds and dogmas. The advent of science changed
the total picture. The test of reality was not faith but experience tested on
the touchstone of reason. There was no private truth. Truth was a common
heritage of all human beings irrespective of creed, caste and religion. The
city of God was replaced by the city of man. There was more emphasis on
suffering than on sin. Religion was changed into human values rather than
ethereal religious experience.

Swami Vivekananda's message to the world was based on comprehensive
Vedantic ideas such as divinity of the soul, unity of experience. Man was
not a bundle of flesh or a cog in a machine. He was a descendant of the
immortal principle. That was his true nature. This grand message was
realized by Swami Vivekananda through the grace of his teacher Sri
Ramakrishna and he promulgated this message to the whole world. He put
these thoughts succinctly in the following words:

> "Each soul is potentially divine. The goal is to manifest this divinity
> within by controlling nature: external and internal. Do this either

by work, or worship, or psychic control, or philosophy – by one, or more, or all of these – and be free. This is the whole of religion. Doctrines, or dogmas, or rituals, or books, or temples, or forms, are but secondary details."

He ushered in a new dawn
– Swami Chidananda Saraswati

Swami Vivekananda came upon the scene of our country's social life, like the great sun rising out of the horizon. For, through his advent in our *rashtra* he brought *jagriti* (awakening) in our *samskriti-devata* and ushered in therefore a *suprabhata,* a new dawn. But then the dawn is the beginning of the day, the day has to proceed and progress and move towards the meridian splendour of mid-day, when the whole world is illumined with the blazing light of the meridian sun.

We, of this fourth quarter of the twentieth century, are almost two generations apart from the one who brought in the *suprabhata* of *Bharatavarsha's punarutthana* and two generations have worked, but they have worked under very very adverse circumstances. The time was not ripe and circumstances not favourable. *Bharatavarsha* was still under subjugation and it did not have the freedom to evolve in the way in which its national urge wished it to evolve. And it is only a quarter of a century ago that our land came into its own. It has now become *swatantra.* Now doors are opened, circumstances have become favourable, the right time has come to work out with full vigour the ideas of this great prophetic patriot of India. And this task, more than on any other generation after his time, devolves upon this present generation, both the elder section and the younger section. I recommend each and every young man to read Swami Vivekananda's *Lectures From Colombo to Almora.* That contains the quintessence of his message to India, most thrilling, most direct and ever relevant. The message that he has given and the awakening which he has inspired is still in the stage of dawn only.

India's inspiration is needed by the whole world today. India can effectively give this great guidance, this light, this inner spiritual nourishment to the starved world, only if it is lived here, if it is revitalized here, if it is made into a living force by the people of India. Then alone can India be a path-shower, *margadarshak,* as well as *loka-uddharaka.* If it is said that this Motherland will be *loka-uddharaka,* it will not be a mis-statement. Therefore, the message of Swami Vivekananda is the most relevant today for *Bharatiya samaj* to accept into its life-strearn, the great and immortal message of the sages and seers of the Upanishadic era.

Two great things Vivekananda has called India to. The first is the recognition or an experiencing of the divinity which you are first and foremost. You are divine and therefore you must be established in divine consciousness. That is your foremost and highest duty. Vivekananda said,

"The central core of religion is worship of God here and now, not of a remote Brahman elsewhere." But religion means realization of presence of Brahman here and now, and a worship of that Brahman through a life of unceasing love, devotion and dedicated service. He said, the greatest worship is the service of living God, the *'sajeeva Bhagavan'* who is enshrined in *manava, Janardhana* who is visible in *janata.* That is the great message of Swami Vivekananda.

A great messenger
– Swami Chidbhavananda

It is the message that makes the messenger what he is. When the messenger happens to be the embodiment of the message that he brings, then his impact on society is irresistible. Such is the personality of Swami Vivekananda.

In this age, when India was immersed in ignorance and sluggishness, Swami Vivekananda has come as a great messenger by the grace of Providence as a dynamic force to awaken the people to their normal state of spiritual greatness.

'Arise, awake, stop not till the goal is reached' is the message that Swami Vivekananda has brought to the erstwhile slumbering India. The country was in dire need of such a forceful personality and Swami Vivekananda has come to fill in that need. His further exhortation to the country is 'They alone live who live for the welfare of mankind, the others are more dead than alive.'

Renunciation and service are the watchwords of his message to his countrymen and women. There was nothing negative in his advice to renounce. There is no place for escape-mentality and quietism in his message. The awakened man ought to renounce everything pertaining to selfishness and embrace an active life for the welfare of society. The more he renounces selfishness the better equipped he becomes for public good. In whatever field the man of selflessness serves the society, there is sacredness and usefulness in his service.

Today, India is in need of a large number of men and women imbued with this great ideal of Swamiji. There is no religion superior to serving man recognizing the divinity enshrined in him.

An international figure
– Swami Durgananda

India is a land of spirituality. The spiritual background has helped her to outlive the civilizations of ancient Greece and Rome.

During the second half of the nineteenth century India rose from her deep slumber under foreign rule, and manifested her real strength. Great leaders arose in the land, in all walks of life. Foremost among them was the saint of Dakshineswar who lived on the banks of the Ganges, near Calcutta.

He was Sri Ramakrishna – the God-realised and God-intoxicated saint, and the spiritual father of Swami Vivekananda. The spiritual genius of Sri Ramakrishna blossomed forth through his great disciple. Swami Vivekananda soon became an international figure in the field of spirituality. He presented himself at the great Parliament of Religions held in America as the representative of Hindu religion from India. He distinguished himself there above all others and established himself, that time onwards, as a great saint-in-action, upholding the tenets of *Sanatana Dharma.* Travelling all over the civilized Western world he delivered the spiritual message of India. By his inspiring oratory backed by the magnificent personality he awakened, in the minds of those he met, the Divine consciousness. He exhorted them to arise and awake and not to stop till the goal of total freedom from the fetters of materialism was reached, and to work for their spiritual emancipation as well as for the emancipation of their fellow-men from material thraldom. He reminded his countrymen that spirituality was India's real strength and devoid of spirituality, India would dwindle away into insignificance.

A dominant feature of Swami Vivekananda's life was his deep love for mankind. He wept bitterly at the appalling poverty and misery of the Indian masses and appealed to his Western admirers and friends to help alleviate this poverty and misery. He asked them to impart to India the secular knowledge of the West in the fields of science and technology and take back in return India's knowledge in the realm of spirituality. To that end he founded the Ramakrishna Mission with its headquarters at Belur, near Calcutta.

His life was one of intense activity and total self-dedication. He completely merged his humble personality in that of Sri Ramakrishna, his Great Master, and through absolute self-surrender to the guru he attained the highest Divine Wisdom and Bliss. This made his speeches and writing vibrant with immense power. They have indeed become as sacred as the scriptures themselves, with an abiding message for humanity. His works have been fortunately made available to us in nine volumes, thanks to the devoted services of his Western disciple and stenographer Goodwin.

Thus in his short but eventful life Swami Vivekananda has bequeathed a lofty spiritual legacy to posterity. "I have given humanity", declared he, "enough for the next fifteen hundred years." Further, he also said, "May I be born again and again, and suffer thousands of miseries, so that I may worship the only God that exists, the only God I believe in, the sum total of all souls."

A dynamic personality
– Swami Ghanananda

In the whole range of religious biography, we hardly come across a personality more dynamic and more virile and forceful than Swami

Vivekananda. He was born on January 12, 1863, and attained *mahasamadhi* (final illumination) on July 4, 1902. In this short life of thirty-nine years, five months and three weeks, he achieved what had not been given to other Indians to achieve for a thousand years after Shankaracharya, and what other Indians after him – with the exception of Mahatma Gandhi – were not privileged to accomplish for the last sixty years. He was the first Hindu monk after the Buddhist missionaries of old to cross the distant seas and spread the unifying gospel of Vedanta in far-off lands.

Three factors contributed to the growth and development of Swami Vivekananda's personality. These were his early education, his spiritual training under Sri Ramakrishna, and his love and knowledge of India and her people.

Vivekananda has been acclaimed as a "paragon of Vedanta", "an apostle of New Dispensation", "a patriot-monk", and "an orator by divine right", and known also by other epithets. He was all these and much more.

What did he teach and preach? To use his own words, he poured the old wine in new bottles: he preached the ancient wisdom of India in a new manner, charged with rare power which came from his own intense spiritual realizations.

Vivekananda fused the varied spiritual disciplines of Hinduism, its different schools of philosophy, its logic, its psychology, its ethics, its metaphysics, and its mysticism into one whole in the fire of his genius and presented it at the Parliament of Religions held in Chicago in 1893. He knew that it would not do to give coats of the same dimensions to Tom, Dick and Harry; he therefore taught jnanayoga for the intellectual and philosophical type of man; bhaktiyoga for the devotee, and karmayoga for those wanting to practise spiritual discipline through right activity. He also taught and preached rajayoga, expounding the science and psychology of religions. He put the whole of religion in practice in these few words: "Each soul is potentially divine. The goal is to manifest this divine within, by controlling nature, external and internal. Do this either by work, or worship, or psychic control, or philosophy, by one or more, or all of these, and be free. This is the whole of religion – doctrines, or dogmas, or rituals, or books, or temples or forms, are but secondary details."

He pointed out that study of philosophy would be quite inadequate without character-building and spiritual practice, for these alone would give the votaries experience of God or self-realization.

Swami Vivekananda taught that when we look upon a suffering man as a manifestation of the Divine, as a being in whom there is the same soul as in us, our service to him becomes transformed into worship. All service goes to the Divine in man, and it is, therefore, a blessing when we are afforded an opportunity to serve the sufferers by removing their needs, physical, mental, moral, or spiritual.

With a view to translating into practice this ideal of service, the Swamiji founded the Ramakrishna Mission, which has numerous branches in India today (and many outside, all working out his programme of all-round service to the needy). The practice of this ideal results not only in objective utility but also in subjective purification, as service to the Divine in man purifies and uplifts the man who serves and also creates a favourable atmosphere for the ennobling and edification of the man who is served.

Swamiji's mission was both national and international. He made no distinction of race, nation, creed, colour, caste or sex. The whole world was his home.

He was a world mover, "What is India or England or America to us? We are the servants of that God who by the ignorant is called man."

It is a surprise that he expressed his wish in the following words: "When will that blessed day dawn when my life will be a sacrifice at the altar of humanity?"

Time has proved the truth of the words he uttered before his death: "It may be that I shall find it good to get outside my body – to cast it off like a worn-out garment. But I shall not cease to work! I shall inspire men everywhere until the world shall know that it is one with God!"

He exerted himself to rouse the nation
– Swami Hiranmayananda

Swami Vivekananda was born in 1863 in an aristocratic family of Calcutta. From his boyhood days, he developed a strong interest in religion. But English Education, which he received in the school and college, gradually shook the foundation of his innate religious faith. A student of Bentham, Mill and Spencer, he found it difficult to reconcile his empirical and rationalist approach with the dogmatic views of religion. He gradually turned agnostic, even atheistic. It was at this period of his life that Swami Vivekananda came in contact with Sri Ramakrishna, and found in him a person who could say boldly that he had seen God. This infused new hope into his mind. From now on, he remained under the training of Sri Ramakrishna till the latter's passing away in 1886. But the surrender to the Master did not come without a severe fight. At every step there were questionings and a demand for proof. In the end the darkness of doubt and unbelief melted away before the illumination of self-realization, and acceptance was complete and unreserved.

Swami Vivekananda could now understand the full implication of his master's life. It was nothing short of the spiritual regeneration of the whole world. Through Buddha, Asia heard the Aryan truths and added a glorious chapter to her life-history. Through Sri Ramakrishna, the world was now to hear the eternal truths of Hinduism, the glory of the Atman and the oneness of existence. This great task demanded the energy of a whole nation. Swami Vivekananda, therefore, exerted himself to rouse the nation to the full height of its manhood. For about six years he wandered about the country

acquainting himself with the condition of the people. Everywhere he met
with squalor, poverty, injustice and callousness. But behind this pervading
gloom he found that the soul of India was young and throbbing with life.
He began to think about the ways and means of reawakening this sleeping
leviathan, and sitting on the last stone of India at Cape Comorin, he hit
upon a plan.

The spell of hypnosis under which India lay unconscious had come
from the West. And the exorcism of this bewitching influence must also
come from that direction. Nothing would be acceptable to India, dazed by
the glamour of the West, unless and until the West admitted its excellence.
So Swami Vivekananda decided to go to America, where a Parliament of
Religions was being held at Chicago, in 1893.

Here, before an august assembly of chosen delegates of different
religions of the world, he spoke as a representative of Hinduism. But his
utterance had a universal appeal. He spoke not on any particular aspect or
sectarian dogma of Hinduism, but on its basic tenets as exemplified in the
life of his master. But not even once did he refer to the personality of Sri
Ramakrishna in his lectures. To him the principles counted more than the
personality, and it was through the principles that the personality would
receive the due recognition and homage in time. His clear and convincing
exposition, combined with his breadth of vision and depth of feeling, found
a ready response not only in the hearts of his audience at the Parliament
but also in those of the wider public of America. It was a sort of cultural
and spiritual conquest of the West by India.

Both in the international and national sphere this event had a
momentous influence. In Swami Vivekananda's message the materialistic
West could find the necessary corrective that was so much needed for
saving it from its mad rush for power and sense-enjoyment. Morever, his
life became the confluence where the Eastern and Western ideals and ideas
could meet, resulting in a vast and universal synthesis that would give
birth to a new moral order for humanity.

In the national sphere, the success of Swami Vivekananda at Chicago
awakened the self-respect of the people and a faith in their own heritage. It
also threw open the floodgate of India's latent dynamism so long kept confined within the four corners of her boundary. A new and glorious chapter
of her history began.

For more than three years Swami Vivekananda carried on his preaching
work in the West, returning to India in 1897. In the meantime, India had
undergone a revolutionary change. Gone was the vegetative insouciance
of the people. There was enthusiasm, and earnestness everywhere. And
all this was due to the re-awakened self-consciousness which the
marvellous achievements of Swami Vivekananda at Chicago had brought
about. After his return from the West, he went about preaching and
teaching from Colombo to Almora. Everywere he was given unprecedented

ovation. The whole nation seemed to rise as one man to honour him, and greet him.

But Swami Vivekananda was not satisified with this outburst of enthusiasm only. He wanted to harness this manifestation of energy and put it on a permanent basis. With this end in view he founded two institutions which would give a practical shape to his and his master's teachings. These institutions are the two wings of the Ramakrishna Movement, and are named the Ramakrishna Math and the Ramakrishna Mission. After having the satisfaction of seeing these institutions in good working order, Swami Vivekananda passed away in 1902.

A world citizen
– Swami Lokeswarananda

In all he said and did, Swami Vivekananda's chief concern was man. He described man as 'the only God I believe in.' 'Man-making is my mission,' he used to say. Man, according to him, has immense possibilities, there being almost no limit to his growth. The task before man is to grow, to keep growing despite constraints. Vivekananda, therefore, preached a philosophy which envisaged that men and women all over the world would keep growing till they reached a state in which they had become completely transformed into gods and goddesses.

What was needed was the right kind of environment, education, and encouragement so that the growth of the individual might go on unhindered. While an ideal state would deem it its obligation to ensure such conditions, religion would accept responsibility to motivate the individual to go on striving till he reached the limit of his growth. Swami Vivekananda thought that religion imparted that quality to man which sustained him all through his trials and tribulations. He called that quality self-confidence. Strength, courage, and self-confidence – these, according to him, are the essence of religion, all other things are peripheral.

By religion Swami Vivekananda never meant any creed or dogma; he meant faith in one's infinite capacity to grow. Anything that weakened an individual's faith in himself or hampered his growth was, according to him, the antithesis of religion. By growth he meant multi-dimensional growth, growth not only materially but also morally and spiritually.

Man's progress, in his view, must include moral and spiritual growth – more and more 'selflessness.' According to him, to be selfish is a sin. The ideal man is 'an infinite circle whose circumference is nowhere but whose centre is everywhere.' He is a free man, uncluttered by race, religion, language, country, society, and family. He belongs everywhere, every home is his home, every man and woman are his brother and sister. This is the ideal before man. Peace will come to earth when men and women vigorously pursue this ideal.

'Each soul is potentially divine', he used to say. That is to say, man is not just man, but also God, God only potentially now but with every chance that this potentiality shall some day be transformed into reality. The goal is to grow, to go on growing, till the divinity that is in man becomes manifest.

But philosophy did not blind Swami Vivekananda to human misery. He found working people everywhere exploited. To end this, he felt the basis of human relationship must be changed to one which recognized that man was essentially divine. The ideal society, according to him, was one with 'Vedanta brain and Islam body', i.e., a classless and casteless society with the philosophy of the highest possible collective and individual growth. Lest the goal be lost sight of, he preached it from every possible forum till it became his world mission. The only God he cared for was man, no matter under what cloak he was found. He was a true humanist, a true world citizen.

He had the practical sense to realize that it would be a vain talk to preach religion and morality to people who starved, people who were neglected, oppressed, and were victims of social injustice. He was a champion of freedom, justice, and eqality everywhere; he welcomed science and technology, because he recognized their potentiality to promote material growth. But he rejected the view that material prosperity was an end in itself. His message was that this should be matched by religion, for religion alone can give man the moral and spiritual tilt which he now lacks and which alone makes him a complete man.

He was an epitome of all that was great and good

– Swami Madhavananda

In his youth, sitting at Dakshineswar, at the feet of his Great Master, Sri Ramakrishna who was the fulfilment of the aspirations of humanity of all ages and climes, he had imbibed the spirit of universality through the realization of the Divine in man. So, though he was born in India, he belonged to the whole world, and India had no exclusive claims on him, His mission in the East and the West was to rouse men and women to an awareness of their divine nature and the unity of man, which alone can bring peace to this world torn with hatred and strife.

And this marvellous union of Sri Ramakrishna and Swami Vivekananda has ushered into the world a flood of spirituality which was never before witnessed on earth. We shall not discuss how much the disciple got from his Master, and what was his own contribution to it, for an ideal disciple is the exact mirror of his guru, he has to assimilate the Master's teachings and make himself the selfless instrument whereby the guru's message is carried from corner to corner of the globe. For practical purposes, it will be best to treat Sri Ramakrishna and Swami Vivekananda as a composite personality, as two facets of the same thing, the two together making the circuit of galvanic spirituality complete.

As in the case of Sri Ramakrishna, so in Swamiji's case also, the realization of Advaita – the One without a second – was the central pivot on which all the other aspects of his personality were balanced. Through the guru's blessings Swami Vivekananda got this highest realization in the very prime of youth, and succeeded in perfectly assimilating it before he attained the age of thirty. As he himself playfully expressed it to one of his brother disciples, "I have finished all that there was to be achieved within twenty-nine years." As soon as he was ripe to deliver his message of uplift to the world, there was field ready for him in the Parliament of Religions held in Chicago in 1893. To move the world a good fulcrum is needed, and the Chicago Parliament served as that point to the Swami.

The Chicago Parliament is one of the turning points of history. It was convened for the glorification of Christianity, but by an irony of Fate the scales were turned, and instead of bringing Christianity to the forefront, it proved a triumph for a pagan religion – Vedanta, and the representative of this religion was no other than Swami Vivekananda. He had made his mark. The doors of the civilised world were thrown open to him. America and Europe listened with admiration to the words of this young scion of the ancient *rishis* of India. Having sown the seeds of world-federation in the West, the Swami came back to the land of his birth and set himself to give out his experiences to his countrymen.

He boldly voiced forth the teachings of the Vedanta, clothing the wonderful truths of unity-in-variety with a forceful and intelligible language, so that the modern man and woman might grasp them with ease.

Swami Vivekananda was an epitome of all that was great and good in the India of the past, and all that is also potentially great and good in her. With Sankara's intellect he combined Buddha's heart, Christ's renunciation, and the Prophet of Arabia's spirit of equality, and the result of this holy confluence will in time flood the whole world. Though he was the most accomplished of men, none possessed greater humility or genuine devotion to the guru than Swamiji, and his lion-heart throbbed with surging emotions whenever Sri Ramakrishna's sacred name was mentioned in his presence. Had Sri Ramakrishna not been born into the world, the world would have worshipped Swami Vivekananda himself with divine honours, so great was Swamiji and of so multi-sided a personality. But he believed from the bottom of his heart, that he owed everything to the divine touch of that wonderful man. To quote his own words: "And if there has ever been a word of truth, a word of spirituality, that I have spoken anywhere in the world, I owe it to my Master, only the mistakes are mine." His love for his brother-disciples also was unique, and was the admiration of the sadhus of Hrishikesh and other places, who could not understand how a paramahamsa of his type could be so full of the spirit of loving service to his gurubhais. But Swamiji was born to beat all record. Well might Sri Ramakrishna say, "There has never been a personality like Noren's, nor will there ever be." Only a jeweller knows the merit of jewels, the laymen will only display their ignorance by trying to value them.

Swamiji himself declared, he wanted to be "a voice without a form," the unattached spokesman of the message of his beloved gurudeva. And if we look into the present literary activities of India and abroad, into what is being given out from the Press and the Platform, do we not find everywhere an echo of the harmony and freedom, of brotherliness and love for which the Swamiji stood pledged and which he so eloquently proclaimed before all the world? Some acknowledge the indebtedness, others may not, but the careful reader never fails to understand where the wind is blowing from. And the spirit of Swamiji must be glad at the phenomenon, for what did he care for personal name and fame so long as his Master's teachings were appreciated all over?

As to his power of eloquence who shall describe it? As one of his brother-disciples put it, "His words seemed to bring the dead back to life!" – So fiery and enthusiastic they were! For he threw his whole soul into the conversation or lecture. He used to carry his audience to the ethereal heights of Advaitic Oneness, where there is neither aught nor naught, where the least breath of duality is an intrusion. Truly has it been remarked by another fellow-disciple of his, "His words are not mere letters, but spirit itself!" Every sincere reader will testify to the truth of this statement from his own experience.

In his comprehensive message, science and religion, reason and faith, the secular and the sacred, the modern and the ancient and the East and the West became unified and he himself was the personification of that union. His life and message have given the necessary impetus for the ushering in of a new era in the history of the civilization of man.

His message of strength, faith, energy, and solidarity is specially needed today in our present crisis.

May the spirit of the great Swami, who awakened India and united the East and West, inspire us all to live and work to this end in the light of the life-giving motto – *'Atmano mokshartham jagaddhitaya cha'* – 'For one's own liberation and welfare of the world.'

The hero of my life
– Swami Madhurananda

While I was studying in the school, I happened to read the comprehensive biography of Swami Vivekananda written by his Eastern and Western disciples. My young mind was completely overwhelmed by the unique personality of Swamiji. His majestic appearance in the Chicago pose, his charming eyes, his versatile genius, and his simple but very forceful language, his burning patriotism breathed out in his *'Lectures From Colombo to Almora '*, his melting heart for the poor and the downtrodden masses, his spirit of selfless service completely won me over and transformed my life. I read no other book with so much zeal and zest as the unique life of Swamiji which appealed to my young mind as an epic, as an engaging novel. I read it through and through and took down long notes of important portions. Swamiji thus became the hero of my life.

'Vivekananda' is a subject which can never be exhausted. And the more the life and teachings of the great Swami are propagated, the more will the world be benefitted both spiritually and materially. His life and words are a tremendous living force, edifying the world slowly and steadily. As Swamiji himself had prophesied, that force will continue to work for centuries to come. In the hearts of men living in the modern world that is being threatened with a nuclear holocaust, the roaring message of this 'Vedanta Kesari' (the lion of Vedanta), will instill absolute fearlessness and perfect calm. Hail Swamiji, the Veereswara Siva! Hail the chroniclers of his life and words! Hail those who follow him devotedly.

One of the greatest prophets
– Swami Mukhyananda

Swami Vivekananda is one of the greatest prophets the world has produced.

The modern world has had some great personalities and prophets, but none represents the spirit of the age so truly and comprehensively and answers to the all-round aspirations of mankind at all levels as does the great Universal Spiritual Power which manifested through the triune personality of Ramakrishna-Sarada Devi-Vivekananda whose composite message to the world was voiced by Swami Vivekananda during the last decade of his life.

All the previous prophets mostly gave their own individual message, and the scope of their message and the field of their activities were limited as per the conditions of the time and their personal equipment. The previous prophets and their immediate disciples were all men, and hence the message was mostly male-oriented. The message of Vivekananda, in contrast, was a combined and composite one issuing from the great lives and divine realisation of his seraphic Master Sri Ramakrishna, the prophet of Religious Harmony, and his Master's illustrious spiritual consort, co-partner, and disciple, the Holy Mother Sarada Devi, both of whom shaped his life and thought, and it was reinforced by his own great intellectual attainments and spiritual illumination. All the three of them had several eminent men and women disciples (some of Vivekananda's brilliant men and women disciples were from the West) who worked to further the composite message along with them. For the first time in history we find both the halves of mankind equally engaging the attention of a prophetic message. Vivekananda was the mouthpiece of this composite message and the message was addressed to both the East and the West, on the spiritual and secular levels, and was launched on a global scale.

And moreover, though Vivekananda had the sublime lives of Sri Ramakrishna and Holy Mother Sarada Devi in the background, he did not place their personalities before the world, nor did he project his own personality or thoughts, nor any particular religion based on personalities, but interpreted the universal, impersonal Truths discovered by the *rishis* (seers) of India and other sages of the world which are rational, scientific, and open to investigation and realization by all. They were illustrated in the lives of his Master and Holy Mother and confirmed by his own realizations and by those of other sages in the past. These realizations and experiences and his studies had revealed to him the profound and sublime Truths lying hidden in the Upanishads, the *Gita*, and other great works, which are the products of the religio-philosophic investigations and realizations of a whole people, a whole culture, and not of any single individual. They had been openly debated, reasoned out thoroughly, formulated in the Vedanta philosophy, and tested and attested by great savants and sages over a long period.

'India is a world in miniature', and if these life-giving Truths tested in its cultural crucible are broadcast to the wide world, Vivekananda felt, they will compose the distractions of mankind and lift it up from the soulless morass of materialism and frustration to an illumined new life of hope and divinity. Theologies are galore in the world but they have ceased to inspire mankind, especially because of the violent records of the extrovert religionists. Man has advanced greatly in knowledge and science and the formalistic theological religions do not attract him. The accounts of miracles do not overwhelm his mind, for, before the natural wonders science had worked and has been working, which are universal and openly and repeatedly applicable, they pale into insignificance. What the modern man wants are solid realizable facts, universal in their import and application and open to rational understanding and investigation. And it is here that the Upanishads are unique in their presentations of the *Atma-vidya,* the science of the Divine Self within, the One Supreme Divinity manifesting in each one as his Self. Hence Vivekananda's message was primarily the message of India, of the Divine Self within all and its infinite possibilities, and of the Oneness of Existence, Unity of all Life and Solidarity of Humanity.

Vivekananda had made a deep and comparative study of world history, modern Western science, and the thought and culture of different countries of the East and the West in general and of India in particular. He had intimate experience of India during his extensive wanderings all over the country, mixing with the masses and the classes, the poor and the rich, the ignorant and the learned, and the peasants and the kings, because of which he possessed a keen and intelligent understanding of the various world forces that operated and the needs of mankind in the East and the West. He had also acquired a deep insight into the significance of the Hindu scriptures and Indian spiritual and philosophical thought in the light of his great Master's life and realizations.

Moreover, besides his giant intellect and the towering catholic spirituality, Vivekananda had an intensely feeling heart which loved mankind.

And this moved him to sacrifice his all for the removal of the sufferings of humanity and its spiritual upliftment.

An unusual phenomenon
– Swami Nikhilananda

Swami Vivekananda is a many-sided genius. An unusual phenomenon of all times, he was a philosopher, a man of action, an introspective yogi. and also a writer, a dynamic speaker, a brilliant conversationalist and a dreamer. But in his inmost heart he was a lover of God. This love, not sentimentalism in any form, was manifest in his love of men. This love captivated the hearts of all who came into contact with him, either in the East or West.

Swami Vivekananda's inspiring personality was well-known both in India and in America during the last decade of the nineteenth century and the first decade of the twentieth. The unknown monk of India suddenly leapt into fame at the Parliament of Religions held in Chicago in 1893, at which he represented Hinduism. His vast knowledge of Eastern and Western culture as well as his deep spiritual insight, fervid eloquence, brilliant conversation, broad human sympathy, colourful personality and handsome figure made an irresistible appeal to the many types of Americans who came into contact with him. People who saw or heard Vivekananda even once still cherish his memory after a lapse of more than half a century.

In America, Vivekananda's mission was the interpretation of India's spiritual culture, especially in its Vedantic setting. He also tried to enrich the religious consciousness of the American through the rational and humanistic teachings of the Vedanta philosophy. In America he became India's spiritual ambassador and pleaded eloquently for better understanding between India and the New World in order to create a healthy synthesis of East and West, of religion and science.... His message of the divinity of the human soul, the unity of existence, harmony of religions has found an abiding place in the thought of America....

In his own motherland Vivekananda is regarded as the patriot-saint of modern India and an awakener of her dormant national consciousness. To the Hindus he preached the ideal of a strength-giving and man-making religion. Service to man as the visible manifestation of the Godhead was the special form of worship he advocated for the Indians, devoted as they were to the rituals and myths of their ancient faith. Many political leaders of India have publicly acknowledged their indebtedness to Swami Vivekananda.

The Swami's mission was both national and international. A lover of mankind, he strove to promote peace and human brotherhood on the spiritual foundation of the Vedantic Oneness of existence. A mystic of the highest order, Vivekananda had a direct and intuitive experience of Reality. He derived his ideas from that unfailing source of wisdom and often presented them in the soul-stirring language of poetry.

The natural tendency of Vivekananda's mind, like that of his Master, Ramakrishna, was to soar above the world and forget itself in contemplation of the Absolute. But another part of his personality bled at the sight of human suffering in East and West alike. It might appear that his mind seldom found a point of rest in its oscillation between contemplation of God and service to man. Be that as it may, he chose, in obedience to a higher call, service to man as his mission on earth; and this choice has endeared him to people in the West, Americans in particular.

In the course of a short life of thirty-nine years (1863-1902), of which only ten were devoted to public activities – and those, too, in the midst of acute physical suffering – he left for posterity his four classics: *Jnana Yoga, Bhakti Yoga, Karma Yoga,* and *Raja Yoga,* all of which are outstanding treatises of Hindu philosophy. In addition, he delivered innumerable lectures, wrote inspired letters in his own hand to his many friends and disciples, composed numerous poems, and acted as spiritual guide to many seekers who came to him for instruction. He also organized the Ramakrishna Order of monks, which is the most outstanding religious organization of modern India. It is devoted to the propagation of Hindu spiritual culture not only in the Swami's native land, but also in America and in other parts of the world.

Swami Vivekananda once spoke of himself as a "Condensed India." His life and teachings are of inestimable value to the West for an understanding of the mind of Asia. William James, the Harvard philosopher, called the Swami the "paragon of Vedantists." Max Muller and Paul Deussen, the famous Orientalists of the nineteenth century, held him in genuine respect and affection. "His words", writes Romain Rolland, "are great music, phrases in the style of Beethoven, stirring rythms like the march of Handel Choruses. I cannot touch these sayings of his, scattered as they are through the pages of books, at thirty years distance, without receiving a thrill through my body like an electric shock and what shocks, what transports, must have been produced when in burning words they issued from the lips of the hero!"

Vivekananda's message is not merely for the hour, but for the modern age; not for a particular nation, but for humanity. Even his message for India does not aim at partial social or religious reform, but at complete rejuvenation of her national life. The reader will be stirred, whether or not he agrees with the Swami; for every word he spoke is charged with power. And what he accomplished in short span of his thirty-nine years will nourish humanity for centuries.

Contemplating the malady of our times one wistfully asks, in the words of the bard of Avon, "When comes such another."

He enlightened the West

– Swami Nirmalananda (Tulasi Maharaj)

In these days when patriotic workers for the welfare of India are required in enormous numbers, there is no greater soul than Swami Vivekananda whose life can be set up as an ideal for honest workers. He was the first sannyasin to break the barriers of the inveterate exclusiveness of the Hindus, to cross the seas and to hold aloft to the outside world the torchlight of the teachings of the Vedanta philosophy, and it was he who raised in a great measure the status of India and its civilization in the eyes of the Westerners. Anyone who has even a superficial idea of his life and work can realize how ardent a patriot the Swami was and how every throb of his heart was for the uplifting of the masses.

He spoke about Hinduism at the World's Parliament of Religions held in America. Before he went there, the Americans had many false notions regarding Indians. They believed that Hindus were an uncivilized people, superstitious, half-naked and little removed from beasts. Swamiji's lectures removed those notions and awakened in them an interest in Hindu Religion. Several eminent persons began to accept Hindu ideas.

The versatility of the Hindu religion was just the reason why the message of Sri Ramakrishna as preached by his devoted disciple, Swami Vivekananda, found such ready favour and instantaneous effect in the highly advanced and intellectual minds of America and Europe, in whose eyes the teachings of modern Christian Missionaries were but exploded theories in the test of scientific analysis and investigation. Swami Vivekananda used to say that the religion in Europe was like a particular kind of coat cut according to one measurement which every man must wear whether it would fit him or not. But the Hindu religion is so vast that it can take any person with any turn of mind into its fold. It is for this reason only, that Hinduism has stood the test of centuries, and it will do so without doubt to the very end of time.

In him Divinity is made manifest

– Swami Parahitananda

The Swami exhorted man to strive for the emancipation of the soul, and for the good of the world. In religious terms the motto of the Order he founded, and equally, he would hold, the proper motto of every serious-minded man and woman, is, "For the realization of God, and for the good of the world." These two maxims find their almost exact parellels in Christ's two great commandments, to love God, and to love one's neighbour. The essential condition of fulfilling Christ's first commandment and

Vivekananda's first precept, is purity of heart, which is nothing more or less than renunciation of selfishness. And the second commandment and second precept may be summed up in the word service, for that is what love of neighbour and the good of the world imply. The motto virtually common to both Christ and Vivekananda may be epitomized in the two words, renunciation and service.

If we take Swami Vivekananda's own actions as a guide, we find the same see-saw between renunciation of action on the one hand, and service on the other, as we find in his teaching. Vivekananda the servant of humanity, the inspired teacher, the fiery preacher, the founder and organizer, the great heart spending in dedicated service of the down-trodden masses: this is one side. Narendra in quest of *Nirvana* at Buddha Gaya; Vivekananda, the beggar, wandering over this face of India, visiting the Alps, making pilgrimage to Amarnath, retiring to Kshir-Bhavani, deliberately departing from earthly life: this is the other side.

Clearly, in the Swami's words and actions we shall find no hard-and-fast guide, independent of the stage of progress and other conditions governing the case of each individual aspirant, to the precise place service is to take in a life of renunciation. What we shall find is the mark at which to aim.... a glance at the relation of the teaching of Swami Vivekananda to that of Ramakrishna is instructive. On a first view, Ramakrishna seems to stress renunciation – "first God, then charity" – and Swami Vivekananda, service. There is surely nothing about Swami Vivekananda which has given rise to discussion as much as the importance he has given to public service in drawing up the plan of the Ramakrishna Order. People have not infrequently made a distinction between master and disciple in this matter. Our best guides here are those saints who knew both Ramakrishna and Swami Vivekananda very intimately – namely the Swami's monastic brother-disciples. Their testimony is of very great weight – the more so when we learn that they also had doubts at first. Their verdict is that Swamiji, as Vivekananda is called by those who love him, alone truly understood. Ramakrishna. Swami Turiyananda, whose words it would be ridiculous to ignore, goes so far as to say, "Swamiji did not preach even a single idea of his own." The mature view, it would seem, is to think in terms of one entity, Ramakrishna-Vivekananda which may be likened to an ocean of truth. In this illustration, Ramakrishna is the ocean when it is calm; Swami Vivekananda is the ocean lashed into waves. It is the same ocean, the same truth, whether it is at rest or moving.... The story of his life, even apart from the success that is attending his undertakings, and apart from what time reveals to have been the effect of his teaching, is a most precious sermon. No less is the manner of his death. It is the type of the Free Man's death, even as Christ's is the type of martyr's death, and Socrates' the type of the philosopher's death. In Vivekananda, God is greatly glorified. The Vedanta says that Divinity is in every man: in Vivekananda It is made manifest.

He could transmit spirituality

– Swami Prabhavananda

It is interesting to note that Buddha preached his first sermon in Benares, the seat of learning of his times, and that Vivekananda preached his first sermon in Chicago at the World's Parliament of Religions, where the Western intellectuals of his day had congregated. There is another similarity between these two great teachers: both Buddha and Vivekananda had a message for their own time as well as for all ages. What was the substance of Vivekananda's message? It was the message of harmony and universality in religion.

Vivekananda had a dream. And his dream was to harmonize the cultures of the East and the West.

The industriousness of the West and contemplativeness of the East must be harmonized. If external achievements are made the goal of life and God the means to reach that goal, there will continue to be suffering and misery. But if God is known to be the supreme purpose of existence, and activity and outward achievements are made the means to fulfil this purpose, then the divinity within man will become manifest, and he will see this divinity everywhere. This is the essence of religion, which Vivekananda summed up as follows: "Do not depend on doctrines, do not depend on dogmas, or sects, or churches or temples; they count for little compared with the essence of existence in man, which is divine; and the more this is developed in man, the more powerful is he for good. Earn that first, acquire that, and criticize no one, for all doctrines and creeds have some good in them. Show by your lives that religion does not mean words, or names, or sects, but that it means spiritual realization. Only those can understand who have experienced it. Only those who have attained spirituality can communicate it to others, can be great teachers of mankind. They alone are the powers of light."

And Vivekananda was such a power of light.

He had the power of transmitting spirituality by a touch. There was a professor of science in Madras, an avowed athiest. One day he had a long argument with Swamiji about the existence of God. Finally, Swamiji gave the professor a touch, saying 'Kidi don't you see God: don't you see God?' The man was completely transformed....

A world renowned personality

– Swami Ramdas

Swami Vivekananda came into contact with Sri Ramakrishna, who gave him all the spiritual wealth which he had gathered during the years of his hard and tremendous austerities. The supreme grace of Sri Ramakrishna illumined the heart of Swami Vivekananda and removed from it all impurities. It raised him to a spiritual eminence which is rare in the world. Swami

Vivekananda became world-renowned personality. He carried out the great mission for which Sri Ramakrishna came to the world, by visiting various countries of the world and propagating the great ideal of Vedanta. He taught that everything is Brahman.... He awakened in the hearts of millions a longing for God, and granted them the strength to realise God.

When Swami Vivekananda went to America to address the Parliament of Religions he virtually electrified the world. At that time Ramdas found that the message of Vedanta which Vivekananda delivered in America was accepted by the world.

He lived an intense life
– Swami Ranganathananda

Swami Vivekananda roused his nation from its sleep of centuries and gave it a man-making and nation-building faith and resolve.... He imparted to the waiting people of the West, the rational and universal messege of India's Vedanta Philosophy.

His span of earthly life was hardly forty years, but within this short period, he lived an intense life, first as a student in school and college, then as the foremost disciple of his Great Master, Sri Ramakrishna, then as a wanderer across the length and breadth of India, and lastly as the spiritual teacher of West and East. His public teaching commenced with the speeches at the World's Parliament of Religions at Chicago in 1893; and he passed away on 4 July, 1902. He spent four intense years in the United States and England, and five equally intense years in India, delivering his message of a universal and practical spirituality and setting in motion a movement as an effective conduit for the furtherance of his message.

Everywhere, he taught man to realize his divine heritage. The innate divinity of man was the constant theme of all his teachings. This teaching cuts across all divisions based on political or religious affiliations. Its assimilation by man will make for a character at once deep and broad. He held that spirituality was the core of every religion; dogmatic exclusiveness and intolerance are no part of the true religion. The more spiritual a man, the more universal he is. He held that the modern age stood in urgent need of this education from religion, by which men will learn to make their love of God flow into the love and service of all men. He worked hard to give this spiritual orientation to the world's religions, so that they may be transformed into wholly constructive forces and become capable of redeeming modern man from his inner impoverishment in the context of external enrichment.

"Be and make" is the motto that Swamiji has given us. Be men yourselves and stand on your feet and make men of others by helping them also to stand on their feet. It is through this human transformation, said Vivekananda, that we shall be able to forge a healthy body-politic for the ever healthy, eternal, soul of our Mother India. Its health is as much an international as a national concern in this post-war age. But our own national responsibility is primary.

There is no greater work for us today than to inspire ourselves with that vision of Vivekananda, the vision of India's greatness and glory, and with the resolve to translate that vision into our special experiment and experience. This is the way by which we can endow our nation with a healthy body-politic; this is the guarantee of the steady moral and spiritual uplift of not only our own people, but of the rest of the world as well.

There is much hunger today in the rest of the world for that bread of spirituality which India has always manufactured and accumulated for the good of mankind. It is true that when we look around us today, we don't see evidences of that spirituality on the surface of our national life. That surface greets us with much that is unspiritual, much that is distressing and depressing. But in the depths of our national consciousness Vivekananda experienced the tangible pulsation of the spiritual energy resources of our nation. We need to master and apply the technical know-how of bringing these spiritual energy resources to the surface of life in order to become available to our people so as to overcome the spiritual and moral malnutrition of our nation, side by side with our mastering and applying the technical know-how of bringing to the surface, the physical energy resources of our nation to overcome our material backwardness.

This technical know-how of the science of spirituality teaches us that it can be mastered and applied by every citizen in every field of life – in the fields and factories, in the home and offices, everywhere. None need to go to a forest or a cave to become spiritual, except to intensify the spirituality gained in life and work, for this science teaches us that spirituality is the birth-right of one and all, that the Atman is our true nature, that the kingdom of heaven is within us, and that life and action are the field for the culture of our spiritual awareness. This is the great message of Practical Vedanta of Swami Vivekananda.

In the simple, humble duties and joys of life, man can cultivate and manifest the divine that is within him, making for compassion, making for social concern, making for love and service. This is the type of practical spirituality which has to become the character-strength of every citizen in our country. Too long have we made a distinction between life in the world and life of religion. And we have been widening that gulf century after century. Ramakrishna and Vivekananda came to bridge this gulf between life and religion.

He inspired most of our national leaders
– Swami Rudratmananda

The life and teachings of Swami Vivekananda have inspired and influenced most of our national leaders. And some of them, in acknowledging the nation's indebtedness to Swami Vivekananda, have left such glowing testimony as may sound hyperbolic to the present generation. To give an instance Sri C. Rajagopalachari, more familiarly known as C.R., had the privilege of harnessing the chariot of Swami Vivekananda as a college student when Swamiji returned a hero from the Chicago Parliament of Religions. That was in 1897. After nearly 70 years, in 1963, when the nation was celebrating the birth-centenary of Swamiji, the octogenarian C.R. most nostalgically remembered how 'Swami Vivekananda saved Hinduism and saved India.' He also recalled, 'but for him we would have lost our religion and would not have gained our freedom. We, therefore, owe everything to Swami Vivekananda.' And finally, he prayed: 'May his faith, his courage and his wisdom inspire us so that we may keep safe the treasure received from him.'

Swamiji was a prophet. And a prophet always lives far ahead of his time. If we go through the pages of his 9-volume *Complete Works* we shall come across many a thought which would add new dimensions to our thinking and impel us to gather fresh strength to face the problems of life. In the words of Romain Rolland, 'Battle and life for him were synonymous.' Hence, what a clarion call we expect from a hero like Vivekananda? It must be the call for a grand march 'onward and forward.' 'Come, be men! Come out of your narrow holes and have a look abroad. See how nations are on the march! Do you love men? Do you love your country? Then come, let us struggle for higher and better things; look not back, no; even if you see the dearest and nearest cry. Look not back, but forward!'

A man of multiple personality
– Swami Sambuddhananda

Swami Vivekananda was a man of multiple personality. Though one could see the traces of the heart of the Buddha, the brain of Sankara, the love of Sri Chaitanya, the spiritual fire of Guru Nanak, the apostolic eloquence of St. Paul, and the mildness of Christ – all harmoniously combined in him, one could hardly miss an eloquent expression of the spirit of renunciation and service in and through all the aspects of his life. Renunciation and service were the *alpha* and *omega* of his life. He, in fact, was the veritable embodiment of renunciation and service.

Nowhere in the history of the human race would one come across a personality that holds aloft these ideals before humanity with a greater urge and emphasis. Nor does it afford us a second personality, whose ideal of renunciation and service makes a more passionate appeal to human minds and sentiments.

In the spirit of selfless service and sacrifice Swami Vivekananda was therefore second to none. He was unparalleled and unique in his type ever since the days of Lord Jesus Christ. None but a hero can understand and appreciate the heroism of another. To understand and appreciate the great and illustrious Swami Vivekananda the world would require a man of his altitude of thought and personality. A Vivekananda can alone understand and appreciate a Vivekananda. But unfortunately the world has not produced a second personality of his type to understand and appreciate him, far from preaching and popularizing his ideals. Swami Vivekananda can better be imagined than described. Very often he is beyond the pale of human comprehension, a man of inconceivable flights in the world of thought and often to many, an enigma. His was a complex personality, whose complexities in his every day life and deed made the confusion of the people all the more confounded, whenever they would make an attempt to understand him in his real perspective with all the enormous conflict and confusion with which any ardent student of his life and character is faced. He was all the same a man of plain living and high thinking to those who could with patience and perseverance, read between the lines of his life and deeds. To others he was, in reality, a paradox – social, intellectual and above all spiritual.

Transformed by the divine touch of Sri Ramakrishna and diving deep into his life and teachings Swamiji broadcasted our heritage all over the civilized world. At the same time his missionary work and preachings gave a tremendous fillip to the Indian renaissance. His inspiration indeed went a long way to mould the spiritual, social and political movements of this country. It is admitted on all hands that the rich and vitalizing stream of spirituality that lay sequestered in Ramakrishna's life was unlocked by Swamiji for the benefit of mankind. And this he did with a spiritual power, abiding faith, erudition and untiring energy that are rarely to be matched in the history of the modern world.

Swamiji's emergence at the Parliament of Religions at Chicago in 1893, his influence as a teacher of Vedanta, the universal religion, in America, Europe and India, consecration of his life for the cause of spiritual uplift of humanity, all go to prove that he was an apostle of rare courage with a divine mission and organizing ability. His achievements in spiritual and cultural spheres have undoubtedly won for him a permanent niche in the hall of immortals of the world.

Remarkably universal

– Swami Satprakashananda

A distinctive characteristic of Swami Vivekananda is the comprehensiveness of his vision. He is remarkably universal. His thought is universal, his love universal, his message universal, his life-work universal. He stands up for mankind in general, without distinction of race or nationality, creed or culture, sex or age. He has in his view all types and grades of human beings, takes into account the various aspects of human life, and dwells on the basic problems of human existence. He sees the divine self of man and looks upon the human form as the very symbol of the Divinity. In Vivekananda the universal spirit has found a loving, dynamic and all-encompassing expression, which is rarely to be found elsewhere. In his scheme of life there is no inherent conflict between faith and reason, between science and religion, between poetry and philosophy, between action and meditation, between social and monastic ideals. His plan is to lead each and every individual at whatever level, or in whatever sphere, of life to the highest goal, to the realization of his innate perfection, along his own line of development.

Like all other great teachers of religion Swami Vivekananda has special interest in man's spiritual life, which leads to the highest goal; yet he has included in his plan of human regeneration the seekers of the temporal values as well as the seekers of the supreme good. The search for the temporal regulated by ethical principles leads to the search for the eternal regulated by spiritual idealism. The one is preparatory to the other. The Vedic religion consists of both the ways. They are called respectively "*pravrtti-marga,* the path of activity characterized by desire" and "*nivrtti-marga,* the path of detachment or renunciation." While stressing the second, which is the direct way to the ultimate goal, Swami Vivekananda has shown due regard for the other way as well.

Swami Vivekananda's universality is rooted in his experience of the spiritual oneness of existence. It is not due simply to his intellectual com- prehension, extensive knowledge, keen interest in human values, and world- wide sympathy or fellow-feeling. It is different in character from humanism, humanitarianism, and universalism. All these value man as man irrespective of creed, colour, rank, or position. Their highest conception of man is from the empirical view-point. But Swami Vivekananda sees God dwelling in human forms. To his spiritual vision man's real self is ever pure, free, immortal, and divine. The same Supreme Being, Pure Consciousness, dwells within each psychophysical organism as the conscious self, more or less manifest. In human individuals He shines distinctly as the knowing self. The One Infinite Self is apparently divided into countless individual selves, even as the moon appears as myriad moons being reflected in innumerable ripples of water. Of all the living creatures man alone is capable of realizing his essential identity with the Divinity and his unity with all living creatures. He who attains this experience feels spiritual relationship with one and all, the only relationship between man and his fellow-creatures that transcends all distinctions of the psychophysical adjuncts and develops universal love.

Swami Vivekananda's all-embracing love was the spontaneous expression of spiritual enlightenment in the highest sense.

He is the standard-bearer of Ramakrishna. Their divine mission is the reconstruction of humanity in the present age on the spiritual foundation, which means the recognition of four fundamental truths. Explicit or implicit, these basic principles underlie all religions. Not only do they sustain the religious life of man but also uphold other human ideals. We may enunciate them as follows:

1. The ever-changing world of phenomena, marked by inter-dependence and consisting of pairs of opposites, is held by one eternal ideal Reality, usually called God, who is self-existent and self-manifest, and answers to man's conception of perfection in every way.

2. Every individual psycho-physical system of ceaseless change is sustained by a central principle, which is constant, self-luminous, ever pure and free.

3. The central principle of the microcosm is not different from the central principle of the macrocosm, that is to say, there is kinship- or unity between the soul of man and the soul of the universe. The truth is, what is innermost in the one is the innermost in the other.

4. To realize this kinship or unity is the goal of life; all human concerns should be regulated with this end in view.

These universal truths have been declared primarily by the world's oldest religious literature, known as the Upanishads or the Vedanta. Swami Vivek- ananda has interpreted them in modern terms in view of modern problems. In so doing he has built a bridge between the ancient and the modern, between the East and West. Today the world is in dire need of a universal message and a comprehensive view of life, both of which Swami Vivekananda has provided.

Swami Vivekananda perceived spiritual unity as the ultimate ground of all diversity. It is the one goal of all human knowledge. It underlies all religious doctrines and experiences, all metaphyscial conceptions, all ethical ideals, and scientific truths. It unites all forms of existence, penetrates all phases of life. Indeed, this imperfect world has perfection as its very basis and being the same ideal existence has varied manifestations through divergent forms. The forms differ, but the substance is one and the same. He who finds this One Self of all abhors none.

Swami Vivekananda's penetrating insight finds no fundamental difference between one section of humanity and another; the Eastern and the Western form one human race struggling for the fulfilment of its highest destiny.

The special contribution of the Orient to world-culture is religion; the special contribution of the Occident to world-culture is science. In Swami Vivekananda's view the present age needs the union of the two; this will bring about a unique civilization. He has explained that there is no contradiction between science and religion, and that modern science has strengthened the position of religion rather than weakening it.

The message of Swami Vivekananda is, indeed, the gospel of universal truth. The religion and philosophy of Vedanta (wrongly called Hinduism), which he expounded, contains the essentials of all the religions of the world.

The central truth of religion is the divinity of man. "The Kingdom of God is within you", says Jesus Christ. To realize this divinity is the goal of spiritual life. As defined by Swami Vivekananda, "Religion is the manifestation of the divinity already in man."

The knowledge of this divinity is the secret of man's development both in individual and collective life, secular as well as spiritual. It finds expression in two distinct ways: "I am divine" and "Thou art divine." As a man becomes aware of his own divinity he becomes aware at the same time of the divinity of his fellow-beings. Along with the development of his faith in himself his regard for others develops. His potentialities grow as his self-faith is intensified. His capacity for serving his fellow-creatures necessarily increases. Says Swami Vivekananda:

"This infinite power of the Spirit brought to bear upon matter evolves material development, made to act upon thought evolves intellectuality, and made to act upon Itself, makes of man a God.... Manifest the divinity within you, and everything will be harmoniously arranged around it."

It is true that Swami Vivekananda had a very deep love for India. He has been called "The Patriot-Saint of India." But it is to be noted that his love for India was a phase of his love for humanity in general. He was primarily a lover of man. His heart bled for the poor, the ignorant, and the down-trodden everywhere. If he felt particularly for the suffering millions of India it was because he had witnessed their condition and because he knew that the spiritual regeneration of the world depended on the regeneration of India. He was convinced that nothing but the supreme spiritual truths, which India had preserved from time immemorial, which had been verified by the mystical experiences of her sages and saints and interpreted in terms of reason by her seer-philosophers throughout the ages, could save the modern world from growing secularism, which threatened her civilization, nay, her very existence.

Swami Vivekananda's interest was neither national nor international, but universal. As an ideal sannyasin (monk of Non-dualistic Order) he ever knew in the depth of his heart that he was one with the Infinite, he did not belong to any particular country, nation, or race.

Swami Vivekananda has also introduced a universal form of worship. Since God dwells in man as the inmost Self, He can be directly worshipped by serving man. All social work and the teaching of religion as well should he carried on in the spirit of worshipping God in man. In this way humanitarian deed turns into spiritual practice. The aspirant's inner development and the amelioration of the world condition can go together.

With this end in view Swami Vivekananda established the Ramakrishna Math and Mission – a religious and philanthropic institution that has developed into a world-wide organization – the monastic and the lay members of which strive to render service to the ignorant, the needy, the distressed, and the diseased as the veritable worship of God dwelling in them.

Swami Vivekananda stresses the importance of man above all. Man's inner nature is much more important than his outer resources. It is man that makes money; money does not make man. The solution of world problems rests basically on the individual's moral and spiritual lives. If these be lacking nothing can save the human situation; no political or economic system, no social order, no world-organization, no advancement of scientific knowledge and technology, no development of arts, no rapidity of transportation and communication, no high standard of living, no defence measures, no subtle ideologies, no metaphysical concepts can establish peace and security in the world. Even education without a sound outlook on life cannot help us in this respect.

Swami Vivekananda was an apostle of strength. His words infuse strength into the recipient immediately. He encouraged the cultivation of strength above all. If he was intolerant of anything, it was weakness. According to him all virtues can be summed up in one word "strength", all vices in one word "weakness." The secret of man's strength is faith in himself. It counteracts fear, which is paralysing. What can give man greater faith than the consciousness of his own divine nature? It is the religion of strength that Swami Vivekananda taught. In his view strength is religion and weakness is irreligion.

Swami Vivekananda had the capacity to appreciate greatness in any form. In judging races as well as individuals his principle was "each is great in his own place." "Each race has a peculiar mission to fulfil in the life of the world", says he. A king or a farmer, a monk or a householder, each has his own status. Each and everything has to be viewed from its particular position. He saw a person's strong points, degraded though he might be, and appraised him accordingly. He would not cut the ground under anybody's feet, loose though it might be, but lead him to firmer ground where he stood.

Like the world's great religious reformers Vivekananda's method was to fulfil and not to destroy. He wanted a country's progress on the basis of her own greatness, past and present.

With this universal, sympathy, with this lively interest in all that is great and good, Swami Vivekananda was completely detached from his surroundings.

As a knower of Brahman, Swami Vivekananda lived on both the transcendental and normal planes. He had only the semblance of the ego. His "I-consciousness" was ever united with Supreme Consciousness. Fully established in the knowledge of the Blissful Self, the ground of all diversity, he moved unaffected from one condition of life to another, no matter how great the difference between the two might be.

The life and the message of Swami Vivekananda point to the fact that there can be unity among men on the widest scale despite all differences. The world-unity which is the crying need of the age has to be achieved not by exclusion or uniformity but by unison, by following the principle of unity in variety. The one and the same – Ideal Reality – Pure Being-Consciousness-Bliss – holds all multiplicity; the same Divine Being who controls the universe, dwells in the hearts of all the individuals as the inmost self. This central truth is the key to the explanation of all facts. To realize the Divinity is the supreme end of human life. From any situation in life a person can proceed towards this Goal following his own line of development according to his or her psycho-physical constitution. One expression of life does not contradict another as long as it is in conformity with the highest ideal. All other ideals of life should be subordinate to this supreme one. Religion promises to lead to it directly. All human values – all that are necessary and desirable – art, literature, science, philosophy, ethics, politics, economics can contribute to the attainment of the highest good, the Divine perfection.

He is still a beacon light
– Swami Shraddhananda

Swami Vivekananda should not be looked upon as a powerful figure belonging to the past history of our country. He is surely a living influence in the history that is being made at present. There was a time when the fiery words of this great sannyasin kindled and sustained in many young men of India the spirit of self-sacrifice for the motherland. Not a few of our leaders who guided the struggle for India's independence were inspired by his life and example. But even today when India is free, the need for Swamiji's message is not gone, for stimulation to political freedom is only a part of that message. Even responsible leaders are realizing now that the attainment of independence has been but one step towards total national well-being. Many more steps remain yet to be covered. Numerous thinkers with different standpoints have been putting forward various views with regard to these steps. Many researches are also being conducted. Those in authority very often hold aloft many hopes and go on appealing to people for help and co-operation. Considerable anxiety and sense of frustration too are expressed from time to time. We believe that the ideas of Swami Vivekananda about national reconstruction can help a great deal toward removing much of our confusion in this regard. In his message can be found the clue to resolving the severe conflict in our mind between stereotyped patterns in our government and society on the one hand and drastically reactionary movements on the other. The modern Indian nation did not have one single 'father' as certain quarters like to proclaim. Modern India was built by the combined genius and efforts of a legion of heroic workers, thinkers and savants. Swami Vivekananda was undoubtedly one of these. The time has not yet come to put these 'fathers' of the nation in a showcase. We have to actively remember each one of them, seek light from their sayings for the solution of our problems. Particularly it is necessary to turn to Swami Vivekananda and try to guide our thoughts and activities according to his directions.

The Swami lived in this world for only thirty-nine years. The powerful personality that was manifested in this short span of life had many striking facets. Equally wonderful is the variety of themes about which he spoke and wrote. For many, therefore, it is as difficult to perceive a complete picture of his character as it is to find a consistent harmony among his different utterances. Sometimes he appears as a great sannyasin with intense renunciation, adept in the yogas of jnana, bhakti and dhyana like his master, Sri Ramakrishna; at other times we find in him the clear image of a self-forgetful servant of his motherland deeply absorbed in the furtherance of the material well-being of the masses. Swamiji may be taken as a serene philosopher with vast wisdom, and it is equally possible to look on him as a sociologist or an educator with unprecedented foresight. To many he is a devoted and dynamic representative of orthodox Hinduism; to others again, his presentation of Hinduism seems to have deviated considerably from the ancient way. Sister Nivedita and Miss Josephine Macleod, two of his famous Western disciples, testify to the deep emotional fervour they used to witness in the face of their Master when he would utter the word 'India.' The same Vivekananda may as well have the claim of being a citizen of the world in the truest sense of the word. When he is seen to discuss China or analyse the mode of living, education and industry of the Japanese, when he is feeling the heartbeat of Europe with a mature historian's insight, when he is mixing in the American society as if he belonged to it, or losing himself in the antiquities of Egypt, Turkey and Greece – who would then say that Vivekananda was only an Indian and his heart was satisfied by counting the well-being of the Indian alone?

And yet through these different traits in Swamiji's personality there must be a thread of unity. Those traits are not mutually contradictory.

When we hear him say, 'For the next fifty years this alone shall be our key-note – this, our great Mother India. Let all other vain gods disappear for the time from our minds. This is the only God that is awake, – our own race. Everywhere His hands, everywhere His feet, everywhere His ears. He covers everything. All other gods are sleeping.... The first of all worship is the worship of the *virat*, of those all around us' (*'The Future of India'*, an address in Madras), the question arises in our mind, is he the same person who elsewhere spoke so passionately about self-knowledge, austerities and renunciation? Sometimes Swamiji pays glowing tribute to the glories of ancient India. At other times his words are full of sharp criticism against many old customs and mores. Now he praises eloquently Western society, education and science. Again he speaks fearlessly about the worthlessness of the material civilization of the Occident. Yet we cannot believe that there is no intrinsic harmony between the apparently conflicting viewpoints.

The dream of a future India which Swami Vivekananda enunciated in his '*Hinduism and Sri Ramakrishna*' is not based on any partial achievement. It is the picture of an all-round expansion of the whole Indian nation. Food, clothing, secure shelter, health, education, industrial progress – these surely are its primary factors, but social freedom, national unity and above all a resuscitation of religious values form vital elements in that national growth. According to Swamiji's imagination, future India is to be a unique model of nations. Each nation has to advance in its own way to its cherished ideal. The advancement of India too must have its own characteristic quality which should not copy that of America or China or Japan or Russia. Vivekananda over and over again warned his countrymen that attempts to cast one nation completely in the pattern of another are sure to jeopardize if not destroy its essential vitality. India must learn many things from the Western nations but must not on that account turn Western.

Swami Vivekananda was not only a saint, religious leader and philosopher of the highest order but he had to function also as a great patriot, educationist, social reformer and a humanist with unparalleled sympathy and understanding. It was natural, therefore, that he manifested different phases of personality in different contexts. But one should never suspect any division in the total make up of his character. His was a wonderfully integrated character tuned to the infinite and turned earthward for the service of God in Man. Absolutely unselfish, dynamic in action and profound in his judgements, he was really a beacon light for humanity in general and for the Indian people in particular.

Since the problems of India were manifold in the different levels of her life, Swamiji had often to speak from diverse angles. Each of his utterances has to be judged with regard to its particular context. There is not really any contradiction between any two of his statements. To Swamiji's thinking, the material progress of India need not have to stand on the ruins of her spiritual culture. Let India move forward in science and technology, but let her not abandon her faith in God, her worship and prayers in temples, her spiritual contemplation and pursuit of the Eternal. Free from the selfishness and superstitions of the past, a new, virile society has to emerge in India, but there will be no place in it for perversities, injustice and unbridled sensuality. In Swamiji's speeches and writings we get a clue as to how the different problems of our country can have a well-balanced solution on these lines. The ideal Indian character of the future should imply a harmony of several contraries – serene calmness and tremendous activity, natural strength and deep humility, profound spiritual wisdom and absorbing concern for the world, intense patriotism and genuine goodwill towards all nations, unshakeable self-confidence and unreserved openness to learning from others. Such a character need not be considered an idle dream. In Swami Vivekananda we can see such a harmony realized.

*   *   *

Swami Vivekananda was as unique in the role of a spiritual teacher as that of a saint, a philosopher, or a patriot. The many qualities of his head, heart and character did no doubt contribute to the power which one felt emanating from him when he taught, but the principal source of this power seems to have been elsewhere. His words and ministrations issued from the depth of a spiritual personality which cannot be evaluated by our normal way of analysis. If we are to believe Ramakrishna, his great Master, Vivekananda brought this spiritual potential with him when he was born. He was a *nityasiddha,* an eternally perfect sage who came on this earth to teach and help mankind. His teaching, therefore, manifested a wonderful glow of light which removed doubt and darkness spontaneously. When he spoke, he convinced the listener, and, upon such conviction, he brought about an inner transformation. Swami Vivekananda was a teacher by divine right. He understood the minds of men with extraordinary clarity and foresight, and the solutions to men's problems which he presented were difficult to challenge. His famous biographer, Romain Rolland, did not exaggerate at all when he wrote in 1932: "I cannot touch these sayings of his, scattered as they are through the pages of books, at thirty years' distance, without receiving a thrill through my body like an electric shock. And what shocks, what transports, must have been produced when in burning words they issued from the lips of the hero!"

Though the power of his teaching came primarily from his vast innate spirituality, yet his profound and wide range of scholarship, penetrating intellect, keen sympathy, and remarkable manliness contributed not a little to the effectiveness of that power. These latter factors were, of course, more easily recognizable than his spirituality, and that is why many persons appraised his teaching role in terms of one or more of these qualities.

A world teacher with infallible vision of the future, he made of himself the link joining the East and the West. Many of his predictions with regard both to India and to the West, though appearing to be far-fetched in his time, have materialized. Thus no one need consider as unrealistic and arrogant his great idea that the East and the West meet in a mutual understanding of each other's needs, each giving help unstintingly to the other. The West has a responsibility toward India; India too, has a sacred obligation to the West as well as the means and the power to fulfil it. Neither should feel superiority or humiliation. Give-and-take, as ancient as creation itself, is the law of life and progress. So let the East and the West wake up to a new consciousness of spiritual brotherhood and work together to bring about an abiding well-being for the one human family all over the world. Vivekananda, the teacher of the new age, holds out his blessings to us.

A multi-faceted personality
– Swami Siddhinathananda

Swami Vivekananda was a man of God; God and the ways of realizing God are his legacy to humanity at large. To the materially advanced West he preached the glories of the Spirit. To the impoverished masses of India whose mortal tenements were finding it hard to sustain the Spirit because of poverty, he preached the gospel of work, work to produce food, raiment and education.

For the preservation and the propagation of our spiritual heritage, and the amelioration of the masses, Swamiji founded the Ramakrishna Math and the Ramakrishna Mission. The former as a means to enable individuals to realize God through renunciation, meditation and service of God in fellow-beings, and the latter to enable laymen also to participate in the service of man and thus make one's own and other's lives happy and blessed.

Innumerable are the channels through which the river of Swami Vivekananda's bequests is flowing. Spiritual, religious, social, political, national, international, literary, artistic and several other fields of human interest have been influenced and nourished by Swami Vivekananda.

He is a multi-faceted personality. And every face of it has innumerable aspects. To deal adequately with any one aspect is beyond even the best of us. In one respect we, who are removed from that great personality by about a century, are in a better position than those who were his contemporaries and companions. We get better revelations of the personality through fuller biographies and fresh discoveries of hitherto unknown materials concerning the man and his message, whereas those of his time could get only partial views which they were given to witness. The impact of such contacts, how- ever, has been tremendous, for many have been aided by the majesty and mystery of the man, inspired by his message and transformed by his example. They have left us an invaluable legacy which they received from their Master and thus we are in possession of a legacy, the worth of which it is impossible to assess. Indeed, as time passes, its worth goes on increasing immeasurably.

The various religions were warring against one another. All spoke in the name of God and fought in the name of God. In this regard, the Indian religions were an exception. Swami Vivekananda defined religion as realization of God and the various religions as only the varied paths that different peoples take towards the self-same goal. Vivekananda called them frogs in the well who could not see the unity of religions. Man travels from truth to truth, from lower truth to higher truth and never from error to truth, he said. Each religion is a proper path for the particular people among whom it is prevalent. There is no need for any conflict among religions. According to the competence, preference and historical background, the path of every seeker is necessarily different; but all are wending their way to the same summit.

The Indian constitution has made the practice of untouchability an offence. What was the main single force that made this happy culmination possible? It was Swami Vivekananda. All our political leaders of the last generation were inspired by Swami Vivekananda's patriotism. Gandhiji in 1943 or 1944, while at the Congress House in Calcutta, told some of our Swamis who visited him that he was only working out Swami Vivekananda's ideas and that he was not bringing in any personality in order to avoid conflicts. Subhas Chandra Bose had openly declared that his place would be at the feet of Swami Vivekananda were he alive now. Pandit Jawaharlal Nehru also has spoken in glowing terms of Swamiji's mission and its influence on him and on men of his generation. The terrorists of Bengal had as their vade-mecum the letters of Swami Vivekananda along with the *Gita*. If Gandhiji is considered the Father of the Nation, Swami Vivekananda is the Grand-Father of the Nation

To Swamiji, India was his object of worship. He asked his countrymen to worship this Goddess, Mother India, through service of the poor and the downtrodden, setting aside all other gods, for the next fifty years. And as destiny would have it, exactly fifty years after his exhortation, India was freed from the yoke of foreign domination. He instilled the sense of universality into his followers. His nationalism was not the narrow love of one's own country of the political patriot. He loved India because India was the light of the world and the mother of religions. India had something precious and lasting to contribute to the common pool for human weal. He was a colossus striding the continents. Verily to him the whole of humanity belonged to one family.

Vivekananda's works are the modern commentary on the Upanishads in English. What Sri Sankara did a thousand years ago through his Sanskrit commentaries, Swami Vivekananda did in modern times through English in propagating the eternal values of our spiritual lore. His words are live and direct; you feel you are hearing him straight and not simply reading his words. They are music to the soul. They go home straight.

Swami Vivekananda's legacy is invaluable and innumerable and it goes on growing. Of his Indian bequests, a lot is about the raising of the masses, and much of the activities of the organization inaugurated is directed to that end.

There are two aspects to his legacy, one temporal, and the other eternal. Philanthropic activities and exhortation therefor may in course of time become out-dated, but the call to seek the Eternal will remain valid for ever. Even the temporal aspect of his message was meant only as a preliminary step to the Eternal. Though the mode of operation of the temporal service may change, the appeal to sympathy for fellow-beings which forms the mainspring of the exhortations will remain relevant for ever. As for the eternal legacy it will remain valid so long as man cares for the welfare of his soul.

Vivekananda was a prophet of unity and his legacy cannot be viewed compartmentally. In fact it is one message taking different shapes to suit different circumstances. His gaze is always fixed on the One, and his legacy is attuned to the attainment of that celestial symphony. His legacy in its totality is for humanity at large. The greatest of Swami Vivekananda's legacy is the revelation he has made of the meaning and magnitude of the advent of Sri Ramakrishna. The world accepted Sri Ramakrishna on the testimony of Swami Vivekananda.

The *Complete Works* form his greatest monument and the priceless treasure of his legacy. They are the Gospel of the future. Swami Vivekananda's works will be considered one of the greatest contributions of India to the world at large.

Great men do not die, especially so is the case with one of such stature as Vivekananda. As time rolls on they grow greater and taller. Take any page of Vivekananda's works and read a paragraph; your brooding spirit will begin to throb with new life.

His message is for eternity; it will never become stale, for, he was a prophet of the Eternal Truth. Verily he was a messenger from God. His life and message are an inspiration for all people, for all times.

A rare preceptor
– Swami Suddhananda

Really, Swamiji never looked into man's failings and weaknesses. On the other hand he used to encourage whatever was good in any one thereby giving him the proper surroundings and facility to manifest his latent possibilities. But our readers need not be under the impression that Swamiji used to praise one and all in every one of his doings. Far from it, many times we have seen him assuming a severe appearance and pointing out one's shortcomings, especially of his *gurubhais* and disciples. But he did that to rid us of our faults, to sound us a note of warning, and never to discourage us in any way. Where could we find another like him to fire us with such enthusiasm, courage and hope? Where could we find such another to write to his disciples, "I want each one of you, my children, to be a hundred times greater than I could ever be. Everyone of you must be a giant – must, that is my word."

His was a positive gospel
– Swami Swahananda

Swami Vivekananda lived only for about forty years. He was born on January 12, 1863 and passed away on July 4, 1902. A very short life indeed! Of those years again he worked for a decade only. Still he left such indelible impression on the latter generations that many writers thought it necessary to include his ideas in their specialized studies. Hence many Universities in India teach and do research on his philosophy, social thought, political thinking and even his literary and anthropological ideas. Several scholars from the West as well as from Russia are specially studying him. Max Muller popularized the teachings of Sri Ramakrishna. Romain Rolland wrote on Swami Vivekananda and his Universal Gospel. In recent days in his book on the life of Mahatma Gandhi entitled, *Lead Kindly Light*, Vincent Shean wrote a chapter on Swami Vivekananda and Sri Ramakrishna. He signifies them as 'Fore-runners of Gandhi.' Another scholar Dr. Brown, in his book on the political thought of India called *The White Umbrella*, devotes a chapter to Vivekananda. In an interesting book *The Inevitable Choice*, the author Dr. Soper finds in the Swami's harmonizing ideas a great challenge to all 'special' revealations.

Many of the leaders of India, including Mahatma Gandhi, Aurobindo and Subhas Chandra Bose felt his impact. Many political, social and even revolutionary workers derived inspiration from his writings. So tremendous has been the influence on the posterity of this great son of Mother India.

To Swami Vivekananda losing faith in one's self means losing faith in God. 'We are the children of the Almighty', he said, 'we are sparks of the infinite, divine fire. How can we be nothing? We are everything, ready to do anything, we can do everything and must do everything.' Thus his was a positive gospel of manliness and self-reliance which put enthusiasm in those who came in touch with his personality or teaching.

Vivekananda preached the glory of the divine nature of human beings and wanted people to manifest their potential divinity. The awareness of one's real nature is a great motive force. Far from making people impractical and irresponsible, it gives man a bold and healthy attitude towards life. It supplies him with a calm, resolute determination to strive for individual and collective perfection. Attachment clouds man's vision; a detached outlook clears it and endows man with a capacity to look at things and issues objectively. Objectivity is the primary virtue for correct estimation. So understanding of one's divine heritage leads to maximum efficiency and minimum waste of mental energy in fretting and fuming, worrying and beating the breast.

A new world order is coming to the old weary world. The eternal spirituality of India is re-interpreted by its modern mouthpiece, Swami Vivekananda, to suit modern conditions....

A spiritual personality like Vivekananda cannot be claimed as the exclusive asset of any particular race or clime. Vivekananda stands for universal religion and world culture, and his sublime message goes for humanity at large. His nationalism is the outcome of India's attempt to express herself in modern times. Yet it has a universal significance for all lands, in as much as it set forth a lofty ideal, gives us a new angle of vision and reveals a spiritual outlook – in brief a rare cultural heritage which can satisfy both the East and the West. We must try to translate this ideal in the life of the individual and society. This is the message of Vivekananda to Modern Youths.

A personality with multifarious endowments
– Swami Tapasynanda

In Swami Vivekananda we get an apostle and world-teacher who has made an impact on the religious history of the world.

As an upholder of the spiritual traditions of India, and as a mighty force awakening India's self-respect, sense of unity and patriotic fervour, Vivekananda stands unique among the great men of India. The speeches he delivered and the lines he wrote more than half a century back remain as powerful, inspiring and relevant today as they were when they were given to the world. Like the scriptures, their inspirational quality is unfading and their wisdom unsurpassed.

Swamiji lived for about 40 years of which 10 years were devoted to works of public significance. He took the world by storm at the Parliament of Religions at Chicago in 1893, and since then spent himself unsparingly in spreading the message of Vedanta among mankind and in working for the uplift of India. The contribution he made in these respects is best put in the words of the noted patriot and statesman-philosopher the late C. Rajagopalachari: "Swami Vivekananda saved Hinduism and saved India. But for him we would have lost our religion and would not have gained our freedom. We therefore owe everything to Swami Vivekananda. May his faith, his courage and his wisdom ever inspire us, so that we may keep safe the treasures we have received from him."

We in India look upon him as the patriot-monk whose clarion call helped our motherland to wake up from her age-long sleep. At the time of his advent, India was groaning under the triumph of a company of English merchants over what was till then considered the invincible might of the Mughal Empire. As a consequence, India of that time was not only in political subjection but also was on the verge of cultural extinction. While the masses were steeped in poverty and ignorance, the elite had come to be convinced that the Indian culture had nothing worth preserving and that India's hope lay in imitating the Western ideals of life. Such a loss of national self-respect leads to national doom. Swami Vivekananda's appearance was the main force that arrested this trend of total self-condemnation and self-denigration.

The great ovation Vivekananda received in the West at and after Parliament of Religions was felt in India of those days as a striking vindication of the greatness of India's spiritual message. His return to India in 1897 witnessed a great enthusiasm and an awakening among the people of this country. Mass meetings of a type that India had never witnessed before were organized in the cities to receive him and present him addresses of welcome. In reply to these addresses the Swami gave thrilling speeches about the cultural greatness of India and the great future awaiting our country. The power of those exhortations, compiled and published as books, can still be felt and will continue to thrill people like any great scripture of the world. Vivekananda brought home to the minds of his listeners that India was not a dead country but was very much alive and young, even though it might be old by the calculations of history.

The enthusiasm that the Swami evoked as he toured India had all the characteristics of a national revival. The whole of India seemed to recognize in him their man, their leader, irrespective of their own regional, linguistic and sectarian affiliations. After India got united into a single political unit under the British rule with a common administrative, educational and judicial system, the process of national integration had begun. This process, hitherto an unconscious and externally stimulated process, now received from the personality of Vivekananda a conscious and vigorous momentum from within.

The role that Vivekananda and his teachings had in the promotion of national integration and patriotic idealism has received recognition from several leaders of Indian national revival. For example, Mahatma Gandhi, speaking at a birthday celebration of Swamji in 1921, said, "I have gone through his works (Swami Vivekananda's) very thoroughly and after having gone through them, the love that I had for my country became thousandfold."

The charm and appeal of Swami Vivekananda to people of diverse temperaments consist in the fact that aspirations and achievements of a varied, and sometimes mutually conflicting nature were harmoniously blended in him, and that, through words and deeds fraught with striking dynamism, he worked for the benefit of all mankind.

He was a great nationalist, but no internationalist had wider sympathies than he. The patriot-saint of India had also declared, along with passages burning with the love of India and its people: "What is England or India to us who are the servants of that God whom the ignorant call man?" He was a great sannyasin, full of the spirit of renunciation, and an adept in yoga and *samadhi,* but the welfare of the world was always his most active concern.

He was a scholar and philosopher, but, he was equally a man of action whom few have excelled in qualities of leadership and capacity for organiztion. He was the teacher of a gospel having renunciation and realization as its watchwords, but no socialist can come anywhere near him in his passion for the uplift of the masses and eradication of poverty, illiteracy, squalor and other social maladies. He was Vedantin, as great a teacher of this spiritual philosophy as any in the past, but few can excel him in advocacy for modernization in all fields of life. He was an ascetic and contemplative to the core, but perhaps no emperor ever had so majestic and imposing a bearing as he. In fact these multifarious endowments, often supposedly contradictory, make his personality so appealing, so universal and confusingly complex.

According to his analysis India has the superiority in the field of spirituality. He held the view that the Indians as a nation have a special capacity to understand and actualize spiritual ideals. In the past ages India has produced all the greatest spiritual giants of the world from whom spiritual seekers all the world over have received light on God, soul and means of spiritual perfection. He believed that in future also India will have to be the spiritual teacher of mankind. According to him each nation has got a national purpose running through its history and the continuity of its life as a nation depends on its proper fulfilment of this purpose. When it fails to do so and through imitativeness becomes thoroughly deflected from its national purpose, Nature eliminates it from its scheme as a superfluous and atrophied entity. So Swamiji warned that if India abandons its spiritual ideal, prefers to follow the capitalistic, communistic and militaristic cultural pattern of the East or the West, and becomes unsuited to play its historic part as the spiritual guide of mankind, then India will perish as a nation. Any national revival, spear-headed by purely worldly minded politicians having no appreciation for the spiritual ideal, will put India on this suicidal path. Swami Vivekananda came as warner to the nation in this respect.

The Swami therefore wanted Indians to be firmly established in a sense of achievement and possibility in the spiritual field, a sense of national mission in this respect, while meeting the vigorous nations of the capitalistic West or of communistic East and receiving whatever there is great and constructive in their cultural life. Failure in these respects in adhering to our cultural roots of the past on the one hand and in keeping ourselves open and receptive to modern influences on the other would result in the stultification of our national life. It was in this sense that the Swami asked us to look into the past, and not because he wanted us to be ante diluvian lotus-eaters. He wanted us essentially to be forward-looking but not as our Anglican imitators wanted us in the past or as our modern communist worshippers of Russia and China want us today.

But has India really got this spiritual aptitude and superiority? Our performance during the past decades of independence seems to belie the estimate and expectations of the great Swamiji. He believed that the cream of Indian youth would take to life of renunciation and service, that knowers of Brahman and bhaktas of exalted type would abound in the country, that competent spiritual teachers would go out of this land to spread the genuine knowledge of Vedanta all the world over, that men dedicated to the ideal of service and non-attachment taught in the *Gita* would hold the reins of power in the land and lead the people, that Indian universities will be filled with professors and students devoted to study and research with one-pointed zeal like the *rishis* of old, that the *vaisya* power (the wealth-producing section) of the country will devote the gains of industry for the service of the nation – for the care of the poor and the sick, for the promotion of religion and holy living, for financing education and research, and that the *Shudra Shakti* (labour) released from old shackles and re-asserting its rights, would none the less work with a proper sense of the new responsibilities that freedom has invested it with and devote itself to the service of national and humanitarian interests rather than sabotaging production by strike and endangering national freedom by alliances with the forces of international depredation. It is the tragedy of modern India that among the nations outside we are considered as the arch-beggars of the world, and within the country itself we call ourselves a race of corrupt people.

The discouraging national predicament in which we find ourselves today is largely due to the fact that our leaders diverted us from the path that Swamiji chalked out for us. Spiritual rejuvenation was neglected and all emphasis was laid on secularism, planning and economic uplift. The consequence has been that the growing generation has lost hold of all spiritual values and has turned into materialism, time-servers and pleasure-seekers of the most ignoble type.

In order to arrest this rot a reverential study of Swami Vivekananda is the most urgent need of our times.

His timely advent
– Swami Tejasananda

Today in the midst of the full blaze of our political independence, we recall with pride and reverence the hallowed memory of Swami Vivekananda who occupies a unique place in the shining galaxy of the illustrious sons of modern India. His advent into the arena of Indian life was a historical necessity. India, then under the political thumb of the British, was passing through a welter of cultural ideals as a result of the influx of occidental thought which, with its sparkling glamour, lured the unwary children of the soil into a position of utter helplessness through a silent process of intellectual, social and economic exploitation. Against such a tragic background, Swami Vivekananda was projected into the nineteenth century by the birth-throes of Nature as a mighty challenge to the ideology of the West. At the clarion-call of this heroic monk, the slumbering soul of India was stirred to its inmost depth and it expressed itself in a magnificent variety of creative activity. The accumulated spiritual forces of three hundred and thirty millions of people compressed themselves, as it were, into the multicoloured life of this towering personality who set himself to the Herculean task of rebuilding the nation on the basis of a synthetic ideal bearing in it the best elements of the cultural contributions of the East and the West. The nation in which the great Swami was born leaped into a full flame of life and regained its long-lost freedom in the course of a few decades, and the rest of the world also did not escape the overmastering influence of his life-giving message. Consciously or unconsciously it has begun to weave into the texture of its cultural life the explosive ideas of this dynamic soul for the reconstruction of a social order in the corporate life of mankind.

Though the great Swami has broken the prison-wall of earthly existence and soared beyond the grasp of Death in *nirvikalpa samadhi,* the words which he spoke long before his passing away, still ring in our ears with a profound significance. "It may be", he said, "that I shall find it good to get outside my body – to cast it off like a worn-out garment. But I shall not cease to work. I shall inspire men everywhere, until the world shall know that it is one with God." And verily his reassuring words have proved to be true. With the roll of years since his passing away, his message of peace and goodwill has been gathering momentum and securing from day to day a firm foothold in the citadel of human thought and action and the conviction is growing in every heart that the spirit of Swamiji will not cease to function as a dynamic force in the society of mankind till the whole world attains to the realization of the highest Truth.

He is so great
– Swami Vimalananda

A small photo-print was set in a frame and hung on the wall of the house where I grew up as a child in the first decade of this century. I was told, it was Sri Sri Swamiji (Swami Vivekananda). Since then, contact with my betters and personal study have no doubt increased my knowledge of this great personality, but I feel I have not understood him in any very great measure as he is so great. But I can say now that his life and teachings can be pointed out in a single statement of his: "We should never try to be guardians of mankind, or to stand on a pedestal as saints reforming sinners. Let us rather purify ourselves, and the result must be that in so doing we shall help others."

My protracted study of Swami Vivekananda's writings impressed on my mind some of his memorable words indelibly. We read his words published in compilations: a) The greatest name man ever gave to God is truth; b) Stand by truth and you have God; c) Everything must be sacrificed for truth but truth cannot be sacrificed for anything; d) Those who think that little sugar-coating of untruth will help the spread of truth are mistaken and will find in the long run ruin.... a single drop of poison poisons the whole; e) Follow truth wherever it may lead, do not be cowardly and hypocritical.

Swami Vivekananda shines forth in the firmament of those epoch-making persons who dedicated their lives to the eternal service of mankind. Great man of heroic compassion and pure from the very birth, he persevered in his action till the dawn of success. He illuminated the whole world with his great lustre assuming the greatness of a universal teacher. The course of action advocated by him for the attainment of greatness would pave the way for the future prosperity of India.

A versatile genius
– Swami Virajananda

Swami Vivekananda's genius reached such great heights of versatility that however much we may talk about him or make him our object of study, we will hardly be able to give proper valuation to even a fraction of the manifold traits of his sublime character. Only those who were fortunate enough to come in direct contact with him, would be able to fully realize the truth of this statement. In the presence of Swamiji's superhumanly powerful personality, a person however great would invariably feel himself a mere boy. In him were harmonized in an unprecedented manner, the characteristic messages and personal qualities of the religious teachers of legend and history. The following remark in Swamiji's English biography is no mere hyperbole but a fact: 'He combined in himself the profundity of Sankara's knowledge, the magnanimity of the Buddha, the fullness of Narada's devotion, the absorption of Sukadeva in Brahman, Brahaspati's polemical faculty, the beauty and grace of Kamadeva, the heroism of Arjuna and the great erudition of Vyasadeva in the *shastras*.'

As days roll on, the full significance of the prophecy of his Master, Bhagavan Sri Ramakrishna, concerning him, is gradually making itself felt. Said he, "Those who pass as 'great men' manifest in themselves one or two *shaktis* (special powers) at best; Naren, however, is the storehouse of eighteen such *shaktis*." He would add, "Naren would be recognized by few. A character of such great potentialities, had never before been revealed in this world."

Swami was a supreme *jnani,* he was an indefatigable karmayogin too. A great yogi who had attained the supreme loneliness of *samadhi,* he was simultaneously a person glowing with compassion for all. A great patriot, he was also a lover of the whole world. He knew that all were his own brethren, no matter what religion and creed they adhered to. His all-embracing love made every one look upon him as one of their very own. The only sin, the only atheism, he counted were weakness, cowardice, selfishness and insincerity. Weakness is the bacillus which causes all sorts of mental troubles. So he would always thus address us in the language of the Gita – 'Oh ye mighty one, weakness, as this of yours, does not become you; shake off this trashy morbidity. Arise and awake. What is there to be afraid of? Are you not a hero?' Of what avail are religion and the Vedanta, if these cannot infuse strength into man – cannot make him free from all his apprehensions – cannot make him a real man? Hence Swamiji would always exclaim thus – "The quintessence of the Vedanta philosophy, as also the keynote of the Upanishads consists in this – 'Fearlessness! Fearlessness! Be fearless, away with all weakness.' If you can do this, then alone you are man indeed. Whom to fear? What to fear? The Atman that shines through you is the same Atman dwelling in all. If you cannot perceive the identity of the Atman in all individuals, if you cannot sympathise with the afflictions of all, if you cannot remove the sufferings of others, if your heart does not well out in love for one and all and you are unable to serve others to the best of your ability – how do you reckon yourself a man? You are no better than a beast. Is it not an absurdity on your part to talk of religion? So, first try to be a man in the true sense of the term – strong, virile, self-relying. You will then see that religion and liberation will be within your easy reach."

If we can attain true manliness, signal success will be ours in our spiritual quest, as also in our everyday walk of life, no matter how and where our energies are employed. Accordingly, Swamiji has given us hints in his lectures entitled *Practical Vedanta* as to how the teachings of the Vedanta can be put in practice in our everyday life.

Each of the prophets in days gone by, was the precursor of one particular epoch.... Swami Vivekananda, too, heralded the dawn of a new era, which is destined to deluge the world in times to come and will raise mankind to the level of divinity. We are now having only some faint glimpses of this great coming event. Let us all be imbued with the Master's life-giving spirit. Let our lives be shaped according to the invaluable message he has left for us and let us consecrate our physical and mental powers for the fulfilment of the great ideal. May Bhagavan Sri Ramakrishna and Swamiji guide us.

He was a man of realization
– Swami Vireswarananda

Swamiji was a multifaceted diamond; from whichever side you look, it appears brilliant. Nowadays some people think of Swamiji as a patriot, some think of him as a great poet, or as a great social reformer or as an educationist, and so on. But the fact is, Swamiji was all these and something more. He was a *rishi*, a man of realization and he had realized the Atman and from that height of realization he looked at the various phases of our national life, and wanted to regenerate and enrich each sphere of our national life by the power, by the light of that Atman He wanted to shed that light of Atman on all the different spheres of our national life, so that the country may be rejuvenated according to that great deal. That was what he tried to do.

If we want to understand Swamiji, we cannot simply do it by reading his books. We have to meditate on him and only in the depth of the meditation, when we are in union with him, can we realize his greatness and his message. Once Swamiji remarked that if there were another Vivekananda then he would have understood what this Vivekananda had done. Our estimation of Swamiji will not at all be complete. Swamiji came into this world to propagate the mission and the message of Sri Ramakrishna, so that this country may again rise up as a great nation. It is only by adopting Swamiji's message, which he imbibed from

Sri Ramakrishna, that India can become great. The sooner we take up this message and try to build our nation according to it, the better it is for the country. Otherwise, we will be only beating about the bush and wasting our energy, time and probably wealth, by all these destructive movements. Only if we take to his path and try to build this nation according to the great ideals that Swamiji preached, is there hope for this country. Swamiji once remarked, "Sri Ramakrishna is India and India is Sri Ramakrishna's." Sri Ramakrishna is the unifying force of the whole country, and under his banner all the various religions, sects, etc, will become united as one great nation. He is the unifying force, the centre of the nation. The great ideals lived by Sri Ramakrishna and preached by Swamiji all over the world will alone help us – to rebuild India. The sooner we take them up the better it is for us. May Swamiji's grace be on all of us so that we may imbibe his message and work for the regeneration of the country on the lines that he has shown to us!

The Ramakrishna Mission, no doubt, has been trying to do its best in implementing Swamiji's message; but I must tell you frankly that what we have been doing – either in the urban area or in the tribal area – is only microscopic compared to the needs of the whole nation. It is therefore necessary that this Ramakrishna-Vivekananda message should be spread all over the country so that the youths of the country instead of wasting their time and energy in useless political processions etc., as at present, would take to this constructive work of educating the masses. Thereby they will be doing greater service to the country than by what they are doing now. That is why we stress on the spread of Swamiji's message.... I wish that this message of Ramakrishna-Vivekananda and Holy Mother spreads throughout the country so that many people, many associations, many societies may come forward, and work for the regeneration of the country on the lines laid by Swamiji. That is why I say that this message should be spread all over the country more than the social work. The message of Ramakrishna-Vivekananda must be spread all over the country, that is more important than having hospitals, schools, etc. Not that these are useless, I don't say that. But if the message is spread and the people take to this message, the work will be a hundred times, or a thousand times more than what the Ramakrishna Mission is now able to do. From that standpoint, the message is more important than the social work done by the Mission.

He came to us with a divine message

– Swami Vishuddhananda

He came to us at a time when we needed him most. His sublime teachings have proved a panacea for many evils in this materialistic age. The glamour of Western civilization has blinded our vision of the glorious past of India and we have long forgotten that we are the children of the Vedic sages and that we still possess the noble heritage of their spiritual treasure. It was Swamiji who had brought home to us the fact that we have the strength and courage to dig out the treasure-trove within ourselves and share the Divine Bliss with one another. Fearless as he always was, he boldly proclaimed the message to the world and illumined many a soul with those lofty and inspired teachings of the Vedanta.

Now Swamiji has been and is being accepted as a Teacher of modern India and his teachings have been gaining ground upon the minds of people who are earnest and sincere about knowing God and religion.

The Swamiji made a comparative study of all religions and found out that to understand the true import of the teachings of other religions the study of the Vedanta was absolutely necessary.

The Swami defines religion as "the manifestation of the Divinity already in man." He says, "Each soul is potentially divine. The goal is to manifest the Divinity within by controlling nature external and internal." To see this Divinity within and to become one with it is the supreme happiness of human life. Religion begins only when we catch a glimpse of the Divine soul. We may talk glibly of religion all our life and study the various scriptures of the world, but that will be of no avail until we realize the Atman, the Divinity within us. To manifest it, the Swamiji lays down the four different methods of spiritual practice and urges us to adopt any one or more of them according as it suits us. He says, "Do this either by work or worship or psychic control or philosophy, by one or more or all of these and be free." Here he chalks out the four paths leading to the emancipation of the soul, viz, karma, bhakti, yoga and jnana. There are men of different tendencies and temperaments and each one is at liberty to choose and practise one or the other of these *sadhana* to see the Divinity within.... When the Divinity within is made manifest, we see Oneness everywhere. Service, love and compassion to all beings are transformed into the worship of God, seeing them as the veritable manifestations of the Divinity.

Swamiji demands of us spiritual boldness. He exhorts us to believe in the effulgent glory of the Atman. He calls him an atheist who does not believe in the pristine purity of his Soul.... To what a miserable state we are driven by forgetting what we really are! We shall have to summon up spiritual boldness, shake off this delusion and recognise the *real man* in us.... How boldly the Swamiji has preached the message of the Vedanta!

We are alone responsible for what we have made of ourselves. The power to undo it is within us. Believing in the infinite glory of the Atman, we have to throw the yoke of *avidya* off our shoulders. It is foolishness to say that we are worked upon by other forces. This shows our lack of faith in the Omnipotence within. "The infinite power of the spirit", says the Swamiji, "brought to bear upon matter evolves material development; made to act upon thought evolves intelligence; made to act upon itself makes man a God." This is indeed a tremendous faith which India needs today. The effulgent Atman is at the back of all these planes of existence – physical, mental and spiritual and manifests Its powers in them. It alone supports the universe. This we must recognize. All differences between man and man, between man and animal, nay between things animate and inanimate will cease to exist when we realize the All-blissful Atman. This is the ideal of our life. We must know it. The Swamiji has made it easy and accessible for us. Each one of us can follow these sublime teachings of the Swamiji and put them into practice in his everyday life and attain the life Divine.

Swami Vivekananda came to us with the Divine message to rouse us from our deep slumber and make us recover our real nature and thus realize the Divinity within.

A mighty spiritual personality
– Swami Yatiswarananda

The greatest of Sri Ramakrishna's disciples was Swami Vivekananda. The Master classed him among the *nityasiddhas,* the ever-perfect souls who are born on earth for the welfare of mankind. Even in his childhood he showed signs of future greatness – uncommon intelligence, courage and power of concentration. Under the influence of college education he became an agnostic for a short lime during his adolescence. But the contact with Sri Ramakrishna at the age of eighteen brought about a great change in his life. Under the Master's guidance he practised intense *sadhana,* and at the age of twenty-three, was blessed with *nirvikalpa samadhi,* the highest state of spiritual experience.

After the Master's passing away and at his bidding, he organized the young disciples of Sri Ramakrishna into a monastic brotherhood and set out on a journey across the seas to America and England and all over the world. He burst upon the American society with his message of Vedanta like a bombshell. After four years of preaching work he returned to his motherland which gave him a hero's welcome. He lectured at several places from Colombo to Kashmir, rousing the sleeping nation to the glories of its ancient heritage, and to the poverty and backwardness of the masses of modern India. His great heart bled at the sufferings of the poor and the ignorant. In India he stressed social service very much, and founded the Ramakrishna Mission with this end in view. His great compassion for humanity made him declare: "May I be born again and again and suffer thousands of miseries, so that I may worship the only God that exists, the only God I believe in, the sum total of all souls – and above all, my God the wicked, my God the miserable, my God the poor of all races, of all species is the special object of my worship."

When as young men, fresh from the college, we joined the monastic Order, we were ardent admirers of Swami Vivekananda. However, some of the other great direct disciples of Sri Ramakrishna who were alive then told us: 'Now you have great admiration for Swamiji. Well, that is good. But you will understand and admire him more as you yourselves progress in spiritual life.' This proved true in our case. We soon came to the understanding that Swami Vivekananda was first and foremost a mighty spiritual personality, and his compassion for humanity was of a higher order: it was based on actual spiritual kinship with all men and women. He saw the Self hidden in all beings, and service of man was for him worship of God. That is the highest form of worship. The great Swami did not live to see his fortieth birthday. His life and message are a great force shaping the destinies of millions of people all over the world.

TRIBUTES FROM SAVANTS AND SAINTS

He united the East and the West
– Dr. Sir. C. P. Ramawami Aiyar

Swami Vivekananda has been the most important link between the East and the West, and has not only done memorable service in rousing the latent energies and the consciousness of Indians and making them realize the innate characteristics of their heritage, but has conveyed in a formative and creative fashion the message of Indian scriptures, enabling the West to take advantage of the spiritual treasures of the East and to utilize them in conjunction with their own dynamic and essentially humanitarian and scientific outlook whose advantages he demonstrated to India in turn.

Vivekananda was one man who really united the East and the West. He brought into play an idea of mass organization of spiritual forces in the world. With his far-sighted vision, he started a great organisation, viz. the Ramakrishna Math and Mission and the organization is the great example of fellowship and harmony. The world of today would greatly benefit by the message of Swami Vivekananda.

His writings are our newest scriptures
– Baba Saheb Apte

The closest disciple of *Yugavatara* Bhagavan Ramakrishna Paramahamsa, Swami Vivekananda has been in recent times an illustrious son of Bharat Mata. They say: *"Atmavai putranamasi."* So also, people have seen in Swami Vivekananda the soul of Bharat. His fame has spread the world over.

True, no one has as yet called him *jagadguru.* But there can be no doubt whatsoever that his life-work fully entitles him to be revered as the *rashtraguru.*

Our chief malady has been oblivion of the national self. Swami Vivekananda swept clean the cobwebs of this oblivion and gave us a consciousness of the national self. Since the last several centuries the flow

TRIBUTES FROM SAVANTS AND SAINTS 251

of the nation's cultural life-stream had been obstructed as it were. Swamiji made it burst forth once again. Expansion is life, that was what Swamiji's own precept taught us. After Vyasa, Valmiki and Manu, it has been Swami Vivekananda who has made a conscious effort to give enlightenment to the entire world and thus do justice to Bharat's role as the preceptor of humanity. It is a matter ot pride for us that this spiritual world-conqueror is today being honoured all over the world.

For the people of Bharat, Swamiji's teachings are invaluable. They spell out for us at length our purpose in life and our duty. We ought to study Swamiji's works thoroughly. Reading articles and listening to speeches about Swamiji is not at all sufficient. It is a matter of good fortune that Swami Vivekananda's speeches and writings are fully available. Let us make the most of this good fortune, and drink deep from the treasure he has bequeathed us and translating his teachings into our lives, mould our conduct in accordance with them.

It still remains to be realized that Swami Vivekananda's works deserve to be adopted as scriptures for regular study.

Vivekananda's books are the *Dasbodh* of today and like the *Dasbodh* embody perennial truths which would continue to guide us for ever. My point is that they need to be read reverently every day even as the *Ramayana* and the *Mahabharata* are read.

The outstanding lesson in Swamiji's works is *"Atmano mokshartham jagaddhitaya cha."* Our ancient texts do not pointedly tell us of duties to our country, our society and our *dharma*. It is therefore perhaps that they are not very effective from this point of view. Sri Vivekananda's on the other hand expound very lucidly these fundamental duties of ours. An average educated person can understand them very well.

Swamiji told his contemporaries: Let *Bharata Mata* be your only God. Worship of this God alone will bring fruits to you.

Swami Vivekananda has written about Advaita Vedanta, so lucidly and interestingly that everyone can follow it. There is in his exposition no haziness, no dry philosophization, no confused definitions. And every word of his exudes inspiration for action.

It can be said that credit for the manifestation of a conscious and integrated *akhil Bharatiya* nationalism goes to Swami Vivekananda much more than can be given to, say, Goswami Tulsidas, Nanak, Kabir, Chaitanya, Gyaneshwar or Ramdas.

It would be no exaggeration to say that after Valmiki's *Ramayana* and Vyasa's *Mahabharata* and the *Gita*, if there can be works which can uniformly inspire the entire country irrespective of province or sect, it is Vivekananda's.

All those engaged in the task of strengthening the national spirit ought to give thought to this matter.

The speciality of Swamiji's literature is that it does not stink of party or sect, does not ridicule, oppose or criticize anybody or anything. The whole discussion is simple and straightforward. All its emphasis is on constructive work. In this literary mirror we can see ourselves clearly, and as we really are. But however effective the medicine is, it has to be taken to cure a disease; similarly we must remember that a mere introduction of Swamiji's thoughts by somebody will not be enough. We must ourselves read the original books. Only when we ponder over, and assimilate these powerful thoughts, will they form a part of our life and conduct.

Remembering that no quick results can be expected, we must keep studying these books with religious zeal. We must make a rule of not taking our food or going to bed unless we read some portion of Swamji's literature every day. The younger generation must partake of this food in ample measure. Parents and teachers must see that children read and assimilate his literature as much as they can.

If crores of children of *Bharata Mata* acquire character through such efforts, and prepare to serve the nation in an organised manner, they can certainly write a glorious chapter in the history of the country, and the Bharata of Swamiji's dreams will come true.

A rare genius
– Mahakavi Kumaran Asan

Prominent among the disciples of Sri Ramakrishna – the saint of Dakshineswar, he was an extremely brilliant man, a rare genius the like of whom was never seen before. Incessantly engaged in disseminating the gospel of Vedanta, he dazzled the world by dint of his powerful oratory. Just as he freely passed across the ocean (to go to the West), so also did he swim across the very ocean of wisdom.

Though no more physically, his world-wide fame and the abiding fragrance of his noble qualities have immortalized his significant name – "Vivekananda."

His influence still working gigantically
– Sri Aurobindo

It was in religion first that the soul of India awoke and triumphed. There were always indications, always great forerunners, but it was when the flower of the educated youth of Calcutta bowed down at the feet of an illiterate Hindu ascetic, a self-illuminated ecstatic and "mystic" without a single trace or touch of the alien thought or education upon him that the battle was won. The going forth of Vivekananda, marked out by the Master as the heroic soul destined to take the world between his two hands and change it, was the first visible sign to the world that India was awake not only to survive but to conquer.... Once the soul of the nation was awake in religion, it was only a matter of time and opportunity for it to throw itself on all spiritual and intellectual activities in the national existence and take possession of them.

Vivekananda was a soul of puissance if ever there was one, a very lion among men, but the definite work he has left behind is quite incommensurate with our impression of his creative might and energy. We perceive his influence still working gigantically. We know not well how, we know not well where, in something that is not yet formed, something leonine, grand, intuitive, upheaving that has entered the soul of India and we say, "Behold, Vivekananda still lives in the soul of his Motherland and in the souls of her children."

The visit of Swami Vivekananda to America and the subsequent work of those who followed him did more for India than a hundred London Congresses could effect. That is the true way of awakening sympathy, – by showing ourselves to the nations as a people with great past and ancient civilization who still possess something of the genius and character of our forefathers, have still something to give the world and therefore deserve freedom, – by proof of our manliness and fitness, not by mendicancy.

[During the jail period, for a short time, Sri Aurobindo used to hear the voice of Swami Vivekananda instructing him on a particular aspect of *sadhana*. "It is a fact" he wrote, "that I was hearing constantly the voice of Vivekananda speaking to me for a fortnight in the jail in my solitary meditation and felt his presence. The voice spoke on a very important field of spiritual experience." Years later he spoke categorically about Vivekananda having been to him the very first messenger to reveal the lore of the Supramental Truth, and added: "It was the spirit of Vivekananda who first gave me a clue in the direction of the Supermind. This clue led me to see how the Truth-consciousness works in every thing.... He did not say 'Supermind.' 'Supermind' is my own word. He just said to me, 'This is this, this is that' and so on. That was how he proceeded by pointing and indicating. He visited me for fifteen days in Alipore jail, and, until I could grasp the whole thing, he went on teaching me and impressed upon my mind the working of the Higher Consciousness – the Truth consciousness in general – which leads towards the Supermind. He would not leave until he had put it all into my head.... I had never expected him and yet he came to teach me. And he was exact and precise even in the minutest details."

Aurobindo had another direct experience of Vivekananda's presence when he was practising hathayoga. He felt this presence standing behind and watching over him.]

His message continues to inspire us
– T. S. Avinashilingam

Swami Vivekananda had a message for India and the world. His message to India was meant to introduce life into her people, to give vigour to our national life, to shake our people out of their age-long lethargy and to make them appreciate the great destiny of our land. He was not superficial in the diagnosis of the reasons for her ills, but went into the causes which were eating into her vitals and which led to her downfall.

He spoke of the urgent need for India to assimilate the spirit of modern science, develop technical efficiency and practical skills and through these build up a healthy and progressive body-politic. Education according to him should be a blend of Vedanta and modern science. Spirituality, he said, must continue to remain the central theme of Indian life. He found no conflict between material well-being and spiritual welfare, both of which he united into a comprehensive spiritual life. He expounded the scope and contents of this spirituality, welding Vedanta to modern science, in the following well-known testament of faith: 'Each soul is potentially divine, having within it all power and perfection.'

Born out of this principle of divinity in every individual was his great message of work as worship. At a time, when men avoided society and work in their search for God, and sought the solitude of the caves and the forests, the Swamiji's message came with significant originality. He said, 'Where are you going to seek God? Is not God present in the living beings around you? God has come in the shape of the poor and the miserable, the sick and the lowly, the suffering, and the downtrodden. Serve them sincerely and with humility. Work for them and that will be the real worship of God.'

To him a proper system of education was the remedy for all our social ills. His message in the field of education was a unique one – based on the divinity of the human soul. He believed that all souls are potentially divine and education should be the manifestation of the divinity already in man. The duty of the teacher is to help in the manifestation of this divinity by positive help and encouragement and by his own high example. As he said: "The Light Divine within is obscured in most people. It is like a lamp in a cask of iron; no gleam of light can shine through it; gradually by purity and unselfishness, we can make the obscuring medium less dense, until at last it becomes as transparent as glass." The duty of the teacher is to help the child by positive guidance to become conscious of his great national and spiritual heritage and strive for it.

Swami Vivekananda is no more with us in body, but his spirit and his message continue to inspire us. That message is as much for the world as for India and will continue to inspire millions of people for all ages to come.

That message, if it can be put in a few words, is: 'Renounce the lower pleasures; Realize the Divine Nature and dedicate yourself to the service of God in the form of the poor and down-trodden. Awake, arise and stop not till the goal is reached!'

It is our proud privilege to live at a time when the message is fresh.... Let us open our hearts and minds to receive this great spiritual message. Let us dive deep into this eternal wisdom and be blessed by it.

A unique personality
– Mahakavi Subramanya Bharati

There is no subject on which Swami Vivekananda has not thought. There is no scripture he is not familiar with. The course of his intellect knows no impediments. His courage knows no limit. After Sri Krishna taught the *Gita*, removed all doubts man is prone to, and established Vedic Knowledge on a firm basis it is Vivekananda who has explained in a language everyone can understand the true import of Hinduism.

It was Vivekananda who was responsible for initiating the renaissance of *Hindu Dharma*.

He roused us
– Acharya Vinoba Bhave

Vivekananda not only made us conscious of our strength, he also pointed out our defects and drawbacks. India was then steeped in *tamas* (ignorance and unwisdom) and mistook weakness for non-attachment and peace. That is why Vivekananda went so far as to say that criminality was preferable to lethargy and indolence. He made people conscious of the *tamasika* state they were in, of the need to break out of it and stand erect so that they might realize in their own lives the power of the Vedanta. Speaking of those who enjoyed the luxury of studying philosophy and the scriptures, in the smugness of their retired life, he said foot-ball-playing was better than that type of indulgence. Through a series of *obiter dicta*, he rehabilitated the prestige of India's soul force and pointed out to the *tamoguna* (unwisdom) that had eclipsed her. He taught us, "The same soul resides in each and all.

If you are convinced of this, it is your duty to treat all as brothers and serve mankind." People were inclined to hold that, though all had equal right to the *tattva-jnana* (knowledge of the Spirit), the difference of high and low should be maintained in the day-to-day dealings and relations. Swamiji made us see the truth that *tattva-jnana*, which had no place in our everyday relationship with our fellow beings, and in our activities was useless and inane. He, therefore, advised us to dedicate ourselves to the service of *'Daridranarayana*, (God manifested in the hungry, destitute millions) to their upliftment and edification. The word *'Daridranarayana'* was coined by Vivekananda and popularised by Gandhiji.

He went and saw and conquered all
– C. C. M

The Swami sailed to Western shores,
Not as Cortes did before,
To conquer with the fire and sword
A dark unillumin'd horde,
His weapons were of other mould
His aim not earthly power or gold;

Bravely he steered athwart the main,
With none to follow in his train;
With not a single shell in hand,
To raise his revered motherland.
In the eyes of people far away,
Of masterminds as bright as day,
He told them in language clear,
They need not shed a drop of tear
For fallen Ind, who still doth own
A precious stone, to them unknown.
The Hindu is by culture mild,
Forebearing, generous and kind;
The Hindu does not take delight
In hawking, hunting or in fight;
For birds and beasts as well as men
He always has a tender vein:
Feels in fact a brotherly love
For insects, worms and all above
Though strongly wedded to his own,
He does not in his heart disown
The merits of another's creed
The piety of a pious deed,
Be it done by a Hindu true
An Arab wild or wand'ring Jew.
How quick did Swami gain his end,
And the ways of 'mericans mend!
When Caesar went to conquer Gaul
He went and saw and conquer'd all.

He preached a universal religion
– M. C. Chagla

Swami Vivekananda was a bridge between the East and the West. He was a great and illustrious son of India, but he was as well-known in the West as he was known in India. He realized that there was much that the East could take from the West, and much that the West could take from the East. He appreciated the material and scientific progress the West had made, he realized the sense of equality which was there in the West, he also admired the democratic institutions of the West, but so far as his own country and the East was concerned, he knew we followed the things of the spirit. He felt that both parts of the world had much to contribute to each other, and that contribution would lead in the long run to bringing about a world which would work for peace and happiness.

He went to the Congress of World Religions in Chicago in 1893, and those who were there and who heard him felt they were hearing the voice of a saint and a seer. He preached a universal religion, and the thing which he emphasized was the value and importance of the individual. His creed was that every individual had the divine spark in him whether the individual was a rich man or a poor man, whether he belonged to a high caste or to a low caste, whether he was a saint or a sinner. All individuals were alike, because each human being had a divine spark in him; that was really the essence of his religion. He also felt that you could find God anywhere, whether in the temple, the church, the mosque or the synagogue. God was omnipresent, and you did not have to resort to rites or rituals or any particular form of religion in order to discover Him.

Now what is the legacy he has left behind? His legacy is first of all the Ramakrishna Missions which you find dotted all over the world. These Missions exist in order to spread the gospel of the Swamiji, and also to bring succour to the poor and the suffering, because one of the important tenets of Swamiji's philosophy was that the best form of prayer, the best form of worship, was service. He did not believe in people retiring and thinking of their own immortal souls. He thought that was a selfish way of showing your religion or your faith in God. The best way to show your faith in God, the best way to practise religion, was to serve: service was the finest form of religion. It is because of that noble message that these Missions that you find everywhere are dedicated to service, and they carry on humanitarian work all over the world.

The other legacy which he has left, and which we should think of today in this troubled world, is that what makes a country great is not an affluent society, not material possessions, not arms and armaments but the things of the spirit. It is the ideals which a country sets before itself, and the values it cherishes.

Today most of us are troubled in spirit; there is fear and suspicion in our heart, there is a sense of frustration. It is wise, it is becoming, it is proper that we should ponder over the message the Swami Vivekananda gave to all of us.

A divinely inspired and God-appointed leader

– Suniti Kumar Chatterji

Vivekananda appeared to me immediately to be a man who was intensely moved by the sufferings of Humanity, and particularly of Humanity in India. Some of his tirades against middle class and upper class societies in this matter moved us to the depths of our being. He discovered for us the greatness of Man, and particularly of men in the humbler walks of life who were the despised and the denied in our Indian society. At the same time, he brought home to us the value of Indian thought at its highest and pristine best, as in the Vedanta. He was able to convince us that what our ancestors had left in the Vedanta Philosophy was of permanent value, not only for us in India but also for the rest of Humanity. This put heart in us, and made us feel a new kind of elation as members of a people who have always had a mission and a sacred task to serve Humanity. The Hindus as a race were losing their nerve, and it was Vivekananda who helped us to regain this nerve which we were losing. There was a lot of unthinking and unsympathetic criticism of our ways and our life, particularly from among Christian missionaries of the older type, and this was demolished by Vivekananda. All this made us hold him very close to our heart, and to think of him as a great master and as a new kind of incarnation who came down to earth to lead us into the good life and the life of the strong man.

Vivekananda, in the first instance, knocked off a lot of nonsense in our Hindu social life, and drew our attention to the Eternal Verities and not to the ephemeral accidentals – social usages and such like – in our life. He was a sworn enemy of what we now call in India casteism. Untouchability was something which he abhorred both as a sannyasin and as a lay Hindu. He coined the word which is very commonly used in our Indian English – "don't-touchism." His heart overflowed with love and sympathy for the masses, whom he wanted to serve with religious zeal – serve as a believer in the Vedanta which sees God in all life. He coined a new word for our Indian languages – *Daridranarayana* or a "God in the poor and the lowly." This word has been accepted by the whole of India, and in a way it brings in a sense of responsibility for the average man. He has to look upon the poor and the humble, the suffering ones and the frustrated ones of society, as if they were deities incarnate or fragments of God, to serve whom was to serve God. Mahatma Gandhi's revival of the old expression which was used in Gujarati by the Vaishnava poets of Gujarat, namely, *Harijana* or "the Men of God" was a very fine expression; but *Daridranarayana* implied or brought in an element of a sense of duty which was enjoined upon man to serve the poor if they wanted to serve God.

Swami Vivekananda is looked upon as a great religious teacher, and indeed he made a definite contribution to the study of both Hindu religion and philosophy, and also in spreading a knowledge and appreciation of this philosophy and religion. His great works on aspects of Vedanta in theory and practice still inspire hundreds and thousands of enquirers all over the world. But it has also been said that he was more a philanthropist, one who dedicated himself to the service of man, than a religious theorist or preacher. One need not seek to analyse Vivekananda's personality in this way. It is best to take the service of man as a form of serving God, for, from the point of view of all practical religion, God and Man are the obverse and reverse of the same medal. Vivekananda may be said to have been an innovator in two matters. As his great disciple Sister Nivedita suggested – he was the first to formulate the basic character of Hinduism as a system of thought and as a way of life in the modern age. This is the first great thing we as Indians may note about Vivekananda. Secondly, Vivekananda may be said to have brought before the Western World a new point of view in religious thinking – a new approach to the problems of faith – which they needed very badly. To this also might be added as a pendant that

Vivekananda, as one of the thought-leaders of modern India, gave the tone to modern Indian culture. He conceived of an integration of all human religion and culture into one entity claiming the homage of all and sundry.

I consider, and many agree with me also, that Swami Vivekananda's participation and his magisterial and at the same time sweet and reasonable pronouncements at the International Congress of Religions at Chicago in 1893 form a very important event in the intellectual history of modern man. There he proclaimed for the first time the necessity for a new and an enlightened kind of religious understanding and toleration, and this was particularly necessary in an America which was advancing so rapidly in science and technology, and in wealth and power, which were not, however, divorced from altruistic aspirations and achievements. But apart from a few of the most outstanding figures, particularly in the New England orbit of the United States, generally the religious background was crude and primitive. It had pinned itself down to a literal interpretation of the Bible, and accepted all the dogmas with a conviction which was pathetic in its combination of sincerity and fanatic faith, of credulity and crudity. This very primitive kind of religion was not satisfying to those who were actuated by the spirit of enquiry in a higher and more cultured plane, and for them Vivekananda's message came like rain on a thirsty soil.... So in this way, we might say that quite a new type of spiritual conversion has taken place in the mind of a considerable portion of intelligent men and women in the West, beginning with America; and here we see the leaven of Vedanta working through Vivekananda. In a novel on Mexican life by D. H. Lawrence – *The Plumed Serpent* – where we have the picture of a revival of the pre-Catholic Aztec religion among a section of political workers in Mexico, the mentality displayed by some of the leaders of this movement is something astoundingly modern. Many of the views expressed by one of the characters in this novel, the hero Ramon talking to Roman Catholic Bishop, might have been taken over bodily from the writings of Vivekananda. In this way, although the ordinary run of people are not conscious of it, the message which was given out by Vivekananda to America and the Western World at Chicago in 1893, and subsequently to people in America, England, and India, has been an effective force in the liberalization of human spirit in its religious approach.

The first point in Vivekananda which I mentioned above, namely, his giving before the world a definition of Hinduism in its essence, was a service which was done not only to India but also in another way to Humanity....

Vivekananda was the lover of all those who had suffered through the injustice of others, and he tried his best to restore them to a sense of human dignity.... It is remarkable how in India in her days of political submission and spiritual inanity, when everything seemed hopeless, and the people had lost all confidence in themselves, a spirit calling us to action like Swami Vivekananda could come into being. That such a person could come at a time when the prospect was bleak, when we seemed to have lost all hope, indicated that God in His mercy never forsakes His people, and this in a way bears out the great idea behind this oft-quoted verse of the *Gita* that whenever righteousness is on the decline and unrighteousness is in the ascendant, God creates Himself as a great *avatara* or Incarnation – as a leader to guide men to the right path of salvation. And in that sense Vivekananda was an *avatara,* a divinely inspired and God-appointed Leader, not only for man in India, but also for the whole of Humanity in the present age.

One of the rare geniuses
– Dr. U. N. Chatterji

Vivekananda was one of those rare geniuses who looked and thought ahead of his times. He passed away in 1902 but in his short span of life of about thirty-nine years, he has left volumes of utterances and recorded thoughts which are relevant to events and happenings of the present-day human affairs.

When one thinks of Swami Vivekananda one is naturally reminded of the great Sankaracharya. For, in action and thought and permanent achievement, the two bear a close comparison. Like Sankaracharya, Vivekananda sought to revive and re-enunciate the Vedantic doctrines. The former roamed throughout the length and breadth of India to give a concrete form to his mission, Vivekananda went further. Like a colossus he strode not only the length and breadth of our vast motherland, but crossed the seas, went to foreign countries and drew the attention of the rest of the world to the perennial philosophy of India and the sublimity of her thoughts and ideals. Again, in a manner similar to Sankaracharya's he organized the monks of the Ramakrishna Order into ascetic societies charged with the mission of propagating Vedantism, but not in this country alone. Vivekananda's thrilling message is for all climes and all times. This blending of the age-old spiritual processes and conceptions of India into an acceptable present-day mental discipline available to every citizen of the world is a unique gift of Vivekananda. His genius moulded the ideas propounded by a long succession of sages and saints culminating in his great Master, Sri Ramakrishna, to give them a name and habitation which have a rare appeal to the modern world.

One is struck with wonder at Vivekananda's unusual power of foreseeing the forces of history shaping human destiny. He grasped the mobility of historical forces and sensed the occurrence of situations which are being identified today.

Vivekananda bestowed particular attention on the youth of the land. He taught them to be fearless, to be and doing and to be daring in their thought. Years later, Pandit Jawaharlal Nehru asked the youth of India to live dangerously. But the ground had already been prepared for him by Vivekananda. In fact, the great Swadeshi Movement initiated in 1905 was to a great extent the direct result of Vivekananda's teachings and exhortations. The youth involved in this movement largely drew inspiration from his utterances. The cult of violence was brought into being by the foolish act of Lord Curzon's partition of Bengal. The young men who propagated the cult, now widely recognized as misguided were imbued with the teachings of Vivekananda. It was not unusual to find persons arrested for their involvement in violent political actions, possessing books written by Vivekananda alongside the *Gita*. They were inspired by his words; they sought from his teachings sustenance for their thought and actions; and they learnt to be fearless and to live dangerously. Indeed the suspicion of intellectual coherence of these youths with the Vivekananda literature and movement was so overwhelming that, years later, Lord Chelmsford even thought of banning the Ramakrishna Mission. However much they were considered as misguided in later years, to them belongs the credit of rousing their countrymen to the consciousness of political subjection and preparing the mental level of the people to receive the seeds of non-co-operation which later sprouted and grew up and ultimately bore the fruit of freedom. Vivekananda has thus been rightly called the *"veer sannyasi"*, the heroic ascetic who acted as a harbinger of the freedom of this country. But at the same time it must be admitted that nowhere in his writings and speeches has Vivekananda ever urged anyone to resort to violent political actions. As a matter of fact, in the preamble to the trust deed of the Ramakrishna Mission he had expressly stated that it should steer clear of any political involvement. But probably, the spirit of fearlessness, born of the sacred incantation eulogizing the conception of the universe as the manifestation of an all-pervading Supreme Power, so much permeated his writings and speeches, that it could without any manifest attempt embolden ordinary human beings to heroic actions.

Vivekananda was of the view that service to fellow-beings was serving God Himself. To him man was a patent manifestation of God. Service to humanity was the behest of his Master. Impelled by this idea he organized relief measures when the plague epidemic was rampant in Calcutta. Later he gave a concrete shape to his plan of service. The Math he established was not meant to be an association or assemblage of hermits escaping from society. Serving the common man was part of the discipline enjoined on the inmates of the Math for the attainment of their spiritual evolution. He once even threatened to sell away the Math, which had been established at Belur, when he was asked to consider the financial aspects of his motto of service. Thus it is that hospital work became increasingly associated with the Ramakrishna movement. Also it is that whenever there occurs any calamity in any part of the country, be it flood, famine, drought or pestilence, the Ramakrishna Math is the foremost non-official organization to come forward to rush help and relief to the suffering humanity. Branches of the organization have been established in every nook and corner of this country and abroad. These Maths have become for the common man the symbols of service and spiritual attainment and God-realization. In this is enshrined, in a nutshell, the idea of the Welfare State which has come to be accepted as the ideal of Governments in most parts of the world.

Thus Vivekananda was not a *sannyasi* in the traditional sense of the term. His thoughts were always progressive; he looked ahead of his times. He was dynamic in his manner of thinking and action. It was because of his wide vision and tireless advocacy of the truths and basic principles underlying his mission, that the Ramakrishna Order has been able to spread out into the remotest parts of the world. At no other time in India's long history have missionaries of peace and progress and service gone out in such large numbers except probably in the ages of Buddhist expansion. But the latter was confined to Asian countries. In the movement initiated by Vivekananda, on the contrary, the East has expanded into the West and substantiated the vision: 'Truth is one; learned men speak of it in different ways.'

He made an indelible impression
– M. Dharmapala

Brother Vivekananda made an indelible impression of his life and learning on the American public. We had great time; and Vivekananda was one of the most favoured of delegates.

A true and beautiful picture of Hinduism has been exhibited to them (Americans) by our friend, Swami Vivekananda, and to him all credit is due for the propagation of the exact idea of Hindu religion in America. In the Parliament of Religions, thousands of intelligent American people listened, for seventeen days, to the able expositions that were made by the distinguished representatives of the different religions. And I can unhesitatingly say that, in the Parliament of Religions, there was no figure that attracted more attention than that great and good Hindu monk, Vivekananda. I think, the time has come when India should again illuminate the spiritually darkened world. Though not advanced in material civilization, yet the people of India are rich in other respects; and could gladly give the spiritual spark to illuminate the countries, at least of America. Our good brother Swami Vivekananda has done a great and inestimable service not only in bringing forward the pure doctrines of Hindu philosophy, but has succeeded in convincing the intelligent and enlightened portion of the American public of the fact that India is the mother and seat of all true philosophy and metaphysics. I would tell you when Swami Vivekananda was advertised to speak, there would always be a rush for seats. The picture of Swami Vivekananda was placarded all over the city of Chicago, with the advertisement announcing that he was to deliver lectures at such and such place on such and such a subject. Wherever he went, the people thronged round him, and great was the interest shown by them in every thing he said. I say, he has rendered great service to this country, and Bengal should be proud that, of all representatives that were present there, he occupied the most conspicuous place in that great assembly, the Parliament of Religions at Chicago.

....You should be grateful to the good people of Madras for having sent Swami Vivekananda to America as a representative from the people of

Hindustan. Now, we see that the efforts of our brother have been crowned with wonderful success. I, therefore, tell you that if men of his character go to America, thousands would be converted into followers of the deep philosophy of the Upahishad. The Swami is the best exponent of the liberalizing doctrine of the Upanishad. If you go and preach sectarianism, the people will not listen to you; they are not trammmelled by any sort of bias or prejudices. Swami Vivekananda had expounded the theory of Hindu philosophy in a liberal and cosmopolitan way which commanded the attention of not only the thoughtful men, but even the simple-minded men were in a position to grasp his expositions of Hindu philosophy. Therefore, I say, that the descendants of the ancient Aryas, who have yet that noble and self-abnegating spirit of charity, will be able to illuminate the land with spiritual light. If you want that this should be carried over to America, then I earnestly say, send on some young men like Swami Vivekananda, who, by their moral excellence and spiritual vigour, will illuminate the sixty millions of people again.... The young men must sacrifice their lives, their wealth, and their parents, and should make themselves free from all earthly cares and anxieties, and go abroad just like their ancestors, crossing the deep ocean with the torch of spiritual light in their hands. I say with all earnestness and entreaty that the young men of today could do this work for India, if they only wished to do so.... My brothers, I, therefore, say, you must sacrifice your comfort, your pleasures, and then you will surely succeed in your noble undertaking. The example has already been set by our brother, Vivekananda.

In the Hall of Columbus, when, in the presence of about 5000 people, I introduced him as my Hindu brother, after speaking about Buddhism and its work, he said, in glowing terms, that when the Buddhists and the Hindus unite with each other, then India would regain her former glory. Brothers, we Buddhists have come back again to this land after 700 years. Now that we are enjoying the peaceful atmosphere, everywhere we see harmony reigning supreme. You must not forget the good services of our brother who learned these high, ennobling and soul-stirring doctrines from his teacher, Sri Ramakrishna Paramahamsa, who always inculcated in his disciple the vital importance and necessity of self-sacrifice. There is not only Swami Vivekananda, I have seen his colleagues in the Dakshineswar Math, and I say if five or six men go abroad with the liberal ideas of that great master Ramakrishna, I am sure, you will soon bring about a great revival of Hinduism among the millions of human beings in this country. If you organize a Missionary propaganda, millions will join in your great work. Send them to all parts of the world. You have got the key, and the success in your hands. The best men of England and Germany are now learning the Indian philosophy.

A Mahayogi
– Prof. S. N. Dhar

Swami Vivekananda was a *mahayogi*, whose life, as such, was not "lived on the surface." Attuned to the Absolute, by far its vaster part as that of the iceberg which is beneath the waves, it is beyond our mortal ken.

Unlike many other saints, Swamiji lived, worked and died for the world. He was, right from the moment of his appearance at the World's Parliament of Religions at Chicago in 1893, a great historical personality in the full view of the world's publicity. He was one of the makers, or, as some hold, the maker of Mother India, and a man with a world mission, who laboured to give the world, conceiving of progress in materialistic terms and rushing headlong with it, new values, or to reiterate old ones.

He was a prophet in the real sense of the term
– Dr. Tapash Sankar Dutta

It is rightly said, prophets come ahead of their times. Hence persons living during their time do not realize their worth nor do they visualize what they (prophets) are going to do. This is especially true in the case of Swami Vivekananda who said to himself: "Had there remained another Vivekananda, he would have understood what I have done."

Soon after Sri Ramakrishna's passing away Swami Vivekananda travelled all over India and was moved at the pitiable condition of the great nation, "battered, bruised and defeated, lying prostrate under the British boots." But Vivekananda was not an ordinary man who lacks foresight, farsight and insight. He was a prophet in the real sense of the term. So with a prophet's unerring insight he made profound discoveries about India. He pointed out that the main cause of India's degradation lay in the neglect of the masses. This may not appear to be a discovery at all in the present day context. But in the latter half of the nineteenth century when Swamiji lived and worked, it was really a discovery. At that time social reformers kept themselves busy talking about widow remarriage etc. But Swamiji went deep into the matter. He was out to root out the problems with which the human society was plagued.

Vivekananda's second discovery about India was that religion was the backbone of this nation.

When Swamiji talked of religion, he took it in a special sense meaning thereby spirituality. For him it meant realization of God.

The life-blood of religion is spirituality. The neglect of this life-blood will virtually lead to the annihilation of the nation.

Swamiji's prediction has come true. India attained independence decades ago but she is facing problem after problem because she has neglected her life-blood. People have managed to forget Swamiji's words of caution, namely, "Religion is as the rice and everything else, is like the curries."

Had we remembered the timely warning of the great prophet Swami Vivekananda, we would not have been riddled with problems even after years of our independence.

Swamiji's third discovery about India is that religion is one, and that is Vedanta. Vedanta teaches that God is in everything. This absolute democracy based on the spiritual oneness of mankind places Vedanta in a privileged position to preach true universal brotherhood.

The future world will require the genius and spirit of Swamiji to save itself from the evils of unadulterated use of Marxism. Already rot has set in and made severe dents into the Marxian materialism or the materialism as practised by the Western world. Vivekananda is at once a challenge and a warning to the entire world which includes India as well. He is the beacon light of the world in this darkest day of materialistic civilization. Here is the future man whom the world must take as its guide in order that it does not get bogged down in general catastrophe. He is the man who gave a new vision to the eyes of humanity, which had got dim, and lost in darkness of selfishness, love of dominance and power, vain boasting and ideology.

Prince of monks

– Prabuddha Bharata (March, 1919)

Among the various facets of the personality of the Swami Vivekananda, there is one which constitutes the very foundation of his being, the bedrock as it were, on which the aggregate of his multiform personality is reared. It is, that he was a monk, first, last and always. Strong, virile, manly, he moved fearlessly among all circumstances of life, standing as the champion of humanity, his mind rising to new heights in defence of the weak, the oppressed, his God, "the poor, the wicked, the poor of all races, of all species."

Vivekananda the preacher, the patriot, the lover of humanity, the metaphysician and philosopher was adventitious superimposition; beneath these cloaks beat the heart of Vivekananda the sannyasin, the Apostle of the spirit of man, disdainful of all dependence on material conditions.

He was an embodiment of the other ideal of the sannyasins, – the ideal of chastity. In the course of his chequered life, passing through different grade of society and diverse types of men, the purity of his heart was a great asset with him. In his dealings with men and women all over the world, some sort of spiritual relationship sprang up. Everywhere the blessed privilege of his relationship was a purifying, chastening and ennobling influence and was sought after eagerly by many who came in touch with his personality. How he was passionately followed by some of his disciples over whom was cast the magic charm of his personality, is narrated in his life.

He had risen above the sex idea, nay, he was born without it. In the Atman, there is no sex and it is only men who have been degraded to the animal, who see the difference of men and women. He rooted out this distinction and it was absolutely obliterated from his mind.

"Brahmacharya should be like a burning fire in the veins", the Swami told his disciples, and he was an embodiment of that. In his holy presence, one felt the burning glow of purity; sin and unholiness hid their heads and shrank away, and the fire of his purity infused into others made new men and women of them. It was the power of purity which gave such force and authority to his words, it was purity which was the sheet-anchor in his life, by the strength of which he defied all powers of the universe and smiled at the form of Death.

Indeed he was the Prince of monks, the Paragon sannyasin who by his unblemished life had shed added lustre on the long line of Indian saints and sannyasins, and enhanced the glory of the time-honoured and glorious institution of sannyasa.

His influence on me
– Mahatma Gandhi

I have come here (to Belur Math) to pay my homage and respect to the revered memory of Swami Vivekananda, whose birthday is being celebrated today (6 February, 1921). I have gone through his works very thoroughly, and after having gone through them, the love that I had for my country became a thousand-fold. I ask you, young men, not to go away empty-handed without imbibing something of the spirit of the place where Swami Vivekananda lived and died.

[During his stay in Calcutta in February 1902, with Gopalakrishna Gokhale, Gandhiji went to Belur Math one day with a keen desire to meet Swami Vivekananda. About this visit Gandhiji recorded later on, in his autobiography as follows: "Having seen enough of Brahma Samaj, it was impossible to be satisfied without seeing Swami Vivekananda. So with great enthusiasm I went to Belur Math, mostly, or may be all the way, on foot. I loved the sequestered site of the Math. I was disappointed and sorry to be told that the Swami was at his Calcutta house, lying ill and could not be seen."

Though unable to meet and talk with Swamiji, Gandhiji was deeply influenced by him. On the occasion of his visit he paid to Belur Math on 6th February, 1921, and being requested to say something on Swamiji, he quietly walked to the upper veranda of the monastery (Belur Math) overlooking the Ganga and addressed the public on the lawn. What he said, in substance, on that occasion is given above].

Man-making was his mission
– Hemachandra Ghosh

The patriot-saint blessed me with a gentle look and said, "Man-making is my mission of life. Hemachandra, you try with your comrades to translate this mission of mine into action and reality...." And we have ever remembered the words of the Great Master. Along with our hosts of friends and compatriots, we have tried in our humble ways to carry out his behests....

Strength and service were the keynotes of his life
– Guruji Golwalkar

It would certainly not do just to speak about Vivekananda, pay verbal tributes to his memory, or only to raise a statue to commemorate him. We must translate into our lives his teachings, the lofty ideals he stood for. Let us strive to change the entire society with the idealism of Vedanta he preached. He never claimed to reform society. He held that once an individual begins to know himself in the light of Vedanta, he would be able by himself to discover the path to Godhead. So no one needed to become the *margadarshak*. When once some one said to Sri Ramakrishna Paramahamsa, "We must reform society", he flared up to ask: "Who are you to reform society?" Not reform, but service of society was what he stressed. And Swami Vivekananda's entire life is imbued with this teaching of Sri Ramakrishna.

Swamiji was a worshipper of strength. Weakness is sin, that was a cardinal precept of his. A look at him would tell us how strong he was, and how fearless. Even his pictures radiate strength. He used to tell everyone to keep the body fit and strong. Great tasks cannot be achieved without a strong physique, he said. "Muscles of iron and nerves of steel", that was what he insisted on. Your patriotism demands from you a sound body, he said.

He went round the world working without respite, disregarding his own food and drink, rest and sleep. Would that have been possible if he had not imbued his body with great strength and vigour in his early life? He had accumulated such great vitality and energy in his body, that he could save the whole humanity from falling into the ditch of materialism....

Though a great saint and ascetic, Swami Vivekananda has placed before us the example of a strong physique. I think we should take this lesson.

But then, merely a strong body won't suffice. By itself, this strength may well become *asuric*. So Swamiji insisted also that the mind be pure which could keep in control strong physique.

....From Swamiji we learn that, however strong our body may be, and however learned we may become, by studying a large number of books, if we do not keep our life absolutely pure, we will not be worthy of being called a human being. The life of Swamiji was supremely pure.... In the life of Swamiji we will not find anything but purity – in body, mind and speech.

Swamiji had divine power in him. People used to sit spellbound when he spoke. An American newspaper observed: "He is an orator by Divine right," That is why foreigners listened to him – listened as they would to a prophet....

He became the uncrowned king of the Parliament of Religions. Wherever he went like an emperor with his retinue, unhindered.... he gave a new life to everybody whom he met.

If we are fortunate enough then we will see that the light that Swami Vivekananda had kindled in Chicago in the midst of dazzling materialism, is spreading all over the world as if it has the brightness of ten million suns, enveloping all human beings and in that well lit path getting all round welfare, man is becoming fit to realize God. I feel that time is getting nearer.

The great soul, the source of that Divine light which Vivekananda carried with him to the foreign land to illumine the whole world, was that epoch- making Incarnation, Bhagavan Sri Ramakrishna. Let us study their teachings and mould our life in the pattern of their noble lives. Let us devote ourselves to the service of man. Let us not allow any selfish interest to come and stand in the path of our service. Let us once again prove this truth, through our lives by making them perfect, that each and every son of Mother India, invigorating himself with the vigour of Swami Vivekananda, is perfectly capable of giving the knowledge of truth to the world.

Swami Vivekananda was a devout worshipper of the Motherland. His first teaching for the people was: worship this Motherland, with intense faith, with ardent devotion. Swamiji held that if there is any country on earth where man may worship God and actually establish communion with Him, it is this land of *Bharatavarsha*. The noble *karmas* of our former births bring us here. In fact, he said, even after all the good acts one may perform in other births, for the attainment of *moksha*, one must take birth in *Bharatavarsha*. In other lands and other climes, one may enjoy; one may achieve scientific distinction, one may even reach to the moon. But one cannot reach God. For that you have to take birth in this country. So Swamiji exhorted the sons of this Mother to venerate this Holy Land.

He said this and then gave a call to educate the people, to disseminate knowledge. In doing so, he said, let there be no running down of our culture, our religion. While he did not deny that there were shortcomings in our social mores and customs, he emphasised that it would serve no purpose if we keep on talking of these shortcomings.

Swamiji repeatedly said that there were many customs and practices which today seemed wrong to us but which in their origin did serve a useful purpose. So there was no use decrying them. While we might suitably change and alter them, let us not cite them to deride our ancestors.

Today we have our own scholars and 'representatives' running down the nation ....Indian students go abroad for education and very often their character and conduct earn contempt for our country. Whether it be for business, or education, or plain enjoyment, whosoever goes abroad must be scrupulously careful to ensure that his conduct secures respect and esteem for the country. Swami Vivekananda is an ideal for them all.

You must be aware that Swamiji's speeches and writings refer frequently to the Hindu Nation. At places, he wants us to emulate Guru Govind Singh, at others Chhatrapati Shivaji. Because according to him it is the society to which these great men belonged that is the natio nal society of this land. In fact a study of his works makes it clear that he has used the words 'Hindu' and 'Indian' as synonymous attributes. Keeping in view this society, he urged that the sublime teachings of *Hindu Dharma* be spread all around. Make the society strong. And serve society.

Strength and service – these were the two keynotes he dwelt on. Swamiji dedicated himself completely to the nation's service. Little wonder that years ago he could foresee a crisis. His vision seemed to penetrate into the future, and in reply to questions put to him in America, he said that China may seem asleep now, but it would soon awake and when it did wake up, it would become a menace. The questioners asked further: Would it be a danger for your country too? And Swamiji replied that it would be a danger even to India. So this was his forecast years ago. What does this prove? That political acumen by itself is not sufficient. With all the acumen that our rulers had, they discovered the fact of Chinese aggression only after aggression had been actually committed! So a life imbued in cultural and religious truths imparts an insight and vision which political experience cannot.

About this aggression. We must understand, that still further aggressions can come. Swami Vivekananda has however confidently affirmed that this land and nation of ours would successfully withstand all attacks, that this society is immortal. Why is that so? Why is this society immortal? People often say that the Hindu has a meek temperament, a mild character. Well, this mild-mannered Hindu has survived many an onslaught of history. Every people after all has a purpose to fulfil in this world. It lives so long as it continues to fulfil that purpose. The Greeks made a contribution, and then disappeared. So also the Romans. Very many other empires too. Numerous have been the powerful empires which have struck against this nation. But this Hindu Nation has braved all those attacks. Why? Because it treasures the great purpose which underlies its existence namely to help humanity work up its way to the Highest Reality, to make the attainment of *moksha* possible for all. So long as human society lives, Hindu society will live also – that seems to be God's scheme of things!

Despite all sorts of impediments and dangers, Swamiji exuded confidence and faith. The sort of determination he thought was needed for the service of society, can be gauged from his own attitude. He said this about himself: "I do not want *moksha*. But I aspire to take birth again and again to serve this society presently steeped in ignorance." This attitude of his was typically Hindu. In the *Mahabharata* also, the same desire is once expressed: "I crave not for any kingdom, I long not for Heaven, I seek not *moksha,* my one desire is to be born again and again, if necessary infinite times, to allay the suffering of the distressed.".

Here is therefore a lesson for us all. What should be the impelling motive of our service to society? Are we to do that to achieve name? No. To secure some office? No. In order that we be lauded and *jayakars* be sounded in our name? Certainly not. Our service of society must be absolutely selfless. Swamiji would refer in this context to Guru Govind Singh's quiet demise far away in the south. Such selfless service does not mind the scorns and scoffs of any. It is unmindful of what would happen when one grows old and when no one cares for him. Let us rather lay down our frame to rest beneath the shade of any tree, than to desire some *quid pro quo* in old age for our years-long-service to society – this was one of Swamiji's greatest teachings.

We too have a great mission to fulfil. In carrying it out let us be extremely vigilant that neither pride nor any longing for power touches us even for a moment. Unfortunately, in this spiritual land of ours, the motivation of most activity around us is selfish. Some want office, others honour. But we need workers who crave for nothing and are inspired by Swamiji's example to devote themselves entirely to building up of an organized, strong, high charactered society.

There are numerous facets of Swamiji's teachings which we need to imbibe. He has, for instance, stressed the importance of Sanskrit. Some said Sanskrit was a dead language. But Swamiji said, "teach Sanskrit to all." We must make a conscious attempt to spread the study of Sanskrit because the purest gems of our wisdom are in Sanskrit. The Philosophy of man's highest good has been expressed in Sanskrit. Our ignorance of this language deprives us of a great treasure. The study of Sanskrit would give us a view of all the religions of the world. And it is not only the *brahmana*, but the *shudra*, the *nishad*, the *vaishya*, the *kshatriya* – in fact all those who look upon this *Bharata Mata* as their mother – who must take to the learning of Sanskrit.

It was only through Sanskrit that we could understand India, Swamiji stressed.

Swamiji used to say: I want just one hundred persons, forceful, steeped in spiritualism and with a spirit of service in their hearts, and the shape of the world can change. Perhaps we may not attain the standards set by Swamiji. So let us have some thousands, be it of slightly less calibre, and let them stand together, exert together, shoulder to shoulder and I am sure with the spiritual energy generated, we would be able to change the world as Swamiji desired. It would be well if we do that. If we don't, we would be ignoring Swamiji's wishes.

There is no doubt that very many of our foremost men today neglect *dharma*. An invaluable ancient legacy is thus being ignored. In the name of progressiveness, whatever is ours is scorned and a servile infatuation for everything foreign is taking root. The calamity which faces the nation cannot be counteracted with this attitude. We must have our *dharmic* moorings restored. All our movements and endeavours would succeed only if undertaken in a spirit of dedication to the Supreme Reality.

It would be tragic if Swamiji's works are not adequately known to his own countrymen. It is known how his writings have been studied abroad. A good lady has taken immense pains to compile all the reports published about his trip to America, his stay there, the press reactions he evoked there etc. etc. and published a book titled *"Swami Vivekananda in America –New Discoveries."* Our ignorance about Vivekananda would indeed be like that of the musk-deer which is stated to roam about all the world over in search of the musk which all the while remains embedded in its navel! This must not be, and the message of Vivekananda is to be taken to his countrymen.

His great contribution
– Dr. M. S. Gore

Swami Vivekananda as an interpreter of Hinduism also made a great contribution and that is why the twentieth century India first came to remember him. He made us feel proud of our past. This was also the contribution of the other Movements – socio-religious movements like the Brahmo Samaj, Arya Samaj, Prarthana Samaj and the Theosophical Society – towards the end of the nineteenth century. All these different movements tried in various ways to contribute to a reawakening of our sense of pride in our own heritage. Vivekananda contributed to this; but he contributed to it with a very conscious, sensitive and open mind. He did not flatter everything of the past. He examined it critically and gave ancient knowledge a new interpretation, more related to what the modern mind needed.

Swami Vivekananda also stands out as an organiser. As the founder of the Ramakrishna Math and Mission, he ushered in the concept of a group of whole-time servants of God and it was for the first time that this idea emerged in modern India. Earlier we had Buddhist monks. But at least for a thousand years prior to Swami Vivekananda, the Buddhist monks had ceased to be an important force in India. He conceived of the activities of individual monks belonging to a religious Order dedicated not merely to their own spiritual discipline and progress, but also to the well-being of the society in which they lived. This direction to the work of the Ramakrishna Mission was given consciously by Swami Vivekananda.

To my knowledge, it was wholly a new direction within the practice of Hinduism.

While Hinduism has all the highest ideals of the spiritual unity of mankind, in our day-to-day life there is no unity. There is not merely diversity, but a great hierarchy in our relationships. Vivekananda wanted to break through this. In doing this, he used the influence of his personality, his understanding of Hinduism, his understanding of other religions, and his capacity to organize. He wanted to develop a tool by which a new kind of awakening could take place.

He says in another place: "For the next fifty years, let all other gods disappear from our minds. The first of all worships is the worship of the *virat* or those all around us. These are all our gods – men and animals, and the first god we have to worship is our own countrymen." This again is a very different kind of acceptance of sannyasa. Our traditional concept of sannyasa was for a person to leave society and go to meditate in the forest. No order of sannyasins except probably the Buddhists had emphasised in India the social service function. This is a wholly different approach to matters spiritual.

Our philosophy was that our sufferings of this life are caused by our actions in a past life, or may be earlier actions in this life itself. This attitude towards human suffering makes you insensitive to other people's suffering. But Swami Vivekananda said – don't bother what may have been the source of a man's suffering or who may have been responsible for it. You are a human being and so you have a responsibility to those who suffer. This is a wholly different approach to matters spiritual and moral. Swami Vivekananda preaches a path of action, or redressing suffering and of spreading education. Earlier saints had expressed compassion for the poor who suffered. The Bhagavata saints of Maharashtra, right from Jnaneswara to Tukaram, had all expressed compassion for the poor; but none of them had shown either an inclination or the ability to organize, to do something about it and advocate action to remove suffering as was done by Swami Vivekananda.... The establishment of a Mission, as distinguished from a Math, was certainly a new type of activity for Hinduism.

Most leaders, political, social or religious, consciously and unconsciously, use the non-rational aspect of human personality to mobilize people for action. Yet, I think, that to recognise the existence of non-rational elements in human behaviour is not the same as accepting the existence of a spiritual order. They are two different things. For Swami Vivekananda, once he had overcome his initial reservations, the world of the spirit in all its diversities, dualistic as well as non-dualistic, was a reality and an experience. It was the corner-stone of his message of service to fellow-beings.

Harbinger of the glorious hour
– Nagendra Nath Gupta

I knew him when he was an unknown and ordinary lad, for I was at College with him; and I knew him when he returned from America in the full blaze of fame and glory. He stayed with me for several days and told me without reserve everything that had happened in the years that we had lost sight of each other. Finally, I met him at the monastery at Belur near Calcutta shortly before his death....

Nearly a quarter of a century (1927) has elapsed since Swami Vivekananda went to his rest; and every year that passes is bringing fresh recognition of his greatness and widening the circle of appreciation. Such of his contemporaries as are left owe it to his memory and to their country to place on record their impression of one who, by universal assent, was one of the greatest Indian as well as one of the world's great men....

....When he arrived in America, without friends, without funds, he had nothing beyond his intellectual and spiritual equipment, and the indomitable courage and will that he had acquired in the course of his purposeful wanderings in India.... How he carried that great assembly of religious men by storm, how pen-pictures of the young Hindu monk in the orange-coloured robe and turban filled the newspapers of America, and how the men and women of America crowded to see him and hear him are now part of history. Slightly varying Caeser's laconic and exultant message, it may be truthfully said of Swami Vivekananda, he went, he was seen and heard, and he conquered. By a single bound as it were he reached from the depth of obscurity to the pinnacle of fame. Is it not remarkable, is it not significant, that of all the distinguished and famous men present at the Parliament of Religions only one name is remembered today and that is the name of Vivekananda? There was, in sober fact, no other man like him in that assembly, composed though it was of the distinguished representatives of all religions. Young in years, the Hindu monk had been disciplined with a thoroughness and severity beyond the experience of the other men who had foregathered at the Parliament of Religions. He had had inestimable advantage of having sat at the feet of a Teacher the like of whom had not been seen in the world for many centuries. He had known poverty and hunger and had moved among and sympathized with the poorest people in India, one of the poorest countries in the world. He had drunk deep at the perennial fountain of the wisdom of the ancient Aryan *rishis*, and he was endowed with a courage which faced the world undismayed. When his voice rang out as a clarion in the Parliament of Religions, slow pulses quickened and thoughtful eyes brightened, for through him spoke voices that had long been silent but never stilled and which awoke again to resonant life. Who in that assembly of the wise held higher credentials than this youthful monk from India with his commanding figure, strong, handsome face, large, flashing eyes and full voice with its deep cadences?

In him was manifested the rejuvenescence of the wisdom and strength of ancient India, and the wide tolerance and sympathy, characteristic of the ancient Aryans. The force and fire in him flashed out at every turn, and dominated and filled with amazement the people around him.

In conversation Vivekananda was brilliant, illuminating, arresting, while the range of his knowledge was exceptionally wide. His country occupied a great deal of his thoughts and his conversation. His deep spiritual experiences were the bedrock of his faith and his luminous expositions are to be found in his lectures, but his patriotism was as deep as his religion. Except those who saw it, few can realize the ascendancy and influence of Swami Vivekananda over his American and English disciples....

His thoughts ranged over every phase of the future of India, and he gave all that was in him to his country and to the world. The world will rank him among the prophets and princes of peace, and his message has been heard in reverence in three continents. For his countrymen he has left a priceless heritage of vitality, and invincible strength of will. Swami Vivekananda stands on the threshold of the dawn of a new day for India, a heroic and dauntless figure, the herald and harbinger of the glorious hour when India shall, once again, sweep forward to the van of nation.

A lion amongst men
– Brahmachari Gurudas

Swamiji was so simple in his behaviour, so like one of the crowd that he did not impress me so much when I first saw him. There was nothing about his ways that would mark him as the lion of New York society, as so often he had been. Simple in dress and behaviour, he was just like one of us. He did not put himself aside on a pedestal, as is so often the case with lionized personages. He walked about the room, sat on the floor, laughed, joked, chatted – nothing formal. Of course, I had noticed his magnificent, brilliant eyes, his beautiful features and majestic bearing, for these were parts of him that no circumstance could hide. But when I saw him for a few minutes standing on a platform surrounded by others it flashed into my mind: 'What a giant, what strength, what manliness, what a personality! Everyone near him looks so insignificant compared with him.' It came to me almost as a shock; it seemed to startle me. What was it that gave Swamiji this distinction? Was it his height? No, there were gentlemen there taller than he was. Was it his build? No, there were near him some very fine specimens of American manhood. It seemed to be more in the expression of the face than anything else. Was it his purity? What was it? I could not analyse it. I remembered what has been said of Lord Buddha, – 'a lion amongst men.' I felt that Swamiji has unlimited power, that he could move heaven and earth if he willed it. This was my strongest and lasting impression of him.

An immortal spiritual personage
– K. Sumdararama Iyer

I met Swami Vivekananda for the first time at Trivandrum in December 1892 and was then privileged to see and know a good deal of him. He came to Trivandrum in the course of an extended Indian tour, fulfilling the time-honoured practice obtaining among Indian monks of paying a visit to, and making *tapas* (spiritual austerities) at the sacred shrines in the four corners of the *punyabhoomi*.....

Within a few minutes conversation, I found that the Swami was a mighty man. Having ascertained from that, since leaving Ernakulam he had taken almost nothing, I asked him what food he was accustomed to. He replied, "anything you like; we sannyasins have no taste."

The Swamiji's presence, his eyes, the flow of is words and ideas were so inspiring that I excused myself that day from attending at the palace of the late Martanda Varma, the First Prince of Travancore, who was prosecuting his M. A. studies under my tuition....

During all the time he stayed, he took captive every heart within the home. To every one of us he was all sweetness, all tenderness, all grace. My sons were frequently in his company, and one of them still swears by him and has the most vivid and endearing recollections of his striking personality.... It hardly seemed as if there was a stranger moving in our midst. When he left, it seemed for a time as if the light had gone out of our home.

....As the Swami was leaving, Vanchiswara Shastri – a master of that most difficult branch of learning, Sanskrit grammar, and highly honoured by all who knew him for his piety, learning, and modesty – made his appearance and implored me to arrange for an interview, however short, even if it be of a few minutes duration. He had heard of the arrival and stay with me of a highly learned sannyasin from North, but had been ill and could not come. He was anxious to have some conversation. The Swami and Mr. Bhattacharya were just then descending the stairs to get into their carriage and drive away. The Pandit entreated me in the most pressing manner to ask the Swami for at least a few minutes delay. On being informed of this, the Swami entered into a brief conversation with him in Sanskrit, which lasted seven or eight minutes only. At that time I knew no Sanskrit, and so I could not understand what they talked about. But the Pandit told that it related to some knotty and controversial point in *vyakarana* (grammar) and that, even during that brief conversation, the Swami showed that he could display his accurate knowledge of Sanskrit grammar and his perfect mastery of the Sanskrit language.

With this the Swami's stay of nine days had come to a close. In my recollection of today, it seems to be somewhat of a nine day's wonder; the impression is one which can never be effaced. The Swami's towering personality and marvellous career must be said to mark an epoch in history whose full significance can become discernible only in some distant future time. But to those who have had the privilege of knowing him intimately, he seems to be only comparable to some of those immortal spiritual personages who have shed an undying lustre on this Holy Land.

He created a Charter of Hindu Faith
– G. M. Jagtiani

Swamiji was an upright and tough man who refused to compromise with his conscience, or tell a truth in a varnished plaster-coated language. He was a veritable thunderbolt of *Shakti,* a human dynamo of energy, Truth personified. He lived like a lion, he died like a lion. And even after his death, his bones continue to work wonders.

He was not only a saint who blazed a new trail in combining Vedas with Volleyball, prayers with power, *mantram* with manliness, and saintliness with *Shakti,* but he was also a nationalist Indian, a patriotic proud Hindu. His heart bled at the captive condition of his motherland which, for him, was the queen of his dreams.

In his very first extempore speech before the Parliament of Religions at Chicago, he publicly, candidly and defiantly said that he was proud to be a Hindu. He was not afraid of publicly calling himself a proud Hindu. He had the guts, the conviction, the uprightness. He said it, boldly. He was taller than any other man living then.

His words pulsate with power; there is punch in them. They can convert sheep into lions, sinners into saints, men into gods, cowards into heroes, lotus-eaters into indomitable soldiers.

In a way, he created a charter of the Hindu Faith. He was an innovator. He was not docile, namby-pamby, feeble. In thought and action, he was an incarnation of *shakti.*

He was the Captain of the Spiritual-Soldiers of India, but he was not the man to take the naked sword in hand to unleash a reign of terror and torture and declare to the world, "Believe or Perish!" How wonderfully and lucidly he explained to us the secularism of Hinduism which embraced the Jews, the Buddhists, the Zoroastrians, the Tibetans, the Christians who came to this Mother of Religions!

No wonder, soldiers, and Swamis, politicians and pundits, revolutionaries and anchorites take his name.

It has become a trite fashion nowadays to praise Swami Vivekananda as a secular man, though he championed the cause of Hinduism. Politicians come forward to praise him and raise him to a lofty ceiling. I am, however, doubtful whether they really speak from their heart. For onething, how many of our public men have read the *Complete Works of Swami Vivekananda* in nine volumes? Next, had Swamiji been alive today, and had he spoken the same words of challenge and defiance as he did in the nineteenth century, would not our secular, progressive, socialist and rationalist men of limelight have branded and condemned him as a communal arch-reactionary revivalist Hindu?

He cleaned and polished Hinduism's dusty and rusty sword, made it resplendent and demonstrated to the prosperous West that the so-called pagan Hindus were a few inches above them. So much dust and mud raised against the Hindus and their religion that the world at large came to believe that the Hindus in Hindustan had either no God to believe in or had millions of gods and goddesses in whom they believed. It was left to Swami Vivekananda to go into the lion's den and rebuff and refute all their mischievous and poisonous propaganda.

Swami Vivekananda exposed all the mudslinging, and character-assassinating barbs of the Western dealer in religion. He expounded Hinduism in such a lofty way that nobody could dare raise an accusing finger at us. Of all the votaries of Hinduism, Swami Vivekananda stands supreme – proud, erect, defiant, lion-like.

Swamiji was not captured by the opulent prosperity of the West, nor dazzled by its eye-blinding and sense-befogging civilization. He was proud to be a Hindu, he was proud to be a descendant of the shining galaxy of saints and soldiers, he was proud to belong to the soil of Hindustan, and he was proud of his Hinduism.

He gave us a Charter of Hindu Faith. Keep the banner flying. Sound the tocsin. Give the trumpet-call: 'Arise, awake, and stop not till the goal is reached.'

He was proud of being a Hindu
– Dr. K. N. Katju

The birth centenary of Swami Vivekananda (1963) is definitely a great event in our national history. Hundred years ago when he has born we were living in India under strange conditions. The suppression of the Indian revolt of 1857 had strengthened the British rule in India. All disgruntled elements had been ruthlessly exterminated by the rulers and the Indians of the day, particularly the landed and the educated classes, were clinging to the British.

It was not merely political subordination which we were accepting and indeed calling a divine dispensation. All our culture, our religious traditions, our noble philosophy of life, all these were being suppressed and were being undermined by western material civilization. It was not merely a case of choice between the two, but the English-educated community of India were looking down upon their own culture, and hoary traditions and religious sentiments, almost with contempt. They were almost ashamed of being Hindus.

Upto 1835 oriental education was in Sanskrit, Persian and Arabic. But thereafter educational policy was completely changed by Macaulay. He thought, and he said so, that all that had come down to us from ages past was unworthy and ignoble, and should be dropped and even rooted out. We were a lot of caste-ridden superstitious people. We were, so to say, mere infants and had to be shaped for our own benefit on another model. Not only Macaulay said so but our leaders of the day also fell under his charm and influence. The charm of Western civilization seems to have completely smothered their own national outlook. Everything that we had inherited in India was to be discarded. Our great religious beliefs and philosophy were all bundles of meaningless doctrines. This was the teaching of the societies that were formed in those days. Then by God's grace great personalities were born in this ancient land of ours. In the Punjab there was Swami Dayanand Saraswati who aroused the masses of Punjab and Uttar Pradesh to the nobility of the doctrines of the Vedas. In Bengal came the divine Ramakrishna Paramahamsa. He taught his countrymen the excellent doctrine of bhakti, devotion to God. Dakshineswar, where he lived became the abode of piety in the eyes of millions of the countrymen. They went there, sat under his shade and learnt great lessons from him, and along with those lessons they learnt also to look upon with pride their own religion and culture and their own ancient traditions. Then came at the nick of time Swami Vivekananda. From his youth he became the disciple of Ramakrishna Paramahamsa and imbibed his teachings and moulded his life according to Ramakrishna's doctrines. He was proud of being a Hindu and he broadcast his faith not only in every nook and corner of India, but went abroad and declared with his matchless eloquence and wonderful personality that he was a Hindu. The speech that he delivered, and the setting under which he delivered it, at Chicago in the Parliament of Religions in 1893 would ever remain a signal in our history of great turn for advancement. It was a national movement. The British rule continued at that time. But the Indian people under Swami Vivekananda, his guidance and influence, had turned the corner. They were no longer ashamed of their past. They ceased to bow their heads before the missionaries and to look down upon themselves. They began to stand on their feet and looked upon themselves with pride and self-respect. This was not only in the religious sphere. This was also in the political sphere. With the increasing influence of Ramakrishna Paramahamsa came the spread of political movement in India. In 1885 the Indian National Congress was founded and its first session was held in Bombay. Ramakrishna Paramahamsa died in 1886, and for another 15 years Swami Vivekananda held the field. He toured all over the country. What was needed for the expansion of the political movement was self-esteem, self-confidence and self-respect of the people for themselves and that was gained by Swami Vivekananda's efforts. He died in 1902, and in 1906 in the Calcutta Session, Dadabhoy Naoroji pleaded for *swarajya* in India.

The debt that we owe to Swami Vivekananda is immeasurable. He on his return from the United States of America in 1897 went round the whole country and after two years he went back to Europe and spent another two years there. He died young. It is our national misfortune. But his was such a dynamic personality that in the course of a few years he unleashed forces in our national life which have borne fruit ever since. To him we owe our national self-respect and it is that self-respect which became the foundation later on of Gandhiji's movement for independence. May Swami Vivekananda's example continue for centuries to guide the youth of the country.

He occupies a unique place amongst our saints and philosophers
– Dr. M. Lakshmi Kumari

On the auspicious *Makarasankranti* Day, 12th of January, 1863, was born Narendranath Dutta, the veritable fire-ball of knowledge and renunciation from his childhood, who, later, under the benign influence of Sri Ramakrishna Paramahamsa, got metamorphosed into the great Swami Vivekananda – foremost among India's Patriots, Saints and Philosophers – a true Master, Mentor and Moulder and Maker of India's destiny. More than eighty years have passed, since this flame, which drew people to him like a magnet, extinguished itself. Yet, the sparks therefrom continue to set aflame the hearts of thousands with fiery ideals of renunciation, dedication and love for Motherland, spreading blazing trails of idealism.

Swami Vivekananda, occupies a unique place amongst our saints and philosophers in that, thanks to him the universal truths of Vedanta philosophy came to find practical application in the day-to-day life of man. Like the legendary Shiva, who took in his head the massive flow of Celestial Ganges and later released it in a trickle for the welfare of humanity, so did Swamiji first absorb unto himself the great wisdom of our Vedas and Upanishads as also the fullest meaning and purpose of the immaculate life of his great Master, Sri Ramakrishna Paramahamsa, and then translate both in simple practical terms for the common man to understand, appreciate and practise in one's own personal life. But for him, India would have by now lost forever her chance to revive the truth, beauty and vitality of her ancient culture and civilization, the oldest in the world today, and an average Indian would have been swept away in the storm of Westernisation that was raging over the country. But for him, the world would not have understood the meaning and import of the advent of Bhagavan Sri Ramakrishna Paramahamsa, which was to demonstrate the compatibility of the ancient wisdom of the Upanishads with the scientific and technological civilization of the modern world and proclaim the immutability and all-time validity of the ultimate truth, the core of not only Hinduism but of all religions and philosophies. Swamiji imbibed the great humanism and the truly universal spirit of his great Master and showed us a new path to establish harmony amongst the warring sections of humanity.

In modern times, he was the first to proclaim to the West, standing on a Western platform, the highest truths of Vedanta, which recognise man himself as God, thus truly transcending barriers of caste, creed, sex and religion. In a moment the world understood India, and the flag of eternal *dharma* was unfurled in the West. Vedanta became the topic of elitist study and discussion. The first sign of India's renaissance showed itself in the hall of the Parliament of Religions. The boat of Indian culture, found her way once again back into the stream of international life – all in a matter of minutes, thanks to the fire and force with which the message came out of the realized Master's mouth.

Out of his declarations, was formed a true wave of Universal Brotherhood, which drew into its vortex, hundreds of men and women with a rare catholicity of ideas and universal vision. Swamiji's appearance on the Western horizon, truly opened a flood-gate of sympathy and understanding for India and her problems. In his own Motherland, it ushered in an era of a new pride and faith, strengthened the currents of nationalism, which were faintly making their appearance here and there and truly laid the foundation of the struggle for Independence that was soon to sweep over the country.

By paying homage to this royal Patriot-saint with the lion's courage but with a heart soft as a petal, we pay homage to all that is best, beautiful and glorious in Indian culture, because, in him was embodied the whole of India's culture. Such a multifaceted personality he was, it is difficult to describe him in a nutshell, as difficult as to describe Indian culture itself. In him was seen a spark of all that was glorious, strong and beautiful in all fields of human endeavour. Yet he transcended all of these. He was a musician par excellence, an orator who kept his audience spell-bound for any length of time, a true disciple, a true Master, a great friend and above all, an intense human being, moved to tears at the thought of suffering in another.

The universal dimension of Swamiji is what makes him truly appealing to the conservative East and the technologically advanced West. The seeker in him could accept no superstitions or super-impositions. He could be satisfied by truth and truth alone. And the search for truth which brought him to his great Master, also compelled him to accept and appreciate the truth in every religion and philosophy. His absolute devotion to truth, helped him to cut asunder layers of superstitious encrustations in his own religion and bring out the pristine purity of Vedanta in all its grandeur and universal application. At the same time, he could intuitively understand and appreciate the truth in other religions and philosophies. What irked him most was man's surrender to his own weaknesses, lack of faith in himself and the consequent 'fear' in the human mind. He traced all the sinful acts of man to this lack of strength and exhorted his countrymen all the time to shake off this great fear and establish the supremacy of their innate divinity. That each soul is potentially divine was not just a verbal assertion for him, but a reality which he lived every moment of his life.

Yet, the sufferings of his fellow countrymen, their poverty and misery moved him immensely and he exhorted his disciples to first feed the poor and then preach Vedanta. Breaking the myth of the traditional role of the Indian monk, who spent his time seeking his personal salvation, Swamiji created a new order of monks based on "Renunciation and Service" where worship of the poor was at par with worship of God. This new concept has since then revolutionized the Indian idea of sannyasis, enjoining upon them to take up service as a mission and thus contribute to the welfare of the poor and the downtrodden. The establishment of Ramakrishna Mission apart from Ramakrishna Math, is thus a glorious tribute to Swamiji's great compassion for suffering humanity.

Today, only the sparks that emanated from his fire, remain with us, each more sublime than the other, messages that are enough to transform one's life and lead a Nation onward in its march....

....'Arise! Awake! Stop not till the Goal is reached'....'Renunciation and Service'....'Each Soul is potentially Divine'....'All expansion is growth, all contraction is death'....'Work is Worship', 'Faith, faith, faith in ourselves, faith in God – this is the secret of greatness'....'Strength is life, weakness is death'....'Be and Make'....'Man-making and Nation-building'....

....Out of the still burning embers of his pyre must we create a new religion and universal tolerance, acceptance, and brotherhood....Out of these sparks, we have to build the fire of the New India....Out of his spirit, should the magic bird of a new faith in our religion and culture take flight....Out of this new awareness and faith alone, can we re-establish our national character, honour and dignity. The time is not far, when Indians-the upholders of the oldest faith and heirs to the great immortal messages of the Upanishads, are called upon to render account to the rest of mankind.

Only then can we claim to be the children of this ancient Motherland of his dreams – "awakened once more, sitting on Her throne, rejuvenated more glorious than ever." Then alone can we "proclaim Her to all the world with voice of peace and benediction."

He breathed a new life into India
– K. P. Leelamma

If India is resurgent today, if it is pulsating with a new life and vigour and if it has been able to make a mark on the modern history of the world, it is because Swami Vivekananda – the Patriot-saint of India, had breathed a new life into it. He had the vision of a prophet and his message is not for the hour, but for the age, not for the nation only, but for humanity. As far as Indian renaissance is concerned, there is no aspect of culture which Swamiji has not touched. He did not care much for little bits of social reforms. He had in view a complete rejuvenation of the national life of India in all its phases. He knew that the solution of any problem cannot be attained on racial or national grounds, for any problem if it has to be solved on a permanent basis will affect the entire world.

During the travel from Kashmir to Cape Comorin, Swami Vivekananda was able to see India, study her history, see with naked eyes to what low depth, she, the once glorious land of the Hindus had gone down and he could clearly visualize the cause of her downfall. And he had finally come to the conclusion that the causes of her present downfall were neglect of the masses and trampling upon women. In his opinion, no amount of politics would be of any avail until the masses were more educated, well fed and well cared for. They were at the root of every prosperity the country enjoyed, but they got in turn only kicks from the authorities. Women who were .considered to be the embodiments of the Divine Mother had been turned into mere manufacturing machines. Laws had been made just to bind them down and nothing had been done to raise their status. And until these two evils were rooted out no amount of reform was going to regenerate India.

Imitating other countries and nurturing their civilization in this country was not good. All attempts to Europeanize India are useless. For, any attempt will not Europeanize India. If India is giving up spirituality and going after the materialistic civilization of the West, the result will be that in three generations the nation will be extinct. Because, he says that "the backbone of the nation will be broken, the foundation upon which the national edifice has been built will be undermined and the result will be annihilation all round."

He did not mean that we should not go out and assimilate anything from outside. We have to assimilate whatever is good in other nations and develop our society on that basis.

A great saint and fervid nationalist
– Dr. R. C. Majumdar

Vivekananda championed the cause of Hinduism in the Parliament of religions held at Chicago (U. S. A.) in 1893 in connection with the celebration of the 400th anniversary of the discovery of America by Columbus, There, in the presence of the representatives of all the religions from almost all the countries in the world, the young monk from India expounded the principles of Vedanta and the greatness of Hinduism with such persuasive eloquence that from the very first he captivated the hearts of the vast audience. It would be hardly an exaggeration to say that Swami Vivekananda made a place for Hinduism in the cultural map of the modern world. The civilized nations of the West had hitherto looked down upon Hinduism as a bundle of superstitions, evil institutions, and immoral customs, unworthy of serious consideration in the progressive world of today. Now, for the first time, they not only greeted, with hearty approval, the lofty principles of Hinduism as expounded by Vivekananda, but accorded a very high place to it in the cultures and civilizations of the world. The repercussion of this on the vast Hindu community can be easily imagined. The Hindu intelligentsia were always very sensitive to the criticism of the Westerners, particularly the missionaries, regarding the many evils and shortcomings of the Hindu society and religion, as with their rational outlook they could not but admit the force of much of this criticism. They had always to be on the defensive and their attitude was mostly apologetic, whenever there was a comparative estimate of the values of the Hindu and Western culture. They had almost taken for granted the inferiority of their culture vis-a-vis that of the West, which was so confidently asserted by the Western scholars. Now, all on a sudden, the table was turned and the representatives of the West joined in a chorus of applause at the hidden virtues of Hinduism which were hitherto unsuspected either by friends or foes. It not only restored the self-confidence of the Hindus in their own culture and civilization, but quickened their sense of national pride and patriotism. This sentiment was echoed and re-echoed in the numerous public addresses which were presented to Swami Vivekananda on his homecoming by the Hindus all over India, almost literally from Cape Comorin to the Himalayas. It was a great contribution to the growing Hindu nationalism.

On his return to India, Swami Vivekananda preached the spiritual basis of Hindu civilization and pointed out in his writings and speeches that the spirituality of India was not less valuable, nor less important for the welfare of humanity, than the much vaunted material greatness of the West which has dazzled our eyes. He was never tired of asking the Indians to turn their eyes, dazed by the splendour of the West, to their own ideals and institutions. By a comparative estimate of the real values of the Hindu ideals and institutions and those of the West he maintained the superiority of the former and asked his countrymen never to exchange gold for tinsel....

But Vivekananda was not prejudiced against the West nor insensitive to the value of her achievements. He frankly admitted that Indian culture was neither spotless nor perfect. It has to learn many things from the West, but without sacrificing its true character.

Swami Vivekananda combined in himself the role of a great saint and fervid nationalist. He placed Indian nationalism on the high pedestal of past glory, and it embraced the teeming millions of India both high and low, rich and poor. He devoted his life to the awakening of national consciousness and many of his eloquent appeals would stir the national sentiments of India even today to their very depths....

Though an ascetic, Vivekananda was a patriot of patriots. The thought of restoring the pristine glory of India by resuscitating among her people the spiritual vitality which was dormant, but not dead, was always the upper- most thought in his mind....

This great sannyasin who had left his hearth and home at the call of his spiritual guru, Sri Ramakrishna, and delved deeply into spiritual mysticism, was never tired of preaching that what India needs today is not so much religion or philosophy, of which she has enough, but food for her hungry millions, social justice for the low classes, strength and energy for her emasculated people and a sense of pride and prestige as a great nation of the world. He made a trumpet call to all Indians to shed fear of all kinds and stand forth as men by imbibing *Shakti* (energy and strength), by reminding them that they were the particles of the Divine according to the eternal truth preached by the Vedanta. The precepts and example of this great sannyasin galvanized the current of national life, infused new hopes and inspirations and placed the service to the motherland on a religious level....

Swami Vivekananda thus gave a spiritual basis to Indian nationalism. The lessons of the Vedanta and *Bhagavad Gita* permeated the lives and activities of many nationalists, and many a martyr, inspired by his teachings, endured extreme sufferings and sacrifices with a cheerful heart, fearlessly embraced death, and calmly bore the inhuman tortures, worse than death, which were sometimes inflicted upon them....

Vivekananda was par excellence a religious devotee – a saint of the highest category gifted with extraordinary spiritual powers.... The most distinctive feature of Swami Vivekananda's teachings is that he applied his philosophic principles to the affairs of everyday life. He laid emphasis on the fact that we shall seek salvation, not so much in the traditional way, by renouncing the world and taking to the life of a recluse, as by serving the God in man.

He could only lay the foundation of the great organization which bears the name of his guru. He never ceased to proclaim that in all that he did he merely followed in the footsteps of his guru.... To give a concrete shape to Ramakrishna's spiritual teachings, to spread his mission all over the world, and place it on a stable basis – these are the greatest achievements to the credit of Vivekananda.

The practical application of his guru's ideal of service, as interpreted by Swami Vivekananda, paved the way for the regeneration of India.

....The development of religion and spirituality and the regeneration of the down-trodden Indian masses formed the two chief planks in Vivekananda's programme for the future of India. It is interesting to note that the two greatest Indians of the twentieth century, Aurobindo Ghosh and Mahatma Gandhi, took up these two aspects of Swamiji's programme as the chief aims of their activities. Some of the poems of Rabindranath indicate that he was also influenced by Swamiji's ideas of living and working among men, and serving the God in man.... Thus the three great Indians of the twentieth century were all inspired by him. And this has been openly admitted by Aurobindo and Gandhi.

Swamiji looked upon the propagation of spiritual teaching in the West as the great task now before India. He laid the foundations of his humanitarian work in America. But he knew that India cannot play an effective role in this direction so long as she occupies only the status of a subject country. Free India should now take up the task which Vivekananda had begun, and should build upon the foundations so well and truly laid by him.

A forceful and dynamic personality

– A. Sreedhara Menon

In the whole range of religious philosophy it is very difficult to come across a personality so forceful and so dynamic as that of Swami Vivekananda. Swami Vivekananda lived only for 39 years, 5 months and 3 weeks. Born on the 12th January, 1863, he died on 4th July, 1902. As he himself had prophesied, he did not live up to the age of 40.

There were four important factors which influenced the life of Swami Vivekananda, viz., his early training and education under his parents, his contact with Sri Ramakrishna, his travels in the country which gave him an intimate knowledge of the problems and aspirations of the people of India and, above all, his own contact with Western science and philosophy.

There are various aspects of his work which deserve notice. He wanted that the people of this country should progress not merely in the moral field but also in other fields as well.... He never wanted India to be a nation which is not physically strong. Bengal in those days was the cradle of Indian Nationalism. In fact, a few years after the death of Swami Vivekananda, there was the partition of Bengal and intense political agitation. The great revolutionaries of Bengal in those days always used to look up to Vivekananda and his teachings for ideological inspiration. Of course, his teachings contained moral exhortations to the people. They emphasized particularly the need for action and work. To the political revolutionaries of those days, there was nothing conservative or reactionary about the teachings of Swami Vivekananda. In fact, every one of them carried in his pocket or kept in his library a book on the speeches and sayings of Swami Vivekananda, because they served to keep alive the spirit of patriotism of the people. It was possible for him to rouse the people from their slumber and awaken their national consciousness. He made them feel a sense of national identity. We speak nowadays of "national integration." Swami Vivekananda was in his days a great exponent of the message of national integration. There were other great contemporaries like Lokamanya Tilak, Aravind Ghosh and others whom he influenced in many ways.

Swami Vivekananda had a progressive social outlook. He has been called the 'cyclonic Hindu', the patriot monk of India. He advocated the cause of radical social reforms. He condemned the caste-system. Vivekananda was also against various social evils that prevailed in this country. He spoke against 'untouchability' or what he called 'don't-touchism.' The campaign against untouchability gained momentum in the days of the struggle for freedom under Mahatma Gandhi. It was a continuation of the fight of Swami Vivekananda against this social evil. The Swami wanted the people of India to feel that they are Indians first and thus rise above the barriers of caste and creed. He wanted every Indian to feel a sense of national pride and also a sense of national identity.

....Swami Vivekananda believed that there is the divine spark in every man. He did not believe in the doctrine that man is a sinner. He thought that to say that man is a sinner is a libel on human nature. He wanted every Indian to serve his poverty-stricken, illiterate and suffering fellowmen by providing medical treatment, educational facilities and other kinds of social service. In fact, the message that work is worship was the most dynamic message given by Swami Vivekananda. The Ramakrishna Mission of which he was the founder is in fact one of his great legacies to the people in this country and elsewhere.

Swami Vivekananda stood for the meeting of the East and West. It is true that he was a citizen of India, a nationalist to the core. But at the same time, as a result of his travels abroad, he had developed a global, universal, or world outlook and blossomed into a citizen of the world. He thought that it should be possible for the world to evolve a happy synthesis of all the best elements in Oriental culture, particularly Indian culture, and the values enshrined in Western science and technology. Though Kipling has sung that "the East is East and the West is West and the twain shall never meet", Swami Vivekananda was never pessimistic in this regard. He honestly believed that there is a meeting ground between the East and the West and that the spirituality of the East and the science and technology of the West can still blend and make a real contribution to the cause of international peace and understanding.

His great help
– The Mother (Mirra Alfassa), Pondicherry.

Between the age of nineteen and twenty, I had achieved conscious and constant union with the Divine Presence, and....I had done so all by myself with absolutely nobody to help me. When I found out, a little later, – Vivekananda's *Raja Yoga* came into my hands – it seemed so marvellous that someone was able to explain something to me. It enabled me to achieve in a few months something which I might have taken years to do.

He changed the direction of Indian nationalism
– Dr. V. K. Sukumaran Nair

Ramakrishna spoke of Vivekananda in these words, "He is not a pond, he is a reservoir; He is not pitcher or jug, he is a veritable barrel; He is not a minnow or sardine, he is a huge red-eyed carp; He is not an ordinary sixteen-petalled lotus, he is a glorious lotus with a thousand petals." Everything about Vivekananda suggested strength and vigour. It was inevitable that a religious and spiritual leader like Vivekananda should identify himself with the political aspects of the Indian renaissance. As Romain Rolland said "Men like Vivekananda are not made to whisper. They can only proclaim." What Vivekananda proclaimed in the loudest tones possible was that a new India, heir to a great cultural and spiritual legacy had been born and demanded a place under the sun.

Like other young men of his time Vivekananda came under the influence of Western science and liberalism. He studied the writings of John Stuart Mill as well as Kant and Hegel. He even entered into correspondence with Herbert Spencer. However, Vivekananda the rationalist was completely converted by Ramakrishna. It was Ramakrishna who introduced him to India's cultural traditions and the strength of its spiritual heritage. At the same time Vivekananda's intellectual interests and his wide travels made him realize India's poverty and social backwardness. Vivekananda was greatly influenced by his visit to America. "The dynamism, social awareness, spirit of adventure, capacity for hard work and concern for practical values" that he saw in the West made a profound impression on his thinking and outlook. While Vivekananda was the first to give India's spiritual message to the West, he was also captivated by the dynamism that activated "Western Civilization." What he did was to forge a link between India's philosophical thinking and the approach of modern science. He made Hinduism a universal religion and rescued it from degenerating into a narrow and ritualistic creed.

Vivekananda's main contribution to political India was to bolster up the self-confidence of the Indian people. The myth of the superiority of Western civilization was demolished when the Parliament of Religions at Chicago hailed the new Messiah from the East. India assumed a new significance in the West as the home of spirituality. That the Western man, in spite of material prosperity and technological superiority, should hunger for Indian spirituality was something new for the Indian who had been forced to accept the superiority of the West.

Vivekananda thus changed the direction of Indian nationalism. In an indirect manner his teachings were responsible for the emergence of a new school of Indian nationalism. This school glorified Indian culture and civilization and demanded immediate withdrawal of British Power. If India had something to teach the world in the matter of spiritual values it was possible for Indian people to govern themselves. Vivekananda can thus be seen as the political *guru* of Lokamanya Tilak and Mahatma Gandhi. These leaders based their appeal on Indian traditional values. While Tilak gave a new and dynamic interpretation to the *Gita*, Mahatma Gandhi based his philosophy on the spiritual foundations of non-violent resistance.

Vivekananda's second major contribution was to spiritualize Indian politics. Until he came on the scene, political activity was directed by politicians and not by spiritual leaders. It was Vivekananda who aimed at the spiritual regeneration of India under the leadership of a dedicated band of missionaries. This was the same thing that Gokhale proposed in creating his "Servants of India Society." Mahatma Gandhi attempted to convert the Congress into a band of dedicated political missionaries.

The third major contribution of Vivekananda was to create a feeling in the minds of Indians that this country had a role to play in the world affairs. Vivekananda proclaimed Hindu culture as a universal culture with a message which could cut across the boundaries of mountain and sea. He was one of the first to break the insularity of India. India's importance in the world today is not due to its military or economic power. It is due to recognition by more powerful nations of India's influence as a centre of culture and civilisation. Vivekananda was one of the first to apreciate the extent of this influence. He made the West conscious of India's strength. He made the Indian people conscious of their own importance.

Though Vivekananda was not a political leader he made immense contributions to Indian political development. In fact he made foreign rule impossible. "Stand up, be bold, be strong. Take the whole responsibility on your shoulders and know that you are the creator of your own destiny." Words like this spoken by Vivekananda inspired an entire generation and made the freedom struggle possible. Vivekananda proclaimed to the Indian people that a great destiny awaited them if they could realise the meaning of this spiritual legacy. It was not a narrow patriotism that Vivekananda preached. He only wanted India to have its due place in the world. Vivekananda thus shaped the political values of India. These values are based on the new interpretation which he gave to Vedanta Philosophy. He declared that spiritual values were bound up with India's destiny.

The universally adored one
– Ottoor Subrahmanya Namboodiripad

अशेषान्तर्भावादमितवितते हैन्दवमते
विवेकानन्दोऽभूत् सकलमतराशेः प्रतिनिधिः ।
समे त्वन्ये दौत्यं निजनिजमतस्यैव विदधुः
प्रसिद्धे चिक्कागोनगरमिलिते धर्मसदसि ॥ १ ॥

In the Parliament of Religions held at Chicago, each one represented his own religion. But Vivekananda representing the Hindu Religion which is verily all-comprehensive, literally became the spokesman of all religions.

महायोगो मेरीतनयमतमानाय घटितो
व्यंरसीदार्षस्य च्युतिरहित धर्मस्य विजये ।
वधार्थं दैत्यारेर्निर्जविरचिते मल्लसमरे
स्वयं कंसो ध्वस्तो निरतिशयवीर्येण हरिणा ।। २ ।।

The great assembly convened to proclaim the greatness of the religion of
Christ – the son of Mary – concluded with a note of victory to the infallible
Arsha Dharma, as the pugilistic combat arranged by Kamsa to destroy the
indomitable Hari, the enemy of demons, proved to be an act of self-
destruction.

समक्षं सर्वेषामभिनवमहाधर्मसमितौ
विवेकानन्दस्य प्रयतवपुराविश्य रहसि ।
गृहीत्वाग्र्यां पूजामधिगतयशो हैन्दवमतं
जयेद्घण्टाकर्णैः कुटिलहृदयैर्भर्त्सितमपि ।। ३ ।।

The religion of the Hindus entering the body of Vivekananda, so to say,
won the highest acclaim in that assemblage of religions though it is often
criticized by the wicked.

विवेकानन्दाख्यसकलसुजनैः कीर्तितयशा-
स्सुगम्भीराकारः श्रुतिवचनसारार्थविदुरः ।
स्वजन्मोर्वीभक्तस्सहृदयमणिर्ब्रह्मविद्या परे
सदामग्रो लोकव्यवहतिविदग्धो विजयताम् ।। ४ ।।

May Vivekananda, whose qualities are sung by the worthy, who is
endowed with great physical charm, who is likened to Vidura for his
knowledge of the scriptures, who is a lover of his motherland, whose mind
is always immersed in the Supreme Soul and one well versed in the affairs
of the world, be victorious.

सुरश्लाघ्यश्लोकोऽप्यपगतमदोत्सेककणिकः
स्वजन्मोर्वीप्रिष्ठोऽप्यखिलजगतां क्षेमनिरतः ।
निजानंदारामोऽप्यगतिषु दयाविध्दहृदयो
विवेकानन्दाख्यो भुवि यतिवरेण्यो विजयताम् ॥ ५ ॥

May Vivekananda, the great saint, who despite divine acceptance remained
unspoiled by the rut of ego, who while remaining a lover of his motherland
sought the welfare of the people of all countries, who all the while immersed
in heavenly bliss was compassionate to the hapless, be victorious.

यतो निर्वेदाग्निर्ज्वलति विषयासक्तिदहनो
यतो ज्ञानादित्यस्तपति हृदयध्वान्तदलनः ।
यतश्च प्रेमेन्दुर्लसति परमानन्दरसदो
विवेकानन्दस्य त्रिभुवनगरिष्ठो विजयताम् ॥ ६ ॥

May Vivekananda, the foremost among the beings of the three worlds, from
whom the fire of renunciation bursts forth razing down the passion for
worldly things, from whom blazes forth the Sun of wisdom dispelling the
inner darkness and from whom shines forth the Moon of love bestowing
Supreme bliss, be victorious.

मूर्तं मुक्तिमहासुखं धृतवपुर्योगाधिरुढस्थितिः
स्वेच्छोपात्ततनुः पविब्रभगवद्धर्मस्वरूपा दया ।
दृश्यो भारतपूर्वपुण्यनिचयस्साङ्गं महापौरुषं
यस्मिन् भान्ति जयेच्चिराय स विवेकानन्द योगीश्वरः ॥ ७ ॥

May that *Yogiswara* Vivekananda who appears to be the personification
of the supreme beatitude of Salvation, the exalted state of yoga assuming
a form, the sacred *Bhagavata Dharma* (i.e. the virtuous actions performed
in the spirit of divine worship) taking a body out of self-will, mercy
personified, and who is the embodiment of the past accumulated virtue of
India, and in whom the great quality of valour is visible in fullness, be
eternally victorious.

स्वच्छन्दं भुवनेश्वरीजठरतो जातः स्वयं जन्मना-
संसिद्धोऽपि मनुष्यभावमनुसृत्यान्वेषयन् सद्गुरूं ।
चन्द्रासूनुमुपेत्य तत्करुणया ब्रह्मावगच्छन् स्फुटं
तज्ज्ञानं जगते वितीर्य गतवान् जेजेतुकाशीश्वरः ॥ ८ ॥

May that Lord of Kasi born from the womb of Bhuvaneswari of his own
will, though possessed of wisdom searching for a preceptor to be true to
his human form, approaching the son of Chandramani and realizing vividly
the Supreme Reality by His grace and imparting that knowledge to the world
before his disappearance, be victorious.

पुत्रत्वेनावतीर्णो निजचरणजुषोर्भक्तयोः काशिनाथ-
स्सिद्धाचार्य विचिन्वन्नतिविविदिषया रामकृष्णं प्रपन्नः ।
तस्माज्ज्ञात्वात्मतत्वं निखिलभुवमटन् भारतं चान्यदेशां-
श्रोद्धृत्याज्ञानकूपाज्जयतु यवनिकान्तर्हितोऽसौ नराख्यः ॥ ९ ॥

May Vivekananda, known as Narendranth who is verily an incarnation of
the Lord of Kashi, born as the son of parents who were His great devotees,
who took shelter in Ramakrishna, the saint, with intense thirst for realization
and who having obtained the Supreme Knowledge travelled all over India
and abroad, uplifting fellow-beings from the deep well of ignorance before
retiring from the scene, be victorious

पाश्चात्यैर्भारतीयैरपि सकलजनैस्सादरं स्तूयमान
कामार्थादैः पुमर्थैरहमहमिकया शश्वदन्वीयमानः ।
नानाशिष्यैस्सतीर्थ्यैः प्रणयजलधिभिः श्रद्धया सेव्यमानो
दर्पं यो नैव भेजे कचन जयतु स ब्रह्मनिष्ठो नरेन्द्रः ॥ १० ॥

May Narendra, adored equally by the West and the East, hunted relentlessly
by both *kama* and *artha*, followed by devoted disciples, bereft of pride
and established in the Supreme Reality, be victorious.

देवानां पुष्पवर्षो न्यपतदविरतं भूरिशो यस्य शीर्षे
मर्त्यानां स्तोत्रघोषो वियदनुरणयन् यस्य कर्णौ बिभेद ।
भक्तानामुत्तमाङ्गान्यनुपदमनमन् यस्य पादारविन्दे
सोऽसौ जीयात्रनरेन्द्रो भरतवसुमतीभाग्यसर्वस्वभूतः ।। ११ ।।

May Narendra, upon whose head the celestials poured forth flowers incessantly and in plenty, whose ears were rent with the eulogies of human beings echoing the sky, whose lotus feet were touched on every step by the heads of devotees prostrating in obeisance, and who is verily the fortune of the country of Bharata, be victorious.

अद्वैतज्ञानभानोरनुपहतगतौ शंकराचार्यतुल्यः
कारूण्यव्योमनद्यास्सरभसपतने बुद्धदेवोपमानः
एकान्तप्रेमभक्तेस्सुरुचिरविहृतौ कृष्णचैतन्यकल्पो
योगत्रय्याः प्रयागो जयतु विजयतां विश्ववन्द्यो नरेन्द्रः ।। १२ ।।

May Vivekananda, worshipped by the whole world, who is an equal to Shankaracharya in radiating the brilliance of the Sun of Advaitic wisdom, who is likened to Buddha for the forceful fall of the celestial Ganges of piety, who is similar to Sri Krishna Chaitanya in the beautiful play of divine love and who symbolizes the Prayaga for the confluence of the three yogas, be victorious.

Most impressive personality
– Dr. Gokul Chand Narang

It was in 1897, when I was student in the Second Year Class of the D. A. V. College, Lahore, that Swami Vivekananda paid a visit to that city. He was received at the railway station by large crowds. He was invited to deliver a lecture and he made his first speech in the fortress-like Haveli of Raja Dhyan Singh, who used to be the Prime Minister of the Punjab during Maharaja Ranjit Singh's reign. The subject of the lecture was: *"Common Bases of Hinduism."* He dealt with various features and aspects of Hinduism. I need hardly say that the lecture, and Swamiji's wonderful oratory made a tremendous impact on the audience. It was heard by the large concourse of admirers with rapt attention.

He delivered another lecture in a college on the philosophy of Vedanta. In this lecture he dealt at length with the various points of Vedantism. This was later published and probably this was one of the most important, if not the most important, of his lectures.

He was also pleased to pay a visit to our college and came to our room when our Professor was lecturing on some subject of physics. Of course, the whole class rose like one man and cheered. Swamiji had a most impressive personality and cheerfulness radiated from his face. He went round the other classes also and had some conversation with our Principal.

Swami Vivekananda was accompanied by some Americans, one of whom if I remember correctly – was one Capt. Sevier. We were told that these Americans were so devoted to the Swami's personality that while the Swami slept on a well-furnished bed, his American disciples slept on the ground out of respect for him as faithful disciples.

Swamiji is said to have been asked why he had brought these white Americans with him and he is reported to have said that as the Indians as a nation suffered from inferiority complex and the white nations look upon them with little regard, he brought them with him so that our people might cast off to a certain extent the feeling of inferiority from which they suffered, as they could see that even white people can show such devoted respect for a brown Indian! This might have been more in a jocular vein but there was great truth in it.

The Swami was indeed one of the greatest Indians.

A multiple personality with a multiple vision
– M. P. Pandit

It was at a meeting of learned pundits in Madras that young Vivekananda was explaining how Dvaita, Visishtadvaita and Advaita were not to be looked upon as contradictory lines of Vedanta but were really successive stages of spiritual realizations. Someone from the audience asked him why, if that was so, none of the Masters had mentioned it so far. The reply was startling: "Because I was born for this, and it was left for me to do."

This attitude was typical of the young monk. He started life as a strong individualist and continued to be so till the very end of his life. Nothing was true to him unless it satisfied his individual tests. Even his renowned Teacher, Sri Ramakrishna, respected this demand of his soul and took care to communicate the experience to him before asking him to believe in it. "Each one", declared Vivekananda, "must preserve his individuality and grow according to his own law of growth." Each individual has a spark of Divinity in him and it is the purpose of life to develop it and manifest it in life. Religion is a means to awaken to this Divine Presence, articulate it and develop one's consciousness Godward. All religions have this truth at their core and men must find their unity at this level instead of fighting over their respective claims. Listen to his faith: "I accept all religions that were in the past and worship them all. I worship God with every one of them, in whatever form they worship Him! I shall go to the mosque of a Mohammedan. I shall enter the Christian Church and kneel before the Crucifix. I shall enter the Buddhist temple and there I shall take refuge in the Buddha and his law. I shall go into the forest and sit down in meditation trying to see the light which enlightens the heart of every one."

And after he found the light and the inner liberation what did the fiery young man do? Merge in the Bliss of Brahman? No, he had heard the call of the disguised Godhead in Humanity. He looked around and in the nobility of his large being, he could not think of saving himself when millions wire groaning in the world. His immediate concern was with the downtrodden masses in India who had been exploited and denied their elementary rights in the name of the religion, under specious pleas of tradition and so on. His spirit rebelled at the travesty that had been made of the truths of the Hindu Religion. He boldly proclaimed that *All is Brahman,* God dwells in every person irrespective of his social or economic or political standing and this Universal Godhead has got to be served before one's own mission in life is completed. He called for dedicated service from awakened men and women to raise the masses from their unrelieved poverty – material, cultural and spiritual – so as to manifest the Divinity in this ancient race inhabiting India. "So long as the millions live in hunger and ignorance, I hold every man a traitor who, having been educated at their expense, pays not the least heed to them." Thus did Vivekananda initiate a social revolution on a spiritual basis. If today we find work for the downtrodden, the suffering and the underprivileged treated as part of religious or spiritual movements in India, the first credit must go to this modern monk. His influence is everywhere. As Sri Aurobindo observes: "We perceive his influence still working gigantically, we know not well how, we know not well where, in something that is not yet formed, something leonine, grand, intuitive, upheaving that has entered the soul of India, and we say, 'Behold Vivekananda still lives in the soul of his Motherland and in the souls of her children.' "

His feeling and his vision were not confined to the boundaries of his motherland. During his extensive travels abroad and by his comprehensive study of the history of nations and their peoples, his heart had learnt to beat in unison with the heart of the whole of humanity. He refused to accept the current geographical and political segmentations of the world and preferred to stress on the underlying oneness of life, oneness of goal notwithstanding the different assignments to different civilizations by the Divine Creator. He said: "I see that each nation, like each individual, has one theme in this life, which is its centre, the principal note round which every other note comes to form this harmony. In one nation, political power is its vitality, as in England. Artistic life in another, and so on. In India, religious life forms the centre." But he was not blind to the failings of societies, whether in India or in Europe. He predicted the collapse of Europe within fifty years unless she changed the material basis of her life to the spiritual – a prophecy that has come true to the letter. He also foresaw the awakening and the rise of the Chinese people and warned the world against a possible peril in that development, He confidently saw the coming of a new wave of civilization, the rule and values of the proletariat.

Vivekananda was thus a multiple personality with a multiple mission and multiple vision. In him fused together the true concerns of the Individual, the Collectivity and the Race. He found in himself the secure base of the manifest Divine on which he could erect the magnificent edifice of a renovated Humanity – '*Atmano mokshartham jagaddhitaya cha*', for the liberation of the self and the weal of the world.

To sum up: he combined in himself the best of modern science in its application to human problems and the tradition of the Vedanta at its widest; to his sturdy spiritual individualism he joined his intense universalism – horizontal and vertical. He brought the East and the West together for a spiritual dialogue which continues to this day.

Unifier of Hindu ideology
– K. M. Panikkar

What gave Indian nationalism its dynamism and ultimately enabled it to weld at least the major part of India into one state was the creation of a sense of community among the Hindus to which the credit should to a very large extent go to Swami Vivekananda. This new Sankaracharya may well be claimed to be a unifier of Hindu ideology. Travelling all over India he not only aroused a sense of Hindu feeling but taught the doctrine of a universal Vedanta as the background of the new Hindu reformation.... The Hindu religious movements before him were local, sectarian and without any all-India impact. The Arya Samaj, the Brahmo Samaj, the Deva Samaj and other movements, very valuable in themselves, only tended further to emphasize the provincial character of the reform movements. It is Vivekananda who first gave to the Hindu movement its sense of nationalism and provided most of the movements with a common all-India outlook.

His impact and influence still live dynamically
– P. Parameswaran

That man is really great, whose relevance outlives him by decades or centuries. Swami Vivekananda is one such....

Vivekananda's appeal is not confined to any particular section of people. Though, as his favourite disciple Sister Nivedita put it, "He was born a lover and the queen of his adoration was his Motherland." His message was universal. Although he was an all-renouncing sannyasi, he was equally an all-embracing patriot, and was known as the 'Patriot-Monk of India.' While he was a philosopher of the highest order, he was a radical revolutionary in his ideas. No wonder, one of the greatest sons of Modem India, himself a thorough-going revolutionary, Subash Chandra Bose said this about Swami Vivekananda: "If Swamiji had been alive today, he would have been my guru; that is to say, I would have accepted him as Master. It is needless to add, however, that as long as I live, I shall be absolutely loyal to Ramakrishna-Vivekananda."

If these are the words of an arch revolutionary, inspired with deep surge of emotions, here is a glorious tribute paid to the great Swamiji, by probably the most balanced, rational and mature statesman of India, C. Rajagopalachari: "Swami Vivekananda saved Hinduism and saved India. But for him, we would have lost our religion, and would not have gained our independence. We therefore owe everything to Swami Vivekananda."

While the capitalist West – England, America and Europe – came under his magnetic spell, Russia of that time, spoke with great admiration about the Swami through her great son Leo Tolstoy. "The reading of such books (Vivekananda's) is more than a pleasure, it is a broadening of the soul."

Why is it that men of such diverse views and temperaments living in any part of the globe, found in Swami Vivekananda an object of admiration? Why is it that poets like Tagore, philosophers like Radhakrishnan, men of action like Gandhiji, statesmen like Rajaji, seers like Aurobindo, Marxist ideologists like Rybakov, scholars like Will Durant, and politicians like Jawaharlal Nehru, found in the great Swami a greatness worthy of equal adoration? What was that spark in Swami Vivekananda, that elicited the spontaneous admiration, bordering on veneration, of these and others, who are by no means men of ordinary stature?

One most dominating factor for this is that the Swamiji was the very epitome of India, of her entire past, present and future, and the very soul of her aspirations. No wonder Rabindranath Tagore acclaimed: "If you want to know India, study Vivekananda. In him everything is positive and nothing negative." That was the unique greatness of the Swamiji. He represented India in her best and the most positive aspects. Maharshi Aurobindo, in his inimitable style, introduced Swamiji to his readers "as a soul of puissance, if ever there was one, a very lion among men, but the definite work he has left behind is quite incommensurate with our impression of his creative might and energy. We perceive his influence still working gigantically, we know not well how, we know not well where, in something that is not yet formed, something leonine, grand, intuitive, upheaving that has entered the soul of India and we say 'Behold, Vivekananda still lives in the soul of his Mother, and in the souls of her children.' "

So Vivekananda's impact and influence still live and live quite dynamically. India's national leaders and freedom fighters, with hardly an exception, had his stamp imprinted on them. From his inexhaustible store of unalloyed patriotism, they gathered their inspiration to dedicate themselves to the cause of the Motherland. "I have gone through his work very thoroughly" says Mahatma Gandhi, "and after having gone through them, the love that I had for my country became a thousand fold." Pandit Nehru had no reservations to admit that "many of my generation were very powerfully influenced by him, and I think it would be a great deal of gift to the present generation if they also went through Swami Vivekananda's writings and speeches, and they would learn much from them." Nehru found in Vivekananda a great man, "rooted in the past and full of pride in India's heritage, Vivekananda was yet modern in his approach to life's problems and was a kind of bridge between the past of India and her present." Nehru almost goes lyrical when he describes the Swamiji thus: "He was a fine figure of a man imposing, full of poise and dignity, sure of himself and his mission and at the same time full of a dynamic and fiery energy and a passion to push India forward. He came as a tonic to the depressed and demoralized Hindu mind and gave it self-reliance and some roots in the past."

So this was Vivekananda, ancient yet modern, a bridge between India's past and present: a beacon-light beckoning her to her destined and glorious goal. He not only bridged India's past with her present, he also bridged the East with West.... While remaining uncompromising in the matter of Hindu nationalism, Swami Vivekananda set in motion the dynamic forces that go to create what we today call "one world."

As the great revolutionary savant, M. N. Roy, has pertinently pointed out, "The reaction of native culture against the introduction of Western education ran wild, so to say, in the person of Vivekananda and the cult of universal religion he formulated. He preached Hinduism – not Indian nationalism – should be aggressive. He called on Young India to believe in the spiritual union of India. This romantic vision of conquering the world by spiritual superiority electrified the young intellectuals."

He initiated a new movement of humanitarianism
– Dr. K. Raghavan Pillai

As in several things, the contact with the West from the 17th century onward rekindled the conscience and impulses of India. The large-scale humanitarian service rendered by Christian missionaries, although very often done with the object of conversion, opened the eyes of the Hindu. He started to look at himself critically and found to his dismay, that he who preached the oneness of all negated it in everyday practice. Swami Vivekananda was the most powerful expression of this self-examination and awakened conscience of India.

In many respects it was inevitable that he represented this new urge in India and gave expression to it. The Swami was the embodiment of youth, pulsating with life, blood and vigour. This vitality was completely free from selfish urges, and in its pure and powerful state it could not but vibrate in unison with life all round him. And what was life around him? It was the very negation of it, frustrated in the mire of poverty, ignorance and misery. The emergence of Vivekananda as the champion of the *Daridranarayanas* of India was an inescapable fact arising from the very constitution of his personality and the impact that the degradation of the country had on it. We may remember in this connection that among Sri Ramakrishna's disciples there were some at least who did not see eye to eye with him in this matter of the diversion of spiritual discipline and power into the path of humanitarian activities. Not that they lacked in love of man; but their nature perhaps was turned to the life of the recluse meditating in isolation and treading their lonely spiritual paths. Vivekananda's modern education, his extrovert-introvert personality, his contact with the Western world, his natural compassion were all factors which made him lead this new movement of humanitarianism in Hindu religious life.

....Over and over again, the Swami declared that the service of man was adequate worship of God. Through the Swamiji's life-work, and the work of those who followed him, Hinduism has expiated for the sin of its long neglect of its own cardinal teaching of the oneness of all life in actual practice.

Looking at the India which was contemporary with the Swamiji, one can see the difficult path he had to tread in creating a new consciousness of active humanitarianism in the country. The rich at that time were like the rich at all times in every country – selfish, smug and indifferent to human suffering. The poor were too crushed to think in terms of upgrading themselves through their own efforts or the efforts of others. They had given up hopes and took refuge in bleak despair and a justification for inaction in fate. Young people with modern education had become cynical and contemptuous of the heritage of the country and ignorant of their own duties to their fellow-men. Running after the glory of the West many of them were blind to their duties at home in their country. It was this almost unresponsive nation that the Swami had to fire with a new humanitarian impulse generated from religion. He did it with his thunderous message repeatedly delivered with authority and sometimes anger and through the organizational activities which he and his associates undertook.

The tradition in Hinduism was to establish temples in the wake of new religious movements. Swami Vivekananda also established temples; they were of two kinds, one, the orthodox temples and another the number of hospitals to treat the sick.

Subsequent to Swami Vivekananda several great men thought in terms of employing religion to serve the poor. Mahatma Gandhi did it on a nationwide scale, Sri Narayana Guru did it in Kerala. In modern times it is to Swami Vivekananda that the credit goes to have first conceived on a large scale the notion of serving God through the service of man.

The foremost leader of mankind
– Dr. P. K. Narayana Pillai

तपस्विनं सप्तमहर्षिमण्डले
ददर्श यं तैजसरूपवान् शिशुः ।
वितप्तलोकोचितसेवने रतं
विवेकमानन्दयुतं प्रणौमि तम् ॥ १

My homage to Vivekananda whom the Divine Child (Sri Ramakrishna) found in the region of *saptarishis* as a sage inclined to render suitable service to those in distress.

प्रसादतः काशिमहेश्वरप्रभोः
प्रकीर्तनैर्मातुरथार्थनाशतैः ।
शिवांशसम्भूतमनर्घमर्भकं
विवेकमानन्दयुतं प्रणौमि तम् ॥ २

My homage to Vivekananda the priceless child born of a part of Shiva Himself as a result of the grace of Lord Vishwanatha who was propitiated by the mother through ceaseless prayers and importunities.

विवित्सया निस्तुलया च मेधया
विशिष्टसौशील्यगुणादिभिश्च यः
.समेषु विध्यार्थिषु मुख्यतां गतो
विवेकमानन्दयुतं प्रणौमि तम् ॥ ३

My homage to Vivekananda who with his great earnestness in study, unparalleled intellect, excellent character and other similar qualities stood topmost in the student community.

गदाधरं विश्वपतेर्दिदृक्षया
समेत्य सर्वादृतदक्षिणेश्वरे
तदीयशिष्योत्तम भावभूषितं
विवेकमानन्दयुतं प्रणौमि तम् ॥ ४

My homage to Vivekananda who in his great aspiration to see God, approached Sri Ramakrishna in Dakshineswar, a place held in reverence by all, and distinguished himself as the foremost among the disciples of that great teacher.

गुरोर्निदेशात्रिजदेशसेवने
कृतादरं भारतदर्शनोत्सुकम् ।
परिव्रजन्तं परिनिष्ठयोगिनं
विवेकमानन्दयुतं प्रणौमि तम् ॥ ५

My homage to Vivekananda the great yogin who undertook a religious wandering to observe India, as he got interested in serving the motherland at the behest of his teacher.

शिलां शिवामेत्य कुमारिकापुरे
सहोदरो द्वारविचिन्तने स्थितम् ।
अमेरिकायानविनिश्चिताशयं
विवेकमानन्दयुतं प्रणौमि तम् ॥ ६

My homage to Vivekananda who having reached the holy rock at Kanyakumari remained there in meditation searching for the means to uplift his brethren and at last came to the decision to go to America.

महात्मनां भिन्नमतानुयायिनां
सभातले धर्मसमन्वयाशयम् ।
समर्प्य विद्योतितविश्वमानसं
विवेकमानन्दयुतं प्रणौमि तम् ॥ ७

My homage to Vivekananda who enlightened the world as a whole by presenting the ideal of religious synthesis at the World's Parliament of Religions in which great men representing different faiths participated.

अमेरिकास्वांगलदेशसीम्न्यपि
प्रसार्य वेदान्तसुधारसं परम् ।
समार्जितागोलयशःप्रभोज्वलं
विवेकमानन्दयुतं प्रणौमि तम् ॥ ८

My homage to Vivekananda who won international glory by popularizing extensively the great Vedanta philosophy in America and England.

विदेशतः सम्प्रतिपद्य भारतं
प्रबुद्धदेशीयपथेन सोदरान् ।
प्रचोदयन्तं जनतैकनायकं
विवेकमानन्दयुतं प्रणौमि तम् ॥ ९

My homage to Vivekananda the foremost among the leaders of our country, who returning to India from the West, led his countrymen on the path of enlightened nationalism.

जगत्कृते देशिकरामकृष्णसं-
स्मृति समादृत्य समाजनिर्मितौ ।
कृतश्रमं प्राप्तसमाधिमिच्छया
विवेकमानन्दयुतं प्रणौमि तम् ॥ १०

My homage to Vivekananda who founded the great Mission in memory of his illustrious teacher, Sri Ramakrishna, for the good of the entire world and finally attained *mahasamadhi* at his pleasure.

Father of modern Indian nationalism
– R. G. Pradhan

Swami Vivekananda might well be called the father of modern Indian Nationalism; he largely created it and also embodied in his own life its highest and noblest elements.

He embodied the spirit of India
– Dr. S. Radhakrishnan

The city of Calcutta has produced many men of genius in education, science, literature and spiritual endeavour and one of the greatest of them all is Swami Vivekananda. He embodied the spirit of this country. He was a symbol of her spiritual aspirations and fulfilment. It is that spirit which was expressed in the songs of our devotees, the philosophies of our seers, the prayers of our common people. He gave articulation and voice to that eternal spirit of India.... He felt the pangs of all human beings and he wanted that every human being should live, should live a decent life. Most of us exist, but do not live. He wanted every one of us to acquire strength, beauty, power, dignity and be a truly human being.... And if there is any call which

Vivekananda made to us, it is to rely on our own spiritual resources. Say that man has inexhaustible spiritual resources. His spirit is supreme, man is unique. There is nothing inevitable in this world, and we can ward off the worst dangers and worst disabilities by which we are faced. Only we should not lose hope. He gave us fortitude in suffering; he gave us hope in distress; he gave us courage in despair.... Renunciation, courage, service, discipline – these are the mottoes which we can learn from his life.

It is essential, therefore, that we should remember what this great soul stood for, what he taught us. It is not merely a question of remembering it but trying to understand what he wished us to do. We shall assimilate his teachings, incorporate them in our own being, and make us worthy to be citizens of the country which produced Vivekananda.

When I was a student in the early years of this century, we used to read Swami Vivekananda's speeches and letters which were then passing from hand to hand in manuscript form and they used to stir us a great deal and make us feel proud of our ancient culture. Though our externals were broken down, the spirit of our country is there and is everlastingly real — that was the message which we gathered from his speeches and writings when I was a young student.

But today we can see a growing tendency among our young men and women to think that all these things are not of date, that they have betrayed us and that we should turn to copying another kind of civilization. We may possess Indian bodies, but we must borrow other souls to inhabit them.

I should like to ask you whether you are so much satisfied with the high-pressure machine civilization that had led us to this tragedy in which we are today.

The question is 'What is man?' Is he a crawling earthworm? Or, is he the most cunning of all animals, or is he an economic being controlled by the laws of supply and demand, or is he, as Swami Vivekananda said, an 'Atman', a universal spirit? However dense, however obstinate, however depraved a human being may be, there is that essential divine spark in him, that can never be surrendered.

Swami Vivekananda has made an appeal to us to realize that a human being is not to be regarded as an earthworm or an economic being, or a political creature, but that he has an inner citadel, a sanctuary of his soul which cannot be penetrated by anything external, and the inner sanctuary of his, will have to be preserved against attacks of economics and politics.... That is the gospel for which Swami Vivekananda stood and that has saved India until the present moment, and that is the gospel to which we have been disloyal.

There are people who say we are contemplative and that we are not sufficiently practical. But that must be regarded as something which is not corroborated by any of our great writers or lives of great personalities. You cannot think of more dynamic personalities in this country than those religious geniuses who have stirred us to incarnate the high ideals of spirit. Buddha, Sankara and the Gitacharya, all these are people who not only dwelt on mountain heights, but returned to the service of the ordinary men, came back to the plane of history. If moments of contemplation are necessary to make us firm in this attitude, moments of actions are equally necessary to put those ideals to practical service. By standing up for the great ideals which alone can save humanity, by standing up for them, Swami Vivekananda tried to lead humanity to a nobler and better path than that which it found itself in.

We are today at a critical period not merely in the history of our country but in the history of the world. There are many people who think we are on the edge of an abyss. There is distortion of values, there is lowering of standards, there is widespread escapism, a good deal of mass hysteria, and people think of it and collapse in despair, frustration, hopelessness. These are the only things which are open to us. Such a kind of lack of faith in the spirit of man is a treason to the dignity of man. It is an insult to human nature. It is human nature that has brought about all the great changes that have taken place in this world.... Swamiji told us: 'Do not be led away by the appearances. Deep down there is a providential will, there is a purpose in this universe. You must try to co-operate with that purpose and try to achieve it.'

Whatever may be your social programme, whatever resolutions you may bring about in the economic and political world, unless you have the dynamic inspiration of religion, you will never succeed in this enterprise. Even if you are radically minded, ask yourself the question whether you are going to reduce human beings to mere political or social creatures or would you give him some inner sanctity which nothing outward can touch? If you really believe in the divine spark in man, do not for a moment hesitate to accept the great tradition which has come to us, of which Vivekananda was the greatest exponent.

His universalism
– Prof. S. S. Raghavachar

Sri Ramakrishna and Swami Vivekananda are the makers of modern India in so far as its philosophy of life is concerned. Sri Ramakrishna is the master, the originating seer of the vision and the Swami is the authenticated and inspired interpreter of his message in the medium of thought and life. Full articulation of what Swamiji stood for as a whole and the nature of the epoch he opened up lies beyond our powers. We can only choose a particular line of devoted approach for our tribute to this mighty heritage.

Swami Vivekananda rescued our philosophical and religious outlook from its conventional and particular form, with all its fixity of loyalty and specificity of historical structure, and liberated it into universality, investing it with power to illumine and guide human life as a whole, breaking down inherited exclusiveness and rigidity. The universalism of the message he delivered is a fascinating theme.

Vedanta in the hands of Swami Vivekananda, passing through the crucible of science and reason in general, ceases to be a particular religious tradition and ascends to its legitimate status of a universal philosophical standpoint.

Spirituality or religion for Sri Ramakrishna and Swami Vivekananda is not a mere matter of belief or assent through even reasoned conviction. It is affirmed time and again that it is essentially realization or an experiential certainty.

Vivekananda, the great Vedantin he is, builds up a strong and invulnerable case for the ethics of humanity and service. His ascetic ethics breaks forth into a tremendous gospel of service. This is the universalism, unlimited and dynamic, that he propounds in his fiery orations to the people of India, broken up into countless fragments by birth, occupation and culture.

The humanism of Vivekananda, springing from his Vedanta, is of many levels.... By service of fellowmen Swami Vivekananda understands the process of this entire revolution and liberation of man in his body, mind and spirit. Alleviation of economical and physical privation, the fostering of intellectual awakening and the release of the inner spiritual self-identity form in their totality Swami Vivekananda's concept of social service. It is to this scheme of work for fellow-men that he exhorts man. He plans for all men in all the levels of their being. It is doubly universal.

In pursuance of this creative humanity, Swami Vivekananda initiated and inspired a multiplicity of institutions appropriately named Maths and Missions in the name of his Master. They cater to the physical and economic life of the masses in the form of industrial schools and hospitals.... The spiritual aspect of development is taken care of by the spread of the universal message of spiritual truth in the footsteps of Sri Ramakrishna and Vivekananda by personal initiation and preaching and by the publication of treasures of wisdom of all faiths and all prophets. Centres have sprung up all over the country and abroad to keep alive and advance the cause of the inner life of man towards the Goal Supreme.

His was an explosive divinity
– Prof. C. S. Ramakrishnan

"Arise, awake and stop not till the goal is reached." What a clarion call to man! And what a majestic and multi-faceted personality behind those thunderous words!

Swami Vivekananda was a phenomenon. He lived for barely forty years, but in that brief span of time he has left us a legacy whose rich and variegated dividends India and the world continue to reap. Saint and savant, orator and patriot, keen critic and ebullient humourist, mellifluous singer and charming raconteur, he did not touch anything which he did not adorn. His athletic frame and glowing eyes dominated the scene wherever he was.

Out of dust he made us into men. At the time he appeared, India was in the doldrums, materially and psychologically. We were under alien rule and the people had been emasculated. Poverty and ignorance stalked the land and the people were groaning in the depths of misery, not knowing in what direction to turn. The various movements functioning at that time were doing only patchwork and the sense of frustration among the masses was in no way assuaged. Swami Vivekananda burst upon the scene and by his thundering words roused the sleepy nation from its lethargy and made us proud of our motherland. And we must remember that he had travelled practically all over the world, and observed with keenness the organizations, customs and habits of different peoples. He was convinced that the renaissance of India can come through only our own strength and not by presenting ourselves as beggars at Western doors.

Strength, was what he preached at every step. He pointed out that the strength of a chain is determined by its weakest link. India has inherited a rich cultural and spiritual heritage, but as long as the masses continue in poverty, ignorance, superstition and ill-health, the nation cannot regain its pristine glory. Therefore he passionately pleaded to the would-be patriots to feel for the masses first.

He coined the phrase "Worship of *Daridranarayana*" to connote the spirit of humility with which social service should be done. Serving the masses should be a pleasure and privilege, and not a status symbol. He insisted on every patriot and social worker remembering that each soul is potentially divine and we should help every man and woman from where he or she is to reach the highest in consonance with human dignity. His was the positive secularism as explained by Sister Nivedita: "To him the workshop, the study, the farm-yard and the field are as true and fit scenes for the meeting of God and man as the cell of the monk or the door of the temple. To him there is no difference between the service of man and worship of God, between manliness and faith, between true righteousness and spirituality."

The Swamiji had travelled all over India from Kashmir to Kanyakumari on foot and mixed with princes and paupers, scholars and ignoramuses, and felt the heart-throb of living India. He was indeed the first integrator of awakened India. He did not preach any sectarianism, either in religion or in political and social life, but saw every Indian as his brother and insisted that in all our thoughts and deeds we must look upon our motherland as single entity.

Swami Vivekananda was a bomb-shell. His was an explosive divinity. "I shall inspire men everywhere until the world shall know that it is one with God", he declared with a verve that only a master-artist can command. Having experienced through the grace of Sri Ramakrishna the ineffable touch of the One in the wondrous play of the many, he made it his life's mission to bring the nectar of Vedanta from mountain caves and ivory towers to the doorsteps of the common man, toiling and moiling in the din and dust of the market place. For him religion was solid realization, and not the froth of academic philosophy or the barren leaves of ritualistic worship. His cosmic mind ranged over all themes under the sun. But the refreshing refrain in all his inspired talks and writings is practicality, the actualization of the ideal.

The richest tribute we can pay to his memory is to practise in our own lives some of the lofty ideas and patriotic ideals for which he lived and died.

His was the message of strength
– Eknath Ranade

A great disciple of Sri Ramakrishna Paramahamsa, he was, in the recent centuries, the first Hindu missionary who went abroad and re-enunciated to the world the Hindu Message of the Universal Religion *(Sanatana Dharma)*. A great patriot, reformer and organizer, he was also the first to set in motion the forces of national revival and put in process the rebuilding. of the country which was scattered and demoralized at the first impact of the British rule. It was he who laid the foundation of the regenerated Bharat by making the country aware of its life-centre which was religion round which alone, he emphasized, could our Hindu Nation be effectively and purposefully reorganized.

His was the message of strength – the strength of the body, the mind and the will. And this strength in all its aspects is the greatest need of the hour. Swami Vivekananda wanted the nation to have "muscles of iron, and nerves of steel inside which dwells a mind of the same material as that of which the thunderbolt is made." He wanted his countrymen to possess and to cultivate "strength, manhood, *kshatra-virya,* plus *Brahma-teja.*" These are precisely the things needed in the present hour of crisis and peril, and these are precisely the qualities which have been neglected by us in the post-independence period under the influence of the imported hedonistic philosophies and materialistic views of life.

If we were to sum up Swamiji's teachings, we could say that he gave us one great *mantra*: the *mantra* of faith in God, faith in ourselves. Faith in oneself is based on the great Upanishadic truth which declares: "I am the Spirit. Me the sword cannot cut; nor any weapon pierce; nor fire burn; nor air dry. I am Omnipotent; I am Omniscient." This is the *mantra* Swami Vivekananda was constantly dinning into the ears of his countrymen. In whatever he spoke and preached, this *mantra* was the refrain of his gospel-song. It is time that we grasped the inner meaning of this Truth and tried to live up to it. If we do that no power on earth could harm us.

He further declares that in aspiring to attain *moksha,* we have to fulfil our *dharma* first. In fact there is no *moksha* without *dharma.* This is a truth which needed re-emphasis at a time when our religion tended to become life-weary. He rehabilitates a house-holder's life and gives it a new dignity. He reminds his countrymen of their *shastras* which declare that only "heroes enjoy the world" and urge them to "show heroism." He asks us to remember that the *shastras* enjoin upon us to accept the moral conditions under which we work and have to function. Only by such acceptance of our conditions and environment can we hope to improve them and raise them. Therefore Swami Vivekananda exhorts his countrymen not to forget the *shastric* injunction: "Apply according to circumstances the fourfold political maxims of conciliation, bribery, sowing dissensions and open war to conquer your adversaries and enjoy the world – then you will be *dharmika.* Otherwise you live a disgraceful life if you pocket your insults, when you are kicked and trodden down by any one who takes it into his head to do so; your life is a veritable hell here and so your life hereafter."

This is a message of great value and efficacy for the purpose of steeling our nerves and strengthening our resolve.

Time and again he preached that "the national union in India must be gathering up of its scattered spiritual forces." He taught that "a nation in India must be a union of those whose hearts beat to the same spiritual tune." This message demands our most careful attention today.

Swamiji has one more message to give to the Hindu Nation. He asks us to give up our *tamas,* for *tamas* gives birth to all the evils such as imbecility, superstition, pettiness of mind, mutual quarrels and bickerings about trivial things. Giving up these evils, we should build up great power on the rock of unity and organization. And thus by co-ordinating our separate wills we should build up a future far more glorious than our past. This message of Swamiji too is timely.

Arresting personality
– D. B. Raghunath Rao

My father, the late D. R. Balaji Rao, was a close friend of Swami Vivekananda. He used to tell us that Swamiji was an arresting personality with handsome features, always smiling and had a robust constitution. His voice had a pleasant ringing tone.

Swamiji would revolt at the impotence of Indian nationhood, express how we have been emasculated politically, economically and otherwise and say that it was still not too late to rise and drive away the foreigner and shed the foreign yoke, even though the country was riven with a narrow minded and communal and jealous outlook. However, it appears, he would also say in a stentorian voice, that all was not lost and that India would have its resurgence and ultimately become independent. He laid great stress on manliness in any form.

Swamiji would say that this part of India (South India) was a blessed land. He had great faith in the strength of Indian Nationhood and said his task was to unify the forces, gone at a tangent, and galvanize the nation to work, strive and succeed.

Swamiji had a beautiful voice and could sing well some of the *kirtans*. Once he was walking on the Marina Beach with father and other friends and was challenged as a bachelor to wrestle with a *pahilwan*. Swamiji accepted the challenge and defeated him on the sands of the Triplicane Beach.

Sometimes he would do hathayoga and show by cutting his finger with a knife that he would not bleed.

Swamiji said to my father that there was ample sympathy for India in America and elsewhere for gaining independence and all that was needed was a unifying force.

Swamiji had a glimpse of divinity. When he used to wait for father in the house, he would close his eyes and say "Om" with a hum vibrant with energy. Mother used to say that the whole house would, so to say, shake with his spiritual power.

A man among men and yet greater than the most
– Dr. V. K. R. V. Rao

Narendranath Datta, later to become and pass into history as Swami Vivekananda, was born in Calcutta on Monday the 12th January, 1863. He did not live to see his fortieth birthday and left this mortal life on Friday the 4th July, 1902. Within this short period of less than forty years, Vivekananda lived a life that would have taken ordinary mortals many times that period to leave an indelible mark not only on his own country but also on many other parts of the world. His voice comes resounding over the years; and it is a voice born of the past, troubled by the present, and looking forward to the future. A young man himself when he started preaching, he was essentially addressing the young. And what he said so many decades ago is still as fresh, as poignant, as inspiring and as relevant today as it was then.

A man among men and yet greater than most, is what one can say about Vivekananda the Man. But because he was a man after all, the strain of his self-conquest ruined his health, shortened his years, and brought about his end in the very prime of his life. Truly, it was himself and his life that the man Vivekananda gave in sacrifice to build Vivekananda the Monk and found the practical Vedanta which was his prescription for the ailing world. In my view this sacrifice was greater than even the greatness of the truth for which he made the sacrifice.

The Vedantic concept that the same divinity is present in every human being – manifest in varying degrees – gives, in my opinion, the strongest base that we can find for the concept of human equality of humanity as one unit irrespective of class, caste, creed, nation or language. And I think this is what we must emphasize.

....We have to rediscover the concept of humanity, that human beings, irrespective of differences in language, colour, caste, creed, ideology, economic status, social status and political status – all these are very important, but irrespective of all these diffetences – human beings constitute one body, and every human being counts with equal value. Now this is the message of Ramakrishna-Vivekananda.

....It may be asked why we always link together the illiterate priest Ramakrishna, and Vivekananda, the scholar, the great orator, the world conqueror in spiritual ideas, and the organizer of a great Mission. Why do we always refer to 'Ramakrishna-Vivekananda'? We never call Vivekananda by himself, or Ramakrishna by himself. Because the power that Vivekananda got was through Ramakrishna. Ramakrishna was the truth and Vivekananda was the expositor. What was the truth? That religion is not to be kept only in the churches, mosques and temples, nor only in monasteries or forest caves in mighty Himalayas, where people pray for their own salvation. Religion is to be brought down into the market place brought down into actual life. This is what Vivekananda calls 'Practical Vedanta.'

If you take the subject of secularism, patriotism, national integration, education, spiritual rediscovery, Practical Vedanta and a positive attitude to science, no obscurantism, no materialism, no going back on human evolution, you can find all that in the Ramakrishna-Vivekananda teachings. Vivekananda was the most comprehensive human being I can think of, and he is the answer to so many problems we are being confronted with in India today.

Strength and fearlessness were the keynote to Vivekananda's approach to life's problems.

He attached more importance to character than to religiosity or other external manifestation of religious discipline.

To him worship of God meant service of man.

Vivekananda was a highly emotional being. Whatever he undertook had behind it not only his intellectual reasoning and his spiritual insight but also the entire force of his emotional strength.

The proudest Hindu
– K. Suryanarayana Rao

Swami Vivekananda was a versatile genius, a multifaceted personality full of wisdom and dedication. He not only inspired and galvanized the people during his lifetime but even after, for ever: ....'I will not cease to work. I will inspire everyone until the world will know that it is one with God', as he put it.

When we read or hear about him and about what he has spoken and written, rather poured out his innermost feelings for the people of our country, our religion, our *dharma* and our culture, we are not only thrilled but spurred on to action. We in R. S. S are working hard to bring into practice the life-giving grand message of Swamiji with regard to the regeneration of our Motherland.

With all his erudition of Vedanta and its Universal application, he was essentially a passionate patriot and an ardent Hindu. He was the proudest Hindu and gave call to everyone of us to be proud of being born as Hindus. He says, "When a man has begun to be ashamed of his ancestors, the end has come. Here am I, one of the least of Hindu race, yet proud of my race, proud of my ancestors. I am proud to call myself a Hindu, I am proud that I am one of your unworthy servants, I am proud that I am a countryman of yours, you the descendants of the sages, you the descendants of the most glorious *rishis* the world ever saw. Therefore, have faith in yourselves; be proud of your ancestors, instead of being ashamed of them. And do not imitate, do not imitate! O ye modern Hindus dehypotize yourselves"! Many of such statements in his speeches and writings would surely scare some of the so-called secular intellectuals of modern times, who will not hesitate to dub him as a rabid communalist and a fanatic. This is the result of Western indoctrination of those English educated, who have lost their roots.

He implored for a man-making education, character-building education, a national education giving strength, courage and self-confidence to the meek and emasculated Hindus. In the rules and regulations of the Ramakrishna Math, in the section 'Plan of work for India', in the very first clause, Swamiji discusses the decline of Hindu population because of conversions to Islam and Christianity and then writes, "It is specially for the preservation of the Hindu race and religion that Bhagavan Sri Ramakrishna, the embodiment of mercy has incarnated himself".

Bhagini Nivedita, the dedicated disciple of Swamiji, in her book *Master as I Saw Him*, in the chapter 'Swamiji's Mission considered as a Whole', writes: "His object as regards India, said the Swami, in a private conversation, had always been 'to make Hinduism aggressive'. The eternal faith must become active and proselytizing, capable of sending out special missions, of making converts, of taking back into her fold those of her own children who have been perverted from her and of the conscious and deliberate assimilation of new elements". This is a repetition of what Swamiji had himself written in the rules and regulations of the Ramakrishna Math and later said to a correspondent of the Ramakrishna Math's monthly magazine *Prabuddha Bharata*, where he has also said "that every man going out of the Hindu pale is not only a man less but an enemy the more". In the same rules and regulations Swamiji has warned about the dangers to Hindu society and *dharma*. He writes: "The life of the Aryan Race is founded on religion. If that is destroyed, the downfall is inevitable. Hence the Hindu society should be broadened by giving *samskaras* to all the castes down to the Chandalas and even to the foreign races.... Great efforts should be made to bring even

Muslims and Christians into the Hindu fold." What a significant and pregnant statement! How much it means in today's context? This is the amount of concern that Swamiji had for the degenerated condition of Hindus and their decline.

How to regenerate the Hindus? Can political power and independence give the solution to the problem? Śri Bhupendranath Dutta, the younger brother of Swami Vivekananda has written a book: *Swami Vivekananda, the Patriot Prophet.* In his Foreword to the book he write, "The year before his death when two of his foreign admirers with the collaboration of some noted citizens of Calcutta started a nationalist group, which later on became the nucleus of the revolutionary movement of Bengal, Swamiji desisted his disciple Nivedita from joining it. Once being asked by Sister Christine as to why he requested Nivedita to keep aloof from Indian politics, he answered, 'What does Nivedita know of Indian conditions and politics? I have done more politics in my life than she! I had the idea of forming a combination of Indian princes for the overthrow of the foreign yoke. For that reason, from the Himalayas to Cape Comorine, I have trampled about all over the country. For that reason, I made friends with the gunmaker Sir Hiram Maxim. But I got no response from the country. The country is dead'." And he narrated further attempt of his at this time in other direction; but he again said, "India is in putrefaction. What I want today is a band of selfless young workers, who will educate and uplift the people". The Swami further narrated of his doings to Sister Christine. Thus it is very clear that Swamiji had come to the conclusion that politics is not the solution for the rejuvenation of a degenerated country. It required something more, a grassroot work to awaken and activate the people. The society should rise from the lowest levels. He has spoken out these ideas very forcefully in his *Lectures from Colombo to Almora.*

He has pleaded for the awakening of Hindu masses, for organization, for young men to come forward, for young men to be physically strong and fearless in their hearts and mind. He says, "Men, Men are wanted. We want fiery young men, intelligent and brave, who dare to go to the jaws of death and are ready to swim the ocean across. A hundred thousand men and women, fired with the zeal of holiness, fortified with eternal faith in the Lord, and nerved to lion's courage by their sympathy for the poor and the fallen and the downtrodden, will go over the length and breadth of the land, preaching the gospel of salvation, the gospel of help, the gospel of social raising up – the gospel of equality".

"....To make a great future India, the whole secret lies in organization, accumulation of power, coordination of wills; bringing them all into one focus". Swamiji desired that all the Hindus should love each other rising above all differences and build up a formidable organization. During his talks many a time he has said our country is a Hindu Nation. He further says – "National Union in India must be a gathering up of its scattered spiritual forces. A nation in India must be a union of those whose hearts beat to the same spiritual tune".

Nivedita further writes in the same chapter quoted above: "At any rate his whole work, from the first consisted, according to his own statement, of a 'Search for the Common Bases of Hinduism.' He has again and again stressed these common bases and aroused the Hindus on these common feelings and appealed for their oneness and unity. In his Lahore speech "The Common Bases of Hinduism", he gives a clarion call: "Mark me, then and then alone you are a Hindu, when the very name sends through you a galvanic shock of strength. Then and then alone you are a Hindu when the distress of any one bearing that name comes to your heart and makes you feel as if your own son were in distress. Then and then alone you are a Hindu when you will be ready to bear everything for them. Mark me! Every one of you will have to be a Guru Gobind Singh if you want to do good to your country. You may see thousands of defects in your countrymen, but mark their Hindu blood. They are the first gods you will have to worship even if they do everything to hurt you. All our hatchets let us bury and send out this grand current of love all round". We can understand the intensity of his love for every Hindu. He was a patriot to the core. In fact he was an inspired Patriot-saint, the watchword of whose heart was Hindu and Bharat. He wanted all his followers and admirers to intensely love the country. Even he wanted the same love from his foreign disciples. When after her arrival in our country Miss Josephine Macleod asked, "How can I best help you"? "Love India" was the answer of Swamiji. Towards the end of his life he writes, "My life's allegiance is to my Motherland, and if I had a thousand lives, every moment of the whole series would be consecrated to your service, my countrymen, my friends".

Swamiji was thus the consummation of thousands of years of Hindu civilization, Hindu culture, *Hindu Dharma* and everything that was noble and glorious in Bharath. Wherever he went he saw to it that the greatness of his Motherland and its progeny was projected and established. He was a champion of dynamic and aggressive Hinduism. His identification with everything that is Hindu was such that he stood totally in defence of Hinduism. He never allowed anyone to deride his religion, *dharma* and country. He was ever eager to clinch and vindicate the superiority of his country, countrymen and their genius. His love for his people and their heritage was intense and his struggle to make them great once again, was passionate. For him the very air and dust of Bharath was holy, sacred, nay heaven, itself. His patriotism was of the highest order. He was the proudest Hindu. Every word he uttered came from the depths of his sincere heart. It at once thrills and will inspire the youth of this land for generations to come. Let us try to imbibe his spirit and vow to fulfil his mission.

He gave equal importance to secular matters also
– Dr. A. V. Rathna Reddy

As a preacher of universal religion, Swami Vivekananda is well-known both in the East and the West. To the common man, he is, first and foremost an exponent of Vedanta and nothing else. But he should not be regarded exclusively as religious prophet. His individuality and thought are too complex to be measured by any rigid classification. Though we find that the chief occupation of his life was religion, he made significant observations on every aspect of life. As a Neo-Vedantin, he did not differentiate the sacred life from secular affairs and he did give equal importance to the secular matters.

As the foremost exponent of universal religion, Swami Vivekananda considered an absolute religion in India best suited for achieving perfection. He advocated a practical religion which could pervade and be a guide in an individual's life. Vivekananda's political ideas being inseparable from religion, he explained the utility of religion in terms of individual, social and political life. Adhering scrupulously to the principle of 'preservation by reconstruction', he offered constructive criticism of the society in India without attacking national faith or institutions.

The Complete Works of Swami Vivekananda, which contain various strands of thought, provide us the glimpse of his social and political ideas. It is on the basis of his works that scholars have systematized his ideas on society and established his place as a social thinker and reformer. His political ideas still need to be systematized.

The political thought of Vivekananda is inextricably linked to his role as an agent of national resurgence and was conditioned and influenced by the prevailing environment. While trying to surmount the problems that confronted him, Vivekananda devised means for national reconstruction on spiritual basis and in the process won for himself a pre-eminent place in the galaxy of modern Indian leaders and thinkers.

He fulfilled the vital need
– A Reviewer (in *Glory of India*)

In Swami Vivekananda, the foremost disciple of Sri Ramakrishna and organizer of the Ramakrishna Math and Mission, the universal spirit has found a loving, dynamic and all encompassing expression which is rarely to be found elsewhere. In his scheme of life there is no inherent conflict between the faith and reason, between science and religion, between poetry and philosophy, between action and meditation, between social and monastic ideals.

He interpreted the fundamental spiritual truths in modern terms; so as to enlighten mankind on the age-old problems of human existence. He built a bridge between the ancient and modern, between the East and West.

In so doing he has fulfilled the vital need of the present-day world for a universal message and a comprehensive view of life.

A dynamic redeemer
– Romeshwadhera

A 'phenomenon' of a human being, his remarkable life and neat style of functioning served and uplifted his downtrodden brethren through abundant and varied avenues of spiritual recovery and regeneration.

He was a mystic par excellence, an incomparable social reformer, an awakener unmatched, and a Hindu savant unrivalled, whose universality and compassion have been classic; whose mission is an unfolding benediction; and whose ceaseless efforts for religious harmony and enlightenment are a landmark of spiritual maturity.

Volcanic in his intensity and immensity, oceanic in his awareness and realization, a voracious worshipper of suffering humanity, his love was boundless and beauteous for the dispossessed, the discriminated and the disheartened. He was a beacon for the despairing, a lighthouse for the ignorant, and a steady guide for the wayward wayfarers for truth and righteousness.

A loving embodiment of humility, Vivekananda was an honourable asset of our religion-suffused dignity, and was a fine representative of resurgent Hindu glory. He was a splendid blend of our noble racial traditions and quintessence of genuine modernity, immune to and beyond the pollutions and pretensions of myths and superstitions. A perfect hero, a true national leader, and an authentic spokesman of the Hindu Heritage and its luminous destiny, Vivekananda is our valid and revered focus of veneration. The 'cyclonic monk' is an abiding echo of Indian greatness, at once stirring and appealing in its inspiration and approach towards purer life and saner society.

His clarion call is so miraculous, mighty and insistent that the essence of universe throbs majestically in it; and it has a deeply ennobling and chastening impact on the course of undemocratic institutions and humane individuals who disdain governmentalization and espouse the benefits of ideal citizenism, tempered with ethical values. He was a grass-roots educationist, a sparkling patriot and a basic revolutionary of a high order, preparing people both for the Kingdom of Heaven and the brotherhood of mankind. A titanic soul, a life supreme by all counts.

He greatly influenced the national movement
– Binoy Kumar Roy

In the history of India's freedom movement a very special position is occupied by Narendranath Dutta, known to the world as Swami Vivekananda.

Formally he was a monk in yellow robes, a religious preacher, founder and organizer of a philosophical-religious movement known as Vedantism or, more correctly, Neo-Vedantism. He was also the founder of the Ramakrishna Mission – a philanthropic organization with centres throughout India as well as in America and England. But his views and teachings gradually influenced the national movement of India especially the revolutionary movement, and many aspects of our national life and culture. Many generations of Indian revolutionaries, beginning with the early 20th century, were practically reared up, inspired and steeled by the fiery speeches and writings of Swami Vivekananda. His call to the youth of the country to fight for the enlightenment of the downtrodden dumb millions, his revolutionary approach to the problem of liquidating the privileges of the propertied classes and giving the toilers their due share in the national wealth, his preachings against untouchability and, above all, his teachings on the purification of the soul were later adopted by different political and social organizations of the country including the Indian National Congress led by M. K. Gandhi.

Narendranath was born in the year 1863, six years after the great national liberation war of 1857. During the very same decade a number of outstanding sons of the country were born, including Rabindranath Tagore and M. K. Gandhi. He appeared at a time when India and the world were at crossroads – critically revaluating old values, searching for a way out from the old, the then existing order.

Vivekananda appeared like a meteor and within a short period of less than a decade of his public life, not only endeared himself to millions of his countrymen and thousands of his admirers and followers in Europe and America, not only dispelled the century-old slanderous notions about India and Indians spread carefully and constantly by the imperialists and their agents in various guises, but made major contributions in many fields of human knowledge which were of far-reaching consequences.

He was an immaculate soul
– Dilip Kumar Rao

Our scriptures say that the father is reborn in the son and lives on through him. Even so, the guru reveals himself and survives through his beloved disciple. So it would not be wrong to aver that Sri Ramakrishna's message came to be fulfilled because it was amplified and complemented by the missionary ardour of Swami Vivekananda. Was not that why the great Messiah of Mother Kali had said just before his passing that he had stowed finally all the treasures of his fecund Realisation in the *adhar* (receptive soul) of his great messenger, Naren?

Vivekananda was an immaculate soul-cum-the sinner's friend; one of the seven *rishis* (sages) – as Sri Ramakrishna put it – and, withal, a devotee of the eternal child, his guru; a Bird of Fire who yet accepted the cage of flesh-bars only to break himself free: in a word, he was a living paradox; a man of God who repudiated: "the worship of the great God of getting-on" and yet made good as one of the most spectacular "go-getter" the world has ever seen – an ambassador of the Elysium who had gone out to America a pauper with no credentials and came out a resplendent victor, aye, to receive ovations which grew into a legend even in his own life-time. For all that, he knew himself as little more than his great Master's nursling who was utterly dependent on him.

And yet there were many honest critics who while sincerely admiring his many-faceted personality, held that Sri Aurobindo had overstressed his greatness when he wrote: "Vivekananda was a soul of puissance if ever there was one, a very lion among men.... We perceive his influence still working gigantically. We know not well how, we know not well where, in something that is not yet formed, something leonine, grand, intuitive, upheaving that has entered the soul of India and we say 'Behold, Vivekananda still lives in the soul of his Motherland and in the souls of her children.' "

I came across such hidebound critics galore in my adolescence and was not a little influenced by their verdict that Vivekananda had deviated not a little from the express injunctions of his great guru whose essentially orthodox outlook he had come to repudiate in his over-enthusiasm for the modern view of life imported from the West. I shed this influence years later only when I came to learn from Sri Aurobindo himself how Vivekananda had once helped him materially. "It is a fact" he wrote, "that I was hearing constantly the voice of Vivekananda speaking to me for a fortnight in the jail in my solitary meditation and felt his presence. The voice spoke on a very important field of spiritual experience." Years later he spoke categorically about Vivekananda having been to him the very first messenger to reveal the lore of the Supramental Truth and added: "I had never expected him and yet he came to teach me. And he was exact and precise even in the minutest details." This came to serve me as an eye-opener after which his messianic role was borne home to me as never before.

Prophet of Hindu nationalism
– Manabendranath Roy

Religious nationalism of the orthodox as well as reformed school had begun to come into evidence in the province of Bengal since the first years of the twentieth century. Although its political philosopher and leader were found subsequently in the persons of Aurobindo Ghose and Bipin Chandra Pal respectively, its fundamental ideology was conceived by a young intellectual.... Narendra Nath Dutta, subsequently known by the religious nomenclature of Swami Vivekananda. While still a student in the University of Calcutta, Dutta felt the rebellious spirit affecting the lower middle class intellectuals. It was in the early nineties. He was moved by the sufferings of the common people. Declassed socially, possessing a keen intellect, he made a spectacular plunge into the philosophical depths of Hindu scriptures and discovered in his cult of Vedantism (religious Monism of the Hindus) a sort of socialistic, humanitarian religion. He decried scathingly orthodoxy in religion as well as in social customs. He was the picturesque, and tremendously vigorous embodiment of the old trying to readjust itself to the new. Like Bal Gangadhar Tilak, Dutta was also a prophet of Hindu nationalism. He also was a firm believer in the cultural superiority of the Indian people, and held that on this cultural basis should be built the future Indian nation. But he was not a partisan of orthodoxy in religion: to social conservatism, he was a veritable iconoclast. He had the courageous foresight, or perhaps instinct, which convinced him that if religion was to be saved, it must be given a modern garb; if the priest was still to hold his sway over the millions of Hindu believers, he must modify his old crude ways; if the intellectual aristocracy of the fortunate few was to retain its social predominance, spiritual knowledge must be democratized. The reaction of native culture against the intrusion of Western education ran wild, so to say, in the person of Vivekananda and the cult of Universal Religion he formulated in the name of his preceptor, Ramakrishna Paramahamsa. He preached that Hinduism, not Indian nationalism, should be aggressive. His nationalism was a spiritual imperialism. He called on Young India to believe in the spiritual mission of India....

This romantic vision of conquering the world by spiritual superiority electrified the young intellectuals..... The British domination stood in the way as the root of all evils. Thus, an intelligently rebellious element.... had to give in to national pre-occupations, and contribute itself to a movement for the immediate overthrow of foreign rule....

A gigantic personality
– V. C. Samuel

A gigantic personality, Swami Vivekananda opened up a new era for Hinduism. Till he came on the scene of history, Hinduism had been considered by its own adherents as a comprehensive name for all Indians who did not want to be grouped under any other religious title. Though Swami Vivekananda did not change this particular state, he put a definite meaning-content into it – a meaning-content derived from the Hindu Scriptures and religious traditions. Having done this, he developed a Hindu mission for the world, and that is what the Ramakrishna Movement is.

With the achievement of India's national freedom, the Movement has entered a new era of progress in India. The unselfish service rendered by the Mission centres in India through Hospitals, Dispensaries, Educational Institutions and various other ways is being increasingly appreciated by the Government and the public. To cope with the growing need, most of the centres expand their work and institutions. One can observe through all these developments the amount of confidence the Indian public as well as sympathizers abroad have vested in the authorities of the Movement.

As Swami Vivekananda has made it clear, one of his great dreams was to make Hinduism "aggressive." The one movement in modern Hinduism which has the dynamism as well as public support in India to try to work out this idea in practice is assuredly the Ramakrishna Movement. In the words of D. S. Sarma:

> "Of all the religious movements that have sprung up in India in recent times, there is none so faithful to our past and so full of possibilities for the future, so rooted in our national consciousness and yet so universal in its outlook, and therefore none so thoroughly representative of the religious spirit of India, as the movement connected with the names of Sri Ramakrishna Paramahamsa and his disciple, Swami Vivekananda."

A world-conqueror of our times
– Prof. Binoy Kumar Sarkar

As a student of world culture and the creator of modern India it is possible to call the attention of scholars to Swami Vivekananda as one of the World-Conquerors of our own times.

It is indeed possible to talk an entire encyclopaedia about Vivekananda's messages and activities. Physically of athletic build, healthy and strong, as a mere man, he knew to be very realistic, how to do justice to the daily meals. He was a lover of art, a poet, a musician and a singer. Wanderlust was in his very blood. He knew every province of India by travel and he was a world tourist. Men and things he knew how to observe shrewdly.

A first-rate orator, he was a writer of the same rank. Bengali literature he has enriched with vigour and Bengali language with expressions picked up from the streets. A researcher and translator, he was no less a commentator and a propagandist. He knew the Buddhist teachings and the Christian Gospels as much as he knew his Hindu texts. His knowledge of Western instituitions and ideals was no less extensive than his familiarity with those of Orient. He studied the antiquities as much as he came into contact with the modern realities.

He was deeply absorbed in religious preachings and social reform. His patriotism also was perennial and of the loftiest type. Nay, he was a socialist too. His socialism, however, was not Marxian, but rather romantic like that of, say, the Frenchman, St. Simon. Or rather, like Fichte, the father of the German youth-movement and exponent of nationalism and socialism, Vivekananda initiated in India the cult of *Daridranarayana* (God as the poor). He was emphatically a nationalist and yet a fervent internationalist. His comparative methodology served to establish the universalistic, cosmopolitan and humane basis of all religious and social values.

As one dying at the age of forty and accomplishing so much for his fatherland and the world, Vivekananda was certainly an *avatar* of youth-force. One may adore him as a man of action, as a man of self-sacrifice, as a man of devotion, as a man of learning, as a man of yoga. He was a hundred per cent idealist, a thorough going mystic, and yet he was a foremost realist and a stern objectivist.

If we look upon Ramakrishna as the Buddha of our times, Vivekananda may pass for one or other of the greatest apostles of yore, say, the scholar Rahula, the constitutional authority Upali, the devoted lieutenant, Ananda, the sage Sariputta, or the master of discourses, Mahakachchayana. One can almost say that Vivekananda was all these great Buddhist preacher-organizers boiled down, as it were, into one personality.

And yet when this whole encyclopaedia has been said about Vivekananda, we have not said all or enough. He was much more than a mere exponent of Vedanta, or Ramakrishna, or Hinduism, or Indian culture. Antiquarian lore, translation of other persons' thoughts, past or present, popularization of some Hindu ideals did not constitute the main function of his life. In all his thoughts and activities he was expressing only *himself.* He always preached his *own* experiences. It is the truths discovered by him in his own life that he propagated through his literature and institutions. As a modern philosopher he can be properly evaluated solely if one places him by the side of Dewey, Russell, Croce, Spranger, and Bergson. It would be doing Vivekananda injustice and misinterpreting him hopelessly if he were placed in the perspective of scholars whose chief or solid merit consists in editing, translating, paraphrasing or popularizing the teachings of Plato Ashvaghosha, Plotinus, Nagarjuna, Aquinas, Sankaracharya and others.

Vivekananda's lecture at Chicago (1893) is a profound masterpiece of modern philosophy. Before the Parliament of Religions this young Bengali of thirty stood as an intellectual facing intellectuals, or rather as whole personality face to face with the combined intelligence of the entire world. And the impression left by him was that of a man who told certain things that were likely to satisfy some great human wants, as one who thus had a message for all mankind. There he shone not as a propagator of Vedanta or Hinduism or any other traditional "ism" but as a creative thinker whose thoughts were bound to prevail.

What, then is Vivekananda's self? What is the personality that he expressed in this speech? The kernel can be discovered in just five words. With five words he conquered the world, so to say, when he addressed men and women as "Ye divinities on earth! – sinners?" The first four words summoned into being the gospel of joy, hope, virility, energy and freedom for the races of men. And yet with the last word, embodying as it did a sarcastic question, he demolished the whole structure of soul-degenerating, cowardice – promoting negative, pessimistic thoughts. On the astonished world the little five-word formula fell like a bomb-shell. The first four words he brought from the East, and the last word he brought from the West. All these are oft-repeated expressions, copy-book phrases both in the East and the West. And yet never in the annals of human thought was the juxtaposition accomplished before Vivekananda did it in this dynamic manner and obtained instantaneous recognition as a world's champion.

Vivekananda's gospel here is that of 'energism', of mastery over the world, over the conditions surrounding life, of human freedom, of individual liberty, of courage trampling down cowardice, of world conquest.

The key to Vivekananda's entire life, his decade-long preparation down to 1893 and his decade-long work down to his death in 1902 is to be found in his Shaktiyoga, 'energism', the vigour and strength of freedom. All his thoughts and activities are expressions of this 'energism'. Like our Pauranic Vishwamitra or the Aeschylean Prometheus he wanted to create new worlds and distribute the fire of freedom, happiness, divinity and immortality among men and women.

In his life-work there is to be found another very striking characteristic. This consists in his emphasis on individuals, on persons, and in his attempt to harness 'energism' to their thoughts and activities. Vivekananda may have ostensibly preached religious reform, social reconstruction as well as crusade against poverty. But it is the making of individuals, the training for manhood, the awakening of personality and individuality, on which his whole soul was focused. Everywhere he wanted men and women who were energetic freedom-loving, courageous, and endowed with personality. The objective of his diverse treatises on yoga is none other than the "chiselling forth" of such individuals as may be depended on as "divinities on earth", as persons who are determined to master the adverse conditions of life and to conquer the world.

Vivekananda deals in Shaktiyoga, human 'energism'. It is above the region, the climate, the space, the environment, in one word, above Nature that he places man and his destiny.

The words that are constantly on Vivekananda's lips are the Upanishads and the Vedanta. These philosophical documents of ancient India appeal to him simply because they can be utilized as texts of his own cult of Shakti, energy, individuality and manhood. We may describe his philosophy as embodying the cult of Neo-Vedantism.

Vivekananda is not a statical fact. He is a going concern. His philosophy compels one to move not only from village to village and region to region but from idea to idea, mores to mores, custom to custom, ideal to ideal. He is to move out of the shackles of the degrading and dehumanising theories to the theories of man-making, or rather, the transformation of nature and man by manhood, the re-making of man.

His originality
– Prof. D. S. Sarma

....Swami Vivekananda did for the gospel of Sri Ramakrishna something similar to what St. Paul did for the gospel of Christ. He took the good seed from the premises of the Dakshineswar temple and scattered it far and wide over three continents. In America, Europe and India, he broadcast the truths of Vedanta, as realized in the experience of Sri Ramakrishna.... And in his own country Swami Vivekananda showed, both by precept and by example, that, if only the ancient Vedanta were reinterpreted in the light of Sri Ramakrishna's unique spiritual experience and applied to modern life, it would enable India to solve all the problems with which she was confronted and rise once again to deliver a message to mankind....

Vivekananda's originality lay in applying his Master's teachings to the problems of national life and in making the Hindu Order of sannyasin an example to the lay public not only in religious practice but also in social service and relief work. His lectures and talks made clear to the students of Hinduism for the first time the essentials and non-essentials of that religion. He pointed out in a thousand ways that Vedanta was the steel frame within that vast structure which goes by the name of Hinduism.

A King of boundless and supreme domain of the soul
– K. S. Ramaswami Sastri

It was given to me to meet Swami Vivekananda and spend many days with him at Trivandrum towards the close of 1892 before he went to Chicago to represent Hinduism at the Parliament of Religions there in September 1893 and also at Madras after he returned from Chicago and landed at Colombo on 15th January 1897 and reached Madras a few days later. My entire life was transformed by those memorable and holy contacts.

....I passed my matriculation in 1892 and joined the Maharaja's college, Trivandrum, for the intermediate class. It was at this juncture, towards the end of 1892 that fate threw me into Swamiji's holy company.

Swamiji was then unknown to fame but felt a great urge to spread Hinduism and spirituality all over the world. One morning while I was in my house he came unexpectedly. I found a person with a beaming face and a tall, commanding figure. He had an orange coloured turban on his head and wore a flowing orange coloured coat which reached down to his feet and round which he wore a girdle at the waist.

Swamiji asked me: "Is Professor Sundararaman here? I have brought a letter to be delivered to him." His voice was rich and full and sounded like a bell. Well does Romain Rolland say about the voice, "He had a beautiful voice like a violincello, grave without violent contrasts, but with deep vibrations that filled both hall and hearts. Once his audience was held he could make it sink to an intense piano piercing his hearers to the soul." I looked up and saw him and somehow in my boyishness and innocence (I was only fourteen years old at that time) I felt that he was a Maharaja. I took the letter which he gave and ran up to my father who was upstairs and told him, "A Maharaja has come and is waiting below. He gave this letter to be given to you." My father laughed and said "Ramaswami! What a naive simple soul you are! Maharaja will not come to houses like ours." I replied, "Please come, I have no doubt that he is a Maharaja." My father came down, saluted Swamiji, and took him upstairs. After a pretty long conversation with Swamiji, my father came down and said to me "He is no doubt a Maharaja, but not a king over a small extent or area of territory. He is a king of boundless and supreme domain of the soul."

An inspired Bohemian with an iron will
– Dr. Brojendranath Seal

When I first met Vivekananda in 1881, we were fellow-students of principal William Hastie, scholar, metaphysician, and poet, at the General Assembly's College. He was my senior in age, though I was his senior in the College by one year. Undeniably a gifted youth, sociable, free and unconventional in manners, a sweet singer, the soul of social circles, a brilliant conversationalist, somewhat bitter and caustic, piercing with the shafts of a keen wit the shows and mummeries of the world, sitting in the scorner's chair but hiding the tenderest of hearts under that garb of cynicism: altogether an inspired Bohemian but possessing what Bohemians lack, an iron will; somewhat peremptory and absolute, speaking with accents of authority and withall possessing a strong power of the eye which could hold his listeners in thrall.

Tears he shed and life-blood he gave
– Basiswar Sen

Swami Vivekananda gave his message with such boldness, such freedom of thought, such directness, and above all with such a burning appeal for the suffering millions that it is unnecessary to make commentaries on them. His spirit seems to speak through his writings. He did not talk platitudes, neither did he pose. Tears he shed and life-blood he gave. To read him makes one sit up and think. Yes, think and soon to work, – work constructive – however humble might be our lot. For in youth we mainly derive our inspiration through love of persons and later in manhood through interest in work and ideas. These he amply fulfils.

After his highest spiritual realization with his Master at Dakshineswar he travelled the length and breadth of India, and this not in an American tourist fashion but in a way which he himself has sung, "with sky thy roof and grass thy bed. And food? What chance may bring." He travelled, and he saw India. He saw her once joyous notes of life now sunk into murmurs and sobs, her once glorious light now waxed dim, her once flaming fires now grown cold. He saw the ignorance that permeates and apathy that exists. He saw the ravages of famine, plague, cholera, small-pox, and malaria and other deities of destruction. He saw how amidst all these the millions are fast decaying losing everything in their bare struggle for existence.

He saw all these. And Vivekananda had a heart. He felt. He realized the crisis – crisis so stupendous, so imminent as to awaken the deepest slumbers of memory. He looked back to the hoary past with love and reverence, and saw the possibility of reviving its glorious traditions. To gaze into the future through the grim realities of the present required the strongest stretch of vision. And Vivekananda's vision of the future was one of hope and not of fear. He says:

"Though whirlwind after whirlwind of foreign invasion has passed over the devoted head of India, though centuries of neglect on our part has visibly dimmed the glories of ancient Aryavarta, though many a stately column on which it rested, many beautiful arches, many marvellous corners have been washed away by the inundation that deluged the land for centuries – the centre is all sound – the key-stone is unimpaired; the spiritual foundation upon which the marvellous monument of glory to God and charity to all beings has been reared, stands unshaken, strong as ever."

Being a sannyasin he had nothing to fear, as he had nothing to lose and nothing to gain. So it was not policy that made him say that. It was the truth he saw and felt. He realized that each country has its dominant tradition and its own special line of evolution. Religion has been our line. The choice glorious, or the choice fateful, as you like, was made in ages long gone by and we cannot alter it now. Inevitable crisis must follow. We could but rise up to the occasion and readjust to suit our new environment, and take this as an opportunity of our own development. Swamiji saw that however priest-ridden, however degenerated, the religious ideas and ideals still govern the life of the people. It is either Sita-Rama, or Radha-Krishna who inspire them and sustain them in their existence. And he tried to revive it, to make it living. He interpreted religion anew. He made it vital, the religion of life, suited to our present needs and future developments, and these at their fullest and best. He begged the ascetic to descend from his Himalayan heights and the devout to come out of his temple and renew their contact with life throbbing, life moving, life evolving. Religion is the vision we hold and its realization in life. It is our relation with the infinite. How we allow ourselves to be acted on by the environment and how we react on the complex, ever changing, ever-evolving environment, for we are not creatures that are finished but creators of our creaturehood, imperishably active. Thus our religion consists not merely of our brief meditative moments, but it comprehends life's every detail, how we act, how we think, how we feel.

Swamiji saw what priceless treasures our forefathers have left us, treasures gathered through centuries of life's experiments and experiences, of heroic deeds and bold speculation – treasures open to labour and merit. He wanted us to enjoy and to be able to enjoy. What good would it be to possess the best of the libraries if we cannot think, much less if we cannot read. And yet he did not blame us. Vivekananda knew that man's physical needs are fundamental and that of the intellect central and only after these are adequately developed, true spirituality can follow. But with bodies half-famished, minds mostly occupied in evading the grasp of starvation, or at best engrossed in litigation, what chance is there for spirituality to develop? For any knowledge we need experience, for experience we have to work, and for work we need food and health. "India is to be raised, the poor are to be fed, education is to be spread." These he indicated as the religion of India at present if she does not want to be wiped off from the face of the earth with all her Vedas and philosophies!

As for the life of a sannyasin, his work and his ideals, we need not recall the past. All that is necessary for us is to remember that Vivekananda was a sannyasin. Critics of life of sannyas must be very unobservant of recent history; Narendranath Dutta as a lawyer might have won laurels in his profession, might have occupied the most coveted position in life. But Vivekananda is quite a different power altogether. What little we see of his life's influence is but a dim beginning.

About himself, he said: "My life's allegiance is to my Motherland, and if I had a thousand lives, every moment of the whole series would be consecrated to your service, my countrymen, my friends." Man he was and work he did. Monk he was and God he preached. His God was the suffering millions, the real living gods of his. Elevation of the depressed classes was not his idea but worshipping God the poor, God the lowly, God the depressed, was his theme. He believed in the power of the Spirit, which is infinite, "made to bear upon matter evolves material development, made to bear upon thought evolves intellectuality, made to act upon itself makes of man a god." For our worship he wanted us to develop all these in a harmonious balance. This was his idea of revival of religion and unless we develop this true religious spirit, of worship of God in the needy, the task of feeding and educating our millions is well-nigh impossible,.

A man in a million
– Norendronath Sen

To Swami Vivekananda belongs the undying honour of being the pioneer in the noble work of Hindu religious revival, consummated by bringing Western thought to bear upon it in appreciation of the beauty and grandeur of its doctrine and discipline. The heroic efforts of the Swami towards uniting the East and West into a fraternal union by the silken ties of spiritual kinship, deservedly met with a considerable measure of success. He dedicated his life to the blessed task of spreading the light of Hindu thought, which attained to the sublimest flights that the mind of man can ever ascend in the Western land and mists and shadows, overshadowed by doubts, perplexities and errors, and steeped in materialism of the grossest type, and the good seed since sown by him in America and Europe promises to germinate and yield in abundant harvest in the fulness of time. It was almost entirely owing to his genial personality, his vast culture and erudition, in the lore of Vedantism, his undoubted sympathy, his simplicity, and unostentatiousness and his earnestness and will, that Hindu philosophy and theology could make such headway, and be appraised at its true worth in Western countries. He devoted himself with the whole force of his gigantic intellect to achieve the regeneration and moral conquest of the world by the illumination of Hindu religion and philosophy and to harmonize the aggressive civilization of the West, against which the trend of religious ideas in Christendom seems to be absolutely impotent in robbing it of its conspicuous character of iron and blood, on lives of harmony, spirituality and bliss.

There is yet another aspect of the surpassing usefulness of the Swami, worthy of the highest commendation, which brings out in prominent relief, the nobility of his character, the loftiness of his aim and the feminine kindness of his heart. Rare indeed, is the example he has so gloriously set of disinterested and almost selfless philanthropy. We all remember with admiration and gratitude the magnificent work of rescue and succour undertaken and accomplished by the noble band of self-sacrificing workers of the Ramakrishna Mission, under the inspiration and guidance of the great Swami. As the accredited head of this earnest band of devoted workers he organized with remarkable success, extensive, philanthropic works in different parts of India for the alleviation of pain, misery and wretchedness. This silent but practical altruism has left a permanent record in the annals of the country and impressed the popular mind with a profound sense of moral duty, with which asceticism can be associated.

Such, indeed, was his character – a man in a million – who has laid down the burden of life to the intense sorrow of his admiring countrymen and passed away after the end of his temporary journey in this fleeting world, into peace eternal. The venerable Swami was in every sense a Prince among men, whose purity of life, loftiness of aim and principles and many-sided activity have entitled him through generations yet unborn, to the admiring gratitude of posterity.

> *"He was a man, take him all in all;*
> *We shall not look upon his like again."*

He heralded the birth of national renaissance
– H.V. Seshadri

Leaders like Vivekananda, Tilak and Gandhi could move the masses because they were inspired with a life-mission. The people too understood them. They felt the inmost chord of their heart touched. Swami Vivekananda, even while pouring out his agony at the suffering and misery of the toiling masses, invoked the sublimest impulses of the hoary spiritual and cultural heritage imbedded in the nation's psyche to set things right. Tilak and Gandhi spoke more of the immediate political and economic serfdom tormenting the body and mind of our nation. Every one of their programmes, actions and utterances, however, was directed towards quickening the spirit of national pride and national identity and charging the people with the spirit of resistance to all opposing forces.

Swami Vivekananda, even before he stepped on our soil, back from his itinerary in the West, had created an unprecedented wave of national response. People, right from the Maharajas to the humblest of the humble, were ready to offer him a thrilling hero's welcome. And the Swami's celebrated *Bharata-yatra* from Colombo to Almora literally heralded the birth of National Renaissance of modern Bharat. He gave to the people a vision of the glorious national destiny and infused them with a sense of national direction to march forward. Thus was lit the fire of national idealism in a thousand hearts, right from fiery revolutionaries to moderates in politics, from wandering monks to social reformers, and in every field of national resurgence.

Indeed, today, the need of the hour is for such men – not merely for one man here or another man there but hundreds and thousands and lakhs covering every tiny part of the country – men who themselves are content with minimum needs of life and find a joy in working without any desire for name or fame or monetary or political gains. They have to toil as disciplined and dedicated soldiers fired with the vision of resuscitating our national life in all its varied aspects – the social, educational, religious, cultural, economic and political.

Towards that end a vast country-wide man-moulding process has to go on steadily and silently year after year, decade after decade, in fulfilment of the man-making mission of Swami Vivekananda.

His was a rich life
– Dr. Karan Singh

Swami Vivekananda lived a very short life, in the normally accepted sense of the term, only 39 years from 1863 to 1902. And yet how much did he achieve in this very short period! His was a rich life.... in the course of this short life, Swami Vivekananda achieved virtually a miracle. He not only formulated the very essence of Hinduism, to meet the requirements of his age, but also of Religion itself, of Universal Religion....

With Swamiji's visit to America and his apperance in the Chicago Parliament of Religions, began a long and continuing process of creative interaction between the highwatermark of Hindu civilization – The Vedanta – and the West. In Chicago Swamiji gave a new perspective of Religion and introduced India to the West.

It seems to me that the message of Swami Vivekananda is even more needed today than it was at the time when he delivered it.... It seems to me that there is no better guide in these troubled times than Swami Vivekananda.... He is a *rishi*, a *drshta*, a seer. He has seen the vision of India. It is for the people like you and me to try to fulfil that vision.... This to my mind is the truest way of paying our homage to Swami Vivekananda.

His gospel marked the awakening of man in fullness
– Rabindranath Tagore

If you want to know India, study Vivekananda. In him everything is positive and nothing negative.

Vivekananda said that there was the power of Brahman in every man, that Narayana (i.e. God) wanted to have our service through the poor. This is what I call real gospel. This gospel showed the path of infinite freedom from man's tiny egocentric self beyond the limits of all selfishness. This was no sermon relating to a particular ritual, nor was it a narrow injunction to be imposed upon one's external life. This naturally contained in it protest against untouchability – not because that would make for political freedom, but because that would do away with the humiliation of man – a curse which in fact puts to shame the self of us all.

Vivekananda's gospel marked the awakening of man in his fullness and that is why it inspired our youth to the diverse courses of liberation through work and sacrifice.

In recent times in India, it was Vivekananda alone who preached a great message which is not tied to any do's and don'ts. Addressing one and all in the nation, he said: 'In every one of you there is the power of Brahman (God); the God in the poor desires you to serve Him.' This message has roused the heart of the youths in a most pervasive way. That is why this message has borne fruit in the service of the nation in diverse ways and in diverse forms of sacrifice. This message has at one and the same time, imparted dignity and respect to man along with energy and power. The strength that this message has imparted to man is not confined to a particular point; nor is it limited to repetitions of some physical movements. It has, indeed, invested his life with a wonderful dynamism in various spheres. There at the source of the adventurous activities of today's youth of Bengal is the message of Vivekananda – which calls the soul of man, not his fingers.

Vivekananda's message lights up for man's consciousness the path to limitless liberation from the trammels and limitations of the self. His message is a call of awakening to the totality of our manhood through work, renunciation and service.

A rich personality
– S. R. Talghatti

Swami Vivekananda is one of the greatest sons of India. His was a rich personality in which the physical, mental, intellectual, and moral qualities fructified into a fine example of a spiritual being. He was a philosopher, a true guide and a devoted friend of the Indian people and nation. As one of the chief architects of the Indian Renaissance, he aroused India to a sense of her cultural and national glory. "Arise, Awake" was the call he gave to her in the words of the Upanishads, "and stop not till the goal is reached." Though the call was addressed to the Indian people, in its spiritual aspect, it was addressed to the whole of humanity. The essence of his teaching is that man bears the spark of divinity in his bosom; and the essence of his lifelong activity consists in setting this spark aglow by reminding man of his divinity and by trying to bring it to the fore. This he calls religion.... It is on this principle of Divinity that his "Religion of Man" is built.... This is Swami Vivekananda's unique contribution to both philosophy and religion.

His nationalistic teachings were meant to awaken the Indians, especially Hindus, to their immediate duties and the true nature of their spiritual heritage. He preached the gospel of strength both in mundane and in spiritual life. By strength, of course, he meant not only physical, but also mental and spiritual; mental strength signifying emotional stability and sound intellect. Swami Vivekananda's life itself is the expression of this 'strength.'

He was convinced of the truth that to serve man is to serve God.

Religion was one dominant theme of his discussions. But his versatile intellect was devoted also to the study and exposition of other philosophical topics and problems in Indian philosophy. He has also given us a scholarly exposition of the basic principles of all the yogas prescribed for God-realization or self-realization, viz., *Jnana Yoga, Karma Yoga, Bhakti Yoga,* and *Raja Yoga,* with an excellent commentary of the *Yoga Sutras* of Patanjali.

Being basically a rationalist, Vivekananda sought rational explanations and justifications for his views and preached these to others. Though a champion of religion, he never thought that science was an impediment to religion, or reason to faith.

Education being the most powerful means of social regeneration, the Swami was very much concerned with it. The very mission of his life was to educate people. He defined education as, "the manifestation of perfection already in man." This short definition contains a whole philosophy of education.

Swami Vivekananda was a prophet of spiritual life who preached and practised universal humanism. He harmonized, in himself, East and West, reason and faith, material values and spiritual ones. He was a brave warrior who fought to the last against ignorance and poverty, discrimination and hatred. He wanted others, especially the intelligentsia, to do the same. Hence the establishment of Ramakrishna Math and Mission.

The distinctive feature of the spiritual renaissance movement started by Swami Vivekananda in the light of the teachings of Sri Ramakrishna was the organization of selfless workers formed into what was called Ramakrishna Mission.

His lofty legacy
– Prof. L. C. Thanu

Swami Vivekananda, one of the greatest sons of India, was the brightest star in the religious firmament of the world in the 19th century. He represented the best in the spiritual traditions of India and gave his best to the world during the nineties of the last century.

Within a brief span of less than forty years, Swamiji compressed an intensity of life, thought and action which had its impact on both the East and the West. His charismatic personality was a blending of the finest traditions of the spirituality of the East and the scholarship of the West. He was a pragmatic transcendentalist who dreamt of a universal religion and preached the Universal message of unity and tolerance and strove for the reconciliation of human contrasts and conflicts. He was a pioneer in modern India in the spheres of philosophy and religion. He was one of the leading torch-bearers who reawakened India and instilled self-confidence in the nation and revived the respect and faith in their glorious past and removed their inferiority complex, brought about by the British rule. Thanks to him, Hinduism attained the pinnacle of its glory, both at home and abroad.

Pandit Jawaharlal Nehru describes the many-splendoured personality of this warrior monk in the following words: "Rooted in the past and full of pride in India's heritage Vivekananda was yet modern in his approach to life's problems. He was a kind of bridge between the past of India and her present." Romain Rolland says: "Equilibrium and synthesis are the two watchwords of the personality of Swami Vivekananda. He was the harmony of all human energy." The Patriot-monk characterized himself as a 'condensed India' and is the symbol of national integration.

Swamiji had his spiritual training under the great master Sri Ramakrishna Paramahamsa. The two between them constituted a single integrated personality, the guru was the inspiration and the sishya, action. As spiritual heir to Sri Ramakrishna he understood fully the message of his guru, namely that of the universality of the supreme, of the essential oneness of the various religions of the world and of the duty to serve man in order to reach God. His mission in life was to find the common bases of Hinduism and to awaken national consciousness among Indians. His message was always the gospel of salvation, of social elevation and of equality for all. His vision was all-embracing, and his outlook 'universal.'

Swami Vivekananda was a man of the masses, his great motto being their elevation. His concern always was for the common man, the poor, the lowly and the lost who were for him the *Daridranarayana*. He realized that it was absurd to preach spirituality before hungry millions; 'an empty stomach is no good for religion.' He pointed out that what people needed first and foremost was food, beside employment; then and only then, could any spirituality be aroused among the masses. He was a patriot. To him, love of the Motherland meant the love of its people and the service of the masses in a spirit of dedication. He embodied in his life the motto: "If you want to find God, serve man." Hence service of the Indian masses was the service of India, was his message to his countrymen. According to him "worship of God is worship of the *virat*, (cosmic form of the Absolute) of those all around us. Let this be our God – men and animals – and the first God we have to worship is our countrymen. He alone is worshipping God who serves all beings. Worship Shiva in the poor, the diseased and the weak.

He enunciated the doctrine of social philosophy and service to the low. He held everyman as a traitor who did not try to alleviate the sufferings of humanity. His concept of brotherhood of man runs thus: What good is it, if we acknowledge in our prayers that God is the Father of us all, and in our daily lives do not treat every man as our brother? He was thus a humanist possessing infinite love towards humanity; he could not restrain tears when he came into contact with the suffering humanity.

His approach to religion is scientific and rational. According to him, "religion is realization, not talk nor doctrine nor theories; it is being and becoming, not hearing and acknowledging." He advocated a man-making religion, a humanistic religion, a religion which looks upon all human beings as kindred, as belonging to one family. He envisaged 'one Universal Religion' because he realized the harmony of all religions. All religions are complementary; they are different forces in the scheme of God working for the good of mankind. Brotherhood, spirituality, renunciation and service are the basic truths behind them all. Hence he exhorted not only toleration, but acceptance of all religions.

Swami Vivekananda wanted the youth to pursue a life-building, man-making, character-building education. He asked them to develop an integrated personality; cultivate *abhaya* (fearlessness) in the pursuit of truth; develop science and rationality in the place of superstition and obscurantism.

He served as a bridge between the East and the West; he was our cultural ambassador to the Occident. As an impartial observer, he appreciated the virtues and condemned the shortcomings of both. He could see both sides of a coin. He saw India's grinding poverty, her social backwardness and the mental inertia into which she had fallen; but he also saw her cultural wealth, the strength of her traditions, her assimilative powers and, above all, her latent spiritual energy. He admired the West for their dynamism, social awareness, spirit of adventure, capacity for hard work and concern for practical values. In the achievement of science, he saw the triumph of the human spirit. But the limitation of Western civilization also became apparent to him. He saw the monumental ignorance, the crushing incomprehension that co-existed with so much progress. The safety of the Western civilization, he pointed out, lay in the tempering of its materialism with spirituality.

He conquered the West by his message of sprituality at the Parliament of Religions held at Chicago in 1893, where his appearance was like the lightning and speech soul-stirring. At a forum specifically got up to proclaim the Western religion and thought, he literally, "went, saw and conquered." "The cyclonic monk from India" addressed the audience as "Sisters and Brothers of America." Unlike those of politicians, those words came from the bottom of his heart and profoundly impressed the audience. He pleaded for universal tolerance and stressed the common basis of all religions presenting the universal aspect of Vedanta. His clarion call to the people of the world through the Parliament was, "Help, and not fight", "Assimilation, and not destruction", "Harmony and peace, and not dissension."

Swami Vivekananda was the morning bird of Indian religious and cultural renaissance. He worked for social emancipation and championed the cause of the poor and the downtrodden. His message, in brief, was "Be and Make." His greatest gift is the Ramakrishna Mission dedicated to the ideals os spiritual regeneration and social emelioration.

Summing up, Swami Vivekananda's contribution may be described as the organizing and consolidation of Hindu ideals. There is, according to him, in reality, no difference between sacred and secular. Every aspect of life is and should be made a part of religion; and man becomes divine by realizing the divine in every aspect of the universe and of life's activities. Swamiji insisted that by expression *Ishtadevata* was meant that each man may seek God in his own way provided that he is sincere and tolerant."

Swami Vivekananda's message has great relevance to us at present as the country is passing through a crisis of character. We also witness the sorry spectacle of poverty, economic inequalities, unemployment, shortage of goods, rising prices, anti-social activities like black marketing, adulteration, smuggling, corruption, fall in moral values, dichotomy in our profession and practice, religious bigotry, untouchability, divisive forces in the shape of communalism, linguism, regionalism, differing political ideologies, lack of national consciousness and character, absence of dedicated leadership, undue emphasis on rights forgetting duties, the mania to become rich quick by any means – fair or foul and the like. All these evils are the result of lack of proper perspective on our part. Vivekananda's teachings can offer us proper guidance and will be a royal remedy to most of these maladies that afflict the land and act as cankers. So let us pay our homage to the great Swamiji by practising in letter and spirit, what he taught us and it is the best way to perpetuate his memory.

A veritable saviour of the whole human race
– Prof. Trilochan Das

Swami Vivekananda was one of the greatest men ever born on earth. He shines like a bright luminary in the spiritual firmament of the world. A beloved and worthy disciple of Sri Ramakrishna, Vivekananda had realized God.

Physically of athletic build, Swami Vivekananda's fiery patriotism, phenomenal knowledge, extraordinary dialectical skill, gifted oratory, together with the charm of his magnetic personality, made him the veritable idol of young men and women and wherever he went, whoever read his speeches and writings, were completely conquered by him. Indeed, his tall commanding figure, his arresting appearance, his magnetic personality with eyes flashing like lightning and a voice militant and dynamic made him the most attractive figure in the Parliament of Religions at Chicago, U. S. A.

A harbinger of the message of Joy Eternal, of Peace and Heavenly Bliss, Vivekananda, in his world-famous Chicago Address hailed mankind as: 'Ye Divinities on Earth' and not as so many 'Sinners.' He has thus divinized every human being on Earth and has enthused millions with the 'fire of freedom' and has roused them from their age-long slumber and morbidity. Vivekananda has thus proved himself to be the veritable saviour of the whole human race.

There was a time when Swami Vivekananda was regarded as one of the greatest saviours of Hinduism. There was also a time when he was regarded as the Prophet of Patriotism – the inspirer of Indian nationalist movement as he was. I feel the time has now come when Swami Vivekananda has to be evaluated as one of the greatest saviours of mankind.

It is a religion of man-making and character-building that Swami Vivekananda has preached. It is a religion of patriotism that he has preached. It is a religion of Universal Love, of Universal Brotherhood, of Universal Tolerance, that he has preached – a religion of love and service for the poor, the lowly, the humble, the down-trodden, exploited miserable masses and hungry millions throughout the length and breadth of the Universe. It is a religion of fearlessness and of Divine Humanism that he has preached – a religion to turn every man and woman on Earth into so many palpable, blissful living gods and goddesses. It is a Religion of self-sacrifice and renunciation for the well-being of millions and millions of under-privileged suffering human beings.

A ruthless crusader against poverty, Vivekananda pleaded strongly not only for moral progress but for the material and economic progress, as well. He wanted to have a social revolution by launching root and branch reform. A bloodless revolution through love, tolerance, renunciation and fraternal feelings was Swami Vivekananda's dream.

His pride for India's glorious past – his pride for India's rich cultural heritage – knew no bounds. He is also the Saint-Patriot of India, inspirer of India's Nationalism as he is. As Netaji Subhas Chandra Bose has aptly observed: "With Swami Vivekananda religion was the inspirer of nationalism. He tried to infuse into the new generation a sense of pride in India's past, of faith in India's future and a spirit of self-confidence and self-respect."

Who is not aware of the fact that Swami Vivekananda revitalized and regenerated the Hindu Religion? He has further led many people to "believe firmly that wonderful spiritual truths lie hidden in the ancient Hindu Scriptures...."

None before Swami Vivekananda ever made an impassioned appeal to the Indians irrespective of their caste, creed or provincial affiliations to love everything Indian – to love all objects, animate and inanimate, to the extent of even loving and venerating every particle of sand and dust of the Indian soil. How sacred is the Indian soil to him! No wonder, Sister Nivedita observes: "But the Queen of his adoration was his Motherland."

Swami Vivekananda has taught us to be one with the teeming millions of India, nay of the whole world – the teeming millions of suffering human beings. Vivekananda has dreamt and worked for a World Religion – for Universal Brotherhood.

All the religions of the world were according to his conception "so many forms of an unending Eternal Religion." He believed not in theological doctrines, dogmas and rituals but in realization and inner illumination. He has identified religion with altruistic service, with Knowledge, with action, with the manifestation of divinity, energy and manliness, and with bravery, morality and fearlessness. Finally, he has reduced religion to a realistic, practical, rational form.

As Benoy Sarkar observed, Swami Vivekananda "wanted to create new worlds and distribute the fire of freedom, happiness, divinity and immortality among men and women."

It may justly be said that India's destiny was changed by Vivekananda and that his teachings re-echoed throughout Huminity. He give birth to a mighty new India – the India of today and India that is yet to be. And what we see today is that behind all the modern movements of India, – political, economic, social, cultural, educational or whatever else it may be, there is Vivekananda's teachings and ideal.

It strikes us with wonder that even after nearly eighty-five years (in 1986) of Swami Vivekananda's death, none has been able so far to evaluate in the proper and true perspective, his unique and invaluable contributions to India and to humanity at large.

It should be the sacred duty of everyone to establish on a strong footing the life, message and thought of Swami Vivekananda throughout the length and breadth of India; nay the whole world. Nothing is more sacred than performing that noble task.

For years to come, generations of boys and girls will be inspired and fascinated by the teachings of Swami Vivekananda. In fact, he has a message of hope for the whole human race. Spiritual path-finder of millions of men and women on earth, Swami Vivekananda is adored and admired not only by the young men and women, he is the symbol of hope for mankind tormented by conflicting ideologies, dissensions and self-interest.

A great spell all around he lent
– Dr. S. B. Varnekar

येनोध्वस्तं जडमतवतां राज्यमेकातपत्रं
सच्चैतन्यं जनगणमनः सर्वथाऽकारि तूर्णम् ।
धर्मग्लानिः प्रवचनमहामन्त्रशक्त्या निरस्ता·
उच्चैर्नीता भुवि भरतभूवैनयन्ती जयन्ती ॥ १ ॥

Oh God, oh God, how shall I dare
To describe Vivekanand of divine glare?
India was in materialism's grip,
She was in slumber deep.
But when Vivekanand appeared
Materialism quivered
And vanished into the air
Like mists before the sun bright and fair;
The masses that had become demoralised
Were awakened and revitalized;
Religion that in a fainting fit lay
Woke up and looked cheerful and gay;
And Vivekanand now unfurled
Among the nations of the world
India's religious banner
In the most glorious manner.

साक्षात् काली शुचिजनमनःकामनाकल्पवल्ली
सा यस्याग्रे स्वयमुपगताऽभीष्टकामप्रपूर्त्यै ।
येनापत्तिक्रथितमनसाऽप्यर्थितार्तस्वरेण
विस्मृत्यान्यन्निजसुखमहो भक्तिरेवातिशुध्दा ॥ २ ॥

It is known to one and all
Whatever a devotee fervently does want
Kalee the Mother Divine does grant.
One day Kalee did appear
To know Vivek's heart's desire.
She assured she would grant

Whatever he would want.
Hard pressed by poverty
Vivekanand and his family starved
And suffered innumerable pains
But he would not pray for material gains.
He prayed to Kalee not for wealth,
Property, Money, success or health.
The world for him had no charm or lure,
So he prayed only for devotion pure.

फुल्लत्रीलाम्बुरुहनयनं निष्कलङ्केन्दुवक्त्रम्
व्यूढोरस्कं दृढतमवृषस्कन्धमुत्तुङ्गकायम् ।
यत्सौन्दर्यं ललितवनिता वीक्ष्य कामेषुविध्दाः
यूना येन प्रथिततपसा मातृवद् वन्दितास्ताः ॥ ३ ॥

Vivek's face was like a spotless moon
And his eyes like lotuses in full bloom,
His chest broad and shoulders thick
His gait majestic and quick.
Wherever, wherever he went
A great spell all around he lent.
When he went to the West
With a religious mission
Many a woman developed passion,
But when they went near him
Vivek's love divine
Flowed like a violent stream
And all that was gross and vile in them
Disappeared as does a dream
When sleep is broken.
And in spiritual dread
They surrendered and bowed their head
As does a cobra wild
To a charmer's music mild.

वन्दे यस्येन्द्रियगणकृतिनैष्ठिकी कर्मयोगं
चेतोवृत्तिर्यमनियमसुस्थापिता राजयोगम् ।
ईशस्तोत्रस्मरणरसिका भावना भक्तियोगं
सःस्वाध्यायप्रवचनरता शेमुषी ज्ञानयोगम् ॥ ४ ॥

All his sense organs –
Nose, skin, tongue, eye and ear
Acted in harmony clear.
His mind was passion free
Like a calm and quiet sea
With its rythmic roll heaving free.
His mind, intellect, heart, emotion
All acted in perfect unison.
They were, as it were,
Wedded together
To help the soul
To reach its goal.

यत्सङ्गीतस्वरमधुरिमापानतृप्तान्तराणां

ब्रह्मानन्दोऽनुभवपदवीं प्राप सद्भावुकानाम् ।

यद्व्याख्यानश्रवणविगलत्सर्ववेद्यान्तराणां

ज्ञानानन्दः प्रतिपदसुधास्वादभाजां जनानाम् ॥ ५ ॥

Vivekanand's voice was as sweet as honey,
And he poured harmony on harmony
When he sang songs divine;
Melody on melody filled the air
And persons who would be near
Would forget the earth gross and vile
And enjoy heavenly bliss for a while.
When he did deliver a lecture
He did a million minds capture.
There was a wizard in his each sound
And it kept the millions spellbound
Anybody who him did listen to
Did have surely a peep into
The joys and bliss of heaven.

दृष्ट्वा विद्याविभवमतुलं यस्य विभ्राजमानं

पाश्चात्यानामतिधनवतामस्तमाप्तो हि गर्वः ।

दिव्यं तेजः शुचितमसुशीलोद्भवं यन्मुखाब्जे

गौरास्यानामशुचिचरितानामभूत् कृष्णभावः ॥ ६ ॥

Proud, haughty and impolite,
And arrogant Western white
Felt small and in fear shrank
To see this Indian monk.
Their pride vanished like the morning mist
Before this brilliant son of the East.
Each member of the white race
Seemed to have no beauty, charm, or grace
Beside the divinely illumined face
Of Swami Vivekanand.

येनानेकोत्तमबुधसभाजिष्णुना पण्डितेन
माद्यन्मेघध्वनितमुखरो हिन्दुभूगौरवाय ।
वाक्सामर्थ्याहत इव यशोदुन्दुभेः सान्द्रनादः
दिङ्मातङ्गैश्चकितचकितं श्रूयतेऽद्यापि नित्यम् ॥ ७ ॥

About a hundred years ago
In the city of Chicago
Vivekanand did attend
The conference of religions,
Attended by legions
From all the world round,
And kept all spellbound.
It was here that he sounded clear
The drum of Victory.
Even after the lapse of a hundred years
That voice of Vivek rings in the ears
Of one and all like a trumpet call
In every part of the world.

शब्दे शब्दे भुवनजयिनी यस्य सन्मन्त्रशक्तिः
पादे पादे सुदृढनिहिते कास्विदुत्साहशक्तिः ।
यद्दृक्पातैर्जनगणमनस्स्वाहिता राष्ट्रशक्तिः
यत्सङ्कारैः प्रथममुदिता भारती धर्मशक्तिः ॥ ८ ॥

In every word he did tell
There did dwell a divine spell;
Every step he did take
Had the power to shake
The lethargy of the land;

And his fiery glance
Was like a divine lance
To send a man into a trance
Of divine ecstasy.
He wandered, wandered, and wandered
Through the country's breadth and length
Stimulating spiritual health.
And blended nationalism
With the broad aims of Hinduism.

यस्योद्गारैः स्थिरपदमभूत् तत्र वेदान्तशास्त्रं
यस्याचारैर्विचलितमभूत् सर्वपाखण्डजातम् ।
यस्याह्वानैर्हतवलमभूद् दुर्मतं नास्तिकानां
सानन्दोऽभूत् प्रथितयशसा यस्य नाम्ना विवेकः ॥ ९ ॥

He casually referred to the Vedanta
In the Western world
And these casual references unfurled
The glory and eternal character
Of the Vedanta literature
In a voice clear and loud
He proclaimed the existence of God
And the agnostics and sceptics
Gathered in a crowd
And their heads bowed
And stricken with terror
Admitted their error.
His voice everybody dreaded,
For he was truly Vivekanand
Which means conscience to gladness wedded,

पीत्वाऽप्यादौ नवमतसुरामाङ्ग्लसाहित्यसूतां
पीता पश्चाद् गुरूचरणसद्भक्तिपीयूषधारा ।
तत्सामर्थ्यव्यवहितमहाशक्तिना येन यूना
पीत्वा रोगद्रवमयजलं धिक्कृतो ह्यन्तकोऽपि ॥ १० ॥

He had deeply read English literature
And was steeped in Western culture.
Then this ascetic of unique power
Met Ramakrishna in Rashmoni's bower
And then sat at the feet of his great preceptor

And enjoyed divine devotional nectar.
This devotional flow at length
Gave him strength and power
To look beyond the temporal hour,
To defy death and disease,
All worldly comfort and ease.

मामाश्रित्य स्वगुरुचरणोपासनाऽसंख्यसंख्यैः
श्रीकृष्णाद्यैरपि सुरवरैः साधिता, नो मया तु ।
इत्येवाद्याश्रम इह नरेन्द्रस्य यस्याप्य रूपं
सच्छिष्यत्वं स्वयमिव गतो रामकृष्णस्य तस्य ॥ ११ ॥

Gods, saints and sages celibacy observed
And thus shelter at their guru's feet deserved.
But celibacy itself remained ever poor,
For it could not enter heaven's door
By worshipping a guru.
Desiring into heaven to step
Celibacy took birth in the concrete shape
Of Narendra, later called Vivekanand
Who is celibacy concretized,
And thus it realized
The ultimate Reality
Through the grace and pity
Of Sri Ramakrishna.

विश्वख्यातं कृतं येन
भारतस्योज्ज्वलं यशः ।
वन्दे विवेकानन्दं तं
सद्धर्मपथदर्शकम् ॥ १२ ॥

Salutations unto Swami Vivekananda, the able guide on the path to true religion, who made universally renowned the resplendent glory of Bharat.

He had a vibrant message
– Prof. K. N. Vaswani

Vivekananda, an *avatar* of both *shakti* and *bhakti,* came to awaken a slumbering people, a nation that had forgotten its past glory and was not facing the challenge of its present problems and was not forging ahead to fashion a worthy and bright future for itself, for its suffering and neglected, diffident and dejected, demoralized and dispirited people who were going down in the field of battle, because they had lost faith in themselves, lost faith in God, faith in values of their civilization, their culture, faith in their forefathers, faith in their ancient heritage, the wisdom of the Vedanta, of the Upanishads, and the ancient sages. To such a people in such a condition, comes, to rouse and revitalise them, the moving message of Swami Vivekananda.

What is this message? What is Swami Vivekananda's message to modern India, to the modern world?

His message to the modern world is the message of harmony and universal brotherhood. He delivered it in his speeches at the World's Parliament of Religions in Chicago. While others had spoken of their separate narrow sects, here was Vivekananda proclaiming the message of Vedanta, the wisdom of the *Gita*, the great truth of the oneness of man; the fact of the brotherhood of man. Here was a man whose heart was as broad as the ocean and here was a religion which embraced all without exception, without any condition. That is why Swami Vivekananda became the most popular figure at the Parliament of Religions. "Sisters and Brothers of America", the very words uttered by him, were spoken with such firm conviction, with such feeling born of real *tapas* that the listeners were lifted up beyond themselves, elevated in the presence of a pure soul and kept clapping for several minutes.... Swami Vivekananda was therefore a voice of vision and wisdom. He was forging a bridge between the East and the West. He was for fraternity, the highest ideal of humanity.

'Why fight, are not all men His children? Potentially Divine? Gods in the making?' That was Vivekananda's Vedantic view. His view could well be put in those memorable words: 'The world is my country, to do good is my religion, all mankind are my brethren.'

And what was his message to modern India? 'We want a man-making religion. We want a character-building education. We all must work hard, to build the nation great and strong. Nation-building needs strong muscles and loving hearts of dedicated men. We want man, man with a Capital 'M'. Men with a will, men with vigour and vitality, men with faith in God and faith in themselves to surmount all obstacles. Men, selfless men, who put the country and the nation above themselves and are willing to serve the nation – to sacrifice for the nation. Men, who have a vision of their ideal and will to pursue it with zeal, determination and dedication.'

Swami Vivekananda's message to modern India is that mere meditation is not enough. Meditation must flower into action, into service, national service. Meditation builds the bridge between man and God and brings in tune the finite with the Infinite. Meditation flowering into action, into service, must bridge the gulf between man and man and create a climate of compassion and a feeling of fraternity and fellowship, and generate the spirit of co-operation and comradeship and inspire the activities of giving or sharing with God's creatures who are in need.

'Give, give with generosity, give out of the goodness of your heart, give with kindness and compassion, true sympathy and love. Give, Give'– is the call of Swami Vivekananda to all. Let us learn to give, for to give is to live, and to give lovingly is to live gloriously, to live truly.

Swami Vivekananda had a vibrant message for young India, the youth of India. His message to youth of India was 'Be simple, be pure and be strong'. Be strong in the service of the nation, our suffering countrymen, sunk in misery and destitution, ignorance or superstition. His message was 'Simplify, Purify, Unify, Sanctify!' To simplify is to observe voluntary poverty, adopt a life of austerity; to purify is to free ourselves from the ego; to unify is to strengthen the unity in the country; and to sanctify is to link ourselves with the divine and have the feeling that God blesses us.

What is Vivekananda's message to us – to you and me?

I hear this message every morning as I sit to greet the sunrise, the beautiful dawn. I hear it every evening as I watch the wonder of the sunset, hear it as I listen to the rythmic roar of the sea waves dashing ceaselessly against the shore. This message comes gently, tenderly, sweetly, and sometimes in moving, stirring, commanding tones: O child of *Bharata Mata*, 'Arise, Awake and stop not till the goal is reached.'

It is a call for awakening to the fact of our Divine Origin, and to arise and march towards our Divine Destiny.

It is a call to *sadhana*, to hard work, to *tapas*, a call to dynamic and dedicated action.

Swami Vivekananda has received countless tributes. Among the best known to me is by Romain Rolland, the great French savant and the Nobel Prize winner in literature, who has written a beautiful Biography of Swami Vivekananda. He has written about "his lion's heart."

Another tribute to the great memory of Swami Vivckananda, very significant indeed, has been the erection of a magnificent National Memorial on the Vivekananda Rock at Kanyakumari, where he meditated and where dawned on him the mission of his life that his meditation must flower into dynamic action and he must spread the message of Vedanta to the West, as well as to his people in India and so he decided to go to America, to the World Congress of Religions in Chicago. The memorial is truly national for it was conceived as the significant programme in the Vivekananda Centenary Celebrations (1963) and has been built by the people of India – the common people from every nook and corner of the country, contributing their little mite towards its cost of over a crore of rupees. Begun by the Vivekananda Centenary Celebrations Committee set-up in 1963, the Memorial was completed in 1970.

A greater tribute than this magnificent national memorial in stone to Swami Vivekananda is certainly, 'the living memorial', Vivekananda Kendra,

. the Service Mission, which trains and transforms the Youth of India, men
and women, into dedicated selfless *sevaks* of the people, seeking and
striving to fulfil Swami Vivekananda's dream of dedicated Youth going over
the length and breadth of the land, serving the poor, the dispossessed and
the downtrodden, assiduously engaged in the task of social raising up and
working towards bringing an era of equality. May their numbers grow more
and more, and also the quality of their service too grow, through the
inspiration of Swami Vivekananda and by the blessings of the Lord.

A great soul
– Sadhu T. L. Vaswani

A marvellous story this – of Vivekananda's life. I see in it the grace of
God. Vivekananda, a keen intellectual of the College meets the great mystic,
Sri Ramakrishna Paramahamsa. The saint loves young Vivekananda. He
hears the saint say in answer to his question: "God can be realized. I see
Him and I speak to Him as I speak to you and see you. But who takes the
trouble to realize Him?.... If a man weeps sincerely for Him, He in His mercy,
will manifest Himself to him."

For some years the struggle within Vivekananda continued when,
suddenly, his eyes were opened. He felt there was around him a Presence.
A new life came pouring into him. Vivekananda was a changed man. His
life was henceforth a dedicated life. He became a sannyasin; – a servant of
God, a servant of man.

"The highest knowledge of life", it has been rightly said, "is to make
contact with a great soul." Vivekananda, the beloved disciple of
Ramakrishna, was, verily, "a great soul."

India heard him; and his rich, rhythmical voice was heard in many places
In Europe and America. He was one of the great leaders of the Indian
Renaissance – one of the inspired interpreters of Hindu culture and Hindu
ideals.

Vivekananda was a man amongst men. He preached a "man-making
religion." Listen to Vivekananda's words: "It is a man-making religion that
we want. Give up all weakening creeds. Be strong!" "Religion", urged
Vivekananda, "is realization. It is awakening of the life of the Spirit in the
heart within. It is not creed."

Vivekananda voiced a faith reaffirmed in our days by Mahatma Gandhi.
Vivekananda says:

'He alone serves God who serves all beings. For the next fifty
years, let all vain gods disappear from our minds.

'Here is the God who is awake, – our Race. Everywhere His hands,
everywhere His feet, everywhere His ears. He covers everything.

'The first of all worships is the worship of those all around us.
These are our gods, – men and animals. And the first gods we
have to worship are our own countrymen!'

Vivekananda preached a virile message which has reminded me, again and again, of the teaching of the *rishis* and Heroes of India.

Vivekananda was a spiritual athlete, a man of *Shakti*. And in the heart of this strong man of *Shakti* was such tender love for the poor and the outcaste!

To Vivekananda, all religions were different paths to the one Eternal God, all religions were sacred as varying expressions of the one Religion of Truth and loving service and manliness.

Truth and courage were the essential elements of Vivekananda's faith which he boldly spoke of as the "Hindu Faith" and which he urged was the 'brother" of all religions. For, all religions, he pointed out, were true; all were God's revelations to man.

Vivekananda elevated work to the status of worship – but only when it is dedicated work, work dedicated to the service of humanity. The service of such a dedicated soul brings us all nearer to the *Ramarajya*, the kingdom of God.

Humility and love, – were two marks of Vivekananda's spiritual life. His soul rejoiced in the One God in all. Vivekananda declared that spiritual life was denied to none. As a true disciple of Ramakrishna,Vivekananda bore witness to the Vision Universal.

Filled with faith in the values of the Hindu Faith, he wished to make it a world-force. "With God," he said, "You can go over the sea! Without Him, you cannot go over the threshold!" With God, Vivekananda went over the sea! With God, Vivekananda crossed the Continents and re-proclaimed the wisdom of the *rishis*. "Arise! Awake!" was Vivekananda's trumpet call to India, England and America. In India, he set on fire the hearts of many with the message to make Hinduism world-dynamic. He interpreted to the world – values of Hindu Culture. He proclaimed the message of the brotherhood of Life to the nations of the world.

Vivekananda's great address at the Parliament of Religions, at Chicago, was full of love for all religions; but it was, also, a bold challenge to the critics of the Hindu Faith. He came; he spoke; he conquered! He captured the "Parliament" by his magnificent presence, his picturesque dress, his eloquence, above all, by his gospel of unity of all religions and by his ethics of the service of the poor and forlorn as the best worship of God. Vivekananda's speech revealed him as a world figure. The "Parliament" crowned him with the crown of glory.

Echoes of his great speech at the "Parliament of Religions" reached me when I was boy, studying in the school. I recall the day when I read the full text of his address; it thrilled me. It has been called the "Charter of the Hindu Faith" – the *Sanatana Dharma*. It delivers, in the words of imperishable beauty, the triple message at once of the spirit of religion, of the gospel of the Veda, the Upanishads, the *Gita*, and the soul of *Bharatavarsha* – the India of Ages – ancient yet ever new.

Every religion is a flower and we "gather all these flowers", Vivekananda said, "binding them together with the cord of love and making them into a wonderful bouquet of worship."

In Vivekananda's speeches at the "Parliament of Religion", you hear the note of his great Master, Ramakrishna Paramahamsa, the note of the Unity of all Religions. I hear in Vivekananda's speeches the notes, too, of India's *rishis* and saints, all blended in the music of Krishna and the Buddha and the sages of the East.

After the Congress, Vivekananda lectured on the Vedanta for over three years in America and Europe, and he studied the social progress of the West. He returned to India in 1897. In May, 1897. he founded the Ramakrishna Mission. Religion, he urged, must be religion of action – a religion of selfless service.

Vivekananda saw the place of technological, scientific and political achievement in the programme of national life. He realized the value of medicine, sanitation, electric power and food for nation-building. But let it not be forgotten that all programmes of social welfare stand in need of a "regulative idea", and that is the Atman, the Spirit. India's regeneration will not be achieved by mere technological discoveries. We must not destroy the "roots" of India's life. India's life is rooted in the Atman, the Spirit.

A dear, departed Russian friend of mine, Nicholas Roerich, who came to India in 1923, wrote – "Vivekananda was not merely an industrious Swami; something lion-like rings in his letters. How he is needed now!" More even than in 1923, India, today, hath need of thee, O Lion-hearted Vivekananda!

The man of the age
– Selvaraj Yesudian

He was my idol in childhood, because he personified the ideal. It was through him that I was able to grasp the abstract or esoteric teachings of the Bible. His was the concrete teaching I held on to till the abstract was in my possession. Then I let go the concrete aspects. In his teachings there was no repentance or regret for our past errors. There was no hell, hell-fire, eternal damnation or such elements of fear that the Christian Church instilled into me as a child. As the rising sun dispels darkness, so did his words dispel all fear in me and awake my crushed dignity. He was fearless in delivering his message to mankind, regardless of caste, creed and nationality. He was outspoken, and he operated like an expert surgeon in eradicating superstition.

The reason we love Vivekananda is because he was so human, and we Indians are prepared to accept any amount of criticisms and reprimands from him, for they were uttered with love. His heart bled for his suffering country- men.

Vivekananda's mission in life was to serve a double purpose. The first purpose was to fulfil the injunction of his revered Master Sri Ramakrishna, which was to work for the regeneration of his motherland, India, to whip it out of its lethargic sleep and to remind it of its first and foremost duty of standing on its feet and being strong as it once was in the past seeing the world on its march and keeping step with the evolution of today. The second was to tell mankind that we are one big family, no matter to what creed, caste, or nation we belong, that we should not quarrel about our religious outlooks, but respect each other's faith and realize that we are all worshipping one and the same God, though called by different names.

The messenger was for the moment more fascinating than his message. He spoke with authority, for he spoke out of experience. His unflinching attachment to truth was reflected in his dominating personality. His huge audiences were spell-bound at the mere appearance of the man and naturally they gave preference to the person rather than to the principles he taught.

I think that Vivekananda is the man of the age. It is as though this age itself had given birth to its leaders and wanted to follow him through thick and thin.

The simplest and most direct approach to Truth I found in the lectures of Vivekananda on the four yogas, for they were realized truths. In studying the lectures of Vivekananda, you will make a remarkable discovery that what he says is nothing new. His words merely confirm what we have come to know through experience in life.

Actually there is no dividing line between the four yogas.... The name given to the four things necessary for the attainment of true happiness are karma, bhakti, raja and jnana. This means that work, love, self-control and discrimination are the paths to the goal of happiness. This is in truth the essence of all the existing religions of the world. The science of yoga transcends all the paraphernalia of dogmas and rituals and teaches simple, plain truth. The Bible also emphasizes: 'It is Truth that shall set thee free.' Truth is not Christian, Hindu, Buddhist, Jewish or Islamic, nor is God a Christian, a Hindu, a Buddhist, Jew or Muslim. The truth is that we are spirit and not matter. For if not spirit, then what are we? The universal expression of the all-pervading, omnipotent and omnipresent spirit is creation. Karma, bhakti, raja and jnana yoga show us the means of experiencing this universal Truth.

Karmayoga tells us that work is one of the most beautiful means of expressing our perfection of spirit.

Bhaktiyoga teaches us to revere the whole of creation as a manifold manifestation of God, appearing before us in the most tangible form.

Rajayoga helps us to discover the legions of forces at our disposal, to bring them under control and make them work for us.

Jnanayoga equips us with the strength of knowledge gained through the power of discrimination. Ultimately we learn that when we wield the sword of discrimination we become invincible.

....I remember as a boy, when I was poor, sickly, weak, even friendless, I used to walk alone along the sea-coast before sunrise and read aloud Vivekananda's passionate and patriotic appeal: "Ninety per cent of human brutes you see are dead, are ghosts – for none lives, my boys, but he who loves. Feel, my children, feel; feel for the poor, the ignorant, the downtrodden, feel till the heart stops and the brain reels and you think you will go mad; then pour the soul out at the feet of the Lord and then will come power, help and indomitable energy. Struggle, struggle, was my motto for the last ten years. Struggle, still I say. When it was all dark I used to say struggle; when light is breaking in, I still say, struggle. Be not afraid, my children. Look not up in that attitude of fear toward that infinite starry vault as if it would crush you. Wait! In a few hours, more than whole of it will be under your feet. Wait, money does not pay, nor name; fame does not pay, nor learning. It is love that pays; it is character that cleaves its way through adamantine walls of difficulty."

Several such messages of this warrior-God were manna dropped into my starved soul, and they filled me. One day I was witness of a hurricane. I was perched on a high rock and far below, the sea was raging in all its fury. The waves rose mountains high, descending like a deluge on the rocky coast for miles. The earth quaked at every onslaught and the sight was at once frightening and fascinating. It was nature enacting the drama of life and death. It was the union of heaven and earth through war. This drama of apparent destruction reminded me of Vivekananda's revolutionary message to effect the evolution of mankind in due time. At once my heart poured itself out in a song of surrender to the great hero:

Thou God of Strength!
To burst upon the world
And grind its fetters into dust!
To come as a comet
And move man's slumbering heart to act!
Thy voice of thunder
Did awaken the dead man's soul!
Thou warrior!
Alone didst thou march on to the battlefield
With legions of gods to sing thy praise.
With lightning as helmet to blind the foe!
With the drum of the Vedas
To sound the eternal march of man!
Thy clarion call from peak to plain:
'Arise! Awake! And stop not till the goal is reached!'

Bharat's most noble son!
Hearing thy children call didst thou come
To lead us by the hand and say:
'Shake off thy slumber and thy sloth!
Shake off thy blinding shackles!
Shake off thy weakness and thy woe!
Bound is he who says he's bound!
Free is he who says he's free!
Arise! Awake! and onward go!'

Thou warrior! Thou blazing torch of light!
A thought of thee suffices,
For courage courses through our veins
And rushes to the heart,
And speaks with action bold,
Thy message we hear through all eternity:
'Be manly!
Be fearless!
Be free!
Stoop not, nor stop! But
Arise! Awake! and onward go!'

Prostrated by slavery, we lay low
Covered by the dust of dark centuries.
But thy touch of power has awakened
Bharat to breathe once more.
What thou didst breathe into her ear
Now throbs in her heart aloud:
'Awake! Awake, *Aryavarta!*
Arise! Awake!
And stop not till the goal is reached!'

Dream's curtain is drawn,
The sleep is over,.
Bharat rises once more
To herald her Hero's message to the world;
His biddings to fulfil
From peak to plain she now proclaims:
'Arise! Awake, O Man!
And stop not till the goal is reached!'

TRIBUTES FROM STATESMEN AND POLITICIANS

Morning bird of Indian renaissance
– M. Bhaktavatsalam

Swami Vivekananda was the mighty man who stemmed the tide towards Westernization by making our people aware of the wealth and variety of their cultural and spiritual heritage and by awakening in them the spirit to serve man and thus serve God truly. Vivekananda can be hailed as the forerunner of Mahatma Gandhi. The work started by him was continued on a wider scale and with greater intensity by Mahatmaji. India will always pay its reverential homage to this Patriot-saint.

His contribution to quicken the dawn that was breaking in the country was immense. With the light and power which he received from his Master, he strode the earth like a colossus, broadcasting the message which ancient India had for the West and rousing his countrymen, from inertia of ages.

Swami Vivekananda was the morning bird of Indian cultural and spiritual renaissance. For sixteen years he toiled.... He condensed the work of a whole epoch within these sixteen years and by the time he passed, he left placid India simmering with new life, new thoughts. The impulses he generated gathered titanic force in the next two decades after his departure. The ideas he broadcasted acquired strength and shape in the years that followed.

Few men have loved India and its people so well and dedicated themselves to their service with such wholehearted devotion as Swami Vivekananda. The saint who had scaled the heights of self-realization was found to be human and intensely human whenever he was confronted by the suffering and misery of people....

Generations of Indians draw inspiration from the life, work and teachings of this king among monks.

A rare personality
– Subhash Chandra Bose

In the eighties of the last century, two prominent religious personalities appeared before the public who were destined to have a great influence on the future course of the new awakening. They were Ramakrishna Paramahamsa, the saint, and his disciple Swami Vivekananda.... Ramakrishna preached the gospel of the unity of all religions and urged the cessation of inter-religious strife.... Before he died, he charged his disciple with the task of propagating his religious teachings in India and abroad and of bringing about an awakening among his countrymen. Swami Vivekananda therefore founded the Ramakrishna Mission, an Order of monks, to live and preach the Hindu religion in its purest form in India and abroad, especially in America, and he took an active part in inspiring every form of healthy national activity. With him religion was the inspirer of nationalism. He tried to infuse into the new generation a sense of pride in India's past, of faith in India's future and a spirit of self-confidence and self-respect. Though the Swami never gave any political message, every one who came into contact with him or his writings developed a spirit of patriotism and a political mentality. So far at least as Bengal is concerned Swami Vivekananda may be regarded as the spiritual father of the modern nationalist movement. He died very young in 1902, but since his death his influence has been even greater.

I cannot write about Vivekananda without going into raptures. Few indeed could comprehend or fathom him – even among those who had the privilege of becoming intimate with him. His personality was rich, profound and complex and it was this personality – as distinct from his teachings and writings – which accounts for the wonderful influence he has exerted on his countrymen and particularly on Bengalees. This is the type of manhood which appeals to the Bengalee as probably none other. Reckless in his sacrifice, unceasing in his activity, boundless in his love, profound and versatile in his wisdom, exuberant in his emotions, merciless in his attacks but yet simple as a child – he was a rare personality in this world of ours....

Swamiji was a full-blooded masculine personality – and a fighter to the core of his being. He was consequently a worshipper of *Shakti* and gave a practical interpretation to the Vedanta for the uplift of his countrymen. Strength, strength is what the Upanishads say – that was a frequent cry of his. He laid the greatest stress on character-building. I can go on for hours and yet fail to do the slightest justice to that great man. He was so great, so profound, so complex. A yogi of the highest spiritual level in direct communion with the truth who had for the time being consecrated his whole life to the moral and spiritual uplift of his nation and of humanity, that is how I would describe him. If he had been alive, I would have been at his feet. Modern Bengal is his creation – if I err not.

How shall I express in words my indebtedness to Sri Ramakrishna and Swami Vivekananda? It is under their sacred influence that my life got first awakened. Like Nivedita I also regard Ramakrishna and Vivekananda as two aspects of one indivisible personality. If Swamiji had been alive today, he would have been my guru, that is to say, I would have accepted him as my Master. It is needless to add, however, that as long as I live, I shall be absolutely loyal and devoted to Ramakrishna-Vivekananda.

It is very difficult to explain the versatile genius of Swami Vivekananda. The impact of Swami Vivekananda made on the students of our times by his works and speeches far outweighed that made by any other leader of the country. He, as it were, expressed fully their hopes and aspirations. (But) Swamiji cannot be appreciated properly if he is not studied along with Sri Sri Paramahamsa Deva. The foundation of the present freedom movement owes its origin to Swamiji's message. If India is to be free, it cannot be a land specially of Hinduism or of Islam – it must be one united land of different religious communities inspired by the ideal of nationalism. (And for that) Indians must accept wholeheartedly the gospel of harmony of religions which is the gospel of Ramakrishna-Vivekananda....

Swamiji harmonized East and West, religion and science past and present. And that is why he is great. Our countrymen have gained unprecedented self-respect, self-confidence and self-assertion from his teachings.

The harmony of all religions which Ramakrishna Paramahamsa accomplished in his life's endeavour, was the keynote of Swamiji's life. And this ideal again is the bed-rock of the nationalism of Future India. Without this concept of harmony of religions and toleration of all creeds, the spirit of national consciousness could not have been built up in this country of ours full of diversities.

The aspiration for freedom manifested itself in various movements since the time of Rammohan Roy. This aspiration was witnessed in the realm of thought and in social reforms during the nineteenth century, but it was never expressed in the political sphere. This was because the people of India still remained sunk in the stupor of subjugation and thought that the conquest of India by the British was an act of Divine Dispensation. The idea of complete freedom is manifest only in Ramakrishna-Vivekananda towards the end of the nineteenth century. "Freedom, freedom is the song of the Soul" – this was the message that burst forth from the inner recesses of Swamiji's heart and captivated and almost maddened the entire nation. This truth was embodied in his works, life, conversations, and speeches.

Swami Vivekananda, on the one hand, called man to be real man freed from all fetters and, on the other, laid the foundation for true nationalism in India by preaching the gospel of the harmony of religions.

....With me it is a firm faith that unless at the beginning we have acquired strength of character, rare in its human quality, there is hardly any hope of redeeming mankind by means of any of these "isms". This was why Swami Vivekananda would say, "Man-making is my mission." Men, true in spirit, were indeed the basic need, for without men, hopes of national reconstruction or the founding 'isms' on any firm ground would be idle dreams. Hence every youth movement should primarily aim at producing men of the truest type; and a man to be true and good must develop on all sides....

Ablest exponent of Hindu philosophy
– Morarji Desai

Swami Vivekananda occupies a very significant place in the realm of Indian Philosophy. His brilliant exposition of Vedanta has not since been equalled, much less excelled, by anybody. He was a chosen and devout disciple of Ramakrishna Paramahamsa as he had a rare vision of the divinity in man. He perceived that human minds were seized with timidity and weakness which crippled their growth. He therefore sought to rouse them from their slumber by a spiritual awakening in human minds and by harnessing it to the service of mankind.

He saw the sufferings of *Daridrinarayana* during his travels through the country and came to the conclusion that mere pursuit of religion was not enough for individual salvation when millions of people suffered in ignorance. He felt, therefore, that unless we helped the people to shed their ignorance and their weaknesses, our spiritual pursuits will not be rewarding.

He interpreted Hindu philosophy to the West and stimulated their interest in the true religion of man. He was a great scholar indeed. His speeches on Hindu philosophy before the World's Parliament of Religions at Chicago in 1893 created a remarkable impression on the audience and stimulated in them a desire to study the Hindu philosophy. These speeches have adorned the pages of the history of philosophy and religion and have been a great achievement for his charismatic personality. These have not only earned for him a name and fame but the Hindu religion found a place of glory in the world of religion.

He was not only one of our ablest exponents of Hindu philosophy but was one who did so much by precept and example to awaken Indians to the need for a well co-ordinated attempt to rebuild the glory of India and her people, for he believed that India had a mission to fulfil and thus enable mankind to live in peace and happiness.

He awakened us to the need for patriotic effort to rebuild our social order on the foundation of social justice and equality in order that India could be what her heritage and culture would entitle her to be.

Religious thoughts and precepts of Swami Vivekananda have imparted a powerful impetus which has not failed to produce a transvaluation of values which govern the life of man.

Swami Vivekananda was one of those sages of India who by virtue of their enlightenment created a tremendous impact on the life of the people and restored the glory of the religion of man. We have need for his message of virility of spirit and rectitude of action in order that mankind may be able to obtain release from the bonds of ignorance which results in misery.

A great sannyasin
– R. R. Diwakar

Some of the greatest religious teachers as well as profound philosophers in India have been sadhus, sannyasins and saints. It is, therefore, not very extraordinary that Swami Vivekananda was a sannyasin to whose credit there is so much of achievement in the way of mystic experience, philosophy and metaphysics, yogic knowledge and leadership in the all-sided Renaissance of India.

It is one of the paradoxes in Indian hagiology that some of the greatest saints and monastic philosophers who preached that the world was an illusion and a passing pageant, were also men of intense action and extraordinary achievement in practical affairs. The paradox has an explanation and that is, some of these great Advaita Vedantins did not neglect the 'illusion or the dream', but acted very much as if the world was a solid reality so long as it was present to them, to their senses, to their mind and to their heart. Thus, for them the relative world of the senses was as much a truth as the transcendental existence beyond relativity. There were, no doubt, many Vedantins who absorbed themselves in the transcendent, were equally aware and actively associated with the immanent.

Swami Vivekananda belonged to this class of Indian Vedantins whose head was high in the heavens while their feet were firmly planted in the earth.

If Swami Vivekananda is to be distinguished from other sadhus and Saints and Vedantins of contemporary India, he is to be distinguished as one who was not satisfied with absorption in the Unqualified Absolute of Vedanta, and as one who gave equal importance to progress of the world in which man lives, moves and has his being.

He aroused and inspired the nation
– Indira Gandhi

Swami Vivekananda's contribution to our national rebirth cannot easily be remeasured. He brought a new awareness of our spiritual inheritance. For the first time the ancient truths were given a modern meaning and expressed in terms relevant to the problems of the day. To him true religion was not merely worship but work. He spoke of *Daridranarayana* and emphasized the importance of lifting our people from poverty. His teaching aroused and inspired the nation during his lifetime. It guides us now and will be cherished by generations to come.

The greatness of Swami Vivekananda was not only due to his great intellectual power and discretion but also his burning passion to do something not only to the whole of india but to the entire world. I think his greatness was that he sought to release our ancient wisdom, to find a sense of individual purpose and to promote social well-being and collective progress. His special intellectual gift was that he was keenly aware of the forces at work in the modern world.... And it was remarkable how he could address himself to the modern world knowing fully well the trends at work in modern days.... We have many words of wisdom and guidance from Swami Vivekananda and other great spiritual leaders. But if there is a lacuna in the thinking of modern man, it is as regards action....

I had the special privilege of being introduced to the writings, sayings, and life of Swami Vivekananda and the Ramakrishna Mission. That was when I was very small. In fact both my parents and specially my mother had very close connections with the Mission. And I can truly say that the words of Swami Vivekananda inspired the whole of my family, in our political work as well as in our daily lives.

He brought about a re-awakening
– V. V. Giri

Swami Vivekananda, as we all know, brought about a reawakening in the outlook and attitude of the people towards religion. He considered religion or faith in God not as a refuge when we face difficulties, but a living inspiration and hope.... He made a healthy synthesis of the best in the East and the West. Deep awareness of the infinite nature of the spirit of the East is happily linked to the material advancement, economic resurgence and social regeneration of the West. This is exactly what he stressed in all his works.

His constant appeal for material progress, bringing up the down-trodden and tackling such problems like poverty, squalor and want, added a new dimension and fresh perspective to the entire outlook about the nature and content of Hinduism which till then was considered to be negative or at best passive, so far as its attitude towards material happiness was concerned. He thus brought about a fresh outlook dispelling all false notions. He reiterated time and again that the need and the ultimate object of every individual is to pursue the path of spiritualism which alone held the key to *mukti* or salvation. The poverty which he himself suffered was not an unmitigated evil in the sense it developed in him a deep feeling for the needy and afflicted.

Swami Vivekananda was a great nationalist who built great traditions for his countrymen but his nationalism was not of the narrow parochial type. It was essentially in spirit internationalism.

He was a modernist and realist. He knew that the fruit of scientific and technological advance could be exploited for human good to the fullest extent, if man's activities could be directed under a proper balance of spiritual and material values.

Vivekananda indeed belongs to the class of great seers of the truth. His intellect was great, but greater still was his heart. He once told his disciples at Belur Math that, if a conflict were to arise between the intellect and heart, they should reject the intellect and follow the heart. This is an evidence of his stress on human approach.

Swamiji was first and foremost a philosopher and a preacher and was not an active political leader. Nevertheless, he was an inspirer of nationalism. While he gave no political message, every one who came into contact with him and his writings developed a spirit of patriotism and political mentality. His mission of service, his constructive role to uplift the masses from the depths to which they have sunk had, and continues to have, a profound effect and significance on individual minds as much as it has on the nation as a whole.

He did not believe in the seekers of truth running to forests and secluded places and working only towards their own self-salvation. He wanted that everyone, be he a householder or a sannyasin, to engage in selfless service towards their less fortunate brethren. Neither did he advocate that the world was an illusion of the mind, which in the earlier times made the people take refuge in inaction and indifference. The world, as we see it, is real. 'Let the body, since perish it must, wear out in action and not rust in inaction.'

Many-faceted personality
– Dr. Balram Jakhar

Swami Vivekananda was a many-faceted personality – an erudite scholar, a poet, an orator, a mystic, a devotee, a yogi, a nation-builder, a social reformer, all in one and had played a vital role in the shaping of modern India. The ideas and principles on universal brotherhood, social service, practice of true religion, universal literacy, woman's emancipation and abolition of untouchability were enunciated by Swamiji. His teachings have great relevance in the present state of things.

Swami Vivekananda remains a perennial source of inspiration for our youth who must translate his preachings into reality while devoting themselves to the task of national reconstruction....

A lion of Vedanta
– B. D. Jatti

I avail this opportunity to join you all in paying homage to a great son of Mother India whose message of spirituality and service has lent a humanistic orientation and significance to the very concept of religion. His thoughts and idealism have stirred the minds and hearts of millions in our country and abroad and equated humanity with God and the sanctity of service to humanity with the sanctity of the worship of God.

Swami Vivekananda lived for less than forty years and he had only about five years to complete his tutelege under Ramakrishna Paramahamsa. Into this brief span he packed missionary activities, writings and lectures of tremendous magnitude and depth, and travelled far and wide as a true *parivrajaka,* dispelling darkness, bringing hope, inspiring action and enlightening millions of minds. Swami Vivekananda has rightly been described as the one who brought down "the celestial fire at God's own command" and utilized it to create a new order of things, and to build up a new world on a foundation of spirituality, universal love, renunciation and service.

Swami Vivekananda thought and spoke in terms of eternity and eternal values. Hence it would be true to say his teachings have a relevance not only to the current age but for all times. His dynamism inspired his Western admirers to hail him as the "cyclonic monk of India." He travelled far and wide like a veritable "lion of Vedanta" roaring to rouse his somnolent countrymen. The Swami made them aware of their present sad state, their physical, spiritual and mental deterioration, their lack of manliness, self-help, seriousness and capacity, and more than all, their lack of love, generous feelings and spirit of service. The Swami called on his countrymen to endeavour to live once again upto the lofty ideals of their original scriptures and to pull down all barriers that divided man from man. He pointed out that the Vedantic ideas about the divinity of the soul would not only unite the people by harmonizing all differences, but they would also infuse enormous strength into the nation and raise it to great new heights.

....Narendra, who was an athiest and agnostic, was transformed by Ramakrishna into Vivekananda, a confirmed believer in the Universal Spirit which is immanent in all creation. Ramakrishna taught his disciple, 'Shivamatmani pasyanti' – the Supreme is in every being. *Jiva* and *Shiva* are one, he revealed, and every creature was God Himself, to be served in a spirit of devotion and gratitude rather than mercy and charity. It was this revelation of "unparalleled significance" that ultimately led the Swami to introduce the scheme of divine worship through the service of humanity as a manifestation of God. The founding of the Ramakrishna Order of monks was thus the logic of events in the continuing propagation of the ideal of rendering humanitarian service as the highest spiritual discipline.

Swami Vivekananda believed not only in universal toleration but in the truth as expounded by all religions. He invested religion with universal acceptability by defining it as the manifestation of the divinity that is immanent in men. The spirit of mutual toleration and respect, which an appreciation of the Swami's message is bound to promote in the world, will be a distinct gain to humanity.

The Swami's life and work shine in a multifaceted splendour. The Swami's message of humanity, compassion and service has special significance to us in our endeavour to bring about social justice to the poor and downtrodden sections of society.

The Swami advocated the importance of the true religious spirit. He warned against using religion as an escape from reality....

If we imbibe the spirit of Swami Vivekananda's message, our country and the world will doubtless move nearer to the dawn of a new life for the people. Technology, linked to ethical and moral norms, will lose its terrors for humanity. Man will discover divinity in his fellow-beings and serve humanity as he would worship God, in a spirit of devotion and dedication. There will be peace and harmony for which people have striven from time immemorial. I would urge you, particularly my young friends, to ponder over the human situation as it stands today and the solution which Swami Vivekananda's message provides. You will find, I am sure, that the Swami's message is what we need today to take our people and the people of the world towards peace, harmony and happiness. I am sure you will find perennial inspiration and guidance in Swami Vivekananda's message of spirituality and service in your endeavours to meet the challenges and opportunities which the future holds for you. May his spirit guide you.

He conquered the minds of men
– M. Karunanidhi

Swami Vivekananda's historic visit to Parliament of Religions at Chicago was an epoch-making one, in the history of the world.

It was the good fortune of Tamil Nadu and Kanyakumari, to have played a notable part in Vivekananda's making up his mind to attend the important world-meet, where he conquered the minds of men.

The name, 'Vivekananda', means, one who can distinguish the right from the wrong. He was a noble sage who had a universal vision which ennobled everyone who came into contact with him or with his teachings.

When this quiet, unknown young man of thirty appeared at the inaugural meeting of the Parliament of Religions at Chicago in September, 1893, his strength and beauty, his grace and the dignity of his bearing, the brilliance of his eyes, his commanding personality and the splendid music of his rich voice took the audience by storm.

Wherever he went he was the first. Though he is not with us today, the flame he lit is still alight and from his teachings have sprung the conscience of India, its faith in her unity, and in his great message, mankind finds solace and confidence.

Swami Vivekananda always had before him the great motto of "elevation of the masses." Many of his speeches were full of sympathy for the poor, the fallen and the downtrodden. His messages were always gospels of salvation, social elevation and equality of every one.

Vivekananda's vision was all-embracing, and his outlook universal. I would advocate that class and caste feelings should be abolished from all of our hearts, and a united India thus created, where every one feels equal in every respect, will be the rightful tribute India could pay to the greatest of her sons.

Let us arise, awake and stop not, till the goal is reached.

A beam of sunshine
– S. L. Khurana

When, in the nineteenth century, a fog of despondency had settled over our land, Swami Vivekananda's message of self-respect and self-realization came through it like a beam of sunshine. With the blessings of Sri Ramakrishna, he transformed the thoughts of our scriptures from an archival curiosity into a living vision of our nation's greatness.

Apostle of renaissance
– K. M. Munshi

Few can understand, unless they belong to my age-group, the great influence which Swami Vivekananda had on us, in the first decade of the

20th century, when we were at College. We were then subject not only to political but also to cultural and religious humiliation. In those days small booklets, very cheap, were issued by missionaries in which our culture and religion were held up to ridicule, scorn and contempt.... We were then at an impressionable age and were not intelligent enough to find an answer to the criticism contained in these books. We felt humiliated.

At that time, the Arya Samaj, founded by Swami Dayanand Saraswati, was the only movement which accepted the challenge of the missionary. But it was only when we began to read the books of Swami Vivekananda that our eyes were opened. Reading these books, we derived considerable knowledge of Hindu culture and religion from the modern point of view.

Swamiji gave us the message of New India; he gave us pride in ourselves. We felt that we were not the uncivilized barbarians which the missionaries were trying to make us out, but a people with great cultural heritage. This gave us back our self-respect.

Indian Renaissance was not merely an artistic and literary movement like the European Renaissance. Nor was it only a religious movement. It was essentially cultural and spiritual. Though Raja Rammohan Roy, Ramakrishna Paramahamsa and Dayanand Saraswati began the work, it was Swami Vivekananda who brought to us, the younger generations, the message of the renaissance.

We knew about *Ramayana* and *Mahabharata* but we found in them fresh inspiration only when we read Swamiji's summaries of his works. Yoga was a word of mystic implication, but it was only when we read his *Raja Yoga* and *Karma Yoga* that we realized what it was.

As one of the great architects of our renaissance, Swami Vivekananda made us 'India-conscious.'

Swami Vivekananda taught us to ignore the excrescences of our culture and to go back to the Upanishads, the *Bhagavad Gita* and to find in them the fundamental truth of our culture. Here again, it was Prof. Aurobindo Ghosh (at the Baroda College) who suggested to me to read *Yoga Sutras* and the works of Swami Vivekananda.

Swami Vivekananda took us back to the fundamental values of our culture and brought God into our life. It is a strange way of putting it, for, we always thought of 'approaching Him', or 'living in Him.' Swami Vivekananda gave us a new message – to bring God into our daily life.

He taught us that religion must necessarily mean that God should come in our life by our living a dedicated life, that is, by consecrating all our actions as an offering to God Himself.

Unless we begin to look upon the whole humanity as part of God, we cannot expand our religious outlook. What is wanted is to live for others, to conquer egoism, to sink our *swartha* in *paramartha*. This can only come by broadening our outlook so as to include in our affection as many people as possible.

This way, Swami Vivekananda laid the foundation of our attitude that service was essential to spiritual life. We cannot lead a spiritual life unless we work for others in utter selflessness, in a spirit of devotion, with a sense of dedication that we are doing it for God's sake.

We celebrated the centenary of Swami Vivekananda as he was a great apostle of our modern renaissance. We offer him our tribute not merely for what he has done, but because it provides us with an opportunity to mobilize our own spiritual aspirations by dwelling on him, his works and his ideas. This way, we light our little lamp from the flaming torch that he was.

He was India's gift to the world. A realized soul himself, he spoke with the authority of direct intuitive experience of the verities of life and that lent to his words a dynamic force which rivetted the attention of his hearers and readers and compelled their conviction.

Vivekananda practised in his life the twin objectives of salvation for oneself and the welfare of the world: *'Atmano mokshartham'* and *'jagaddhitaya cha.'* He was as much concerned with the betterment of the world as with individual liberation. All the pages of his immortal writings breathe this twin purpose, justifying his reputation as the patriot-saint of India. A pioneer of Indian renaissance, he raised our religion to a pedestal of worshipful dignity, at the same time warning his countrymen of the unfortunate excrescences which have dimmed it.

His impact on Indians
– E. M. S. Namboodiripad

The soul of India ground down under foreign imperialism rose up ready to challenge the foreign domination. The speech delivered by Swami Vivekananda in the Parliament of Religions at Chicago and the welcome that it received at the hands of Western intellectuals served to do away with the inferiority complex of the Indians and made them feel that they were the inheritors of a cultural legacy capable of challenging the foreign rulers.

His powerful influence
– Jawaharlal Nehru

Rooted in the past and full of pride in India's prestige, Vivekananda was yet modern in his approach to life's problems and was a kind of bridge between the past of India and her present.... He was a fine figure of a man, imposing, full of poise and dignity, sure of himself and his mission, and at the same time full of dynamic and fiery energy and a passion to push India forward. He came as a tonic to the depressed and demoralized Hindu mind and gave it self-reliance and some roots in the past.

Wherever he went he created a sensation, not only by his presence but by what he said and how he said it. Having seen this Hindu sannyasin once, it was difficult to forget him or his message. In America he was called the "cyclonic Hindu".... "America is the best field in the world to carry on any idea", he wrote to a friend in India. But he was not impressed by the manifestations of religion in the West, and his faith in the Indian philosophical and spiritual background became firmer. India, in spite of her degradation, still represented to him the light.... He thundered from Cape Comorin on the southern tip of India to the Himalayas, and he wore himself out in the process.

He started new movements of thought. While he drank from the rich streams of English literature, his mind was full of ancient sages and heroes of India, his thoughts and deeds and the myths and traditions which he had imbibed from his childhood....

I do not know how many of the younger generation read the speeches and the writings of Swami Vivekananda. But I can tell you that many of my generation were very powerfully influenced by him and I think that it would do a great deal of good to the present generation if they also went through Swami Vivekananda's writings and speeches, and they would learn much from them. That would, perhaps, as some of us did, enable us to catch a glimpse of that fire that raged in Swami Vivekananda's mind and heart and which ultimately consumed him at an early age. Because there was fire in his heart – the fire of a great personality coming out in eloquent and ennobling language – it was no empty talk that he was indulging in. He was putting his heart and soul into the words he uttered. Therefore he became a great orator, not with the orators' flashes and flourishes but with a deep conviction and earnestness of spirit. And so he influenced powerfully the minds of many in India and two or three generations of young men and women have no doubt been influenced by him....

Much has happened which perhaps makes some forget those who came before and who prepared and shaped India in those early and difficult days. If you read Swami Vivekananda's writings and speeches, the curious thing you will find is that they are not old. It was told decades ago, and they are fresh today because, what he wrote or spoke about dealt with certain fundamental matters and aspects of our problems or the world's problems. Therefore they do not become old. They are fresh even though you read them now.

He gave us something which brings us, if I may use the word, a certain pride in our inheritance. He did not spare us. He talked of our weaknesses and our failings too. He did not wish to hide anything. Indeed he should not. Because we have to correct those failings, he deals with those failings also. Sometimes he strikes hard at us, but sometimes points out the great things for which India stood and which even in the days of India's downfall made her, in some measure, continue to be great.

So what Swamiji has written and said is of interest and must interest us and is likely to influence us for a long time to come. He was no politician in

the ordinary sense of the word and yet he was, I think, one of the great
founders – if you like you may use any other word – of the national modern
movement of India, and a great number of people who took more or less an
active part in the movement in a later date drew their inspirations from Swami
Vivekananda.... Directly or indirectly, he has powerfully influenced the India
of today. And I think that our younger generation will take advantage of
this fountain of wisdom, of spirit and fire, that flows through Swami
Vivekananda.

....Men like Sri Ramakrishna Paramahamsa, men like Swami Vivekananda
and men like Mahatma Gandhi are great unifying forces, great constructive
geniuses of the world not only in regard to the particular teachings that
they taught, but their approach to the world and their conscious and
unconscious influence on it is of the most vital importance to us.

Instrument of a great master
– Bipin Chandra Pal

Vivekananda, however, does not stand alone. He is indissolubly bound
up with his Master, Paramahamsa Ramakrishna. The two stand almost
organically bound up, so far as the modern man, not only in India but in
the larger world of our day, is concerned. The modern man can only
understand Paramahamsa in and through Vivekananda, even as Vivekananda
can be understood only in the light of his Master.

It was given to Vivekananda to interpret and present the soul of
Paramahamsa Ramakrishna and the message of his life to this generation
in such terms as would he comprehended by them.

Vivekananda clothed the spiritual realization of His Master in the
language of modern Humanism.

Paramahamsa Ramakrishna, like Jesus Christ, needed an interpreter to
explain him and deliver his message to his age. Jesus found such an interpreter in St. Paul; Ramakrishna found him in Vivekananda. Vivekananda therefore must be understood in the light of the realizations of Paramahamsa
Ramakrishna.

Paramahamsa Ramakrishna saw into the innermost composition of
Vivekananda's nature and spirit and recognized in him a fit instrument for
delivering the message of his own life. This is the real story of
Vivekananda's conversion. Vivekananda felt drawn to his Master by what
he hardly knew. It was the operation of what is now called soul-force.
Vivekananda worked after his conversion under the inspiration of his
Master.

The Message of Vivekananda, though delivered in the term of the
popular Vedantic speculation, was really the message of his Master to the
modern man. Vivekananda's message was really the message of modern
humanity. His appeal to his own people was, "Be men."

To help man to realize his essential divinity is the object of all religious
culture. This is what Vivekananda really meant when he appealed to his

people to be men.... "I am Divine. I am none other. I am not subject to grief and bereavement. I am of the form of True, the Self-conscious and the Eternally Present. I am by nature eternally free." This was the message really of his Master as delivered to the modern world by Vivekananda.

It is the message of freedom, not in a negative sense, but in its positive and most comprehensive implications.... from personal freedom, through social freedom including political freedom, man must attain his real freedom. And when he attains it, he realizes that he and God are one. This is the message of the Vedanta as interpreted by Vivekananda. This is really the message of his Master to the modern world.

Some people in India think that very little fruit has come of the lectures that Swami Vivekananda delivered in England, and that his friends and admirers exaggerate his work. But on coming here I see that he has exerted a marked influence everywhere. In many parts of England I have met with men who deeply regard and venerate Vivekananda. Though I do not belong to his sect, and though it is true that I have differences of opinion with him, I must say that Vivekananda has opened the eyes of a great many here and broadened their hearts. Owing to his teaching, most people here now believe firmly that wonderful spiritual truths lie hidden in the ancient Hindu scriptures. Not only has he brought about this feeling, but he succeeded in establishing a golden relation between England and India. From what I quoted on "Vivekanandism" from *The Dead Pulpit* by Mr. Haweis, you have already understood that owing to the spread of Vivekananda's doctrines, many hundreds of people have seceded from Christianity.

He was a practical man
– Vijayalakshmi Pandit

Swami Vivekananda gave new strength and new purpose to an old message, and in himself combined the highest qualities which any human being can hope to possess. He was a practical man and approached life in a practical fashion; but the deep spiritual content of his nature and his wide vision made it possible for him to give nourishment to the dying roots of India's religion and culture and reawaken thinking people to a sense of India's true mission.

Swami Vivekananda was a patriot. The political subjection of the country as well as the social degradation into which she had fallen was a challenge which he met with complete fearlessness. In his time, as again in our own, India stood at an important cross-road in her history. He warned them of the danger we faced by trying to seize the shadow and letting the substance go. Now, living in an age of speed and great scientific developments, we have opportunities greater than ever before to build society and the world, and Swamiji's message today is that man must begin with himself. The tremendous scientific and political power now in our hands must be allied to the strength of the spirit if it is to give happiness to the individual and peace to the world. The best form of homage we can pay today is to dedicate ourselves to the values for which Swami Vivekananda stood and for which he worked.

The spiritual path-finder
– Dr. Rajendra Prasad

Men who lead their fellow-beings in any sphere of life are rare and those that lead the leaders are rarer still. These super guides come not very often upon this earth to uplift the sinking section of humanity. Swami Vivekananda was one of these super souls. Well, may the land of Bharat feel ennobled by the memory of such great one having sprung on its soil to serve humanity at large, to be the spiritual path-finder of many a suffering soul, and to shine in the spiritual firmament with the lustre of the glory of Vedic civilization enlightening the world. It was he who could set the sceptic mind of the West at rest in the spiritual area. Ambassadors of spiritual mission had risen before him in the East, but none could speak to the West as he did with that voice of conviction, keeping audiences spellbound and enthralled. The worthy disciple of the worthy Master rose to the pinnacle of spiritual eminence, preaching the gospel of the innate oneness of the human race, and preaching universal love and the affinity of all human souls. Like the story of the seed and the tree each sustaining the other's existence, personifying the two essential stages of spiritual sublimity, the centenary (1963) of this great scion of the spiritual world reminds us of the greatness of the human soul, for there could be no better interpreter of the heritage of the Vedic civilization than he. Not only Indians but Westerners too stand indebted to Swami Vivekananda for his bequest of 'viveka' (wisdom) to posterity.

We owe everything to him
– C. Rajagopalachari

I was a law student living in Castle Kernan on the Madras beach, when Swami Vivekananda arrived back from Chicago in 1897, after becoming world-famous by then. He stayed for nine days about a month in Castle Kernan then, and I look back to those days with pride and joy. *Prabuddha Bharata* was started then and Madras was thrilled by Swamiji's lectures. Hinduism arose from the grave as Jesus did.

Swami Vivekananda saved Hinduism and saved India. But for him we would have lost our religion and would not have gained our freedom. We therefore owe everything to Swami Vivekananda. May his faith, his courage and his wisdom ever inspire us so that we may keep safe the treasure we have received from him.

A great spiritual leader
– M. G. Ramachandran

India's history is inseparable from the history of spirituality and religion. This great country even today holds the torch of spirituality to the rest of the world which is ridden by fear of annihilation on account of racial strife, greed for territory and power. If the various civilizations of the world, particularly that of the materialistic West, now look upon India as the only source of hope for peace and love, it is because of the fact that our great religious leaders have meticulously preserved the spiritual character of our civilization and our culture. In spite of the strong influence of the Western civilization on the Indian mind, its core remains spiritual.

Foremost among our spiritual leaders is Swami Vivekananda who found that spirituality could solve the problems confronting the humanity. It was he who made the Westerners turn towards India and to realize the greatness of its religion and its faith. His eloquent speech at the Chicago Parliament of Religions advocating universal brotherhood opened the eyes of the entire world and made them look upon India as a spiritual leader among nations. Thus, Swami Vivekananda made himself as one belonging to the entire humanity. His life and teachings are a source of inspiration to the mankind. He gave a new dimension to the Indian philosophy.

Swami Vivekananda was responsible for the awakening of the soul of this great country. He reminded our people of our hoary cultural heritage and exhorted them to preserve the spiritual values in life. He preached that the best and sincerest way of worship of God is to love the fellow-beings; especially the poor and the weak and alleviate their distress. He strongly urged that our country should first become free from ignorance, poverty and disease.

His teachings seem to be more relevant to the present world situation. We can say that the answer to the various complex problems confronting the world today lies within the life and teachings of Swami Vivekananda.

First to hold aloft the banner of Hinduism
– Bal Gangadhar Tilak

It is doubtful if there is any Hindu who does not know the name of Sri Vivekananda Swami. There has been extraordinary advancement of material science in the nineteenth century. Under the circumstances, to present the spiritual science prevailing in India for thousands of years by wonderful exposition and then to kindle admiration and respect among the Western scholars, and, at the same time, to create a sympathetic attitude for India, the mother of spiritual science, can only be an achievement of superhuman power. With English education, the flood of material science spread so fast that it required extraordinary courage and extraordinary genius to stand against that phenomenon and change its direction. Before Swami Vivekananda, the Theosophical Society began this work. But it is an undisputed fact that it was Swami Vivekananda who first held aloft the banner of Hinduism as a challenge against the material science of the West.... It was Swami Vivekananda who took on his shoulders this stupendous task of establishing the glory of Hinduism in different countries across the borders. And he, with his erudition, oratorical power, enthusiasm and inner force, laid that work upon a solid foundation.... Twelve centuries ago, Sankaracharya was the only great personality, who not only spoke of the purity of our religion, not only uttered in words that this religion was our strength and wealth, not only said that it was our sacred duty to preach this religion in the length and breadth of the world – but also brought all this into action. Swami Vivekananda is a person of that stature – who appeared towards the last half of the nineteenth century.

His greatness surpasses my power of assessment
– Brahmabandhav Upadhyay

For a few days I went on a trip to Bolpur. On my return as I stepped down at the Howrah Station, someone said, 'Swami Vivekananda passed away yesterday.' At once an acute pain, sharp like a razor – not the least exaggerated – thrust into my heart. When the intensity of the pain subsided, I wondered, 'How will Vivekananda's work go on? He has, of course, well-trained and educated brother-disciples. Why, they will do his work!' Yet an inspiration flickered in me; 'You give your best with whatever you possess by trying to translate into action Vivekananda's dream of conquest of the West.' That very moment I vowed I would sail to England. So long I never even dreamt of visiting England. But on that day in Howrah Station I decided I must go to England and establish Vedanta there. Then I understood who Vivekananda was. He whose inspiration can drive a humble person like me across the seas, is not, really, an ordinary man. Shortly afterwards I left Calcutta and sailed for England with a sum of only twenty-seven rupees in my pocket. Finally, I reached England and delivered lectures at the Oxford and Cambridge Universities on Vedanta. Celebrated (British) scholars listened to my expositions and expressed their desire to learn the science of Vedanta by appointing Hindu scholars. I did not publish the letters of appreciation which those scholars wrote to me. How profound was the influence of Vedanta in England could be understood if I had published those letters. I am just an ordinary man. It was all like a dream that such a great work was accomplished by me. All these were miracles brought about by the inspiration and power of Vivekananda behind me – this is what I believe. That is why sometimes I think, who is Vivekananda? The greatness of Vivekananda surpasses my power of assessment as I think of the stupendous programme of work he had boldly initiated.

On another occasion I came across Vivekananda by the side of Hedua Park in Calcutta. I said to him, 'Brother, why are you keeping silent? Come, raise a stir of Vedanta in Calcutta. I will make all arrangements. You just come and appear before the public.' Vivekananda's voice grew heavy with pathos. He said, 'Brother Bhavani, I will not live long (it was just six months before his death). I am busy now with the construction of my Math, and making, arrangements for its proper upkeep. I have no leisure now.' At the pathetic earnestness of his words I understood that day that his heart was tormented with a passion and pain. Passion for whom? Pain for whom? Passion for the country, pain for the country. The knowledge and culture of the Aryans were being destroyed and crushed. What was gross and un-Aryan was deflating what was finer and Aryan. And yet there is no response, no pain in your heart? – this (callous indifference of his countrymen) evoked a painful response in Vivekananda's heart. The response was so deep that it struck at the root of the conscience of America and Europe. I think of that pain and passion in Vivekananda, and ask, who is Vivekananda? Is it ever possible that passion for the motherland becomes embodied? If it is, then only one can understand Vivekananda.

Swamiji! I was your friend in youth. How much of merry-making I have enjoyed with you! With you I went on picnics and spent hours in talks and conversations. But then I never knew that there was a lion's strength in your soul, a volcanic pain and passion for India in your heart. Today with all my humble strength I have come to follow your way.... In the midst of this fierce struggle, whenever I get torn and tossed, whenever despondency comes and overwhelms my heart, I look up to the great ideal you set forth, I recollect your leonine strength, meditate on the profound depths of your agony – then all at once my weariness withers away. A divine light and a divine strength comes from somewhere and fulfils my mind and heart.

PART TWO

A CHRONICLE OF IMPORTANT EVENTS IN THE LIFE AND TIMES OF VIVEKANANDA (1863-1902)

What is most fascinating about this book is the Chronicle, for it brings to the reader in vivid terms the atmosphere of the times in which Vivekananda lived. It tells us a great deal about the events that took place during forty years of the Swami's life. It has been rightly said that the significance of a man's life and activities is best understood in the context of the times in which he lived. The Chronicle that Swami Jyotirmayananda has compiled is fascinating on its own. It is really an excellent background to Vivekananda's life and times. That life is nailed to its historical perspective.

Swami Jyotirmayananda has chosen world and domestic events wisely to provide the background to Vivekananda's own development which took place at a time when western materialism was progressing by leaps and bounds. India, too, was touching peoples minds.

The Chronicle is a magnificent way of placing Vivekananda against his times and the Editor has to be congratulated for the pains that he took. It has involved a great deal of research. Newspaper accounts make fascinating reading. And the compiler has provided us long quotes from a variety of sources, both Indian and Foriegn. They paint between them such a vivid picture of Vivekananda that he comes through in all his vibrancy. Vivekananda's last days are recalled meticulously and compels one to take a sharp breath. There is drama here, unconcious and not forced. Then come the obituaries. In compiling, these, the editor's task is done.

– M. V. Kamath

PART TWO

CONTENTS:

COMMENDATION

This book is a welcome and valuable addition to the growing stream of Ramakrishna-Vivekananda literature, specially because its second part, "*A Chronicle of Important Events in the Life and Times of Vivekananda (1863-1902)*", presents the message of Swami Vivekananda in world perspective, outlining and underlining the events and achievements, the trends, the trials and tribulations of the times (1863-1902), the discoveries and the inventions, the significant publications, the prominent contemporary personalities, the atmosphere – cultural, educational, ethical, social, economic, commercial, scientific and religious – which puts it in a class by itself. Readable for the common people, the book at the same time, is of special interest to the serious student, the research worker and the scholar.

Swami Jyotirmayananda deserves the congratulations and compliments of all, for his continuous, sustained hard work undertaken as a labour of love, in the noble cause of spreading the message of Swami Vivekananda to more and more people, in an enlightened way, with adequate background of world events during the era of Swamiji's brief but bright sojourn among us in the East and the West.

I have no hesitation in commending this book, because of its valuable contents and even more for its invaluable background of a comprehensive Chronology of the times, to both the general reader and the research worker as worthy of their perusal and study. More comprehensive than similar Chronologies of Mahatma Gandhi's life and that of Jawaharlal Nehru, this book which covers the Chronology of not only the life but also the times of Swami Vivekananda will, I have no doubt, find a well-deserved place in every library, for it will serve very well as a reference work also.

NATIONAL YOUTH DAY   Prof. K N. VASWANI
Vivekananda Jayanti   Vice-President
Kanyakumari   Vivekananda Rock Momorial
12th January, 1985.   and Vivekananda Kendra

A WORD ABOUT THE CHRONICLE

In order to grasp the significance and importance of Swami Vivekananda's personality, life and work, it would be helpful to bestow some attention on his contemporaneous environment. Compiled, with this end in view, from various authentic sources, "*A Chronicle of Important Events in the Life and Times of Vivekananda (1863-1902)*", Part II, is the first of its kind and a distinctive feature of this volume.

An attempt has been made in the Chronicle to present the important events in the life of the Swamiji and, side by side, the salient features of the significant developments that took place during his times (1863-1902) in India and abroad. Thus the chronicle includes the religious events and the political developments of the period; the various organisations – social, political, religious and cultural – whether existing or established during the time; the pioneering work done in the realms of science, technology and medicine; the series of inventions and discoveries that took place during the period; the galaxy of inventors and discoverers from different walks of life and climes; the explorations and expeditions undertaken; the institutions – educational and philanthropic – and commercial enterprises that flourished during the period; the developments in transport and communication; the several notable publications by the leading personalities of the time; and the several "firsts" which occurred during the period.

In sum, the Chronicle seeks to provide a vista of the principal events in the life and times of Swami Vivekananda, and brings together some of the items which might aid the reader in understanding Swamiji's historic environs and some of the forces which were at work, moulding human consciousness during his period. Also provided is information relating to the contributions made by the leading contemporary personages in India and abroad. Besides, interspersed in the Chronicle are the significant excerpts from Swami Vivekananda and the eminent contemporaries as also from various other quarters such as the leading Indian and Foreign Newspapers which regularly carried significant news items, reports and editorials about the movements and the missionary activities of Swami Vivekananda both in India and abroad. These excerpts not only serve as a pointer to the contemporary thought-current but also present to the reader the impact of Vivekananda the world over. The Chronicle concludes with extracts from several touching obituaries that appeared in the leading Indian newspapers and periodicals soon after the *mahasamadhi* of the great Swami.

A General Index at the end of the chronicle is followed by a subject index. While the former enables easy and immediate location of any particular information contained in the Chronicle, the latter provides, in a short compass and under different heads, various information of kindred nature found scattered in the Chronicle. A Bibliography of the books referred in the compilation of this Chronicle is also given at the end.

In the Chronicle, events and information about Swami Vivekananda are naturally found scattered all through besides the events and information of his times. Hence a Special Index to Swami Vivekananda under the caption: 'Vivekananda at a Glance', is provided at the very outset to enable easy and immediate location of any desired events or information about Swamiji right from his advent into the world to the final departure.

No originality is claimed for this compilation, nor is the Chronicle an exhaustive one. Some important items might have been missed while others not so important might have found a place here. The compiler can only say that he has done his best to bring together as many items as possible.

According to the dictionary, a chronicle is a detailed and continuous record of events in order of time; a historial record especially one in which the facts are narrated without philosophic treatment, or any attempt in literary style. So strictly speaking a chronicle does not attempt to interpret events. But in the case of the present one, liberty has been taken to add comments wherever necessary. In some cases information which might not be immediately connected with the particular event but all the same present the back-drop or the subsequent developments has also been provided so as to give a clear and comprehensive picture of the event.

In a work like this compiled over a period of about five years and for which material was collected from various sources, it is almost impossible to thank everybody by name, but the compiler is grateful to all the authors of books, editors of newspapers and periodicals whose books and archives he has made use of. But he is particularly indebted to Swami Vimalanandaji Maharaj (1903-1985), a senior monk of the Ramakrishna Order, Sri Ramakrishna Ashrama, Trivandrum-13, for encouragement to carry on the work. In fact it was he who gave the idea of preparing this Chronicle when the compiler met him in August, 1981, with a typescript of the first part of the book. He asked the compiler to append a Chronology of the important events in the life and times of Swami Vivekananda. Initially when the Swami gave the suggestion, the compiler felt unequal to the task. However, with the guidance, encouragement and benediction of the revered Swami, he made bold to embark upon this venture. After a lot of labour the Chronicle is now before the readers. The compiler does not know how he has fared in the venture, and whether he has done justice to the Chronicle. Nevertheless he has the satisfaction of having made at least a humble beginning in that direction. The compiler will be thankful if any discrepancies found by the reader are brought to his notice. Comments and suggestions from the readers for improving the work will be gratefully received.

– S. J.

SWAMI VIVEKANANDA
A Brief Life-sketch

"Narendranath is really a genius. I have travelled far and wide, but I have never yet come across a lad of his talents and possibilities, even in German Universities, among philosophical students. He is bound to make his mark in life!"

– Prof. William Hastie

Narendranath Dutta, afterwards known by the immortal name of Swami Vivekananda was born in 1863. His birth-place, Calcutta – the metropolis of British India then – was under the deluge of Westernization. In fact, the whole of Bengal was then in the throes of a revolutionary religious convulsion. Missionary propaganda under the enthusiastic leadership of its Hebers and Duffs was reaping a rich harvest. The missionaries criticized Hindu beliefs most unjustly while preaching the message of Jesus Christ. They carried on their fanatical tirade in season and out of season. Consequently, the educated youths were turning agnostic and losing faith in their hoary cultural heritage.

Young Narendranath entered adult life in Calcutta much as an actor steps on a busy stage. He encountered the strong tides of social change at the time of his entry into Calcutta's Presidency College in 1880. He joined many other young contemporaries who were equally and inevitably prodded by the prevailing intellectual climate to find solutions to the problems that transcended the individual sphere of life. The crucial needs of society were many, and the responses of sensitive individuals diverse.

As a youth, the future Swami displayed a keen intelligence in school and broad interests that made him a lover of music and an adept in sports. He was a voracious reader with a prodigious memory. To his mastery of the Hindu classics, begun under the tutelage of his mother, he later added an often verbatim familiarity with the *Encyclopaedia Britannica* to his store of knowledge. Rev. W. W. Hastie, his principal at General Assembly's Institution (now Scottish Church College) where he studied European philosophy, was once moved to remark, "Narendranath is really a genius. He is bound to make his mark in life".

And it was from Hastie that Narendranath first came to hear about the famed spiritual leader and mystic Sri Ramakrishna, to whom the Principal had referred while lecturing on the mystical experiences of the poet Wordsworth.

Clearly the young man was equipping his intellect for great efforts to come. He soon took a step that added heightened spiritual motivation to his resources. Responding to his growing urge for divine enlightenment, Narendranath went to Sri Ramakrishna in whose teachings he had developed a mounting interest following a first brief meeting in 1881.

During the ensuing five or six years of association with Sri Ramakrishna, in the secluded exchange between teacher and disciple, spiritual growth wrought a transformation in the young intellectual – and as from a chrysalis, Narendranath emerged as Vivekananda. Spiritual shape and size now supplemented knowledge, insight and wisdom were wedded to man's vast worldly horizon. The discipline of meditation could underlie the urge to action.

After the death of Sri Ramakrishna in 1886, Vivekananda rallied the departed master's disciples and eventually organized them into the illustrious Ramakrishna Mission and later founded the chief monastery of the Order, Belur Math. In the interim he also plunged into the main task of his life; from his own successful fusion of Eastern Spirituality and Western learning he was powerfully imbued with the desire to show the way to his fellowmen everywhere.

Vivekananda had known personal adversity in his younger years, and in his wanderings through India his enlightened mind experienced the anguish of witnessing the plight of the country's impoverished multitudes. His goal of service to humanity and his inspiring national ideas, derived from living incentives.

The Swami's travels are among the best known features of his career. He devoted most of the last fifteen years of his strenuous life to the effort of communicating, through personal appearance, his universal message of unity and tolerance. The impact of his dynamic personality and skilful oratory was often overwhelming. He travelled to all corners of India and visited much of Eastern Asia, Europe and the United States. His triumphs were achieved amongst vast audiences and small groups of devotees. He taught in the city buildings of Chicago in the United States and in his remote Ashram in the Himalayas. It was in Chicago, with his discourses at the Parliament of Religions in 1893, that Vivekananda first gained international attention. His efforts culminated in the establishment of many Vedanta Centres in the world, the first of which he himself founded in New York in 1894,

The great Swami to his last days strove for the reconciliation of human contrasts and conflicts. He never spared himself in his work of projecting his own clear vision that the brotherhood of man demanded social as well as spiritual well-being. His selfless labours sapped his once boundless vitality, and the renowned Swami wound up his earthly career in 1902 at the age of thirty-nine. It was a sublime death, a fitting close to the life that had preceded and one in harmony with the grand philosophy of Vedanta that he had loved so well and taught so faithfully. A world teacher that he was, he had given his light fully, unstintingly to man; he had given enough, as he had said, for fifteen hundred years.

Though the great Swami has broken the prison-wall of earthly existence and soared beyond the grasp of Death in *nirvikalpa samadhi,* the words which he spoke long before his passing away still ring in our ears with a profound significance. "It may be," he said, "that I shall find it good to get outside my body – to cast it off like a worn-out garment. But I shall not cease to work. I shall inspire men everywhere, until the world shall know that it is one with God." And verily his reassuring words have proved to be true. With the roll of years since his passing away his message of peace and goodwill has been gathering momentum and securing from day to day a foot-hold in the citadel of human thought and action, and the conviction is growing in every heart that the spirit of Swamiji will not cease to function as a dynamic force in the society of mankind till the whole world attains to the realization of the highest Truth.

Vivekananda is today a voice without form. He has transcended the limitation of human personality. He has become concretized into an impersonal institution. He is a system of thought, an attitude of men and things, an approach to life, a tradition which has woven itself inextricably into the world. His spirit is more alive today than his body was decades ago. It permeates a network of organizations spread over the whole world, it has expressed itself in diverse activities which have become insitutionalized. His invisible evangelic personality works as a dynamic spiritual force. It permeates the re-awakening India. It revitalizes man. It infuses new life and strength. Acquaintance with him opens a new portal to life. Accepting his message and applying it in full makes one's life exalted.

In the words of Sri Aurobindo, "Vivekananda was a soul of puissance if ever thére was one, a very lion among men, but the definite work he has left behind is quite incommensurate with our impression of his creative might and energy. We perceive his influence still working gigantically, we know not well how, we know not well where, in something that is not yet formed, something leonine, grand, intuitive, upheaving that has entered the soul of India and we say, 'Behold Vivekananda still lives in the soul of his Motherland and in the souls of here children"

VIVEKA-SUTRAS
(Inspiring Aphorisms of Vivekananda)

Arise! Awake! and stop not till the goal is reached.
Bless men when they revile you.
Conquer yourself and the whole universe is yours.
Do not merely endure, but be unattached.
Eat to Him, drink to Him, sleep to Him, see Him in all.
First get rid of the delusion, 'I am the body'.
Give everything, and look for no return.
Homogeneity, sameness is God.
Incarnations like Jesus, Buddha, Ramakrishna, can give religion.
Jnanayoga tells man that he is essentially divine.
Knowledge exists, man only discovers it.
Look at the Ocean, and not at the wave.
Man as the Atman is really free, as man he is bound.
Never turn back to see the result of what you have done.
Out of purity and silence comes the word of power.
Perception is our only real knowledge or religion.
Quarrels in religion are always. over the husks.
Religion without philosophy runs into superstition.
See no difference between man and angel.
The more our bliss is within, the more spiritual we are.
Unchaste imagination is as bad as unchaste action.
Vedas cannot show you Brahman, you are That already.
We are human coverings over the Divine.
Xian you will be when you see Christ. Look only for realization.
You are good, but be better.
Zeal with faith *(shraddha)*: Have this, and everything else is bound to follow.

'VIVEKANANDA AT A GLANCE'

Instructions:

In the **Chronicle of Important Events in the Life and Times of Vivekananda**, *events and information about Swamiji* are naturally found scattered all through besides the *events and information of his times*. Hence a Special Index to Swami Vivekananda under caption: 'Vivekananda at a Glance', is provided at the very outset to enable easy and immediate location of any desired *event or information about Swamiji right from his advent into the world to the final departure.*

1. For events and information conneted with Ramakrishna-Vivekananda, the General Index may be referred to under 'Ramakrishna'.

2. A General Index to the *events and information of Swamiji's times* is given at the end of this book.

3. Please note that in the Index, page numbers have been substituted by the year, month and date of the events in order to make it easier to locate the entry about the events and information in the Chronicle.

4. Every entry in the Index is followed by year, month and date indicating thereby that, for details, reference should be made to that partiular year, month and date in the Chronicle.

5. Where the date of an event or information is not known, only the year and month are mentioned; where even the month is not known, only the year is mentioned.

6. Where the months and dates of more than one event or information transpiring in the same year could not be indicated, a letter of the alphabet (in bracket) has been appended to the year to enable identification and location.

This is a Special Index to enable easy and immediate location of any desired *event or information about Swami Vivekananda* in the Chronicle right from his advent into the world to the final departure.

The following is a guide to the Special Index:

I   Narendranath
     — Pre-monastic Life
II   Swami Vivekananda
     — References to the name occurring in the Chronicle
III Swami Vivekananda
     — Post-monastic Life
IV   Swami Vivekananda
     — Obituaries
V   Swami Vivekananda
     — Tributes
VI   Swami Vivekananda
     — In Western Newspapers
VII Swami Vivekananda
     — In Indian Newspapers
VIII Swami Vivekananda
     — And other events, connected persons, organizations etc.
IX   Swami Vivekananda
     — And his physical features, talents, spiritual experiences etc.
X   Swami Vivekananda
     — On significant persons, places, topics etc.
XI   Swami Vivekananda
     — Miscellanea

I NARENDRANATH
(Pre-monastic Life)

1894 Aug. 8 (a), 1894 Aug. 15 (a); Birth of, 1863 Jan.12; — entered Primary Class, 1871 (a); — his admiration for wandering monks, 1871 (a); — his wish 'I must become a monk', 1871 (a); — a member of Brahma Samaj, 1878 May 15; — entered college, 1879 (a); — challenged a *padre* who abused Hinduism, 1879 (a); — heard about Ramakrishna from his principal, 1881; — saw Ramakrishna first time at Calcutta, 1881 Nov.; — met Ramakrishna first time at Dakshineswar, 1881 Dec.; — Prof. Hastie's remark about, 1881; — passed B. A. Examination, 1884 Jan. 30; — initiated into Freemasonry, 1884 Feb.19; — death of his father, financial distress and privation at home, 1884 Feb. 25; — sent by Ramakrishna to meet Bankim, 1884 Dec.; — in deep meditation, 1885 Sept.; — initiated into *Rama Mantra* by Ramakrishna, 1886 Apr.; — disciples of Ramakrishna under the leadership of, 1886 Aug.16; — Ramakrishna transmitted his spiritual powers to, 1886 Aug.; — took to monastic life with his brother disciples, 1887 Jan.

II SWAMI VIVEKANANDA
(References to the name occurring in the Chronicle).

1893 Sept. 11, 1893 Sept. 11 (a), 1893 Sept. 19, 1893 Sept. 28, 1893 Oct. 1, 1893 Oct. 11, 1893 Nov. 18, 1893 Nov. 30, 1893 Dec. 6, 1893 Dec. 27, 1893 Dec., 1894 Feb. 21 (b), 1894 Mar. 9, 1894 Mar. 14, 1894 Mar. 21, 1894 Apr. 10, 1894 Apr. 11, 1894 Apr. 13, 1894 Apr. 22, 1894, June, 1894 Aug. 8, 1894 Aug. 8 (a), 1894 Aug. 15, 1894 Aug. 15 (a), 1894 Sept. 1, 1894 Sept. 5, 1894 Sept. 7, 1894 Sept. 25, 1894 Nov. 4, 1894 Nov. 7, 1894 Dec. 10, 1895 Mar. 4, 1895 Apr. 19, 1895 May 19, 1895 May 31, 1895 Jul. 27, 1895 Sept., 1895 Oct. 5, 1895 Nov. 3, 1895 Nov. 23, 1895 Dec. 22, 1896 Jan. 18, 1896 Feb. 29, 1896 Mar. 25 (a), 1896 Mar. 28, 1896 Apr. 2, 1896 Apr. 11, 1896 Apr. 11 (a), 1896 June 3, 1896 June 14, 1896 June 14 (a), 1896 June 18, 1896 May 23, 1896 June 27, 1896 Jul. 9, 1896 Jul. 17, 1896 Jul. 18, 1896 Aug. 4, 1896 Aug. 27, 1896 Nov. 21, 1897 Jan. 11, 1897 Jan. 21, 1897 Feb. 4, 1897 Feb. 6, 1897 Feb. 6 (a), 1897 Feb. 6 (b), 1897 Feb., 1897 Mar. 8, 1897 Mar. 17, 1897 June 23, 1897 Aug. 22, 1897 Apr. 5, 1898 Jan. 15, 1898 June, 1898 Sept. 30, 1899 Jan., 1899 Mar. 19, 1899 Mar. 19 (a), 1899 Apr. 30, 1899 Apr., 1899 June 2, 1899 June 25, 1899 Jul. 9, 1899 Aug. 17, 1899 Sept. 27, 1900 June 10, 1900 June 24, 1900 Jul. 8, 1902 Jan., 1902 Mar. 22, 1902 Jul. 1, 1902 Jul. 6, 1902 Jul. 6 (a), 1902 Jul. 6 (b), 1902 Jul. 7 (a), 1902 Jul. 9, 1902 Jul. 9 (a), 1902 Jul. 10, 1902 Jul. 10 (a), 1902 Jul. 10 (b), 1902 Jul. 11, 1902 Jul. 13, 1902 Jul.13 (a), 1902 Jul. 13 (b), 1902 Jul. 13 (c), 1902 Jul. 14, 1902 Jul. 20, 1902 Jul. 25, 1902 Jul. 25 (a), 1902 Jul. (a), 1902 Jul. (d), 1902 Jul. (e), 1902 Jul. (f), 1902 Jul. (g), 1902 Jul. (j), 1902 Jul. (k), 1902 Jul. (1), 1902 Aug. (a), 1902 Aug. (b), 1902 Oct. 17, 1902 Oct. 26, 1902 Dec. 16, 1903 Feb.

III SWAMI VIVEKANANDA
(Post-monastic Life)

— on a pilgrimage to holy places, 1888 (early part); — his second pilgrimage, 1888 Jun. - Nov.; — his extraordinary way of reading, 1888 Jun. - Nov.; — with Pawahari Baba, 1890 Feb. 4; — into the treadmill of hard spiritual discipline, 1890 Jul.; — began his historic itinerary, 1891 Jan.; — in the clutches of the practitioners of black magic at Limbdi, 1891 Nov. (first week); — with B. G. Tilak at Poona, 1892 June; — with Chattambi Swamigal at Ernakulam, 1892 Nov.; — perturbed over the mass conversion spree of the *padres* in Travancore, 1892 Nov.; — at Trivandrum, 1892 Dec. 13-22; — the epoch making *tapasya* at Kanyakumari, 1892 Dec. (last week); — at Hyderabad, 1893 Feb.; — witnessed an incident testifying the powers of human mind, 1893 Feb.; — sailed for America, 1893 May

31; — wrote his first letter from America referring to the financial panic there and the ill-treatment of the Negroes, 1893; — with Prof. John H. Wright, 1893 Aug. 25-28; — spoke at the World's Parliament of Religions during the first day's afternoon session, 1893 Sept.11 (a); — read his celebrated paper on Hinduism, 1893 Sept. 19; — his telling reply (extempore) to the Christian delegates who made a concerted attack on Hinduism, 1893 Sept. 19, 1893 Sept. 29; — denounced religious intolerance and bloody wars of the Christian nations, 1893 Sept. 19; — in the final session of the Parliament, 1893 Sept. 27; — Yogic powers in, 1894 Feb.; — demonstration of materialization by, 1894 Feb. (a); — "The Christian Missions in India"; — a lecture by, 1894 Mar. 11; — "The Women of India"; — a lecture by, 1894 Mar. 25; — John D. Rockefeller calls on, 1894 Mar. - Apr.; — public meetings at Madras and Calcutta to thank Vivekananda for his grand success in America, 1894 Apr. 28, 1894 Sept. 5; — organized 'The Vedanta Society of New York', 1894 Nov.; — report about his ill-treatment as a 'nigger'at Baltimore,1894 Dec. 10; — wrote to Alasinga giving an idea of his task in America, 1895 Feb.17; — began Vedanta classes at New York, 1895 Feb.; — at Percy, passed into *nirvikalpa samadhi*, 1895 June; — at Thousand Island Park, 1895 June 18-Aug.7; — composed "*The Song of the sannyasin*", 1895 June. 18-Aug.7; — "*The Inspired Talks*", 1895 June 18-Aug. 7; — dictated "*Raja Yoga*", 1895 June 18-Aug.7, 1895 June (a); — entered into *nirvikalpa samadhi* on the bank of St. Lawrence, 1895 June 18-Aug. 7; — publication of "*Raja Yoga*" in America, 1895 July; — with Prof. William James at New York, 1895 July; — his first visit to England, 1895 Oct.-Nov.; — his public lecture at Piccadilly, 1895 Oct. 22; — in British Newspapers, 1895 Oct. 22; — met Margaret Noble in England, 1895 Nov.; — his schedule of class lectures at New York, 1895-96; — spoke on "*Soul and God*" at the Metaphysical Society at Hartford, 1896 Feb.; — lectured before the 'Ethical Society of Brooklyn', 1896 Feb. (a); — spoke at the Harvard University on philosophy of Vedanta, 1896 Mar. 25; — was offered a chair of Eastern philosophy at the Harvard University and a Chair of Sanskrit in the Columbia University, 1896 Mar. 25; — visited London, second time, took regular classes, 1896 Apr.; — met Prof. Max Muller at the Oxford University, 1896 May 28; — on a Continental tour, 1896 Sept.; — met Paul Deussen at Kiel, 1896 Sept.; — back in London and continued the lectures, 1896 Oct.-Dec.; — a farewell meeting at London, I896 Oct.-Dec.; — left for India, 1896 Oct-Dec.; — humbled the missionaries who abused Hinduism, 1867 Jan. (first week); — arrived at Colombo, 1897 Jan. 15; — given a grand reception, 1897 Jan.15; — welcome address and his reply, 1897 Jan. 15; — his first public lecture in the East (at Colombo) "*India the Punyabboomi*", 1897 Jan. 16; — at Pamban, 1897 Jan. 26; — welcome address by Raja of Ramnad and reply by Swamiji, 1897 Jan. 26; — taken in a State carriage drawn by the Raja himself, 1897 Jan. 26; — visited Rameswaram temple and delivered a stirring address, 1897 Jan. 27; — a

monument of victory was erected at Ramnad in honour of, 1897 Jan. 27;
— reply to the address of welcome presented by the Raja of Ramnad,
1897 Jan. 29; — reply to the address of welcome presented by the citizens
of Paramakudi, 1897 Feb. 1; arrived at Madras, 1897 Feb. 6 (b); wrestles
with a *pahilwan,* 1897 Feb. 6 (b); — his last public lecture at Madras:
"The Future of India", 1897 Feb. 14; — was given a grand public reception
by the citizens of Calcutta, 1897 Feb. 28; — address of welcome and his
reply, 1897 Feb. 28; — deputed Swami Ramakrishnananda to Madras, 1897
Apr. 5; — founded the Ramakrishna Math in Calcutta, 1897 May 1; — at
Kashmir on tour, 1897 Sept.10; — at Punjab: reception at Lahore and his
first lecture, 1897 Nov. 5-15; — his third lecture at Lahore on *"Vedanta",*
met Prof. Thirtha Ram Goswami, 1897 Nov. 12; — ordained Margaret Noble,
1898 Jan. 28; — purchased a plot of land for Belur Math, 1898 Mar. 5; —
consecration of the newly purchased Math grounds, 1898 Mar. 5; — carried
on shoulder the sacred urn, 1898 Mar. 5; — organized Plague Relief at
Calcutta 1898 Apr.; — the R. K. Mission plague service managed by Sister
Nivedita, 1898 Apr.; — wrote at the news of Mr. Goodwin's premature
death,1898 June 2; — observed the Anniversary of American Declaration
of Independence, 1898 July 4; — composed *"To the Fourth July",* 1898
Jul. 4; — undertook pilgrimage to Amarnath with Sister Nivedita, 1898
Aug. 2; — had a great mystic experience at Amarnath, 1898 Aug. 2; —
attended the opening ceremony of Nivedita school at Calcutta, 1898 Nov.
13; — consecrated the Belur Math, with the installation of Ramakrishna's
image in chapel, 1898 Dec. 9; — Ramakrishna Math was finally removed
to the new monastery at Belur and was occupied by the members of the R.
K. Order, 1898 Dec. 9; — founded Advaita Ashrama at Mayavati,
Himalayas, 1899 Mar. 19; — left for the West on his mission for the second
time, 1899 June 20; — at Ridgely Manor, U. S. A., 1899 Oct. 30; — delivered
a lecture on *"Mahabharata"* at Pasadena, California, 1900 Feb.1; —
referred to the *Gita* and its influence on the American mind, 1900 Feb.1; —
wrote to Swami Akhandananda, "Tell me where your Congressmen are",
1900 Feb. 21; — at California, 1900 Feb.-May; — received a gift of 160
acres of land situated on the eastern slope of Mt. Hamilton for 'Shanti
Ashram', 1900 Feb.-May; — participated in the Congress of History of
Religions, met Dr. J. C. Bose at Paris, 1900Aug.-Oct.; — arrived at Belur
Math after his second trip to the West, 1900 Dec. 9; — scaled the Math
compound wall gate to be promptly present for the dinner, 1900 Dec. 9; —
at the Advaita Ashram, Mayavati, 1901 Jan. 7; — "The old man had
already established himself even there", 1901 Jan. 7; — at Belur Math,
1901 Nov. — with the two learned Buddhists from Japan, 1901 Nov.; —
with B. G. Tilak at Belur Math, 1901 Dec. (last week); — his love for the
poor Santal labourers employed at the Belur Math, served a hearty meal to
them, 1901 Dec. (a); — wept on hearing that nobody came forward to
preside over the *Shivaji Utsav* organized by the nationalists of Bengal, 1901

(b); "I will not live long", 1902 Jan.; — Gandhiji who was at Calcutta, went to Belur Math desiring to meet, 1902 Feb.; — News of his serious illness, 1902 Mar. 22; — *"Nirvana* is before me", 1902 May. 15; — *Mahasamadhi*, 1902 Jul. 4; his room at Belur Math, 1902 Jul. 5; "passed away yesterday", 1902 Jul. 5 (a).

IV SWAMI VIVEKANANDA
(Obituaries)

The Indian Mirror, 1902 Jul. 6, 1902 Jul. 25, 1902 Jul. 10 (b); — *The Bengali,* 1902, Jul. 6 (a), 1902 Dec. 16; — *The Statesman and Friend of India,* 1902 Jul. 6 (b); — *The Times of India,* 1902 Jul. 7; — *The Indian Nation,* 1902 Jul. 7 (a), 1902 Oct. 17; — *Native Opinion,* 1902 Jul. 9 (a); — *The Tribune,* 1902 Jul. 10; — *The New India,* 1902 Jul. 10 (a); — *The Behar Times,* 1902 Jul. 11; — *The Hindu,* 1902 Jul. 13; — *The Indian Social Reformer,* 1902 Jul. 13 (a); — *The Mahratta,* 1902 Jul. 13 (b); — *The Native States,* 1902 Jul. 13 (c); — *The Mysore Herald,* 1902 Jul. 14; — *The Hindu Organ,* 1902 Jul. 16; — *The Gujarati,* 1902 Jul. 20; — *Advocate,* 1902 Jul. (a); — *Prabuddha Bharata,* 1902 Jul. (b), 1902 Jul. (1); — *East and West,* 1902 Jul. (c); — *The Journal of the Maha Bodhi Society,* 1902 Jul. (e); — *The Kayastha Samachar,*1902 Jul. (f); — *The Indian Review,* 1902 Jul. (g); — *The Brahmacharin,* 1902 Jul. (h); — *The Brahmavadin,* 1902 Jul. (i), 1902 Oct. 26, 1903 Feb., 1903 Feb. (a); — *The South Indian Times,*1902 Jul. (j); — *The Theosophist,* 1902 Aug. (a); — *Malbar Mail,* 1902 Aug, (b); — *The Illustrated Buffalo Express,* 1902 Dec. 16; — *The Anubis,* 1903 Feb.

V SWAMI VIVEKANANDA
(Tributes)

Dr. J. C. Bose, 1902 Jul. 9; — Babu Romesh Chandra Dutt, 1902 Jul. (d); — Norendranath Sen, 1902 Jul. (k); — A Western Disciple, 1902 Jul. (l); — San Francisco class of Vedantic Philosophy, 1902 Oct. 17; — A Memorial Service held by the Vedanta Society of New York, 1902 Oct. 26; — S. E. Waldo, 1903 Feb.; — Dr. John C. Wyman, 1903 Feb. (a); — A letter to the Editor, 1902 Jul. 25

VI SWAMI VIVEKANANDA
(In Western Newspapers)

Chicago Daily Tribune, 1893 Sept. 19, 1893 Dec., 1897 Jan. 30; — *Daily Chronicle,* 1893 Sept. 19; — *Boston Evening Transcript,* 1893 Sept. 30, 1894 Aug. 8; — *New York Critic,* 1893 Oct. 7, 1893 Dec. 27; — *Evanston Index,* 1893 Oct. 7 (a); — *Wisconsin State Journal,* 1893 Nov. 21; — *Minneapolis Star,* 1893 Nov. 25; — *Des Moines News,* 1893 Nov. 28; — *Press of America,* 1893 Nov. 30; — *New York Herald,* 1893 Dec. 27,

1896 Jan. 19, 1896 Mar. 25 (a); — *Appeal Avalanche,* 1894 Jan. 16, 1894 Jan. 21; — *Memphis Commercial,* 1894 Jan. 17; — *Detroit Tribune,* 1894 Feb. 15, 1894 Feb. 16, 1894 Feb. 18 (a); — *Detroit Evening News,* 1894 Feb. 17, 1894 Aug. 8, 1896 Apr. 11 (a); — *Detroit Free Press,* 1894 Feb. 18, 1894 Feb. 18 (a), 1894 Feb. 21 (a), 1894 Mar. 25; — *Pioneer,* 1894 Mar. 14 — *The London Standard,* 1895 Oct. 22, 1895 Oct.-Nov.; — *New York Independent,* 1894 Dec. 5, 1894 Dec. 10; — *Hartford's Daily Times,* 1895 Apr. 19 *Westminister Gazette,* 1895 Nov. 19; — *London Daily Chronicle,* 1896 Jul. 17; — *Sunday Times,* 1896 Jul. 18; — *India* (London), 1896 Aug. 27; — *New York Tribune,*1897 Jan.11; — *Detroit Journal,* 1894 Feb. 21; — *Unity,* 1900 June 24

VII SWAMI VIVEKANANDA
(In Indian Newspapers)

Amrita Bazar Patrika, 1894 Mar. 14, 1894 Aug. 15 (a); — *Brahmavadin,* 1895 Nov. 23, 1896 Feb. 29, 1896 Mar. 28, 1896 Apr. 11, 1896 Apr. 11 (a), 1896 May 23, 1896 Nov. 21, 1897 Jan. 11, 1897 Jan. 30 — *The Hindu,* 1895 Nov. 3, 1899 June 2; — *Hindu Patriot,* 1894 Nov. 7, 1894 Dec. 5, 1896 Jul. 18; — *Indian Daily News,* 1894 Sept. 7; — *Indian Mirror,*1893 Nov. 30, 1893 Dec. 6, 1893 Dec. 27, 1893 Dec., 1894 Feb. 21(b), 1894 Mar. 9, 1894 Mar. 21, 1894 Apr. 10, 1894 Apr. 12, 1894 Apr. 13, 1894 Apr. 22, 1894 June, 1894 Aug. 8, 1894 Aug. 8 (a), 1894 Aug. 15, 1894 Sep. 5, 1894 Nov. 4, 1895 Mar. 1, 1895 Mar. 4, 1895 Apr. 19, 1895 May 19, 1895 May 31, 1895 Oct. 5, 1895 Nov. 3, 1895 Nov. 19, 1895 Dec. 22, 1896 Jan. 18, 1896 Mar. 25 (a), 1896 Apr. 2, 1896 Jun. 3, 1896 Jun.14, 1896 Jun. 18, 1896 Jun. 27, 1896 Jul. 9, 1896 Jul. 17, 1896 Aug. 4, 1896 Aug. 27, 1897 Jan. 21, 1897 Feb. 7, 1897 Feb. 23, 1897 Jun. 23, 1899 Jun. 2, 1899 Aug. 17, 1899 Sep. 27, 1902 Mar. 22; — *Indian Nation,* 1894 Dec. 10, 1897 Mar. 8; — *Indian Social Reformer,* 1899 May; — *Madras Mail,* 1897 Feb. 4, 1897 Feb. 6; — *Madras Times* 1895 Mar. 1, 1897 Feb. 7; — *The Mahratta,* 1899 Apr. 30, 1899 Jun. 25, 1899 Jul. 9, 1900 Jun. 24, 1900 Jul. 8; — *Prabuddha Bharata,* 1899 Apr., 1899 Jun. 25; — *Tribune* 1895 May 19

VIII SWAMI VIVEKANANDA AND....
(Other events, connected persons, organizations etc).

— Advita Ashram, 1899 Mar. 19, 1901 Jan. 7; — Ajitsingh, Raja, 1895 Mar. 4; — Alasinga Perumal, 1863 (c); — Akhandananda, Swami, 1888 Jun. - Nov., 1900 Feb. 21; — American Independence Day, 1898 Jul. 4; — Belur Math, 1898 Mar. 5, 1898 Dec. 9; — Bose, Dr. J. C., 1900 Aug.-Oct.; — *Brahmavadin,* 1895 Jul. 27, 1895 Sep.; — Buddhists from Japan, 1901 Nov.; — Chattambi Swamigal, 1892 Nov.; — Christian delegates, 1893 Sep. 19, 1893 Sep. 29; — Christian Literature Society, 1895 May 19; — Christian

Missionaries, 1893 Dec., 1894 Mar. 9, 1894 Apr. 22, 1894 Aug. 8 (a), 1894 Nov. 7, 1894 Dec. 5, 1894 Dec. 10, 1895 May 19,1895 May 31, 1897 Jan., 1897 Feb. 6, 1897 Feb. 7, 1897 Jun. 23, 1898 Sep. 30, 1899 Mar. 19, 1899 Aug. 17, 1899 Sep. 27; — Christian students, 1895 Jun. 18-Aug. 7; — Deussen, Paul, 1896 Sep.; — Encyclopedia Britannica,1901 May; — England, 1895 Oct. - Nov., 1895 Oct. 22, 1896 Apr., 1896 Oct. - Dec.; — Ethical Society of Brooklyn, 1896 Feb. (a); — Gandhi, M. K., 1902 Feb.; — Goodwin, 1898 Jun. 2; — Harvard University, 1896 Mar. 25; — Hiram Maxim, 1884 (j); — Ingersol, Robert, 1899 Jul. 21; —"Imitation of Christ", 1889 (q); — Kashmir, 1897 Sep. 10; — Max Muller, Prof., 1896 May 28; — Merwin-Marie Snell, 1894 Mar. 9; — Nivedita, Sister, 1867 Oct. 28, 1898 Jan. 28, 1900 Jun. 10; — Paris, 1900 Aug. - Oct.; — Parliament of Religions, 1893 Sep. 11; — Pavabari Baba, 1890 Feb. 4, 1898 Jun.; — Phrenological Society , 1895 Oct. 5; — Plague relief, Calcutta, 1898 Apr.; — Prabuddha Bharata, 1896 Jul., 1896 Jun. 14; — Punjab, 1897 Nov. 5 - 15; — Raja of Ramnad, 1897 Jan. 29, 1897 Jan. 26, 1897 Jan. 27; — Ramakrishna, Sri, 1881 Nov., 1881 Dec., 1884 Dec., 1886 Apr., 1886 Aug.; — Ramakrishnananda, Swami, 1897 Apr. 5; — Ramakrishna Math, 1897 May 1; — Ramathirtha, Swami, 1873 Oct. 22, 1897 Nov. 12; — Rockefeller, 1894 Mar. - Apr.; — Shanthi Ashram, 1900 Feb. - May; — Shivaji Utsav, Calcutta, 1901 (b); J. N. Tata, 1893 May 31 (a); — Tesla, Nikola, 1883 (c), 1896 Mar. 28; — Thousand Island Park,1895 Jun. 18-Aug. 7; — Tilak, B. G., 1892 Jun. 1900 Feb. 21, 1901 Dec.; — Udbodhan, 1899 Jan.; — Vedanta Society of New York, 1894 Nov.; — William James, Prof., 1895 Jul.; — Wright. Prof. John H., 1893 Aug. 25 - 28.

IX SWAMI VIVEKANANDA AND....

(His physical features, talents, spiritual experiences etc).

— his physiognomy, 1895 Oct. 5; — his physical features, 1893 Sept. 28 — his prodigious retentive power, 1901 May; — his love for Santal labourers, 1901 Dec. (a); — his tribute to the 'ever trampled labouring class of India', 1900 (a); — his spiritual humanism, 1895 Aug. 9; — his popularity, 1894 Apr. 11, 1894 Sep. 1; — his mystic experience at Amarnath, 1898 Aug. 2; — his yogic powers, 1894 Feb., 1894 Feb. (a); — his oratory at its best, 1897 Feb. 14; — his experience at the Parliament of Religions, 1896 (b); — his noteworthy experience at Baltimore, 1894 Dec. 5; — his success in America spreads consternation through the ranks of Missionaries, 1895 May 31; — his ipse dixits regarding Christ, Christianity and Christian Missionaries, 1895 Jun. - Aug.; — his warning about the critical situation in the West, 1896 (a); — his prediction about the shudra dominance, 1896 (a); — his appeal for harmony of religious faiths, 1893 Sep. 27; — his views on reconversion, 1899 Apr., 1899 May, 1899 Jun. 25; — his remarks about conversion and bigotry, 1894 Feb. 18; — his views on occultism, 1897 Feb.; — his advice to monks, 1901 (a); — his lectures at the Vedanta Society of New York, 1900 June 10; — his letter to Raja Peary Mohan Mukherji, 1895 Apr. 18; — his letter from America, 1895 (p); — his letter to the Editor of *East and West,* 1897 Feb.; — his four *yogas,* 1896 (c); — his book, *The Philosophy of Yoga,* 1896 (n); — his *Lectures From Colombo to Almora,* reviewed, 1897 Aug. 22; — his *Lectures on Raja Yoga,* reviewed, 1897 Jan. 30; — his influence on Gandhiji, 1902 Feb.; — his influence on Tolstoy, 1894 (e); — his affinity with America,1898 Jul. 14; — his second visit to the West, 1899 Jun. 20; — his continental tour, 1896 Sep.; — his study of Encyclopedia, 1901 May; — "his religion has eclipsed the beauty of the old time Christianity", 1894 Jan. 21.

X SWAMI VIVEKANANDA ON ....

(Significant persons, places, topics etc).

— on Max Muller, 1900 Oct. 28; — on Pavahari Baba, 1898 Jun., 1890 Feb. 4; — on J. J. Goodwin, 1898 Jun. 2; — on *The Future of India,* 1897 Feb.; — on *Hindus and Christians,* 1894 Feb. 21 (a); — on *Vedanta,* 1897 Nov. 12; — on *Mahabharata,* 1900 Feb. 1; — on the *Gita,* 1900 Feb.; — on *The Crying Evil in the East,* 1893 Dec.; — on *Brahmacharya,* 1901 May; — on his motherland, 1896 Oct. - Dec.; — on India's need for socialism, 1896 Nov. 1; — on 'Christian Science', 1894 Sep. 25; — on 'New Dispensation', 1881 Jan. 25; — on Christian Missionaries, 1893 Dec.; — on Mass conversions in Travancore, 1892 Nov.; — on reconversion to Hinduism, 1899 May, 1899 Jun. 25; — on the religion of the future in the West, 1896 (a); — on the dangers facing the West, 1897 Feb. 1; — on the financial panic in America, 1893; — on the ill-treatment of Negroes in America, 1893; — on evils of British rule in India, 1899 Oct. 30; — on the dominance of proletariat, 1896 (a); — on plague preventive measures, 1899 Apr. 30; — on Kashmir, 1897 Sep. 10; — on Punjab, 1897 Nov. 5 - 15

XI SWAMI VIVEKANANDA

(Miscellanea)

— Gandhiji's desire to meet, 1902 Feb.; — Bipin Chandra Pal on the influence of, 1898 Jan.15; — Raja Ajit Singh's address to, 1895 Mar. 4; — Dr. J. C. Bose's tribute to, 1902 Jul. 9; — Babu Romesh Chandra Dutt's tribute to, 1902 Jul. (d); — Prof. Sundararama Iyer's tribute to, 1892 Dec. 13-22; — Tolstoy's interest in, 1894 (e), 1896 (n); — Merwin-Marie Snell on, 1894 Mar. 9; — John H. Wright's remark about, 1893 Aug. 25 - 28; — Tesla's admiration for, 1863 (c); — Sister Nivedita in appreciation of the lecture of, 1900 Jun. 10; — Dr. John C. Wyman's tribute to, 1903 Feb. (a); — S. E. Waldo's obituary of, 1903 Feb.; — A Western Disciple's obituary of, 1902 Jul. (l); — The tribute of the San Francisco Class of Vedantic

Philosophy 1902 Oct. 17; — New York Vedanta Society's Memorial Service to, 1902 Oct. 26; — in defence of Hinduism, 1893 Sep. 19,1893 Sep. 29, 1897 Jan; — in appreciation of Alasinga, 1863 (c); — ill-treated as 'nigger' at Baltirnore, 1894 Dec. 10; — Christian Missionary crusade against, 1894 Mar. 9, 1894 Apr. 22, 1894 Dec. 5, 1894 Dec. 10, 1895 May 31, 1898 Sep. 30, 1899 Mar. 19 (a), 1899 Aug. 17, 1899 Sep. 27; — Christian missionaries jealous of, 1894 Aug. 8 (a); — Christian missionaries rage and fume over the success of, 1897 June 23; — Christian Literature Society's tirade against, 1895 May 19; — versus Christian Missionaries, 1893 Sep. 29, 1893 Oct. 11, 1893 Dec.,1894 Mar. 9, 1894 Nov. 7, 1897 Jan., 1897 Feb. 6, 1897 Feb. 7; — interviewed by The Madras Times, 1897-Feb. 7; — interviewed by The Madras Mail, 1897 Feb. 6; — thrilled at the success of the Indian painter in America, 1893 (a) — examination of his physiognomy by the Phrenological Society, America, 1895 Oct. 5; — a letter to, 1894 Sep. 5; — an address to, 1894 Jun.; — an illuminated address presented to, 1896 Oct.-Dec., — at Belur Math, 1902 May 15— the name, 1887 Jan.; —"I am proud to call myself a Hindu", 1897 Nov. 5; — "plain living and high thinking", 1902 Jul. 11; — "wept tears bitter as blood", 1902 Jul. 10 (b); — "Religion not the crying need of India", 1893 Oct. 11; — "an extraordinary man", 1895 Mar. 1; — "That is all nonsense", 1866 Apr. 10.

A CHRONICLE OF IMPORTANT EVENTS
IN THE LIFE AND TIMES OF
VIVEKANANDA (1863-1902)

1863 JAN. 12: SWAMI VIVEKANANDA, the great soul, loved and revered in East and West alike as the rejuvenator of Hinduism in India and the preacher of its eternal truths abroad, was born at 6.45, a few minutes after sunrise. It was the day of the great Hindu festival *Makarasankranti* (symbolising a major transformation or the birth of a new era) when special worship is offered to the Ganga by millions of devotees. Thus the future Vivekananda first drew breath when the air above the sacred river not far from the house was reverberating with the prayer, worship, and religious music of thousands of Hindu men and women.

"His advent into the arena of Indian life was a historical necessity. India, then under the political thumb of the British, was passing through a welter of cultural ideals as a result of the influx of Occidental thought which, with its sparkling glamour, lured unwary children of the soil into a position of utter helplessness through a silent process of intellectual, social and economic exploitation. Against such a tragic background, Swami Vivekananda was projected into the nineteenth century by the birth-throes of nature as a mighty challenge to the ideology of the West."

1863 JUL. 1-3: The **Battle of Gettysburg** in Pennsylvania, a major engagement in the American Civil War. [see 1865 Apr. 14 and 26]

90,000 Northerners battled against 75,000 Confederates, on the first, second and third days of the month. By the night of July 3 when the battle was over, the South had 20,000 casualties and the North 17,500. Southern troops were routed and the Confederate advance into North was doomed.

On November 19, **Abraham Lincoln** (1809-1865), the 16th American President, dedicated a national cemetery on the battlefield of Gettysburg. On this occasion he made an eloquent address which is popularly known as the 'Gettysburg Address.' It has come to be regarded as one of the most profound expressions of the democratic ideals in the English language.

1863 JUL. 30: Birth of **Henry Ford** (d. 1947), American pioneer of the automobile industry and the founder of the world's largest philanthropic trust, 'The Ford Foundation.' [see 1893 Dec. 24].

1863 NOV. 14: Birth of **Leo. H. Backeland** (d.1944), American Chemist and inventor and manufacturer.

By the time he was 36, he was a millionaire, having sold his invention, a slow-developing photographic paper called 'Velox', to the Eastman Kodak Co. In 1909, Backeland announced the development of a material called Bakelite – the first man-made plastic which formed the foundation of the modern plastic industry. [see 1893 (i)]

1863 DEC. 13: Birth of **W. H. Parker** (d. 1939), American physician and public health official, who was the first to systematically apply bacteriology to diagnosis, prevention and treatment of the common infectious diseases.

1863 (A): Under the guidance of a sannyasini named Bhairavi Brahmani who was an expert in *Tantra shastra,* **SRI RAMAKRISHNA** (1836-1886), the saint of Dakshineswar, Calcutta, completed the most difficeilt *Tantrika sadhana,* and became established in the realization of the Divine Mother.

In the course of his *sadhana,* he performed profound and delicate ceremonies in the Panchavati and under the bel-tree at the northern extremity of the Dakshineswar temple compound. He practised all the disciplines of the sixty-four principal *Tantra* books, and it took him never more than three days to achieve the result promised in any one of them. This is how he described those practices: "The Brahmani would go during the day to places far from Dakshinewsar and collect the various rare things mentioned in the *Tantric* scriptures. At night fall she would ask me to come to one of the meditation seats. I would go, and after performing the worship of Mother Kali, I would begin to medîtate according to her directions. As soon as I would begin to tell my beads, 1 would be always overwhelmed with divine fervour and fall into a deep trance. I cannot relate all the varieties of wonderful visions I used to have. They followed one another in quick succession and I could feel the most tangible effects of those practices. The Brahmani put me through all the exercises mentioned in the sixty-four principal Tantra books. Most of these were extremely difficult *sadhanas* – some of them so dangerous that they often cause the devotee to lose his footing and sink into moral turpitude. But the infinite grace of the Mother carried me through them unscathed."

1863 (B): **Alexander Duff** (1806-1878), Scottish Presbyterian missionary, left for Scotland after more than thirty years of his evangelical and educational activities in India.

He came to Calcutta in 1830, and chose to work amongst the upper caste (Brahmins), with a plan for creation of an Indian Christian elite to become the source of the evangelization of the Indian subcontinent. He hoped that his new style of education might "undermine" Hindu society. But his method did not produce large number of converts.

The conversion of a student of Duff School and his wife to Christianity created a great commotion in Calcutta, and the orthodox Hindus rallied round Devendranath Tagore who had launched a vigorous campaign against such forcible conversion. These efforts of the Indians were successful to a large extent and considerably reduced the number of conversions to Christianity. An indirect result of this anti-conversion campaign was the establishment of English schools by the Indians in order to draw away the students from the mission schools. Thus, as a result of the campaign mentioned above, a school was established (1845) providing free instruction to about one thousand Hindu students.

The most disconcerting feature of the activities of Christian missionaries then in India was the rabid tone of their criticism – rather abuse of Hinduism. Even Alexander Duff lost all balance while assailing Hinduism. The following extract from his book *India and Indian Missions* gives us a fair specimen of missionary mentality: "Of all systems of false religion ever fabricated by the perverse ingenuity of fallen men, Hlinduism is surely the most stupendous.... Of all systems of false religion it is that which seems to embody the largest amount and variety of semblances and counterfeits of divinely revealed facts and doctrines." Duff's book was criticised in the most scathing terms by *The Tattvabodhini Patrika,* the organ of the Brahma Samaj (Bharathiya Vidya Bhavan's *History and Culture of the Indian People,* Vol. X, Part II, p.155).

English education by missionaries began in Bengal in Serampore in 1800. The names associated with it are Carey, Marshman and Ward. The following are extracts from an account of the Danish Mission: "William Carey, an English Baptist, arrived in Calcutta on the 11th November, 1793.... He studied Bengali and Sanskrit, began the work of translating the Bible into Bengali, gained his experience and developed his methods. In 1800 he settled in Serampore under the Danish flag and in the same year he began to teach Sanskrit and Bengali in Lord Wellesley's College in Calcutta. It was chiefly by the winning of actual converts from Hinduism by his schools, newspapers and literature that he was able to bring Christian thought effectively to bear on the Indian spirit.... Their methods of work were partly those which had been developed by Danish missionaries in South India in the 18th century, and partly new.... They had a printing press and in it Indian type was first founded and used. They laid great stress on education and opened numerous schools around them for both boys and girls. They opened boarding schools and orphanages. They even attempted medical work and did not neglect the lepers" (Farquhar's *Modern Religious Movements in India).*

1863 (C): Birth of **Alasinga Perumal** (d.1909), one of the most ardent admirers and devoted disciples of Swami Vivekananda.

Alasinga was the foremost in making house-to-house collections in Madras to send the Swami to the West to participate in the World's Parliament of Religions held at Chicago, U. S. A., in September 1893. About Alasinga, Swamiji wrote: "One rarely finds men like our Alasinga in the world – one so unselfish, so hardworking and so devoted to his guru, and such an obedient disciple is indeed very rare on earth."

1863 (D): **Henry Clifton Sorby** (1826-1908), English geologist, discovered the **microstructure of steel,** marking the beginning of modern metallurgical science. In the same year the **open-hearth process** for manufacture of steel was developed by **Martin brothers** in France.

1863 (E): **Thomas Henry Huxley** (1825-1895), British biologist and the champion of Darwin's (1809-1882) theory of evolution, wrote *Evidence as to Man's Place in Nature,* supporting the great debate with **Samuel Wilberforce** (1805-1873), the Bishop of Oxford.

When Darwin published his theory of evolution in *The Origin of Species* in 1859, Victorian society was incensed. The challenge to the Biblical account of creation threatened man's view of his God-given superiority, and the clergy took it up at a famous meeting of the British Association at Oxford in June 1860. Samuel Wilberforce, Bishop of Oxford, led the concerted attack and declared beforehand that he was out to 'smash Darwin'. He told a packed and hushed hall that the theory was 'casual', 'sensational' and contrary to the Divine revelations of the Bible. He then turned on the biologist, T. H. Huxley, a champion of Darwin's theory, and demanded to know whether it was through his grandmother or grandfather that he claimed to be descended from the apes. Huxley was infuriated by the insolence of the question, and heatedly replied that he would prefer to be descended from an ape than from a cultivated man who prostituted his culture and eloquence to prejudice and falsehood. During the uproar that followed one woman fainted, and Wilberforce's supporters angrily demanded an apology.

In his book *Evidence as to Man's Place in Nature,* Thomas Huxley emphasized that the differences in the foot, hand, and brain between man and higher apes were no greater than those between the higher and lower apes. To Thomas Huxley, by comparison, the old doctrine that each species was an immutable special creation of God seemed "a barren virgin". For his part in the open clash which resulted between science and Church, Huxley became a famous public figure. The controversy over Darwin's seemingly heretic theories of evolution and natural selection raged throughout the late Victorian era – till the overwhelming weight of subsequent findings put his basic premise beyond question.

1863 (F): The world's **first underground railway system** opened in London, by Metropolitan railway. This early underground line ran from Bishops Road to Farrington Street (about six kilometres); the lines were in cuttings beneath the street, roofed over to take the road surface.

The first underground rail service on the European continent began at Budapest where a 2.5 mile electric sub-way went into operation in 1896. The Paris Metro underground rail service began operation in 1900. It was the world's third largest subway.

1863 (G): lvan M. Sechenov (1829-1905), Russian physiologist, published *Reflexes of the Brain,* one of the earliest attempts to establish the physiological basis of psychic processes.

His teaching and research had a decisive influence on the development of physiology in Russia.

1863 (H): The United States Congress approved creation of a **National Academy of Sciences** to advise the U. S. Government in scientific matters, and to promote scientific research.

1863 (I): Ferdinand Reich (1799-1882), German minerologist, discovered a new element called 'indium' while he was spectroscopically examining a yellow precipitate he had obtained from a zinc ore.

1863 (J): Capt. E. Carlsen, German explorer, first circumnavigated **Spitsbergen** group of polar islands at the Arctic region.

1864 JUN. 29: Birth of **Sir Asutosh Mukherjec** (d.1924), eminent Indian jurist, educationist and social reformer.

1864 AUG. : **Red Cross,** national and international body, founded in Geneva for the protection and care of war casualties.

It was inspired by **Jean Henri Dunant** (1828-1910), Swiss humanitarian, who had been deeply moved by the plight of the wounded in the Battle of Solferino, in June 1859, where there were nearly 40,000 casualties. Dunant had been horrified to learn that soldiers were left to die in open battle fields, with no medical attention. In 1862 he published a booklet urging people to set up voluntary societies that would help the sick and wounded in time of war. Dunant's appeal had immediate result. An international conference took place in Geneva, Switzerland, in 1864 and twenty-six governments were represented. The Conference led to the 'Geneva Convention' where the Red Cross Society was founded. The emblem of a Red Cross on a white background was adopted, as well as the motto 'Charity in War'.

1864 OCT. 1: A **cyclone** destroyed most of Calcutta and killed an estimated 70,000.

1864 DEC. 8: When the ternporal power of the papacy was tottering to its fall, **Pope Pius IX** (1792-1878) flung down the gauntlet of defiance to the new social and political order in the encyclical **Quanta Cura,** with the appended syllabus errorum. He condemned modern political doctrines and liberal catholicism in Quanta Cura. The syllabus listing 80 of the 'Principal errors of our times', specially repudiated the notion that the Pope would ever ally himself with progress of modern civilization.

The Pope censured the 'errors' of pantheism, naturalism, indifferentism, socialism, communism, freemasonry and various other 19th century views. He claimed for the Church the control of all cultures and sciences and the whole educational system; denounced the enjoyment of liberty of conscience and worship, and the idea of tolerance; claimed the complete independence of the church from state control; upheld the necessity of a continuance of the temporal power of the Roman See, and declared that "It is an error to believe that the Roman Pontiff can and ought to reconcile himself to, and agree with progress, liberalism, and contemporary civilization."

The ultramontane party was loud in its praise of the syllabus, but the liberals were amazed and treated it as a declaration of war by the Church on modern civilization. The syllabus undermined the liberal catholics' position, for it destroyed their following among the intellectuals and placed their progress irrevocably out of court. It was also a mortal blow aimed at the liberal catholics, who were reconciled to religious liberty and democratic government. [see 1870 Jul. 18]

1864 (A): Towards the end of the year, **Totapuri,** an itinerant monk of the highest Vedantic realization, came to Dakshineswar and initiated **SRI RAMAKRISHNA** into sannyasa and set him on the path of Advaita (non-dualism).

Under his guidance, Ramakrishna attained to *nirvikalpa samadhi,* a state in which the soul realizes its identity with Brahman, the highest Impersonal Truth. Sri Ramakrishna remained completely absorbed in *samadhi* for three days. With breathless wonder Totapuri stood before, this august spectacle. Ramakrishna had attained in a single day what it took Totapuri forty years of strenuous practice to achieve! A monk of the most orthodox type, Totapuri never stayed at a place more than three days, for fear of creating attachment. But he remained at

Dakshineswar for eleven months, and in turn learnt many things from his own disciple. [see 1866 (a)]

1864 (B): Satyendranath Tagore (1842-1923), brother of Rabindranath Tagore (1861-1941), was the first Indian to pass into the **Indian Civil Service.** [see 1869 (b)]

1864 (C): Dr. Clough came to India as a missionary to the Telugus. Like his contemporary Christian missionaries, he looked upon India as a heathen and uncivilized country waiting to be saved by him. His enthusiasm both in evangelization and spreading English education was equally bubbling.

In his book *Social Christianity in the Orient,* he wrote. "At that time (1864), little was known of the Oriental races. Christian people took it for granted that the older religions were wholly bad and their sciptures contained nothing but evil. There was no sympathetic approach, no feeling that perhaps God had not left Himself unrevealed to the heathen world. It distressed many thoughtful men and women in Christian lands at that time to think that unless the heathens heard the Gospel of Jesus Christ and accepted it, they would be eternally lost. This was my opinion, too, when I went to India. It formed my missionary motive. I looked upon the Hindus as simply heathens; I wanted to see them converted. As the years passed I grew tolerant and often told the caste people, if they could not or would not receive Jesus Christ as their Saviour, to serve their own Gods faithfully. During my visits to America I sometimes told American audiences that the Hindus were in some respects better than they."

1864 (D): The First Socialist International (Working Men's Association) founded in London by **Karl Marx** (1818-1883), Prussian born political philosopher and prophet of International revolutionary communism.

The association, later known as the First Communist International, was designated to unite the workmen of all countries in support of Marxian Socialism. But after the anarchists joined the movement in 1869 conflict arose between the Marxist concept of socialism as an authoritarian, centralized movement and the anarchist's dislike of organization and discipline. Mikhail Bakunin (1814-1876), the leading anarchist, was Marx's most vigorous opponent. He believed that instead of a government, a self-controlling system of little societies, undisturbed by outside forces, would form the ideal basis for society. Marx believed in the 'dictatorship of the proletariat', a belief which forms the basis of modern communism. This theory advocated a situation where the proletariat (the industrial working class) makes and controls a new state of its own. Bakunin, however, rejected the idea of the state altogether. He was expelled in 1872, but the International had lost its impetus and was dissolved in 1876. Its failure encouraged the participation of Marxists in national politics, first evident in the growth of the Social Democratic Party in Germany. [see 1889 (o)]

1864 (E) Thomas Alva Edison (1847-1931), American inventor, the most prolific inventor of his times, developed an **automatic Telegraph repeater** which sent messages from one wire to the next. It was the first of the series of his inventions which revolutionized man's way of life.

In his lifetime, Edison had acquired more than 1,300 U. S. and foreign patents on his inventions; most of the patents were for electrical devices and electric light and power. His most original invention was phonograph (1877) and his most significant, the incandescent electric lamp which he perfected in 1879.

Edison developed an electric generating system to make the electric light practicable and constructed the first central power station in 1882. A decade later, he made the first commercial motion pictures and later worked effectively in other fields. His greatest invention was organized research.

It was Edison who said that genius was one per cent inspiration and 99 per cent perspiration. [see 1877 Nov. 29, 1878 (h), 1882 (e), 1883 (d), 1889 (h), 1891 Dec. 29, 1893 (h)]

1864 (F): James Clerk Maxwell (1831-1879), Scottish mathematician and physicist, read out to the Royal Society of London a great paper entitled, *A Dynamic Theory of the Electromagnetic Field,* in which he first fully set out his **electromagnetic theory.**

The paper was later expanded into his classic *Treatise on Electricity and Magnetism* (1873) in which the best exposition on his theory is to be found. His theory was strikingly confirmed by the experiments of Heinrich Hertz (1857-1894), German physicist, some years later, when he demonstrated the production of electromagnetic waves. Maxwell's theory led to advances in science and technology that have transformed the modern world. [see 1873 (f)]

1864-69: Sir John Lawrence (1811-1879), the Viceroy of India.

It is he who declared: "We have not been elected or placed in power by the people, but we are here through our moral superiority, by the force of circumstances, by the will of Providence. This alone constitutes our charter to govern India. In doing the best we can for the people, we are bound by our conscience and not theirs."

In consonance with the "Divide and Rule" policy of the British, Sir John Lawrence once said: "Among the defects of the pre-mutiny army, unquestionably the worst, and the one that operated most fatally against us, was the brotherhood and homogeneity of the Bengal army, and for this purpose the remedy is counterpoise; firstly the great counterpoise of the Europeans, and secondly of the native races."

As far back as 1858 Sayed Ahmed Khan, an Indian Muslim leader, had deplored the fact (and regarded it as a cause of the Mutiny) that the two antagonistic races, Hindus and Muslims, were put into the same regiment of the British army and thus a feeling of friendship and brotherhood sprang up between them. He significantly added: "If separate regiments of Hindus and separate regiments of Mohammedans had been raised this feeling of brotherhood would not have arisen." Later the British took the lesson to heart and carried into practice the suggestion hinted by Sayed Ahmed.

1865 JAN. 28: Birth of **Lala Lajpath Rai** (d. 1928), Indian nationalist, educationist and a great social reformer, popularly known as 'Lion of the Punjab'.

In one of the demonstrations against the Simon Commission in Lahore, he was beaten up by the police with lathis. He died as a result of his injuries. Bhagat Singh (1909-1931), a great Indian patriot, and his comrade shot dead J. P. Saunders, a police official who was alleged to have assaulted the 'Lion of the Punjab'. They had felt that the murder of a great leader at the hands of an ordinary police official was an insult to the nation and that it was their duly to avenge his death.

1865 APR. 14: **Abraham Lincoln** (b.1809), the 16th American President, was **assassinated** while attending a performance at Ford's Theatre in Washington D. C.

Actor John Wilkes Booth who shot the President in the head, cried out: "The South is avenged" and escaped. Mortally wounded, Lincoln died the next day. A vigorous opponent of Negro Slavery, he had led the Northern States in the American Civil War which began on April 12, 1861. [see 1863 Jul. 1-3]

1865 APR. 26: The American Civil War – a conflict that pitted the Northern States of the American union against the Southern States – ended.

The war raged for four years and was marked by some of the fiercest military campaigns of modern history. Large armies were involved in large movements, and the entire population were engaged in supporting the war efforts of both sides. The war had international impact. It had cost the Southern States 260,000 dead and hundreds of millions of Dollars in property damaged, and had left the region with a ravaged economy. For the victorious North, 360,000 men had died, and the nation had been strained to the utmost to preserve the union and eliminate the cancer of slavery. [see 1863. Jul. 1-3]

1865 JUL. 15: Birth of **Lord Northcliff** (d. 1922), the most successful publisher in the history of British press and the creator of popular modern journalism.

1865 DEC. 18: The **13th Amendment** to the U. S. Constitution finally **abolished slavery throughout America.**

The emancipation proclamation had been issued on September 22, 1862, by President Lincoln, and when it took effect on January 1, 1863, nearly 4 million Negro slaves had been freed in U. S. A. The proclamation was instrumented in 1865 through the 13th Amendment. Later on, the U. S. Congress adopted series of laws – the Civil Rights Acts of 1866 and 1875, and the Enforcements Acts of 1870, 1871 - and the 14th and 15th Amendments that were ratified in 1868 and 1870. These laws and amendments gave the Negroes federal and state citizenship, the right to vote, to enforce contracts, to sue, to give evidence, to deal with the real and personal property. They protected the Negroes from violence, assured them accommodation without discrimination in public places and guaranteed them due process of law and equal protection of laws.

1865 DEC. 24: The **Ku Klux Klan,** one of the most notorious secret societies of modern times, was organized at Pulaski, Tenesse, after the American Civil War, in protest against the emancipation of Negroes in order to prevent their voting.

The members of this secret society, enraged at seeing former slaves in position of power while they themselves were forbidden to hold public office under Reconstruction, resorted to terror and violence to subdue the newly enfranchised Negroes and keep them from polls.

1865 DEC. 30: Birth of **Rudyard Kipling** (d. 1936), British poet and one of the first masters of the short story in English.

In 1907, he became the first English writer to receive the Nobel Prize for literature. [See. 1894 (f)].

1865 (A): **William Booth** (1829-1912), British evangelist, brought into existence **'Salvation Army'** in London.

His zeal for outdoor evangelism took him out of ordinary denominational work and into independent evangelism in London. It was this that led him to his founding the Army, with himself as 'General'. His organization, modelled along the lines of the army, was devoted to bringing people to salvation. He believed that unconverted people would be eternally damned. Writing to his son 'General' Booth said:

"The social work is like a bait, but it is salvation that is the hook that lands the fish."

William Booth began his evangelic ministry in the East End of London in 1865, and formed the East London Revival Society which later became the Christian Mission. In 1878 he changed the name of his organization to the 'Salvation Army'. As its 'General', William Booth served the Salvation Army until his death. Despite many setbacks, the Salvation Army grew into an international organization.

1865 (B): Natural laws of heredity were elucidated in a paper read to the Brunn Society for the Study of Natural Science by **Gregor Johann Mendel** (1822-1884), Austrian Augustinian monk and botanist, who had studied the genetics of garden peas over a period of a decade.

Subsequently, Mendel published his paper entitled *Experiments with Plant Hybrids,* in the journal of the Brunn Natural Science Society. In his paper, Mendel summarized the results of his extensive programme of hybridizing experiments started in 1854. Established scientists did not begin to appreciate Mendel's work until the turn of the century. In 1900 it was rediscovered independently by three other scientists (viz. Correns of Germany, De Vries of Holland and Tschermak of Austria) when his theory was generalized as Mendel's Laws of Heredity.That date also marked, the beginning of the science of heredity, which in 1906 was named 'genetics' by William Bateson. [see 1900 (c)]

1865 (C): Joseph Lister (1827-1912), English surgeon, initiated **antiseptic surgery** by using carbolic acid (phenol). He revolutionized modern surgery when he performed the first surgical operation (1867) under antiseptic conditions on his sister, Isabella, at Glasgow's Royal Infirmary.

He made the first experiment upon a compound fracture applying carbolic mist created by a sprayer specially developed by him. The value of carbolic acid as an antiseptic in treating compound fractures was discovered by Lister at Glasgow after he read a paper on germ theory of disease, published in 1861 by Louis Pasteur (1822-1895). The paper contained Pasteur's findings in France. According to Pasteur's research, diseases were caused by micro-organisms. On learning this it occured to Lister to kill germs in surgical wounds by chemical treatment. This discovery of antiseptic technique represented the beginning of modern surgery. [see 1877 Oct.]

1865 (D): William A. Bullock (1813-1867), American inventor, devised **the first web press,** which printed from a continuous roll, or web of paper. It was the first to print on both sides of paper simultaneously and to cut and fold. His machine delivered 10,000 impressions an hour.

In 1871, another U. S. inventor and manufacturer, Richard March Hoe (1812-1886) who had earlier perfected and patented the Hoe rotary press, improved on Bullocks's invention with a high speed web press that could produce 18,000 papers an hour. It was this machine – plus an 1881 Hoe company invention, a triangular folder, which creased the paper as they came off the press – that made the newspaper a true mass-communication medium. The modern rotary press, which has evolved from this revolutionary innovation, makes more than 50,000 impressions per hour.

1865 (E): The first Women's Suffrage Committee was formed at Manchester, England, with a view to secure women their **right to vote.**

After a long, sustained struggle, in 1918, married women over 30 achieved right to vote, and in 1928 the age of women electors was lowered to 21, to place the women voters on an equality with male voters.

In America, a National Women's Suffrage Association was organized at New York in 1869. Representatives of 19 States were present and its objectives declared by resolution to be to secure the ballot for women by a 16th Amendment to the Federal Constitution. In 1918 they acquired equal suffrage with men in 15 States, offering the only instance in the world where the voters themselves gave the franchise to women. The World War – I accelerated progress leading to 19th Amendment (1920) making denial of women's right to vote unconstitutional.

In 1893 women's suffrage was adopted in New Zealand which became the first country in the world to give women the right to vote.

1865 (F): **Thaddeus Lowe** (1832-1913), U. S. inventor, developed a **compression ice machine.**

As early as in 1834, an American Engineer living in London had patented a practical ice-making machine, a volatile-liquid refrigerator using a compressor that operated in a closed cycle and conserved the fluid for reuse. In 1844, a U. S. physician, John Gorrie, had successfully developed a **refrigerator machine.** His machine consisted of a compressor that compressed air, which was then cooled by circulating water. In 1856, another American, Alexander C. Twinning, had produced first commercial ice by means of a vapour compression machine. Another type of machine was developed by Ferdinand Carre in France, between 1850 and 1859. Methyl refrigerator and an ammonia refrigerator were developed by a German Engineer, Carl Linde (1842-1934) in 1874 and 1876 respectively. The basic principles on which refrigeration machine operates were thus developed by 19th century inventors. Subsequent inventions involved only modifications and improvements in the machines and processes. [see 1895 (b)]

1865 (G): *Alice's Adventures in Wonderland,* by **Lewis Caroll,** and its sequel, *Through the Looking Glass* (1871) were the most famous children's books written in English.

The former was made into an animated film by Walt Disney in 1951, and has been the subject of numerous plays.

1866 JAN. 29: Birth of **Romain Rolland** (d. 1944), French man of letters and Nobel Laureate, who produced many critical and historical works, reflecting the conscience of a great humanist.

In 1930, he was attracted to Ramakrishna-Vivekananda whom he called the "Prophets of New India". He wrote biographies of them in French, the English translations of which are even today highly popular.

1866 APR. 10: A secret meeting was held in the Royal Asiatic Society, London, when a conspiracy was hatched to induct the **theory of Aryan invasion of India,** so that no Indian may say that the English are foreigners. "India was ruled all along by outsiders and so the country must remain a slave under the Christian benign rule." (The British wanted to justify their rule in India. To that end they tried to show all people here as outsiders.)

"A clever clergyman Edward Thomas spelled the theory with Lord Strangford in the chair. Slowly and slowly it was suggested that the so-called aborigines, Dravidians, Aryans, Hunas, Sakas, Rajaputas and the Muslims came at different epochs and ruled the country. Thus it was suggested that the country had been ruled by the foreign invaders and so there is nothing wrong if the Britishers are ruling the country. And, therefore, Indians had no right to demand independence." (Dr. D. S. Triveda, Professor, Prakrit Research Institute, Vaisali, Bihar).

Swami Vivekananda was the first to challenge the theory of Aryan invasion of India. He said: "That is all nonsense."

"In what Veda, in what *sukta,* do you find that the Aryans came into India from a foreign country? Where do you get the idea that they slaughtered the wild aborigines? What do you gain by talking such nonsense? Vain has been your study of the *Ramayana*; why manufacture a big fine story out of it?"

"Well, what is the *Ramayana*? The conquest of the savage aborigines of Southern India by the Aryans! Indeed! Ramachandra is a civilized Aryan King, and with whom is he fighting? With King Ravana of Lanka. Just read the *Ramayana*, and you will find that Ravana was rather more and not less civilized than Ramachandra. The civilization of Lanka was rather higher and surely not lower, than that of Ayodhya."

"And then, when were these *vanaras* (monkeys) and other southern Indians conquered? They were all, on the other hand Ramachandra's friends and allies. Say which kingdom of Vali and Guhaka were annexed by Ramachandra?...."

"And may I ask you, Europeans, what country you have ever raised to better conditions? Wherever you have found weaker races, you have exterminated them by the roots, at it were. You have settled on their lands and they are gone forever. What is the history of your America, your Australia, and New Zealand, your Pacific Islands and South Africa? Where are those aboriginal races today? They are all exterminated, you have killed them outright, as if they were wild beasts. It is only where you have not the power to do so, and there only, that other nations are still alive."

"The object of the peoples of Europe is to exterminate all in order to live themselves. The aim of the Aryans is to raise all up to their own level, nay, even to a higher level than themselves. The means of European civilization is the sword; of the Aryans, the division into different *varnas*. This system of division into different *varnas* is the stepping stone to civilization, making one rise higher and higher in proportion to one's learning and culture. In Europe, it is everywhere victory to the strong, and death to the weak. In the land of Bharatha, every social rule is for the protection of the weak."

1866 MAY 9: Birth of **Gopalakrishna Gokhale** (d.1915), Indian nationalist leader, humanitarian and social reformer.

In 1905 he founded the famed 'Servants of India Society' dedicated to advancement of the nation's welfare and to the "spiritualization" of politics.

1866 JUL. 27: The first successful trans-Atlantic Cable, between Newfoundland (United States) and Ireland (Britain) was finally completed, thereby enabling transmission of telegraphic signals across the Atlantic.

Two previous attempts to link North America and Europe by a submarine telegraphic cable, had failed because of weather conditions and cable construction. Cyrus W. Field (1819-1892) an American businessman, was the guiding genius whose persisting faith in its possibility made it a success in spite of great adversity.

1866 SEP. 21: Birth of **H. G. Wells** (d. 1946), English novelist, journalist, sociologist, and popular historian.

He exerted a powerful influence in the early 20th century movement toward change in society, morals and religious beliefs.

1866 NOV. 11: Keshab Chandra Sen (1838-1884), and his followers who desired more rapid social reform, seceded from the 'Brahma Samaj' led by

Maharshi Devendranath Tagore (1817-1905) and formed a new organization called **"The Brahmo Samaj of India,"** which addressed itself to various social and spiritual reforms.

Keshab brought to the Brahma Samaj a dynamic force which it never possessed before. He made Brahmaism a real force all over Bengal and was the first to inaugurate an All-India movement of religious and social reforms.

The first Samaj, henceforth known as the 'Adi Brahmo Samaj' was founded in 1828 by Raja Rammohan Roy (1774-1833), the great Indian social and religious reformer, who believed in a formless God and deprecated the worship of idols. The Samaj gathered strength in the hands of Devendranath Tagore from 1839 onwards, and Keshab joined it in 1857.

The Brahma Samaj effectively helped the progress of Hindu society, first by stemming the tide of conversion to Christianity; secondly by holding a living example of society based on progressive and liberal views; and thirdly, by supplying eminent persons who advanced liberal ideas in other spheres of life such as politics.

1866 (A): SRI RAMAKRISHNA remained in the Advaita plane for six months.

Earlier he had been initiated into Advaita (non-dualism) by Totapuri who left Dakshineswar after a sojourn. Since then Ramakrishna remained always in a state of absolute identity with Brahman, far above all subjective and objective experiences. Looking back at this period of his life in his later days Sri Ramakrishna said: "I remained for six months in the state of perfect union which people seldom reach, and if they reach it, they cannot return to their individual consciousness again. Their bodies and minds could not bear it. But this (my body) is made up of *sattva* particles (pure elements) and can bear much stress. In those days I was quite unconscious of the outer world. My body would have died for want of nourishment, but for a sadhu who came at that time to Dakshineswar and stayed there for my sake. He recognized my state of *samadhi* and took much trouble to preserve this body, while I was unconscious of its very existence".

This *Advaita siddhi* was the culmination of Ramakrishna's spiritual sadhana. The disciplines that he practised after this were more for proving to himself and to the world through actual experience that all religious paths lead to one God. [see 1864 (a)]

1866 (B): Towards the end of the year, **SRI RAMAKRISHNA** practised the discipline of **Islam**.

With *Advaita sadhana,* he had already reached the acme of spiritual endeavour. But his desire to go through as many different courses of *sadhana* as possible led him to practise Islam. He got initiated by a Sufi mystic who was at that time living in the premises of the Dakshineswar temple. With characteristic single mindedness and sincerity he plunged into that *sadhana.* He described his own attitude in those days: "Then I used to repeat the name of Allah, wear my cloth in the fashion of the Mohammedans and recite the Namaz regularly. All Hindu ideas having been wholly banished from my mind, not only did I not salute the Hindu gods, but also I had no inclination even to visit them. After three days I realized the goal of that form of devotion." The path that he followed under the guidance of the Sufi mystic led him in no time to the same God, though the name and language were different. [see 1874 Nov.]

1866 (C): In a prospectus issued with a view to the establishment of a 'Society for the Promotion of National Feeling Among the Educated Natives of Bengal', Rajnarain Bose wrote:-

"Now that European ideas have penetrated Bengal, the Bengaleĕ mind has been moved from the sleep of ages. A restless fermentation is going on in Bengalee Society. A desire for change and progress is everywhere visible. People discontented with old customs and institutions are panting for reform. Already a band of young men have expressed a desire to sever themselves at once from Hindu society and to renounce even the Hindu name. It is to be feared that the tide of revolution may sweep away whatever good we have inherited from our ancestors. To prevent this catastrophe and to give a national shape to reforms it is proposed that a Society be established by the influential members of native society for the promotion of national feeling among the educated natives of Bengal. Without due cultivation of national feeling no nation can be eventually great. This is a fact testified to by all history." [see 1871 (b)]

1866 (D): A **cholera epidemic** took a toll of 120,000 lives in Prussia and 110,000 in Austria. Cholera killed some 50,000 Americans with 2,000 of the fatalities occurring at New York which created the first U. S. Municipal Board of Health.

1866 (E): In order to harness the power of nitroglycerine discovered by an Italian chemist Ascanio Sobrero (1812-1888) in 1847, **Alfred Nobel** (1833-1896), Swedish Chemist and engineer, experimented with the nitroglycerine/diatomaceous combination and invented **'dynamite'**, a safe blasting powder. The sticks of dynamite replaced the dangerous nitroglycerine as a blasting compound.

The new invention was vigorously exploited and a worldwide industry established. Nobel further experimented and developed a more powerful form of dynamite, blasting gelatine, in 1875, and in 1887 he produced ballistite, a smokeless, slow-burning projectile propellant. This was Nobel's last major invention. He made a fortune from dynamite and other explosives, with which he established five annual awards known as 'Nobel Prizes'. [see 1888 (g), 1896 Dec. 10, 1901 (g)]

1866 (F): *War and Peace,* a masterpiece of the Russian novelist and moral philosopher, **Leo Tolstoy** (1828-1910), was published in its first instalment. Tolstoy completed his long novel about the 1812 Napoleonic invasion in three years. [see 1882 (g), 1894 (e)]

In the same year, another Russian novelist, **Fedor Dostoevski** (1821-1881), and the French author **Victor Hugo** (1802-1885) brought out their works – *Crime and Punishment,* and *Toilers of the Sea,* respectively.

1866 (G): **Robert Whitehead** (1823-1905), British Engineer, developed the **underwater torpedo,** the first guided missile.

The weapon's effectiveness was demonstrated by the Japanese during their attack on the Russian Fleet of Port Arthur in 1904.

1866 (H): The **clinical thermometer** was invented by English physician **Thomas Clifford Albert.**

1866-67: **Orissa famine;** one million dead.

The famine affected different parts of the east coast from Calcutta to Madras. But its effects were most dreadful in Orissa. Referring to the "extreme severity" of the Orissa famine, Sir George Campbell (who led the enquiry commission regarding the Orissa famine) remarked: "We were shocked by the human remains we saw all around.... it was, I think, by far the most acute famine experienced in any part of India in the present (19th) century."

The causes of the Orissa famine were "the failure of the later rains of 1865, and consequently of the autumn crops of the last year, together with the almost entire absence of importation of food from outside". Proper steps were not taken by the Government to avert its devastating effects. (Bharatiya Vidya Bhavan's *History and Culture of Indian People,* Vol. IX Part I, p. 829 and 830).

In Bengal 1,50,000 people died (May-Nov.) during the course of this famine.

During the period of 50 years from 1860 to 1909 India experienced 20 famines and scarcities, an average of one famine and scarcity every two and half years. There is no greater proof needed of the conditions of extreme poverty and want under which the people of India, especially the agricultural classes lived, than the figures of mortality caused by these famines. [see 1868-69, 1873 (b), 1874 (a), 1876-78, 1877 Jan.1, 1878 (b), 1896-97, 1897 Jan. 13, 1897 May 16, 1899-1900]

Terrible famines began for the first time with the British rule in India. In 1770 there was a terrible famine in the district of Purnea, in Bengal, in which above one-third of the population died of starvation; but the revenue from land-tax was exacted with such tyranny and oppression that even during that famine it was larger than in previous years. On the 9th of May, 1770, the Calcutta Council wrote to the Court of Directors: "The famine which has ensued, the mortality, the beggary, exceed all description. Above one-third of the inhabitants have perished in the once plentiful province of Purnea, and in other parts the misery is equal." On the 12th of February, 1771, they wrote: "Notwithstanding the great severity of the late famine, and the great reduction of the people thereby, some increase has been made in the settlements (of taxes) both of the Bengal and Bihar Provinces for the present year." Mr. Dutt says in his *Economic History of India*: "Famines in India are directly due to a deficiency in the annual rain-falls; but the intensity of such famines and the loss of lives caused by them are largely due to the chronic poverty of the people. If the people were generally in a prosperous condition, they could make up for local failure of crops by purchases from neighbouring provinces, and there would be no loss of life. But when the people are absolutely resourceless, they cannot buy from surrounding tracts, and they perish in hundreds of thousands, or in millions, whenever there is a local failure of crops." *(Complete Works of Swami Abhedananda,* Vol. II, p. 78, 79 & 80)

1867 FEB. 26: In a letter to Dr. Milan, the Dean of St. Paul's **Max Muller** (1823-1900), the Orientalist and philologist, wrote that India was ripe for Christianity.

"I have myself the strongest belief in the growth of Christianity in India", he stated, "There is no other country so ripe for Christianity as India, and yet the diffculties seem enormous" *(The Life and Letters of Max Muller,* edited by his wife Georgina Max Muller, Vol. I, p. 350).

A decade earlier (on 20 Aug. 1856) Max Muller had written to Bunsen from Oxford: "India is much riper for Christianity than Rome or Greece were at the time of St. Paul.... I should like to live for ten years quite quietly and learn the language, try to make friends and then see whether I was fit to take part in a work, by means of which the old mischief of Indian priestcraft could be overthrown and the way opened for the entrance of simple Christian teaching." [see 1868 Dec. 16]

In connection with the "mischief of Indian priestcraft" Upendranath Mukhopadhyaya in his *Life of Raja Rammohan Roy* in Bengali has observed as follows:

"Among the Hindus of the time the brahmins were all in all. In fact, Hindu society regarded and worshipped the brahmins as very gods. People thought that their path to heaven would be free if they could appease the brahmins. One regarded with disfavour by the brahmin was ostracized and had to lead a life of abject misery. No one would accept water from his hands and even the services of the barber would be denied to him. It did not matter whether one had those virtues that alone would entitle one to be called a brahmin, or whether one had the faith and the force of character befitting a brahmin. To command consideration, respect, and even reverence of all people, what was necessary was just to bear the sacred thread. 'He who knows brahman is a true brahmin' is a saying which the brahmin of the time had completely forgotten. They had nothing to do with religion or morality. It is the duty of the brahmin to instruct the people in morals and religion, but they had forgotten and forsaken all these for their mess of pottage. They were content with the gold and silver which they earned by offering the dust of their feet to the shudras.

"The shudras were excluded from the study not only of the Vedas but of all scriptures. The brahmins took every opportunity to impress and enjoin on the shudras that they would be thrown into hell if they dared touch the Vedas and the shudras with bowed head obeyed the injunction and acted accordingly."

1867 MAR. 31: 'Prarthana Samaj', a religious body similar to 'Brahma Samaj' was founded in Bombay, under the influence of **Keshab Chandra Sen** (1838-1884), the celebrated Brahmo leader, who paid a visit to Bombay in 1864.

The main planks of the Prarthana Samaj, led by **Dr. Atmaram Pandurang** (1823-1898), were theistic worship and social reform. The members of the Samaj considered themselves, unlike the earlier Brahmas, as Hindus. They were devoted theists and adhered to the great religious tradition of the Maharashtra saints.

1867 AUG. 25: Death of **Michael Faraday** (b. 1791), English physicist and Chemist, who was one of the greatest experimentalists of all time.

Convinced of the interrelation of electricity and magnetism, he discovered the phenomenon of electromagnetic induction – the production of electric current by a change in magnetic intensity. He also discovered the principle of the electric motor and built a primitive model of one. He produced the first dynamo and was the first to liquefy chlorine. He stated the basic laws of electrolysis and studied dielectrics.

1867 OCT. 28: Birth of **Sister Nivedita** (d. 1911) alias Margaret Elizabeth Noble, an Irish teacher, who became the disciple of Swami Vivekananda.

Since childhood Christian religious doctrines were instilled into her. But search for 'Truth' led her in 1895-96 to Swami Vivekananda's teachings of the Vedanta. She came to India and dedicated her life for the cause of Hinduism and India.

1867 NOV. 7: Birth of **Marie Curie** (d. 1934), Polish-French physicist, who pioneered radioactive research by her part in the discovery of Radium and Polonium, and in determination of their chemical properties. [see 1898 (a)]

1867 DEC. 9: In a letter to his wife, **Max Muller** (1823-1900) whose life-work was translating of the *Rig Veda,* revealed the motive behind his venture:

"I hope I shall finish that work, and I feel convinced though I shall not live to see it, that this edition of mine and the translation of the Veda will hereafter tell a great extent on the fate of India and on the growth of millions of souls in that country. It is the root of their religion, and to show them what that root is, is I feel the only way of uprooting all that has sprung from it during the last 3000 years." *(The Life and Letters of Max Muller,* Vol. I, p. 346). [see, 1874 Nov. (a), 1874 Dec., 1875 Dec. 13]

1867 (A): **Nabagopal Mitra,** editor of the *National Paper* (founded by Devendranath Tagore in 1865) started in Calcutta an institution known as **"Hindu Mela"** to promote the national feelings, sense of patriotism, and a spirit of self-help among the Hindus.

It was an annual public gathering on the last day of the Bengali year. The special features of the annual gathering were patriotic songs, poems and lectures, a detailed review of the political, social, economic, and religious condition of India, an exhibition of indigenous arts and crafts, and performance of different forms of physical exercises and feats of physical strength. It had an all-India outlook and specimens of arts and crafts were collected from Banaras, Kashmir, Jaipur, Lucknow, and Patna. Rewards were also offered for good books written in Bengali and Sanskrit, which were calculated to promote the welfare of the country. Thus intellectual development through fine arts and literature, and economic progress by means of industrial development formed the main planks of the Hindu Mela. It met altogether fourteen times from 1867 to 1880.

1867 (B): The first-ever English translation of the *Bhagavad Gita* (London Edition of 1784), one of the most popular texts among the world's scriptures, was reprinted in New York, for the first time, reflecting the growing American awareness of and the interest in Hindu religion and philosophy.

The tremendous general appeal of the *Bhagavad Gita* was voiced forth in prophetic words by Warren Hastings, the first British Governor-General of India (1773-85) – a personality one would least expect to deal with such a subject. In his introduction to the translation by Charles Wilkin, Hastings remarked that "Works as the *Gita* would live long after the British domination in India has ceased to exist," and that it contains passages "elevated to a track of sublimity into which our habit of judgement will find it difficult to pursue."

1867 (C): **Karl Marx** (1818-1883), Prussian-born political philosopher and prophet of international revolutionary Communism, published the first volume of his most impotant work, *Das Kapital,* the second and third volumes (1885, 1894) of which were edited by Friedrich Engels (1820-1895) after his death

This well-known book, described as the "Communist Bible", gives an elaborate analysis of economic and social history and at the same time the basic exposition of what is known as "scientific" socialism.

Das Kapital was written in London where Karl Marx lived for a period and studied economics and history in the Reading Room of the British Museum, and developed his theories of class struggle and inevitable revolution, coloured by his observation of the mid-19th century industrial England.

Earlier, on the eve of the February Revolution in Paris (1848), Marx had written with Engels, the *Communist Manifesto,* a masterpiece of political propaganda. It advocated the expropriation of landed property, a high, graded income tax, abolition of the right of inheritance, the establishment of a State Bank to centralize credit, nationalisation of transport, increasing State ownership of factories, State education, the ending of children's factory labour and the duty of all to work. *The Communist Manifesto* attacked the State as an instrument of oppression, and religion and culture as capitalist ideologies in a system whose competition would lead to over-population and downfall. It summoned the working classes of Europe to rebel against their capitalist masters. Its argument is clearly stated, neatly summed up in the sentence: "The history of all hitherto existing society is the history of class struggle". "Workers of the world unite! You have nothing to lose but your chains!" became the revolutionary slogan.

1867 (D): **Christopher Latham Sholes** (1818-1890), American journalist, invented the **first practical typewriter.**

In 1868, the first commercially feasible typewriting machine was patented by Sholes, and two associates, Samuel W. Soule and Carlos G. Glidden.

An improved model of Shole's machine was manufactured by Remington and Sons, Gunsmiths of Illinois, New York, and first marketed in 1874. It featured the present-day arrangement of keys but printed only in capital letters. The typed line was not visible to the typist, and the carriage return was operated by a foot-pedal.

Thomas Alva Edison (1847-1931), American inventor, was granted the first patent for an electric typewriter in 1872. The machine proved impractical, and nearly half a century passed before modern electric typewriter was developed in 1920s. From the late 19th century the typewriter revolutionized office procedure throughout U. S. A.

1867 (E): **Lord Kelvin** (William Thomson) (1824-1907), Scottish engineer, mathematician, and physicist who profoundly influenced the scientific thought of his generation, invented a **receiver for the submarine telegraph**.

He superintended the successful laying of the first submarine cable across the Atlantic [see 1866 Jul. 27] studied, the capacity of the cable to carry an electric signal, and invented improvements in cables and galvanometers, without which the Atlantic cable would have been useless. Thomson's contributions include a major role in the development of the law of conservation of energy, the absolute temperature scale, the dynamical theory of heat; the mathematical analysis of electricity, and magnetism, including basic ideas for the electromagnetic theory of light; the geographical determination of the Earth's age; and fundamental work in hydrodynamics.

1867 (F): **Joseph Monier** (1823-1906), French gardener, discovered **reinforced concrete.**

He made garden pots and tubs of concrete reinforced with iron mesh and obtained his first patent on July 16, 1867. He exhibited his invention the same year at the Paris Exposition. It soon occurred to him to extend its application to railway sleepers, to pipes, and to floors, arches, and bridges. In Monier's patented design the basic principle of reinforced concrete structural members was clearly established.

The practical development of reinforced concrete was initiated in 1880s primarily by G. A. Wayss of Berlin, Francois Hennebique of France and Johan Bauschinger of Austria. In the 1890's the reinforced concrete was utilized for pipes, aquaducts, bridges and tunnels. Later it was also employed extensively in building construction. Design methods based on scientific principles of engineering mechanics were developed shortly after 1900.

Since that time vast improvements in reinforced concrete design and construction practice have resulted from research and experience.

1867 (G): An **International Exhibition** was held at **Paris.**

The site of the exhibition covered 41 acres; about 7 million people visited the exhibition to view 43,217 exhibits costing £ 800,000. One of the ominous exhibits was the new 50 ton steel cannon made by Krupps of Prussia. [see 1878 (d), 1900 Aug.-Oct.]

1867 (H): **Thomas Bernardo** (1845-1905), British philanthropist, opened the first of his famous Children's Homes ('Bernardo Homes') at Stepney, London, to shelter destitute children.

1867 (I): **Diamonds** were discovered in **South Africa** near the junction of the Orang and Vaal rivers and were rapidly exploited.

1867 (J): The **sulphite process** for producing wood pulp for paper making was devised by U. S. inventor **Benjamin Chew Tilghman.**

1867 (K): Sri **Vishnu Bhava Brahmachari** (1825-1871), the 'Indian Marx' brought out his Marathi publication: *Sukhadayak Rajyakarani Nibandh* (a treatise on welfare oriented Government) containing modern revolutionary and basic ideas in the political, social and economic spheres. (Its English edition appeared in 1870 in three volumes; Hindi and Gujarathi editions followed later on.)

Vishnu Bhava's book, the advent of which coincided with that of the *'Das Kapital'* by Karl Marx, was widely discussed in the Press the world over; it became a point of discussion in many countries. Though Vishnu Bhava and Marx did not meet one another, their ideologies were evidently identical. The only difference was that Vishnu Bhava did not despise religion as opiate, perhaps because he, unlike Marx, had the opportunity to be in touch with all-embracing religious life, pointing to the path of perfection. *(Aarti Alok Ki,* by Hari Vinayak Dattye, pp. 254 & 255.)

1868 MAR. 16: Birth of **Maxim Gorky** (d. 1936), Russian novelist and story writer.

1868 MAR. 28: Birth of **Robert A. Millikan** (d. 1953), American physicist, who helped bring about the 20th century revolution in physics.

In 1911 Millikan measured the charge of the electron, and later proved the validity of Albert Einstein's photoelectric effect equation, and carried out pioneering cosmic-ray experiments. A firm believer in the ultimate reconciliation of religion and science, he held that the existence of cosmic-rays offered evidence that "the Creator is still on the job".

1868 JUL. 15: Death of **William T. G. Morton** (b.1819) American Surgeon, who first demonstrated publicly the use of ether to produce insensibility to pain during surgical operations (Oct. 16, 1846).

Before that time there had been, from the beginning of history a search for means of relieving pain. On March 30, 1842, Crawford W. Long (1815-1878) used ether to produce surgical anesthesia, but did not publicize his discovery. Horace Wells, in Dec. 1844, had Nitrous Oxide administered to himself for extraction of a tooth. A public demonstration by him of its use for a surgical operation ended in a fiasco. Later demonstrations proved successful. In 1847, Sir James Simpson (1811-1870) discovered the anesthetic properties of chloroform and was the first to use anesthesia in childbirth and this met with considerable criticism from ardent souls who believed that the pain of childbirth was decreed by God as a part of the curse of Eve. Simpson pointed out that God did not rejoice in pain and that when he extracted a rib from Adam to make Eve, he, first caused a 'deep sleep" to fall upon him. Simpson's victory was clear when he was appointed Queen Victoria's official physician. Many people were against the use of chloroform, but Queen Victoria, who bore nine children, had no patience with them; 'That blessed chloroform!' she gratefully called it.

1868 DEC. 16: In a letter to the Duke of Argyl, soon after his appointment as Secretary of State for India, **Max Muller** (1823-1900) pleaded that the second conquest of India should be through Western type of education, and that the ancient religion of India – Hinduism – was doomed:

"India has been conquered once, but India must be conquered again, and that second conquest should be a conquest by education.... As for religion, that will take care of itself. The missionaries have done far more than they themselves seem to be aware, nay much of the work which is theirs they would probably disclaim. The Christianity of our nineteenth century will hardly be the Christianity of India. But the ancient religion of India is doomed – and if Christianity does not step in, whose fault will it be?" (*The Life and Letters of Max Muller,* Vol. I, p. 377). [see 1867 Feb. 26]

1868 (A): According to the *Holy Bible* printed this year, it was in 4004 B. C. that the world was created for the first time by God.

"But the History of the world presents a different picture. Egypt, Mesopotamia, Syria and China were highly civilized at that time. The Vedic India preceded all these civilisations. At least fifteen thousand years before the Biblical God thought of creating the world Vedanta Philosophy was in its perfection." *(Bible In the Light of Vedanta* – by Swami Chidbhavananda).

1868 (B). **John Wesley Hyatt** (1837-1920), American printer, developed **Celluloid, the first successful plastic,** in an attempt to win a $10,000 prize for creating a substitute for ivory in billiard balls,

A similar composition developed in the 1850s by Alexander Parker (1813-1890), English Chemist, had lacked durability. Hyatt, a self-trained chemist, combined nitrocellulose, camphor, and alchohol to form a mixture that he moulded under heat in a hydraulic press. At first used to make solid objects, celluloid found its principal use 20 years later in the photographic film invented by George Eastman (1854-1932).

1868 (C): **George Westinghouse** (1846-1914), American engineer, inventor and manufacturer, developed the **air-brake,** first used on passenger trains this year.

He patented his first air-brake invention in 1869 and organized the Westinghouse Air Brake Company. This device, which was soon adopted, greatly increased the safe speed of trains, as it enabled the driver to apply simultaneously the individual brakes on all coaches and wagons. A number of patented improvements followed, including the truly revolutionary automatic air-brake for trains (1872). With the additional automatic features incorporated into its design, the air-brake became widely accepted. Westinghouse also worked to make all air-brake apparatus standardized and inter-changeable and later developed a complete signal system for railroads.

1868 (D): **Tungsten Steel** was invented by English metallurgist, **Robert Forester Mushet,** whose alloy was much harder than ordinary steel.

Manganese steel was invented by English metallurgist Robert Abbot Hadfield in 1882. Nickel Steel was invented in France in 1888.

1868 (E): **Sir William Huggins** (1824-1910), English astronomer, calculated the **radial velocity of a star** for the first time.

He pioneered in applying the techniques of spectrum analysis; or spectroscopy to the study of the stars; with it he revolutionized the observation of celestial bodies.

1868 (F): **Badminton** was invented at England's Badminton Hall, Gloucestershire residence of the Duke of Beaufort Henry Charles Fitzroy Somerset, 44, whose late father promoted the Badminton Hunt. The new race-quest game was played with a feathered shuttle-cock which was batted back and forth across a net.

1868 (G): *Chamber's Encyclopedia* was published In 10 volumes.

1868 (H): The first recorded **bicycle race** was held at Paris over a 2-kilometre course at the Parc de St. Cloud.

1868 (I): Railway opened from Ambala (Punjab) to Delhi

1868-69: Failure of rains caused an **intense famine** in Rajputana and also affected parts of the North-western provinces and Punjab. 1.5 million people died. The Government took some steps to relieve distress of the sufferers. [see 1866-67, 1873 (b), 1874 (a), 1876-78, 1877 Jan. 1, 1878 (b), 1896-97, 1897 Jan. 13, 1897 May 16, 1899-1900]

1869 JAN. 12: Birth of **Bhagvan Das** (d. 1958), Indian nationalist, educationist and philosopher, and the founder-member of Central Hindu College and Benaras Hindu University and Kashi Vidyapith.

1869 MAY. 10: America's **first transcontinental railroad** (2,957 km.) came into being, at Promontory Point, Utah, when a gold spike was driven joining the Union Pacific Railroad with the Central Pacific Railroad.

1869 OCT. 2: Birth of **M. K. Gandhi** (d. 1948), apostle of non-violence, and Indian nationalist leader, whose distinguished leadership won for India liberation from British domination.

1869 NOV. 17: Suez Canal (103 miles long, more than 196 feet wide at its narrowest point, and 38 feet deep) officially opened.

It provided the shortest sea-route from Europe to East. Built by a French engineer, Ferdinand de Lesseps (1805-1894), the canal cost £ 20 million. Economically the canal was important in stimulating the export of bulk cargoes of foodstuffs and raw materials from Asia and Australia to Europe, and the export of manufactured goods from Europe. The canal was, thus, the key to trade with the East, by-passing the lengthy route round the Cape. It brought oriental ports 5,000 miles closer to Europe, 3,600 miles closer to America.

1869 NOV. 17 (A): Swami Dayananda Saraswati (1824-1883), a vital force in the Indian renaissance movement, engaged himself in a mighty disputation with the leaders of the Hindu theology and orthodoxy at Benaras, in the presence of several thousand people, on whether or not the Vedas advocated idolatry. [see 1874 June 12]

1869 DEC. : The Government of India sanctioned the establishment of the **Lahore University College,**

The specific objects of this college were "to promote the diffusion of European Science, as far as possible, through the medium of vernacular languages of Punjab, and the improvement and extension of vernacular literature generally", and to "afford encouragement to the enlightened study of Eastern Classical languages and literature." It was at the same time declared that "every encouragement would be afforded to the study of the English language and literature; and in all subjects which cannot be completely taught in the vernacular, the English language would be regarded as the medium of instruction and examination." A large number of institutions were affiliated to the Lahore University College and its activities expanded for a decade before another demand for a University in the Punjab was put forth by the "British Indian Association" of the North-Western provinces.

1869 (A): Keshab Chandra Sen (1838-1884), the celebrated Brahmo leader, tried to win over **Swami Dayananda Saraswati** (1824-1883), the founder of Arya Samaj, when the latter stayed in Calcutta. But the Swami did not agree to give up the infallibility of the Vedas and the belief in the transmigration of souls.

The founders of the Theosophical Society, **Madame Blavatsky** and **Colonel Olcott,** in order to woo Dayananda, went to the extent of recognizing that their own society was a branch of Arya Samaj. For some years, certificates of fellowship were issued jointly. But at last Swamiji dropped the society and condemned it.

1869 (B): Surendranath Banerjee (1848-1925), a major figure in early Indian nationalism, became the second Indian to succeed in the **Indian Civil Service** competitive examination. [see 1864 (b)]

1869 (C): Dmitri Ivanovich Mendeleev (1834-1907), Russian Chemistry professor, brought out (at St. Petersburg) his renowned text-book of Chemistry entitled, *The Principles of Chemistry,* containing the periodic table of chemical elements, which arranged the 63 known elements in the order of increasing atomic weight (valency), noted the periodic recurrence of similar properties in groups of elements, and successfully predicted the properties of elements yet to be discovered.

In his text book of Chemistry, Mendeleev attempted to systematize the properties of the elements he described and as a result, he formulated an important scientific generalization, the **'Periodic law of Elements'.** This law brought order to existing information and directed further research towards the existence and properties of elements then unknown, predictions of which were soon fulfilled.

1869 (D): The first college for women, **Girton,** was founded at **Cambridge.**

In 1878 women became eligible to take degrees at London University for the first time. In 1880 England's first high school for girls opened. In 1870 women entered the University of Michigan for the first time since its founding at Ann Arbor (U. S. A.) in 1817.

1869 (E): The Germans, inspired **by Dr. A. Petermann,** explorer, organized a great **Greenland expedition** under **Capt. Karl Koldewey,** German leader.

1869 (F): The **All-England Croquet Club,** which was founded this year introduced **lawn tennis** as an added attraction to augment its dwindling resources.

The club had to pay the enhanced rent of £ 100 for its four acre tract, adjacent to the London and South Western Railway line near Worpole road. The game became so popular that the club had to be renamed the All-England Croquet and Lawn Tennis Club in 1877. It was then that the idea of the first **Wimbledon tennis tournament** dawned upon the club's members. [see 1877 Jul. 9-16]

1869-72: **Lord Mayo** (1822-1872), the Viceroy of India.

1870 JAN. 10: John D. Rockefeller (1838-1937), U. S. industrialist and philanthropist, founded the **Standard Oil Company** of Ohio, with a capital of one million dollars. [see 1882 (c)]

His oil business absorbed many Cleveland refineries and expanded into Pennsylvania oil fields to become the world's largest refining concern. The division of the operations into 18 companies – later to include more than 30 corporations – under the umbrella of Standard Oil of New Jersey (1899) helped him to accumulate a personal fortune of over one billion dollars. After his retirement in 1911, he expanded his efforts in philanthropy, which claimed about one-half of his vast fortune. Rockefeller's career is often regarded as a prime example of the American self-made man.

1870 FEB. 7: Birth of **Alfred Adler** (d.1937), Austrian physician and psychologist, who created a socially oriented personality theory and system of psychotherapy called individual psychology.

His school of thought stressed the influence of inferiority feelings on human behaviour.

Adler was an early follower of Sigmund Freud [see 1895 (n)] but split with him over differences in their approach to psychology.

1870 MAR. 21: Keshab Chandra Sen (1838-1884), the celebrated Brahmo leader, left for England for an intimate study of the Western civilization, as he himself stated.

He was given a grand ovation in England. He was also invited to meet Queen Victoria. During his sojourn of six months he spoke in London, and all the principal towns, and produced deep impression on all his hearers from all classes of society.

Christianity in England appeared to Keshab too sectarian and narrow. Christian life, in England, he considered more materialistic and outward than spiritual and inward. In one of his speeches in England he observed: "I found Christ spoke one language and Christianity another. I went to him prepared to hear what he had to say, and was immensely gratified when he told me, 'Love the Lord thy God with all thy heart, with all thy mind, and all thy soul, and with all thy strength, and love thy neighbour as thyself'. Christ never demanded from me worship or adoration that is due to God, the Creator of the Universe. He placed Himself before me as the spirit I must imbibe in order to approach the Divine Father, as the great Teacher and guide who will lead me to God. Christ demands of us absolute sanctification and purification of heart. In this also I see Christ on the one side, and Christian sects on the other. To be a Christian then is to be Christlike. Christianity means becoming like Christ, not acceptance of Christ as a proposition or as an outward representation, but the spiritual conformity with the life and character of Christ. By Christ I understand one who said, 'Thy will be done.' " *(Scholar Extraordinary* by Nirad C. Choudhary, p. 330)

1870 MAR. : Kesbab Chandra Sen (1838-1884), the Brahmo leader, met **Max Muller** (1823-1900) for the first time in London.

Referring to this meeting, Max Muller wrote to his wife in a letter dated 1st April 1870: "We soon got into a warm discussion, and it was curious to see how we almost made him confess himself a Christian." *(The Life and Letters of Max Muller,* Vol. I, p. 395)

Keshab held Christ and Christianity in greater veneration than his two predecessors, Ram Mohan and Devendranath. He allowed the Western culture and Christian influences to play fully on his mind. His publication of *Jesus Christ, Europe and Asia* in 1865, clearly indicated the trend of his mind. Brahmos became more Christian in their belief and outlook and enthusiastically studied the Bible and hailed Jesus as the Prince of Prophets. Keshab's chief lieutenant, P. C. Majumdar, depicted Christ as an Eastern prophet in his *Oriental Christ.*

At this crisis of our national life, "when Keshab and his progressive Brahmos developed unmistakable tendencies towards the modern European or Christian ethics and rationalism" the tide was turned by Rajnarain Bose, (who succeeded Devendranath Tagore as the president of Adi Brahma Samaj) himself a product of the Western education. He boldly proclaimed "the superiority of Hindu religion and culture over European and Christian theology and civilization." The Hindus, said he, had forgotten their past to such an extent that they had no recollection of the fact that rational thinking and ideas of social and personal freedom were not wanting in the history of their own culture.

Rajnarain Bose boldly asserted that "not only have we the most perfect system of theism or monotheism in our ancient theology and religion, but Hinduism presented also a much higher social idealism, all its outer distinctions of caste notwithstanding, than has yet been reached by Christendom.... These ideas were catching up and his clarion call rallied round his banner a number of Hindus who accepted his views with enthusiasm, and probably without argument or discussion. Rajnarain held before them a complete ideal of nationalism to be realized in every department of life. (Bharatiya Vidya Bhavan's *History and Culture of the Indian People,* Vol. X, Part II, p. 469 and 470.)

1870 MAR. (A): **Railway between Calcutta and Bombay** completed.

1870 APR. 22: Birth of **Lenin** (d. 1924), Russian statesman, the creator of the Bolshevik party, the Soviet State, and the Third International.

He was a successful revolutionary leader and an important contributor to revolutionary socialist theory.

1870 JUNE 9: Death of **Charles Dickens** (b.1812), English author and the most widely read Victorian novelist. His childhood experience of poverty and family debt, and his knowledge of London, influenced his writing.

In numerous novels he portrayed conditions of living among the poor and defenceless in the new urban society of the Industrial Revolution. He made a major contribution to the exposure of the 19th century social evils and their redress by Parliamentary legislation.

1870 JUL. 18: The first Vatican Council convened by **Pope Pius IX** (1792-1878), endorsed **papal infallibility.**

Infallibility was confined to those occasions upon which the Pope made pronouncements *ex cathedra* (from his throne), but these pronouncements were to take their authority from God and not from any other authority existing in the Church except that of the Pope. This endorsement that Pope is infallible when he defines doctrines of faith or morals *ex cathedra* and that such dicta are "irreformable" and require no "consent of the church", was attended by important results. It marked the final triumph of the papacy over the episcopal and conciliar tendencies of the church. It attempted to exalt Pope above all secular states and to extend "faith and morals" to political domain. As a result, church and state were finally separated, authority in church was centralized in Rome and Church was ranged in opposition to the dominant political forces. The action produced a wave of anti-church legislation in the German States. [see 1864 Dec. 8]

1870 OCT. 1: The British Post Office issued **the world's first post cards.**

1870 NOV. 5: Birth of **Chittaranjan Das** (d.1929), Indian National Congress leader and an apostle of Indian nationalism, well-known as 'Deshabandhu' ('friend of the country').

His main aim was Swaraj, or self-rule for India.

1870 (A): **James Starley,** an Englishman, made a **bicycle** with a large front wheel and a small rear wheel, derisively nicknamed "pennyfarthing" after the largest and smallest English copper coins of the period.

In 1877 a safety-type of machine with two wheels of the same type was introduced by H. J. Lawson.

The first foot-pedalled bicycle had been built in 1839 by a Scottish blacksmith, Kirpatrick Macmilan. Subsequent improvements included wire-spoked wheels, gears and chains, brakes, and pneumatic tyres. James Starley improved the safety bicycle, adding to the popularity of bicycling and increasing its safety. He built and patented the first light-weight all-metal bicycle (and the first with wire-spoked tension wheels).

In 1885, the Rover Company of Coventry, England, introduced the safety bicycle designed by J. K. Starley whose vehicle had wheels of equal size, a departure from the "ordinary" whose front wheel was much larger than its rear wheel. In the same year, the bicycle designed by French engineer, G. Juzan, had two wheels o' equal size with chain-driven wheel. The new French and English models made the bicycle suitable for general use.

The greatest revolution in bicycle history was the introduction of the pneumatic rubber tyres (patented on Oct. 31, 1881) by John Boyd Dunlop (1840-1921), Scottish Veterinary Surgeon and inventor. [vide 1881 Oct. 31]. Although received with a scepticism at first, it was quickly appreciated at its true worth, riders finding that it gave an enormous increase of comfort and speed. The combination of safety bicycle and pneumatic tyre placed the bicyle on an unassailable foundation and since that date its use has rapidly spread.

In 1889 safety bicycles were manufactured for the first time on a large scale in U. S. A. The safety bicycle of 1893 was the modern bicycle in general outline. In 1901 the Raleigh Cycle Company introduced its All Steel Safety Bicycle. The invention of the internal combustion engine led to attempts to motorise the bicycle, and Gottlieb Daimler (1834-1900), developed the motorcycle in 1885 [see 1885 (b)].

1870 (B): **The Education Act** of 1870 (Forster's Education Act) laid the cornerstone of the modern system of national education in England.

Recognizing that the voluntary schools could no longer satisfy the national need, the Act afforded the means of further provision through the new school boards and was gradually followed by compulsory attendance, a broadened curriculum and a longer school life. Thus elementary education for children from the ages of 5 to 10 first became free and mandatory after the passage of the Act. Compulsory education was extended by law to 11-year-olds in 1893 and to 12-year-olds in 1899. After 1870 local school boards were established to assume control of the existing voluntary schools and to found new ones. In 1902 these independent boards were abolished, and their functions were taken over by the Local Education Authorities who are still responsible for all education in Britain except in Universities.

1870-71: The Franco-Prussian war (July 19, 1870 – May 10, 1871), brought on the fall of the second French Empire, created the situation that enabled Bismarck (1815-1898) to establish the German Empire. It was the first European war in which both principal adversaries used railroads, the electrical telegraph, rifles, and rifled and breech-loading artillery – technological innovations that revolutionized warfare in the 19th century.

The two nations (French and Prussia) went to war (declared by the former, on July 19, 1870) nominally over the candidacy of a Hohenzollern prince for the Spanish throne but actually over Prussia's growing power in Germany which Napolean III saw as a threat to French security. The war was almost over within three months with French surrender at Sedan (Sept. 2) and Metz, but Paris held out under seige (began on Sept. 19, 1870) from Sept. 23, 1870, to Jan. 28, 1871 and for the last 23 days was bombarded by German artillery.

A most dramatic episode in the history of Paris, the seige brought Parisians to the verge of starvation. "By the time they surrendered on Jan. 28, 1871, the beleaguered citizens of Paris had been reduced to eating dogs, cats and even rats." *(365 Days to Remember, p. 159)*. The war was ended by Frankfurt treaty (May 10, 1871). **German Empire** was formally proclaimed in the Hall of Mirrors of the Palace of Versailles on Jan. 18, 1871, after the defeat of France. Thus the Franco-Prussian war marked the end of French hegemony in continental Europe and the formation of the Prussian-dominated German empire. It was to survive only until Germany's defeat in World War – I, when France recovered its lost territories. The forty years period between the Franco-Prussian war and the beginning of World War – I was marked by extremely unstable peace between the major powers of Europe.

1871 AUG. 30: Birth of **Lord Rutherford** (d. 1937), British physicist, who was the founder of nuclear physics.

As a result of an outstanding series of experiments (1893-1909) he determined the nature of alpha particles, one of the three types of radiation given off by radioactive substances, and evolved the theory of both the radioactive disintegration of elements and the nuclear atom. For this work he was awarded the 1908 Nobel Prize for Physics. In 1919 he demonstrated the first artificial splitting of atoms with the transmutation of one element into another.

1871 AUG. 30 (A): A **devastating fire** broke out in **Chicago,** U. S. A. engulfing an area of 3.5 miles, destroying seventeen thousand structures and property worth 299 million dollars.

1871 (A): NARENDRANATH who was eight years old entered the ninth class (equivalent to the present primary class two) of Pandit Ishwarachandra Vidyasagar Metropolitan Institution at Calcutta.

Naren retained his admiration for the wandering monk. "I must become a sannyasin", he would tell his friends, "a palmist predicted it", and he would show a certain straight line on the palm of his hand which indicated the tendency to the monastic life.

1871 (B): An association, called the **'National Society'** was founded in Calcutta. Its avowed object was the promotion of unity and national feeling among the Hindus.

The National Society arranged a monthly discourse. In one of these monthly meetings, presided over by Devendranath Tagore, Rajnarain Bose delivered an address on the "Superiority of Hinduism".... It evoked a keen controversy and meetings were held not only by Christians but also by advanced Brahmos to oppose his views. As the society was confined to the Hindus, objection was taken to the use of the word 'National'. Against this, the *National Paper,* the organ of the Hindu Mela, observed as follows: 'We do not understand why our correspondent takes exception to the Hindus who certainly form a nation themselves, and as such a society established by them can very properly be called a 'National Society.' " In this context, Nabagopal elaborated his view on Hindu nationalism through his writings. He maintained that the basis of national unity in India has been the Hindu religion. "Hindu nationality is not confined to Bengal. It embraces all of Hindu name and Hindu faith throughout the length and breadth of Hindustan; neither geographical position, nor the language is counted a disability. The Hindus are destined to be a religious nation." (Bharatiya Vidya Bhavan's *History and Culture of the Indian People,* Vol. X, Part II, p. 472 and 473) [see 1866 (c)]

1871 (C): Charles Darwin (1809-1882), British naturalist, brought out *The Descent of Man,* which was the natural sequel to the *Origin of Species* (1859).

While the latter established the fact of evolution and provided the explanation by the mechanism of natural selection which did away with all ideas of design, the former applied Darwin's conclusions to human evolution. His convincing arguments as to how humanity developed from earlier creatures and remained just one part of a complex and evolving animal kingdom clearly undermined belief in the literal truth of Genesis as explained in the Bible, and brought attacks on Darwin from many sides. [see 1882 Apr. 19]

1871 (D): Trade Unions were fully legalized in Britain – the **Trade Union Act of 1871** recognized the Trade Unions as legal associations. The act also granted workers the right to strike and the right to picket.

Trade unionism grew into a movement of political and social significance, in the climate of Industrial Revolution and, after repression in the early part of the 19th century, achieved legal and social acceptance in 1870s by which time it had also begun to develop in the continent of Europe. In 1869 the British Trade Unions took part in forming Labour Representation League to send workmen to parliament, and two miners were elected MPs in 1874.

1871 (E): **James Freeman Clarke** (1810-1888), U. S. Unitarian clergyman, reformer and author, brought out his most notable work in the field of comparative religion, *Ten Great Religions* (2 Vols., 1871-73).

This publication reflected growing American awareness of religions other than Christianity. Written from a liberal view point and free from bigotry, this work included substantial chapters on Hinduism and Buddhism. By 1886, Clarke's book had run through 21 editions.

1871-74: Discovery of **Franz Josef Land** (in the Arctic region) by the Austrian Julius Payer and Carl Wezprecht.

1872 APR. 2: Death of **Samuel Morse** (b. 1791), U. S. artist, who invented the most widely used telegraph (1835).

The idea of an electromagnetic recording telegraph came to him as he was on a ship returning to New York to take up his job as professor of painting. In 1838 he also devised the system of dots and the dashes, now called, 'Morse Code', for sending message.

1872 MAY 12: Birth of **Bertrand Russell** (d. 1970), British philosopher, mathematician and social reformer.

He made original and decisive contributions to logic and mathematics and wrote with distinction in all fields of philosophy. His work *Principia Mathematica* (1910, with A. N. Whitehead) is the foundation of the Calculus of proposition and modem symbolic logic.

1872 MAY: On the auspicious night of new moon, at Dakshineswar, **SRI RAMAKRISHNA** (1836-1886) worshipped his immaculate consort **Sarada Devi** (1853-1920), the Holy Mother, as the embodiment of the Divine Mother.

With the help of an assistant, he went through the regular form of worship in which the Holy Mother took the place of the Deity. During the ceremony she passed into *samadhi.* Sri Ramakrishna too, when he had finished the *mantras,* went into the superconscious state. Priest and Goddess were joined in a transcendental union in the self. At the dead of night Sri Ramakrishna partially recovered consciousness, then with the appropriate *mantra* he surrendered himself and the fruits of his life-long *sadhana,* together with his rosary, at the feet of the Holy Mother and saluted her. With this sacred ceremony, called in the Tantra the *'Shodashi Puja' (shodashi* – of the age of sixteen – is one of the names of Kali) was completed the long series of Sri Ramakrishna's spiritual practices.

1872 AUG. 15: Birth of **Sri Aurobindo** (d.1950), the celebrated yogi, and one of the most dominant figures in the history of the Indian renaissance and Indian nationalism.

After studying classical philosophy at Cambridge University and a career as teacher, poet, publicist, and radical politician, he devoted himself in his Ashram in the then French Pondicherry, to spiritual realization, urging the necessity of spiritual emancipation of Mother India, whom he identified with the divine Mother, and teaching a yoga by which to transform ordinary human being into a divine being possessing love, wisdom and power for the good and so to achieve a transformation of material existence.

The emphasis of his teaching was on spiritualization of the phenomenal world and all human activity through emergence of a disciplined religious elite extending widely to touch all mankind.

1872 NOV. 9: A **devastating fire** which began with an explosion in a four-storey warehouse in **Boston,** destroyed $ 75,000,000 in property.

It engulfed 65 acres, and raged for three days, destroying the richest part of the city, burning 776 buildings including warehouses filled with merchandise; within four years (1876) the area was rebuilt more substantially than ever.

1872 DEC. : The first public stage was opened in Calcutta. It was named **'National Theatre',** according to the prevailing spirit of the time.

1872 (A): At the request of **Keshab Chandra Sen** (1838-1884), the celebrated Brahmo leader, the Government of India passed a special legislation for legalising Brahmo marriage.

The new legislation was called the **Native Marriage Act,** popularly known as the Civil Marriage Act. It was applicable to any one who declared 'I am not a Hindu, not a Mussalman, not a Christian'. The passing of the Act was strongly resented by the Hindus and gave an impetus to the Hindu renaissance movement.

1872 (B): The first All India Census, though not synchronously taken, was completed. It essentially represented the pooling of results of the census taken round about that time in various parts of the country.

In 1801, England had begun her census series and the British were anxious to ascertain the population of the dependencies and territories of their vast Empire. Consequently statistical studies on population were conducted in the Indian sub-continent also between 1816 and 1930. As desired in the Statistical Despatch No. 2 of 23rd July, 1856, of the Home Government, the Government of India considered the means of conducting a general census of the population of India in 1861. But after a postponement, the census were taken up in North Western Provinces (1865), Central Provinces (1866), Bihar (1867) and in Punjab (1868). Census of the cities of Madras (1863), Bombay (1864) and Calcutta (1866) were also taken. In 1865, the Government of India and the Home Government agreed on principle that a census should be conducted in 1871. Between 1867 and 1872, census were conducted in as much of the country as was practicable. Though these were based on a uniform set of schedules they were not certainly supervised or compiled. This series of census conducted during the period 1867-72 is commonly known as the census of 1872 but it was not a synchronous one nor did it cover all the areas of India. [see 1881 (a), 1891 (a), 1901 (c)]

1872 (C): *A Sanskrit English Dictionary* (etymologically and philologically arranged with special reference to Greek, Latin, Gothic, German, Anglo-Saxon and other cognate Indo-European languages) by **Sir Monier-Williams** (1819-1899), professor of Sanskrit in Oxford University, was brought out by the Oxford University Press, with the support of the Secretary of State for India in Council. The second enlarged and improved work (1899) also enjoyed the same privileges.

In his preface to the Dictionary, Monier-Williams wrote: "....In explanation I must draw attention to the fact that I am only the second occupant of the Boden chair, and that its founder Colonel Boden, stated most explicitly in his will (dated August 15, 1811) that the special object of his munificent bequest was to promote the translation of Scriptures into Sanskrit so as 'to enable his countrymen to proceed in the conversion of the natives of India to the Christian Religion.' "

The following excerpts are from his lengthy and learned introduction to his monumental work:

"The Hindus are perhaps the only nation, except the Greeks, who have investigated, independently and in a true scientific manner, the general laws which govern the evolution of languages."

"By Sanskrit is meant the learned language of India – the language of its cultured inhabitants – the language of its religion, its literature, and Science – not by any means a dead language, but one still spoken and written by educated men in all parts of the country, from Kashmir to Cape Comorin, from Bombay to Calcutta and Madras."

"We are appalled by the length of some of India's literary productions as compared with those of European countries. For instance, Virgil's *Aeneid* is said to consist of 9,000 lines, Homer's *Illiad* of 12,000 lines, and the *Odyssey* of 15,000 whereas the Sanskrit Epic Poem called *Mahabharata* contains at least 200,000 lines, without reckoning the supplement called *Hari-Vamsha*. In some subjects too, especially in poetical descriptions of nature and domestic affections, Indian works do not suffer by a comparison with the best specimens of Greece and Rome, while in wisdom, depth, and shrewdness of their moral apophthegms they are unrivalled."

"More than this, the Hindus had made considerable advances in astronomy, algebra, arithmetic, botany, and medicine, not to mention their superiority in grammar, long before some of these sciences were cultivated by the most ancient nations of Europe." [see 1899 Apr. 11]

1872 (D): **Oceanography** was pioneered by the British vessel HMS Challenger which set out on a four year-old voyage of 69,000 nautical miles to collect specimens and extend human knowledge of animal and plant life in the sea.

HMS 'Challenger' was the first steam propelled vessel to cross the Antarctic circle. Her biologists collected an immense number of specimens from the sea floor. They found nothing to support the notion that some primitive forms of life survived in the deep sea that would throw light on the early history of life. Their results were published in fifty large volumes, over a period of 20 years.

1872 (E): A system of **automatic electric signalling** for railroads patented by Irish-American engineer **William Robinson.**

It is the basis for all modern automatic rail-road block signalling systems.

1872 (F): The **Farquharson Rifle** patented by English Gunsmith **John Far quharson,** was a single-shot rifle with a falling-block action.

George Gibbs of Bristol began production of the rifle. Later it was produced in numerous variations by Webley, Bland, Westley Richards and various European firms.

1872 (G): The world's first industrial dynamo was perfected by Belgian electrician **Zenobe Theohile Gramme,** who employed a ring winding of the same type invented independently by Italian Physicist, Antonio Pacinotti in 1860.

1872 (H): Sir **James Dewar** (1842-1923), Scottish physicist and chemist, who was pioneer of low-temperature studies, invented (Dewar) **flask,** which was adapted for domestic use and as such is better known as a thermos flask. The first vacuum flask was constructed by Dewar in 1892.

1872 (I): Louis **Pasteur,** French Chemist, published a classic paper on *Fermentation* showing that it was caused by micro-organisms.

1872 (J): German botanist, **Ferdinand Julius Collins,** published the first major work on **bacteriology.**

1872 (K): Opening of the **telegraphic line** across the Australian continent from Adelaide to Port Darwin, which was soon afterwards connected with Java and so with the lines of India and Europe.

1872-76: Lord Northbrook, the Viceroy of India.

1873 MAY 1: Death of **David Livingstone** (b.1813), Scottish missionary, who explored Africa's interior in an attempt to introduce Christianity and eliminate slavery by developing channels of commerce.

By a series of journeys in the mid-19th century, David Livingstone contributed more than any other single person to the opening of Africa to the West. His explorations furnished Great Britain with claims to parts of Africa. He was the first European to sight the Zambezi River (1851) and Victoria Falls (1855), which he named. He was the first non-African to cross the African continent from west to east. Livingstone's accounts of his travels in Africa – *Missionary Travels,* (1857), and *The Zambezi and its Tributaries* (1865) were best sellers and he achieved widespread fame.

1873 MAY 8: Death of **John Stuart Mill** (b.1806), British philosopher, economist and exponent of utilitarianism.

He was the most influential British thinker of the 19th century. His works contain major strands of 19th century philosophy, logic, and economic thought. His Autobiography (1873) is a document of great importance in the history of utilitarian and liberal ideas. He was a humanitarian who felt that the greatest good was to serve the society, and he is best remembered for his brilliant essay '*On Liberty*' (1859). His belief in votes for women and the freedom of thought and speech influenced both his own and future generations.

1873 AUG. 26: Birth of **Lee De Forest** (d. 1961) U. S. inventor of the audion (1906), the elementary form of the modern radio tube.

His invention paved the way for the development of broadcasting.

In 1910 De Forest transmitted the singing voice of Enrico Caruso and thus was one of the pioneers of radio broadcasting. In 1916 he established a radio station and was broadcasting news. He also helped to develop sound film, television and radio-therapy.

1873 OCT. 22: Birth of **Swami Ram Tirtha** (d. 1906) in Punjab.

In his pre-monastic life, when he was a professor at Lahore, he met Swami Vivekananda who had come there to deliver a lecture on Vedanta. Contact with the Swami greatly influenced him and brought a turning point in his life. [see 1897 Nov. 12].

1873 DEC. 3: **Max Muller** openly voiced his unfavourable opinion as to the beliefs and practices of contemporary Hindus. He considered Hinduism to be dead, and said so, in plain language, in **Westminister lecture on Missions.**

Referring to the Hindu Religion, he said:

"That religion is still professed by at least 110,000,000 of human souls, and, to judge from the last census, even that enormous number falls much short of the real truth and yet I do not shrink from saying that their religion is dying or dead. And why? Because it cannot stand the light of day.

"The worship of Shiva, of Vishnu, and the other popular deities, is the same, nay, in many cases a more degraded and savage character, than the worship of Jupiter, Apollo, and Minerva; it belongs to a stratum of thought which is long buried under our feet; it may live on, like the lion and tiger, but the mere air of free thought and civilized life will extinguish it. A religion may linger on for a long time, it may be accepted by the large masses of the people because it is there, and there is nothing better. But when a religion has ceased to produce defenders of the faith, prophets, champions, martyrs, it has ceased to live, in the true sense of the word; and in that sense the old, orthodox Brahminism has ceased to live for more than a thousand years.

"It is true there are millions of children, women, and men in India who fall down before the stone image of Vishnu, with his four arms, riding on a creature half bird, half man, or sleeping on the serpent, who worship Shiva, a monster with three eyes, riding naked on a bull, with a necklace of skull for his ornaments. There are human beings who still believe in a god of war, Karthikeya, with six faces, riding on a peacock, and holding bow and arrow in his hand, and who invoke a God of success, Ganesha, with four hands and an elephant's head sitting on a rat. Nay, it is true that, in the broad daylight of the nineteenth century, the figure of the goddess Kali is carried through the streets of her own city, Calcutta, her wild dishevelled hair reaching to her feet, with a necklace of human heads, her tongue protruded from her mouth, her girdle stained with blood. All this is true; but ask any Hindu who can read and write and think, whether these are the gods he believes, and he will smile at your credulity. How long this death of national religion in India may last no one can tell; for our purposes, however, for gaining an idea of the issue of the great religious struggle of the future, that religion too is dead and gone."

Max Muller's view that Hinduism was dead led him to a controversy with Sir Alfred Lyall, whose knowledge of India was both wide and deep. He replied to Muller in an article in the *Fortnightly Review* (July 1, 1874), and contended that so far from being dead Hinduism was very much alive.

1873 (A): SRI RAMAKRISHNA (1836-1886) met **Swami Dayananda Saraswati** (1824-1883), the founder of the Arya Samaj, when the latter paid a brief visit to Calcutta and stayed at a garden in the suburb. [see 1875 Mar.]

Though already known as a great scholar, the Swami had not yet made known his doctrines or founded his Samaj. Referring to him Sri Ramakrishna said to some of his disciples later on, "I went to see him at the Garden of Sinthi. He had a little power. I found his chest always red owing to congestion. Day and night he discussed the scriptures.... He seemed to have the ambition of doing something original – starting a new sect." [see 1875 Apr. 10]

1873 (B): The Bihar famine.

The monsoon failed prematurely from September in North Bihar, "quite the most populous part in India" and to a lesser extent in certain other parts, producing disastrous effect on the winter rice crop and making the prospects for spring crops bad. Sir George Campbell, then Lieutenant-Governor of Bengal, came to Patna for making inquiries and on the 23rd October, officially reported "the gravest apprehension of general scarcity throughout the country, and of worse evils in large parts of it". [see 1866-67, 1868-69, 1874 (a), 1876-78, 1877 Jan-1, 1878 (b), 1896-97, 1897 Jan. 13, 1897 May 16, 1899-1900]

1873 (C): An **International Exhibition** was held at **Vienna.**

The site of the exhibition covered 40 acres: about 7 million people visited the exhibition to view 25,760 exhibits costing £. 2,200,000.

The Vienna exhibition had an atmosphere of glamour and eclat only equalled by the Parisian Displays (1863). Its special characteristic was the large number of exhibits from countries in the Near, Middle and Far East.

Electricity drove machinery for the first time in history at Vienna.

1873 (D): **Father Damien** (1840-1889), Belgian Roman Catholic missionary, went to the government hospital for lepers on the Hawaiin island of Molokai to care for victims of the disease (that was later called Hansen's disease).

He not only ministered to the spiritual needs of the lepers but also dressed their sores, provided shelter and food, and buried them. Even after he had contracted leprosy, Father Damien continued his work until he became too ill to do so.

1873 (E): **DDT** (Dichloro diphenyl-trichloroethane) was prepared for the first time by German Chemistry student, **Othmar Zeidler,** at Strasburg.

Zeidler described DDT the following year in the *Proceedings of the German Chemical Society,* but he had no idea of the significance of his discovery. It was only in 1939 that DDT was developed and introduced
as a persistent low-cost hydrocarbon pesticide by Swiss Chemist Paul Muller of Geigy Company and was applied almost immediately and with great success against the Colarado potato beetle which was threatening Switzerland's potato crop.

1873 (F): **James Clerk Maxwell** (1831-1879), Scottish Mathematician and physicist, published his *Treatise on Electricity and Magnetism* in which he postulated the identity of light as an **electromagnetic phenomenon.**

He described the properties of the electromagnetic field in a series of equations, which entailed the electromagnetic theory of light. The test of this theory in various experimental forms occupied the time of a large number of physicists throughout the world for the remainder of the century. [see 1864 (f)]

1873 (G): Introduction of compulsory, secular schooling in Victoria, Australia.

In the same year the **first Australian Factory Act** was passed by the Victorian Government at Melbourne to protect female and juvenile millhands and to maintain safe and sanitary working conditions.

1873 (H): **A Fine Art Exhibition** was conducted at **Madras** with Lord Hobart, the Governor of Madras, as the patron.

Raja Ravi Varma (1848-1906), the celebrated artist of Travancore, encouraged by the popularity acclaimed for the picture "Nair Lady", sent it as an entry to the above exhibition. This picture won for him the Governor's Gold Medal. Thus Ravi Varma made his debut in the field of art with a prize-winning picture. This picture was subsequently sent to the Great International Exhibition at Vienna where it fetched him a gold medal and a certificate.

Ravi Varma again won the gold medal at the exhibition at Madras in the subsequent year. This time it was for the painting of "A Tamil Lady playing on Sarabat". When king Edward VII visited India in 1875, this picture was presented to him. The king expressed his appreciation of the work and was surprised to see European techniques used even though Ravi Varma had no training from abroad. It was by sheer merit and research that he had succeeded in designing from experiences of his own which had a mingling of Indian and European styles unknown to India till that time. [see 1893 (a)].

1874 JAN. 30: **Swami Ramalingam** (b. 1823), popularly known as 'Vallalar' – the great Benevolent and Munificent – a great yogi and *siddha* of South India, (who lived in Vadalur, about 35 miles from Pondicherry, who had attained integral realization of the Divine, and the transformation of his nature and body into their deathless states of glorious perfection) sacrificed his deathless body by dematerialisation, for the universal manifestation of the Divine Light of Supreme Grace directly on the earth, and with a view to enter into all the physical bodies universally and fix its deathless substances and powers into the earth-nature for the benefit of a divine evolution of the earthly life.

The Swami is considered to be the fore-runner of Sri Aurobindo and the Mother.

1874 FEB. 13: **Communal riots in Bombay.**

There was a brutal and unwarranted attack on Parsis by a mob of Mohammedans. They invaded Parsi place of worship, tore up prayer books, extinguished the sacred fires and subjected the fire temples to various indignities. Parsis were attacked in the streets and in their houses and free fights took place all over the city of Bombay. Thanks to the weakness and supineness of the Police and the Government, hooliganism had full play and considerable loss of life and damage to property were caused. The riot continued for several days till the military was called out (Bharatiya Vidya Bhavan's *History and Culture of the Indian People,* Vol. X, Part II, p. 326 and 327). [see 1877 Sept., 1885 (a), 1886 (c), 1889 (m), 1891 (b), 1893 (c), 1897 June]

1874 APR. 25: Birth of **Guglielmo Marconi** (d.1937), Italian electrical engineer, who invented the wireless telegraph (1895) and who was the first to transmit a radio signal across the Atlantic. [see 1895 (b), 1901 Dec. 12]

1874 JUN. 12: At the suggestion of some of his devotees and admirers, **Swami Dayananda** (1824-1883), founder of Arya Samaj, who agreed to write down his lectures in the form of a book, started his work, and when completed, it came to be known as the *Satyartha Prakasha* and its English translation as the *Light of Truth.*

The preliminary outline of this book was drawn at Varanasi, and, imbued with ideas, the Swami reached Allahabad (on July 1, 1874) where he stayed for over three months to complete the book, his *magnum opus* which was printed in 1875 as the first tentative edition. It was later on thoroughly revised and enlarged by the author at Udaipur (1882), and it came out as the posthumous publication from the Vedic Yantralaya, Allahabad, in 1884. This is the only book of Hindi prose that has been translated into so many languages in India and abroad. The work created a stir in the world of theology, creeds, cults and religions. It aimed at a crusade against credulities and superstitions.

1874 OCT. : When **Max Muller** went to stay with Mr. Grand Duff, formerly under-Secretary for India, he met **Charles Darwin,** the English naturalist.

The conversation turning on apes as the progenitors of man, Max Muller asserted that if speech were left out of consideration, there was a fatal flaw in the line of facts. "You are a dangerous man", said Darwin laughingly (*The Life and Letters of Max Muller,* Vol. I, p. 494).

1874 NOV. 30: Birth of **Sir Winston Churchill** (d. 1965), British statesman, prime minister and historian.

Churchill's forceful, aggressive leadership played a major part in the victory of Britain and her Allies in World War II. During the War, when Britain and her Allies were facing defeat, Churchill, through his broadcast speeches, lifted morale from its lowest abyss. Thereafter he planned relentlessly for victory. His leadership, co-operation with the U. S. and Russia, and tireless energy accomplished this by 1945.

1874 NOV. : SRI RAMAKRISHNA followed the path of **Christianity**.

A devotee read the Bible to him on occasions, and he appreciated it very much. Soon after, a strong desire to try the Christian way of

approach to God took hold of Ramakrishna's mind. One day, in a devotee's house, while he was looking attentively at the picture of the Ma-
donna with the Divine Child, and was reflecting on the wonderful life
of Christ, he felt as though the picture had become animated, and that
rays of light were emanating from the figures of Mary and Christ and
entering into him.... Deep respect for Christ and Christian Church filled
his heart. He saw the vision of Christian devotees burning incense and
candles before the figure of Jesus in the churches and offering unto
him the eager and prayerful out-pourings of their hearts. After a couple
of days, when Ramakrishna was walking in the Panchavati he saw an
extraordinary looking person of serene aspect approaching him with his
gaze intently fixed on him. He knew him at once to be a man of foreign
extraction. Ramakrishna was charmed and wondered who he might be.
Presently the figure drew near, and from the innermost recesses of
Ramakrishna's heart went up the note, "This is Christ who poured out
his heart's blood for the redemption of mankind and suffered agonies
for its sake. It is none else but the Master yogin Jesus, the embodiment
of love." Then the Son of Man embraced Ramakrishna and became
merged in him. At this Ramakrishna went into *samadhi* and lost all
outward consciousness. [see 1866 (b)]

1874 NOV. (A): **Max Muller** (1823-1900) completed the long piece of work
– the translation of the sixth and the last volume of *Rig Veda* – which he
started after he settled at Oxford in 1849.

In the preface to the last volume of his great work, he wrote: "When I
had written the last line of the *Rig Veda* and Sayana's commentary, and
put down my pen, I felt as if I parted with an old, old friend. For thirty
years scarcely a day has passed on which my thoughts have not dwelt
on this work, and for many a day, and many a night too, the old poets
of Veda, and still more their orthodox and painstaking exposition, have
been my never failing companions. I am happy, no doubt, that the work
is done, and after having seen so many called away, in the midst of
their labours, I feel deeply grateful that I have been spared to finish the
work of my life." [see 1867 Dec. 9]

1874 DEC. : In reply to Sir Lewis Mallet, the Secretary of State for India in
Council, who had thanked Max Muller for the satisfactory manner in which
he had carried out the important work entrusted to him, **Max Muller** wrote:

"The *Rig Veda,* though for the last 3,000 years it has formed the
foundation of religious life in India, had never before been rendered
accessible to the people at large, and its publication will produce, nay,
has already produced, in India an effect similar to that which the first
printing of the Bible produced on the minds of Europe. Beyond the

frontiers of India also, the first edition of the oldest book of the whole Aryan race, has not been without its effect, and as long as men value the history of their language, mythology and religion, I feel confident that this work will hold its place in the permanent library of mankind." (*The Life and Letters of Max Muller,* Vol. I, p. 496). [see 1867 Dec. 9]

1874 (A): Severe **famine** throughout **Bengal.** [see 1866-67, 1868-69, 1873 (b), 1876-78, 1877 Jan. 1, 1878 (b), 1896-97, 1897 Jan. 13, 1897 May 16, 1899-1900]

1874 (B): Joseph F. **Glidden,** an Illinois farmer, patented the **barbed wire** – a form of cattle fencing made of steel wire strands into which sharp wire barbs were twisted or welded.

It was also used in warfare as a defence against the advance of infantry units. Its widespread use, often, violently opposed by cattle ranchers, ended the era of the open range in the West.

1874 (C): The **leprosy bacillus** (Mycobacterium leprae) was discovered by Norwegian physician, **Armauer Gerhard Hansen** (1841-1912).

1874 (D): NewYork got its **first electric street car** invented by **Stephen Dudley Field** (1846-1913). It replaced the horse carrier introduced in 1832.

In 1884, electric street cars employing overhead wires appeared in Germany.

1874 (E): George Cantor (1845-1918), German mathematician, published his major work, founding **set theory,** one of the greatest achievements of 19th century mathematics.

Later he also developed the theory of trans-infinite numbers. By devising original techniques for treating the infinite in mathematics, he contributed substantially to the development of analysis and logic; and by drawing on ideas of the infinite in the writings of ancient and medieval philosophy, he introduced new modes of thinking concerning the nature of number.

1875 JAN. 14: Birth of **Albert Schweitzer** (d. 1965), Austrian-German theologian and philosopher and medical missionary.

He was known specially for founding the Schweitzer Hospital, which provided unprecedented medical care for the natives of Lambarene in Gabon, Africa.

1875 MAR. : SRI RAMAKRISHNA (1836-1886), the saint of Dakshineswar, and **Keshab Chandra Sen** (1838-1884), the celebrated Brahmo leader and preacher, met for the first time. [see 1873 (a)]

Sri Ramakrishna had heard of Keshab's piety and spiritual attainments, and wished to meet him. Keshab was then staying with some of his followers in the garden house of Jayagopal Sen at Belgharia, a couple of miles from Dakshineswar. On meeting Keshab, Sri Ramakrishna said: "I hear that you have seen God: so I have come to hear about Him." Then followed a conversation on matters spiritual, which held Keshab and his followers under its spell. They were greatly attracted to this man of God and listened to the inspiring words that fell from his lips. Sri Ramakrishna spoke to them of immeasurable revelations of God and illustrated them with some parables. The uplifting force of his words of wisdom convinced Keshab that Sri Ramakrishna had seen God. Keshab was awed and amazed by the extraordinary spirituality of this man of realization and received unforeseen light from his personality and utterances. The contact with Sri Ramakrishna left an indelible impression on Keshab's mind: nay, it proved a turning point in his life. He visited Sri Ramakrishna frequently and spent long hours in his holy company. Gradually they became very intimate.

Keshab wrote about the saint of Dakshineswar in high terms in his journals. And as a result, English educated urbanized Bengal turned its steps towards this unlettered man from a village and began to draw inspiration. In fact this was the beginning of the real self-knowledge for Westernized minds. They could see in Sri Ramakrishna the embodiment of the spiritual wisdom of the ages.

1875 APR. 10: Arya Samaj, a powerful religious and social reformist movement which played an important role in the awakening of Indian national consciousness founded in Bombay by **Swami Dayananda Saraswati** (1824-1883), a great scholar of the Vedas.

The Arya Samaj fought as much against the evils in orthodox Hinduism as against Christianity and Islam, which were taking advantage of those evils to propagate their own religion and get converts. Soon the influence of this movement was felt throughout Western India. It gave birth to national spirit and organized social and educational reforms.

1875 JUL. 26: Birth of **Carl Jung** (d. 1961), Swiss psychologist and psychiatrist, and the founder of analytic psychology. [see 1895 (n)]

1875 OCT. 31: Birth of **Sardar Vallabhbhai Patel** (d. 1950), Indian nationalist, and political leader who was the dominant figure of the first post-Independence Government of India.

He helped organize the Indian nationalist movement and after independence (1947), succeeded in integrating several princely states into the Republic of India.

1875 NOV. 15: **Theosophical Society** of America founded in New York city by a Russian lady, **Madame H. P. Blavatsky** (1831-1891) and an American Colonel, named **H. S. Olcott** (1832-1907).

> The chief objects of the society when formed were: to unite humanity in universal brotherhood without race or creed distinctions; to encourage the study of Eastern cultures; and to make a systematic investigation into unexplained laws of nature and psychical powers latent in man, which is usually called Occultism.

> In 1879 Madame Blavatsky and Colonel Olcott came to India and established their headquarters at Adyar, a suburb of Madras, in 1882. Here they came into contact with Buddhism and Hinduism. Colonel Olcott remained President of the Society till his death in 1907, when Mrs. Annie Besant succeeded him.

1875 DEC. 13: In a letter to the Duke of Albany, **Max Muller** (1823-1900) pointed out the importance of the Veda:

> "Now I believe that the Veda is an extremely important book, in fact the only book in Indian literature which is important, not only for India, but for the early history of the whole Aryan race, including Greeks, Romans and ourselves. It contains the first attempt at expressing religious thought and feeling and it alone can help us to solve many of the most critical problems in the science of Religion." (*The Life and Letters of Max Muller,* Vol. I, p. 530) [see 1867 Dec. 9]

1875 (A): **Sir Sayed Ahmed Khan** (1817-1898), Indian Muslim leader, educationist and politician, founded a school at Aligarh.

> This school later (1877) developed into the **Mohammedan Anglo-Oriental College** which prospered and became the key intellectual centre for Indian Muslims, Aligarh University. Sayed Ahmed who wanted that his co-religionists should be progressive people, stressed the importance of liberal education on Western pattern.

1875 (B): **Max Muller** (1823-1900) took up the editorship of a gigantic corpus of the scriptures under the title, *The Sacred Books of the East.*

> Soon after he had published the sixth and the last volume of his *Rig Veda* (1874), the idea of supplementing this work with translations from the sacred writings of other religions as a comprehensive source for the study of religion, entered his mind. The first reference by him to such a project is to be found in a letter to the Sinologist Legge, which he wrote on February 1875. The same year the project became more concrete. It finally ran into forty-nine volumes and occupied him over the last 25 years of his life in collaboration with specialists and fellow-workers in many countries. It was his major editing work.

1875 (C): **Gallium,** a chemical element, was discovered by
L. De Boisbaudran (France).

1876 MAR. 3: **Alexander Graham Bell** (1847-1922), Scottish-American
physicist and inventor, patented an apparatus embodying the results of
his studies in the transmission of sound by electricity – the basis of modern
telephone.

The first telephone message transmitted (on March 10), was from Bell
to his assistant: "Mr. Watson, please come here; I want you." The first
demonstration of his telephone occurred at the American Academy of
Arts and Science Convention in Boston two months later. Bell's display
at Philadelphia Centennial Exposition a month later gained more
publicity.

In 1877, the first telephone was installed in a private house in U. S. A.
The first telephone exchange for facilitating the conversations of any
user with any other was commissioned in New Haven, Connecticut,
U. S. A. in 1878. Since then telephone exchanges came up in all parts of
the world. Three telephone exchanges were placed in service by private
companies in Bombay, Calcutta and Madras on January 28, 1882.

1876 Jul. 26: **Surendranath Banerjee** (1848-1925), a major figure in early
Indian nationalism, founded **'The Indian Association'** in Calcutta.

It aimed at organization of public opinion on an All-India level and
unification of the people of India on the basis of common political
interests and aspirations and the inclusion of the masses in the great
public movement of the day.

An outstanding public speaker and a master parliamentarian, Banerjee
now embarked on a political career to organize Indian public opinion,
to redress wrongs and protect rights, and to give Indians a serious role
in the administration of their country and voice in the counsels of their
government. His tours (1877) in different parts of India were acclaimed
as 'the first successful attempt of its kind at uniting India on a political
basis.' [see 1877 (b)]

1876 OCT. 6: **American Library Association** established in Philadelphia
by a group of leading public and university librarians for the purpose of
supplying "the best reading for the largest number at the least expense."

1876 OCT. 20: Birth of **Mohammed Ali Jinnah** (d. 1948), the Indian Muslim
politician whose demand for a separate state for the Muslims culminated
in the creation of Pakistan.

Jinnah insisted that Hindus and Muslims constituted two separate
nations and that the partition of India on August 15, 1947, into India

and Pakistan, was the fruit of his argument that Muslims must have their own homeland. Earlier (Aug. 16, 1946), Jinnah and Muslim League launched 'Direct Action'; violent riots broke out in Calcutta. A chain reaction set in and the riots spread to Naokali District in Bengal, Bihar and U. P.

1876 (A): Sayed Amir Ali (1849-1928), an Indian muslim politician, founded the **Central National Muslim Association** at Calcutta. He continued to be its Secretary for a quarter of a century.

1876 (B): Sir Dugald Clerk (1854-1932), Scottish engineer, built his first **gas engine.**

His researches on the explosive pressure and specific heat of gases advanced the science of thermodynamics and brought him international fame.

1876 (C): Nicholas August Otto (1832-1891), German engineer, who had patented a decade ago crude internal combustion engine (1866), built the first practical **internal combustion petrol engine** in which he introduced the four-stroke cycle operation.

This principle was also used in the petrol engine invented (1882) and perfected (1885) by Gottlieb Daimler (1834-1900), another German inventor. Otto's work was based upon previous engines of Etienne Lenoir (1822-1900), Belgian-French engineer, and Alphonse Beau de Rochas (1815-1891). More than 30,000 engines were sold by Otto's company during the following decade. It was the Otto engine that made the automobile and the airplane possible. [see 1883 (e), 1885 (b)]

1876 (D): Samuel Langhorne Clemens (1835-1910), pen name 'Mark Twain', published his famous novel: *Tom Sawyer.*

In 1884 *The Adventures of Huckleberry Finn* was brought out. These two novels have become world classics and give a wonderful picture of life in and around the Mississippi.

1876 (E): In America, the rise of great modern University – complete with graduate and professional school – started with the establishment of **John Hopkins** in Baltimore with a grant of 3.5 million dollars from philanthropist John Hopkins.

The trend towards philanthropic underwriting of private education accelerated when **Cornelius Vanderbilt** in 1873, gave 1 million dollars for the establishment of Vanderbilt University, later to be toppled by **Leland Stanford's** grant of 20 million dollars in 1885 for Stanford University [see 1885 (k)] and **John D. Rockefeller's** 30 million dollars in 1890 for the University of Chicago. [see 1891 (j)]

1876 (F): **Melville Dewey** (1851-1931), U. S. Librarian and the author of *A Classification and Subject Index for Cataloguing and Arranging the Books and Pamphlets of Library,* evolved the **Dewey Decimal system** for classifying books.

The system was initially intended for use by the American Library Association, which was established in the same year, Dewey being one of the original founders. In 1887, Dewey founded the first Library School in the U. S. and was Director of the New York State Library (1888-1905).

1876 (G): A **'World Fair'** (officially called the 'International Exhibition of Arts, Manufacturers and Products of the Soil and Mine') was held in **Philadelphia,** U. S. A. to celebrate the centennial of American Independence.

It was opened by President Grant in the presence of the Emperor of Brazil. The President and the Emperor ceremonially turned on the steam of the giant Corlis Engine which worked the mechanical exhibits, a feature of this impressive display of American technology.

37 foreign nations and 26 states were represented along with innumerables private exhibitors. The site of the exposition covered 60 acres. About 10 million people visited the Fair to view 60,000 exhibits costing $ 7,680,000.

It was in this Fair that Alexander Graham Bell's invention (the Telephone) was exhibited for the first time. The other important exhibit was the first sewing machine. Also, the Remington Typewriter was first introduced at this Fair.

1876 (H): In **Northern China famine** killed 9.6 million people.

1876 (I): *Life and Letters of Lord Macaulay* brought out by Longman, London, contained a letter (dated 12th October 1836) in which **Lord Macaulay** wrote: "Our English schools are flourishing wonderfully. If our plans of education are followed up there will not be a single idolator (Hindu) among the respectable classes in Bengal thirty years hence." [see 1882 (b)]

"Perhaps to laugh at Lord Macaulay and to shatter his imperialistic dreams the Providence produced in the same Bengal and in the same year (1836) a unique personality, Ramakrishna (1836-1886), who not only enlivened Hinduism in Bengal and India but also spread it in Macaulay's West – amazing indeed. And the phenomenon is gaining strength every day."

1876-78: Severe **famine in Deccan** and the adjacent areas took over 5 million lives.

The famine affected part of Native States of Hyderabad, Madras and almost the whole of Mysore and the Bombay Deccan, and later, the North-Western Provinces, Awadh and the Punjab. In this famine "relief was to a large extent insufficient and to a large extent imperfectly organized." "The system adopted in 1876-77", remarked Sir George Campbell, "was not successful in combating famine and preventing mortality; on the contrary, mortality was enormous while the expenditure was at the same time very great." [see 1866-67, 1868-69, 1873 (b), 1874 (a), 1877 Jan. 1, 1878 (b), 1896-97, 1897 Jan. 13, 1897 May 16, 1899-1900]

1876-80: Lord Lytton (1831-1891), the Viceroy of India.

1877 JAN. 1: Even as millions were dying of famine in South India, **Queen Victoria** (1819-1901) was proclaimed, amidst great pomp and ceremony, the 'Empress of India' at Delhi.

The expenses of this magnificent **'Delhi Durbar'** had to be borne by the famished people of India which had already come under the direct Government of the Crown, in 1858, when the East India Company ceased to be the ruler. Since then, till the end of the nineteenth century, there was a series of famines in British India. The principal victims of the famines were agricultural labourers, artisans, particularly weavers and small cultivators. Official indifference and lack of sympathy combined with natural causes like droughts and floods, accentuated the frightful suffering of the people.

During about a century of the East India Company's rule, India suffered in one part of it or another, several famines and scarcities. In the first half of the nineteenth century, there were seven famines, with an estimated total of 1.5 million deaths from famine. In the second half of the nineteenth century there were twenty-four famines (six between 1851 and 1875 and eighteen between 1876 and 1900), with an estimated total, according to official records, of over 20 million deaths. (Bharatiya Vidya Bhavan's *History and Culture of the Indian People,* Vol. IX, Part I, pp. 828, 829, 836 and 837). [see 1866-67, 1868-69, 1873 (b), 1874 (a), 1876-78, 1878 (b), 1896-97, 1897 Jan. 13, 1897 May 16, 1899-1900]

1877 JAN. 1 (A): At the time of **'Delhi Durbar'** held by Lord Lytton to declare Queen Victoria as 'Empress of India', an attempt was made to formulate a set of doctrines acceptable to all Indians – Hindus, Muslims, Christians and Parsis. **Swami Dayananda Saraswati, Sayed Ahmed Khan, Kesbah Chandra Sen** and others took part in the discussion. But it came to nothing. Swami Dayananda Saraswati held fast to the infallibility of Vedas.

1877 JAN. 4: Death of **Cornelius Vanderbilt** (b. 1794), U. S. business entrepreneur and financier, who made a fortune in the competitive steamboat business in the New York area after 1812.

He endowed Vanderbilt University [see 1876 (e)] At the time of his death Vanderbilt controlled many railroads and his fortune was estimated at $105 million, the bulk of which went to his son William Henry Vanderbilt (1821-1885)

1877 JUL. 9-16: The first **Wimbledon Tennis Tournament** was held.

There were 200 spectators at the first men's final staged on a slushy and slippery court and the entries for the first championship were just 22. At stake was a silver Challenge Cup worth 25 guineas, offered by the Proprietors of the daily, *The Field,* at the persuasion of its editor, J. H. Walsh. The players who were asked to "provide their own racquets and wear shoes without heels", were encouraged to play diagonally from corner to corner as the net was high at the ends and low in the centre. The rules of Major Walte C. Wingfield, British Army Officer, who is considered to be the inventor of this game, were used during the first championship.

The honour of staging the first championship was shared by J. H. Walsh along with three others – C. C. Heathcot, Julian Marshall and Henry Jones all men of eminence. The Challenge Cup, however, was won outright by William Renshaw, who was the undisputed Wimbledon King for a six-year spell from 1881 to 1886.

The first men's doubles was staged in Scotland and to Ireland goes the distinction of staging the first Women's championship in 1878. The number of entrants to the 1878 championships had swelled to 34 and after World War II, the All-England Club, which conducted the tournament, had outgrown itself.

1877 JUL. 16: The last and the eventful day of **Wimbledon tennis tournament.**

Spencer W. Gore, in the traditional attire of a British croquet player, entered the slippery court and his opponent Marshall served the first ball. The first set was over within 15 minutes, with Gore winning it at 6-1. The second set, won at 6-2 by Gore, lasted just 13 minutes and the third set too was won by Gore in 20 minutes (6-4). Thus emerged Wimbledon's first men's singles champion.

1877 SEP. 11: Birth of **Sir James Jeans** (d. 1946), English mathematician and physicist, who made important contributions to the development of quantum theory and to theoretical astrophysics especially to the theory of stellar structures.

1877 SEP: Hindu Muslim riots at Janjira.

The Muslims prevented Hindus from playing music in the public, during Ganapathi festival. This led to riots. Several disturbances took place. In some cases, Muslims took the offensive, entering Hindu houses and breaking idols. [see 1874 Feb. 13, 1885 (a), 1886 (c), 1889 (m), 1891 (b), 1893 (c), 1897 June]

1877 OCT. : **Joseph Lister** (1827-1912), British surgeon and medical scientist, who pioneered in the use of chemicals for the prevention of surgical infection, demonstrated conclusively that his method of **antisepsis** reduced danger from surgery. [see 1865 (c)]

1877 NOV. 29: **Thomas Alva Edison** (1847-1931), American inventor, demonstrated his most celebrated invention, the **phonograph.**

Edison's device used a tin-foil-covered drum which was hand cranked while a stylus traced a groove on it. The first recording ever made was of Edison's own voice reciting 'Mary had a little lamb'. His device was patented on 19th February 1878. Later, Edison improved his phonograph by substituting wax for tin-foil-coated cylinders, and by adding a loudspeaker to amplify the sounds produced by the diaphragm (1889-90). A decade later [see 1887 (g)] Emile Berliner (1851-1929), German-American inventor, carried out further improvements to the phonograph. [see 1864 (e), 1878 (h), 1882 (e), 1883 (d), 1889 (h), 1891 Dec. 29, 1893 (h)]

1877 (A) : After a private education in india, the young **Rabindranath Tagore** (1861-1941) was sent to England for prosecuting studies there.

He studied English literature for sometime under Henry Morley at the University College, London, and soon returned to India. While still quite young, he commenced writing for Bengali periodicals and in due course became the most highly gifted poet of renaissance of India. In 1913, he won the Nobel Prize for literature.

1877 (B): **Surendranath Banerjee** (1848-1925), the founder of **'The Indian Association',** toured India, propagating the message of unity. [see 1876 Jul. 26]

"The propagation tour of Surendranath Banerjee from one end of India to the other, constitutes a definite landmark in the history of India's political progress. It clearly demonstrated that in spite of differences in language, creed and social institutions, the people of this great sub-continent were bound by a common tie of ideals and interests, creating a sense of underlying unity which enabled them to combine for a common political objective. For the first time within living memory, or even historical tradition, there emerged the idea of India over and above the Congress of states and provinces, into which it was divided." (Bharatiya Vidya Bhavan's *History and Culture of the Indian People,* Vol. X, Part II, p. 502).

1877 (C): The **cystoscope** for examining the inside of the urinary bladder and introducing medication into the bladder was constructed by German Surgeon-urologist, **Max Nitz,** with the help from an instrument-maker named Leiter.

1877 (D): A loose-contact **telephone transmitter,** superior to Bell's telephone was developed by German-American inventor **Emile Berliner,** 26.

1877 (E): The germicidal qualities of **ultraviolet rays** were discovered by Englishmen **A. Downes** and **T. P. Blunt,** whose findings led to new techniques for sterilization.

1877 (F): Carl Gustav Patrick de Laval (1845-1913), Swedish engineer, invented a centrifugal **cream separator** which eliminated the need of space-consuming shallow pans and the labour of skimming the cream that rises to the top.

By reducing the cost of producing butter, Laval's invention led to a vast expansion of Danish, Dutch and Wisconsin butter industries.

1877-93: Sir Francis Galton (1822-1911), British social scientist, and **Karl Pearson** (1857-1936), British mathematician and one of the founders of modern statistics, developed the major **statistical tools** of present-day social science, e.g., regression (Galton, 1877), correlation coefficients (Galton, 1888), moments and standard deviation (Pearson, 1893) [see 1885 (f)]

1878 MAR. 14: The **Vernacular Press Act** was passed by Lord Lytton's Government in India.

Its object was to muzzle the newspapers in Indian languages which spread the message of nationality and the newly awakened sense of political consciousness.

Under the provisions of this Act, "the Government was given the power to work and to confiscate the plant, deposit, etc. in the event of the publication of undesirable matter." This "Gagging Act" did not permit any appeal against the orders of a Magistrate.

There was a strong opposition to this Act all over India, especially in Bengal where it was more strictly enforced. A large meeting was held in

Calcutta Town Hall, attended by about 5,000 persons to protest against the repressive measure and to appeal to the House of Commons for its repeal. The agitation was continued both in India and England till the Act was repealed by Lord Ripon in 1882.

1878 MAY 13: Death of **Joseph Henry** (b. 1797), U. S. Physicist, who devised and constructed the first **electromagnetic motor.**

1878 MAY 15: A band of Keshab Chandra Sen's followers who seceded from him due to differences, organized a new Samaj named **'Sadharan Brahmo Samaj',** under the leadership of Pandit Shivnath Shastri (1847-1925).

NARENDRATH (age 15 years) who had joined Brahmo Samaj, attracted by the magnetic personality of Keshab, identified himself with the new organization.

The founders of the new body framed a democratic constitution based on universal adult franchise. This new body proved to be the most powerful and active branch of the Brahmo Samaj.

1878 SEP. 20: *'The Hindu'* was founded in Madras, as a weekly by a group of six young men of Madras, all of them in their twenties, and still fresh from college.

They had little capital and no experience of running a newspaper. They all belonged to a Society called "The Triplicane Literary Society" which was then an important forum for native opinion and which they utilised to discuss current topics. What gave them the idea of starting a journal was the feeling that there was no Indian newspaper to represent Indian opinion. At the time *The Hindu* appeared on the scene public opinion in Madras Presidency was stagnant and there were very few recognized forum to voice the feelings and grievances of the Indian population. And when *The Hindu* made its appearance it became the sole representative of Indian opinion.

The first issue appeared on September 20, 1878, and was well received. On October 1, 1883, the Weekly was turned into tri-weekly and it became a daily from April 1, 1889, as it found that people who had been imbued with the new spirit of nationalism could not wait for two days to read the news of the day.

The Hindu had as its contemporaries two strong British-owned papers with whom it was to be in perpetual conflict for over two decades. They were *Madras Times* (Morning) and *The Madras Mail. The Madras Times,* founded in 1860 and the *Madras Mail* in 1867, were intended to protect and further the interests of the European community.

When Bipin Chandra Pal, who was later *The Hindu* correspondent in Calcutta, visited Madras in 1881, he found *The Hindu* had "already become a great power and an influence for good in that Presidency". He noted that during that period the emphasis of English educated people in India "was not on our respective provincialities but almost exclusively on India's national unity. And this helped *The Hindu* to be accepted from its very birth as an All-India paper even though it could not claim any large All-India circulation."

"The Birth of *The Hindu*", B. C. Pal said, "opened a new chapter in the history of Indo-English journalism not only in Madras but in some sense all over India. *The Hindu* was the first English journal owned and edited by Indians which represented the opinions and aspirations of the English educated community directly in Madras and indirectly of the other Indian provinces also."

1878 OCT. 16: Birth of **Vallathol Narayana Menon** (d. 1958), nationalist and versatile poet.

He was the best representative of the cultural renaissance in modern Kerala.

1878 (a): First publication *of Sayings of Ramakrishna, (Paramahamser Ukti)* by **Brahmo Samaj.**

Keshab Chandra Sen, the celebrated.Brahmo leader, and his colleagues heartily loved and respected **SRI RAMAKRISHNA** and were profoundly influenced by his life and teachings. Keshab, with a view to share with others the wisdom he learned from Sri Ramakrishna, disseminated from 1875 onwards the teachings of the Master through sermons from the pulpit, lectures from platform as well as through writings in the English and Bengali newspapers, such as *Sulabha Samachar, Sunday Mirror, Theistic Quarterly Review,* etc. Pratap Chandra Majumdar, Keshab's chief lieutenant and successor, wrote an excellent article on Sri Ramakrishna in the *Sunday Mirror* of 16th April, 1876. In that article Pratap Chandra writes how, in spite of his English education and culture, he was completely enchanted like many others by Sri Ramakrishna.

1878 (B): In the wake of a **severe famine in Deccan** (1876-77), the Indian Governor General, Lord Lytton, realized the need of deciding general principles of famine relief, and appointed a Commission for this purpose under the chairmanship of General Sir Richard Strachey.

Reporting in 1880, the Strachey Commission formulated some general principles of famine relief, and also suggested certain measures of a preventive or protective nature. It 'recognised to the full the obligation imposed on the state to offer to the necessitous the means of relief in times of famine.'

In the spirit of the recommendations of the Strachey Commission, a Provincial **Famine code** was framed in 1883 and the lines on which famine relief would be administered were determined. The principles of the famine code were put to a 'crucial test' in the famines in different parts of India that occurred in subsequent years.

In the wake of acute famines of 1896-97 and 1898-1900, another Commission was appointed, with Sir James Lyall ex lieutenant Governor of the Punjab, as its President. It conducted an elaborate enquiry into the causes of the famines and endorsed the principles enunciated by the Commission of 1880 suggesting certain changes in their acutal working. [see 1866-67, 1868-69, 1873 (b), 1874 (a), 1876-78, 1877 Jan. 1, 1896- 97, 1897 Jan. 13, 1897 May 16, 1899-1900]

1878 (C): The **worst famine** in history killed at least 10 million Chinese and possibly twice that number as drought continued in much of Asia as it had since 1876.

1878 (D): An **International Exhibition** was held at **Paris.**

The site of the exhibition covered 66 acres; more than 16 million people visited the exhibition to view 52,835 exhibits costing 55,400,000, Francs [see 1867 (f-1), 1900 Aug-Oct]

1878 (E): The world's first birth-control clinic was opened at Amsterdam by Dutch Suffragist leader **Aletta Jacobs** 29, who was the first woman physician to practise in Holland.

1878 (F): Conflict of **refigious fundamentalism** and the new scientific attitude reflected in dismissal of American geologist Alexander Winchell from Methodist-sponsored Vanderbilt University (U. S. A.) for scientific contradiction of Biblical Chronology.

1878 (G): Birth of **Glenn Curtiss** (d. 1930), American aviation pioneer, who developed the first successful sea-plane and manufactured the famous World War I Jenny training plane.

1878(H): **Thomas Alva Edison**, American inventor, produced **the first incandescent lamp,** fore-runner of the electric light bulb.

In this lamp, which produced a glow for 45 hours, Edison had used a filament made from a length of carbonised sewing thread, mounted on an evacuated glass tube. Earlier he had tried filament of platinum, carbonized paper, bamboo thread, and thousands of other substances before finding the solution in a loop of cotton thread.

On December 31, 1879, Edison gave the first public demonstration of his incandescent lamp. It was patented the following year. In 1878,

Edison also worked out methods for cheap production and transmission of electrical current and succeeded in subdividing current to make it adaptable to household use. [see 1864 (e), 1877 Nov. 29, 1882 (e), 1883 (d), 1889 (h), 1891 Dec. 29, 1893 (h)]

1878 (I): **William Crookes** (1832-1919), English chemist and physicist, devised **'Cathode Ray Tube'** (Crookes Tube) with the help of which the radiation could be more efficiently studied.

Crookes showed that cathode rays proceed in straight lines, and are capable of turning a small wheel, can be deflected by a magnet, excite fluorescence in certain substances, and heat and sometimes even melt some metals.

In 1897 Karl Ferdinand Braun (1850-1918), German physicist, modified Crooke's cathode-ray tube, so that the spot of green fluorescence shifted in accordance with the electromagnetic field set up by a varying current. Thus was invented the Oscillograph by means of which time variation in electric currents could be studied and which was the first step, as it turned out, towards television .

1878 (J): The first commercial milking machines were produced at Auburn, New York, by **Albert Durant,** who introduced the machine invented by L. O. Colvin.

1878 (K): **J. W. Gibbs** (1839-l903), American mathematical physicist, in his rigorously mathematical thermodynamic study *On the Equilibrium of Heterogeneous Substances,* used the concept of chemical potential and introduced the phase rule.

His pioneering work in statistical mechanics laid the basis for the development of physical chemistry as science. [see 1902 (e)]

1879 JAN. 28: The first commercial **telephone exchange** opened at **New Haven,** Conn., U. S. A.

The exchange had 21 subscribers and after 6 weeks it operated at night as well as during the day. A telephone exchange was also opened at Manchester, London.

1879 FEB. 13: Birth of **Smt. Sarojini Naidu** (d. 1949), the Indian poetess and nationalist leader, who became famous after her 3 small volumes of verses, published between 1905 and 1917, won critical acclaim in England.

She was the first woman President of the Indian National Congress.

1879 MAR. 14: Birth of **Albert Einstein** (d. 1955), German physicist, who revolutioniz ed the science of physics by his theory of relativity.

He had the distinction of being recognized in his lifetime as one of the most creative minds in the history of mankind.

When in 1939, the potentialities of atomic fission were recognized, it was Einstein who, urged by other leading physicists, wrote to President Roosevelt, explaining the need for immediate investigation of its possible application to weapons of destruction. In a letter, he informed the President of the possibility of building an 'extremely powerful' new weapon. It was the first move towards the development of Atomic Bomb; and in 1945 the bomb proved his theories about matter and energy which he had published in 1905 and 1916.

1879 NOV. 5: Death of **James Clerk Maxwell** (b. 1831), Scottish Physicist, remembered for his great researches in electricity.

He formulated important mathematical expressions describing electric and magnetic phenomenon and postulated the identity of light as an electromagnetic action. His work on **electricity and magnetism** constitutes his supreme achievement. [see 1864 (f), 1873 (f)]

1879 NOV. 12: Birth of **C. P. Ramaswamy Aiyer**, statesman, educationist and an eminent lawyer.

As a Diwan of the erstwhile Travancore, he was responsible for the famous Temple Entry Proclamation of 10 November, 1936, opening the temples of the Kerala State to Harijans, showing the way to the rest of India.

1879 NOV. 25: Birth of **Sadhu T. L. Vaswani** (d. 1966), popularly known as 'Dada' who longed to dedicate his life to the service of God and His suffering children.

Under his ever-loving guidance and inspiration a number of humanitarian activities were initiated at Poona.

Sadhu Vaswani was one of India's representatives to the Welt Congress, the World Congress of Religions held at Berlin (1910). His speeches there and his subsequent lectures in different parts of Europe aroused deep interest in Indian thought and religion and linked many with him in India's mission of help and healing. The Mira Movement in Education founded by him in 1933 attempts at enriching students with vital truths of modern life and at the same time, making them lover of the Indian ideal and India's culture, at once idealistic and spiritual.

1879 DEC. 21: Birth of **Joseph Stalin** (d. 1953), leader of the Communist Party of the Soviet Union and the dictator of the U. S. S. R.

1879 DEC. 30: Birth of **Ramana Maharshi** (d. 1950), 'The sage of Arunachala' whose original contribution to yogic philosophy is the technique of 'self-enquiry' (*Atma-vichara*), that is knowing oneself (one's true nature) through the enquiry 'who am I?'

1879 (A): NARENDRANATH who was sixteen, passed the Entrance Examination and entered the Presidency College of Calcutta for higher education.

He had grown up into a handsome young man, possessing presence of mind, keen intelligence and prodigious memory, a passion for truth and devotion to purity in thought, word and deed.

Calcutta, the metropolis of British India then, was under the deluge of Westernization. The educated youths were turning agnostic and losing faith in their hoary cultural heritage. Christian missionaries criticized Hindu beliefs most unjustly while preaching the message of Jesus Christ. They preached in the market places and to the passers by at the street corners. They distributed hundreds of copies of Bible among English reading people for leisurely perusal. The *padres* (clergymen) publicly decried bathing in the Ganges, worshipping of images and other Hindu religious customs as meaningless superstitions. The missionaries carried on their fanatical tirade in season and out of season, but the public dared not fight them as they belonged to the ruling race, and were patronized by the rulers. Young Narendranath, however, one day boldly faced a *padre* who was abusing Hinduism and challenged him. In this context, Mahendranath Datta (1869-1956), Narendranath's younger brother, writes: "The few religious books that were available in those days are related to the life of Jesus Christ. Taking advantage of this, the Christian missionaries would stand up at the road-crossings, or in the market places and preach. Every Sunday morning one could see Bengali *padres* standing near Hedo (Cornwallis Square, now re-named Azad Bagh) preaching Christianity and abusing Hindu gods and goddesses. One day my brother (Narendranath) was passing that way at 9 a.m. He listened to them for a while and then engaged himself in a heated discussion with them. The discussion developed into a quarrel, in which passers by joined, ranging themselves on the two sides, till a riot was apprehended. Both sides eventually calmed down, and the crowd dispersed. The Christian missionaries fanned themselves out in all directions, their ranks being swelled on account of natives who had been converted to Christianity collaborating with them. They misrepresented, vilified and ridiculed the Hindu faith without let or hindrance. They said – bathing in the Ganges was sinful, bathing after besmearing the body with mustard oil (as Bengalis even now, specially in winter frequently do, and more frequently did in those days) was a superstitious practice, and even to shave the beard was a superstitious practice. So we gave up shaving. They said – everything that the Hindus

have, everything that they do is synonymous with superstition, the only
things which are in accordance with reason were what they themselves
said. Few people in those days knew what Hinduism was, or its essential
is; fewer still had read the scriptures, which were rarely available in those
days. Hence, people found it difficult to refute the arguments of the
missionaries. It was risky also to enter into arguments with them; so
people did not dare argue with them. Such courage as Narendranath
showed when he had an argumentation with the *padres* near Hedo was
indeed rarely to be met with. We feared the missionaries and had no
respect for them – they were capable of doing any mischief to those
who they fancied were their opponents," (*A Comprehensive Biography
of Swami Vivekananda,*   Part I, p. 62 and 64). Mahendranath Datta
narrates this incident while giving an account of the conditions of social
life in Calcutta at the time of Narendranath's early youth.

On another occasion, a certain *padre* in the course of his preaching
threw a clincher at the Hindu audience, "What can your idol do if I strike
it with my stick?" he asked. An enraged listener promptly retorted,
"What could your Christ do when he was crucified?" The evangelical
crusade of the missionaries gave rise in Bengal to a general feeling that
'The *padres* had come to destroy our caste and religion'. This cultural
invasion had an appalling effect on the mind of the subject race.

1879 (B): Lectures delivered by **W. Adam** on '*suttee*' at Boston, U. S. A.,
in 1838, were printed and published at Calcutta by G. P. Roy and Co.

The following extract from the book spot-lights the custom of *suttee*
which seems to have been prevalent more in Bengal than elsewhere:
"The extent to which human life was annually sacrificed may be estimated
from the returns made by the police to the Bengal Government for a
single year. Those returns show that in the year 1823, the number of
widows who burned on the funeral piles of their husbands within the
Bengal Presidency was, of the brahmin caste 234, of the kshatriya caste
35, of the vaishya caste 14, of the shudra caste 292, total 575. Of this
total, 340 widows perished thus within the limits of the Calcutta court
of circuit, which shows that the returns were given with accuracy only
for the immediate neighbourhood of Calcutta, and suggests the inference
that the number sacrificed beyond that limit was much greater than that
actually reported, besides that the returns profess to extend only to the
Bengal Presidency, leaving entirely out of view the two other Indian
Presidencies where, although the practice was certainly not so prevalent
as in Bengal, it was by no means wholly unknown. The ages of the
different individuals are also included in the returns to which I have
referred and they exhibit another feature of this horrible picture. Of these
575 victims of 1823, 109 were above sixty years of age, 226 were from
forty to sixty, 208 were from twenty to forty, and 32 were under twenty

years of age. Thus the tenderness and beauty of youth, the ripened years and affection of the venerable matron, and the feebleness and decripitude of old age alike fell victims."

1879 (C): The Church of Christ, Scientist, was founded at Boston, U. S. A., by **Mrs. Mary Baker Eddy** (1820-1910) to propagate the spiritual and metaphysical system of **Christian Science.**

In 1866 Mrs. Eddy suffered a fall on the ice in Lynn, Mass.; and was carried home seriously injured. Shortly afterwards, she read a passage of the Bible in which Christ spiritually healed a man afflicted with palsy and she enjoyed a similar immediate recovery. Out of her own experience came the basic tenets of the Christian Science – that man is a spiritual being made in God's likeness, while all forms of sickness are illusions to be corrected through spiritual education and understanding. Mrs. Eddy saw her recovery as a result of a fusion of spiritual and mental powers; she had previously observed faith healing in her role as a patient and later assistant to a mesmerist.

Earlier Mrs. Eddy had published the main text of the movement, *Science and Health,* in 1875; In 1883 she established the *Christian Science Journal* for the education of members. The movement has successfully established branches in many parts of the world.

"The salient features of Christian Science have been depicted in her book, *Science and Health.* Mrs. Eddy was mostly influenced by the book, *Song Celestial* which is the English translation of the *Bhagavad Gita* by Sir Edwin Arnold, and also by the English translation of the *Bhagavad Gita* by Charles Wilkins, published in London in 1785, and in New York in 1867. Mrs. Eddy quoted certain passages from the English edition of the *Bhagavad Gita,* but unfortunately, for some reason, those passages of the *Gita* were omitted in the 34th edition of the book, *Science and Health.* If we closely study Mrs. Eddy's book, *Science and Health,* we find that Mrs. Eddy has incorporated in her book most of the salient features of Vedanta philosophy, but she denied the debt flatly." – *The Philosophical Ideas of Swami Abbedananda,* by Swami Prajnanananda, p. 164.

"In the earliest edition of *Science and Health,* Mrs. Eddy had the courage to quote certain passages from one of the most authentic books of the Vedanta philosophy, thus herself acknowledging the harmony that exists between the basic principles of the Vedanta philosophy and Christian Science. Unfortunately, for some reason, since the publication of the 34th edition, these passages have been omitted." – Swami Abhedananda, vide *Complete Works of Swami Abhedananda,* (Vol. II, p. 223.) [see 1886 (o), 1894 Mar. 9, 1894 Sept. 25]

1879 (D): **Sri Aurobindo** (1872-1950), was sent to England with his brother for higher education to prepare for the **Indian Civil Service.** [see 1893 Feb. (a)]

1879 (E): India had a poor crop and much of the harvest was consumed by rats which plagued many districts in the following two years and which consumed a significant portion of the nation's grain stores.

1879 (G): An **International Exposition** was held at **Sydney.**

The site of the exposition covered 15 acres; more than one million people visited the exposition to view, 9,345 exhibits costing £ 313,987.

1879 (H): Birth of **C. Rajagopalachari** (d.1972), prominent Indian nationalist leader and the first Governor General of Independent India.

1879 (I): U. S. electrical wizard **Elmer Amrose Sperry,** 19, invented an improved **dynamo** and a new type of **arc lamp.**

1879 (J): The **gonococcus bacterium** *"Neisseria Gonorrhea"* that transmits the venereal infection gonorrhea was discovered by German physician **Albert Ludwig Siegmund Neisser.**

1879 (K): **John Philip Holland** (1841-1914), U. S. inventor, built the first **submarine** which operated submerged successfully. [scc 1900 (g)]

1879 (L): The **multiple switchboard** invented by U. S. engineer **Leroy B. Firman** made the telephone a commercial success and helped increase the number of U. S. Telephone subscribers from 50,000 in 1880 to 250,000 in 1890.

1879 (M): **Saccharin,** a non-caloric, non-nutritive sweetener, was discovered accidentally at Baltimore's New John Hopkins University by Chemist **Ira Remsen,** 33, and his German student **Constantin Fahlberg** who were investigating the reactions of a class of coal tar derivates.

They published a scientific description of the new compound in February 1880, calling special attention to its sweetness (in dilute solution, saccharin is 500 to 700 times sweeter than cane sugar).

1879 (N): **Percy Gilchrist** (1851-1935), and **Sidney G. Thomas** (1850- 1885), two British inventors, developed a method for making **steel** from phosphoric iron ores, thereby doubling in effect the world's potential steel production.

1879 (O): **L. F. Nilson** (1840-1899), Swedish chemist, discovered a hitherto unknown element, which he named **scandium.**

1879 (P): **Per Teodor Cleve** (1840-1905), Swedish chemist and geologist, discovered two new elements among the rare earth minerals – **thulium** and **holmium.**

1879 (Q): **Samarium,** a metallic element belonging to the rare-earth group, was discovered by a French Chemist, **L. De. Boisbaudran** (1838-1912).

In 1886 he separated dysprosium – another new element, from crude holmium.

1879 (R): **William Whitney** (1827-1894), American linguist and one of the foremost Sanskrit scholars of his time, brought out *Sanskrit Grammar* which is a classic work that has remained unrivalled for completeness and clarity. [see 1884 (d)]

1879 (S): **Electricity** was used to draw a **railroad locomotive** for the first time at Berlin.

1879 (T): The British who, along with Dutch, had already taken over and annexed (1843) portion of Zulu territory in South Africa, confronted the Zulu People of the Bantu tribes with a view to conquer them completely.

The Zulus strongly resisted the British encroachment. In the course of this **Zulu war,** the British breachloading rifles killed some 8000 Zulu warriors and wounded more than 16,000. Despite stiff resistance, the British defeated the poorly armed Zulus in July 1879, occupied the remainder of their country and divided Zululand into 13 separate kingdoms. Thus ended the Zulu nation founded by Zulu leader Shaka (ruled 1816-1828) in 1916. In 1887 Zululand (now part of South Africa) became a British crown colony.

1879 (U): At the University of Leipzig, **Wilhelm Max Wundt** (1832-1920), German psychologist, established the **first laboratory** to be devoted entirely to **experimental psychology**, thus bringing the human being into the realm of science.

He also founded in 1881 the first journal to be devoted to the subject. From Wundt's monumental work *Fundamentals of Physiological Psychology* flowed the various movements that had significant effects on education in the 20th century.

Among Wundt's pupils was the American psychologist and philosopher, William James, often considered the father of Amercan psychology of education. In 1878 he established the first course in psychology in the United States and in 1890 he pioneered physiological psychology in the *Principles of Psychology* [see 1890 (h)]. In this famous book James argued that man should be thought as a living organism with instinctive tendencies to react with his environment. A child's mind, therefore, is that aspect of his being that enables him to adapt to the world, and the purpose of education is to organize the child's powers of conduct so as to fit him to his social and physical environment. Interests must be awakened and broadened as the natural starting points of institution. Religious study absorbed James from 1893 to 1903 and produced *The Varieties of Religious Experience* (1902) [see 1901 (1), 1902 (b)].

1879-83: **War of Pacific** fought between Bolivia, Chile and Peru for control of the nitrate-producing fields in the Atacama desert where the three states meet.

The war ended on April 4, 1883, with the treaty of Valparaiso that deprived Bolivia of access to the sea. Victorious Chile gained the Peruvian province of Tarpaca in the treaty of Ancona, and she gained Bolivian territories that are rich in nitrates.

1880 MAR. 4: The first **photographic reproduction** in a newspaper appeared in the *New York Daily Graphic*.

The picture of a shanty-town was printed from a half-tone produced by photographing through a fine screen with dots in the photograph through representing shadows.

1880 MAY 8: Death of **Gustav Flaubert** (b. 1821), French novelist, whose work constitutes an epoch in the history of the art of fiction.

1880 SEP. 13: The first **Employer's Liability Act** passed by the British Parliament, made mandatory on the part of the employers to pay compensation to injured workers or if they died, to their relations.

1880 (A): **Sir William Hunter** (1840-1900), British Publicist, who was asked by the Governor General of India (in 1869) to submit a scheme for a comprehensive statistical survey of the Indian empire, observed that '40 million Indian population go through life on insufficient food.'

Sir Charles Elliot (1862-1931), British Colonial official, wrote (1887) that 'half of our agricultural population never know from year's end to year's end what it is to have their hunger fully satisfied.'

economic enquiry ordered by Lord Dufferin in 1887 to 'ascertain the truth behind the general assertion that the greater proportion of the population of India suffer from daily insufficiency of food' confirmed the correctness of the view expressed by the two officers.

1880 (B): **Sir Jagdish Chandra Bose** (1858-1937), Indian physicist and plant physiologist, went to the University of London to study medicine. [see 1894 (a), 1900 Aug-Oct, 1900 Jul. 8, 1902 Jul. 9]

1880 (C): An **International Exposition** was held at **Melbourne.**

The site of the exposition covered 20 acres, more than one million people visited the exposition to view 12,792 exhibits costing £ 330,330.

1880 (D): The **bacillus of typhoid fever** *(Eberthella typhi)* was identified simultaneously by German bacteriologist **Karl Joseph Eberth** 45, and **Robert Koch.**

1880 (E): **Adolf Von Baeyer** (1835-1917), German Chemist, did **research on Indigo** and succeeded in preparing it artificially.

He received Nobel Prize in Chemistry in 1905.

1880 (F): **Alexander Graham Bell** (1847-1922), Scottish-American physicist and inventor, invented **photophone,** an instrument for transmitting sound by vibrations in a beam of light. On June 3, the first wireless telephone message was transmitted by Bell on his photophone. [see 1873 Mar. 3, 1892 (m)]

1880 (G): **John Milne** (1850-1913), British geologist, developed the first accurate **seismograph,** permitting the careful study of earthquakes and opening the way to new knowledge of the earth's interior.

1880 (H): **J. C. G. Marignac** discovered a metallic element belonging to the rare earth group. He gave it the name **godolinium.**

1880-81: **Boer Struggle** for Independence in **South Africa.**

Led by Paul Kruger (1825-1904), South African statesman, the descendants of Dutch settlers at Transvaal and Orange Free States known as Boers, rose against the British in an attempt to regain the independence they had previously given up in return for protection against the danger from Zulus. In a brief war, the British were defeated on February 27th, 1881, and Boers were restored independence under the British suzerainity. Kruger became the President of the Boer Republic.

1880-84: **Lord Rippon** (1827-1909), the Viceroy of India.

1881 JAN. 25: **Kesbah Chandra Sen,** the celebrated Brahmo leader, who had assimilated the universal teachings of **SRI RAMAKRISHNA** for nearly two years proclaimed his new creed which he called **'New Dispensation'** *(Nava Vidhana).* It signified the harmony of religions, and was fundamentally, a presentation of Sri Ramakrishna's teachings – as far as Keshab was able to understand them.

In this regard Swami Vivekananda wrote later on: " ....A strong and deep love grew between the two, and Keshab's whole life became changed, till, a few years later, he proclaimed his views of religion as the New Dispensation, which was nothing but a partial representation of the truths which Ramakrishna had taught for a long time."

The main principles of New Dispensation, enunciated by Keshab, are: a) Harmony of all scriptures, saints and sects; b) Harmony of reason and faiths, of devotion and duty, of yoga and bhakti; c) The Church of the Samaj stands for One Supreme God, to be worshipped without form. No idolatry in any form may enter the precincts of the Church; and d) the Church stands for Universal Brotherhood without distinction of caste or creed or sect.

In order to illustrate the idea of the harmony of all religions and of the part played by Ramakrishna in introducing it to Keshab Chandra Sen, a pupil of his caused to be painted a symbolical picture in which a Christian Church, a Mohammedan Mosque, and a Hindu Temple appear in the background, while on one side, in front, Ramakrishna is pointing out to Keshab a group in which Christ and Cliaitanya are dancing together and a Mohammedan, a Confucianist, a Sikh, a Parsi, an Anglican, and various Hindus are standing around, each carrying a symbol of his faith.

1881 JAN. 28: Death of **Fedor Dostoevski** (b. 1821), Russian writer, who was one of the greatest novelists of all times. [see 1866 (f)]

1881 FEB. 5: Death of **Thomas Carlyle** (b. 1795), British essayist, historian and philosopher.

A leading social critic of early Victorian England, Carlyle preached against materialism and mechanism during the industrial revolution.

1881 APR 19: Death of **Benjamin Disrael** (b. 1804), English statesman and the leader of the Conservative Party. He served as Prime Minister of England in 1868 and from 1874 to 1880.

1881 AUG. 16: Birth of **Sir Alexander Fleming** (d. 1955), Scottish bacteriologist, best known for his discovery of penicillin.

His discovery, which paved the way for antibiotic therapy for infectious diseases, has been hailed as "the greatest contribution medical science ever made to humanity."

1881: NARENDRANATH heard of his future Master, **SRI RAMAKRISHNA,** for the first time from **Professor William Hastie,** the great scholar and the then Principal of the General Assembly's Institution (now known as the Scottish Church College) at Calcutta, where Narendranath was studying in F. A. Class.

Prof. Hastie introduced Sri Ramakrishna by way of an illustration to bring home the concept of 'a momentary trance' in Wordsworth's poem 'Excursion'. The Professor said, "Such an experience is the result of purity of mind and concentration on some particular object and it is rare indeed, particularly in these days. I have seen only one person who has experienced that blessed state of mind, and he is Ramakrishna Paramahamsa of Dakshineswar. You can understand if you go there and see for yourself."

Prof. Hastie, an Englishman, regarded the culture of India with unusual reverence and understanding. He also had the distinction of being one of the very few non-Indians who had met Sri Ramakrishna. He was once moved to remark, "Narendranath is really a genius. I have travelled far and wide, but I have never yet come across a lad of his talents and possibilities, even in German Universities, amongst philosophical students. He is bound to make his mark in life!"

1881 NOV. : NARENDRANATH, who was preparing for the final F. A. Examination of the Calcutta University met **SRI RAMAKRISHNA** for the first time at the house of **Surendranath Mitra,** a lay devotee of Sri Ramakrishna, who had asked Narendranath to, treat the audience to devotional songs, on the occasion of the saint's visit to his house. It served as a prelude to the 'historic meeting' of the two at Dakshineswar.

1881 DEC. : NARENDRANATH, who was eighteen years of age and had been in college two years, met **SRI RAMAKRISHNA** at Dakshineswar.

'It was a historic meeting of two great souls, the Prophet of Modern India and the carrier of his message.'

Nurtured in English education and European thought, Narendranath had turned agnostic. He had approached some religious luminaries of his time but none could speak of God to him with the authority that comes of direct experience. At last he came to Sri Ramakrishna and asked him straight the question, "Have you seen God?" "Not only have I seen God but I can also show him to you: I see him more intensely than I see you," came the spontaneous and unequivocal reply from the great seer. Astonished and awed beyond words by his revelations, Narendranath surrendered himself to this prophet of God. At last, he had found one who could assure him from his own experience that God existed. His doubts dispelled, and the meeting proved a turning point in the life of young Narendranath. At the second meeting with Sri Ramakrishna, Narendranath underwent a mystical experience at the touch of the Master.

1881 (A): The first synchronous census was conducted in India. According to this census, community-wise, Hindus were 74.32 per cent of the total population of India; Muslims 19.74 per cent, Christians 0.73 per cent and others 5.21 percent.

The census committee consisting of W. C. Plowdin (President) with H. Beverley and W. R. Cornish as members, set up in 1877 had submitted a detailed report on 29th January 1878, on the conduct of a general census in India in 1881. This report paved the way for the first synchronous census in India in 1881. From then onwards, India has had regular synchronous census every ten years. The census of India has been providing an uninterrupted chain of demographic data on the people of India ever since 1881. [see 1872 (b), 1891 (a), 1901 (c)]

1881 (B): Rendition of Mysore.

The decision had been hanging fire since 1868, when the Original Ruler, whose maladministration was the ostensible cause of the introduction of British administration in the State, had passed away. The alarm caused in the minds of the Princes by the action against the Ruler of Baroda and the failure of the Imperial Durbar to quieten that alarm, led to a final decision by which Mysore was restored to its legitimate sovereign. The British, however, continued to assert their right of interference in the internal affairs of the State.

1881 (C): The U. S. **Population** reached 53 million, Great Britain had 29.7 million, Ireland 5.1, Germany 45.2, France 37.6, Italy 28.4., India had a population of some 265 million, up from 203.4 million in 1850.

1881 (D): Death of **James Kamp Starley,** inventor of the sewing machine.

He also designed the bicycle that had wheels 30 inches in diameter with solid rubber tyres, a chain driven rear wheel.

1881 (E): U. S. President **Garfield's assassination,** the second in 15 years, followed that of the Russian Czar (Alexander II) by less than 16 weeks.

1881 (F): Formation of the **American Institute of Christian Philosophy** in New York represented an attempt to integrate science with the Bible by the dissemination of appropriate literature.

1881 (G): Edward Hale (1822-1909), American clergyman and author, brought out the revised edition of *The Age of Fable* (1855) written by **Thomas Bulfinch** (1796-1867).

This book was for decades a very popular family and school book in America and its material on Hindu mythology and Budhism fascinated thousands of readers who were far from being erudite scholars. In the revised edition, Edward Hale included a part of the chapter on Hinduism from *Ten Great Religions* (2 Vols. 1871-1873) written by the unitarian minister, theologian and author, **James Freeman Clarke** (1810-1888). [see 1871 (e)].

1881 (H): Herbert Spencer (1820-1903), British philosopher, sociologist, and educationist who pioneered evolutionary theory brought out his work: *Descriptive Sociology.*

In 1890s he returned to philosophical writing in which his influence on individualism, pacifism, and biological thinking was profound and worldwide. In his day, his works were important in popularizing the concept of evolution and played an important part in the development of economics, political science, biology and philosophy.

1881 (I): Scottish bacteriologist **Jaime Ferran** discovered serum effective against **Cholera.**

1881 (J): The **pneumococcus bacterium** that caused pneumonia was found by U. S. Army bacteriologist-physician **George Miller Sternberg.**

1881 (K): Louis Pasteur (1822-1895), French Chemist, made **vaccine for anthrax** and proved its value in a sensational public demonstration on sheep and goats.

1882 JAN. 30: Birth of **Franklin D. Roosevelt** (d. 1945), U. S. Statesman and 32nd President.

He led the American people through the grave economic crisis of 1930s and through the Second World War. Before he died, he cleared the way for peace, including establishment of the United Nations.

1882 MAR. 24: Robert Koch (1843-1910), German physician and bacteriologist and Nobel Prize Winner in Medicine (1905), made a most remarkable discovery of **tubercle bacillus,** the causative factor of the dreaded disease tuberculosis.

He devised many bacteriological techniques and established the bacterial causes of a number of infectious diseases. One of the first diseases Koch studied was anthrax, an ancient and highly fatal cattle disease. He discovered the bacterial origin of anthrax in 1876, and developed a preventive inoculation against it in 1883. Within about a decade a whole series of specific pathogens – including the causal agents of cholera, typhoid fever and diphtheria; common pyogenic bacteria which caused suppuration in wounds; and varieties of intestinal flora – were isolated by Koch and others.

1882 MAR. 24 (A): Death of **H. W. Longfellow** (b. 1807), the most popular of U. S. Poets in the 19th century.

The well-known stanza of his poem *A Psalm of Life* is:

"Lives of great men all remind us
We can make our lives subline,
And, departing, leave behind us,
Footprints on the sands of time."

1882 APR. 19: Death of **Charles Darwin** (b.1809), British Naturalist renowned for his documentation of evolution and for a theory of its operation. His influence on the scientific and religious tenor of his time was immense and provocative.

After a five-year sea-voyage (1831-1836) involving detailed observations of different animals and fossils at the West Coast of South America and some Pacific Islands, he was convinced of the gradual evolution of species; and after 20 years' careful research in England, he brought out his findings in his monumental work: *Origin of Species* (1859) [see 1871 (c)] wherein he soundly established the theory of organic evolution. Within a few years this book set off a great philosophical debate. Darwin's meticulously researched theory that present species are evolved from extinct ones, that species that survive are those that can adapt to changing environment and that man and ape share a common ancestor represented a direct challenge to the Biblical interpretation of creation. Because Darwin's theory cast doubt upon the Biblical account of the origin of man (as found in the *Book of Genesis),* theological conservatives abhorred it and sought to combat it through all available means, including suppression. However Darwin's theory of natural selection finally won the day and when he died he was buried in Westminster Abbey.

While scientists in general embraced Darwinism, the liberal Protestant clergymen and philosophers sought a philosophical synthesis between evolution and Christianity. Today scientists remain almost unanimous, in their acceptance of Darwin's basic thesis, modified by recent discoveries in genetics.

1882 APR. 27: Death of **Ralph Waldo Emerson** (b.1803), U. S. Essayist, poet and philosopher. He was the most thought-provoking American cultural leader of the mid-19th century.

Emerson was one of the earliest Americans to introduce Indian thought into America. He was for a number of years a neighbour of Thoreau, an ardent 'Asiatist' whose great work, *A Week on the Concord and Merrimack Rivers,* is an enthusiastic eulogy of the *Bhagavad Gita,* and of other great Indian poems and philosophies.

Shortly after the death of his wife in 1832, Emerson resigned his post as a minister of the Unitarian Church in Boston and left for Europe. While in England, Emerson met T. Carlyle, the British social critic and historian. It was Carlyle who made a parting gift – the English translation of the *Bhagavad Gita,* to his friend. He read the classic thoroughly which left a profound influence on his mind. The Unitarian Church adopted in great measure the philosophical thoughts of Emerson.

A copy of the first English translation of the *Bhagavad Gita* has been carefully preserved in Concord, Massachussets, where Emerson lived his last years.

1882 MAY 20: **The St. Gothard Tunnel** (9.25 miles) opened in **Switzerland,** was the first of the great railway tunnels through the Alps.

1882 MAY: **Max Muller** delivered a course of lectures before the University of Cambridge in which he expressed his idea of India and the Hindu religion most succinctly and clearly.

In the very first of the lectures to which he gave the title, *'What can India teach us?'* Max Muller said: "If we are asked under what sky the human mind has most fully developed some of its choicest gifts, has most deeply pondered on the greatest problems of life, and has found solutions of some of them which well deserve the attention even of those who have studied Plato and Kant – I should point out to India. And if I were to ask myself from what literature we, here in Europe, we, who have been nurtured almost exclusively on the thoughts of Greeks and Romans, and of one Semetic race, the Jewish, may draw that corrective which is most wanted in order to make our inner life more perfect, more comprehensive, more universal, in fact more truly human, a life, not for this life only, but a transfigured and eternal life – again I should point to India."

1882 JUN. 2: Death of **Giuseppe Garibaldi** (b. 1801), an important Italian patriot and liberator.

His most spectacular achievement was in 1860, when the nationalists were busy unifying the small states of Northern Italy. He was the key military figure in the creation of the Kingdom of Italy. An unflagging foe of all tyranny, he devoted his life to fighting oppression.

1882 JUL. 11: **Alexandria** was **bombarded** by the British forces and subsequently occupied by them as a prelude to the occupation of Egypt itself.

1882 AUG. 1: Birth of **Purushottamdas Tandon** (d. 1962), Indian nationalist leader.

1882 AUG. 5: SRI RAMAKRISHNA (1836-1886), the saint of Dakshineswar met **Pandit Ishwarchandra Vidyasagar** (1820-1898), the Indian educationist and social reformer, at the latter's residence in Calcutta.

The Pundit was far-famed for his great scholarship. But even greater than his scholarship was his compassion for suffering humanity. Sri Ramakrishna had heard about Vidyasagar's rare qualities since his boyhood and was naturally attracted towards him. The Pundit, though learned, was yet a humble man. Well-known for his philanthropic acts, he could not but be moved by the saint of Dakshineswar. Sri Ramakrishna's spiritual ecstasies and talks made a deep impression on him.

1882 DEC. 11: Birth of **Max Born** (d. 1970), German Physicist, who made most outstanding contribution to modern physics in showing the inherently probable nature of the basic laws of quantum mechanics.

In 1954 he received the Nobel Prize for physics.

1882 DEC. 11 (A): Birth of **Mahakavi Subramania Bharati** (d. 1921), Indian revolutionary poet.

1882 DEC. 28: Birth of **Arthur S. Eddington** (d. 1944), English Astronomer, who greatly advanced theoretical astrophysics as a consequence of his original contributions to the theory of relativity and his studies on the internal constitution of stars.

1882 (A): Bankim Chandra Chatterjee (1838-1894), Bengali novelist, wrote his best-known novel, *Anandmath*.

It contained the famous hymn *'Vande Mataram'*, which inspired the people to sacrifice all for their motherland. It later became the *mantra* and slogan in India's struggle for independence. It charged the whole of India with patriotic emotion.

1882 (B): The University of Punjab was established.

The University of Allahabad came five years later, meeting the needs of Northern and Central India. The three Universities of Calcutta, Madras and Bombay were founded in 1857. Schools and Colleges multiplied rapidly thereafter in India.

Western education was introduced in India after Macaulay's Minutes on Education (1835) had come as a corollary to the policy of admitting Indians to the administration under the Charter Act of 1833. Macaulay believed that English education was sure to destroy the faith of the young students in their past. He, therefore, strongly recommended the introduction of English education. In this context he wrote (12 Oct.,

1836) to his father: "Our English Schools are flourishing wonderfully. It is my firm belief that if our plans of education are followed up, there will not be a single idolator (Hindu) among the respectable classes in Bengal thirty years hence. And this will be effected without efforts to proselytize; without the smallest interference with religious liberty; merely by the natural operation of knowledge and reflection." [see 1876 (i)]

English education brought to India political ideas of the West along with knowledge of Western Science. These ideas produced the great intellectual ferment of the 19th Century. They ultimately found political expression in the national awakening of the eighties.

1882 (C): **John D. Rockefeller** (1839-1937), American industrialist, philanthropist and the founder of Standard Oil Company (1870), created **America's first great 'Trust'.** It had a capital of about 70 million dollars and was the world's largest and richest industrial organization.

1882 (D): The **'Indian Education Commission'** was appointed by the Government of India, in the wake of an agitation started by the Christian missionaries who complained that the Government Schools were competing with missionary schools to such an extent that the latter was threatened with extinction.

The missionaries also held that the educational institutions of Government were "secular", that is, "Godless" or heathen. Such Schools were positively harmful and, therefore, the Bible must be taught in all the Government schools in India. If this were not possible on political grounds, they argued that the Government should withdraw from direct educational enterprise and leave them the field clear for the mission schools.

1882 (E): **Thomas Alva Edison** (1847-1931) developed the world's first **public electricity system.**

He designed and installed the first large central power station on Pearl Street in New York; its steam-driven generators of 900 Horse Power provided enough power for 7,200 lamps; Edison also designed the first English power station, which was opened in Holborn, London, in 1882. The success of these power stations led to the construction of many other central power stations. [see 1864 (e), 1877 Nov. 29, 1878 (h), 1883 (d), 1889 (h), 1891 Dec. 29, 1893 (h)].

1882 (F): The world's first **electric fan** was devised by the Chief Engineer of New York's Crocker and Curtis Electric Motor Company. This two-bladed desk fan was the work of 22-year old **Schuzler Skats Wheeler.** The world's first electric flat iron was patented by H.W. Seely in the same year.

1882 (G): **Leo Tolstoy** (1828-1910), Russian author, moralist and social critic brought out his work *A Confession.*[see 1866 (f), 1894 (e)]

When he was completing *Anna Karenina,* in the 1870's, he experienced a **spiritual crisis,** the history of which was set down in the *Confession.* Thereupon he embraced a rationalist variety of evangelical Christianity, the cardinal principles of which were brotherly love and non-resistance to evil. He aimed primarily at the achievement of inner freedom and personal righteousness, but he also applied his ethical doctrine to the solution of social problems. He rejected the Church, believing that it had corrupted Christ's teachings. He set forth his views in numerous tracts, in private letters and also in the stories and plays he produced after his conversion.

1882 (H): **Psycho-analysis** was pioneered by Viennese physician, **Josef Breuer,** who discovered the value of hypnosis in treating a girl suffering from severe hysteria.

Breuer induced the patient to relive certain scenes that occurred while she was nursing her sick father and he succeeded thereby in relieving her permanently of her hysteria symptoms, a success he communicated to his colleague Sigmund Freud. [see 1895 (n)]

1883 JAN. 23: Birth of **Clement Atlee** (d. 1967), leader of the British Labour Party (1935-55) and Prime Minister of England from 1945 to 1951.

Atlee led the Labour Party in the electoral victory of 1945 and led the Labour Government that established the welfare state in Great Britain. His Government was responsible for a series of measures, notably the creation of a national health service, and the extension of national insurance.

1883 MAR. 14: Death of **Karl Marx** (b. 1818), German political philosopher, radical economist, and revolutionary leader who authored *The Communist Manifesto,* the most celebrated pamphlet in the history of the Socialist Movement, as well as of its most important book, *Das Kapital.*

His basic idea – known as Marxism – forms the foundation of socialist and communist movement.

Marx's masterpiece, *Das Kapital,* the 'Bible of the Working Class', as it was officially described in a resolution of the International Working Men's Association, was published in 1867 in Berlin. Only the first volume was completed and published in Marx's lifetime. The second and third volumes edited by Engels were published in 1885 and 1894. [see 1867 (c)].

1883 MAR. 26: The most lavish party yet held in America was staged at the $ 2 million Gothic mansion of railroad magnate, **William Kissam Vanderbilt,** 34, on the north-west corner of New York's Fifth Avenue at 53rd Street.

Vanderbilt was the Chairman of the Lake Shore and Michigan Southern, and it was estimated by the *New York World* that his wife had spent $ 155,730 for costumes, $ 11,000 for flowers, $ 4,000 for hired carriages, $ 4,000 for hair dressers, and $ 65,270 for catering, champagne, music and the like to make the $ 250,000 fancy-dress ball a success.

1883 MAY 28: Birth of **Vinayaka Damodar Savarkar** (d. 1966), the fierce patriot, popularly known as Veer Savarkar.

He was one of the most active Indian revolutionaries and a militant nationalist. A fighter ready to dare and act in the case of Mother India, he became a legend in his own life time.

1883 JUL. 29: Birth of **Benito Mussolini** (d. 1945), the Fascist dictator, who was the head of the Italian Government from 1922-1943 and led Italy into 3 successive wars, the last of which overturned his regime.

1883 OCT. 30: Death of **Swami Dayananda Saraswati** (b. 1824), the founder of Arya Samaj, a religious movement which played an important part in the awakening of Indian national consciousness. [see 1875 Apr. 10, 1874 June 12]

The Swami was one of the great personalities of Indian Renaissance and the reviver of Indian culture. Well-versed in the interpretation of the Vedas, he was a fearless critic of all dogmas and superstitions and all the evils of rituals and custom. His vehement campaign against the evils of his days had excited many attacks on his life.

For his courageous crusade against orthodoxy and superstitions, Daya- nanda was poisoned a number of times, and as a result of the last one he died. The crowning act of his life was that he not only pardoned his poisoner but also gave money to him to go away and save himself.

Swami Dayananda was the first religious reformer of modern India, who based himself entirely on the light which he had received from his own sacred lore. Before he died, about one hundred branches of Arya Samaj had been established in Punjab, Utter Pradesh, Rajasthan and Bombay.

1883 DEC. 28-30: Under the auspices of the **Indian Association,** an **All India National Conference** met in Calcutta with representatives from all over India.

It was an important landmark in the history of the evaluation of political organization, as it was the first All-India political conference which offered a model to Indian National Congress inaugurated two years later. In 1885, when the Indian National Congress was founded in Bombay, the Indian National Conference merged into it without any difficulty. It soon grew into a significant national body with representatives from all parts of the country and all sections of the people. The Muslims, however, under the leadership of Sir Sayed Ahmed Khan (1818-1898), held aloof from the nationalist agitations of the 19th Century.

1883 (A): In his book, *Asia's Message to Europe,* **Keshab Chandra Sen,** the celebrated Brahmo leader exhorted:

"Sectarian and carnal Europe, put up into the scabbard the sword of your narrow faith! Abjure it and join the true catholic and universal church in the name of Christ, the son of God!...."

"Christian Europe has not understood one half of Christ's words. She has comprehended that Christ and God are one, but not Christ and humanity are one. That is the greatest mystery, which the New Dispensation [see 1881 Jan. 25] reveals to the world: 'not only the reconciliation of man with God, but the reconciliation of man with man!' .... Asia says to Europe: 'Sister, be one in Christ.... All that is good and true and beautiful – the meekness of Hindu Asia, the truthfulness of Mussalman, and the charity of the Buddhist – all that is holy is of Christ....'
"

1883 (B): **Pratap Chandra Majumdar** (1840-1905), writer, orator and the chief lieutenant of Keshab Chandra Sen, brought out his book: *Oriental Christ,* in which he depicted Christ as an Eastern prophet.

This book has been compared by Dr. Barrows to *Imitation of Christ* by Thomas a Kempis.

1883 (C): **Nikola Tesla** (1856-1943), Croatian-American inventor and electrical engineer, constructed his first **induction motor,** utilizing the rotating magnetic field principle discovered by him.

He also produced other electrical motors, new forms of generators and transformers, and a system for alternating-current power transmission. Later he invented the transformer known as the Tesla coil (1891) and made basic discoveries concerning wireless communication. Tesla also invented fluorescent lamps and a new type of steam turbine. His alternating-current electrical system was used by George Westinghouse for a major lighting project (the World's Columbian Exposition at Chicago in 1893). The system was also used for a major power project (Niagara Falls).

A controversy between alternating-current and direct-current advocates raged in 1880s and 1890s, featuring Tesla and Edison as leaders in the rival camps. The advantages of the polyphase alternating-current system as developed by Tesla, soon became apparent, however, particularly for long distance power transmission. The rotating magnetic principle discovered by Tesla, is the basis of practically all alternating-current machinery.

1883 (D): **Thomas Alva Edison** (1847-1931) made a significant discovery in pure science, **'the Edison Effect'** – electron flowed from incandescent filaments, with a metal plate insert, the lamp could serve as a valve emitting only negative electricity.

Although "etheric force" had been recognized in 1875 and "the Edison Effect" was patented in 1883, the phenomenon was little known outside the Edison laboratory. This "force" underlies radio broadcasting [see 1891 Dec. 29], long-distance telephony, sound pictures, television, electric eyes, X-rays, high frequency surgery and electronic musical instruments. In 1885 Edison patented a method to transmit telegraphic "aerial", which worked over short distances, and later sold this "wireless" patent to the Italian electrical engineer Guglielmo Marconi (1874-1937). [see 1864 (e), 1877 Nov. 29, 1878 (h), 1882 (e), 1889 (h), 1891 Dec. 29, 1893 (h)]

1883 (C): **Gottlieb Daimler** (1834-1900), German inventor, constructed a **high speed engine,** making it lighter and more efficient than ever before and adapting it for the use of gasoline vapour as fuel. He fitted the engine to a boat in his first attempt to make practical use of it.

In 1885, Daimler installed one of his modified engines on a bicycle and drove it over the cobbled roads of Mannheim, Baden. That was the world's first motor cycle [see 1884 (h), 1885 (b)]. In 1887, Daimler built the first automobile. [see 1876 (e), 1885 (b)]

1883 (F): **J. W. Swan** (1828-1914), English physicist and chemist, patented a process for producing artificial fibre called **rayon.** In the same year an **artificial silk** was developed from nitrocellulose by French Chemist **Hilaire Berniguad.**

1883 (G): **Robert Louis Stevenson** (1850-1894), Scottish novelist, who was one of the most popular and highly regarded British writers of the end of the 19th century, brought out *Treasure Island,* his first popular romantic thriller.

His other well-known works include *Kidnapped* (an adventure story of the Scottish highlands) and *The Strange Case of Dr. Jekyll and Mr. Hyde.* In the latter, he dealt directly with the nature of evil in man and the hideous effects of a hypocrisy that seeks to deny it.

1883 (H): The **volcano of Krakatoa** (between Java and Sumatra), which had been dormant for hundred years, burst into violent eruptions that could be heard from West Australia. Dense, volcanic clouds and ash were hurled into the air as huge waves, over thirty-six metres high, swamped the coasts of Java and Sumatra, drowning 36,000 people.

1884 JAN. 6: Death of **Gregor Mendel** (b. 1822), Austrian Augustinian monk, who laid the foundation of modern genetics (heredity) with his paper dealing with the hybridization of peas.

The results of his investigations were communicated by him to a Natural History Society in Brunn, in the proceedings of which they were published in 1865. In 1900, nearly twenty years after Mendel's death, his paper was rapidly appreciated. Mendel's success was largely due to the fact that he planned his experiments on lines different from those of any of his predecessors. His invaluable contributions have made his name immortal in the annals of genetical literature. [see 1865 (b), 1900 (c)]

1884 JAN: Death of **Keshab Chandra Sen** (b. 1838), the celebrated Brahmo leader, and a stormy petrel in the history of Indian social and religious reformation.

From March 1875 onward to the end of his life, Keshab remained under the powerful influence of **SRI RAMAKRISHNA**, the saint of Dakshineswar, who met the former for the first time at a garden house, a few miles to the North of Calcutta. Being deeply impressed by his devotion and conversation, Keshab went to see Ramakrishna often, accompanied by a number of his adherents, and drew public attention to his merits both by talking and by writing about him. The result was that Ramakrishna was visited at his temple by many educated Hindus from Calcutta and also made the acquaintance of the young men who became his attached pupils. At the news of Keshab's death, Sri Ramakrishna was overwhelmed; he would not speak to anyone and remained in bed for three days. Later he said 'When I heard of Keshab's death, I felt as if one of my limbs were paralysed.' And again, 'Oh, how happy we used to be together! How we used to sing and dance!' Throughout the rest of his life, Ramakrishna would speak often of Keshab – sometimes critically or humorously, but always with profound affection.

1884 JAN. 30: B. A. examination results of Calcutta University were published in *The Calcutta Gazette*, **NARENDRANATH** passing the examination in the second division.

After graduation, Narendranath started studying law in Metropolitan

Institution (now Vidyasagar College), completed the course in 1886, but did not appear in the final examination.

1884 JAN. (A): The Fabian Society was founded by a small group in London, to promote the advancement of socialism by gradual and non-revolutionary means and so gradually to reconstruct society in accordance with the highest moral possibilities.

The fabians were influenced by Marxism but they based their economic philosophy not on Marx but on John Stuart Mill [see 1873, May 8]. They rejected the Marxist view of the capitalist state as instrument of domination which ought to be overthrown, and hoped instead to capture and use the state for the general welfare. They also advocated state control of the conditions of labour.

Among the many distinguished members of the society were Sidney and Beatrice Webb, George Bernard Shaw, H. G. Wells and Annie Besant. After the publication of *Fabian Essays* [see 1889 (j)] edited by Shaw, the society became an influential political force. Its influence on socialist movement in Britain was profound. In 1892 the first two avowed socialists were elected to Parliament. In 1900 the Fabians took an important part in the formation of the Labour Representation Committee, which subsequently became the British Labour Party.

1884 FEB. 19: NARENDRANATH , 21, was initiated into Freemasonry, passed as a Fellow Craft on 15 April and raised as a Master Mason on 20 May but did not become Master of Lodge.

In quick succession he went through the ceremonies of the three degrees of Freemasonary and within three months only he became a full-fledged member of the Craft *(Brother Vivekananda,* by Dr. P. C. Chunder, p.14).

"Freemasonry is a particular system of morality veiled in allegory, illustrated symbols. Any person who comes to join this fratemity must strongly and absolutely believe in Fatherhood of God and brotherhood of man. He must come of his own free will and accord, freely and voluntarily. Also his approach must be unbiased of improper solicitation of friends and uninfluenced by mercenary or other unworthy motives."

1884 FEB. 25: Death of Narendranath's father, **Vishwanath Dutta,** (b. 1835). Consequently Narendranath's family was plunged into dire financial distress and suffered many troubles and privations. Vishwanath, a spendthrift, had spent more than he earned.

Immediately after his demise it was discovered that the family was over head and ears in debt. The creditors knocked at the door; the erstwhile friends turned enemies and the nearest relatives, taking advantage of this helpless condition, filed a suit to oust them all from the house. Nothing daunted, **NARENDRANATH** fought manfully, and ultimately triumphed in the litigation in which he had to get himself involved in spite of himself under circumstances over which he had no control.

1884 MAR. : Birth of **H. H. Jagadguru Swami Bharati Krishna Tirtha** (d. 1960), the divine personality that gracefully adorned the famous Govardhan Math, Puri.

Renowned for his vast versatile learning, spiritual and educational attainments, wonderful research achievements in the field of Vedic Mathematics, Sri Jagadguru went on a tour to America, the first tour outside India by a Shankaracharya in the history of the said Order, with a view to promote the cause of world peace and to spread the lofty Vedantic ideals even outside India.

1884 JUL: **Ottmar Mergenthler** (b. 1854) German-American mechanic, constructed the first direct-casting **Linotype;** it was patented in August and in December the National Typographic Co., was organized to manufacture it. [see 1885 (e)].

On July 3, 1886, a Linotype was used to compose part of that day's issue of the *New York Tribune*. The machine's use spread quickly throughout the United States and abroad. In 1886, Linotype machines were installed by the *New York Tribune,* and it became the first newspaper to use the machine.

1884 OCT. 14: Birth of **Lala Hardayal** (d. 1938), the great Indian patriot, revolutionary and genius.

1884 NOV. 25: English Surgeon **Rickman John Godlee** performed the **first operation** for the removal of a brain tumour.

1884 DEC. 3: Birth of **Dr. Rajendra Prasad** (d. 1963), Indian nationalist and the first President of Independent India.

He was also an important leader of the Indian National Congress and a close co-worker of Gandhiji.

1884 DEC. 6 : **Bankim Chandra Chatterjee,** the great Bengali novelist, met **SRI RAMAKRISHNA** in the house of Adhar Chandra Sen.

Adhar had invited several of his brother officers, of whom Bankim was one, to meet Sri Ramakrishna. Bankim took up a sceptical attitude and put to Sri Ramakrishna various complicated questions on religion. After giving proper replies to those questions, Sri Ramakrishna said to Bankim Chandra, by way of a joke, "You are Bankim (literally means bent) by name and also by actions." Pleased with the answers which touched him to the heart, Bankim said, "Sir, you must come to our Kanthalpara house some day; there are arrangements about the service of the Divine Lord and all of us take the name of Hari." Sri Ramakrishna replied in fun "How do you take the name of Hari? Is it as the goldsmiths took it?" Saying so, Sri Ramakrishna told an amusing story about some swindling goldsmiths posing as devotees, which was much appreciated. Sri Ramakrishna did not forget Bankim, though they never met again. And he listened to portions of one of his famous novels, *Devi Chaudhurani,* and made apposite comments theron. He also sent **NARENDRANATH** and one or two of his other brilliant disciples to meet and have a talk with him.

1884 (A): *Thus Spake Zarathustra* by German philosopher, **Friedrich Wilhelm Nietzsche** (1844-1900), was published in the first of its four parts and introduced the idea of the Superman. [see 1900 Aug. 25]

Nietzsche's theories influenced German thinking 30 years thence.

1884 (B): **J. H. Van't Hoff** (1852-1911), Dutch Physical Chemist, who pioneered in the development of stereo chemistry, published the results of his research in **chemical thermodynamics** in *Studies in Chemical Dynamics.*

In 1901, he received the first Nobel Prize in Chemistry.

1884 (C): **Italian forces established themselves at Massawa** with British encouragement and began to expand their holdings in the East African highlands.

Germany annexed Tanganyika and Zanzibar.

Britain established protectorates in the Niger River region in North Bechuanaland, and in southern New Guinea. **British troops occupied Port Hamilton,** Korea. Two years later **Britain annexed Upper Burma** following a Third Anglo-Burmese War. In 1887, it **annexed Zululand** to block the Transval Government from establishing a link to the sea.

1884 (D): Charles Rockwell Lanman (1850-1941) of Harvard, who is usually considered among the great Sanskritists of the West, brought out his work: *Sanskrit Reader.* [see 1879 (r)]

It was re-issued many times and became a familiar text to several generations of students in America.

1884 (E): George Eastman (1854-1932), U. S. Inventor, introduced the first successful **flexible roll film,** which permitted development of cameras more convenient to use than plate cameras. Earlier in 1880, he had perfected the process for making photographic plates, and had also begun to manufacture them.

Eastman produced his first Kodak box camera (the first simple, inexpensive camera) in 1888, marketing it on a large scale. His mass production methods helped to make photography a universal hobby. It made amateur photography feasible and widely popular. The Eastman Kodak Company, founded in 1892, rapidly achieved a dominant position in the industry. Large investments in research led further innovations in cameras and equipment, including day-light loading film (1891) and pocket camera (1895). Brownie box camera introduced by Eastman Kodak Co. in 1900 and priced at $ 1, put the photography within reach of every one, and it made Kodak a household name. [see 1888 (i), 1892 (b), 1895 (e)]

1884 (F): Lewis Edson Waterman (1837-1901), U. S. inventor, produced the first practical **fountain pen** with a capillary feed.

He patented it and founded the Ideal Pen Company and had 200 of the pens produced by hand, but the end of the pen must he removed and ink squirted in with an eye-dropper. The venture was so successful that he incorporated it in 1887 as L. E. Waterman and Company

In 1888 **Parker Pen Company** was started at U. S. A. (Jannesville, Wis.) by local telegraph teacher, George Safford Parker, 24, whose firm became the world's largest producer of fountain pens. Parker developed a pen of his own with a superior feed, and in 1904 he obtained a patent for a level mechanism that made it easier to fill his pen's rubber sac.

1884 (G): Television was pioneered by German inventor, **Paul Gottlieb Nipkov,** 26, who devised a rotating scanning disk (a rapidly spinning perforated wheel with an illuminated screen behind it) and patented a picture-sending device based on it.

With this mechanical scanning priniciple all experiments in television began; and in 1923, the invention of modern camera tube by a Russian named Zworykin (b. 1889), marked the beginning of modern picture transmission. [see 1888 (e), 1897 (e)]

1884 (H): The first **motor cycle** was built by an Englishman, **Edward Butler.** The first gasoline-engined motor cycle to appear publicly was built by Gottlieb Daimler (1834-1900) German mechanical engineer, in 1885. The first practical engines and motor cycles were designed by the French and Belgian, followed by Britain, German, Italian and U. S. Makes. [see 1883 (e), 1885 (b)]

1884 (I): The anesthetic properties of **cocaine** in medical practice were discovered by New York Surgeon **William Stewart Halsted,** who injected the drug to pioneer the practice of local anesthesia.

1884 (J): **Sir Hiram Stevens Maxim** (1840-1916), American-born British inventor, produced the first practical automatic **machine gun,** (the Maxim gun) which used the force of the barrel's recoil to eject the spent cartridge and reload cordite, a smokeless powder. Maxim guns were first adopted in 1889 by the British army and thereafter it became a standard equipment for every army.

Before Maxim had left United States for England, a friend had advised him: "Hang your chemistry and electricity! If you really want to make a pile of money, invent something that will enable those Europeans to cut each other's throats with greater facility." And his first invention was the machine gun.

Maxim came to know Swami Vivekananda and became his ardent admirer.

1884 (K): The **diphtheria bacillus** was isolated and cultured at Berlin by **F. A. J. Loffler.**

1884 (M): Death of **J. B. Dumas** (b. 1800), French chemist, who worked in the field of organic chemistry and developed the "type" theory of organic structure.

1884 (N): **Sir Charles Parsons** (1854-1931), British Engineer, first constructed a multistage **steam turbine** which revolutionized marine propulsion. [see 1892 (h)]

In 1894, Parsons took out a patent to use the turbine in ship propulsion; the first ship to be driven in this way was the Turbina (1897).

1884-88: **Lord Dufferin** (1826-1902) the Viceroy of India.

1885 MAY 22: Death of **Victor Hugo** (b.1802) French author, who was the supreme poet of French romanticism.

1885 JUL. 6: **Louis Pasteur** (1822-1895) French chemist and microbiologist, administered the first **anti-rabies vaccine** to a 9 year old Alsatian School boy who had been bitten by a rabid dog.

Pasteur had developed the vaccine from weakened viruses that had developed on the desiccated spinal cords of rabbits that had died from rabies. The young boy Joseph Meister was saved from an agonizing death. The experiment was thus successful. Victims of bites from rabid animals flocked from all over the world to be treated. Since then thousands of persons throughout the world have been kept from develop- ing hydrophobia by being given Pasteur vaccine and being exposed to rabies.

1885 SEP. : One evening **NARENDRANATH** and **Girish Chandra Ghosh** (a house-holder disciple of Sri Ramakrishna) were sitting together in meditation, at Panchavati (Dakshineswar). Girish could not concentrate his mind because of mosquito bites. He found Narendranath's body covered with the mosquitoes as if with a thick blanket but Narendranath was unmindful of it.

He called him but he did not hear, touched him but did not feel. Worried and anxious, Girish pushed him aside. Narendranath's frame fell on the ground but in the same meditating posture, as if a statue. It was only with great difficulty that Girish could restore the 'statue' to consciousness. But later when Girish narrated this episode, Narendranath told that he did not remember anything that had happened.

1885 OCT. 7: Birth of **Niels Bohr** (d. 1962), Danish physicist, known primarily for his pioneering work in the field of atomic theory.

Founder of the modern quantum theory of matter, Bohr was one of the most ingenious interpreters of his generation of the problems in modern theoretical physics, and was among the first to recognise the implications of nuclear bombs. His theory of atoms has become the foundation of modern atomic physics. For his investigations of atomic structure and radiation, Bohr won the 1922 Nobel Prize for Physics.

1885 NOV. 5: Birth of **Will Durant** (d. 1981) American author and lecturer, whose books, *The Story of Philosophy* (1926) and *The Story of Civilization* (1935-67) established him as one of the best known writers of popular philosophy and history.

He devoted more than half a century to write the II volume *"Story of Civilization"*, a massive world history. A teacher for many years he had a tremendous success at the age of 40 with the publication of his first book, *The Story of Philosophy,* which provided enough money for him to devote full time to writing.

1885 DEC. 28: The first session of the **Indian National Congress** was held in Bombay, under the presidentship of W. C. Banerjee (1844-1906).

Founded by a retired member of the Indian Civil Service, A. O. Hume, the Indian National Congress gradually developed into a powerful political organization with an All-India character. Initially it focussed the political ideas of English-educated Indians and gave them a definite shape and form. Its whole endeavour was to rouse British consciousness to the inherent justice of the Indian claims. The annual gatherings of leading representatives from different parts of India gave reality to the ideal of Indian unity, developed patriotic feelings and awakened political consciousness among the steadily increasing circle of English educated Indians. Between 1885 and 1947 fifty-four annual sessions of the Indian National Congress were held at different major cities of India. As a major political party, the Indian National Congress, later under the leadership of Mahatma Gandhi, won for India complete freedom on 15th August 1947.

1885 (A): Hindu-Muslims riots at Lahore and Karnal. [see 1874 Feb. 13, 1877 Sept., 1886 (e), 1889 (m), 1891 (b), 1893 (c), 1897 June] .

1885 (B): Karl Benz (1844-1929), German mechanical engineer, completed his **motor vehicle** (a three-wheeled vehicle) which reached a speed of 9 miles per hour. It was the world's first successful automobile powered by an internal combustion petrol engine. The Benz car was patented on January 26, 1886. Benz and Company (founded in 1883 to build stationary internal-combustion engines), completed its first four-wheeled automobile in 1893, and in 1899 produced the first of a series of racing cars.

In 1885, another German mechanical engineer and inventor, named **Gottlieb Daimler** (1834-1900), who was a major figure in the history of the automotive industry, patented one of the first successful high-speed **internal combustion engines,** and developed a carburettor that made possible the use of gasoline (petrol) as fuel. Adopting his early gasoline engine, Daimler made his first two-wheeled motor cycle in 1885. It was the world's first **motor cycle.** [see 1883 (e), 1884 (h)]. Daimler also used his gasoline engine on a four-wheeled horse-drawn carriage (1886), a boat (1887) and a four-wheeled vehicle originally designed as an automobile (1889). This four-wheeled vehicle was exhibited at the 1889 Paris Exhibition. Though the public took little notice of the vehicle, it did attract R. Panhard and E. Lavassor, who developed the engine in France and began automobile manufacture in 1891. In 1890 Daimler Motor Co. was founded at Canstatt., and in 1899 the firm built the first Mercedes car. In 1926 the Benz Co. merged with the Daimler Motor Co., to form Daimler-Benz, maker of Mercedes-Benz car.

1885 (C): Paul Vieille (1854-1934), French scientist, invented smokeless high **explosives.**

1885 (D): Gas lighting got a new lease of life from Austrian chemist, **Carl Auer Von Welsbach** (1858-1929) who patented a **gas mantle** of woven cotton mesh impregnated with thorium and cerium oxides, rare earths obtained from Indian (Travancore) sands. The Welsbach mantle was fitted over a gas jet to increase its brilliance. Welsbach also discovered (1885) two rare earth elements which he named 'praseodymium' and 'neodymium'.

1885 (E): **Tolbert Lanston** (1844-1913) of U. S. A., invented **Mono-typesetting** machine. In 1897, it was made practicable for book-publishers than the Merganthler Linotype machine of 1884. [see 1884 Jul.]

1885 (F): **Sir Francis Galton** (1822-1911), English social scientist, explorer and anthropometrist, devised new statistical methods, culminating in the **correlational calculus,** his greatest scientific achievement. [see 1877-93]

1885 (G): The world's first **electric trolley** line was installed at Baltimore by English-American electrical engineer, **Leo Daft.**

1885 (H): **Single-shot rifle** designed by U. S. gunsmith, **John M. Browning,** was introduced by Winchester Repeating Arms Company. The rifle became enormously successful.

1885 (I): An identification system based on **fingerprints** was devised by English social scientist, **Francis Galton,** who had founded the science of eugenics with his 1869 book *Hereditary Genius* and subsequent books. Galton proved that finger prints were permanent and that no two people ever have the same finger prints.

1885 (J): **Sir Edwin Arnold** (1832-1904), British poet, scholar, and journalist, brought out *The Song Celestial,* being the English version of the *Bhagavad Gita* occurring in the great Indian epic, the *Mahabharata.*

His epic poem, *The Light of Asia,* that tells in elaborate language the life and teachings of the Buddha, went through sixty editions in England and eighty in America in the course of a few years of its first publication in 1879 and sold in millions. Arnold's other works include: *The Book of Good Counsels,* from the Sanskrit of the *Hitopadesha* (1861), *The Indian Song of Songs* from the Sanskrit of the *Gita Govinda* of Jayadeva (1875); *Indian Idylls* (1883) from the *Mahabharata*; and *Pearls of the Faith* and other translations.

1885 (K): As a memorial to his only child, **A. L. Stanford** (1824-1893), U. S. multimillionaire railroad promoter and philanthropist, founded **Leland Stanford Jr. University** in Palo Alto, Cal., with an original endowment of 20 million dollars. [see 1876 (e)]

1886 JAN. 1: **'Kalpatharu Day'** – the day on which **SRI RAMAKRISHNA** showered his grace and benediction upon his disciples who were with him at Cossipore Garden House.

In an exalted mood Ramakrishna said "I bless you all, be illumined." This was a mass blessing and all felt elevated. He fell into a state of semi-consciousness. All of them touched his feet. He touched everyone of them and blessed them. This powerful touch revolutionized their minds, and the devotees so blessed by Sri Ramakrishna, had wonderful spiritual experiences. Referring to his experience after the magic touch, Ramlal, Ramakrishna's nephew, said, "Formerly I could see in meditation only portions of my chosen ideal's form. But that day, His entire form flashed before my vision and I saw Him seated in my heart as a distinct living presence." Vaikuntha said, "After two or three devotees had been blessed, I too stepped forward and saluting him asked his blessings. He said, 'You have already everything'. 'Then please make me feel it', I said. He said, 'All right', and lightly touched my chest. That worked a strong transformation within me. I saw the blissful form of the Master in everything I saw. I was beside myself with joy and shouted to all to come and share in the blessing. That vision haunted me for days and my work suffered in consequence. Unable to bear the tension I had to pray to Sri Ramakrishna to lessen its intensity after which it became intermittent."

1886 APR. 6: Death of **William Edward Forster** (b. 1818) British statesman and Quaker Vice-President of the Privy Council's Committee for Education in Gladstone's Ministry (1868-74).

As Vice-President of the Council, Forster inaugurated a national system of education by directing debates on the Endowed Schools Act (1869) and the Education Act (1870). The latter was the greatest landmark in the history of English education. [see 1870 (b)]

1886 APR. : At Cossipore Garden House, where **SRI RAMAKRISHNA** was undergoing treatment for his throat illness, **NARENDRA** was engaged in intense *sadhana*. Sri Ramakrishna had initiated him with the *Ramamantra,* telling him it was the *mantra* which he had received from his own guru.

One night, at about 9 O'clock Narendranath was seized with *Mahavirabhava* (he was transformed into Hanuman, Sri Ramachandra's great devotee). He began suddenly to shout *"Jai Ram" "Jai Ram"*, and after some time rushed out of the house with a pair of tongs in his hands. Sri Ramakrishna who heard his shouts, was worried but none dared confront him. But Gopal Ghosh, who was a strong bodied man, pursued him. As there were few street lamps in those parts, he could hardly see him and ran after him in the direction from which his shouts, *"Jai Ram"*, *"Jai Ram"* came. At last after a chase of a few miles, Gopal overtook Narendra who was heading towards Dakshineswar and, clasping him from behind, took away the tongs. Narendra became unconscious. Gopal then brought him back to consciousness by sprinkling water on his face and eyes. They then returned to Cossipore and met Sri Ramakrishna.

1886 MAY 23: **The Canadian Pacific Railway** was formally opened. It was the first single Company trans-continental rail-road in America. Built by James. J. Hill and W. C. Van Horne with 2,095 miles of track, the Canadian Pacific Railway joined the east and west coasts of Canada and spurred migration to Canada's western provinces.

1886: NARENDRANATH who was at Cossipore Garden House, practised spiritual disciplines with unabating intensity. Sometimes he felt an awakening of a spiritual power that he could transmit to others.

One night, Narendranath asked a brother disciple to touch his right knee, and then entered into deep meditation. The brother disciple's hand began to tremble; He felt a kind of electric shock. Afterwards Narendranath was rebuked by his Master, **SRI RAMAKRISHNA**, for frittering away spiritual powers before accumulating them in sufficient measure.

Narendranath had *nirvikalpa samadhi* while at Cossipore Garden House. In the depth of his meditation he felt as though a lamp were burning at the back of his head. Suddenly he lost consciousness. It was the yearned for, all effacing experience of *nirvikalpa samadhi*, when embodied soul realizes his unity with the Absolute. After a very long period he regained full consciousness; his heart was still filled to overflowing with ineffable ecstasy. After a while when Narendranath prostrated himself before Sri Ramakrishna, he tenderly said to him "Now then, the Mother has shown you everything. Just as a treasure is locked up in a box, so will this realization you have just had lie locked up and the key shall remain with me. You have work to do. When you will have finished my work, the treasure box will be unlocked again and you will know everything then just as you do now." Afterwards Sri Ramakrishna said to the other disciples that the moment Narendranath would realize who he was, he would pass away of his own will.

1886 AUG. (second week): Knowing that his end was imminent, **SRI RAMAKRISHNA,** in order to endow **NARENDRANATH** with the spiritual wealth which he himself had acquired after years of super-human efforts and unprecedented austerities, called him to his side. Having seated him in front and looking intently into the eyes of his dear disciple, he fell into a deep trance. Narendranath felt a powerful impact of a tremendous force passing into his own body and soon lost all body consciousness. When, after a while, Narendranath came to himself, Sri Ramakrishna was found shedding tears. When interrogated, Sri Ramakrishna softly replied, **"Oh Naren, today I have given you my all and have become a *fakir* (beggar).... By the force of power transmitted by me, great things will be done by you; only after that, will you go to whence you came."**

Another incident of deep spiritual significance also occurred only a couple of days before the final deliverance of Sri Ramakrishna. Standing by the bedside of Sri Ramakrishna, Narendranth thought that he would accept him as an incarnation of God if he could declare in the midst of this excruciating physical suffering that he was God incarnate. Scarcely had this idea flashed across his mind when Sri Ramakrishna distinctly said, "O My Naren, are you not yet convinced? He who was Rama and Krishna is now Ramakrishna in this body, – but not from the standpoint of your Vedanta." Narendranath was extremely abashed and stung with self-reproach to think that he still doubted the Master even after so much experiment and revelation.

1886 AUG. 16: **SRI RAMAKRISHNA** who had the satisfaction of seeing his young disciples united under the leadership of **NARENDRANTH,** into spiritual fraternity with one common resolve to dedicate themselves to the service of humanity, peacefully, entered into *mahasamadhi,* from which there was no return into normal consciousness. On the bank of the Ganges the mortal remains of the great soul were consigned to fire.

"The devotees realized that from then on they did not have to take recourse to physical means to contact their guru. The released soul of their Master broke the limitations of time and space. Their human guru became the God of their hearts; Out of the ashes of Ramakrishna, the Man, was born 'Ramakrishna, the Power.' "

1886 OCT. 19: **The disciples of SRI RAMAKRISHNA established a Math** (monastery) in an old dilapidated house of Baranagore, midway between Dakshineswar and Calcutta.

This was followed by all the would-be monks taking to a life of very strict austerities to which they submitted themselves most cheerfully for months. The whole place throbbed in no time with an unprecedented vivacity and spiritual power. The fire of enthusiasm thus kindled in them and constantly fed by their ever deepening yearning for the realization of the Truth as also by their whole-souled earnestness for the fulfilment of the mission of their Master spurred them on to face the travail of a new birth and meet the challenges of internal and external nature with indomitable courage and confidence.

The life of severest spiritual austerities lived, the hardship and direst poverty endured and the spirit of unique self-denial exhibited in the Baranagore monastery by this heroic band of sannyasins form a thrilling episode in the history of the Ramakrishna Movement. **SWAMI VIVEKANANDA** himself in a reminiscent mood once spoke to a disciple: "There were days at the Baranagore Math when we had nothing to eat. If there was rice, salt was lacking some days; that was all we had, but nobody cared. Leaves of the Bimba creeper boiled, salt and rice – this was our diet for months! Come what would, we were indifferent. We were being carried on in a strong tide of religious practices and meditation. Oh, what days! Demons would have run away at the sight of such austerities, to say nothing of men!"

1886 OCT. 28: **Statue of Liberty unveiled** and dedicated by U. S. President Cleveland in a ceremony on Bedloe's island in New York Harbour.

Designed by French sculptor, Frederic Auguste Bartholdi, 52, the 225 ton, 152 feet high, copper statue was presented to U. S. by France in commemoration of 100 years of American Independence.

1886 (see after 1886 May 23)

1886 (A): **Devendranath Tagore** (1817-1905), the religious leader of Calcutta, founded **'Shantiniketan'** (Abode of Peace), a retreat in rural Bengal, later made famous by his poet-son Rabindranath Tagore (1861-1941), whose educational centre there became an international university. [see 1901 Dec. 22]

1886 (B): **D. A. V. College** was founded at Lahore in memory of **Swami Dayananda Saraswati** (1824-1883), the founder of Arya Samaj.

Under Lala Hansraj, who remained its principal for 28 years, "it became the foremost agency for planting a sturdy and independent nationalism in the Punjab."

1886 (C): **Hindu-Muslim riots at Delhi,** where military had to be requisitioned. [see 1874 Feb. 13, 1877 Sept, 1885 (a), 1889 (m), 1891 (b), 1893 (c)]

1886 (D): **Discovery of Gold** on the Witwaters Rand in the Southern Transval at **South Africa.**

There was a wild rush to the Rand from all parts of the world. Diamond King, **Cecil Rhodes,** founded Consolidated Gold Fields Ltd., Johannesburg, in South Africa's Transval was laid out and soon a population of 100,000 migrated, as the world's largest gold mines began operations. By 1890, there were 450 mining companies on the Rand (capitalized at £ 11,000,000). The output was almost 500,000 ounces in 1890, and 1,210,865 ounces in 1892.

The discovery of gold in California (1848) had sent thousands of Americans rushing westwards, the population had soared and California was on its way to becoming one of the world's richest – the most violent places. Other great gold rushes include in Victoria, Australia (1851) and Klondike in Alaska and North-West Canada (1897).

1886 (E): George Westinghouse (1846-1914), U. S. Engineer, inventor and manufacturer, organized the **Westinghouse Electric Company** and developed a single-phase, high voltage, alternating-current system for light and power, particularly using the equipment designed by Nikola Tesla (1856-1943). [see 1883 (c)]

Tesla motor and polyphase alternator made it economically feasible to transmit power over long distances. In the same year, a practical transformer for large electricity supply networks was perfected by U. S. Electrical Engineer, William Stanley and George Westinghouse. The following year the two gave the first practical demonstration of an alternating-current system in favour of direct current. Westinghouse Company exploited the alternating-current over long wires, employing transformers to step down the voltage for local distribution to houses, stores, factories and the like. In early 1890s, Westinghouse received contracts to illuminate the World's Columbian Exposition in Chicago and developed a system at Niagara Falls.

The principle of the rotary magnetic field that led to the development of polyphase motors (and of Italy's hydroelectric industry) was discovered by Italian-Physicist Electrical Engineer, Galileo Ferraris, who devised transformers for alternating-current. An American inventor, Elihu Thompson also invented a transformer that stepped down high voltage alternating current.

1886 (F): ElihuThompson (1853-1937), U. S. Electrical Pioneer invented the system of **arc welding.**

1886 (G): The element **germanium** was discovered at Freiburg in Saxony by German physicist **C. A. Winkler** in a silver thiogermanate.

1886 (H): A process for **halftone engraving** that used small raised dots of varying sizes was developed by U. S. inventor **Frederick Eugene Ives** (1856-1937), 30, who 5 years ago pioneered in colour photography by making the first trichromatic halftone process printing plates. In 1892, he introduced the process of **colour photography.**

1886 (I): Commercial **aluminium** production was pioneered by **Charles Martin Hall** (1863-1914), U. S. scientist, who used methods developed by Humphry Davy in 1807 to liberate aluminium electrolytically from aluminium oxide (bauxite).

Hall found that a solution of aluminium oxide in a molten mixture of cryolite (Sodium aluminium fluoride) behaved as an electrolyte, and, when electrolyzed, the pure metal could be isolated. Hall was joined by a French metallurgist, Paul Louis Heroult, 23, and they both developed eventually the Hall-Heroult process that was later used in the aluminium industry.

1886 (J): **Fluorine,** a chemical elemetnt, was first isolated by **Henri Moissan** (1852-1907), French Chemist.

1886 (K): The **machine a calculer** invented by French engineer student, **Leon Bolle,** 18, was the first machine to automate multiplication using a direct method. Bolle's machine had a multitongued plate that constituted a multiplication table and represents a marked advance over calculators that employed multiple additions for multiplication.

The Comptometer introduced by the New Filt and Tarrant manufacturing Company of Chicago was the first multiple-column calculating machine to be operated entirely by keys and to be absolutely accurate at all times. Local inventor Dorr Eugine Felt, 25, had gone into partnership with Robert Tarrant to produce the machine. It was the only multiple-column key-operated calculator on the market until 1902. The Burrough's adding machine developed (1888) and patented by inventor Louis William Seward Burrough (1857-1898) was the first successful key-set recording and adding machine. In 1893, he was granted patents for the first practical adding machine.

1886 (L): Labour agitation for an 8-hours day and better working conditions made this the peak-year for strikes in 19th century **America.** Some 610,000 U. S. workers went on strike and monetary losses exceeded $ 33.5 million. In the same year, the American Federation of Labour was organized.

1886 (M): The Hay Market Massacre (that grew out of a police assault on strikers) at Chicago gave the U. S. Labour Movement its first martyrs and made the beginnings of **May Day** as a world-wide revolutionary memorial day.

1886 (N): An International Exposition was held at London.

The site of the exposition covered 13 acres; 5,550,745 people visited the exposition to view the exhibits costing £ 215,218.

1886 (O): The 24th edition of *Science and Health* by **Mrs. Mary Baker G. Eddy** was published.

The 8th chapter of the book was devoted to Imposition and Demonstration. It begins with four quotations. The second is from Sir Edwin Arnold's translation of the *Bhagavad Gita,* entitled *Song Celestial.* The passage runs thus:

Never the Spirit was born; the Spirit will cease to be never;
Never was time it was not; End and beginning are dreams;
Birthless and Deathless and Changeless remaineth the Spirit forever;
Death has not touched it at all, dead though the house of it seems.

Again, in the same chapter Mrs. Eddy says: "The ancient Hindoo philosophers understood something of this principle when they said in the *Song Celestial,* according to an old prose translation: 'The wise neither grieve for the dead nor for the living. I myself never was not, nor thou, nor all the princes of the earth; nor shall we ever hereafter cease and old age, so in some future frame will it find the like. One who is confirmed in this belief is not disturbed by anything that may come to pass. The sensibility of the faculties giveth heat and cold, pleasure and pain; which come and go and are transient and inconstant. Bear with patience, for the wise man whom these disturb not, and to whom pain and pleasure are the same, is formed for immortality' " (p. 259). This is a quotation from one of the old translations of the *Bhagavad Gita* by Charles Wilkins, published in London in 1785 and in New York in 1867.

"In the later editions of *Science and Health,* the 8th chapter was entirely suppressed and the above quotation was omitted, perhaps to show that the founder of Christian Science did not draw the water of truth from any other fountain than the Christian Bible.... But Mrs. Eddy, herself, was fully aware that the truths which she claimed to have discovered were discovered and taught in India by the Hindu sages and philosophers centuries before Jesus the Christ appeared on earth."– Swami Abhedananda, vide *Complete Works of Swami Abhedananda,* (Vol. II, p. 223, 224). [see 1879 (c), 1894 Mar. 9, 1894 Sept. 25]

1887 JAN. (third week): **NARENDRANATH**, along with his brother disciples performed the sacred *viraja homa* (a sacred ceremony which is gone through on the occasion of taking the vow of monastic life) at Baranagore Monastery and formally took the vows of lifelong celibacy and poverty.

They dedicated their lives to the realization of God and the service of men and assumed new names to signify their utter severance from the former ways of life. (Narendranath who changed his name several times, finally took the name of **SWAMI VIVEKANANDA** according to the suggestion of his own disciple, the Maharaja of Khetri, a few days before his starting for the West).

1887 JUN 22: Birth of **Sir Julian Huxley** (d. 1975), English Biologist and philosopher.

1887 AUG. 12: Birth of **Irwin Schrodinger** (d.1961), Austrian physicist, who contributed to the fundamentals of quantum mechanics by discovering its basic equation.

One of the most creative theoretical physicists of the 20th century, Schrödinger developed (in 1926, at Zurich) the wave equation that describes the behaviour of electrons and other sub-atomic particles. For that work, he won a Nobel Prize in physics in 1933.

1887 DEC. 22: Birth of **Srinivasa Ramanujam** (d. 1920), wizard of mathematics and first Indian to be elected to the Royal Society of London.

He is best known for his work on hypergeometric series and continued fractions. No scientist in India achieved fame so early as did Srinivasa Ramanujam at the age of 27. Prof. Hardy, a famous English Mathematician, wrote about Ramanujam: "It is sufficiently marvellous that he should have even dreamt of problems such as those which it had taken the first mathematicians of Europe a hundred years to solve."

1887 (A): Birth of **K. M. Munshi** (d. 1971), Indian nationalist and eminent jurist.

By his versatility, he made his contribution in all fields of life – political, social, educational, cultural and religious. By far the greatest of Munshi's contributions to the academic and cultural life of the country is the foundation of the Bharatiya Vidya Bhavan in 1938, a centre with many branches in many places.

1887 (B): **Sir Sayed Ahmed Khan** (1817-1898), Indian Muslim politician, led the conservative Muslim opposition to the Indian National Congress, organizing **Muslim Education Conference.** In 1895 he organized the Upper India Muslim Defence Association.

1887 (C): "Power tends to corrupt, and absolute power corrupts absolutely", writes **John Emerich Edward Dalberg Acton,** to Cambridge University professor Mandell Creighton.

Lord Acton was a liberal Roman Catholic and leader of the opposition to the papal dogma of infallibility [see 1870 Jul. 18] on which is based Church resistance to most forms of birth-control.

1887 (D): **Svante August Arhenius** (1859-1927), Swedish chemist and physicist, announced his **theory of electrolytic dissociation,** according to which most of the molecules of an electrolyte (substance that conducts electricity) are immediately dissociated into ions (electricity charged particles) when dissolved.

1887 (E): **Heinrich Hertz** (1857-1894), German physicist, who had been investigating James Clerk Maxwell's 1873 electromagnetic theory of light, [see 1864 (f), 1873 (f)] first demonstrated the existence of **electromagnetic waves.**

Hertz found that the waves were propagated with the velocity of light as Maxwell had predicted. He sent them through space, and measured their length and velocity. He showed that the nature of their liberation and their susceptibility to reflection and refraction were the same as those of light and heat waves. As a result he established beyond any doubt that light and heat are electromagnetic radiations. Hertz's work led to modern radio communications. [see 1895 (b)]

1887 (F): **Albert Michelson** (1852-1931), American physicist, established the **speed of light** as a fundamental constant in a celebrated experiment.

He worked with optical interferometers and using one of those instruments he and a colleague, Edward E. Morley (1838-1929), discovered that light has a constant speed in vacuo. With another interferometer he was able to measure accurately the diameter of a star.

1887 (G): The **gramophone** patented by the German-American inventor, **Emile Berliner** (1851-1929), improved on Edison's phonograph by substituting a disk and a horizontally moving needle for Edison's cylinder and vertically moving needle [see 1877 Nov. 29].

Three years later, Berliner improved the quality of sound reproduction by utilizing disc-recording and better cutting techniques. His improvement was eventually adopted universally.

1887 (H): Using the capillary electrometer invented by Gabriel Lippmann (in 1873), English physiologist **Augustus Waller** recorded the **electric curents generated by the heart**.

To overcome inadequacies of Waller's device, in 1901, **Willem Einthoven** (1860-1927), Indonesian-born physiologist of Leiden invented a recording system using a string galvanometer. The current generated by the heart was led to this recording insturment to obtain a curve that was later called an **electrocardiogram (ECG)**. By 1913, Einthoven had worked out the interpretation of the normal tracing and was able to use ECG as a diagnostic tool. Einthoven was awarded the 1924 Nobel prize for medicine for the development of the electrocardiogram.

1888 (early part): **SWAMI VIVEKANANDA set out on pilgrimage.** He proceeded towards the Himalayas, visiting on the way the notable religious and historical places like Varanasi, Ayodhya, Lucknow, Agra and Brindaban.

It was during this period that the Station Master of the Railway Station at Hathras, Sri Sarat Chandra Gupta (afterwards became known in the Ramakrishna Order as Swami Sadananda) became the disciple of Swamiji and accompanied him in his pilgrimage. This very first journey brought ancient India vividly before his eyes – eternal India – the India of the Vedas, with its race of heroes and gods, clothed in the glory of legend and history, Aryans, Moghuls and Dravidians – all one. At the first impact he realized the spiritual unity of India and Asia and he communicated this discovery to the brethren of Baranagore.

1888 APR. 15: Death of **Matthew Arnold** (b. 1822), English poet and critic, whose most characteristic work *Culture and Anarchy* (1869) deals with the difficulty of preserving personal values in a world drastically transformed by industrialism and democracy.

1888 JUN. - NOV. : During his second pilgrimage to holy places in North India, **SWAMI VIVEKANANDA** was staying at **Meerut,** along with some of his *gurubhais* (brother disciples). One of the latter, viz., Gangadhar (Swami Akhandananda) used to bring him from a library some books, which he read quickly and returned. When he was thus finishing and returning the volumes of Sir John Lubbock, the Librarian became sceptical and asked Gangadhar whether his friend really read the books, or simply looked at the gilded bindings. Swamiji asked Gangadhar to request the librarian to come and ask him any questions about the books he had finished reading. His curiosity roused, the librarian came, asked him some questions and was convinced that he had been wrong.

Later during Swamiji's travels, when he was staying with Haripada Mitra at Belgaum, the latter was filled with astonishment when he found Swamiji quoting some two or three pages from *Pickwick Papers* by Charles Dickens. Mitra asked Swamiji whether he had read the book quite a number of times. Swamiji said that he had read it twice during his school days and once again some six months back.

Swamiji's way of reading was extraordinary. Much of his scholarship and learning was the result of his vast study.

1888 SEP. 4: **M. K. Gandhi,** who had passed his matriculation examination (1887), sailed from Bombay to London, to study Law.

On 10th January, 1891, he passed the Law Examination and was admitted to the Bar.

1888 SEP. 5: Birth of **Sir S. Radhakrishnan** (d. 1975), philosopher, educationalist, and statesman.

He was a great authority on Hindu Philosophy. In his lectures and books he tried to interpret Indian thought for Westerners.

1888 OCT. 30: The first patent for a **ball-pen** invented by **John H. Loud,** was issued in U. S. A.

1888 OCT. 31: The first patent for a pneumatic bicycles tyre was awarded to Scottish veterinary surgeon **John Boyd Dunlop,** 47, at Belfast, Ireland.

The first motor car to be equipped with pneumatic tyres was produced by French, automakers Rene Panhard and E. C. Lavassor, in 1892. In 1893 pneumatic tyres were put in motor cars for the first time [see 1893 (k)] by France's Andre Michelin, 42, and his brother, Edourd, 36, whose Michelin and Co. became the larger tyre producer and one of the world's three leading tyre companies. In 1895, the first U. S. pneumatic tyres were produced by the bicycle maker Pope Manufacturing Company.

1888 NOV. 7: Birth of **Sir C. V. Raman** (d. 1970), Indian physicist who received Nobel Prize for Physics in 1930 for his work on diffusion of fight and discovery of **'Raman Effect'** .

1888 (A): **Sri Narayana Guru** (1856-1928), the harbinger of peaceful revolution in the conditions of the depressed people in Kerala, founded a **Shiva temple** (at Aruvipuram, near Trivandrum,) where they enjoyed freedom of worship.

This was at a time when they were prevented from entering or even going anywhere near such temples, let alone worshipping in them. The founding of Shiva temple was a big challenge hurled against outworn traditions. It was prelude to a great socio-religious revolution which was both constructive and peaceful.

1888 (B): **Sir Sayed Ahmed Khan** (1817-1898), Indian Muslim politician, who never supported the programme of the Indian National Congress, formed an anti-Congress organization – the **United Patriotic Association –** and called on co-religionists to withdraw from Congress.

In a speech delivered at Meerut on March 14, 1888, Sayed Ahmed referred to the Hindus and Muslims not only as two nations, but also two warring nations who could not lead a common political life if ever the British left India. He said: "Now suppose that all English were to leave India, then who would be rulers of India? Is it possible that under these circumstances two nations, the Muhammedan and Hindu, could sit on the same throne and remain equal in power. Most certainly not. It is necessary that one of them should conquer the other and thrust it down. To hope that both could remain equal is to desire the impossible and incredible." (Bharatiya Vidya Bhavan's *History and Culture of Indian People,* Vol. X, Part II, p. 309).

Syed Ahmed who looked upon the system of representative government demanded by the Indian National Congress as dangerous to the interests of Muslims, broadly hinted that if the demand were conceded, the Muslim minority might be forced to take up sword to prevent the tyranny of the majority. He said: "In a country like India where homogeneity does not exist in any one of these fields (nationality, religion, ways of living, custom, mores, culture, and historical tradition), the introduction of representative government cannot produce any beneficial results; it can only result in interfering with the peace and prosperity of the land.... The aim and objects of the Indian National Congress are based upon an ignorance of history and present-day realities; they do not take into consideration that India is inhabited by different nationalities.... I consider the experiment which the Indian National Congress wants to make fraught with dangers and suffering for all the nationalities of India, specially for the Muslims. The Muslims are in a minority, but they are a highly united minority. At least traditionally they are prone to take the sword in hand when the majority oppresses them. If this happens, it will bring about disaster greater than the ones which came in the wake of the happenings of 1857. The Congress cannot rationally prove its claim to represent the opinions, ideals and aspirations of the Muslims. (Ibid., p. 310).

Decades later (1936), in the Bombay Session of the Muslim League, Sir Wazir Hussain also openly declared that the Hindus and Muslims inhabiting the vast continent were not two communities but they should be considered as two nations in many respects. Mr. M. A. Jinnah later developed this theory and saw to it that India was partitioned so as to create a separate homeland for the Muslims.

The demand for a separate homeland for Muslims was first made in a resolution of the Muslim League at its Lahore session held on March 23, 1940, which runs as follows: "Resolved that it is the considered view of this session of All India Muslim League that no constitutional scheme will be workable in this country and acceptable to Muslims unless it is designed on the following lines: viz., that geographically contiguous units are demarcated into regions which should be constituted with such territorial readjustments as may be necessary that the areas in which the Muslims are numerically in majority should be grouped to constitute
independent States." Ultimately this resolution was implemented and Pakistan was carved out of India, to be a separate country for Muslims in 1947.

1888 (C): Birth of **J. B. Kripalani** (d. 1982), a devoted nationalist, and veteran Gandhian, and one of the most outspoken, honest and sincere statesmen of India.

1888 (D): Birth of **Abul Kalam Azad** (d.1958), scholar, and Indian nationalist Muslim.

1888 (E): Birth of **John L. Baird** (d. 1946), Scottish Inventor who successfully demonstrated television in England (1926).

Baird's mechanical system of television, similar to that of C. F. Jenkins in the United States, was based on Paul Von Nipkov's rotating disc (1886), but had technical limitations; modern electronic television developed from the cathode-ray tube (1897) of Karl Ferdinand Braun and A. A. Campbell-Swinton's proposals (1911) for use of a cathode-ray, to scan an image. [see 1884 (g), 1897 (e)]

1888 (F): An alternating-current **electric motor** was developed by Croatian-American inventor **Nikola Tesla,** 31, who applied a variation of the rotary magnetic field principle discovered three years ago by the Italian Galileo Ferraris to a practical induction motor that largely supplanted direct-current motor for most uses. [see 1886 (e)]

A former Edison Company employee at West Orange, N. J. Tesla made possible the production and distribution of alternating-current with his induction, synchronous and split-phase motors. He also developed systems of polyphase transmission of power over distances and pioneered the invention of radio.

1888 (G): **Ballistite,** a smokeless explosive powder, made of nitrocellulose and nitroglycerin, was introduced by **Alfred Nobel** (1833-1896), who had earlier invented dynamite. [see 1866 (e)]

This year a bizarre incident rocked the very nerves of Alfred Nobel. It was in the morning papers that he read his own obituary. In fact his brother Ludwig had died but the press had mistakenly written his obituary. The papers had branded him as a "merchant of death", because his fortune had been amassed through the manufacturing of arms and ammunitions. It left an indelible mark upon his conscience. He resolved to change his "dead image" while he was still alive. He turned a philanthropist. He gave millions of dollars to the poor and those in despair. At the time of his death (1896) his immense fortune amounted to 9 million dollars. In his will, he desired that the money be spent in awarding annual international awards, for outstanding achievements in five domains, namely, Physics, Chemistry, Physiology or Medicine, Literature and the promotion of Peace (awarded since 1901). [see 1866 (e), 1896 Dec. 10, 1901 (g)]

1888 (H): The first **typewriter stencil** was introduced at London by immigrant Hungarian inventor, **David Gestetner,** who, seven years ago, had introduced the first wax stencil duplicating machine to be marketed commercially. Chicago's A. B. Dick Company introduced its first typewriter stencil in 1890.

1888 (I): George Eastman (1854-1932), U. S. Inventor and manufacturer of photographic materials, perfected and introduced the **hand camera (Kodak)**. He had previously invented the first successful roll film (1880).

The Kodak Camera revolutionized photography by making it possible for any amateur to take satisfactory snapshots. [see 1884 (e), 1892 (b), 1895 (e)]

1888 (J): Mme. Blavatsky (1831-1891), theosophist and social reformer, wrote the *Secret Doctrine,* which purports to incorporate the *Book of Dzyan,* a work she affirmed to be a mysterious oriental source expounding the occult origins of the earth.

1888-94: Lord Lansdowne (1845-1927), the Viceroy of India.

1889 JAN. 2: Birth of **Sorokin** (d. 1968), Russian sociologist.

1889 APR: Birth of **Dr. Keshav Baliram Hedgewar** (d. 1940), a champion of Hindu cultural and nationalist renaissance and the founder of Rashtriya Swayamsevak Sangh (R. S. S.), a cultural force for national reorganization in India.

He was a lifelong celibate who had dedicated himself to the cause of national emancipation since his boyhood.

His successor, Sri M. S. Golwalkar (Sri Guruji) (1906-1973) – a highly learned and intensely spiritual personality, spread the organization to every nook and corner of the country and built it up as a powerful national instrument for the rejuvenation of India and its culture.

1889 APR. 14: Birth of **Arnold Joseph Toynbee** (d. 1975), British historian, best known for his comparative study of civilization.

His monumental work, *A Study of History* (1934-1954, 10 Vols.), constitutes an exhaustive re-examination of human development in the light of an idealist philosophy of history.

1889 APR. 20: Birth of **Adolf Hitler** (d. 1945), Austrian-born politician, who became the dictator of Germany in 1933.

1889 JUL. 30: Birth of **Zworykin,** Russian-American physicist and radio engineer who made important contributions to the development of television as well as the new field of electromier.

1889 NOV. 14: Birth of **Jawaharlal Nehru** (d. 1964), the first Prime Minister of Independent India.

An agnostic, he later on wrote in his Autobiography referring to his childhood days: "Of religion I had very hazy notions. It seemed to be a woman's affair. Father and my elder cousins treated the question humorously and refused to take it seriously." (p. 8). "Great as he (father) was in many ways in my eyes, I felt that he was lacking in spirituality." (p. 15). No wonder the son emulated the father.

1889 (A): Birth of **Nandalal Bose** (d. 1966), distinguished Indian artist.

1889 (B): **Almon B. Strowger,** invented an **automatic system of telephone** which was installed at La Porti, Ind., in 1892, the first automatic telephone exchange in the world.

1889 (C): A **coin-operated telephone** was patented by U. S. inventor **William Gray,** and was installed in the Hartford Bank, Conn., U. S. A.

1889 (D): **I. M. Singer Company** introduced the first **electric sewing machine** and sold a million machines, up from 539,000 in 1880.

1889 (E): The **bacilli of tetanus** and of symptomatic **anthrax** were isolated by Japanese bacteriologist **Shibasaburo Kitasato,** who worked with **Robert Koch** at Berlin.

1889 (F): **Diabetes research** was advanced by German physiologists **J. Von Mering** and **O. Minkowski** who removed the pancreas of a dog and observed that although the animal survived, it urinated more frequently, and the urine attracted flies and wasps. When they analysed the urine, they found the dog had a canine equivalent of diabetes, which ultimately caused it to go into a coma and die.

In 1922, the hormone insulin isolated from canine pancreatic juices gave diabetics a new cease of life, the first treatment for the disease other than diet restrictions. Fredrick Grant Banting and Charles Herbert Best, had isolated insulin; they used it to save the life of 14-year old Leonard Thompson who was dying in Toronto General Hospital.

1889 (G): The world's first **electric elevators** were installed by the **Otis Company** in New York's Demarest building of Fifth Avenue at 33rd Street.

1889 (H): **Thomas Edison** patented a form of **peep-show machine** for showing photographic moving pictures to one viewer at a time. [see 1864 (e), 1871 Nov. 29, 1878 (h), 1882 (e), 1883 (d), 1891 Dec. 29, 1893 (h)]

The Lumiere brothers then began to manufacture films for the Edison peep-show and by 1895 they patented a device which would both photograph and project films. This followed by a year the opening of Edison's Kinetoscope Parlour (in New York city) where pictures (peep-show) could be viewed by but one person at a time.

Prototype of the modern film projection was the Vitascope (1896) devised by Charles Francis Jenkins (1867-1934) and Thomas Armat on the basis of Edison's Kinetoscope.

1889 (I): Cordite – the first smokeless, slow-burning explosive powder made of nitroglycerin, nitrocellulose and mineral jelly – was patented by English Chemist, **Frederick Auguste Abel** (1827-1902) and Scottish physicist, **James Dewar** (1842-1923). It was developed to replace gun powder.

1889 (J): Henri Louis Bergson (1859-1942), French philosopher, who opposed mechanism and determinism and vigorously asserted the importance of pure reason, duration and liberty, brought out his work, *Time and Free Will,* in which he suggested that the distinction of philosophy from science indicates that there may be different modes of knowledge.

1889 (K): Fabian Society, London, published *Fabian Essays on Socialism,* which emphasized the importance of economics and class structure. It was edited by **George Bernard Shaw** (1856-1950), British playwright and critic, for whom the economics was "the basis of society".

Believing in permeation, not Marxist revolution, the members of the Fabian Society, at first, aimed to achieve municipal socialism and the collectivist state by influencing liberal and conservative politicians. They assisted in the birth of the Labour Party. Besides publishing *Fabian Essays,* they used the results of their Bureau's research into economic and social problems to educate the public through pamphlets, lectures and summer schools.

New Fabian Essays (edited by R. H. S. Crossman, 1952), outlined fresh paths to socialism since much of early Fabian policy had been effected in the welfare state policy of 20th century Governments. [see 1884 Jan. (a)]

1889 (L): The Eiffel Tower, designed by French engineer **Alexandre Gustave Eiffel,** (1832-1923), was completed in Paris.

Built as the central feature for the Paris Exhibition of 1889, the soaring tower (1,056 ft. high, including a 55 ft. television antenna), had a wrought-iron superstructure on a reinforced concrete base; it contained more than 7000 tons of iron, 18,038 girders and plates, 1,050,846 rivets, and had three hydraulic elevators. The total cost of construction of this tower was £ 260,000. It was a landmark in the building construction history and on the skyline of Paris. It was in this tower that the potentialities of steel construction were strikingly revealed. The Paris Exhibition, opened on May 6, centred around the Eiffel tower.

1889 (M): The **Paris Exhibition** was held in commemoration of the Centenary of the French Revolution.

It was visited by over 32 million people and cost over 144 million Francs. Spread over an area of 72 acres, the Fair had 61,722 exhibits. It was in this exhibition that **Gottlieb Daimler** (1834-1900), German mechanical engineer, exhibited his first motor car (a four-wheeled vehicle). On the occasion of the Paris Exhibition, the Eiffel Tower, the tallest structure in the world, was first opened to public view. [see 1889 (k)]

1889 (N): Hindu-Muslim riots at Hoshiarpur, Ludhiana, Ambala and Dera Ghazikhan. [see 1874 Feb 13, 1877 Sept, 1885 (a), 1886 (c), 1891 (b), 1893 (c), 1897 June]

1889 (O): "The man who dies rich dies disgraceful", wrote U. S. Steel Magnate, **Andrew Carnegie** (1835-1919), in an article on *The Gospel of Wealth.*

He was praised for his philanthropy by U. S. oil magnate John D. Rockefeller (1839-1937).

In 1901 Andrew Carnegie sold his interest in the Carnegie Steel Company and spent the rest of his life distributing his wealth in benefactions amounting to 350 million dollars.

In 1881 Carnegie donated funds for a Pittsburg Library and began a series of library gifts. In 1900 Carnegie's Institute of Technology was founded at Pittsburg with a donation from him. The first extensive public library system in New York city (1901) made possible by his gift of $ 5,200,000, providing for 39 branches. With a gift of $ 10 million each, the Carnegie Institute of Washington (devoted to scientific research) and the Carnegie Foundation for the Advancement of the Technology were founded in 1902 and 1905, respectively. In 1911, the Carnegie Corporation of New York was created with a $ 125 million gift from Carnegie to encourage education.

1889 (P): The Second Socialist International (Working Mens' Association) set up in Paris was a second attempt at the organization of International Socialism, the first being in 1864.

The Association arose from the large assembly of socialists in Paris for the Centenary of the French Revolution (1789). Anarchists were excluded and the International embarked on a long series of congresses, providing an effective forum for debate, the exchange of information and the promotion of international understanding. By 1910, with a permanent base in the international Socialist Bureau in Brussels, the movement had 896 delegates representing 23 nationalities. But its support for the Russian Revolution in 1905 was the nearest it came to true international solidarity. The International's most enduring decision was its proclamation of May 1, as Labour Day. [see 1864 (d)]

1889 (Q): The five issues of *Sahitya Kalpadruma* (a monthly magazine in Bengali) carried **SWAMI VIVEKANANDA'S selections from the *Imitation of Christ*** by Thomas a Kempis.

As footnotes Swamiji appended selections from Hindu scriptures which he felt paralleled the idea expressed by the Christian mystic; or his explanation of the underlying Christian theology; or occasionally, his own comment or interpretation. The selections from the 'Imitation' are from the Book I, Ch. 1-6. It was originally intended to publish selections from the entire book, but the Swamiji did not complete the project *(Prabuddha Bharata,* Sep. 1982, p. 320).

1890 FEB. 4: In the course of his pilgrimage to the holy places in North India, **SWAMI VIVEKANANDA met the illustrious saint, Pavahari Baba, at Ghazipur.**

Swamiji held Baba in high respect for his yogic powers and extreme form of self-denial, and had a mind to learn hathayoga from him. For this he was prepared to go to such lengths as to be ready to accept him as guru. On the night preceding the day fixed for the initiation ceremony he saw the form of Sri Ramakrishna standing before him on the right side, looking steadfastly at him, as if very much grieved. The Master did not say anything but through the mist of tears with which they were covered, the disciple saw words of power, divinity, love and insight. When, after a day or two, the idea again rose in his mind, there was again the appearance of Sri Ramakrishna at night. After he had thus the vision of Sri Ramakrishna for several nights, he gave up the idea of initiation altogether, and returned to the monastery at Baranagore. Later, Swamiji told his disciples, "Mixing with Pavahari Baba, I liked him very much and he also came to love me deeply. One day I thought that I did not learn any art for making this weak body strong, after living with Sri Ramakrishna for many years. I had heard that Pavahari Baba knew this science of hathayoga. So I thought that I would learn the practices of hathayoga from him and through them strengthen the body." [see 1898 June]

1890 JUL. (middle): **SWAMI VIVEKANANDA set out on his pilgrimage to the Himalayas.**

His mind pined for penetrating again into the depths of the snow-clad Himalayas to equip himself by means of meditation and mental discipline, with a tremendous spiritual power to carry on his Master's work without let or hindrance. Before starting for the journey he met the Holy Mother Sarada Devi and received her hearty blessings for the success of his mission. He told his *gurubhais,* "**I shall not return until I acquire such realizations that my very touch will transform a man.**" Elsewhere he told one of his friends, "**I am going away; but I shall never come back until I can burst on society like a bomb, and make it follow me like a dog.**"

Whether at Almora, a beauty spot in the heart of the Himalayas, or, in a lonely cottage by the banks of the holy Alakananda at Srinagar, whether at Tehri and Rajpur, at Hardwar or Rishikesh, the holy seat of saints and sages – everywhere the Swami put himseif into the treadmill of hard spiritual discipline to get ready for the great task ahead.

1890 (A): **Java man fossils** of a prehistoric human ancestor were found at Kedung Brebus, Java, by Dutch Palaeontologist, **Eugene Dubois,** who was serving as a military surgeon in the East Indies. The fossil evidence of Pithecanthus erectus was found in an earth stratum dating from the pleistocene era of 700,000 B. C.

1890 (B): **The first complete steel frame structure** was built in Chicago; steel made possible skyscrapers, as did the earlier invention (1854) of the elevator by Elisha G. Otis (1811-1861).

1890 (C): **The first commercial dry cell battery** was introduced under the name 'Ever Ready' by National Carbon Company.

1890 (D): **Cyanide process** of extracting gold from low grade ore invented by two U. S. metallurgists, **MacArthur** and **Forrest.** As a result, the annual production of gold in U. S. more than doubled within 8 years.

1890 (E): **Emil Von Behring** (1854-1917), German hygienist and physicist, and **Shibasaburo Kitasato** (1856-1931), Japanese bacteriologist, demonstrated that the serum of immunized rabbits neutralized the toxin of **tetanus.** [see 1889 (e)]

This discovery opened the possibility that disease could be prevented through the stimulation of specific antibody production.

The first Diphtheria antitoxin was produced by Behring, who worked with Robert Koch's Laboratory and whose discovery won him the first Nobel Prize for Medicine in 1901.

1890 (F): Publication of *The Golden Bough* (first volume) by Scottish anthropologist **James George Frazer,** 36, who published 15 further volumes in the next 25 years in a monumental exploration of the cults, legends, myths and rites of the world and their influence on the development of religion; a one-volume abridged version was published in 1922.

1890 (G): **Charles Rockwell Lanman** (1850-1941), American Sanskrit scholar, brought out his work: *Beginnings of Hindu Pantheism.*

In 1889 Lanman travelled in India collecting valuable manuscripts for Harvard Library. He was particularly attracted to Indian religion.

Lanman is chiefly remembered for his editorship of the *Harvard Oriental Series,* which he began in 1891, and for which he enlisted the talents of a wide range of scholars in America and abroad. No other American has yet done to provide the West with an accurate knowledge of ancient India.

1890 (H): William James (1842-1910), American psychologist and philosopher, brought out his work: *Principles of Psychology,* which revolutionized study of psychology in America.

1890 (I): Gabriel Tarde (1843-1903), French social psychologist, published *Les Lois D'imitation,* a pioneer work in the field of **social psychology.** At the same time, Pierre Jenet (1845-1949), another French psychologist, carried on studies of hypnosis and hysteria.

1890 (J): Gottlieb Daimler (1834-1900), German inventor, founded the **Daimler Motor Company,** which produced the Mercedes automobiles. [see 1885 (b)]

1891 JAN. (end): SWAMI VIVEKANANDA began his historic itinerary of two years through the vast expanse of his motherland.

A grim struggle had so long been raging within the great Swami between the two apparently conflicting forces – one to dive into the bottomless depth of the ocean of Reality to pick up gems of supreme spiritual wisdom, and the other to jump into the fray of life to mitigate the untold miseries of the inarticulate millions and to liquidate the illiteracy and untouchability that were eating the vitals of the race. The latter ideal now loomed so large before his vision that he snapped the golden ties of love and affection of his monastic brothers, and plunged into the trackless ocean of India to do the bidding of the Master. In the words of Romain Rolland, "He wandered free from plan, caste, home, constantly alone with God. And there was no single hour of his life when he was not brought into contact with the sorrows, the desires, the abuses and feverishness of living men, rich and poor, in town and field; he became one with their lives; the great book of life revealed to him what all the books in the libraries could not have.... the tragic face of the present-day, the God struggling in humanity, the cry of the people of India, and of the world, for help and the heroic duty of the new Oedipus, whose task it was to deliver Thebes from the talons of the sphinx or to perish with Thebes." This memorable sojourn, replete as it was with many a thrilling incident and experience was significant in a variety of ways.

1891 APR. 14: Birth of **Dr. B. R. Ambedkar** (d. 1956), Indian social reformer and politician, and the leader of the depressed classes, who devoted himself to improve the life of his 'untouchable' fellowmen.

1891 MAY 15: The papal encyclical on labour questions, **Rerum movarum,** issued by **Pope Leo XIII,** pointed out that the possessing classes, including the employees, have important moral duties to fulfil; that it is one of the first duties of society (state and church collaborating) to improve the position of the workers. Leo expressed in his encylicals the same condemnation of many phases of liberalism and nationalism, and reiterated the view that the church should superintend and direct every form of secular life.

1891 NOV. (first week)**:** During his itinerary in Kathiawar, (Gujarat), when **SWAMI VIVEKANANDA** visited Limbdi, the headquarters of a cotton-growing state of that name, he had to undergo an ordeal.

> After wandering about here and there in the streets in search of a shelter and living on alms, he came to a place which seemed to be a heaven. The site was removed from the hustle and bustle of the city and the Swami was warmly received by the 'sadhus' who dwelt there. They assigned him a decent room, where, they said, he was free to stay as long as he wished. The place, as a matter of fact, was a den of some practitioners of black magic who, finding that he was a *brahmacharin* with a magnetic personality, wanted to break his *brahmacharya* with a view to achieving psychic powers for themselves through a notorious *'sadhana'*. His suspicions roused, the Swami decided to leave the place immediately but to his bewilderment found that he was locked in. With wonderful presence of mind he at once devised a means of escape. Through a boy who used to come to him and had become very fond of him he sent a message, written with charcoal on a broken piece of water jug, to the Thakore Saheb, informing him about his plight and requesting him to save him. The Prince immediately sent a guard to the place to rescue him. Thereafter, at the earnest request of the Prince, whose name was Bhimia Chand, he stayed at the palace. The Prince became his disciple and soon so very attached to him that he requested him to spend the rest of his days at Limbdi (*A Comprehensive Biography of Swami Vivekananda,* Part I, p. 323).

1891 DEC. 29: First important **radio patent** awarded to **Thomas Edison** for a "means of transmitting signals electrically.... without the use of wires." In the same year Edison made the first commercial motion picture. [see 1864 (e), 1877 Nov. 19, 1878 (h), 1882 (e), 1883 (d), 1889 (h)]

1891 (A): According to the **second All India Census,** Hindus were 72.32 per cent of the total population, Muslims 19.96 per cent, Christians 0.76 per cent and others 6.93 per cent. [see 1872 (b), 1881 (a), 1901 (c)]

1891 (B): Hindu-Muslim riots at Palakod in the Salem District of Madras. [see 1874 Feb. 13, 1877 Sept, 1885 (a), 1886 (c), 1889 (m), 1893 (c), 1897 June]

1891 (C): Russian crops failed, millions were reduced to **starvation** and the rural peasantry raided towns in search of food. In the following year (1892), **famine crippled Russia** by late January, some 3 million barrels of U. S. flour were en route to relieve the starvation that was killing millions.

1891 (D): Thousands rushed to **Cripple Creek** on the slopes of Pike's Peak in Colarado, following the **discovery of gold** there.

By 1900, the Cripple Creek gold field yielded $ 20 million worth of gold per year and was second only to South Africa's Transval Gold Field discovered in 1886. It was far larger than the Klondike Field discovered four years before in Alaska and North West Canada. The Cripple Creek mines grew in the next 20 years and became the fifth larger producer in the world history; they yielded nearly $ 1 billion in the yellow metal.

1891 (E): Death of **Mme. Blavatsky**, the founder of the **Theosophical Society**. [see 1875 Nov. 15]

1891 (F): First **sun photography** in America made possible by the invention of the **spectro-heliograph** by **George E. Hale** of University of Chicago.

1891 (G): **Oscar Wilde** (1854-1900), Irish writer and poet, brought out his novel *The Picture of Dorian Gray* which was the mirror of the new aesthete. He achieved immortality with plays such as *Lady Windermere's Fan* (1893) and *The Importance of Being Earnest* (1894), which are masterpieces of humour. Wilde became a notorious figure in London society for his witty epigrams and unconventional behaviour.

1891 (H): Publication of *Gospel Criticism and Historical Christianity* by **Pres. Orello Cone** of Buchtel College (U. S. A.) reflected new liberal interpretations of the Bible and Christianity, interpretations that came into conflict with the views of fundamental religious leaders in America. Publication of Washington Gladden's *Who Wrote the Bible* also reflected new liberal approach to the scriptures. Although questioning the absolute infallibility of the Bible, Gladden's work discovered the hitherto neglected literary, spiritual and ethical values in the Bible and served to rekindle popular interest in it.

The Fundamentalist's crusade of the early 1900 grew out of conservative protestants' insistence on the liberal truth of the Bible and their increasing alarm at the emergence of liberal theology, which attempted to reconcile Christian teachings with modern scientific thought, particularly Darwin's theories.

1891 (I): German **factory workers won the right** (June 1) **to form Committees** that would negotiate with employers on conditions of employment, and factory inspection was made more efficient. In the same year, **the world's first old age pension plan** went into effect in Germany. Introduced by **Prince Yon Bismarck** in the **Old Age Insurance Act** of June 1889, the plan compelled all workers to contribute if they were over the age 16, were fully employed, and earned more than 2000 marks ($ 500) per year. Employers must contribute equal amounts and the pension was payable at the age of 70 to persons who had paid premium for a minimum of 30 years.

1891 (J): University of Chicago founded with a munificent donation of 30 million dollars from **John D. Rockefeller** (1839-1937) American industrialist and philanthropist.

He gave it over 80 million dollars during his life time. Marshall Field, U. S. merchant gave 25 acres of land on which the University buildings were erected. He also contributed one million dollars the following year.

1891 (K): The **diphtheria vaccine** was given its first human application on a child dying in a Berlin Hospital, the child recovered and was discharged a week later.

1891 (L): Basket ball was invented at Springfield, Mass. by Canadian-American physical Education Director **James Naismith** 30, who was taking a course at the YMCA training School in Springfield and who had been assigned with his classmates the project of inventing a game that would occupy students between the football and base ball season.

1892 MAR. 15: The Reno Inclined Elevator patented by New York inventor James W. Reno, was **the world's first escalator.** The flat step moving staircase patented by U. S. inventor **Charles A. Wheeler** (Aug. 2) was the first practical escalator.

1892 MAR. 26: Death of **Walt Whitman** (b. 1819), who is generally considered to be most important poet of the 19th century.

His *Leaves of Grass* was a landmark in the history of American literature. It was at Lahore towards the end of 1897, a short time after his return from America, that **SWAMI VIVEKANANDA** read *'Leaves of Grass'*, and he called Whitman "the sannyasin of America." *Leaves of Grass* was described by Emerson as 'a mixture' of the *Bhagavad Gita* and *The New York Herald.*

1892 APR. 13: Birth of **Sir Robert Watson Watt,** Scottish physicist, who developed **RADAR.**

In 1935 while working at the National Physical Laboratory at Teddington, not far from London, he perfected a method for locating distant objects in space by the use of radio waves. This device, which was later to become known as RADAR (Radio Detecting And Ranging), provided early warning of an air attack, since enemy aircraft could be detected while they were still many miles away.

1892 JUN. : As an itinerant monk **SWAMI VIVEKANANDA** visited Poona, he was the guest for several days of **Bal Gangadhar Tilak**, (1856-1920), the renowned scholar and patriot, with whom the Swami had many interesting conversations on various topics.

The Swami avoided mixing with society and did not make any public speeches but once, when he accompanied Tilak to the Deccan Club, rose to reply to a speech made by one of the Members on a philosophical subject. He then pointed out, in fluent English, the other aspect of the subject. As Tilak said, at home the Swami talked frequently – about Advaita philosophy and Vedanta.

The Swami had remained anonymous during his stay at Mr. Tilak's house, for, when they first met in the railway carriage at Bombay, the Swami, being asked his name, had said that he was just a *sannyasin*, and courtesy forbade Mr. Tilak to put the question again to him. A couple of years later when Swami Vivekananda returned to India with world-wide fame owing to his grand success at the Parliament of Religions Tilak happened to see his likeness in some of the newspapers, and from a similarity of features thought that the Swami who had resided in his house must have been the same. He wrote to him accordingly, enquiring if his inference was correct and requesting him to kindly pay a visit to Poona on his way to Calcutta. The Swami sent a "fervent reply", frankly admitting that he was the same sannyasin and expressing his regret that he was not able to visit Poona then. It was not till about four years later when Mr. Tilak came to Calcutta to attend a session of the Indian National Congress that another meeting between the two persons took place. [see 1901 Dec. (last week)]

1892 SEP. : The first U. S. motor car was produced by **Charles and Franklin Duryea,** bicycle designers and tool makers, at Chicopee. Mass. It had a four-cycle water-cooled engine and rubber and leather transmission. In the same month an electric automobile, made by William Morrison of Des Moines, Iowa, appeared on streets of Chicago. The owner had to call the police to help him make his way through crowds of curious spectators.

1892 OCT. 6: Death of **Alfred Tennyson** (b 1801), the English poet, regarded by his contemporaries as the greatest poet of Victorian England.

1892 OCT. 20-23: Magnificent ceremonies dedicated the **World's Columbian Exposition at Chicago**.

In pursuance of a public demand for some fitting commemoration of the discovery of America, the U. S. Congress had passed an Act (April 25, 1890) authorizing an "Exhibition of the arts, industries, manufactures and products of the soil, mine and sea" The American President, Harrison, had recommended a sum of "not less than 10 million dollars" be allotted for the Fair. The estimated expenditure was given as over 22 million dollars. The exposition officially opened on May 1, 1893.

1892 NOV. : As a wandering monk, **SWAMI VIVEKANANDA** visited Kerala. He stayed at Trichur for a few days before he went to Ernakularn, the capital of the Cochin State.

While at Ernakulam, Swamiji met **Chattambi Swamigal** (1853-1924) the scholar-saint of Travancore, and a close associate (and according to some the guru) of Sri Narayana Guru (1856-1928). A great soul and an equally brilliant mind Chattambi Swamigal was a remarkable peripatetic. On the day of meeting, he was at the residence of Rama lyer, the Dewan Secretary, who was himself a great admirer of Chattambi Swamigal. The two great sannyasins spoke in Sanskrit. Swami Vivekananda introduced the topic of *chinmudra* in the discussion, and the illuminating way in which Chattambi Swamigal discoursed on the subject enabled Swamiji to have a glimpse of *'Kerala Pratibha'*. They had another edifying discussion on the next day. Swamiji is reported to have described Chattambi Swamigal as a "wonderful man".

While passing through Travancore, Swami Vivekananda saw with his own eyes how Christian missionaries had taken advantage of caste tyranny to convert vast numbers of the people into Christianity. After having witnessed the shocking extent of untouchability in Travancore State the Swami was impelled to remark that the entire state had turned into a "lunatic asylum". In a letter, Swamiji wrote, "come and see what the *padres* (Christian missionaries) are doing in *Dakshin* (South). They are converting by lakhs the lower classes of Travancore – the most priest-ridden country in India, nearly one fourth of the population has become Christians."

According to later census (1901), 6.97 lakhs out of 29.52 lakhs of population of the Travancore State, i.e., 23.60% were Christians. By 1941 the percentage of Christian population in Travancore State shot up to 32.29%. That is 20 lakhs out of 50 lakhs of the population of the State were Christians.

1892 DEC. 6: Death of **W. V. Siemens** (b.1816) German born engineer, inventor and the chief founder of the electrical firm, 'Siemens and Halske'

1892 DEC. 13-22: While at Trivandrum, **SWAMI VIVEKANANDA** was the guest of the learned Professor **Sri Sundararama lyer,** tutor to the nephew of the Maharaja of Travancore.

There he came in contact with a distinguished scholar named Sri Rangachariar of Madras, the Professor of Chemistry at the Maharaja's College. Both the savants were so deeply impressed by the versatility of the genius of Swamiji and also by the sublimity and simplicity of his personality that they spent hour after hour in illuminating conversation with him on a variety of subjects ranging from the highest metaphysical flights of the Vedanta philosophy to modern Kant and Hegel, from the splendid achievements of science to the glories of art and music, both ancient and modern, and from the sublimities of ancient yoga to the complex problems of education and sociology, and they were amazed and enraptured by the vast range of his mental horizon. Prof. S. Iyer, while paying an eloquent and respectful tribute to thd Swamiji in his personal reminiscences, said: "During all the time he stayed, he took captive every heart within the home. To every one of us, he was all sweetness, all tenderness, all grace. My sons were frequently in his company, and one of them still swears by him and has the most vivid and endearing recollections of his visit and of his stirring personality.... When he left, it seemed for a time as if the light had gone out of our home."

1892 DEC: (last week): After travelling the length and breadth of India for three years as a mendicant friar, **SWAMI VIVEKANANDA** arrived at Kanyakumari, the southernmost tip of the country.

This place of pilgrimage contains a temple to Goddess Kanyakumari, an aspect of the Universal Mother. About 0.25 mile from shore, twin rocks jut out from the sea. After worshipping at Mother's temple, Vivekananda swam through the turbulent, shark-infested waters to the farther of the two rocks. He remained for three days and nights on the solitary rock, meditating intensely on the condition of India – her present degradation and the misery of the people, her past glory and future potentialities. In this meditation his ideas for the regeneration of the nation took shape, ideas which eventually found concrete expression in the Ramakrishna Mission. At the same time, he decided to accept the advice of several of his followers to go to America the following year to attend the World's Parliament of Religions in Chicago. He would seek material aid for his country while sharing India's spiritual wealth with the Western World.

1892 (A): **Dadabbai Naoroji** (1825-1917), Parsi businesman resident in England elected to British Parliament on the Liberal ticket. A leading nationalist, author and spokesman, he was the **first Indian to be elected to the House of Commons** (1892-1895).

His example of a selfless service to India inspired many younger compatriots, notably M. K. Gandhi, during their visit to London.

Dadabhai Naoroji was one of the founders of the Indian National Congress and its President in 1886, 1893 and 1906.

1892 (B): George Eastman (1854-1932), U. S. inventor and manufacturer of photographic equipment, founded the **Eastman Kodak Company of New York**. His success at making **photography** easy and inexpensive brought him huge wealth. From 1892 onwards Eastman devoted much of his time to philanthropy. He donated enormous sums (more than 75 million dollars) to educational institutions and in his company introduced the first employees' profit-sharing system in U. S. A. [see 1884 (e), 1888 (i),1895 (e)]

1892 (C): Economic depression began in the **United States** but the country had 4,000 millionaires, up from fewer than 20 in 1940. [see 1893]

1892 (D): A clamp-on tin-plated steel **bottle cap** with an inner seal disc of natural cork and a flanged edge was patented by Baltimore machine-shop foreman **William Painter** 54, who also patented a capping machine for beer and soft drinks bottles. Later Painter designed an automatic filler and capper with a capacity of 60 to 100 bottles per minute, and he established the Crown Cork and seal Company at Baltimore to market his bottle caps and machines.

1892 (E): The science of **virology** was pioneered by Russian botanist, **Dmitri Iosifovich Ivanovski,** 28, who discovered filterable viruses.

1892 (F): The first successful **petrol tractor** was produced by Waterloo, Iowa, farmer **John Froelich** who organized the Waterloo Gasoline Traction Engine Company early the following year.

1892 (G): The **Addressograph** invented by Sioux City, Iowa, engineer **Joseph Smith Duncan** printed mailing addresses automatically. Duncan obtained a patent for his 'addressing machine', in 1896.

1892 (H): Carl G. P. De Laval of Sweden, built a 15 h. p. **steam turbine** for marine application [see 1884 (n)]. An early model similar to this was exhibited at the World's Fair held in Chicago in 1893.

1892 (J): A new **method of producing viscose rayon** patented by English Chemist, **Charles Frederick Cross,** 37, and **Edward John Bevan,** was safer than Chardonnet nitrocellulose process of 1883 and cheaper than the cuprammonium process.

1892 (K): An improved **carburettor** that mixed vaporized fuel with air to create a combustible or explosive gas, was invented by Germany's **Daimler.** The following year a float feed carburettor for gasoline engines was developed by German engineer **William Maybach,** 46, who was an associate of Gottlieb Daimler.

1892 (L): First comprehensive work on bacteriology in U. S. A. : A *Manual* of *Bacteriology,* published by Lt. Col. George Miler Sternberg.

1892 (M): Alexander Graham Bell (1847-1922), Scottish-born American inventor, best known for perfecting the telephone to transmit vocal message by electricity, made the **first call from New York to Chicago**. [see 1873 March 3]

1893 JAN. 5: Birth of **Paramahamsa Yogananda** (d. 1952), an enlightened exponent of the science of yoga and the first Indian yogi to live in the West for a long period of over a quarter of a century initiating over a lakh of students in yoga, scientific techniques for awakening the divine consciousness in man.

Through 'Yogoda Satsanga Society' (1917) and 'Self-Realization Fellowship, (1925), established in India and America respectively, the wisdom of the great yogi is made available to seekers of Truth in all parts of the world.

1893 FEB. : As an itinerant monk when **SWAMI VIVEKANANDA** visited Hyderabad, an incident happened that set him thinking about the powers of the human mind, (a subject which deeply interested him and on which he spoke at length in a lecture he delivered at Los Angeles, California, on 8th January, 1900).

Hearing that there was a Brahmin in the city who produced, as if from the air, anything that was asked for, he went to see him. He found the man suffering from fever – with a high temperature – lying on a cot. Being requested to touch him, he did so, whereupon the man's fever immediately left him and he sat up. Asked to show some of his "tricks", he requested the Swami and his companions to write on a piece of paper the names of the things that they wanted him to produce. The latter wrote down names of such things as either did not grow in that season, or were not locally available. They stripped him of all his clothing, leaving only a blanket with which to cover his body. They then gave him the piece of paper, when, lo, there came from under the blanket all that they had ordered for – bunches of grapes, oranges and what not, which, if they had been weighed, would be found to be twice the weight of the man. He asked them to eat the fruits and finding that they were hesitating to do, began to eat some of them himself, whereupon they also ate and found that they were fresh and of excellent quality. The man finished by producing a bunch of roses – each perfect, with dew-drops on the petals, not one crushed, not one injured. When the Swami asked the man for an explanation, he said it was all sleight of hand. The Swami could not believe that it was merely that. (*A Comprehensive Biography of Swami Vivekananda,* Part I, p. 384).

1893 FEB. (A): **Sri Aurobindo** (1872-1950) returned to India, completing his studies in England. The moment he set foot on the Indian soil at Apollo Bunder, Bombay, he had the first notable spiritual experience of infinite calm.

1893 MAR. 10: **Devastating fire in Boston**, U. S. A., destroyed nearly $ 5,000,000 in property. Several lives were lost.

On August 13, $ 2,000,000 in property destroyed and some 1500 persons made homeless by fire in Minneapolis.

On Aug. 24, 1000 lives lost and a great deal of property damage inflicted by a **terrible cyclone** which ripped through Savannah and Charleston.

On Oct. 2, some 2000 persons killed by a **disastrous cyclone** which raged along the Gulf coast of Louisiana.

1893 APR. : **M. K. Gandhi** (1869-1948) sailed for Durban, readily grasping an opportunity of legal work there.

During his stay in South Africa, when the Natal Indians were deprived of franchise, consequent on the introduction of Disenfranchisement Act of 1896 by the British rulers, M. K. Gandhi became a vigorous champion of the-rights of Indian settlers. By the time he returned to India, in January 1915, he had become known as "Mahatmaji", a title given to him by the poet Rabindranath Tagore (1861-1941).

1893 MAY 1. : **World's Columbian Exposition (World Fair)** officially opened in Chicago, U. S. A. by President Cleveland. It was an international exposition to observe the 400th anniversary of discovery of America, by Christopher Columbus (1461-1506) in 1492. It was also a demonstration of the growth of America to world status as an economic power. [see 1892 Oct. 20-23]

The site of the exposition covered 200 acres and extended about 2 miles along the shores of lake Michigan. More than 21 million people visited the fair to view some 60,000 exhibits costing about 30 million dollars. After a period of six months, the exposition was formally closed on 30th October.

Built largely on reclaimed swamp land, the World's Columbian Exposition was a spectacular "White City" of classically designed plaster structures. (One major building – 600,000 sq.ft. – of the exposition, is now housing the Museum of Science and Industry, a great public educational exhibition which has been called a permanent World Fair).

For the first time. electric lighting was lavishly used. George Westinghouse (1846-1914) U. S. engineer, displayed at the World's Columbian Exposition, for the first time, the alternating current generator, later to become the basis of lighting and electric power.

An interesting feature of the World's Columbian Exposition was the Congress held at the grounds under the auspices of the World's Congress Auxiliary. The Congress discussed the leading phases of professional, scientific, economic, educational and religious thought; the World's Parliament of Religions (held from 11th to 27th September and attended by Swami Vivekananda) attracted the most general attention.

1893 MAY 3I: SWAMI VIVEKANANDA sailed for America to attend the World's Parliament of Religions.

He was helped by a group of brilliant students of the Madras University, who energetically took steps to organize ways and means of his going to America to represent Hinduism at the proposed World's Parliament of Religions at Chicago [see 1863 (c)]. He was also aided by a few of the enlightened native princes. And armed with the blessings of Sarada Devi, the Holy Mother, he set sail for the United States, from Bombay. Passing Colombo, Penang, Singapore, Hongkong, Canton, Nagasaki, Kobe, Osaka, Kyoto, Tokyo and Yokohama, he landed at Vancouver and thence reached Chicago by train on 28th July, 1893. From there on up to his first speech at the Parliament of Religions at Chicago on 11th September 1893, he had to face many hardships and sharp moments of despair.

1893 MAY 31 (A): Sir Jamsetji N. Tata (1839-1904) met SWAMI VIVEKANANDA during his voyage to America.

This meeting opened a new vista for Jamsetji, the potential industraialist. In fact it proved a turning point in his life. Coming under the inductive effect of Swamiji and being blessed by him, Jamsetji became an enlightened industrialist.

Swamiji was on his way to attend the Chicago Parliament of Religions as an unknown monk without any credentials. Swamiji enquired of Jamsetji why he exported matches from Japan for sales in India; for it meant a heavy drain on national wealth. Swamji then pleaded with Jamsetji that if, instead, he set up a match factory in India, that would not only give him a handsome profit, but also employment to quite a number of men and prevent the national wealth from going out of the country. The admonition of an anguished sannyasin did not miss the target, and the potential industruialist immediately realized that here was an uncommon sannyasin with a sure professional approach towards the economic ills of the society. Though a Vedantist to the core, his approach to life was never negative. He was very much concerned about the basic needs of the lowly placed, oppressed humanity. He was always after doing something concrete for the betterment of the condition of the poor and downtrodden.

It was the dynamic inspiration of Swami Vivekananda that moved Jamsetji to come forward in 1898 with a significant announcement about his scheme for promotion of basic scientific research for industrial development and economic resurgence of India. Since he valued higher education as a preparation for industrial and commercial vocation, and visualized the establishment of a post-graduate research institute of science, he made a magnificient gift of Rs. 30 laksh for the purpose. The whole India greeted him in a chorus of commendation. The proposed institute was admirably   calculated to hasten the dawn of that industrial revival in India, upon which depends the salvation of her teeming millions. When founded, the Insitute initially, was called the Indian Institute of Science and also propularaly known as Tata Institute.

Jamsetji sought the spiritual wisdom of Swamiji for the smooth functioning of such an institution. Swamji evinced keen   interest in the Tata-scheme. His friends and disciples undertook to work behind the scene to secure fulfilment of his desire. In this project, however, the role of Sister Nivedita was the more important. Tata-scheme being the embodiment of a cherished desire of her Master, Swami Vivekananda, she devoted every ounce of her energy for its   implementation. Although Swamiji and Jamsetji did not live to see the scheme materialize, Sister Nivedita must have been happy when the institute started functioning from July 1911.

1893: America in the grip of severe financial panic, Wall Street stock prices took a sudden drop (May 5). The market collapsed (June 27), 600 banks closed their doors, more than 15,000 business firms failed, and 74 rail roads went into receivership in a depression that continued for four years.

In the very first letter that **SWAMI VIVEKANANDA** wrote to India after reaching America, he referred to this financial panic which, he said, was created by the raising of the Rupee in India. (In 1892 on the recommendation of the Herschel Committee, the value of the Rupee was fixed at 1s. 4d. gold, and to achieve this mints were closed to the free coinage of silver). Swamiji wrote that many mills had closed down. He was considerably hampered by this, he said. The crisis began with the failure of the leading Railway and the collapse of the National Cardage Company in Spring of 1893. The New York banks suspended specie payments in August, many banks failed; 2300 m. of railways passed under receiverships; construction almost ceased. The panic in many ways proved to be a turning point in American history; it produced an industrial chaos, out of which big business emerged with greater strength which, of course, meant "the rich getting richer and the poor poorer", and social disharmony.

Speaking about the treatment of the Negroes in America, Swami Vivekananda observed that their lot had become worse after the abolition of slavery. "Today", said he, "they are the property of nobody. Their lives are of no value; they are burnt alive on mere pretences. They are shot down without any law for they are murderers; for they are niggers, they are not human beings, they are not even animals...." During the decade, 1889-1899, the total number of Negroes lynched, according to official estimates, was 1460. "Prejudice against the Negroes was equally strong in the North; and the main body of Northern opinion believed, as the South did, that the Negro was an inferior being; that he could never be fully assimilated into the American system, and that he was best kept subordinate to the white man. Segregation, discrimination and 'Jim Crow' customs received the tacit approval even of such Northern liberals as Godkin of *'The Nation'* ". (*A Comprehensive Biography of Swami Vivekananda*, Part I, p. 449, 451 and 452).

1893 JUNE 29: Birth of **P. C. Mahalnobis** (d. 1972), doyen of Indian Mathematics.

1893 AUG. 25-28: SWAMI VIVEKANANDA met **Professor John H. Wright** of Harvard University, at Annisquam (Mass).

The Professor had invited the Swami to spend the week-end at his place. Swamiji promptly responded to this invitation from a reputed scholar. Prof. Wright was so deeply impressed with the profundity of scholarship and the versatility of genius of this young Hindu monk that he himself insisted that he should represent Hinduism in the Parliament of Religions. Swamiji explained the peculiar difficulties that stood in his way in the fulfilment of this objective, and said that he did not possess any credentials whereby to introduce himself to the organizers of the Parliament. Prof. Wright, who had already discovered the sparkling intelligence and the rare ability of the Swami, said, "To ask you, Swami, for your credentials is like asking the Sun to state its right to shine." Prof. Wright, who was well-known to the elite of the city of Chicago and also to many distinguished personages connected with the Parliament, wrote at once to his friend, the chairman of the Committee on the selection of delegates, stating, "Here is a man who is more learned than all our learned professors put together." Moreover, he gave letters of introduction to the Committee which had the responsibility of providing accommodation for Oriental delegates. Knowing that the Swami was short of funds, he himself purchased a ticket for him to enable him to go to Chicago.

1893 SEP. 11: The World's Parliament of Religions opened in the morning, in the great Hall of Columbus, Art institute, Michigan Avenue, Chicago, U. S. A.

A notable event in mankind's long search for spiritual harmony, it emphasised the accord between "Unity in Diversity" and "Diversity in Unity" of outlook and urged a cultural fellowship and mutual understanding between Western and Eastern worlds. The stated objectives of the Parliament were, briefly:

"To bring together in Conference, for the first time in history, leading representatives of the great historic religions of the world; to demonstrate in the most impressive way, what and how many important truths the various religions held and taught in common; to set forth, by those most competent to speak, what are deemed the important distinctive truths held and taught by such each religion and by the various branches of Christendom; to enquire into the mimesis of religions; to discover what light religion can shed on the great problems of the time especially temperance, labour, education, wealth and poverty; to bring the nations of the earth into more friendly fellowship in the hope of securing permanent international peace."

At 10 a. m., ten solemn strokes of the New Liberty bell on which was inserted, "A new commandment I give unto you, that ye love one another", proclaimed the opening of the Congress – each stroke representing one of the chief ten religions, listed by President Bonney as Judaism, Mohammedanism, Hinduism, Buddhism, Taoism, Confucianism, Shintoism, Zoroastrianism, Catholicism, the Greek Church and Protestantism. "The sight", says Houghton, "was most remarkable. There were strange robes, turbans and tunics, crosses and crescents, flowing hairs and tonsured heads". In the midst of this sat **SWAMI VIVEKANANDA** conspicuous in his orange turban and robe or as Rev. Mr. Wente put it, for his "gorgeous red apparel, his bronze face surmounted with a turban of yellow" The auditorium was jam-packed with men and women, intellectuals of the day, both clerical and secular. "Such a scene", writes Houghton again, "was never witnessed before in the world's history". Of this scene and the moment Swamiji later wrote, "My heart was fluttering and my tongue nearly dried up."

Of what followed Marie Louise Burke says: "Suddenly the great organ of the gallery burst forth with the strains of the 'Doxology' and the entire assembly rose to sing, 'Praise God from whom all blessings flow; Praise Him, all creatures here below; Praise Him above ye heavenly hosts; Praise Father, Son and Holy Ghost'. At the end of the hymn, a deep silence was sustained by the uplifted hand of the Cardinal. Then into this impressive hush, he began the words of the Lord's prayer, 'Our Father who art in heaven' – and every voice in the hall joined his." "The supreme moment of the nineteenth century", says Houghton, "was reached".

1893 SEP. 11 (A): SWAMI VIVEKANANDA spoke at the World's Parliament of Religions during the first day's afternoon session, after four delegates had read their prepared speeches.

The spacious hall at the Art Institute of Chicago was packed with nearly 7000 people, representing the best of culture of the country. On the plat- form every organized religion from all corners of the world had its representative. Conspicuous among them was Swami Vivekananda who, with his bright countenance, crimson robe, and yellow turban, easily attracted the attention of the assembled thousands. When he addressed the gathering as "Sisters and Brothers of America" the entire audience broke into prolonged applause and greeted him with unprecedented enthusiasm – not merely because he addressed them as "Sisters and Brothers", for they had already heard many speak on the themes of Universal Brotherhood, but because his words, completely free from platitudes, reflected spontaneous realization of the spiritual oneness of mankind.

In fact there was an electric effect on the audience when Swamiji spoke the first five words of his address. Both Barrows and Houghton comment on the fact that "when Mr. Vivekananda addressed the audience as 'Sisters and Brothers of America', there arose a peal of applause for several minutes" and Swamiji himself tells that "a deafening applause for several minutes followed...." Another reference to this incident comes from Mrs. S. K. Blodgett, who later became Swamiji's hostess in Los Angeles, "I was at the Parliament of Religions in Chicago in 1893", she once told. "When the young man got up and said, 'Sisters and Brothers of America', seven thousand people rose to their feet as a tribute to something they knew not what." In this way, in the words of *Chicago Inter Ocean,* Swamiji "with an eloquence and power not only won admiration for himself but consideration of his own teachings."

It was a brief but intense speech which the Swamiji delivered in the afternoon session. Its spirit of universality, earnestness, and breadth of outlook completely captured the whole assembly. He cast off the formalism of the Parliament and spoke to the people in the language of the heart. The Parliament gave him a tremendous ovation that afternoon, and the American nation, infused by the streamer headlines of the newspapers of his contribution at the Parliament, gave him its silent ovation the next day morning.

During the ensuing seventeen sessions of the Parliament, Swami Vivekananda, in the course of his illuminating address, laid particular stress on the requirements of the day in the domain of religion and culture.

1893 SEP. 19: SWAMI VIVEKANANDA read his celebrated paper on Hinduism at the World's Parliament of Religions at Chicago.

Chicago Inter Ocean depicted a picture of the tremendous excitement that prevailed that day. It reported "great crowds of people, most of whom were women, pressed around the doors leading to the Hall of Columbus, an hour before the time stated for opening the afternoon session, for it had been announced that Swami Vivekananda, the popular Hindu monk who looks so much like Macullough's Othello, was to speak."

As reported by the *Chicago Daily Tribune,* "Dr. Noble presided at the afternoon session of the Parliament of Religions in Chicago. The Hall of Columbus was badly crowded.... Dr. Noble then presented Swami Vivekananda, the Hindu monk, who was applauded loudly as he stepped forward to the centre of the platform. He wore an orange robe bound with a scarlet sash, and a pale yellow turban. The customary smile was on his handsome face and his eyes shone with animation.... When the applause had ceased, Swami Vivekananda, went to read his paper on 'Hinduism' ".

It was a fairly long document, being a masterly summary of the philosophy, psychology, and general ideas and statements on Hinduism, in its all-inclusive aspects. On this day the Hall was crowded to its fullest capacity, women vastly out-numbering the men, and many had to be turned away. In the morning sessions, the Christian delegates, alarmed at the hearing that the Oriental religions were receiving in every meeting, made a concerted attack on Hinduism. Swami Vivekananda made a telling reply, just before he read his paper on Hinduism in the afternoon session. His basic idea was that religion had nothing to do with the material prosperity of Western nations like England, which was brought about by the use of brute force. Said he on this occasion, "We, who have come from East, have sat here on the platform day after day and have been told in a patronizing way that we ought to accept Christianity because Christian nations are the most prosperous. We look about us and we see England, the most prosperous Christian nation in the world, with her foot on the neck of 250,000,000 Asiatics. We look back into history and see that the prosperity of Christian Europe began with Spain. Spain's prosperity began with the invasion of Mexico. Christianity wins its prosperity by cutting the throat of its fellowmen. At such a price the Hindu will not have prosperity. I have sat here and heard the height of intolerance. I have heard the creeds of moslems applauded, when the muslim sword is carrying destruction into India. Blood and sword are not for the Hindu, whose religion is based on the laws of love." (Reported in the *Chicago Daily Tribune,* of 20 Sept. 1893, and quoted by Dr. R. C. Majumdar in Bharatiya Vidya Bhavan's *History and Culture of Indian People*, Vol. X, Part II, p. 127).

In an article entitled *The Parliament of Religions*, appeared in the *Daily Chronicle*, H. R. Haweis, gives a better account of what Swamiji said on this day: "Vivekananda, the popular Hindu monk, whose physiognomy bore the most striking resemblance to the classic figure of the Buddha, denounced our commercial prosperity, our bloody wars, and our religious intolerance, declaring that at such a price 'the mild Hindu' would have none of our vaunted civilization. The recurrent and rhetorical use of the phrase, 'mild Hindu', produced a funny impression upon the audience, as the furious monk waved his arms and almost foamed at the mouth. 'You come', he cried, 'with the Bible in one hand and the conqueror's sword in the other – you, with your religion of yesterday, to us, who were taught thousands of years ago by our *rishis* precepts as noble and lives as holy as your Christ's. You trample on us and treat us like the dust beneath your feet. You destroy precious life in animals. You are carnivorous. You degraded our people with drink. You insult our women. You scorn our religion – in many points like yours, only better, because more humane. And then you wonder why Christianity makes such slow progress in India. I tell you it is because you are not like your Christ whom we could honour and reverence. Do you think, if you came to our doors like him, meek and lowly, with a message of love, living and working and suffering for others, as he did, we should turn a deaf ear? Oh! No. We should receive him and listen to him, and as we have done to our own inspired *rishis*". (*A Comprehensive Biography of Swami Vivekananda*, Part I, p. 485; also p. 464 and 465.) [see 1893. Sept. 29]

1893 SEP. 22: Fridtjof Nansen (1861-1930), Norwegian Arctic explorer, who had earlier successfully crossed the unknown interior of Greenland and studied its Eskimo inhabitants (1888-89), set out on his **voyage to the North Pole.**

He sailed from Christina with a crew of thirteen and thirty sledge dogs. In his ship 'Fram', he explored (1893-96), the North Pole regions, verifying the hypothesis about the westward drift of the polar ice-pack. After more than three years of successful exploration, he returned to Norway, and wrote an account of his adventures in his book *Farthest North*.

1893 SEP. 27: In the final session of the Parliament, **SWAMI VIVEKANANDA** made a grand appeal for the harmony of religious faiths.

He said: "The Christian is not to become a Hindu or Buddhist, nor is a Buddhist or a Hindu to become a Christian. But each must assimilate the spirit of the others and yet preserve his individuality and grow according to his own law of growth. If the Parliament has shown anything to the world, it is this: It has proved to the world that holiness, purity and charity are not the exclusive possessions of any Church in the world, and that every system has produced men and women of the most exalted character. In the face of this evidence, if anybody dreams of the exclusive survival of his own religion and the destruction of the others, I pity him from the bottom of my heart."

The mighty words which were addressed by the Swami to the entire humanity over the heads of the official representatives in the Parliament made a tremendous appeal to the conscience of the people at large. *The New York Herald,* one of the most popular and widely circulated news- papers, editorially remarked, "He is undoubtedly the greatest figure in the Parliament of Religions. After hearing him we feel how foolish it is to send missionaries to his learned nation."

Soon after the termination of the historic sessions of the Parliament of Religions, it became the main object of Swami Vivekananda to acquaint the peoples of the West with the ideals of the civilization and the religious consciousness of his own race, to learn the secret of the material greatness of the Occident and also to collect adequate funds wherewith to provide his countrymen with scientific methods for the improvement of their economic condition. With this dual purpose in view he visited the important cities of America and delivered a series of illuminating lectures on a variety of subjects which comprised not only the history of the Indian people, the religion of the Vedanta and his future plan of work in India, but also the cardinal teachings of the other leading faiths of the world and a comparative study of the cultures and civilization of the East and the West.

1893 SEP. 28: *The Chicago Advocate* gave a picture of **SWAMI VIVEKANANDA** on the opening day at the World's Parliament of Religions:

"In certain respects, the most fascinating personality was the Brahmin monk Swami Vivekananda with his flowing orange robe, saffron turban, smooth shaven, shapely, handsome face, large, dark, subtle, penetrating eyes, and with the air of one being only pleased, with the consciousness of being easily the master of his situation. His knowledge of English is as though it were his mother tongue...."

1893 SEP. 29: Referring to many Christian delegates' open attack on Hinduism, on the very day that **SWAMI VIVEKANANDA** was scheduled to read his famous paper on 'Hinduism' the *Iowa Times* said:

"The Parliament of Religions reached a point where sharp acerbities develop. The thin veil of courtesy was maintained of course, but behind it was ill feeling. Rev. Jospeh Cook criticized the Hindus sharply and was more sharply criticised in turn." Of Swamiji's addres the paper reported: "He was out of humour, or soon became so, apparently. He wore an orange robe and a pale yellow turban and dashed at once into a savage attack on Christian nations." [see 1893 Sept. 19]

The Catholics received Swamiji's criticism with hearty enthusiasm. In Barrow's history, *Introduction to Parliarnent Papers,* it is reported that "On the eleventh day, Bishop Keane said, 'I endorse the denunciation that was hurled forth last night against the system of pretended charity that offered food to the hungry Hindus at the cost of their conscience and faith. It is a shame and a disgrace to those who call themselves Christians....' "

1893 SEP. 30: *Boston Evening Transcript* reported:

"The most striking figure one meets in this afternoon is **SWAMI VIVEKANANDA,** the Brahmin monk. He is a large, well built man, with the superb carriage of the Hindustanis, his face clean shaven, squarely moulded, regular features, white teeth and with well-chiselled lips that are usually parted in a benevolent smile while he is conversing. His finely poised head is crowned with either a lemon coloured or a red turban, and his cassock (not the technical name for this garment), belted in at the waist and falling below the knees, alternates in a bright orange and rich crimson. He speaks excellent English and replied readily to any questions asked in sincerity.

"Vivekananda's address before the Parliament was broad as the heavens above us, embracing the best in all religions, as the ultimate universal religion – charity to all mankind, good works for the love of God, not for fear of punishment or hope of reward. He is a great favourite at the Parliament, from the grandeur of his sentiments and his appearance as well. If he merely crosses the platform he is applauded and this marked approval of thousands he accepts in a childlike spirit of gratification, without a trace of conceit."

1893 OCT. 1: To a request of the *New York World* of date, for "a sentiment of expression regarding the significance of the great meeting (Parliament of Religions) from each representative", **SWAMI VIVEKANANDA** replied with two quotations, one from *Gita* and the other from Vyasa.   "I am He that is in every religion – like the thread that passes through a string of pearls." "Holy, perfect and pure men are seen in all creeds; therefore they all lead to the same birth – for how can nectar be the outcome of poison?" (And this certainly was the lesson learned through the Parliament of Religions at Chicago).

1893 OCT. 7: *New York Critic* reported:

"The most impressive figure of the Parliament was the Hindoo monk,
SWAMI VIVEKANANDA.... No one expressed so well the spirit of
Parliament, its limitations and its finest influence, as did the Hindoo
monk.... He is an orator by divine right and his strong, intelligent face
in its picturesque setting of yellow and orange, was hardly less
interesting than his earnest words and the rich, rhythmical utterance he
gave them....

"Perhaps the most tangible result of the congress was the feeling it
aroused in regard to foreign missions. The impertinence of sending half-
educated theological students to instruct the wise and erudite Orientals
was never brought home to an English speaking audience more forcibly.
It is only in the spirit of tolerance and sympathy that we are at liberty
to touch their faith, and the exhorters who possess these qualities are
rare....

"It was an outgrowth of the Parliament of Religions, which opened our
eyes to the fact that the philosophy of the ancient creeds contains much
beauty for the moderns. When we had once clearly perceived this, our
interest in their exponents quickened, and with characteristic eagerness
we set out in pursuit of knowledge. The most available means of
obtaining it, after the close of the Parliament, was through the address
and lectures of Swami Vivekananda, who is still in this City
(Chicago)....

".... His culture, his eloquence, and his fascinating personality have
given us a new idea of Hindu Civilization; he is an interesting figure,
his fine, intelligent, mobile face in its setting of yellow, and deep musical
voice prepossessing one, at once in his favour. So, it is not strange
that he has been taken up by the literary clubs, has preached and
lectured in churches, until the life of Buddha and the doctrines of his
faith have grown familiar to us. He speaks without notes, presenting
his facts and his conclusions with the greatest art and the most
convincing sincerity; and rising at times to a rich, inspiring eloquence....
At present he contents himself with enlightening us in regard to his
religion and the words of its philosophers."

1893 OCT. 7(A): *Evanston Index* reported:

"**SWAMI VIVEKANANDA** is a representative from India to the
Parliament of Religions. He has attracted a great deal of attention on
account of his unique attire in Mandarin colours, by his magnetic
presence and by his brilliant oratory and wonderful exposition of Hindu
philosophy. His stay in Chicago has been a continual ovation."

1893 OCT. 11: "Christian missionaries", said **SWAMI VIVEKANANDA** (in the course of a brief but soul-stirring speech – *Religion not the crying need of India* – delivered in the evening session of the tenth day of the Parliament of Religions) according to *Christian Herald* of date, "come to offer life but only on condition that the Hindus become christians, abandoning the faith of their fathers and forefathers. Is it right?.... If you wish to illustrate the meaning of 'brotherhood', treat Hindus more kindly, even though he be a Hindu and is faithful to his religion. Send missionaries to teach them how better to earn a piece of bread, and not teach them metaphysical nonsense."

1893 NOV. 16: **Mrs. Annie Besant** (1847-1933), the British social reformer and theosophist, arrived at Madras to take charge of the growing **Theosophical movement.** (In 1907, she succeeded Colonel Olcott and became the President of the Theosophical Society).

Mrs. Besant believed that a revival and reintroduction of India's ancient ideals and institutions could solve most of her problems. With a view to providing Hindu religious instruction, she founded the Central Hindu School of Varanasi in 1898, and this developed later into the Banaras Hindu University. She rose to fame as the creator of Home Rule League in 1916, and the next year she was elected President of the Indian National Congress. Mrs. Besant was a leader among Europeans in reviving and disseminating of Hindu Religion and Culture.

1893 NOV. 18: **Rev. Mr. W. H. Thomas** in a letter published in *Wisconsin State Journal* wrote of **SWAMI VIVEKANANDA:**

"Of the many learned men in the East, who took part in the great World's Parliament of Religions, Vivekananda was the most popular favourite, add when it was known that he was to speak, thousands were turned away for want of room. Nor was it curiosity that drew the masses; but for those who heard him once were so impressed by the magnetism of his fine presence, the charm and power of his eloquence, his perfect command of the English language and the deep interest in what he had to say, that they desired all the more to hear him again. It will be opportunity of a lifetime for the cities of our land to see and hear this noble, earnest, loving Brahmin, dressed in the costume of his order, telling the true story of the religion and customs of his far off country."

1893 NOV. 21: *Wisconsin State Journal* reported:

"The lecture at Congregational Church (Madison), last night by the celebrated Hindoo monk, **VIVEKANANDA** was an extremely interesting one, and contained much of sound philosophy and good religion. Pagan though he be, Christianity may well follow many of his teachings. His creed is as wide as the Universe, taking in all religions, and accepting truth wherever it may be found. Bigotry and superstition and idle ceremony, he declared, have no place in 'the religions of India.' "

1893 NOV. 25: *Minneapolis Star* reported:

"Brahminism" in all its subtle attraction, because of its embodiment of ancient and truthful principles, was the subject which held an audience in closest attention last evening at the first Unitarian Church (Minneapolis) while **SWAMI VIVEKANANDA** expounded the Hindoo faith. It was an audience which included thougtful women and men, for the lecturer had been invited by the 'Peripatetics' and among the friends who shared the privilege with them were ministers of varied denominations, as well as students and scholars. Vivekananda is a Brahmin priest, and he occupied the platform in his native garb, with kaftan on head, orange coloured coat confined at the waist with a red sash, and red nether garments.

"He presented his faith in all sincerity, speaking slowly and clearly, convincing his hearers by quietness of speech rather than by rapid action. His words were carefully weighed and each carried its meaning direct. He offered the simplest truths of the Hindu religion and while he said nothing harsh about Christianity, he touched upon it in such a manner as to place the faith of Brahma before all. The all-pervading thought and leading principle of the Hindu religion is the inherent divinity already existing in man...."

1893 NOV. 28: *Des Moines News,* reported:

"**SWAMI VIVEKANANDA,** the talented scholar from the far off India spoke at the Central Church last night (Nov. 27). He was a representative of his country and creed at the recent Parliament of Religions assembled in Chicago during the World's Fair. Rev. H. O. Breeden introduced the speaker to the audience. He arose, and after bowing to his audience, commenced his lecture, the subject of which was *Hindu Religion.* His lecture was not confined to any line of thought but consisted more of some of his own philosophical views relative to his religion and others. He holds that one must embrace all the religions to become the perfect Christian. What is not found in one religion is supplied by another: They are all right and necessary for the true Christian.... 'I have often been asked in this country if I am going to try to convert the people here. I take this for an insult. I do not believe in this idea of conversion... We tolerate everything but intolerance.' "

1893 NOV. 30: The *Indian Mirror* reproduced the following report published in *The Press of America*:

"One of the most interesting personages to the multitude, is Professor

SWAMI VIVEKANANDA, a Hindu theologian of great learning. Professor Vivekananda, who is of pleasing appearance, and young he be so well filled with the ancient lore of India, made an address which captured the Congress, so to speak. There were bishops and ministers of nearly every Christian Church present, and they were all taken by storm. The eloquence of the man with intellect beaming from his yellow face, his splendid English in describing the beauties of his time-honoured faith, all conspired to make a deep impression on the audience. From the day the wonderful Professor delivered his speech, which was followed by other addresses, he was followed by a crowd wherever he went. In going in and coming out of the building, he was daily beset by hundreds of women who almost fought with each other for a chance to get near him, and shake his hand. It may safely be set down that there were women of every denomination among his worshippers. Some of them were votaries of fashion who did not care what became of their fine toilets in the struggle, while others were the 'mothers in Israel' of the various churches of Chicago and elsewhere. The Professor seemed surprised at this homage, but he received it graciously enough until it became tiresome from repetition, and then he made his entries and exits at times when there were no crowds of women in the vestibule and corridors. Other strangers from the far East, in picturesque garb, and with a Midways plaisance flavor about them, were also much sought after, but in a less degree. This talk in the sessions of the Congress was a revelation to many people, even of education and much reading. That men so well endowed with brains, astute thinkers, should adhere to those heathenish religions, was a surprise to many people, more thoughtful than the women who made a lion of Professor Vivekananda. It was from the Christian theologians on the platform, however, that the women took their cue."

1893 DEC. 6: *The Indian Mirror* in its Editorial:

"Among the representatives from India was....SWAMI VIVEKANANDA, a Bengali Hindu, better known in Madras and Bombay than in Bengal.... But the one figure among the audience, the one Indian representative, on whom were riveted all eyes, and who conquered as he went, was Swami Vivekananda, who appeared in the robes of the sannyasi, of handsome presence, somewhat portly form, and with eyes glittering like large brilliants, even ladies acknowledged the fascination of the mere outward man. But when he spoke, when the inner man emerged from the shell, then the power was doubled, and the vast audience heard his fervid exposition of the Vedic faith of the Hindus with rapture. We can well understand the enthusiasm of the Americans over Swami Vivekananda...."

1893 DEC. 24: **Henry Ford** (1863-1947), American pioneer of automobile industry, completed the construction of his **first gasoline engine** that ran successfully.

His first motor car – tiller-steered quadricycle – was assembled in 1896 and was driven through the streets of Detroit in the early hours of June 4, 1896. In 1903 Henry Ford founded the Ford Motor Company and developed a system of mass production based on the assembly line and conveyor belt which produced a low-priced car within the reach of middle class Americans. [see 1893 Jul. 30]

1893 DEC. 27: In a letter to the Editor of the *Indian Mirror,* a reader wrote:

"The following extracts from two of the leading American papers, viz., *The New York Critic,* and *The New York Herald,* regarding **VIVEKANANDA,** the great disciple of Sri Ramakrishna, will, I am sure, prove interesting to your many readers. After going through them, one cannot but mark the fulfilment of the prophecy regarding him, made by his guru, Sri Ramakrishna, as published in one of your latest issues, viz., that Vivekananda is destined to shake the earth to its foundations.

"The New York Critic says: 'But eloquent as were many of the brief speeches, no one expressed so well the spirit of the Parliament of Religions and its limitations, as the Hindu monk. I copy his address in full, but I can only suggest its effect upon the audience, for he is an orator by Divine right and his strong intelligent face in its picturesque setting of yellow orange was hardly less interesting than earnest words, and the rich rythmical utterance he gave them.' "

"Again, says the same paper: 'His culture, his eloquence and his fascinating personality have given us a new idea of Hindu civilization. His fine intelligent face and his deep muscial voice, pre-possessing one at once in his favour, has preached in clubs and churches until his faith has become familiar to us. He speaks without notes, presenting his facts and his conclusions with the greatest art, the most convincing sincerity and rising often to reach inspiring eloquence.' "

"The New York Herald says: 'Vivekananda is undoubtedly the greatest figure in the Parliament of Religions. After hearing him, we feel, how foolish it is to send Missionaries to this learned nation."

1893 DEC. : *The Indian Mirror* quoted the *Chicago Tribune*:

"**SWAMI VIVEKANANDA** was the last speaker of the evening. He says Missionaries go hungry. He spoke extemporaneously, and said in part – 'Christians must always be ready for good criticism, and I hardly think that you will care if I make a little criticism. You, Christians, who are so fond of sending out missionaries to save the souls of the heathen, why do you not try to save their bodies from starvation? In India during the terrible famines thousands died from hunger, yet you, Christians, did nothing. You erect churches all through India, but the crying evil in the East is not religion – they have religion enough – but it is bread that these suffering millions of burning India cry out for with parched throats. They ask for bread, but we give them stones. It is an insult to a starving, people to offer them religion; it is an insult to a starving man to teach him metaphysics. In India a priest that preached for money would lose caste, and be spat upon by the people. I came here to seek aid for my impoverished people, and I fully realized how difficult it was to get help for heathens from Christians in a Christian land.' "

1893 (see after 1893 May 31)

1893 (A): Raja Ravi Varma (1848-1906) the celebrated artist of Travancore, contributed a set of ten pictures for exhibition at the **World Art Festival** at Chicago and gained two medals and diplomas. The American press spoke very highly of these pictures. **SWAMI VIVEKANANDA,** who was at Chicago at that time was thrilled at the success of this Indian painter.

According to the Chairman of the Executive Committee of Awards at the Chicago Exhibition, "The series of well-executed paintings (of Ravi Varma) give a good idea of the progress of instruction in Art. They are true to nature in form and colour and preserve the costumes, current fashion and social features." According to a contemporary art critic, "Ravi Varma's art makes the mind retire within to see God. His mind was divine, his art is divine and his theme is divine. His art lifts the mind to a serene sky of spirituality. We bathe in it and are baptised by it." [see 1873 (h)]

1893 (B): Bal Gangadhar Tilak (1856-1920) Indian nationalist leader and a major force in the Indian nationalist movement (1890-1920), transformed the traditional **worship of Ganapathy** in Maharashtra, into an altogether, new form and inaugurated the **Shivaji festival** (1896), with the sole motto of bringing people together to ensure their awakening and involvement in the freedom struggle. He used the 'national opportunity' that these festivals provided for the spread of national feeling among the Hindu masses.

It was at the celebration of Shivaji Utsav that Tilak uttered the very memorable historical truth: "God has not given India to the *mlecchas* by a deed of grant written in a copper plate." This cost Tilak a rigorous imprisonment in jail for a certain period.

Tilak sought to mobilise popular support and create a militant, nationalist ideology. His emphasis was on 'Hindutva' (Hinduness), the organic links between Hindus in all parts of India. He was disappointed with the

Congress Party, and anxious either to reform it or to replace it with a more millitant organization which would preserve rather than weaken the cultural basis of the Hindu Nation. Tilak made it the great object of his life to diffuse the spirit of patriotism and nationalism among masses. It was he who declared, "Home Rule is my birth-right and I will have it."

1893 (C): Communal riots broke out over a large area in Azamgarh district (U. P.), Bombay town (lasted six days) and interior, and Isakhel (Mianwalli district, Punjab). [see 1874 Feb 13, 1877 Sept, 1885 (a), 1886 (c), 1889 (m), 1891 (b), 1897 June]

Muharram and Dusserah procession and cow-killing at Bakrid were the causes, and murders, demolition of mosques and temples and looting of shops, the chief characteristics of these riots.

1893 (D): West Africa was explored by English naturalist, **Mary Kingsley,** 30, who was taken down the Ogowe River through Cannibal country by Fang Tribesmen.

1893 (E): The **basal metabolism test** that is used to measure human metabolic rates was devised by German physiologist **Adolf Magnus Levey,** 28.

1893 (F): The world's first open heart surgery operation was performed by Chicago Surgeon **Daniel Hale Williams** who saved the life of a street fighter with a knife wound in an artery near his heart.

1893 (G): Cultured pearl cultivation was pioneered by Japanese entrepreneur **Kokichi Mikimoto,** 35, who five years ago had established the first pearl farm in the Shinmee inlet.

1893 (H): Thomas Alva Edison (1847-1931), American inventor, patented an **electric locomotive.**

In 1896, he patented the fluorescent lamp. In 1902 he improved the copper oxide battery, which resembled modern dry cells. In 1904, his cinema phone appeared, adjusting film speed to phonograph speed. In 1913, his kineto phone projected talking pictures. The universal motor which used alternating or direct current, appeared in 1907; and the electric safety lantern, patented in 1914, greatly reduced casualties among miners. That year Edison invented the telescribe, which combined features of the telephone and dictating phonograph. [see 1864 (e),1877 Nov. 29, 1878 (h), 1882 (e), 1883 (d), 1889 (h), 1891 Dec 29]

1893 (I): Leo H. Backeland (1863-1944), American chemist, and inventor, perfected a process for manufacturing a slow-developing photographic paper called **Velox.** He sold his invention to the Eastman Kodak Co., and became a millionaire.

1893 (J): Francis H. Bradley (1846-1924), British philosopher, brought out his most ambitious work *Appearance and Reality,* which rejected utilitarianism and attempted a return to absolute idealism.

1893 (K): Pneumatic tyres were first applied to motor vehicles by the French rubber manufacturers **Edourd** and **Michalin.**

The principle of pneumatic tyre had been patented as long back as in 1845 by a Scottish engineer, Robert William Thompson (1822-1873) in England. Thompson's patent substantially covers the tyre as it is known today. It showed a non-stretchable outer cover and an inner tube of rubber to hold air. An early set of tyres made on this basis covered 1,200 miles, when placed on an English brougham (a four-wheeled closed carriage). Almost half a century later, when the bicycle became popular, pneumatic tyres were revived by John Boyd Dunlop (1840-1921) of Belfast, Ireland [see 1888 Oct. 31]. He obtained patents in England in 1888 and 1889 on bicycle tyres which served as the foundation of the Dunlop Company.

1893 (L): Otto Lilienthal (1849-1896), German aviation pioneer successfully conducted **glider flights** from an artificially made hill near Berlin.

Earlier he had studied birds in flight with the idea of building a heavier-than-air flying machine. After making thousands of flights, he crashed (on Aug. 9, 1896) while attempting to extend the length of his flight beyond 320 m. (1050 ft.) and died the next day. Following in Lilienthal's footsteps, the American brothers **Orville** (1871-1948) and **Wilbur Wright** (1867-1912) began building and flying gliders. From 1900 to 1902, they tested their machine at their camp near Kitty Hawk, and at their home in Dayton, Ohio, where they analysed their results. They experimented with over 200 wing shapes in a crude wind tunnel of their own design. They used their findings to build a controllable, man-carrying glider. They had made more than 700 flights in the new glider off Kill Devil Hill, near Kitty Hawk, and felt that they were ready to move on to a powered flight. In 1903 they built a 10 h.p. petrol engine and installed it in their modified glider at Kitty Hawk and (on Dec. 17, 1903) made the **world's first controlled flight in an airplane.** The craft was piloted by Orville, and lasted 12 seconds. Later, in 1905, with an improved plane and engine, they made circular flights of more than 38 kms. (24 miles) lasting about 35 minutes. By the middle of 1909, dozens of European designers had planes in the air. Manned flight had become a reality, but so far it was only an exciting novelty without significant purpose. World War I, however, triggered a period of intense research and development.

1893 (M): Britain's **Labour Party** was founded by Socialists who included the Scottish politician **Keir Hardie** (1856-1915).

A miner from age 10 to 22, Keir Hardie organized a labour union among his fellow miners. He headed a new Scottish Labour Party in 1888 and he was elected first Labour M. P., in 1892 to Parliament.

1894 JAN 1: Death of **Heinrich Hertz** (b. 1857), German physicist, who first demonstrated the physical existence of radio waves. [see 1887 (e)]

1894 JAN. 16: *Appeal Avalanche,* reported:

"**SWAMI VIVEKANANDA,** the Hindoo monk, who is to lecture at the auditorium (Memphis) tonight, is one of the most eloquent men who has ever appeared on the religious or lecture platform in this country. His matchless oratory, deep penetration into things occult, his cleverness in debate, and great earnestness captured the closest attention of the world's thinking men at the World's Fair Parliament of Religions, and the admiration of thousands of people who have since heard him during his lecture tour through many of the States of the Union.

"In conversation he is a most pleasant gentleman; his choice of words are the gems of the English language and his general bearing ranks him with the most cultured people of western etiquette and custom. As a companion he is a most charming man, and as a conversationalist he is, perhaps not surpassed in the drawing-rooms of any city in the western world. He speaks English not only distinctly, but fluently, and his ideas, as new as sparkling, drop from his tongue in a perfectly bewildering overflow of ornamental language.

"His wonderful first address before the members of the World's Fair Parliament stamped him   at once as a leader in that great body of religious thinkers. During the session he was frequently heard in defence of his religion, and some of the most beautiful and philosophical gems that grace the English language rolled from his lips there in picturing the higher duties that man owed to man and to his creator. He is an artist in thought, an idealist in belief and a dramatist on the platform.

"Yesterday afternoon he lectured before a large and fashionable audience composed of the members of the Nineteenth Century Club, in the rooms of the club, in the Randolph Building. Tonight he will be heard at the Auditorium on 'Hindooism.' "

1894 JAN. 17: *Memphis Commercial,* reported:

"An audience of fair proportions gathered last night at the auditorium to greet the celebrated Hindu monk, **SWAMI VIVEKANANDA,** in his lecture on Hinduism.

"The eminent oriental was received with liberal applause and heard with attentive interest throughout. He is a man of fine physical presence, with regular bronze features and form of fine proportions. He wore a robe of pink silk, fastened at the waist with a black sash, black trousers and about his head was gracefully draped a turban of yellow Indian silk. His delivery is very good, his use of English being perfect as regards choice of words and correctness of grammar and construction.... Attentive listeners, however, probably lost few words and their attention was well rewarded by an address full of original thought, information and broad wisdom. The address might fitly be called a plea for universal tolerance, illustrated by remarks concerning the religion of India. This spirit, he contended, the spirit of tolerance and love, is the central inspiration of all religions which are worthy and this, he thinks, is the end to be secured by any form of faith.

"His entire lecture cannot be sketched here but it was a masterly appeal for brotherly love, and an eloquent defence of a beautiful faith...."

1894 JAN. 21: *Appeal Avalanche* reported:

"SWAMI VIVEKANANDA, the Hindoo monk delivered a lecture at La Salette Academy (Memphis) yesterday afternoon. Owing to the pouring rain, a very small audience was present.

"The subject discussed was *'Manners and Customs of India'*. Vivekananda is advancing theories of religious thought which find ready, lodgement in the minds of some of the most advanced thinkers of this as well as other cities of America.

"His theory is fatal to the orthodox belief, as taught by the Christian teachers. It has been the supreme effort of Christian America to enlighten the beclouded minds of heathen India, but it seems that the oriental splendour of Vivekananda's religion has eclipsed the beauty of the old time Christianity, as taught by our parents and will find a rich field in which to thrive in the minds of some of the better educated of America.

"This is a day of 'fads' and Vivekananda seems to be filling a 'long felt want'. He is, perhaps, one of the most learned men of his country, and possesses a wonderful amount of personal magnetism, and his hearers are charmed by his eloquence. While he is liberal in his views, he sees very little to admire in the orthodox Christianity. Vivekananda has received more marked attention in Memphis than almost any lecturer or minister that has ever visited the city."

1894 FEB. 15: *Detroit Tribune* reported:

"Last evening a good sized audience had the privilege of seeing and listening to the famous Hindoo Monk **SWAMI VIVEKANANDA,** as he lectured at the Unitarian Church under the auspices of the Unity Club. He appeared in native costume and made, with his handsome face and stalwart figure, a distinguished appearance. His eloquence held the audience in rapt attention and brought out applause at frequent intervals. He spoke of the *'Manners and Customs of India'*, and presented the subject in the most perfect English."

1894 FEB. 16: *Detroit Tribune* reported:

"The Brahmin monk, **SWAMI VIVEKANANDA,** again lectured last evening at the Unitarian Church, his topic being *Hindu Philosophy.* The speaker dealt for a time with general philosophy and metaphysics, but said that he would devote the lecture to that part pertaining to religion....

"Vivekananda was glad he was a Hindu. When Jerusalem was destroyed by the Romans several thousands (Jews) settled in India. When the Persians were driven from their country by the Arabs several thousand found refuge in the same country and none were molested. The Hindus believe all religions are true, but theirs antedates all others. Missionaries are never molested by the Hindus. The first English missionaries were prevented from landing in the country by the English and it was a Hindu that interceded for them and gave them the first hand.... Persecution is unknown in Buddhism. They sent out the first missionaries and are the only ones who can say they have converted millions without the shedding of a single drop of blood. Hindus, with all their faults and superstitions never persecuted.The speaker wanted to know how it was the Christians allowed such iniquities as are everywhere present in Christian countries."

1894 FEB. 17: *Detroit Evening News* reported:

"I cannot comply with the request of the news to work a miracle in proof of my religion", said **VIVEKANANDA** to a representative of this paper, after being shown the News Editorial on the subject. "In the first place, I am no miracle worker, and in the second place the pure Hindoo religion I profess is not based on miracles. We do not recognize such a thing as miracles. There are wonders wrought beyond our five senses, but they are operated by some law. Our religion has nothing to do with them. Most of the strange things which are done in India and reported in the foreign papers are sleight-of-hand tricks or hypnotic illusions. They are not the performances of the wise men....These do not go about the country performing their wonders in the market place for pay. They can be seen and known only by those who seek to know the truth, and not moved by childish curiosity".

1894 FEB. 18: *Detroit Free Press* reported:

"SWAMI VIVEKANANDA, Hindoo philosopher and priest, concluded his series of lectures, or rather, sermons, at the Unitarian Church last night, speaking on *The Divinity of Man.* In spite of bad weather, the Church was crowded almost to the doors half an hour before the eastern brother – as he likes to be called – appeared. All professions and business occupations were represented in the attentive audience – lawyers, judges, ministers of the gospel, merchants, rabbi – not to speak of many ladies who have by their repeated attendance and rapt attention shown a decided inclination to shower adulation upon the dusky visitor whose drawing-room attraction is as great as his ability in the rostrum.

"The lecture last night was less descriptive than preceding ones, and for nearly two hours Vivekananda wove a metaphysical texture on affairs human and divine, so logical that he made science appear like common sense. It was a beautiful logical garment that he wove, replete with as many bright colours and attractive and pleasing to contemplate as one of the many-hued fabrics made by hand in his native land and scented with the most seductive fragrance of the Orient. This dusky gentleman uses poetical imagery as an artist uses colours, and the hues are laid on just where they belong, the result being somewhat bizarre in effect, and yet having a peculiar fascination. Kaleidoscopic were the swiftly succeeding logical conclusions, and the deft manipulator was rewarded for his effort from time to time by enthusiastic applause."

1894 FEB. 18 (A): Regarding SWAMI VIVEKANANDA'S remarks about conversion and bigotry which he made in the course of his lecture on *The Divinity of Man* at the Unitarian Church on the previous day, the *Detroit Tribune* reported:

"Hindus, he said did not believe in conversion, calling it perversion. Associations, surroundings, and educations were responsible for the great number of religions, and how foolish it was for an exponent of one religion to declare that another man's belief was wrong. It was as reasonable as a man from Asia coming to America and after viewing the course of the Mississippi to say to it: 'You are running entirely wrong. You will have to go back to the starting place and commence it all over again.' It would be just as foolish for a man in America to visit the Alps and after following the course of a river to the German sea to inform it that its course was too tortuous and that the only remedy would be to flow as directed.... He thought the hell-fire theory was all nonsense. There could not be perfect happiness when it was known that suffering existed.... The Hindu, he said, closed his eyes and communed with the inner spirit, while some Christians he had seen had seemed to stare at some point as if they saw God seated upon his heavenly throne. In the matter of religion there were two extremes, the bigot and the atheist. There was some good in the atheist, but the bigot lived only for his own little-self...."

Detroit Free Press, another American newspaper, reported in this connection:

"Vivekananda emphasised his opinion that all was well and had no desire to convert Christians. They were Christians it was well. He was a Hindoo, that also was well. In his country different creeds were formulated for the needs of people of different grades of intelligence, all this marking the progress of spiritual evolution.... This system of bribing men to become Christians, alleged to have come from God, who manifested himself to certain men on earth, is atrocious. It is horribly demoralizing and the Christian creed, accepted literally, has a shameful effect upon the moral natures of the bigots who accept it...."

1894 FEB. 21: *Detroit Journal* reported:

"If **VIVEKANANDA**, the Brahmin monk, who is delivering a lecture course in this city could be induced to remain for a week longer, the largest hall in Detroit would not hold the crowds which would be anxious to hear him. He has become a veritable fad, as last evening every seat in the Unitarian Church was occupied, and many were compelled to   stand throughout the entire lecture."

"The speaker's subject was, *The Love of God.* His definition of love was 'something absolutely unselfish, that which has no thought beyond the glorification and adoration of the object upon which our affections are bestowed'. Love, he said, is a quality which bows down and worships and asks nothing in return. Love of God, he thought, was different. God is not accepted, he said, because we rarely need him, except for selfish purposes. His lecture was replete with story and anecdote, all going to show the selfish motive underlying the motive of love for God. The songs of Solomon were cited by the lecturer as the most beautiful portion of the Christian Bible and yet he had heard with deep regret that there was a possibility of their being removed. In fact, he declared, as a sort of clinching argument at the close, the love of God appears to be based upon a theory of 'what can I get out of it?' Christians are so selfish in their love that they are continually asking God to give them something, including all manner of selfish things. Modern religion is therefore, nothing but a mere hobby and fashion and people flock to Church like a lot of sheep."

1894 FEB. 21 (A): SWAMI VIVEKANANDA delivered the fifth lecture at Detroit, the subject being *Hindus and Christians.* It was reported in the *Detroit Free Press:*

In the course of his lecture Swamiji told the audience about the Christian missionaries who came to India and indulged in abusing Hindus and Hindu Religion: "You train and educate and clothe and pay men to do what? To come over to my country to curse and abuse all my forefathers, my religion, and everything. They walk near a temple and say: 'You idolators, you will go to hell'. But they dare not do that to the Mohammedans of India; the sword would be out. But the Hindu is too mild; he smiles and passes on, and says, 'let the fools talk'. That is the attitude. And then you who train men to abuse and criticize, if I just touch you with the least bit of criticism, with the kindest purpose, you shrink and cry: 'Don't touch us; we are Americans. We criticize all the people in the world, curse them and abuse them, say anything, but do not touch us, we are sensitive plants.' ....And whenever your ministers criticize us let them remember this: If all India stands up and takes all the mud that is at the bottom of the Indian Ocean and throw it up against the Western countries, it will not be doing an infinitesimal part of that which you are doing to us. And what for? Did we ever send one missionary to convert anybody in the world? We say to you: 'Welcome to your religion, but allow me to have mine. "

Swamiji asserted that Christianity never succeeded except with the sword and he challenged his audience to show him one place, not two, where it had been otherwise: "....with all your brags and boastings, where has your Christianity succeeded without the sword? Show me one place in the whole world. One I say, throughout the history of the Christian religion – one: I do not want two. I know how your forefathers were converted. They had to be converted or killed; that was all. What can you do better than Mohammedanism, with all your bragging...."

Referring to the part played by the Christian Missionaries in the colonial adventures of some of the European nations, Swamiji said: "Such things tumble down; they are built upon sand; they cannot remain long. Everything that has selfishness for its basis, competition for its right hand and enjoyment as its goal, must die sooner or later. If you want to live, if you really want your nation to live, go back to Christ. You are not Christians. No, as a nation you are not. Go back to Christ. Go back to him who had nowhere to lay his head. 'The birds have their nests and the beasts their lairs, but the son of man has nowhere to lay his head.' Yours is a religion preached in the name of luxury. What an irony of fate! Reverse this if you want to live, reverse this. It is all hypocrisy that I have beard in this country. If this nation is going to live, let it go back to Him. You cannot serve God and mammon at the same time. All this prosperity, all this from Christ! Christ would have denied all such heresies. All prosperity which comes with mammon is transient, is only for a moment. Real permanence is in Him. If you can join these two, this wonderful prosperity with the ideal of Christ, it is well. But if you cannot, better go back to Him and give this up. Better be ready to live in rags with Christ than to live in palaces without Him."

1894 FEB. 21 (B): *The Indian Mirror* in its Editorial:

"When the Executive Committee of the Parliament of Religions, held in connection with the World's Fair at Chicago, issued its invitation to the members of every creed and church in the world to send their representatives to its meetings, we felt an anxiety as to the possibility of finding a man who would be a Hindu of Hindus, and yet would not have scruples to cross the ocean, and must at the same time, be competent to enlighten the Parliament on the subject of Hinduism as might not only justify it in the eyes of the civilized world, but also win for it the respect and admiration of the spiritual-minded and religiously disposed among the followers of every other system of faith. But when reliable reports reached us of the ability, wisdom and eloquence with which **SWAMI VIVEKANANDA** was expounding Hinduism at the Parliament, not only all our anxiety about the matter was at an end, but we felt thankful to the Great Disposer of all events who, it seemed, in his inscrutable ways, had found the right man for the right place. It was a demand of the time, and of the age that Hinduism, which has been so cruelly misjudged and imperfectly apprehended by the Christians in particular, and the followers of other religions in general, should be represented in its true aspect before all the world. The platform of the Parliament of Religions was indeed the fittest place from which Hinduism could be effectively defended against the many false charges, repeatedly brought about against it by interested persons and communities, and also from which its' merits could be expounded to enable people to accord to it its just position in the ranks of the world's great religions. It is a matter of national congratulation that the representative of Hinduism at the great Parliament was equal to his task, and discharged his duties in a manner that has earned for him the gratitude of the entire Hindu community.

"Dr. Barrows characterizes the Swami's address as 'noble and sublime', and it was so much appreciated for its breadth, its sincerity and its excellent spirit of toleration, that the Hindu representative soon came to be as much liked outside the Parliament as within it. His fame, as an eloquent preacher of sublime Hindu doctrines, spread fast through the American cities and towns, and we learn that ever since the Parliament dissolved, the Swami has been eagerly sought for by numerous persons, invitations have poured upon him from various places to deliver lectures, and he has been strongly pressed to prolong his stay in America. Mr. A. Wann, an American gentleman of standing, writing under date the 27th December to a friend in Calcutta says: 'Swami Vivekananda has been delivering splendid lectures all over the country. He is very popular here.'

"As might be expected, some American priests, driven to desperation, as they were, by the sudden lift Hinduism was given to by its expositions by the Swami, made an effort to discredit him in the eyes of the American public, an effort in which they were aided, we are sorry to be told, by a member of the Hindu race. But the opponents failed to find a single flaw either in his life or his teachings, and the Swami has steadily risen in the estimation of the people in the United States, and in Canada, till his popularity has grown to such a high pitch that we are told, he is now in a manner idolized.

"Now, it is a question of no little moment, what is it that has contributed to this unexpected and splendid popularity of a preacher of Hinduism in a far-off Christian country? It is apparent that it is the deep, lofty and all pervading spirituality of the Hindu ideal of a religious life, represented by the Swami that, forming a striking contrast to the material existence, lived by people in the Western world, has taken them by surprise, and awakened a genuine and enthusiastic admiration for it in their hearts. Man even in America is not all senses, not all matter. However addicted to material pursuits a Yankee may be, the divinity within him must at times assert itself. Swami Vivekananda, it appears, has, by his discourses on the spirituality of Hindu religion, succeeded in stirring to their depths the slumbering spiritual aspirations of many an American soul.

"The American ladies, we ate told, have specially manifested a keen interest in the Swami's teachings, and he has come to entertain a high opinion of their religiousness. It is, indeed, a rare phenomenon that American women, reputed to be only votaries of fashion and flippancy, should turn into admirers of a Hindu sannyasin and his teachings.

"With facts before us of this outburst of enthusiasm and admiration for the teachings of Hinduism by hundreds of Americans, shall we not be justified in advancing the opinion that these Christian people have found in the essence of Hinduism a higher and truer ideal of religious life that Christianity could not supply them ?

"Whatever may be the practical outcome of Swami Vivekananda's mission in America there can be no question that it has already had the effect of immediately raising the credit of true Hinduism in the eyes of the civilized world, and that is, indeed, a work for which the whole Hindu community should feel grateful to the Swami."

1894 FEB. : During this time and at certain subsequent periods of his stay in the West, **SWAMI VIVEKANANDA** felt that certain yogic powers had spontaneously developed in him. He rarely used them, and in the few cases that he did so, it was not for name or fame, but to help a truly good soul, too feeble to rise above some weaknesses and evil influence. He could change, if he so wished, the whole trend of man's life by his mere touch. He could see things occurring at great distance.

By the mercy of Sri Ramakrishna, as he wrote (to Mrs. Bull, 25 April 1895), he distinctly "sized up" almost infallibly a human face as soon as he saw it. On many occasions his students would find him answering and solving those very doubts and questions that they would be thinking of at the moment. The story is told how one day at Chicago a man spoke flippantly about yogic powers and challenged him, if he could, to tell him something of his mental make-up, or his past. The Swami hesitated for a moment, and then fixed his eyes on those of the man, whereupon the latter felt some irresistible power piercing through his body to his soul, as it were, and in alarm he cried out, "O Swami, what are you doing to me? It seems as if my whole soul is being churned and all the secrets of my life called up in strong colours." (*A Comprehensive Biography of Swami Vivekananda*, Part I, p. 499 and 500).

1894 FEB. (A): **SWAMI VIVEKANANDA** is said to have given a demonstration of materialization at Detroit, at the house of Mrs. J. B. Bagley where he stayed as a guest.

The following story was narrated by Mrs. J. B. Bagley's granddaughter, Mrs. Frances Bagley Wallace: "I was only nine years old at that time, but I remember that after being locked in grandfather's study at one end of the house, the Swami materialized in the centre of the big parlour at the other end of the house where the guests were. When the prominent gentleman who had locked him in the study and had pocketed the key returned and unlocked the door, there sat the Swami in the same position as he had been when they had locked him in there." (*A Comprehensive Biography of Swami Vivekananda*, Part I, p. 498).

1894 MAR. 9: In a letter to the Editor of *The Indian Mirror* Mr. **Merwin-Marie Snell**, President of the Scientific Section of the Parliament of Religions, Chicago, wrote:

"There having been an occasional note of discord in the chorus of praise which the delegates from India in the World's Parliament of Religions – and especially **SWAMI VIVEKANANDA** – elicited from the American Press and People, I have felt inspired to acquaint your people with the true state of the case, to voice the unanimous and heartfelt gratitude and appreciation of the cultured and broad-minded portion of our public, and to give my personal testimony, as the President of the Scientific Section of the Parliament and all the conference connected with the latter, and therefore an eye-witness, to the esteem in which he is held here, the influence that he is wielding and the good that he is doing.

"The World's Parliament of Religions, held in the city of Chicago last September, may well be considered for many reasons, as marking an event in the history of religions. One of its chief advantages has been in the great lesson which it has taught the Christian world, and especially the people of the United States, namely, that there are other religions, more venerable than Christianity, which surpass it in philosophical depth, in spiritual intensity, in independent vigour of thought, and in breadth and sincerity of human sympathy, while not yielding to it a single hair's-breadth in ethical beauty and efficiency. Eight great non-Christian religious groups were represented in its deliberations – Hinduism, Jainism, Buddhism, Judaism, Confucianism, Shintoism, Mohammedanism and Mazdaism.

"....But no religious body made so profound an impression upon the Parliament, and the American people at large as did Hinduism.

"By far the most important and typical representative of Hinduism was Swami Vivekananda, who, in fact, was beyond question the most popular and influential man in Parliament. He frequently spoke, both on the floor of the Parliament itself and in the meetings of the Scientific Section, over which I had the honour to preside, and on all occasions he was received with greater enthusiasm than any other speaker, Christian or 'Pagan'. The people thronged him wherever he went and hung with eagerness on his every word. Since the Parliament he has been lecturing before audiences in the principal cities of the United States and has received an ovation wherever he went. He has often been invited to preach in Christian pulpits and has by all who have heard him on any occasion, and still more by those who have made his personal acquaintance, been always spoken of in terms of the highest admiration. The most rigid or orthodox Christians say of him, 'He is indeed a prince among men', even when they find it necessary, for the sake of their time-honoured prejudices, to add, 'but he must be altogether an exception; of course there are no other Hindus like him'.

"As intense is the astonished admiration which the personal presence and bearing and language of Paramahamsa Vivekananda have wrung from a public accustomed to think of Hindus – thanks to the fables and half-truths of the missionaries – as ignorant and degraded 'heathen'; there is no doubt that the continued interest is largely due to a genuine hunger for the spiritual truths which India through him has offered to the American people.

"America is starving for spiritual nourishment in spite of its absorption in material things, in spite of the ignorance and provincialism of its upper classes and the savagery of its lower, there are many souls scattered everywhere throughout its great population who are thirsting for higher things. Europe has always been indebted to India for its spiritual inspirations. There is little, very little of high thought and aspiration in Christendom which cannot be traced to one or another of the successive influx of Hindu ideas: either to the Hinduised Hellenism of Pythogoras and Plato, to the Hinduised Mazdaism of the Gnostic, to the Hinduised Judaism of the Kabbalists, or to the Hinduised Mohammedanism of the Moorish philosophers; to say nothing of the Hinduised occultism of the theosophists, the Hinduised Socialism of the New England Transcendentalists and the many other new streams of Orientalizing influence which are fertilising the soil of contemporary Christendom.

"The most illumined men and women therefore in Europe and America have a natural drawing towards Hinduism, the chief historic source of their light and life as soon as they are brought into close contact with it under circumstances all favourable to its just appreciation. In the United States particularly there are several widespread and influential movements which are distinctly Hindu in their character and tendencies. Not only is all the scientific and liberal thought monistic in its trend, but the so-called 'Christian Science' movement (mostly egregiously misnamed), is admittedly based upon the Vedanta philosophy. [see 1879 (c), 1886 (o), 1894 Sept. 25]. America is well-sprinkled with Advaitins, of all three schools, even though they would not always, in the absence of any direct knowledge of Hindu thought, know how to define their position. Even Christian mythology is not so very different from the Hindu, and the latter is gradually becoming familiar to the American people, through the medium of translations, books and articles by scientists and dilettanti, and the writings and personal labours of liberal sects.

"All the Hinduizing forces hitherto at work have received a notable impulse from the labours of Swami Vivekananda. Never before has so authoritative a representative of genuine Hinduism – as opposed to the emasculated and Anglicized versions of it so common in these days – been accessible to American enquirers; and it is certain, beyond peradventure, that the American people at large will, when he is gone, look forward with eagerness to his return, or the advent of some of his confreres of the Institute of Shankaracharya.

"A few, and only a few, representatives of the extreme orthodox wing of the Protestant Christian community have been provoked into hostile criticism by jealousy of his success. But this has come exclusively from religionists of an abnormal type, and, as a rule, jealousy and sectarian animosity even from this quarter have been silenced by the uniform kindness and goodwill, as well as the learning and dignity and personal charm, of the orange-robed monk from the land of Bharata.

"America thanks India for sending him, and begs her to send many more like him; if such there are, to teach by their example those of her own children who have not learned the lessons of universal fraternity and openness of mind and heart; and, by their precepts those who have not yet come to see Divinity in all things and a Oneness transcending all."

1894 MAR. 11: SWAMI VIVEKANANDA delivered a lecture, *The Christian Missions in India,* in the local Opera Club (at Detroit) which was considered as the most eloquent lecture he had ever delivered at the city, and was spoken of by himself as the best lecture he had delivered so far in America.

His speech of nearly two hours and a half was a smashing rejoinder to the criticism levelled (mostly by Christian missionaries) against him, besides being full of sublime thoughts, and was highly applauded by thousands. It seems to have had the effect of silencing his critics for the time – at least so far as vocal denunciation was concerned. However, another (and despicable) form of attack on him, viz., maligning his personal character by inventing scandals, at first in whispers and then in the open, soon began, and an attempt was even made to murder him by poisoning his coffee at a dinner party. "They went to the length", as the Swami said, "of tempting him with young women, promising them recompense if they succeeded." (*A Comprehensive Biography of Swami Vivekananda,* Part I, p. 549).

Vivekananda faced abroad fanatic opposition from the Theosophists and Christian missionaries. "There is not one black lie imaginable that these latter did not invent against me. They blackened my character from city to city, poor and friendless though I was in a foreign country. They tried to oust me from every house, and to make every man who became my friend my enemy. They tried to starve me out; and I am sorry to say that one of my own countrymen took part against one in this.... And this gentleman I knew from my childhood, he was one of my best friends." (*The Complete Works of Swami Vivekananda,* Vol. III, p. 210)

1894 MAR. 14: *The Amrita Bazar Patrika* in its Editorial:

"The letter of **Mr. Mervin-Marie Snell** of Chicago, published in Indian papers, in which he said that America would be converted, if Hindus could send some missionaries like **VIVEKANANDA SWAMI,** has led the *Pioneer* to claim in verse and bewilderment thus:

Do I sleep? Do I Dream?
Do I wonder or doubt?
Are things what they seem?
Or visions about?
Is our civilization a failure?
Or is the Caucasian played out?

"And the cause of this bewilderment of mind is thus described by the paper:

'Here is an educated citizen of the greatest republic the world has ever seen, of the nation founded by the stern Calvinists who took refuge in New England from Popery and the Stuarts, of the people who blazon cuteness and superiority to dogma and superstition on their star-spangled banner – here is such an one confessing that his countrymen have been lying in gross spiritual darkness and had most probably lain there but for the 'Parliament of Religions' at Chicago and the advent of an orange-robed Swami from Hindustan, who have shown the benighted Yankee a great light.'

"But if the letter of Mr. Merwin-Marie Snell has thrown *'Pioneer'* into a state of amazement, it has not at all surprised us; for, we have been saying the same thing for a score of years, as our readers very well know. We have often made the suggestion in our columns, that if the Hindus had sent properly educated missionaries, they could have converted the West, which is day by day getting dry and stiff under the blaze of the artificial civilization which it has developed...."

1894 MAR. 18: An article by **O. P. Deldoc**, appeared in the *Detroit Critic* carried a description of the **religious bigotry existing in the United States**:

"....There were patriarchs, prophets, saints and martyrs; men who 'walked with God'; law givers and high priests, good, wise and holy men, whose bones had crumbled to dust ages before the Star of Bethlehem arose....

"Was there no love, no hope, no joy, no religion then?....

"Were all the noble souls abiding before Christ doomed to perdition?....

"The question is not whether Christianity is true, but are we true to Christianity as professed Christians?

"I claim that the vast majority of so-called Christians are not true, but false to the precepts and practices of their Lord and Master. They are only chimerical Christians, who roar with the lion's head, disguise their body in the form of a goat, and a scapegoat at that, and then wiggle the tail of a venomous dragon. They are continually belching forth flames of fire (hell-fire) upon all who differ from their favourite dogmas, creeds and sects.... Some of their pet and petrified dogmas are comprised in Quarto of beautiful specimens, 'The fall of man in Eden'; 'The sin of unbelief'; 'An atonement by proxy', and 'The eternal punishment of the damned'. If they encounter an individual with manhood, moral courage and wisdom.... they proceed at once to damn him.

"These mongrel specimens love to sing 'This world is all fleeting show', and so it is, veritable wonderland menagerie; filled with curious, incongruous monstrosities and deformities, such as Baptist barnacles, petrified Presbyterians, and Methodist mummeries....

"I am speaking of the vaster body of chimerical Christians. 'By their works ye shall know them'. Intolerance, bigotry, superstition, envy, malice and falsehood are their prominent features.... They evade the truth, and are false even unto themselves.... They delight to prate of missionary work among the heathen, thanking God 'they are not as other men are.'

"The pagan, so-called, could teach them more of the fundamental truth of religion than they ever dreamed of in their philosophy. Better far to be like the heathen worshipping even a false god, than to be false to the God they pretend to worship....

"There is but one religion, one philosophy, One God over all. Religion is love; not love of self, but love of God and all His creatures. Religious people preach for it, write for it, fight for it, die for it, do everything but live for it....

"A religious Hindu comes to us and talks of love, asking for bread and they give him a stone. He tells them he gladly accepts their Christ with his religion which is old to them as the 'rock of ages' upon the eternal hills, but they will accept neither his word, his philosophy or his religion.... They claim Christianity has caused all advancement, all civilization. Whence came all the grandeur and all the wisdom existing before the Nazarene Reformer was born among men and became one of the Sons of God?.... It is falsely ridiculous to claim such chimerical Christianity has been the cause of civilization as it would be to say that it was due to plug hats and suspenders....

"All nations and all eras have had their reformers and their saviours, and there are more to follow, until even the despised Jew may yet have his long-looked-for Messiah....

"Since the advent of the Hindu Monk (**SWAMI VIVEKANANDA**), over-zealous and bigoted preachers have tried to defame him and denounce his pure philosophy. They have pointed out the ungodly conditions of India; they have claimed her women were slaves, the law corrupt and vile. A sapient lawyer has quoted whole volume of the laws of India with sneering sarcasm; as well might he have quoted the ancient Mosaic Codes, or the blue laws of Connecticut or pointed out our own laws with regard to licentiousness, women and prohibition. India never had drunkards until Christian lands carried them liquor.

"As well point out our barbarous treatment of the Western Indian, our old slave laws or the records of vice and crime as found in the slums of our modern civilization....

"Truth is mighty and must prevail. This world or any other God's unlimited universe doesn't stand upon a turtle, nor is it supported upon any Hercules. Its cornerstones are light, liberty, love and law, and it is the chimerical Christians who would knock away these four corner stones of the universe....

"Let the Star of Bethlehem be the true Christian's polar star; let it arise and shine with all its ancient glory, as beheld by the wise men of the east; let its splendid light banish the mist of error and the darkness that befog men's brains. Let it light up the dark and narrow aisles in Christian lands, until the monster chimera, the false deformity of Christianity, shall hide its hideous head forever more."

1894 MAR. 21: *The Indian Mirror* in its Editorial:

"Although the Anglican Church, in its haughty and imperious exclusiveness, and with its characteristic narrowness and bigotry, did not approve of the aims and objects of the Parliament of Religions, that great assembly did not thereby lose a whit of its representative character, as it nevertheless attracted to it the representatives of almost every form of religion and faith, now prevailing in the world. The idea of the Religious Parliament was as noble as it was bold. Dr. John Henry Barrows, who is believed to be the originator, and known to be the most active promoter of this grand movement, must be ranked among the great religious geniuses of the world. The world has almost bled to death by religious animosities and strifes between nations; mankind have been sorely troubled over their differences on the question of life, death and immortality, and the wise and the great of almost every people have racked their brains almost to madness to solve the problem of the consummation of the brotherhood of man and fatherhood of God. This universal unrest and agitation, and longing for love and peace undisturbed, holiness and salvation, have, it seems, at last impelled representatives of races and communities, separated from one another, by birth and language and distance, to unite, and strive to discover the underlying principles of harmony of contending faiths, so that all mankind may come to possess, as it were, one heart, beating with love profound, and moved by the same emotions, ennobled by the same aspirations and sanctified by the same hopes. This was the object – the sublime and almost divine object – of the Parliament of Religions, and we can unhesitatingly declare, judging from the proceedings of the body, that foundations have been already laid for the achievement of this object.

"The spirit that reigned over the Parliament and dominated the soul of almost every religious representative present, was that of universal toleration and universal deliverance, and it ought to be a matter of pride to India, to all Hindus specially, that no one expressed as the American papers say, this spirit so well as the Hindu representative, **SWAMI VIVEKANANDA.** His address, in every way worthy of representative of a religion, such as Hinduism is, struck the keynote of the Parliament of Religions.

"The prospect of a universal religion, binding all nations as brothers, and as sons of the same God, was never made more vivid in the mind of a body of representative religious men of different views, than in the meetings of this unparalleled gathering at Chicago, and the Hindu representative showed himself to be eminently true and loyal to his refined Hindu instincts, when he concluded his address with the following sketch of the ideal of a universal religion....

"The spirit of catholicity and toleration, which distinguishes Hinduism, forming one of its broad features, was never before so prominently brought to the notice of the world, as it has been by Swami Vivekananda, and we make no doubt that the Swami's address will have an effect on other religions, whose teachers, preachers and missionaries heard him, and were impressed by his utterances....

"This great religious convention, held at Chicago, is the flower of the tree of religion which mankind have so long watered and pruned and pruned and watered. It is the crowning work of the nineteenth century. It is the dawn of a new era in religious thought and culture. It is the highest expression yet given to the divinity in the human race. Our chief pride is that it is a thing, quite in accord with Hindu religious thought and aspiration, and that this fact was testified to at the Parliament of Religions by the noble address which the singularly qualified Hindu representative delivered before it."

1894 MAR. 25: *Detroit Free Press* reported:

"**VIVEKANANDA** lectured last night at the Unitarian Church on *The Women of India.* The speaker reverted to the women of ancient India, showing in what high regard they are held in the holy books, where women were prophetesses. Their spirituality then was admirable. It is unfair to judge women in the East by the Western standards. In the

West, woman is the wife; in the East she is the mother. The Hindoos worship the idea of mother, and even the monks are required to touch the earth with their foreheads before their mothers. Chastity is much esteemed.

"The lecture was one of the most interesting Vivekananda has delivered and he was warmly received."

1894 MAR. : Max Muller (1823-1900) delivered three lectures at the Royal Institute, London, on the **Vedanta Philosophy.**

The lectures were an attempt to interest an English audience in the philosophy of the leading school of the thinkers of ancient India – the school that appealed most to the mind and heart of the lecturer so that he could, as the result of his own experience during a long life devoted to the study of many philosophies and many religions, endorse the words of Schopenhauer, "In the whole world there is no study so beneficial and elevating as that of Vedanta philosophy, as contained in the Upanishads. It has been the solace of my life, it will be the solace of death."

Max Muller was most anxious to impress on his hearers that there was nothing esoteric in the Vedanta Philosophy, that it was open to all; and he closed his lecture by repeating the Sanskrit line in which a native philosopher formulated the whole teaching of the Vedanta philosophy, which Max Muller translated, 'God is true, the world is fleeting, man's soul is God and nothing else'. Then giving the old philosopher's deduction from this teaching, he rendered it: 'What shall it profit a man, if he shall gain the whole world, and lose his own soul' (*The Life and Letters of Max Muller,* Vol. I, p. 330).

1894 MAR-APR: John D. Rockefeller (1839-1937), U. S. industrialist and world's wealthiest man, called on **SWAMI VIVEKANANDA** who was then resting for a while at a house at Chicago, after going through his two strenuous and triumphant lecture programmes at Detroit and elsewhere.

Swamiji made Rockefeller understand that "he was only a channel and that his duty was to do good to the world – that God had given him all his wealth in order that he might have an opportunity to help and do good to people." About a week later, when Rockefeller met Swamiji again the second time, he told Swamiji of his plan to donate an enormous sum of money towards the financing of a public institution. Three years hence (1897) Rockefeller devoted himself completely to philanthropy. He spoke his philosophy as follows: "There is more to life than the accumulation of money. Money is only a trust in one's hand. To use it improperly is a great sin. The best way to prepare for the end of life is to live for others. This is what I am trying to do."

Rockefeller is believed to have given away some 550 million dollars in his lifetime, including major endowments to the University of Chicago (1890) [see 1876 (e), 1891 (j)], the Rockefeller Institute for Medical Research (1901), and the General Education Board (1902). He also established the Rockefeller Foundation in 1913, to promote well-being of mankind throughout world. His and his sons's benefactions totalled more than $ 3,000,000,000.

1894 APR. 5: Birth of **G. D. Birla** (d. 1983), doyen of Indian Industry, who pioneered the industrialization of the country.

A deeply religious person, he was also a philanthropist, a promoter of education, a patron of religious and cultural activities, an economic thinker and planner and a visionary with undying faith in the country's future. At his instance, numerous temples – some of them exquisite specimens of architecture – were built in different parts of the country. Many institutions in the country owe their establishment and existence to the charity of the Birla family.

1894 APR. 10: *The Indian Mirror* wrote:-

"That a prophet is not honoured in his country is a commonplace which is often illustrated in life. It is doubtful whether **SWAMI VIVEKANANDA** would have become so widely known, if he had not visited America. The broad-hearted Americans are to be thanked for whatever success the Swami met with in his exposition of Hinduism in the Parliament of Religions at Chicago. How far Swami Vivekananda succeeded in impressing his American hearers with the intrinsic worth of Hinduism, is well-known to us. There is, at the present moment, an unusual commotion in American society about the young Swami, and the religion which he professes.... Swami Vivekananda was pre-eminently the central figure in the Religious Parliament, and the honour which was paid to him by religionists of all persuasions was an honour to the whole Hindu race.... In view of the glorious success, achieved by Swami Vivekananda in his missionary tour in America, we think that Hindus will be doing a grateful duty by presenting an address to the Swami, and also to the organizers of the Parliament of Religions but for whose help the Swami would have found it difficult to obtain such a strong footing in America. We hope, our Hindu brethren all over the country will heartily join the movement. Swami Vivekananda is still in America, and the address ought to be sent to him there without delay. We must also let our American friends know that we are not ungrateful for the good offices which they rendered to our Hindu brother. There should be no loss of time to get up the address, and we should like to have the views of our Hindu brethren in all parts of the country on the subject."

1894 APR. 11: *Northampton Daily Herald* stamped **SWAMI VIVEKANANDA'S popularity** beyond doubt. It reported:

"At the Parliament of Religions, Vivekananda was not allowed to speak until the close of the programmes, the purpose being to make the people stay until the end of the session. On a warm day when some prosy professor talked too long, and people would leave the hall by hundreds, it only needed the announcement that Vivekananda would give a short address before the benediction was pronounced to hold the vast audience. In fact, the thousands would wait for hours to hear a fifteen minute talk from this remarkable man."

1894 APR. 12: *The Indian Mirror* reported:

"We understand that **SWAMI VIVEKANANDA** has succeeded by his eloquent lectures and sermons on the doctrines and principles of Hinduism, in setting a large number of people in America athinking on the subject of Hindu religion, and that a number of persons have so completely accepted his teachings as true, that they are already being regarded as converts to the Hindu faith, as preached by the Swami.

"A Hindu friend writes: 'Mr. Dharmapala (of Mahabodhi Society) speaks highly of the Parliament and its work. He is full of admiration for the Hindu representative at the Parliament, Swami Vivekananda. The account he gives of the Swami, and of the popularity enjoyed by him in the United States, is most interesting and cheering, and cannot fail to gladen the heart of every true Hindu, who wished to see his religion and his race faithfully represented before those representative religionists of the world who gathered together at Chicago. Mr. Dharmapala says that life-size portraits of Swami Vivekananda are found hung up in the streets of Chicago with the words, 'Monk Vivekananda' beneath them, and thousands of passers by, comprising men of all classes, are observed to do obeisance to these portraits, in the most reverential way. The Buddhist representative truly remarks that all Hindus should be proud of the honour accorded to their representative by the American people, and that blessings and good wishes should be sent to him from every Hindu home. Mr. Dharmapala is of the opinion that the success of the Religious Parliament was to a great extent, due to Swami Vivekananda.' "

1894 APR. 13: In a letter to the Editor of *The Indian Mirror,* a reader wrote:

"A copy of **SWAMI VIVEKANANDA'S Lecture on Hinduism** came unexpectedly to my hand, and I had the pleasure of going through it. No sooner had I read a few sentences than my attention was entirely arrested by the pamphlet. After I had gone through it, I could not resist the temptation of reading it over and over again. The appropriate use of every word that he uttered in the course of his lecture justifies us to come to the conclusion that he has gained a thorough mastery over the English language. The way in which he explained what was implicitly meant by the authors of the Vedantic philosophy, indicates his power of penetration into the subject. He is fairly entitled to the epithet 'Vivekananda'. It appears that the knowledge which he now possesses, has been gained by absolute devotion to God. Through the medium of your paper, I wish to draw the particular attention of English missionaries to the pamphlet, refered to before, and advise them to study it, because I often find them, with but rare exceptions, labouring under deep-rooted prejudices against Hinduism. If they take the trouble of reading the pamphlet, they will be greatly benefited, in as much as they will be able to find out the main cause on account of which their attempts to propagate the religion which they profess often prove futile. I am glad to find that the Americans entertain great respect for him, and have unanimously showered praise upon him. One of them had made such just appreciation of his merits, and has been fully convinced of the superiority of Hinduism that he goes to the length – of course, not beyond legitimate limits – of saying, 'it is an act of foolishness on our part to send missionaries to such a learned nation.' "

1894 APR. 22: In a letter to the Editor of *The Indian Mirror* a reader wrote:

"I am extremely sorry to see that the unprecedented success of **SWAMI VIVEKANANDA** has created a strong jealousy and heart-burning among the Christians and Brahmos, who are trying their best to damage his reputation. They have commenced regular warfare in writing and in speaking against the Swami in his absence. But they are fighting a losing battle. Swami Vivekananda is a mighty power now. His culture, his eloquence and his fascinating personality have given to the world a new idea of Hindu religion. All the American papers unanimously declare him to be the foremost delegate in the religious Congress, and none surpassed him in philosophical depth and clearness of thought of what he said. Every Indian ought to be grateful for his most able and quite disinterested advocacy of Hinduism. This is for the first time in the annals of the Indian History that the true and genuine spirit of Hinduism has been expounded in foreign lands, where the Hindus have all along been described as worshippers of 'hideous devils' by the worthy Christian Missionaries. The Swami's address on Hinduism, which has been printed and circulated, is a precious gem. It should be read, pondered over and thoroughly grasped. Every sentence uttered by him is a museum of thoughts, and it is a wonder how he succeeded in giving such a remarkable picture within half an hour's time.

"Vivekananda's religion is as broad as heaven above, and his cause is the cause of the Hindus. But it was sad and strange thing that one of the delegates to the Congress, a preacher of morality among the rising generation, tried his utmost, to spread false report, and we have seen how they were proved to be pure falsehoods by Mr. Dharmapala, the Buddhist representative. Vivekananda has presented within the narrow compass a clear, lucid exposition of every philosophical sect of Hinduism. Every Hindu who has any knowledge of the *Hindu shastras*, will at once perceive the wonderful depth of Vedantic learning which the Swami possesses. Mr. Dharmapala truly says that his uncommon command of the English language and supreme tolerance of religion and his wonderful renunciation electrify the audience.

"The other day Brahmo organ was pouring its venom on revered Swami for his attack on Christianity. It was a sad spectacle that the Editor of that paper thought it fit to sit in judgement without taking the trouble of going to the lecture. There is not a single word in Swami's speech wherein he attacked any religion. He was universal toleration. He accepts all religions as true; and his address was the death-knell of bigotry and fanaticism. People may speak what they like from jealousy and malice, but their attempt to vilify the Swami, will be like knocking their heads against rocks. Madras and Bombay have appreciated the greatness of Vivekananda and America now worships him. It is now the turn of Bengal to join hands with them in their national glory. Every Hindu should be proud of the splendid reception accorded to Vivekananda. I think who has once gone through his lectures will not hesistate to join in giving an address to Swami Vivekananda. I am glad to see that you, Mr. Editor, have taken the initiative in such a laudable religious cause."

1894 APR. 28: A Public meeting was held at Madras to express to **SWAMI VIVEKANANDA** the grateful thanks of the citizens for representing India at the Parliament of Religions at Chicago, as also for his lucid exposition of Hinduism there. [see 1894 June]

The citizens of Calcutta also organized a great representative meeting in the Town Hall on September 5, 1894, to thank the Swami and the American people. The meeting was organized by the most representative members of the Hindu community, and attended by people of all shades of opinion. Some of the most well-known pandits as well as the landed aristocracy, the High Court Judges, noted public men, pleaders, politicians, professors and prominent men in many other walks of life took part in the meeting. [see 1894 Sept. 5]

On November 18, 1894, in his formal reply to the welcome he received from the citizens of Calcutta, the Swami wrote from America, "Give and take is the law, and if India wants to raise herself once more, it is absolutely necessary that she brings out her treasures and throws them broadcast among the nations of the earth, and in return be ready to receive what others have to give her." [see 1895 Apr. 18]

1894 JUN: The Hindus of Madras who held a public meeting to tender their thanks to **SWAMI VIVEKANANDA** for having represented India at the Parliament of Religion at Chicago, and for his lucid exposition of Hinduism before the same, voted the following address and sent it to the Swami in America:

To Sri Swami Vivekananda –

"Sir, – In forwarding to you the accompanying Resolution, conveying the thanks of the Hindu community of Madras, in a public meeting assembled, for representing India at the Chicago Parliament of Religions, I (the Chairman) have the honour to state that I give expression to the general feeling, both in our Presidency town and throughout Southern India, that you have laid the entire Hindu community under immense obligations of gratitude by your powerful, telling and authoritative exposition of the religion of the sages and prophets of India. We, your Hindu co-religionists, who have had the privilege of knowing you personally, never for a moment doubted that your Mission would prove an entire success; your sacred calling, your noble nature, your high intellect, and your devotion to the cause of the *rishis* combined to make that success for us a foregone conclusion. But I wish to be permitted to say that the success, you have actually achieved, has certainly exceeded our most sanguine expectations, and we beg to assure you that this is due quite as much to your mighty enthusiasm and noble oratory, as it is to the greatness and sacredness of the cause which found in you so powerful a spokesman and representative. I need hardly point out here at length, how dear and near that cause is to the hearts of us all. In expounding and enunciating before the great American nation the fundamental principles of the Hindu religious system, you have not only insisted that India is the home of spiritual excellence and the cradle of the world's civilization, but have also demonstrated the insufficiency of a purely materialistic civilization. We admire the convincing thoroughness of your demonstration that our holy scriptures enunciate universal and unchanging spiritual laws; that their central conception lies in the truth that man is to become divine by realizing the divine, 'not by believing but by being and becoming'; and that all religious systems are with the Hindus so many different paths to that heaven to Supreme Bliss and Peace, which is freedom from the bondage of matter, and from the change and mutation which, while it continues, prevents the soul from realizing its truly divine nature. Your exposition of Sri Krishna's ethical teaching has also been thorough and appropriate, and must necessarily bear fruit in making humanity realize the truth and wisdom of His message to mankind.

"We have also watched with pride and pleasure your success among the great American people subsequently to the Chicago convention, and offer you our hearty congratulations on the achievement, within so short a period of, results so brilliant, and so full of promise for the cause of the world's spiritual progress and religious harmony. We feel daily more and more that your cause could not have found a better and more gifted champion; and while all of us are looking forward with hearts full of love, and eager with expectation to your speedy return to your labours among us here, we pray for your continued success, and wish you health and strength to carry your holy Mission in the West to its destined goal." (*The Indian Mirror,* 8 Aug. 1894)

1894 JUL. 26: Birth of **Aldous Huxley** (d. 1963), English author, whose novels, short stories, and essays explore crucial questions of science, religion and philosophy.

1894 AUG. 8: *The Indian Mirror* quoted *The Boston Evening Transcript*:

"**SWAMI VIVEKANANDA** is coming to Boston in all the glory of his gorgeous orange turban and his advanced views on all topics intellectual and moral. Everybody who had any interest in the Parliament of Religions while in Chicago, knows of brother Vivekananda, as he likes to be called. He had come to America on a missionary tour, to see what he could do to aid in the return to spiritual conviction for this material and dollar worshipping land. He is really a great man, noble, sincere, simple and learned beyond comparison with most of our scholars. They say that a professor at Harvard wrote to the people in charge of the Religious Congress to get him invited to Chicago, saying, "He is more learned than all of us together'. He is coming to Boston with letters to a dozen of the best known people here from the leaders of thought, action and fashion for there is a fashion in these things too, in Chicago.

"Swami Vivekananda has been in Detroit recently and made a profound impression there. All classes flocked to hear him, and professional men in particular were greatly interested in his logic and soundness of thought. The Opera House alone was large enough for his audience. He speaks English excellently well, and he is as handsome as he is good. The Detroit newspapers have devoted much space to the reports of his lectures. An editorial in the *Detroit Evening News* says, 'Most people will be inclined to think that Swami Vivekananda did better last night in his Opera House lecture than he did in any of his former lectures in this city'.

"....What Mr. Mazoomdar began might worthily be ended by brother Vivekananda. This new visitor was by far the most interesting personality, although in the Hindu philosophy, of course, personality is not to be taken into consideration. At the Parliament of Religions they used to keep Vivekananda until the end of the programme to make people stay until the end of the session. On a warm day when a prosy speaker talked too long and people began going home by hundreds, the Chairman would get up and announce that Swami Vivekananda would make a short address just before the benediction. Then he would have the peaceable hundreds perfectly in tether. The four thousand fanning people in the Hall of Columbus would sit smiling and expectant, waiting for an hour or two of other men's speeches to listen to Vivekananda for 15 minutes. The Chairman knew the old rule of keeping the best until the last."

1894 AUG. 8 (A): *The Indian Mirror* in its Editorial:

"....Our columns have been recently filled with glowing accounts of the heroic career of a young Bengali, Suresh Chunder Biswas, in the Brazilian Army. But it is another Hindu of Bengal who may be said to have set the Missisippi on fire. Babu Narendra Nath Dutt of Calcutta, now universally known as **SWAMI VIVEKANANDA,** was selected by the Hindu community of Madras to represent them at the Parliament of Religions at Chicago. The Swami had only put in appearance and spoke of the faith of his nation for five minutes to conquer the minds of the Americans, assembled in the Parliament, by the nobleness of the word he preached to an expectant people. The immense excitement he created at Chicago will not be easily forgotten. Since then he has been in universal request in America, and the interest in his preaching on behalf of Hinduism remains unabated today. He has been invited from city to city, and town to town. Truly, it may be said of Swami Vivekananda's work in America, that he went, spoke, and conquered. The influence that this gifted Hindu youth is exercising is something wonderful. His teaching has been so tolerant, unsectarian, lucid, logical, free from resentful invective, and so truly representative of the higher ideals of ancient Hinduism that, his audiences have bowed down before him in astonished gratitude. The American journals are full of descriptions of his personal appearance, of his talk, of his visits from place to place, of interviews between him and local men of note, and of his public homilies. Some idea of Swami Vivekananda's present position in America may be gathered from a lengthy extract we give today from the *Boston Evening Transcript.* Every Hindu who reads this extract will find a glow of delight and pride at his heart and cry out across the seas to the Swami – Well done, thou good and faithful servant! And yet there are some men among us, calling themselves Hindus, who are attempting to belittle the Swami and his work in America, and we have actually been informed of the existence of a shameful cabal among Missionaries and Unitarians to blast Swami Vivekananda's character, and injure his reputation among the American people. We can understand Christian Missionaries getting jealous of a Hindu influence among a people, professing Christianity, though we do not see why they should be intolerant of the doctrines he has been preaching, while he himself has been so very tolerant to true Christianity. But if those Missionaries have any excuse for what they are doing, there is none for those Hindus who have either initiated or joined a league to harm a man who has done so much to raise the Hindu race and their religion so high in the estimation of so large a section of Christendom. We can have no feeling but those of contempt for such Hindus as have grown jealous of Swami Vivekananda and his monumental work in America, But the Hindus, as a nation, will sharply resent all efforts to injure the Swami. All true Hindus will ever stand by him. We rejoice that the Hindus of Madras have, in public meeting assembled, voted an address, which we publish in another column and sent it to the Swami in America. The address is as much a vote of gratitude and continued confidence. But Bengal is the orginal home of Swami Vivekananda, and our Hindu countrymen in these provinces should hold public meetings and vote similar addresses to him, so that he and the Americans may know how highly we appreciate his great work in America. Hindus also from all parts of this country should subscribe to a fund to enable Swami Vivekananda to prolong his stay, and continue his work on so fruitful a soil as the American continent."

1894 AUG. 15: *The Indian Mirror* in its Editorial:

"Hinduism is, at present, not only actively reviving in India, but also engaging the serious attention of all the civilized nations of the earth. **SWAMI VIVEKANANDA** and Mr. Virchand Raghowji, the Jain representative from Bombay, are still addressing crowded audiences in America. Theosophical activities in Europe and America have been, for years past, familiarizing the Western people with the higher truths of the Hindu religious philosophy. But even before that, the great and venerable savant, Prof. Max Muller, had been unfolding to European scholars the glories of the Sanskrit language, and the riches hidden in Sanskrit manuscripts.... Prof. Max Muller's translations, the work of the Theosophical Society, the discussions in the Parliament at Chicago, Swami Vivekananda's lectures, and numerous other activities have increased the interest felt for Hinduism in the West, and we are certain as we are of our own existence this moment, that this interest will continue to grow from year to year, from month to month, from day to day, till Hindusim has its grip over all living people, and becomes the greatest power of the age. Let the prophecy stand; some of us may live to see it approaching realization."

1894 AUG. 15 (A): *The Amrita Bazar Patrika* in its Editorial:

"The Madras Times says what is now felt by Englishmen generally, that Hinduism has been 'revived, spiritualized and modernized....'

"That Hinduism is making its existence felt more and more all over the world, is a spectacle which is now too patent to be ignored. Professor Max Muller has admited, to the infinite wonder of learned Europe, that the Vedanta philosophy has realized the highest aspirations of humanity. The miracle of an intellectually great English lady like Mrs. Besant, with such pronounced free-thinking tendencies, kneeling before the image of Sri Krishna, has produced no little wonder in the world. It was only the other day that Dr. Pentecost was pleased to call the Bengalees monumental liars. This cruel and unworthy attack, on the Bengalees by the celebrated English Missionary, was followed by the presence of a Bengalee, Narendra Nath (**VIVEKANANDA**) in America, as an honoured guest and teacher!....

"That man has body and a soul, that soul is the man and not the body, and that the object of culture is the subordination of the body to the soul, are truths simple enough. But the Hindus practised them, while the civilization, which the Europeans have developed, teaches quite opposite doctrines. When Vivekananda said, that 'what is self is bad and what is unself is good', the saying created great impression in American society. And this is the sole basis upon which the whole of Hinduism is based. But European civilization teaches that 'there must be reciprocity in society'. 'I have no right to your things and you have no right to mine. If I pay you 16 annas, you must pay me something in return which is at least worth that amount'. This is the highest principle taught by European philosophy."

1894 SEP. 1: *The Chicago Inter Ocean*, almost a year following the Parliament, recalling **SWAMI VIVEKANANDA'S unquestionable popularity**, said:

"There was no delegate to the Parliament of Religions who attracted more courteous attention in Chicago by his winning ways, his ability, and his fearless discussion of all questions relating to his religion than Swami Vivekananda. This distinguished Hindu was enthusiastic in his admiration of the greatness of the Western world and its material development, eager in his efforts to learn of those things that might be beneficial to his people, earnest in his desire to recognize the religions of all people as related to each other, and all sincere efforts on behalf of virtue and holiness, but at the same time he defended the Hindu religion and philosophy with an eloquence and power that not only won admiration for himself but also consideration for his own teachings."

1894 SEP. 5: A public meeting of the Hindu community of Calcutta was held at the Town Hall to express their gratitude to **SWAMI VIVEKANANDA** for his able representation of Hinduism at the Parliament of Religions at Chicago, and to thank the American people for the cordial reception they had accorded to him. There was a very large attendance of Hindus. [see 1894 Apr. 28]

The following resolutions were passed unanimously:

a) "That this meeting desires to record its grateful appreciation of the great services rendered to the cause of Hinduism by Swami Vivekananda at the Parliament of Religions at Chicago and of his subsequent work in America."

b) "That this meeting tenders its best thanks to Dr. J. H. Barrows, the Chairman of the Parliament of Religions at Chicago, Mr. Merwin-Marie Snell, Secretary of the Scientific Section of the Parliament of Religions at Chicago, and the American people for the cordial and sympathetic reception they have accorded to Swami Vivekananda."

c) "That this meeting requests the chairman to forward to Swami Vivekananda and Dr. Barrows, copies of the foregoing Resolutions together with the following letter, addressed to Vivekananda:

To Swami Vivekananda –

"Dear Sir, – As Chairman of a large, representative and influential meeting of the Hindu inhabitants of Calcutta and the suburbs, held in the Town Hall of Calcutta, on the 5th of September, 1894, I have the pleasure to convey to you the thanks of the local Hindu community for your able representation of their religion at the Parliament of Religions that met at Chicago in September, 1893.

"The trouble and sacrifice you have incurred by your visit to America as a representative of the Hindu religion are profoundly appreciated by all whom you have done the honour to represent. But their special acknowledgements are due to you for the services you have rendered to the cause they hold so dear, their sacred *Arya Dharma*, by your speeches and your ready responses to the questions of inquirers. No exposition of the general principles of the Hindu Religion could, within the limits of a lecture, be more accurate and lucid than you gave in your address to the Parliament of Religions on Tuesday, the 19th September, 1893. And your subsequent utterances on the same subject on other occasions have been equally clear and precise. It has been the misfortune of Hindus to have their religion misunderstood and misrepresented through ages, and therefore they cannot but feel specially grateful to one of them who has had the courage and the ability to speak the truth about it, and dispel illusions among a strange people,

THE CHRONICLE (1863-1902)

in a strange land, professing a different religion. Their thanks are due no less to the audiences and the organizers of meetings, who have received you kindly, given you opportunities for speaking, encouraged you in your work, and heard you in a patient and charitable spirit. Hinduism has for the first time in its history, found a Missionary, and by a rare good fortune it has found one so able and accomplished as yourself. Your fellow-countrymen, fellow-citizens and fellow-Hindus feel that they would be wanting in an obvious duty if they did not convey to you their hearty sympathy and earnest gratitude for all your labours in spreading a true knowledge of their ancient faith. May God grant you strength and energy to carry on the good work you have begun!" (*The Indian Mirror,* 1894 Sept. 6). [see 1895 Apr. 18]

1894 SEP. 7: In appreciation of SWAMI VIVEKANANDA'S work in the West, *The Indian Daily News* wrote:

"There are unmistakable signs that India is waking up out of her long sleep. But to send a Hindoo monk to America to preach Hindooism is simply taking the bull by the horns. Just fancy, this monk, Swami Vivekananda, is only thirty years of age, has studied philosophy and religion, and on a public platform, in a foreign tongue, is able to captivate an American audience; temperately, wisely, and humorously informing the people of the Western Republic that this mild Hindu is not such a fool as he looks; that his venerable religion is not a farrago of old women's fables but consists of truths of a sublime character. The poor *sannyasin* is a nearer approach to the figure of Christ than my Lord Bishop in his apron and in his palace. The poor, despised Indian does not care for money, clothes, and fine houses, nor does he think the way to Heaven is via Paris. The Indian pagan has never yet tried to localize his God by means of a dozen lighted candles. Let a few more of the B.As and M.As study their old religion and go to Europe, and they will be welcomed. The people are proud of Vivekananda, and so they ought to be."

1894 SEP. 25: In a letter to his *gurubhais* (brother disciples) written from New York, **SWAMI VIVEKANANDA** spoke about the Christian Science people as follows:

"They are Vedantins; I mean they have picked up a few doctrines of the Advaita and grafted them upon the Bible. And they cure diseases, by proclaiming 'Soham, Soham' 'I am He! I am He!' – through strength of mind.... The Christian Science is exactly like our *Kartabhaja* sect: Say, 'I have no disease', and you are whole; and say, 'I am He'– 'Soham'– and you are quits – be at large. This is a thoroughly materialistic country. The people of this Christian land will recognize religion only if you can cure diseases, work miracles and open up avenues to money; and they understand little else. But there are honourable exceptions."

In a letter to Isabelle Mckindley (dt. 25 February, 1895), he makes fun at her expense for writing to him that she was unwell, for Christian Scientists did not confess to sickness. A long letter written by him to the Hale Sisters, dated 31st July, 1894, contains humorous description of a session which the Christian Scientists were holding at Greenacre, which he had joined and greatly enjoyed.

During his stay in America Swami Vivekananda saw a good deal of the Christian Science people.

Swami Abhedananda, a brother disciple of Swami Vivekananda says: "The ideals of New Thought as well as of Christian Science, you will find, are based not upon the doctrines and dogmas of orthodox Christianity, but upon the eternal principles of Vedanta or *Sanatana Dharma*. They do not regard Christ as a personality but as a principle which they have learned from the teachings of Vedanta introduced by us in Europe and America during the last thirty years. The founder of Christian Science, Mrs. Mary Baker G. Eddy, studied the *Bhagavad Gita* and incorporated its ideals in her text-book, entitled *Science and Health*. In my printed lecture on *"Christian Science and Vedanta"*, delivered in New York city, I have quoted from her own writings passages where she said that the ancient Hindu philosophers understood the fundamental principles of Christian Science. Here you should remember that the *Bhagavad Gita,* or *Song Celestial* as Sir Edwin Arnold calls it, contains the teachings of Sri Krishna given about 1500 B. C. The majority of the thinking classes in Europe and America are following today Christian Science which has many Churches in London and different cities of the United States. Today Christian Science is making more converts than the orthodox Christianity has done in the past...." (Swami Abhedananda in his lecture delivered at Kuala Lumpur on 2nd Oct.1921, vide *Inspiring Speeches by Eminent Indians,* p. 146 & 147). [see 1879 (c), 1886 (o), 1894 Mar. 9]

1894 NOV. 4: *The Indian Mirror* wrote an editorial highlighting the significance of **SWAMI VIVEKANANDA'S reply** to the address of the Madras Hindus:

"We published yesterday the reply of Swami Vivekananda to the address of the Hindus of Madras, which, we trust, has been studied by our readers with the attention it deserves. The reply is a most remarkable document, and may be called as a sort of manifesto of the religious views, held by the illustrious Swami. For our part, we feel sure that wherever the paper is read, it will create profound admiration, not unmixed with astonishment that young as the Swami is in years, he should be master of so much learning. Every line of the document bears witness to his erudition, and shows his perfect familiarity with not only the sacred books of India, but also with the beliefs, held by the numerous religious orders and sects of this country at the present time. We would earnestly request every Hindu to peruse Swami Vivekananda's reply over and over again.... We need not recapitulate the leading points of the reply. They cannot be put in better language or more aptly illustrated than Swami Vivekananda has done. But of one thing every reader will feel convinced at every line, as his eyes run over the document, we mean the writer's intense love for the land of his birth, his passionate attachment to India. But while love for country and his religion forces glowing words and imagery from his facile pen, he is calm as to everything else. Nothing moves him to anger, and he can speak of missionary outrages against his faith and his race only as facts which have come within his own cognizance and nothing more. He has been called names by missionaries preaching Christ. But this young Hindu monk has absolutely abjured the language of *tu quo que*. The Swami's doctrine is not that of the jealous God in the Christian Scriptures, which requires an eye for an eye or a tooth for a tooth. Neither retort nor revenge, but return of good for evil. What a splendid ideal, and how should we revere a man who can illustrate so well in his own person, the *tyaga* – renunciation – that he preaches.... So long as we have men like Swami Vivekananda, preaching holy doctrines and living holy lives of renunciation and self-sacrifice for the elevation of the nation to which they belong, and for the salvation of all mankind, so long, we say, we shall not be wanting in materials for spiritual development and growth.

"....Swami Vivekananda is, as we all know, engaged in teaching the truths of the Hindu religion to the American people. Again we have all heard of his phenomenal success. But all of us are certainly not aware that a large number of Americans have become Hindus to all intents and purposes, not only in theory and intellectually, but actually in their physical bodies. We should not be surprised to hear before long that Hindu religious services are conducted in many American homes. Thus we have our own beloved India with us, and may have another India beyond the seas, should He in His wisdom grant it.... Swami Vivekananda has now been in America over a year, and after a while proposes to go to Europe. Besides giving public lectures, he is deeply engaged in writing a moumental work on Hinduism. His time is thus fully occupied; the strain on his health is too severe; he feels it, and would gladly welcome help from India. Have we no men sufficiently gifted and patriotic to continue Swami Vivekananda's work in America? It is believed that when the opportunity comes, the man also is found. Well, we have the opportunity now. Where are the men to be found that we need?"

1894 NOV. 7: *The Hindu Patriot* in its Editorial:

"SWAMI VIVEKANANDA throws a queer sidelight on the method pursued by American Missionaries to instill into the minds of little children attending schools a deep-seated hatred of the Hindus. It would appear that in some of the school books read by American children, there are pictures in which Hinduism is monstrously caricatured in a spirit of uncharitableness which, we think, is anything but Christian. In one of these pictures a Hindu mother is painted as throwing her child into the Ganges to be banquetted upon by crocodiles which are shown as prowling about the banks in anxious expectation of the appetizing offerings. In another, a Hindu husband is represented as burning his wife at a stake with his own hands, his motive being, so the letter-press explains, that the incinerated woman may become a ghost and then employ her time to good purpose by tormenting her husband's enemy. Such is the savage superstition and diabolical vindictiveness of the Hindu! Nor is this all. In another picture a huge car is shown as crushing in its headlong career countless human victims. It is by such means that the young Yankee is taught to hate the Hindus. And all this happens in America which boasts of equality between man and man and is supposed to make no distinctions of race, colour or creed." [see 1899 Mar. 19]

1894 NOV: As a result of the inspiring lectures delivered, by **SWAMI VIVEKANANDA** who created an unprecedented enthusiasm in the United States for Vedantic ideals, **The Vedanta Society of New York** – a non-sectarian body with the distinct purpose of preaching and practising the Vedanta and applying its principles to all religions – came into existence with toleration and acceptance of all religions as its watchwords.

People belonging to the various religious creeds and organizations were cordially invited to enlist themselves as members of the Society without change of faith. This catholicity and universality of outlook had a tremendous appeal to the truth-seekers who enthusiastically rallied under the banner of this Universal Ideal of Vedanta at the New York Centre.

One of the principal objects of Swamiji in organizing a Vedanta Society in New York was to open a suitable Centre for an exchange of ideas between the East and the West for the well-being of both.

From the beginning made in New York, the Vedanta movement gradually spread from coast to coast. At present there are nearly a dozen Vedantic organizations in different parts of the United States. All are monuments of Swami Vivekananda's work in America.

1894 DEC. 5: Referring to a noteworthy experience reported in *The New York Independent* which befell **SWAMI VIVEKANANDA** on his visit to

Baltimore where he was refused admission to first class hotels on account of his colour, *The Hindu Patriot* commented in its editorial:

"Now, if such things happen at the 'headquarters of the largest Christian denomination' in America, then what becomes of that equality and brotherhood of man which is said to be the very cornerstone of society in that progressive land? The 'largest Christian denomination' has, we are afraid, the least Christian traits about it and if Christ were to present himself attired in the habiliments of an Indian ascetic, before a hotel keeper at Baltimore, we are sure that Prophet of Syria would meet with no better fate than what is stated to have befallen the Indian youth who by the way comes much nearer the ideal of Christ than these so-called Christians of the type of the writer in the New York religious journal themselves." [see 1894 Dec. 10]

1894 DEC. 10: *The Indian Nation* wrote:

"A Mr. Hudson, full of the feeling of brotherly kindness, was indignant that a pagan, **SWAMI VIVEKANANDA**, had encroached upon a Christian monopoly and dared to address the Chicago assembly as 'Brothers'. The Swami has been receiving more practical proofs of the Christian doctrine of brotherhood than Rev. Hudson's declamation, and must by this time have been altogether convinced. Christianity of the pulpit is not Always the Christianity of the people, and the Swami is having an experience of every phase of it. *The New York Independent* writes: 'Mr. Vivekananda, the high priest from India, who made quite a sensation at the Parliament of Religions, and who has since remained in the country to expound Brahminism and accuse Christianity, can now go back to his own land with a genuine grievance against Christendom; for having occasion lately to visit Baltimore, the headquarters of the largest Christian denomination in this country, he was refused admission to every first class hotel to which he applied but one, on account of his colour. They looked at him, were puzzled at his straight hair, but convinced by his swarthy skin that he was some sort of a 'nigger', and they would not admit him to sleep in a gentleman's bed or sit at a gentleman's table.' Certain cuticular qualifications are necessary for admission to the Christian brotherhood. Men are brothers, niggers excluded."

1894 (A): **Sir Jagdish Chandra Bose** (1858-1937), Indian physicist and plant physiologist, started his research career.

His research on electrical waves won him recognition in 1897, and he was thereafter engaged in the research on the living and non-living. His invention of highly sensitive instruments for the detection of minute responses by living organisms to external stimuli enabled him to anticipate the parallelism between animal and plant tissues noted by later bio-physicists. He revolutionized the entire concept of Botanical Science through his discoveries. [see 1880 (b), 1900 Aug-Oct, 1900 Jul. 8, 1902 Jul. 9]

1894 (B): S. Kitasato (1852-1931), Japanese physician and bacteriologist, discovered the **bacillus** *Pasteurella Pestis,* the infectious agent of **bubonic plague,** during an epidemic in Hongkong.

1894 (C): The first public demonstration by **Sir Oliver Lodge** in England that electromagnetic waves (radio waves) were able to carry messages over a few hundred yards. [see 1864 (f), 1873 (f), 1887 (e), 1895 (b)]

1894 (D): English physicist **Lord Raleigh** (1842-1919), and a chemist Sir **William Ramsay** (1852-1916), discovered a chemically inert gaseous element which they called "**argon**". They announced their discovery in early 1895.

In the same year Ramsay isolated helium from the uranium mineral cleveite and later (1903) demonstrated that this lightest of the inert gases is continually produced during the radioactive decay of radium, a discovery of crucial importance to a modern understanding of nuclear reactions. In 1898 Ramsay and his colleague Morris W. Travers isolated three more gaseous elements – called neon, krypton, and xenon – from air brought to a liquid state at a low temperature and high pressure. In 1910 Ramsay detected the presence of the last of the noble gas series, called nitron (now known as radon), in the radioactive emissions of radium. In 1904 both Raleigh and Ramsay received Nobel Prizes for physics and chemistry respectively.

1894 (E): Leo Tolstoy (1828-1910), Russian writer and thinker, wrote his book, *The Kingdom of God is Within You,* presenting the Vedantic truths as the central truths of Christianity, in the place of 'original sin' and 'devil'. [see 1866 (f), 1882 (g)]

Tolstoy was fascinated by Indian thought. He first studied Vivekananda's book on *Raja Yoga* and was deeply affected by Vivekananda's spirituality and humanism. After reading the Swami's writing *'God and Soul'*, Tolstoy wrote in his diary on July 4, 1908, 'I read the wonderful writings of Vivekananda on God; this should be translated; intend to do this myself.' (*Swami Vivekananda – His Humanism,* Swami Ranganathananda's Lecture at Moscow University, p. 145). [see 1896 (n)]

1894 (F): Rudyard Kipling (1865-1936), English writer, brought out his best-loved books *Jungle Books* (1894-95) and *The Just-so Stories* (1902) which display his great genius for story-telling.

The Story of Mowgli, the man-child brought up in the jungle by the wolf family is read by children all over the world. Kipling's experiences in India as a child and later as a journalist, influenced his view of British Empire.

1894 (G): London's Tower Bridge opened to span the Thames. The £ 1.5 million bridge had a 200 ft. centre span that could he raised to permit passage of vessels; its chain suspension side spans were each 270 ft. long.

1894-95: The Sino-Japanese War, which was the direct outcome of the rivalry of the two powers for control of Korea. It was the first major conflict between the two nations.

1894-99: Lord Elgin II, the Viceroy of India.

1895 FEB. 17: In a letter of date written from America, **SWAMI VIVEKANANDA gave Alasinga Perumal an idea of the difficulties he had to face in accomplishing his task.**

Said he, "To put the Hindu ideas into English and then make out a dry philosophy and intricate mythology and queer startling psychology, a religion which shall be easy, simple, popular, and at the same time meet the requirements of the highest minds – is a task only those can understand who have attempted it. The abstract Advaita must become living, poetic – in everyday life; out of hopelessly intricate mythology must come concrete moral forms; and out of bewildering yogism must come the most scientific and practical psychology – and all this must be put in a form that a child may grasp it. That is my life's work. The Lord only knows how far I shall succeed. 'To work we have the right, not to the fruits thereof'. It is hard work, my boy, hard work. To keep one's own self steady in the midst of this whirl of *kama-kanchana* (lust and gold) and hold on to one's own ideals, until disciples are moulded to conceive of the ideals of realization and perfect renunciation, is indeed difficult work, my boy. Thank God, already there is great success."

1895 FEB: SWAMI VIVEKANANDA who had delivered a series of learned lectures in almost every part of the U. S. A., now settled down in a comparatively secluded part of the New York city and began Vedanta classes for the earnest-minded devotees.

He considered these class talks more valuable and effective than mere platform speeches in moulding the lives of the genuine seekers after truth. He felt convinced that no substantial work could be built in America unless he were able to form an intimate circle of sincere souls who would devote themselves most seriously to the practice of spiritual exercises which he inculcated in the course of enlightened discourses.

From now on he wholeheartedly threw himself into this responsible task and began to teach the earnest devotees meditation and the process of yoga by a practical demonstration of the same along with his discourses. This served to bring about a wonderful transformation in the lives of a good number of souls who came within the ambit of his spiritual influence.

1895 MAR. 1: *The Indian Mirror* quoted *The Madras Times* which concluded an article on **VIVEKANANDA'S mission** with the following words:

"Independently of religion, the Swami is an extraordinary man and undoubtedly he is one of those amongst us whom men of a future age will look back to as a prophet."

1895 MAR. 4: Address of **Raja Ajitsingh Bahadur,** Maharaja of Khetri, to **SWAMI VIVEKANANDA** in America:

"My Dear Swamiji, as a head of this *durbar* (a formal Stately Assembly) held today for this special purpose, I have much pleasure in conveying to you, in my own name and that of my subjects, the heartfelt thanks of this State for your worthy representation of Hinduism at the Parliament of Religions, held at Chicago, in America.

"I do not think the general principles of Hinduism could be expressed more accurately and clearly in English than what you have done with all the restrictions imposed by the very natural shortcomings of language itself.

"The influence of your speech and behaviour in foreign land, is not only spread with a sense of admiration among men of countries and religions different, but has also served to familiarize you with them, to help in the furtherance of your unselfish cause. This is very highly and inexpressibly appreciated by us all, and we should feel to be failing in our duty, were I not to write to you formally at least these few lines, expressing our sincere gratitude for all the trouble you have taken in going to foreign countries, and to expound in the American Parliament the truths of our ancient religion, which we ever since hold so dear. It is certainly applicable to the pride of India that it has been fortunate in possessing the privilege of having secured so able a representative as yourself.

"Thanks are also due to those noble souls, whose efforts succeeded in organizing the Parliament of Religions, and who accorded to you a very enthusiastic reception. As you were quite a foreigner in that continent, their kind treatment to you is due to their love of the several qualifications you possess, and this speaks highly of their noble nature.

"I herewith enclose twenty printed copies of this letter, and have to request that, keeping this one with yourself, you will kindly distribute the other copies among your friends." *(The Indian Mirror,* May 7, 1895.)

1895 MAR. 22: The first demonstration of **motion pictures** at 44 Rue de Rennes, Paris, by the cinematograph inventors, **Louis** (1864-1948) and **Auguste Lumiere** (1862-1954). Their cinematograph was a vast improvement over the kinetoscope peepshow introduced a year ago by **Thomas Edison,** whose film could be viewed by only one person at a time [see 1889 (h)]. The 16 frame per second mechanism devised by the Lumiere · brothers was the standard for films for decades. The design of their equipments, which was both a camera and a projector, incorporated a claw movement with a 35 mm. film . They introduced (1907) the Autochrome process, the first commercially successful direct colour photographic process. [see 1886 (h)]

A cine projector patented by U. S. Inventor Charles Francis Jenkins, 28, had an intermittent motion. The first commercial presentation of a film on a screen took place on May 20 at New York.

1895 APR. 8: Death of **Bankim Chandra Chatterice** (b. 1838), Bengali novelist and essayist, and the prophet of Indian nationalism.

Bankim's best known novel *Anandmath,* contains the famous hymn '*Vande Mataram*', which exhorted the people to sacrifice all for their motherland. It was sung for the first time in the 1896 session of the Indian National Congress and was a source of inspiration to Indians in their struggle for freedom.

1895 APR. 18: *The Indian Mirror* reproduced the following letter written by **SWAMI VIVEKANANDA** (from New York, on 18th Nov. 1894) to **Rajah Peary Mohan Mukherji,** C. S. I., who presided at the public meeting in Calcutta in honour of the Swami:

"Dear Sir, – I am in receipt of the Resolutions that were passed in a recent Town Hall Meeting in Calcutta, and the kind words my fellow citizens sent over to me .

"Accept, Sir, my most heartfelt gratitude for your appreciation of my insignificant service.

"I am thoroughly convinced that no individual or nation can live by holding itself apart from the community of others, and wherever such an attempt has been made, under false ideas of greatness or policy or holiness – the result has always been disastrous to the secluding one.

"To my mind, the one great cause of the downfall and degeneration of India is this building of a wall of custom round the nation whose real aim in ancient times was to prevent the Hindus from coming in contact with the surrounding Buddhistic nations, whose foundation was hatred of others.

"Whatever cloak, ancient or modern sophistry, may try to throw over it, and whose inevitable result – the vindication of the moral law that none can hate others without degenerating himself – is that the race that was foremost amongst the ancient races – is now a byword and a scorn among nations.

"We are the object-lessons of the violation of that law which our ancestors were the first to discover and discriminate.

"Give and receive is the law, and if India wants to raise herself once more, it is absolutely necessary that she should bring out her treasures and throw them broadcast among the nations of the earth, and be ready to receive what others have to give her in return. Expansion is life, contraction is death. Love is life; hatred is death. We began to die, the day we began to contract – to hate other races – and nothing can prevent our death until we come back to life, to expansion. We must mix, therefore, with all the races of the earth – and every Hindu that goes out to travel in foreign parts, does more benefit to this country than hundreds of those bundles of superstition and selfishness whose one aim in life is to be the dog in the manger. These wonderful structures of national life which the Western nations have raised are supported by pillars of characters – and until we can produce such by hundreds, it is useless to fret and fume against this power or that power.

"Does any one deserve liberty who is not ready to give it to others? Let us calmly and in manly fashion go to work – instead of dissipating our energies in unnecessary frettings and fumings and I, for one, thoroughly believe, that no power in the universe can withhold from any one any- thing he really deserves. The past was great no doubt, but I sincerely believe that the future in store is glorious still. May Lord Shankar always keep us steady in purity, patience and perseverance." [see 1894 Sept. 5]

1895 APR. 19: From the *Hartford's Daily Times*:
"**VIVEKANANDA** was greeted by a fine house last night and all who went will be glad they did, for talks by high caste Brahmins are not a common occurrence in this latitude. The Brahmins seldom leave their native land; they lose caste by crossing the ocean. But Vivekananda was willing to submit to that to get to Christian lands, for his views are more in consonance with those of Christ than those of many so-called Christians. His broad charity takes in all religions and all nations. The simplicity of his talk last night was charming, and in his long red gown

and yellow turban, with his handsome Asiatic face, he was picturesque to the eye as well as fascinating to the ear through his high spiritual ideas. He speaks excellent English with an accent that gives an added zest to his talk...." (*The Indian Mirror*)

1895 APR. 23: Death of **Karl Ludwig** (b. 1816), one of the leading experimental physiologists of the 19th century.

He invented a number of important pieces of laboratory equipment. **Kymograph**, an instrument developed by him became an invaluable measuring instrument for physiology.

1895 APR. 24: **Joshua Slocum** of Nova Scotia, Canada, set out from Boston, Massachusetts, in a three mast topsail schooner on the **first solo circumnavigation of earth.**

1895 MAY 19: *The Tribune* of Lahore wrote:

"We have had occasion before this to refer to some publications of the Christian Literature Society of Madras. The Society published educational books and religious tracts. The former are compilations of little merit and the latter controversial writings of scarcely any literary merit but full of a narrow bigotry.... The latest tract, issued by the Society, is on **SWAMI VIVEKANANDA** and professes to be an examination of his address at the Chicago Parliament of Religions. The method followed in the examination of his speech is novel. The secret of the attracting of such a large audiences in America is explained thus – 'Any great novelty....attention. Crowd would flock to see tattooed New Zealander....the Swami was the first Indian who visited America in the dress of a sannyasin'. In another place we read: 'Swami Vivekananda availed himself of the accommodation of first class hotel. Did he eschew their delicacies and remain a vegetarian? Chicago is noted for its pork. Did he leave the city without once tasting it? Was he not tempted by the savoury roast beef? Did he abstain from wine? What does the Swami think of the quality of Havana cigars?' This is the spirit in which Swami's speech is examined. Is it necessary to say that writings of this kind while doing Swami Vivekananda and the views he represent harm, may injure the cause of Christianity in India?" (*The Indian Mirror*) [see 1895 May 31, 1899 Aug. 17]

1895 MAY 22: Birth of **J. Krishnamurthy,** (d. 1986), Indian mystic and philosopher, whose teachings stress universal religious values, personal insight and autonomous self-discipline, synthesizing both Indian and Western philosophical and psychological principles.

According to him the world and society can change only when there is a fundamental revolution in the depths of man's mind and heart.

1895 MAY 31: *The Indian Mirror* reported:

"The success of **SWAMI VIVEKANANDA** in the United States has spread consternation through the ranks of Christian Missionaries who have chosen India as their field of work. But although it is about two years ago that the Swami delivered his memorable lectures on Hinduism in the Parliament of Religions, it is only recently that a serious attempt has been made by the Christians to give a reply to the Swami's dissertation from the Christian missionary's standpoint.... But if we have Dr. Murdoch essaying to refute Vivekananda, we have on the other hand, Rev. Dr. William Miller, a Christian Missionary of far greater experience, learning, erudition and higher position in the Church, joining the Swami in declaring that Hinduism has a mission in the world, and that it has to teach great lessons to the Christian nations of the world." [see 1895 May 19, 1899 Aug. 17]

1895 JUN 29: Death of **Thomas Henry Huxley** (b. 1825), English biologist, who was most famous as 'Darwin's bulldog', that is, the man who led the fight for the acceptance of Darwin's theory of evolution.

To Huxley, Darwin's theory was a "well-founded working hypothesis", and a "powerful instrument of research". By comparison, the old doctrine that each species was an immutable special creation of God seemed "a barren virgin". For his part in the open clash which resulted between science and church Huxley became a famous public figure [see 1863 (e)]

1895 JUN: Having almost exhausted himself by the uninterrupted work of class and public lecturing, **SWAMI VIVEKANANDA** in the beginning of the month accepted the invitation of one of his friends and went to Percy, New Hampshire, for a period of rest in the silence of the pine woods.

The ten days he spent with his friends at Percy refreshed him spiritually, mentally, physically. So intense was Swamiji's meditation at Percy that he passed into *nirvikalpa samadhi* (union with the Absolute).

On this occasion (June 7) Swami was discovered by a gardener on the shore of the lake – to all appearances dead. Rushing to the scene, his friends did everything in their power to rouse their beloved friend and teacher. Failing to bring him back to consciousness, they were about to accept the incredible fact of his death when signs of life appeared in his body and he returned gradually to normal consciousness. Swamiji had been in *nirvikalapa samadhi,* a state of superconsciousness, from which only the great spiritual teachers can descend to relative world *(Swami Vivekananda in America: New Discoveries.* p. 617)

1895 JUN. 18 to AUG. 7: SWAMI VIVEKANANDA had a memorable sojourn at Thousand Island Park, the largest island in the St. Lawrence River, about 300 miles from New York.

Swamiji had been invited there by one of his students to live in solitude, in a small cottage. He had accepted it gladly as that would afford him an opportunity not only to give some rest to his tired limbs but also to provide a suitable and congenial forum for those who would devote themselves wholeheartedly to the study of the Vedanta and mould their lives in the light of its lofty teachings.

In the uninterrrupted stillness of the Island-retreat, Swamiji spent seven weeks with a devoted batch of Christian students who were deeply inspired by listening to the pregnant lessons of their spiritual preceptor. They were taken through a prescribed programme of meditation, study and prayer for their spiritual unfoldment.

The subjects dealt with during Swamiji's stay in this peaceful retreat were gleaned from the sacred books of the East such as the *Bhagavad Gita,* the Upanishads and *Brahma Sutras* of Vyasa, and he presented them with as much lucidity as possible, the various systems of Indian philosophy including the Dualism (*Dvaita*) of Sri Madhva, qualified non-dualism (*Vishishtadvaita*) of Sri Ramanuja and the Absolute Monism (*Advaita*) of Sri Sankara. Besides, he presented to them for the first time a vivid picture of his own Guru Sri Ramakrishna, his spiritual austerities and practice of all the leading faiths of mankind, harmonization of the apparently contradictory systems of thought and also his universality of outlook on life. The Swami threw light upon all manner of subjects, historical and philosophical, spiritual and temporal.

It was at the Thousand Island Park in an inspiring atmosphere Swami Vivekananda penned his famous poem *The Song of the Sannyasin,* a poetical masterpiece which is vibrant with a resounding note of renunciation and deep spiritual fervour and also gives a glimpse of the depths of his Advaita realization.

One of the students, Miss Waldo successfully took down Swamiji's dictation on *Raja Yoga* and in a diary she summarized the talks from day-to-day mostly in Swamiji's words. She was able to take down quite a lot of what the Master .said in his hours of lofty spiritual heights in the realm of the spirit. They were later published in book form, under the appropriate title *The Inspired Talks.*

During his sojourn at the Thousand Island Park, one day, Swami Vivekananda entered while meditating, into the *nirvikalpa samadhi* on the banks of the St. Lawrence. The incident is described by Mrs. Funke as follows: "This morning there was no class. He asked C. and me to take a walk as he wished to be along with us. (The others had been with him all summer, and he felt we should have a talk). We went up a hill about half a mile away. All was woods and solitude. Finally he selected a low branched tree, and we sat under the low spreading branches. Instead of the expected talk, he suddenly said, 'Now we shall meditate. We shall be like Buddha under the Bo-tree'. He seemed to turn to bronze, so still was he. Then I raised my umbrella and protected him as much as possible. Completely absorbed in his meditation, he was oblivious of everything. Soon we heard shouts in the distance. The others had come out after us with raincoats and umbrellas. Swamiji looked around regretfully, for we had to go, and said, 'once more I am in Calcutta in the rains.' "

1895 JUN. (A): SWAMI VIVEKANANDA finished writing his famous book *Raja-Yoga,* which attracted the attention of Harvard Philosopher **William James** [see 1895 July] and was later to rouse the enthusiasm of Tolstoy.

The book is a translation of Patanjali's yoga aphorisms, the Swami adding his own explanations; the introductory chapters written by him are especially illuminating. Patanjali expounded, through these aphorisms, the philosophy of yoga, the main purpose of which is to show the way of the soul's attaining freedom from the bondage of matter. Various methods of concentration are discussed. The book will serve two purposes. First, the Swami demonstrated that religious experience could stand on the same footing as scientific truths, being based on experimentation, observation, and verification. Therefore genuine spiritual experience must not be dogmatically discarded as lacking rational evidence. Secondly, the Swami explained lucidly various disciplines of concentration, with the warning, however, that they should not be pursued without the help of a qualified teacher.

Miss. S. Ellen Waldo of Brooklyn, a disciple and an amanuensis of the Swami, described the manner in which he dictated the book: "In delivering his commentaries on the aphorisms, he would leave me waiting while he entered into deep states of meditation or self-contemplation, to emerge therefrom with some luminous interpretation. I had always to keep the pen dipped in the ink. He might be absorbed for long periods of time, and then suddenly his silence would be broken by some eager expression or some long, deliberate teaching."

1895 JUN. - AUG. : **Sister Christine** (Miss Christina Greenstidel), an American disciple of **SWAMI VIVEKANANDA,** who had attended his lectures in Detroit, and later attended the classes at Thousand Island Park, recorded in her reminiscences of Swamiji some of his *ipse dixits* regarding Christ, Christianity and Christian missionaries:

"He believed that Jesus Christ was the Son of God, a divine incarnation. He worshipped and adored him, but not as the only incarnation. In other ages and in other climes, God had vouchsafed this mercy to others also.

"Christianity, he told us, was first introduced into India by the apostle Thomas, about twenty-five years after the crucifixion. There has never been any religious persecution in India, and there are even to this day descendants of the first converts to Christianity living in Southern India. Christianity in its purest form was practised in India at a time when Europe was in a state of savagery. They now number scarcely one million though at one time there were almost three times as many.

"When asked why he (Vivekananda) did not defend himself against machinations of a family of missionaries long connected with Calcutta who threatened to 'hound him out of Detroit', he said, 'The dog barks at the elephant, is the elephant affected? What does the elephant care?'

"The one with whom the Swami lived had a violent temper. 'Why do you live with him' some one asked. 'Ah', he replied, 'I bless him. He gave me the opportunity to practise self-control.' " *(Reminiscences of Swami Vivekananda, p. 201 and 202)*

1895 JUN. (see after 1895 June 29).

1895 JUL. 27: In a letter to the Editor of *The Mirror* three prominent devotees of **SWAMI VIVEKANANDA** including **Sri M. C. Alasinga Perumal** wrote from Madras:

"Under the advice and with the encouragement of Swami Vivekananda, it is proposed to start a weekly journal to be named the *Brahmavadin*. The main object of the journal is to propagate the principles of the Vedantic religion of India, and to work towards the improvement of the social and moral conditions of man by steadily holding aloft the sublime and universal ideal of Hinduism. The power of any ideal in filling human hearts with inspiration and the love of the good and the beautiful, is dependent on how high and pure it is; and it shall be the endeavour of the *Brahmavadin* to portray the Hindu ideal in the best and truest light in which it is found recorded in the historical sacred literature of the Hindus. Mindful of the fact that between the ideal of the Hindu scriptures and the practical life of the Hindu peoples, there is a wide gulf of separation, the proposed new journal will constantly have in view how best to try to bridge that gulf, and make the social and religious institutions of the country accord more and more with the spirit of that lofty divine ideal.

"To preach the truth and proclaim the ideal is work that is always, and in itself, of great value. It is even more so in India where all social elevation and improvement of human conduct have been invariably brought about by means of essentially religious influences. Utilitarian considerations of convenience, and of justice based thereon, have never held sway over man's heart here to the same extent as faith in religion and its commandments. The New India of today is, in many respects, far different from the old India of centuries ago, and all our old institutions have to get themselves re-adjusted, so as to be in consonance with the altered conditions of modern life. For this purpose, it is highly necessary to see that the Hindu religion is more than ever earnestly engaged in the services of man in this ancient land of ours, wherein the sacred light from above has shone always on suffering humanity, offering guidance, and the consolation of immortal bliss. As Hinduism believes in the gradual evolution of human perfection and in the harmony of religions, the *Brahmavadin* shall have no quarrel with other religions, but shall always try to do its best to uphold the work of strengthening and ennobling man, under the banner of whatsoever religion such work may be accomplished. All truth is one, and must be perfectly concordant, and the only thing that any religion has to hate is vice.

"It is under contemplation to bring out the first issue not later than the 1st September next. All communications are to be addressed to the Manager of the *Brahmavadin,* Triplicane, Madras." [see 1895 Sept.]

1895 JUL. : SWAMI VIVEKANANDA'S *Raja Yoga* was published in America.

The book was enthusiastically received by American intelligentsia and the demand became so great that it ran into three editions within a few weeks of its publication.

Even the eminent psychologist **Prof. William James** of the Harvard University got so much interested on the subject after the perusal of this treatise that he personally came to meet the great Swami at his residence at New York, became one of his ardent admirers and began to look upon him as a paragon of Vedantists. In his classical work, *The Varieties of Religious Experience,* he specially refers to the Swami, while dealing with monistic mysticism. [see 1895 June (a), 1901 (1), 1902 (b)]

Swami Abhedananda, a brother disciple of Swami Vivekananda says: "I have met many people in this country (U. S. A) who regard *Raja Yoga* in the same light as the most devout Christian regards his own Scriptures. It has been a revelation to many agnostic and sceptical minds; it has transformed the characters of many. Every passage of this wonderful book is charged, as it were with the soul-stirring power generated by the gigantic battery of the pure soul of our great yogi. This wonderful book, which has been translated into several languages and published in three different countries, has commanded respect among the intelligent, educated classes and the sincere seekers of truth in the three continents – America, Europe and Asia." (*Complete Works of Swami Abhedananda,* Vol. 5, p. 583.)

1895 AUG. 9: In a letter of date to an English friend, written from America, **SWAMI VIVEKANANDA** expressed his international interests and sympathies and his broad spiritual humanism:

"Doubtless, I do love India. But everyday my sight grows clearer. What is India or England or America to us? We are the servants of that God who by the ignorant is called man. He who pours water at the root, does he not water the whole tree?

"There is but one basis of well-being – social, political, or spiritual – to know that I and my brother are one. This is true of all countries and all people. And Westerners, let me say, will realize it more quickly than orientals, who have almost exhausted themselves in formulating the idea and producing a few cases of individual realization.

1895 AUG. 26: **The first commercial electric power** from Niagara Falls was transmitted by the Niagara Falls Power Company incorporated in 1889.

The Company employed the 5000 horsepower. Westinghouse electric generators that delivered two-phase currents at 2,200 volts, 23 cycles and the power was used by the Pittsburg Reduction Company, to reduce aluminium ore.

1895 AUG. 30: **Instruction in Catholic religion made compulsory** in all public schools in England.

1895 SEP. 11: Birth of **Acharya Vinoba Bbave** (d. 1982), Gandhian social worker, founder of the *Sarvodaya* ('Welfare of All,') and *Bhoodan* ('Land Gift') Movements.

At the age of ten, he took the vow of celibacy and dedicated his life to the service of the country. A trusted disciple of Gandhiji, he devoted himself to Gandhiji's village welfare programme, making a significant and original contribution of his own by starting the Bhoodan Movement. He successfully persuaded the landlords to donate land, for the landless poor.

1895 SEP. 28: Death of **Louis Pasteur** (b. 1822), French chemist and micro-biologist who was responsible for revolutionizing medical science.

His researches regarding fermentation [see 1872 (a)] and the consequent findings led to the modern study of bacteriology. He investigated several types of micro-organisms to advance the germ theory of disease. His proof of existence of atmospheric germs encouraged Joseph Lister (1827-1912), British surgeon, to initiate the practice of antiseptic surgery (1865) [see 1865 (e), 1877 Oct.]. Louis Pasteur originated the process known as 'pasteurization' for preservation of liquid foods, and of vaccination of sheep and cows against anthrax. His triumph was the development of rabies vaccination, [see 1885 Jul. 6] and in 1888 the Pasteur Institute was founded in Paris to produce this vaccine. (There are now over sixty Pasteur Research Institutes in the world.)

1895 SEP. : At the insistence of **SWAMI VIVEKANANDA** and with his financial support from America, **Alasinga Perumal** (1863-1909), an ardent Madrasi disciple of Swamiji, started publishing the *Brahmavadin* – a monthly journal in English (he later edited it).

It helped spread the ideas of the new movement initiated by the Swami and prepared the ground for his work after his return to India. [see 1895 Jul. 27]

1895 OCT. 5: In a letter to the editor of *The Indian Mirror* a reader wrote:

"Whoever has seen **SWAMI VIVEKANANDA** even in a photo, must have been struck, with the charming appearance of the Hindu monk. For this attractiveness of his feature, he was subjected to an examination of his physiognomy by the phrenological Society of America; and the phrenological journal of New York gives in detail the result of the examination in the following words:

'The Swami Vivekananda is in many respects an excellent specimen of his race. He is five feet eight and a half inches in height, and weighs one hundred and seventy pounds. His head measures 21 inches in circumference by 14 from ear to ear across the top. He is thus very well proportioned as regards both body and brain. His temperament is mental-vital or vital-mental with considerably more of the lymphatic phase of the vital than the sanguine. In the old classification he would probably be called tymphatico-bilious. One of the most striking peculiarities of this man is the familiarity indicated in nearly every contour of the figure, face, head and hands. He has probably as perfect a conic hand as could be imagined, although it should be described further as a refined rather than a heavy instance of the type. The oriental nations generally have been noted for the conic hand. These extremely tapering fingers are ill-adapted for mechanical work. They serve the orator and the opera singer in manipulating the atmosphere, but the points are too narrow to contain the number of nerves which are so essential to success in dealing directly with material things.

'It would be difficult to find a woman in this country with a more typically feminine hand than that of this young monk. This means a great deal as a key to his temperament and the general direction of his mind. The form of his head is also in keeping with the qualities to be inferred from the more general outlines of the figure, with the exception perhaps of the occiput. His back head is decidedly short. There is very little social adhesiveness of any kind, and the pleasure he finds in social life is due to the exercise of other faculties. He will be able to make his home wherever he can find agreeable employment for his intellectual powers, and such friendship as he manifests is chiefly the expression of gratitude for encouragement and appreciation of his missionary work. His instincts are too feminine to be compatible with much conjugal sentiment. Indeed he says himself that he never had the slightest feeling of love for any woman.

'He is opposed to war, and teaches a religion of unmixed gentleness, we should expect his head to be narrow in the region of the ears at the seat of combativeness and destructiveness and such is the case. The same deficiency is very marked in the diameters a little farther up at secretiveness and acquisitiveness. He dismisses the whole subject of finance and ownership by saying that he has no property and does not want to be bothered with any. While such a sentiment sounds odd to American ears, it must be confessed that his face, at least, shows more marks of contentment and familiarity with gustatory delights than visages of Russel Sage, Hetty Green, and many other of our multi-millionaires. The upper back head is wide at caution and over of approbation. The latter is very strongly developed, and as self-esteem is moderate he will exhibit the negative rather than the positive phase of ambition; that is to say, he will be more sensitive to adverse criticism than eager for fame. Firmness and conscientiousness are fairly developed. The central top head is somewhat depressed at reverence. Spirituality and hope are also but little above average. Benevolence however, is quite conspicuous. The temples are narrow at constructiveness, which agrees with the form of his hand. He is not a mechanic, and will find but little to interest him in the arts of manufacturing. Imitation, which adjoins benevolence, helps greatly to expand the frontal top head.

'The forehead is compact and gives evidence that the frontal brain convulsions are dense in texture and closely folded. The space between the eyes denotes accurate judgement of form, and the central arch of the eyebrow bespeaks a fine sense of colour. He has only ordinary ability to estimate size, weight, time and number. The flattened outer angle of the eyebrow is an unmistakable sign of deficient order. This is also coroborated by smooth, tapering fingers. Music is well indicated in the width of the temples. The prominent eyes betoken superior memory of words and explain much of the eloquence he has displayed in his lectures. The upper forehead is well developed at causality and comparison to which is added a fine endowment of suavity and sense of human nature.

'Summing up the organization, it will be seen that kindness, sympathy and philosophical intelligence, with ambition to achieve success in the direction of higher educational work, are his predominant characteristics.' "

1895 OCT. - NOV. : In response to the invitations from Miss Henrietta Muller and Mr. E. T. Sturdy, **SWAMI VIVEKANANDA** paid the first visit to England.

His friends and admirers arranged evening classes and talks in private houses. Also numerous distinguished visitors including Lady Isabel Margesson and several of the nobility sought interviews and crowded into his class rooms to listen to his inspiring discourses. The representatives of leading journals like *The Westminster Gazette,* and *The Standard,* publicized his learned talks in the editorial columns and thus made Swamiji the focus of attention of the persons of light and leading in London.

In the course of three months which Swami Vivekananda spent on the occasion of his first visit to England, he succeeded in conquering the hearts of many enlightened persons of high eminence, distinguished educationists and even learned clerical and Church dignitaries.

1895 OCT. 22: In response to the requests of his friends, **SWAMI VIVEKANANDA** delivered a public lecture in the evening, at Princes' Hall, Piccadilly, one of the most fashionable places in the metropolis of London. It was a tremendous success.

The press acclaimed him with one voice. *The London Standard* wrote:

"Since days of Ram Mohan Roy, with the single exception of Keshab Chandra Sen, there has not appeared on an English platform a more interesting Indian figure than the Hindu who lectured in Prince's Hall.... In the course of his lecture, he made remorselessly disparaging criticism on the work that the factories, engines and other inventions and books doing for man, compared with half-a-dozen words spoken by Buddha or Jesus. The lecture was evidently quite extemporaneous and was delivered in a pleasing voice free from any kind of hesitation."

The Press welcomed Swamiji's religious and philosophical ideas which were based mainly on the universal principles of the Vedanta and the *Gita*; some of the most enlightened clubs of the city and even leaders of its prominent educational institutions invited him and received him with marked admiration. A correspondent of a daily journal who attended the class lectures of Swami wrote: "It is indeed a rare sight to see some of the most fashionable ladies in London seated on the floor cross-legged, of course, for want of chairs, listening with all the *bhakti* of an Indian *chela* towards his *guru*. The love and sympathy for India that

the Swamiji is creating in the minds of the English speaking race is sure
to be a tower of strength for the progress of India."

1895 NOV. 3: The London correspondent of *The Hindu* wrote:

"SWAMI VIVEKANANDA, the famous Hindu monk, is now in England.
He came here from America a week ago. The Swami is now the guest of
Mr. E. T. Sturdy, sometimes back a Theosophist, but now true Advaiti.
Arrangements are being made to enable the Swami to deliver a series of
lectures on the Hindu religion and its philosophy. I am told that Swami
Vivekananda has had a splendid time of it in America. He has, I am told,
established several branches in America, and has actually converted a
good many of the Yankee men and women to Hinduism; and given
'sannyasinism' or monk-hood, to not a few." (*The Indian Mirror*)

1895 NOV. 19: From the *Westminister Gazette*:

"Indian philosophy has in recent years had a deep and growing
fascination for many minds, though up to the present time its exponents
in this country have been entirely Western in their thought and training
with the result that very little is really known of the deeper mysteries of
the Vedanta wisdom, and that little only by a select few. Not many have
the courage or the intuition to seek in heavy translations, made greatly
in the interests of philologists, for that sublime knowledge which they
really reveal to an able exponent brought up in all the traditions of the
East.

It was therefore with interest and not without some curiosity, writes a
correspondent, that proceeded to interview an exponent entirely novel
to Western people, in the person of the **SWAMI VIVEKANANDA,** an
actual Indian yogi, who has boldly undertaken to visit the Western world
to expound the traditional teaching which has been handed down by
ascetics and yogis through many ages, and who in pursuance of this
object, delivered a lecture last night in the Princes' Hall.

"Swami Vivekananda is a striking figure with his turban and his calm
but kindly features...." (*The Indian Mirror*)

1895 NOV. 23: In a letter to the Editor of the *Brahmavadin*, a reader wrote:

"....Before the birth of Buddhism, Christianity and Mohammedanism,
Hinduism was a propagandistic religion, the diffusive influence of its
universal principles working amongst the Hindus of the different parts
of India. After Buddhism arose Hinduism stretched forth its mighty arms
among the Buddhists and collected them once again into the Hindu
fold. When Mohammedans came to India, no doubt some of the Hindus
embraced the faith of Islam; but why? – Because the Mohammedans

preached the faith of Islam by taking sword in one hand and the Koran
in the other. And when the time came the Hindu Vedanta influenced
even Mohammedanism, and its old converts accepted again the
teachings of Hindu preachers. Islam softened and beautified by the
Vedanta is the religion of the Sufis.

"After such conversions and reconversions Hindusim has been silently
working among its followers and gathering for them strength and light.
A new religious wave has now come from foreign lands, which is, in all
possibility, simply a reflected wave recoiling upon the original shore
whose "prophet winds" gave rise to it at the first instance. This new
wave is called Christianity and its historic relation to the Vedantism of
India is sure to be made out sooner or later. Faint voices are already
heard pointing to the Indian origin of Christianity, and the true Hindu
can have nothing but sympathy for all sorts and conditions of converts.
All religion is the conversion of the obdurate heart of man and in
inclining him to virtue and to devotion to God. But do all converts know
this?

"Mercenary preachers of any religion can nowhere do any real good,
for their mission in life is to any how increase the numbers of converts.
With such preachers religion becomes a commercial article. They are
ever in search of new markets for its sale, and often much of what is
not good for home consumption is sold abroad, and very naturally the
figures in the account books swell. Is this religious progress? We are
living in a curiously mercantile age, which has, in a remarkably wonderful
way, made not only religion and philosophy but also philanthropy itself
a paying profession. Indulging in habits of luxury and endeavouring to
satisfy their wordly desire for pleasure and for fame, these mercenary
diffusers of religion do not care so much for the spiritual development
of man as for making numerous converts from other religions. They will
not allow religions and religious men to live at peace with one another.
If they did so their own occupation would be gone.

"Hinduism has in recent years suffered much owing to want of proper
preachers. Though the sannyasins were formerly the real preachers of
religion in India, most of them have now become illiterate and luxury-
loving in their habits, and do not feel the practice of renuciation and
the teaching and preaching of religion to be their daily duty. Hence it is
now necessary that well-educated sannyasins, animated by the sincerest
piety and the most austere spirit of humanity and self-denial, should
rise from the Hindu community to make themselves all in all to the
people, to set before them, examples of perfect righteousness and to
devote their lives with zeal to popular instructions and the office of
preaching religion. Men of real sanctity and high-minded freedom, and

gifted with high intellectual powers should now enter upon this path of religious zeal, and remove the abuses and the moral corruption that are daily working mischief in our society and in our homes. Spiritual strength comes to all, as usual, by the door of renunciation, and resignation can alone be the undisturbed home of the serene life of religious bliss. Heroic Hindus! Take up the begging bowl and go from door to door spreading the love of righteousness and peace among mankind.

"Moreover, it is now high time for us to send Hindu missionaries like **SWAMI VIVEKANANDA** to distant lands for diffusing widely the highest doctrines of the Hindu religion, and for bringing men of all creeds under its benign influence...."

1895 NOV. : **Miss Margaret Noble** (afterwards known as Sister Nivedita) came into personal touch with **SWAMI VIVEKANANDA** in London.

She was the Headmistress of a school and an important member of the Sesame Club founded for the furtherance of educational purpose. The first meeting with Swamiji, her future spiritual master, left on her mind an indelible impression of the profound sanctity and purity of the life and message of this great Swami, and Miss Noble did not from now miss an opportunity to attend Swamiji's thrilling and interesting lectures and talks.

Two years later she dedicated herself to the service of India in answer to the call of Swamiji. He named her as 'Nivedita'– the dedicated one.

1895 DEC. 22: *The Indian Mirror* wrote:

"**SWAMI VIVEKANANDA** had all these times been actively engaged in his propaganda work in the West; now he has turned his attention towards his own country. His most significant act has been the publication of a new religious periodical called *The Brahmavadin*. It is conducted by some Madras friends of the Swami. The main object of the journal is 'to propagate the Vedantic religion of India and to work towards the improvement of the social and moral condition of man by steadily holding aloft the sublime and universal ideas of Hinduism'. A new era of religious thought and aspiration is everywhere, and it is hoped that *The Brahmavadin* in its catholicity and unsectarian spirit will be in accord with the spirit of the age. The ability and originality with which some of the articles are discussed establish its writers on the list of the strongest thinkers. The writings are weighty with sound reflection, lucidly and forcibly expressed. The journal is a notable contribution to the religious literature of the day." [see 1895 Jul. 27, 1895 Sept.]

1895 (A). : Guglielmo Marconi (1874-1937), Italian physicist, designed and developed the first practical system of wireless telegraphy based on the discovery of radio waves [see 1887 (e)] by Heinrich Hertz (1857-1894), the German physicist. Existence of these waves had been detected in 1873 by James Clerk Maxwell (1831-1879), a Scottish mathematician and physicist. [see 1864 (f), 1873 (f)]

In September Marconi transmitted a message to his brother who was out of sight beyond a hill. The following year (June 1896) he patented his invention, and in the same year demonstrated wireless communication in England; he sent the first recorded message through space by electrornagnetic waves. In 1898 he managed to arrange wireless communication between ships and the shore. In 1899, signals across the English Channel, created a sensation.

Marconi's greatest triumph was in 1901 when he successfully transmitted wireless signals across the Atlantic Ocean between England (Cornwall) and America (Newfoundland) – a distance of about 3,200 kms. The rest of his life was spent in the scientific and commercial development of wireless telegraphy, telephony and broadcasting. He was awarded (1909) the Nobel Prize for physics.

1895 (B): Carl Linde (1842-1934), German engineer, set up a large-scale plant for the production of liquid air.

He had previously developed a methyl ether **refrigerator** (1874) and an ammonia refrigerator (1876). Though other refrigeration units had been developed earlier, Linde's were the first to be designed by precise calculations of efficiency. Six years later (in 1901), Linde developed a method of separating pure liquid oxygen from liquid air that resulted in widespread industrial conversion to processes utilizing oxygen; for example, in steel manufacture. Linde's invention of the continuous process of liquefying gases in large quantities formed a basis for the science of refrigeration and provided impetus for modern physics research in low temperatures and very high vacuums. [see 1865 (f)]

1895 (C): King Camp Gillette (1855-1932) of U. S. invented **safety razor** with a disposable blade. It was patented in U. S. in 1901. Gillette's boss, William Painter, had advised him to "invent something which would be used once and thrown away" so that the customer will come back for more.

1895 (D): George Eastman (1854-1932), American inventor, produced the first **'Brownie Camera'**, using daylight loading film. This type of camera marked the beginning of modern snapshot photography. [see 1884 (e), 1888 (i), 1892 (b)]

1895 (E): An **internal combustion engine** (diesel engine) that operated on petroleum fuel less highly refined and less costly than gasoline was invented by German engineer **Rudolf Diesel** (1858-1913) whose engine had no electrical ignition system and was simpler than a petrol engine and motor trouble free. [see 1885 (b)]

Diesel worked with Fried Krupp of Essen and the Augsburg-Nuremberg Machine Tool Factory to build a successful engine (1897) in which the fuel was ignited by the heat produced by the compression of the fuel-air mixture to a high pressure. It was displayed at Munich Exhibition in 1898. Because of its size and weight this engine has proved to be most suitable for heavy-transport vehicles. Heavy oil used as the fuel and the engines are remarkably economic to operate. Today diesel engines are commonly used for buses, taxis and lorries.

1895 (F): *Studies in Hysteria* by Viennese physician, **Sigmund Freud,** was published in collaboration *with* **Joseph Breuer.**

Sigmund Freud worked with Joseph Breuer in treating hysteria with hypnosis, but he developed a new treatment that became the basis of scientific **psycho-analysis.** [see 1895 (l)]

1895 (G): A young mathematics teacher in Borovsk, Russia, published his **first article on space travel.** In the following year, **Konstantin Tsiolkovsky** (1857-1935), Russian research scientist in aeronautics and astronautics, who pioneered the development of rocket and space research, began to write his largest and most serious work on astronautics, *Exploration of Cosmic Space by means of Reaction Devices,* which dealt with theoretical problems of using rocket engines in space, including heat transfer, a navigating mechanism, heating resulting from air friction and maintenance of fuel supply.

Tsiolkovsky was among the first to study the aerodynamics airfoils with a wind tunnel and to work out the theoretical problem of rocket travel in space. His contributions on stratospheric exploration and inter planetary flight were particularly noteworthy and played a significant role in contemporary astronautics. The German scientist, Hermann Oberth, wrote to Tsiolkovsky, "You have lighted the flame and we will not permit it to go out, but will try to accomplish the great dream of mankind."

Further development of rocket theory came in the 1920s from Hermann Oberth, and also from Robert Hutchings Goddard of America, who fired liquid-fuelled rocket. In the Second World War the Germans developed the V-2 rocket, used to, bomb London, and after war, both the U. S. A. and the U. S. S. R. used German scientists and technology to found their space programmes of the 1950s.

1895 (H): **Herbert George Wells** (1866-1946) English novelist, published his first novel, *The Time Machine,* which tells of a machine that could travel into the remote future.

H. G. Wells was writing at a time when science and engineering were changing the face of the world. The novel *Time Machine* was successful at once, and soon he began to produce a series of scientific romances which established him as a writer of startling originality. H. G. Wells was a powerful influence, in the movement which worked towards the breakdown of the 19th century outlook in economics, moral and religious belief.

1895 (I): **Kiel Canal** linking Baltic and North Sea, was opened.

Over one hundred kilometres long and fourteen metres deep, the construction of this canal was started in 1887, and took eight years and at one point eighty thousand men were working on the canal. The Kiel canal proved to be of strategic importance in both World Wars.

1895 (J): **The Lanchester Motor Car** introduced by English engineer **Frederick W. Lanchester** of Lanchester Engine Company, was the first British four-wheel gasoline-powered motor car. It had epicyclic gearing, worm-drive and pneumatic tyres.

1895 (K): **The League of Struggle** for the emancipation of the working class was founded at St. Petersburg by Russian revolutionary, **Vladimir Ilyich Ulyanov,** 25, who later adopted the pseudonym, Nikolai Lenin. He had read the works of Karl Marx. His older brother had been executed 4 years ago for plotting against the life of the Czar. [see.1899 (c)]

1895 (L): After meticulous clinical observations, **Sigmund Freud** (1856-1939), Viennese founder of psycho-analysis, developed his **psycho-analytical method** using the technique of free-association.

Freud had studied (together with Joseph Breuer, an outstanding Viennese physician) neurotic patients under hypnosis and had observed that when the source of patient's ideas and impulses were brought into consciousness during hypnotic state, the patient showed improvement. Observing that most of his patients talked freely without being under hypnosis, Freud evolved the technique of free association of ideas. The patient was encouraged to say anything that came into his mind, without regard to its assumed relevancy or propriety. This method of drawing memories from unconscious to the conscious mind was termed by Freud as **Psycho-analysis** [see 1882 (h)]. Together with Breuer he published *Studies in Hysteria* [see 1895 (f)] which included several theoretical chapters, a series of Freud's cases and Breuer's initial case. In his major work, *The Interpretation of Dreams,* (1899), Freud demonstrated that dreams of every man, just like the symptoms of a hysterical or a otherwise neurotic person, serve as a "royal road" to the understanding of unconscious mental processes, which have great importance in determining human behaviour. Freud had many great followers including Carl Jung (1875-1961) and Alfred Adler (1870-1937).

1895 (M): Henri Poincare (1854-1912) French mathematician, founded **algebraic topology.** He made lasting contribution to mathematical analysis, celestial mechanics and the philosophy of science.

1895 (N): In a Bengali letter from England to one of his friends, **SWAMI VIVEKANANDA** wrote:

"Your suggestion to me to go back to India is no doubt right, but a seed has been sown in this country, and there is the possibility of its being nipped in the bud if I go away all on a sudden. Hence I have to wait for some time. Moreover it will be possible to manage everything nicely from here. Everybody requests me to return to India. It is all right, but don't you see it is not wise to depend upon others. A wise man should stand firm on his own legs and act. Everything will come about, slowly. For the present don't forget to be on the look-out for a site. We want a big plot, – of about ten to twenty thousand rupees, – it must be right on the Ganges [see 1898 Mar. 5]. Though my capital is small, I am exceedingly bold. Have an eye on securing the land. At present we shall have to work three centres, one in New York, another in Calcutta and a third in Madras. Then by degrees, as the Lord will arrange...."

1895-96: How hard **SWAMI VIVEKANANDA** had to work in the United States in order to inculcate the spiritual ideas of India in the Americans may be understood to some extent from the following schedule of class lectures he gave at 228 West 39th Street, New York, during the winter:

Mondays	: Bhaktiyoga	–	11 a.m. and 8 p.m.
Wednesdays	: Jnanayoga	–	11 a.m. and 8 p.m.
Fridays	: Question Class –		8 p.m.
Saturdays	: Rajayoga	–	11 a.m. and 8 p.m.

Besides this programme, the Swami had to give public lectures and numerous interviews, and also carry on a heavy correspondence. All his letters had to be written in his own hand.

1896 JAN. 18: *The Indian Mirror* reported:

"We are glad to note that **SWAMI VIVEKANANDA** has been attracting in London the attention of a distinguished company of ladies and gentlemen. The classes that he holds on Hindu Philosophy and yoga are said to be enthusiastically and devotedly attended. "It is indeed a rare sight", says a London correspondent, "to see some of the most fashionable ladies in London seated on the floor cross-legged, of course, for want of chairs, listening with all the *bhakti* of an Indian *chela* towards his *guru*." [see 1895 Oct. 22]

"The Swami, we are told, has been well-received and honourably mentioned by such distinguished divines as Canon Wilberforce, Hayes, and others. At the former's residence, there was a levee in honour of the Swami to which some of the distinguished ladies and gentlemen in London were invited. The Swami has by this time gone back to America, but he is expected to return in the spring to establish a permanent home in London. The same London correspondent whom we have quoted above observes, and we hope, with much truth, that "the love and sympathy for India that the Swamiji is creating in the minds of the English-speaking race is sure to be a tower of strength for the progress of India."

1896 JAN. 19: Reporting on the character of **SWAMI VIVEKANANDA'S work in America**, the *New York Herald* said:

"Swami Vivekananda is a name to conjure with in certain circles of New York society today – and those not the least wealthy or intellectual. It is borne by a dusky gentleman from India, who, for the last twelve months, has been making name and fame for himself in this metropolis by the propagation of certain forms of Oriental religion philosophy and practice. Last winter his campaign centred in the reception room of a prominent hotel on Fifth Avenue. Having gained for his teaching and himself a certain vogue in society, he now aims to reach the common people and for that reason is giving a series of free lectures on Sunday afternoons at Hardman Hall.

"Sufficient success has attended the efforts of Swami Vivekananda to justify a description of the man and his work in the United States.... Of his early life he never speaks, save to talk in general way about the great Master who taught him the doctrines and practices he is now trying to introduce in this country.

"....His manner is undoubtedly attractive, and he is possessed of a large amount of personal magnetism. One has but to glance at the grave, attentive faces of the men and women who attend his classes to be convinced that it is not the man's subject alone that attracts and holds his disciples....

The New York Herald reporter, after giving a description of the Swami and his work in the United States continues as follows:

"When I visited one of the Swami's classes recently, I found present a well-dressed audience of intellectual appearance. Doctors and lawyers, professional men and society ladies were among those in the room.

"Swami Vivekananda sat in the centre, clad in an ochre-coloured robe. The Hindu had his audience divided on either side of him and there were between fifty and a hundred persons present. The class was on karmayoga....

"Following the lecture on instruction, the Swami held an informal reception, and the magnetism of the man was shown by the eager manner in which those who had been listening to him, hastened to shake hands or begged for the favour of an introduction. But concerning himself the Swami will not say more than is absolutely necessary. Contrary to the claim made by his pupils, he declares that he has come to this country alone and not as officially representing any Order of Hindu monks. He belongs to the *sannyasins*, he will say, and is hence free to travel without losing his caste ....."

1896 FEB. 29: In a letter to the Editor of *The Brahmavadin* a devotee of **SWAMI VIVEKANANDA** wrote from London:-

"The visit of Swami Vivekananda to England has demonstrated that there exists a thoughtful, educated body of people here which has only to be found and properly approached to benefit very largely from the life-giving stream of Indian thought....

"Swami Vivekananda's classes drew together considerable numbers from the various ranks of English life. The great majority of these carried away with them a clear conviction of his capacity as a teacher.

"....Great are the possibilities for the Indian peoples by the conquering of the heads and hearts of their rulers...."

1896 FEB: **SWAMI VIVEKANANDA** was invited to lecture before the Metaphysical Society at Hartford, Conn. He accepted, and spoke on *'Soul and God'*.

Of his lecture the *Hartford Daily Times* wrote: 'His lectures are more in consonance with those of Christ than those of many so-called Christians. His broad charity takes in all religions and all nations. The simplicity of his talk last night was charming.'

1896 FEB. (A): Many famous philosophers and scientists, and the very best of New York's social representatives attended **SWAMI VIVEKANANDA'S** lectures or came to his room to see him and went away filled with a new spiritual vision and a luminous insight.

The great electrical scientist, **Nikola Tesla**, hearing the Swami's exposition of the Sankhya philosophy, was much interested in its cosmogony and its rational theories of the *kalpas* (cycles), *prana,* and *akasha,* to which, he said, modern science might well look for the solution of cosmological problems. He told the Swami that he thought he could prove them mathematically. The Swami wrote on February 13, to E. T. Sturdy: "Mr. Tesla was charmed to hear about the Vedantic *prana* and *akasha* and the *kalpas,* which according to him are the only theories modern science can entertain. Now both *akasha* and *prana* again are produced from the cosmic *mahat,* the Universal Mind, the *Brahma* or *Ishvara.* Mr. Tesla thinks he can demonstrate mathematically that force and matter are reducible to potential energy. I am to go and see him next week, to get this new mathematical demonstration. In that case, the Vedantic cosmology will be placed on the surest foundations.... (*The Life of Swami Vivekananda,* Vol. 2, p. 68). [see 1896 Mar. 28]

"Swami Vivekananda asked Nikola Tesla if he could show that what we call matter (mass) was simply potential energy. Tesla apparently failed to show it and it was not shown till 1905 by Albert Einstein who, at that time, was an in unknown physicist working as clerk in a patent office in Berne, Switzerland." (*Prabuddha Bharata,* January, 1985).

1896 MAR. 25: By special invitation, **SWAMI VIVEKANANDA** spoke before the graduate students of the Philosophy Department of the **Harvard University** on the *Philosophy of the Vedanta.* It was a masterly presentation of the Indian philosophy of non-dualism.

At the end of the lecture there were questions and answers in course of which Swamiji gave, extempore, short but illuminating elucidations of topics arising out of the lecture.... His lecture created such a profound impression upon the minds of the professors that he was offered even a Chair of Eastern Philosophy in the University. He was also invited to accept the chair of Sanskrit in the Columbia University. But as a *sannyasin* he could not accept them and so he declined the offers with thanks.

1896 MAR. 25 (A): *The Indian Mirror* quoted the *New York Herald:*

"Many well-known persons are seeking to follow the teachings of **SWAMI VIVEKANANDA'S philosophy**.

"The personality of the Swami may be gathered in great measure from his picture. He is of dark complexion, of rather more than average height and heavily built.....

"The work of the Hindu in this country consists at present in giving free lectures and holding free classes, initiating disciples and conducting a large correspondence.

"At present while the lectures and classes are popular, and the number of pupils daily increases, the Swami has only two proclaimed disciples.

Both of these have changed their names.... Both of these disciples are Americans of foreign extraction and one at least is well-known in New York...."

1896 MAR. 28: In a letter (dated February 19, 1896) to the Editor of The *Brahmavadin,* Swami Kripananda described the influence exercised by **SWAMI VIVEKANANDA** at New York.

"Since my last letter (of January 31) an immense amount of work has been acomplished by our beloved teacher in the furtherance of our great cause. The wide interest awakened by his teachings, is shown in the ever increasing number of those who attend the class lessons, and the large crowds that come to hear his public Sunday lectures. The physical and mental energy he displays in disseminating true Hindu spirituality in this country which, in spite of its much vaunted Christianity, is a through and through materialistic land, seems exhaustless, and fills with awe and admiration all those who have occasion to witness his gigantic efforts; lecturing twice a day, carrying on a vast correspondence, giving inter- views and private instructions and preparing literature for the guidance of his followers – all this fills his time from the early morning till late at night, and would have long ago broken down his iron constitution, were it not for his powerful will, nourished by his love for mankind, that gives him the strength to cheerfully carry on his difficult task.

"This incessant, untiring activity, to which he is impelled by no other motive than the good of mankind is, indeed, the best object-lesson to illustrate his teachings of unselfish work, especially to the Americans who, though ever active know no higher motive power for his activity than the interest of his petty little self. Thus, our teacher gives us in his own person, the example of a true *karmayogin,* just as in other respects, he proves himself a perfect *bhakta* and *jnanin,* and as such, a worthy disciple of his great master Ramakrishna Paramahamsa, whose ideal was the harmonious union in one character of these three great types of humanity.

"To supply the great demand for some literature on the Swami's teachings, several of his Sunday lectures have been published in pamphlet form at a nominal price hardly sufficient to cover the expenses. They sell very rapidly, and thus help to carry the Vedanta into regions where the existence of this wonderful system of thought was, perhaps, never before dreamed of. Eight of the Swami's class-lessons on karmayoga are in print to be published in book form, a sufficient number of copies to pay the cost being already subscribed for in advance. In this work the Swami was greatly assisted by several of his *grhastha* followers whose unselfish efforts, in behalf of the furtherance of our movement, cannot be commended enough.

"On Thursday, the 13th of this month, another soul joined the children of Ramakrishna: Dr. Street took the vow of renunciation, and thus became a *sannyasin*. The impressive ceremony was performed by the Swami at the headquarters, in the presence of the other *sannyasins* and a number of *brahmacharins*. The name given on this occasion to Dr. Street was Yogananda. Besides the numerous *brahmacharins* who are preparing themselves for the definite step, this is the third *sannyasin* created by the Swami in this land. It shows that the idea of renunciation is coming up slowly, it is true, but surely, the people at last are coming to realize that to be religious, it is not sufficient to merely believe, but they must live in accordance with what they believe to be true, and that there are even in this country, where everybody clings so strongly to the world and all its vanities, these few at least, to whom the Swami has brought home a strong conviction of the necessity of renunciation as the only means of attaining liberation....the fact of these people giving up the world for the sake of God and truth, and joining the ranks of your glorious order of *sannyasins* must be regarded as one of the most marvellous evidence of the Swami's powerful influence for good, and should fill with joy the hearts of all true Vedantins....

"This, however, is not the only result brought about by our beloved teacher. The strong current of religious thought sent out in his lectures and writings, the powerful impetus given by his teachings to the purest of truth without regard to inherited superstitions and prejudices, though working silently and unconsciously, is still exercising a beneficial and lasting effect on the popular mind and so becoming an important factor in the spiritual uplifting of society. Its most palpable manifestation is shown in the growing demand for Vedantic literature and the frequent use of Sanskrit terms by people from whom one would least expect to hear them: *Atman, Purusha, moksha,* and similar expressions have acquired full citizenship, and the names of Shankaracharya, and Ramanuja are becoming with many almost as familiar as Huxley and Spencer. The public libraries are running after everything that has reference to India: the books of Max Muller, Colebrooke, Deussen, Burnouf, and of all the authors that have ever written in English on Hindu philosophy find a ready sale; and even the dry and tiresome, Schopenhauer, on account of his Vedantic background, is being studied with great eagerness.

"People are quick to appreciate the grandeur and beauty of a system which equally, as a philosophy and a religion appeals to the heart as well as to the reason, and satisfies all the religious cravings of the human nature; especially so, when it is being expounded by one who, like our teacher, with his wonderful oratory is able to rouse at will the dormant love of the divinely sublime in the human soul, and with his sharp and irrefutable logic to easily convince the most stubborn mind of the most scientific matter-of-fact man. No wonder, therefore, that this interest in Hindu thought is to be met with among all classes of society. To give only the opinion of two representatives, an emotional nature, and a scientific mind: Sarah Bernhardt, the 'divine Sarah' as people are pleased to call her, the greatest actress of modern times, sought an interview with the Swami, and expressed to him her admiration for an interest in the sublime doctrines of Hinduism; while Nikola Tesla the greatest electrician of this day, when hearing an exposition of the Sankhya system given by the Swami a few days ago, candidly admitted the superiority of its cosmogony, to all other accounts, and declared that its teachings as to *kalpas, prana,* and *akasha* offered the only rational theory modern science can take, to explain the cosmological problem. [see 1896 Feb. (a)]

"By the way, India better at once make clear her title to the ownership of the Swami (Vivekananda). They are about writing his biography for the *National Encyclopaedia* of the United States of America, thus making of him an American *"malgre lui"*. The time may come, when, even as seven cities disputed with each other for the honour of having given birth to Homer, seven countries may claim our master as theirs, and then rob India of the honour of having produced one of the noblest of her children."

1896 APR. 2: *The Indian Mirror* reported:

"From the latest information that reaches us we learn that the work of **SWAMI VIVEKANANDA** in America has assumed gigantic proportions 'hardly possible for a single man to cope with'. Hitherto the Swami has been working silently, steadily, and with wonderful success. His first object was to assert the further spread of materialistic tendency, and in this he has been remarkably successful. By his ardent love and great enthusiasm, this great apostle of Hinduism has achieved great results. It is a matter of great satisfaction that Hinduism has got such an able exponent. The high ideal of Hindu doctrines which he holds before his audience is scarcely to be met anywhere else. He holds his classes twice daily, one for the beginners and the other for the advanced pupils. His class lectures are masterpieces of logic and philosophy. In course of a lecture of the Vedanta Philosophy he held up the ideal of a universal religion, which he learnt at the feet of his great master. He lectured on *Atman, Bhaktiyoga,* and *Karmayoga.* These lectures, when published in a book form in India, prove a great treasure-house of Hindu Theology and Philosophy."

1896 APR. 11: **Helen Huntington** of Brooklyn, America, wrote (on March 2, 1896) to the Editor of *The Brahamavadin*:

"Sir, Next to **SWAMI VIVEKANANDA'S** presence *The Brahmavadin* [see 1895 Jul. 27] is the most excellent and comforting thing we could desire; my fervent wish is that its circulation may extend to the utmost limits of our country, and carry its message of peace and good-will to thousands of hungry souls, to those upon whom 'thirst has come though they stand in the midst of the waters.'

"From long association with the Christian Press and regular attendance at Orthodox Churches, we have become accustomed to speak of 'our missionary work among the poor heathens of India', until we have come to think of India as a land of spiritual darkness only lighted at intervals by rays from our Gospel lamps. Tens of thousands of civilized, tolerably well-educated people listen with awe and sorrowful wonder, Sunday after Sunday, to tales of many millions of the benighted heathens condemned by our Orthodox Clergy to total and everlasting annihilation, because they have never heard Christ preached. How utterly impossible to conceive of and worship a God whose sovereignty admits of such injustice.

"But it has pleased God to send to us out of India a spiritual guide, a teacher whose sublime philosophy is slowly permeating the ethical atmosphere of our country; a man of extraordinary power and purity who has demonstrated to us a very high plane of spiritual being, a religion of universal unfailing charity, self-renunciation and the purest sentiments conceivable by the human intellect. Swami Vivekananda has preached to us a religion that knows no bounds of creeds or dogmas, is uplifting, purifying, infinitely comforting, and altogether without blemish; based on the love of God and man and on absolute chastity. By accepting his teachings we do not refute the Christian religion (as some think we must and are, therefore, ready to denounce the Vedanta), we only break through the barriers of creeds and old superstitions that ignorant men have raised to shut us off from God's ineffable presence.

"I will not admit the faintest doubt of our progress along the lines laid out for us, but if we do not go forward quickly as we could desire, it is because we are beset by difficulties of education and long habit, which cannot be shaken off in a day or many days. If we could have the Swami with us always, the nature of our progress would be different, it would be easier, for while we believe in him implicitly and are his devoted followers, we are also woefully human – we know that spirit is not bound by time or space and that though he is far away, his spirit is still with us; nevertheless we greatly desire his bodily presence in our midst.

"Swami Vivekananda has made many friends outside the circle of his followers; he has met all phases of society on equal terms of friendship and brotherhood; his classes and lectures have been attended by the most intellectual people and advanced thinkers of our cities; and his influence has already grown into a deep, strong under-current of spiritual awakening. No praise or blame has moved him to either approbation or expostulation; neither money nor position has influenced or prejudiced him. Towards demonstrations of undue favouritism he has invariably maintained a priestly attitude of inattention checking foolish advances with a dignity impossible to resist – blaming not any, but wrong doers and evil thinkers, exhorting only to purity and right living. He is altogether such a main as kings delight to honour."

1896 APR. 11 (A): *The Brahmavadin* quoted *Detroit Evening News*:

"**Swami Kripananda,** the advanced disciple of **SWAMI VIVEKANANDA,** has been in the city two days, stopping at the Utopia. He talked enthusiastically of his brother (Vivekananda) and of the work he has been doing in New York, and hopes to do here.

"I have always been a seeker of truth", said he. "I studied many religions and found some truth in all, but all too much encrusted with superstition, until I became a materialist, and remained so until I met the Swami in New York just after he came here, and was helped to find the truth. I have lived with him three years since, and learned to know that religious experiences are capable of demonstration as any other fact in science, that they can be proved, that we may see God. I am an American citizen, and was educated in Germany and France. I have lived in this country for years. I used to have a paper in the South myself, and was later connected with one of the largest dailies in New York.

"The Swami will remain here about two weeks, holding classes at 240, Second Avenue, at 11 a.m. and 8 p.m., every day, beginning Wednesday. They will be free. Religious teachings cannot be sold for dollars and cents. He had had great success in New York for the last three months, holding daily classes with large attendance, and bringing many to the truth. He will go to Boston from here and will address the philosophy students, at Harvard, then after a week in Chicago he goes to England, where Lady Dudley and others have long been interested.

"He will spend the summer there and then return to India, where he will retire to a cave for may be two or three years for contemplation and introspection, as pious monks do. I was initiated by him into the Order of *sannyasins*, or announcers of the truth, and will remain here after he goes, to continue his work.

"How will I live? I will get some work to earn enough to keep body and soul together. We take three vows before we are initiated – poverty, chastity and homelessness. 'Not I, but you,' is the watchword of *sannyasin*. We work for the love of the good. Religion should not be made a profession."

1896 APR. : Having consolidated his work in New York, **SWAMI VIVEKANANDA** visited London for the second time and soon began his regular classes on jnanayoga.

His Sunday lectures comprised such subjects as *The Necessity of Religion, A Universal Religion, The Real and Apparent Man, Renunciation, Realization,* and the like which strongly appealed to the intellectually gifted people of England and prepared the ground for a steady march of Hindu thought and culture throughout the length and breadth of the country. Swamiji carried on his Vedantic activity in London till the end of July 1896.

During this second visit to England, Swamiji was able to gather to his fold some most diligent and devout workers who proved martyrs to his noble cause.

1896 MAY. 23: In a letter to the Editor of *The Brahmavadin* a reader wrote:

"....In a land, where a man's worth is measured by his capacity to earn money, where man's brain and intellect are chiefly employed in devising means to add to physical comforts and pleasures, where the scuffle and scramble for money, place and position make men blind to and forgetful of what is due to those whom nature has not given sufficient strength to run swift in the race of competition, where the cultivation of science and philosophy breeds disbelief in God, in a land such as this for **SWAMI VIVEKANANDA'S mission** to meet with success is what strikes me as nothing short of a miracle. Helpless, friendless and penniless did Swami Vivekananda find himself when he first set foot on the American soil. The message he felt called upon to deliver to the American people had an appearance extremely distasteful to the Americans; but he felt the truth and holiness of his message and – deliver it he must – and he did deliver it and has been delivering it since, with what result readers of *The Brahmavadin* need not be told. Americans in large numbers, gather round him, surprised now to learn that the teachings of religion are not altogether opposed to the principles of science and philosophy and more surprised to see that Hinduism, a religion which has all along been represented to them by Christian Missionaries as another name for barbarism and superstition, contains such solutions of the problems of life and death as properly understood will be found to stand the test of even modern science and philosophy.

Among those in America who have learned to admire and appreciate the Swami and through him, the noble cause he represents, are men and women of note and sufficient pretensions to culture and learning. Just imagine a man of Indian complexion preaching Hinduism, regarded and revered as a *guru* by a number of educated and well-reputed Americans. Just fancy an American lady who would sooner part with her life than cease to indulge in fashionable tastes in respect of dress and outward appearance and worldly enjoyments and comforts, seriously taking upon herself the vow of poverty and devoting her life to preaching what she has till recently considered to be the religion of the heathens. Do not these achievements of the Swami outshine the miraculous performances of many prophets, ancient or modern, of the East or the West?

"....Unfortunately for us, we do not notice the beauty and sublimity of our religion unless they are pointed out to us by men of the West, and when Western opinion expresses itself in favour of our religion it invariably finds an echo in the Indian heart. The extent to which the acceptance by the Americans of the principles of Hindu religion and philosophy through Swami Vivekananda has affected Hindu India furnishes one more proof of the fact above referred to. Since the report for the first time, reached India of the Swami's success in the Parliament of Religions, many young men have taken to studying for themselves the various *Hindu shastras*, some in the original and others, ignorant of the Sanskrit language, through translations. A thirst eager, is noticeable in many quarters, for an acquaintance with the life and teachings of Bhagavan Sri Ramakrishna – the illustrious *guru* of Swami Vivekananda. People daily look into the newspapers for reports of the Swami's doings and lectures. Young men eagerly look forward to the return of the Swami to India to hear religious discourses. And last but not least the publication of a paper like *The Brahmavadin* and the heartiness with which it is welcomed by the public, show the extent of the appreciation by India of Swami Vivekananda's work in America."

1896 MAY 28. : At London, **SWAMI VIVEKANANDA** met the celebrated Indologist, **Professor Max Muller** of the Oxford University, by special invitation.

Swamiji was deeply impressed to see the profundity of the scholarship of the great Orientalist. Max Muller who was then 73, had given the world all his greatest productions in Indology, Comparative Philology, and the Science of Religion. His hands were still full, and he was in a desperate hurry to complete editing the remaining volumes of the *Sacred Books of the East* – a task he had commenced in 1875, and which he had by then, nearly completed.

Swamiji considered it as a rare privilege to be invited by the professor to his residence at Oxford and to converse with him on many subjects of Indian philosophy and above all, on his Master Sri Ramakrishna.

The Professor, who had already gathered some facts about the life and teachings of Sri Ramakrishna from India and written a pamphlet entitled *A Real Mahatman,* was now extremely anxious after his talk with Swamiji to know more about Sri Ramakrishna so as to bring out a larger and fuller account of his life and gospels. Swamiji at once commissioned his brother disciple, Swami Saradananda to collect from India greater details regarding the life and teachings of Sri Ramakrishna. The materials thus gathered were placed at the disposal of the learned Professor who set to work at once and embodied them in a book which was published under the title *The Life and Sayings of Sri Ramakrishna* (1898). This treatise created a great sensation in England and materially helped the Swami in carrying on his mission in the English-speaking world with greater ease and success.

1896 JUN. 3: *The Indian Mirror* reported:

"The following news has been received, by yesterday's mail, from London, regarding Swami Vivekananda's present work there:

"Here in London, **SWAMI VIVEKANANDA** has been holding class lectures, 63, St. George's Road, S. W., every Tuesday and Thursday both in the morning and evening. The number of his students has been increasing very rapidly. He has, therefore, opened a question class which he holds every Friday, at 8.30 P. M. It is a great wonder, indeed, that the Swami has been able to attract, from the very commencement of the course of his lectures, so many men in a materialistic city like London, where none cares a fig for religion, where politics reigns supreme in the minds of the people, especially now at the time of the London season – the season of balls, feasts, and all sorts of entertainments. He, who has once listened to the Great Swami, is tempted to attend every lecture that he delivers. We cannot but own that the man possesses a great magnetic power or some power divine by which he even draws so many Londoners towards him. Many a lady and many a learned man here have become his students. Today Rev. Canon Haweis, a very learned man, came to his class. He has at once marvelled at his lectures."

1896 JUN. 14: In a lettert to the Editor of *The Indian Mirror* four devotees of **SWAMI VIVEKANANDA** (from Madras) wrote:

"A monthly journal (devoted to religion and philosophy) in English from Madras under the title of *The Prabuddha Bharata* or 'Awakened India' will make its appearance on 1st July, 1896.... It will be a sort of supplement to the *Brahmavadin* and seek to do for students, young men and others, what that is already doing so successfully for the more advanced classes. It will, with that view, endeavour to present the sacred truths of Hindu Religion and the sublime and beautiful ideal of the Vedanta in as simple, homely and interesting a manner as possible and amongst others, will contain the lives and teachings of great sages and bhaktas irrespective of caste, creed or nationality, who are and ever will be the beacon lights of humanity.

The conductors of the magazine undertake the work purely as a labour of love and they have secured the sympathy and support of some of the eminent thinkers of the day including Swami Vivekananda now in America. They look for no personal gains from the concern and their only aim is to get for the truths of the Hindu Religion as wide a circulation as possible.... To our youths who are misled by the glamour of materialism, *The Prabuddha Bharata* will ever be a continual warning voice and religious instructor, and to our more advanced brethren its pages will afford a pleasant and healthy spiritual recreation...."
[see 1896 July]

1896 JUN. 14 (A): *The Indian Mirror* in its Editorial:

"Whether our political reforms take any interest in religious matters or not, it is certain that the country is going through a slow religious awakening, and we hope to see in near future the wave of religious reform sweeping over all the land. As a result of this temper of the times, we find that a new magazine is about to be published from Madras, under the appropriate title of *Awakened India.* Madras has already got a very good religious journal in the one, called *The Brahmavadin,* which is a recognized organ of **SWAMI VIVEKANANDA** and his party. *Awakened India,* it is announced, will be 'a sort of supplement' to *The Brahmavadin.* From the few numbers of *The Brahmavadin* issued so far we judge, that they must have been read with much interest by all religious-minded Hindus. The magazine has from time to time published valuable lectures, delivered by Swami Vivekananda in America, and some able and original articles on the Vedanta philosophy. The value of *Brahmavadin* is further increased by the fact of its attempt to diffuse the truths of Vedantism, which is yet another word for Advaitism, far and wide, and we think, it is rendering in this respect excellent service to the Hindu race....

"....We are pleased to find, that Swami Vivekananda is so thoroughly absorbed in the work of reviving the Vedantic philosophy and spreading a knowledge of its truths among the advanced thinkers of Europe and America, and we do not know how sufficiently to thank him for his labours. We believe, therefore, that the more we have such journals as *The Brahmavadin* and *Awakened India,* the better it will be for us....

"....We publish in another column the prospectus of *Awakened India,* from which it may be gathered how Vedantic truths have begun to be appreciated, of late, both at home and abroad. But our chief object in inviting the attention of our readers to the subject is to impress on their minds our own conviction, that Vedanta is destined, in course of time, to spread throughout the world, and that from the day of its revival in India is to be dated her renaissance. We regard Advaitism as the most precious treasure which the ancient Hindu sages bequeathed us, and we ought to make the very best possible use of that treasure. We ought to be thankful that deprived of everything else, we have still that treasure with us. We would appeal to our educated Hindu countrymen to set their hearts on the study of the Upanishads, especially those chapters in them which treat of Vedantism."

1896 JUN. 18: *The Indian Mirror* reported:

"We received the following news regarding **SWAMI VIVEKANANDA** by yesterday's mail:

"Since his arrival in London, Swami Vivekananda has been doing much work here. Besides his regular class lectures, which are in number no less than 5 every week, he has to address several meetings here and there. He intends to stay here for 5 or 6 months more, and after that he will return to India. In America, the Swami has converted nearly 4000 persons to Hinduism who have since been disciplining their minds spiritually according to his directions."

1896 JUN. 27: *The Indian Mirror* published the following letter received from the warmest American disciples of **SWAMI VIVEKANANDA** at the Ramakrishna Math, at Alambazar, Baranagore:

"....We believe with you that a strong bond of union now exists between your land and ours, established by Swami Vivekananda.

"The grand truths of the Vedanta, as presented by him, interested thinking minds of all classes, and met with a ready acceptance by many of those, who had the privilege of hearing them.

"Swami Vivekananda sailed for England on the 5th April. In his farewell address to his friends and pupils in New York, he spoke highly of the Americans, and the freedom of their institutions, which made them peculiarly accessible to the Vedantic Philosophy.

"We did not realize until now, that the Hindus, so distant and so ancient, held so much wisdom and knowledge in trust for us, the youngest among nations...."

1896 JUL. 9: *The Indian Mirror* reported:

"We learn by the last mail that the American followers of **SWAMI VIVEKANANDA** are going to start a magazine, from 168, Brottle Street, Cambridge, Mass. U. S. A, in order to keep up the work, which Swami Vivekananda has begun there. They have requested the Swami of the Alambazar monastery (Ramakrishna Math) at Baranagore, to contribute to each number of paper. It will treat chiefly on bhakti and karmayoga."

1896 JUL. 17: *The Indian Mirror* reported:

"It is now only a little over two months that **SWAMI VIVEKANANDA** has been in England, and we are glad to notice that within this short time, his work has attracted the attention of the English public. His class lectures are attended by men of all classes. Even the members of the Royal Household attend them.

The London Daily Chronicle writes:

"The gentleman, known as the Swami Vivekananda who was one of the most striking figures at the Chicago Parliament of Religions, and who went there to expound the ancient teachings of India to the newest of Western nations, is at present in England, returning to his own land in September.

"The Swami is one of the greatest living exponents of the Vedantic philosophy, his calm manner, distinguished appearance, the ease with which he expounds a profound philosophy, his mastery of the English tongue, explain the great cordiality with which the Americans received him, and the fact that they almost compelled him to remain a year or two among them. The Swami has taken the vow of complete renunciation of worldly position, property, and name. He cannot be said to belong to any religion, since his life is one of the independent thought which draws from all religions. Those who desire that his teachings may be made known, arrange the entire business-part of the work, and the lectures are, so far, made free. They may be heard at 63, St. George's Road, on Tuesday and Thursday, at half past eleven a.m., and half past eight p. m., upto the end of July. It is also announced that the Swami will lecture in one of the rooms of the Royal Institute of Water Colours, 191, Piccadilly, at half past three p. m., on Sundays."

1896 JUL. 18: From *The Sunday Times:*

"English people are well acquainted with the fact that they send missionaries to India's 'coral stand'; indeed, so thoroughly do they obey the behest: 'Go ye forth into all the world and preach the Gospel,' that none of the chief British sects are behind hand in obedience to the call to spread Christ's teachings. People are not so well aware that India also sends missionaries to England.

"By accident, if the term may be allowed, I fell across **SWAMI VIVEKANANDA** in his temporary home at 63, St. George's Road, S. W., and as he did not object to discuss the nature of his work and visit to England, I sought him there, and began our talk with an expression of surprise at his assent to my request....

"The Swami is a picturesque figure in his Eastern dress. His simple and cordial manner, savouring of anything but the popular idea of asceticism, an unusual command of English and great conversational powers add not a little to an interesting personality." *(The Hindu Patriot)*

1896 JUL. : *Prabuddha Bharata* an English monthly was started at Madras, by the disciples of **SWAMI VIVEKANANDA**, under the able editorship of Sri B. R. Rajam Iyer, a true Vedantist. [see 1896 June 14]

But after the death of its gifted editor in May 1898, its publication remained suspended till it was resumed through the inspiration of Swamiji at the Thompson House at Almora with Swami Swarupananda (a disciple of Swamiji) as Manager, in August, 1898. When the Advaita Ashram was founded at Mayavati (May 19, 1899), the office of the *Prabuddha Bharata* was shifted from Almora to this new Ashram.

1896 JUL. (A): Death of **Harriet Beecher Stowe** (b.1811), U. S. writer and philanthropist, whose novel *Uncle Tom's Cabin* helped to intensify anti-slavery sentiment in the United States. (Abraham Lincoln said that the book started the Civil War: 1861-65. It was translated into at least 23 languages.)

1896 AUG. 4: *The Indian Mirror* reported:

"We are sure, every Hindu will be glad to learn that a number of men, who generally attend **SWAMI VIVEKANANDA'S class lectures** in London, have taken upon themselves the task of raising a sum of money necessary to obtain, quarters for the exposition of the Hindu Philosophy in London. The proposal includes a large room for regular lectures, a library of books on Eastern Philosophy, including all translations of Sanskrit literature, and a monthly magazine. It will be an encouraging news to all who are interested in the spread of the Hindu religion that the necessary funds are already forthcoming for this object."

1896 AUG. 27: In the course of a report of an interview with **SWAMI VIVEKANANDA**, the representative of India, London, wrote:

"Swami Vivekananda is a man of distinguished appearance. Tall, broad with fine features enhanced by his picturesque Eastern dress, his personality is very striking. Swami is a title, meaning master; Vivekananda is an assumed name implying the bliss of discrimination.

By birth, he is a Bengali and by education, a graduate of the Calcutta University. The Swami has taken the vow of *sannyasa*, renunciation of all property, position and name. His gifts as an orator are high. He can speak for an hour and a-half without a note, or the slightest pause for a word. Towards the end of September his lectures at St. George's Road will be resumed for a few weeks before his departure for Calcutta,." (*The Indian Mirror*)

1896 SEP. 9: **Cardiac surgery** was first successfully undertaken in Frankfurt, Germany, by **Louis Rehn**, German surgeon, upon a patient who had been stabbed in the heart during a travel brawl.

1896 SEP. : By special invitation, **SWAMI VIVEKANANDA** (who was on a Continental tour) met the illustrious German orientalist, **Paul Deussen** (Professor of Philosophy at the University of Kiel in Germany) at his residence in Kiel.

On return from his recent Indian tour, the Professor had become acquainted with the lectures and utterances of the Swami, and having found in him an original thinker and a spiritual genius, had felt a strong desire to meet him to discuss intricate philosophical problems with him. Though brief, their meeting was eventful.

Later, Prof. Deussen met the Swami again at Hamburg and proceeded with him to London. For two whole weeks during his stay in London, Prof. Deussen frequently visited Swamiji and held discussions on the most recondite principle of the Vedanta which enabled him to have a much clear conception of the whole system of Vedanta Philosophy. He was convinced that a person who wants to go deeper into the very core of Indian philosophy must divest himself of all preconceived notions and then come to grips with the lofty philosophical system of the Hindus.

1896 SEP. (A): During his stay at Kiel at the house of **Prof. Paul Deussen, SWAMI VIVEKANANDA** was once found by the Professor poring over the pages of a poetical work. The latter spoke to him but got no response. When Swamiji came to know of it later, he apologized, saying that he was so absorbed in reading the book that he had not heard him. Dr. Deussen was not satisfied with the explanation until in the course of the conversation, the Swami quoted and interpreted some verses from the book. Dr. Deussen was dumbfounded and asked the Swami how he came to acquire such a power of memory. Thereupon the conversation turned upon the subject of the concentration of the mind as practised by the Indian yogi, and that with so much perfection that the Swami said from personal knowledge, in that state he would be unconscious even if a piece of burning charcoal were placed on his body.

1896 OCT. - DEC. : SWAMI VIVEKANANDA who returned to London after the continental tour, resumed his learned lectures which mostly covered the philosophical portions of the Vedanta known as jnanayoga.

The effect of these lectures was so deep and penetrating that many celebrities including Mr. Frederick H. Myers, the well-known author of several psychological works; Hopps, the non-conformist minister; Mr. Moncure D. Conway, the positivist and peace advocate, Mr. Edward Carpenter, the author of *Towards Democracy,* Canon Wilberforce, the great orator, became very much interested in Indian thought and culture.

Leaving **Swami Abhedananda,** a brother disciple, in charge of the Vedanta work in England, Swami Vivekananda bade adieu to London on December 16. Just before his departure for India, an English friend incidentally put the poser to the Swami: "Swami, how do you like your motherland now after four years' experience of the luxurious, glorious, powerful West?" The great Patriot-saint of India replied with his characteristic frankness and the emphasis he could command: "India I loved before I came away. Now the very dust of India has become holy to me, the very air is now to me holy, it is now the holy land, the place of pilgrimage, the *thirtha!"*

On the eve of Swami Vivekananda's departure from England for India, (Dec.13, 1896) a farewell meeting was organized by his friends, students, and admirers, at the galleries of Royal Institute of Painters in Water-Colours, in London. An illuminated address, the text of which is given below, was presented to the Swami:

"The students of the Vedanta philosophy in London under your remarkably able instruction feel that they would be lacking in their duty and privilege if they failed to record their warm heartfelt appreciation of the noble and unselfish work you have set yourself to do, and the great help you have been to them in their study of religion.

"We feel the very deepest regret that you are so soon to leave England, but we should not be true students of the very beautiful philosophy you have taught us to regard so highly if we did not recognize that there are claims upon your work from our brothers and sisters in India. That you may prosper very greatly in that work is the united prayer of all who have come under the elevating influence of your teaching, and no less of your personal attributes, which, as a living example of Vedanta, we recognize as the most helpful encouragement to us one and all to become real lovers of God, in practice as well as in theory.

"We look forward with great interest and keen anticipation to your speedy return to this country, but, at the same time, we feel real pleasure that India, which you have taught us to regard in an altogether new light, and we should like to add, to love, is to share with us the generous service which you are giving to the world.

"In conclusion we could especially beg of you to convey our loving sympathy to the Indian people and to accept from us our assurance that we regard their cause as ours, realizing as we do from you that we are all One in God."

1896 NOV. 1: In a letter of date written to Miss Mary Hale of Chicago from London, **SWAMI VIVEKANANDA** spoke of India's need of socialism for the development of her millions of oppressed humanity, and expressed his own faith in socialism.

"I am a socialist", he wrote, "not because I think it is a perfect system, but half a loaf is better than no bread.

"The other systems have been tried and found wanting. Let this one be tried – if for nothing else, for the novelty of the thing. A redistribution of pain and pleasure is better than always the same persons having pains and pleasures. The sum total of good and evil in the world remains ever the same. The yoke will be lifted from shoulder to shoulder by new systems, that is all.

"Let every dog have his day in this miserable world, so that after this experience of so-called happiness they may all come to the Lord and give up this vanity of a world and governments and all other botherations."

1896 NOV. 21: In a letter to the Editor of The Brahmavadin, **Helen F. Huntington** wrote from America:

"I am sure that you will be glad to know that the peaceable fruits of **SWAMI VIVEKANANDA'S teachings** have been all the while increasing; his influence is like sunrise – so quiet, so potent and far reaching. It will always be a marvel to us that an Oriental could take such a firm hold on us Occidentals, trained as we have been by long habit of thought and education to opposing views. Yet we, busy materialists, who rush through life with nerves strained to their utmost tension in the march of Western civilization, paused to listen intently to the first message of peace from the Orient; and from that time to this we have been eagerly searching after the true Light 'which lighteth every man that cometh into the world'. Our interest is not of the noisy effervescent quality often incited by passing fads; – today it is stronger and deeper than ever before, and all of the Swami's followers endeavour earnestly to spread the truth according to the various opportunities afforded to them, – some quietly within domestic circles, others more prominently, as the case may be. And who is able to estimate the measure of man's silent influence?

"We are not without opposition from the very men to whom we are accustomed to look for spiritual guidance. The clergy here have not yet been brought to realize that the study of Indian Philosophy, instead of being antagonistic to their belief, gives the student a deeper insight into the life and teachings of our great guide and teacher, Jesus of Nazareth: we as his followers, cannot honour him more than by a life of renunciation and purity as taught by the Vedanta.

"....We need awakening – not so much the stereotyped revival of our orthodox Churches, but a real awakening of spiritual desire and heavenly aspiration.... How I should love to bear the precepts of Vedanta expounded from every pulpit from shore to shore of our big prosperous country, to level the creeds and dogmas men have raised to shut us from God's ineffable presence, and gather our millions of truth-seekers together under the strong bond of universal brotherhood! Universal brotherhood! The God within us manifested towards all mankind every hour of our lives! I love the grand old theme as expounded to us by Swami Vivekananda – not the unsatisfying orthodox acceptation with more or less of limitations, but the wholehearted love and goodwill to all created beings irrespective of race or creed or condition.

"It is impossible not to wish for Swami Vivekananda's return to our midst because he has endeared himself so deeply to all of us. As he said of the *guru*, Ramakrishna Paramahamsa, 'His presence was a blessing to everyone, saint and sinner'. So was his own life among us; for he influenced us to better living and brotherly kindness to all men. If there be found any among his so-called enemies who speak of him otherwise – and I may truthfully say that they are very few – we all feel sure the Swami will freely forgive them realizing that the wrong comes through error rather than through evil intent."

__1896 NOV. :__ **The world's first permanent wireless installation** was established by Marconi's Wireless Telegraph Co. Ltd., at the Needles on the Isle of Wright, Hampshire, England.

__1896 DEC. 10:__ Death of **Alfred Nobel** (b.1833) Swedish chemist, industrialist, and the inventor of dynamite and other more powerful explosives. He made a fortune from his inventions and left a bulk of it in trust to establish international awards. His will directed that his estate, above 33 million Kroner, should endow annual prizes for those who, in the preceding year, had most benefitted mankind in five subjects: Physics, Chemistry, Physiology or Medicine; literature and peace. His will was proved within four years and Nobel Foundation was created. A Nobel Prize is the highest honour men can bestow on any man. The first prizes were awarded in 1901. [See 1866 (e), 1888 (g), 1901 (g)]

1896 (A): SWAMI VIVEKANANDA predicted the coming of the *shudra* (the proletariat) dominance in the modern age:

In a broad survey of the progress of mankind through the ages he pointed out how the society was dominated successively by the priests, the Nobility and the merchants corresponding to the first three castes of India, namely the *brahmana*, *khshatriya* and *vaishya*. Then he observed that the next or fourth epoch will be 'under the domination of *shudra*', the fourth caste. This upheaval, he asserted, "will come from Russia or from China." "Perhaps", said he, "Russia will be the first proletarian state in the world." – a prophecy that was fulfilled in twenty years' time. (Bharatiya Vidya Bhavan's *History and Culture of the Indian People,* Vol. X, Part II, p. 131).

Swami Vivekananda also realized that a very critical situation would arise in the West, threatening its total destruction, owing to the rapid growth of material power and scientific inventions, unaccompanied by the corresponding growth of spiritual insight. Said he "Europe is on the edge of a volcano. Unless the fires are extinguished by a flood of spirituality, it will be blown up." This was said of Europe in 1895 when it was prosperous and at peace. Twenty years later came the first explosion!

The Swami with his prophetic vision indicated the religion of the future in the West: "Materialism prevails in Europe today. The salvation of Europe depends on a rationalistic religion, and Advaita – the non-duality, the Oneness, the idea of Impersonal God, – is the only religion that can have any hold on any intellectual people. It comes whenever religion seems to disappear and irreligion seems to prevail, and that is why it has taken ground in Europe and America."

1896 (B): In telling of his experience at the Parliament of Religions, **SWAMI VIVEKANANDA** said to **Sister Christine** (an American disciple):

"I had never given a lecture before. True I had spoken to small groups of people sitting around me, but in an informal way, usually only answering questions. Moreover, I had not written out any speech as the others had done. I called upon my Master, and upon Saraswati, giver of '*vak*' and stood upon my feet. I began: 'Sisters and Brothers of America', – but I got no further. I was stopped by thunders of applause."

"It seems", writes Sister Christine, "the audience broke all bonds. He described the emotions which, this amazing reception stirred in him – the thrill amounting to awe. He felt as never before the power behind him. From that time not a shadow of doubt assailed his mind as to his commission from on high. He was the pioneer, the first preacher of

Vedanta. His spirituality caused astonishment. People began to ask, 'Why send missionaries to a country which produced men like this?'

1896 (C): SWAMI VIVEKANANDA'S lectures were published in the book form, for the first time.

Karma Yoga was published in New York, in February. Earlier *Raja Yoga* was published in July 1895. *Bhakti Yoga* which was originally published serially in *Brahmavadin* was printed as book in Madras. *Jnana Yoga,* containing the lectures delivered in London, was published from America.

1896 (D): Janab R. M. Sayani delivered the presidential address at the 12th session of the **Indian National Congress** at Allahabad.

Summing up the psychology of Mussalmans he said: "Before the advent of the British in India, the Mussalmans were the true rulers of the country. Mussalmans had therefore all the advantages appertaining to it as the ruling class. The sovereigns and the chiefs were their co-religionists, and so were the great landlords and great officials. The court language was their own. Every place of trust and responsibility or carrying influence and high emoluments was by birthright theirs. The Hindus did occupy some position, but the Hindus were tenants-at-will of the Mussalmans. The Hindus stood in awe of them. Enjoyment and influence and all good things of the world were theirs.... By a stroke of misfortune, the Musalmans had to abdicate their position and descend to the level of their Hindu fellow-countrymen. The Hindus, from a subservient state came into land, offices and other worldly advantages of their former masters. The Mussalmans would have nothing to do with anything in which they might have to come into contact with the Hindus." (*History and Culture of the Indian* People, Vol. X, p. 296-297).

1896 (E): 'Indian Educational Services', was created by the Government of India.

This was an All-India Service, and the candidates were recruited in England by the Secretary of State for India and was given a handsome scale of pay. Consequently, most of the posts in the service were held by Englishmen, although it was theoretically open to Indians to go to England and seek entrance to it in open competition. Its avowed purpose was to attract capable persons from England to work in India.

1896 (F): The Olympic Games were revived after a very long interval, more than two and half millennia, after the first one held c.776 B. C.

The original games were held amid the mountains of north-western Asia in the sacred city Olympia in Greece, taking place every fifth year at the full moon after the summer solistice. But since A. D. 394, they had not been held. It was through the efforts of **Baron Pierre de Courbetin** (1863-1937), a Greek nationalist and a brilliant French scholar that the olympic games were revived. Courbetin felt that nothing but good could result if amateur athletes from throughout the world were to meet once every four years. For the first cycle of the game, a new marble stadium was specially constructed at Athens.

1896 (G): A **Trade Fair** – unusually large and imposing – was held at **Germany**. It provided an impressive demonstration of Germany's industrial greatness.

1896 (H): **Almroth Edward Wright** (1861-1947), British pathologist, discovered the system of **inoculation against typhoid.**

1896 (I): E. A. **Demarcay** (1852-1904), French chemist, discovered a new rare-earth element **Europium.**

1896 (J): **Antoine Henri Becquerel** (1852-1908), French physicist, discovered **natural radioactivity** in uranium compounds.

In 1903 he was awarded a Nobel Prize jointly with Marie and Pierre Currie.

1896 (K): **The Hayness-Duryea Motor Car** produced by the Duryea Motor Wagon Company of Springfield, Mass., was **the first U. S. motor car to be offered for public sale.**

The British-Leyland had its beginnings in the Leyland Motors firm founded at the town of Leyland in Lancashire. The first vertiele four-cylinder motor car engine was introduced by France's Panhard and Lavassor, which also introduced sliding gears with a cone clutch.

1896 (L): **Aviation** was pioncered by U. S. astronomer **Samuel Pierpont Langley** 62, of Smithsonian Institution at Washington D. C. Langley sent a steam-powered model airplane on a 3000 ft. flight along the Potomac (May 6). It was the first flight of a mechanically propelled flying machine, and he sent an improved model on a 4,200 ft. flight in November.

1896 (M): Birth of **Ma Anandamayi** (d.1982) who occupied a unique position in the spiritual milieu of India.

A mystic sage who had got at the heart of things, Ma Anandamayi travelled widely and set up Ashrams all over the country.

1896 (N): For the first time **Leo Tolstoy** noted in his diary that he had read "a charming book on Indian wisdom" which had been sent to him. This was a series of lectures on ancient Indian philosophy delivered by **SWAMI VIVEKANANDA** in New York in the winter of 1895-96.

A. K. Datt, the Indian scholar, who sent to Tolstoy this book, wrote to him: "You will be pleased to know that your doctrines are in complete agreement with the Indian philosophy at the period of its highest achievement, the most ancient to reach us." The name of the book is *The Philosophy of Yoga* (*Raja Yoga*) by Swami Vivekananda, New York, 1896.

Tolstoy wrote in reply to this letter that he liked the book and he noted with approval the reasoning on what was man's 'self'.

The second book by Vivekananda which Tolstoy read was a collection of *Speeches and Articles* (in English) sent to him in 1907 by his acquaintance I. F. Nazhivin. When Nazhivin asked him whether he would like to have this book, Tolstoy replied on 7 July 1907: "Please send me the book by the Brahmin. The reading of such books is more than a pleasure, it is a broadening of the soul."

In 1908, I. F. Nazhivin published a collection of articles, *Voice of Peoples*, which included Vivekananda's articles '*The Hymn of the Peoples*' and '*God and Man*'. The latter article made a strong impression on Tolstoy. "This is unusually good", he wrote to Nazhivin, after reading it.

In March 1909, preparing a list of new popular books for the people, Tolstoy also included in the plan of publication '*The Sayings of Ramakrishna and Vivekananda*', and, in April of the same year, he informed the Orientalist N. O. Einhorn: "We are preparing a publication of selected thoughts of Vivekananda whom I appreciate very much." But this publication did not materialize.

Alexander Shifman wrote: "Among the Indian Philosophers of medieval period he (Tolstoy) studied more thoroughly Shankara and , among the more recent, Ramakrishna Paramahamsa and his pupil Swami Vivekananda.... During his last years Tolstoy did not concern himself with Ramakrishna except selecting from his works passages for the inclusion in his new collections of ancient sayings which he had compiled previously. At this time he was considerably more interested in Vivekananda's teachings...." [see 1894 (e) and 1896 Feb.]

1896-97: Famine all over India cost 4.5 million lives.

The famine was caused by failure of rains, and affected in varying degrees, the North-Western provinces and Awadh, Bihar, the Central Provinces, Madras and Bombay; the area in which sufferings of the people were extreme extending over 125,000 square miles with a population of thirty-four millions. [see 1866-67, 1868-69, 1873 (b), 1874 (a), 1876-78, 1877 Jan. 1, 1878 (b), 1897 Jan. 13, 1897 May 16, 1899-1900]

1897 JAN. (first week): During his sea-voyage back to India, **SWAMI VIVEKANANDA** humbled two Christian missionaries who abused Hinduism.

The ship in which Swami Vivekananda left England on 16 December 1896, had passed through Naples (30 December) and Suez Canal. In the same ship there were two Christian *padres* (missionaries) who, in season and out of season, insisted on having conversation with him. They had only one topic, the relative merits of Hinduism and Christianity, and the superiority of the latter. They were beaten on every point and then they became violent and abusive. The Swami stood it so long as possible but one day, they passed the limits of ordinary decency, whereupon he suddenly walked close to one of them, seized him quietly and firmly by the collar, and said, half humorously and half grimly, "If you abuse my religion again, I will throw you overboard." The man shook in his boots in fright and said "Let me go, sir, I shall never do it again." During the rest of the journey, he and his friend behaved like gentlemen.

Later narrating this story to Priyanath Sinha, a friend of his boyhood, the Swami asked, "If a man insulted your mother what would you do?" "I shall fall upon him and teach him a lesson", Sinha replied. The Swami said, "I wish you had the same positive feeling for the true mother of our country – our religion. Every day the Christian missionaries are abusing Hinduism to your faces and your brothers are being converted into Christianity. How can you bear to see all this? Where is your faith? Where is your patriotism?" (*A Comprehensive Biography of Swami Vivekananda*, Vol. II, p. 855).

1897 JAN. 11: Referring to the first of a series of lectures by **Swami Saradananda,** a brother disciple of **SWAMI VIVEKANANDA**, *The New York Tribune* said:

"Swami Vivekananda, the delegate from India to the Parliament of Religions in Chicago, who taught the principles of the Vedanta philosophy for two years in this city, recently returned to India, and is now succeeded by another teacher of the same faith, the Swami Saradananda. This new teacher delivered his first Sunday discourse in the New Century Hall, No. 509, Fifth Ave., yesterday morning on the general subject of the Vedanta philosophy....

"The Swami Saradananda is about twenty-eight years old, a *sannyasin*, or teacher, who renounces all property and accepts no pay. He had the classic features characteristic of his countrymen, is above medium height, with fine shoulders and chest. He speaks English well. There are free classes on Monday, Wednesday and Friday evenings, and he will also speak next Sunday evening in the same hall." (*The Brahmavadin*, March, 1897).

1897 JAN. 12: Death of **Sir Isaac Pitman** (b. 1813) founder of the Pitman System of Shorthand.

1897 JAN. 13: Famine Relief Fund was organized at Calcutta.

Periodic recurrence of famine was one of the toughest rural problems of the time. The government was seriously concerned, and after years of experimentation evolved a policy which was embodied in the **Famine Code.** It recommended the creation of a special fund for providing relief and employment in the famine affected areas. It also urged the full utilization of railway facilities for the transportation of grains from unaffected areas. [see 1866-67, 1868-69, 1873 (b), 1874 (a), 1876-78, 1877 Jan. 1, 1878 (b), 1896-97, 1897 May 16, 1899-1900]

1897 JAN. 15: SWAMI VIVEKANANDA arrived at Colombo after his three and half years spiritual ministry in the West. He had been successful in planting the seeds of India's spiritual ideas in the very heart of the English-speaking world – in New York and London.

At Colombo Port Swamiji was greeted with deafening jubilant cheers from the seething mass of humanity that had gathered at the quays. A big multitude rushed towards him to touch his holy feet. He was profusely garlanded and taken in a huge procession like a great victor to the accompaniment of an Indian band playing select airs through the thoroughfare bedecked with triumphal arches and festoons and strewn with flowers. A reception function was held. The Hon. Mr. P. C. Coomaraswamy, Member of Legislative Council of Ceylon, garlanded Swamiji and bowed to him in oriental fashion and read an address of welcome which was responded to by the Swami in a most eloquent and impressive speech.

The welcome address expressed thankfulness to Swamiji for his true exposition of the truths contained in India's sacred books, thus disabusing the minds of Westerners of their prejudices and bringing home to his fellow countrymen the value of their glorious heritage. The address also expressed thankfulness in particular for having drawn the attention of the West to the characteristic Hindu ideal of a Universal Religion, and above all, best wishes for the success of the great movement initiated by him for the propagation and revival of Indian religion and philosophy. References were also made to the success achieved by the Swami as the result of having proved the capacity of Hinduism to provide a basis for a Universal Religion, in bringing the West and the East nearer to each other and thus even paving the path for human brotherhood.

In the course of his reply, the Swami disclaimed any personal character in the welcome he had received, and pointed out that it had been acccorded not to a great politician, or to a great soldier, or to a millionaire, but to a begging *sannyasin*. This, said he, was possible only in India, and there because Indians considered religion in India to have the highest value in life. He concluded by urging them to make religion the backbone of their lives. Those who listened to the Swami were so captivated that they hung on outside the bungalow which he entered after his speech and dispersed only after he came out and after the manner of *sannyasins* saluted them and blessed them.

1897 JAN. 16: SWAMI VIVEKANANDA delivered his first public lecture in the East (at Colombo), the theme of which was *India – The Punyabhoomi.*

He began with saying that if there was a land on earth which could lay claim to be the blessed *Punyabhoomi,* it was India. He asserted, "Hence have proceeded the tidal waves of philosophy that have covered the earth, East or West, North or South, and hence again must start the wave which is going to spiritualize the material civilization of the West." The vastness of scholarship, the loftiness of thought, the command of the English language and the eloquence of the great Swami thrilled the listeners.

From Colombo in Sri Lanka, in the far South, to Almora in the Himalayas, in the far North, Swami Vivekananda burst forth like a spiritual avalanche, giving a stirring message of 'Man-making' and 'Nation-building' to his people, in a series of lectures which created a great national awakening. His main theme was the awakening of the Indian humanity and strengthening it to meet the modern challenges, and utilize the vast opportunities of the modern age to evolve a truly humanist social order. The real renaissance began in India after this. A new wave of nationalism swept over Bengal and Maharashtra. The most significant feature of this nationalism was an intense love of the Motherland, based on a conception of its past greatness and future potentialities.

1897 JAN. 21: Referring to the grand success of **SWAMI VIVEKANANDA** in the West *The Indian Mirror* editorial said:

"....He has raised the Hindu Nation in the estimation of the Western World, and has created for the Hindu faith an interest, which would last through all times. It is impossible to over-estimate the value of his service in America to the cause of Hinduism. Hundreds of men and women have enlisted themselves under the standard, which he unfolded in America and some of them have even taken to the bowl and the yellow-robes. The work, that he had to do, speedily assumed such proportions as to necessitate despatch of fresh re-inforcements from India to keep it alive in America.... The classes, opened in several places in America, and even in England, for the teaching of Hinduism in its

purer form, are a sufficient token of the leaning towards Vedantism, which
the West has begun to manifest under the inspiring and soul-stirring
eloquence of Swami Vivekananda.... He made a tour of almost all the
principal places in the United States, and wherever he went, he won
fresh converts to his faith, and left behind him a lasting impression of
his visit. The charming presence, the impassioned eloquence, the
extraordinary strength of will, and tenacity of purpose that he brought
to bear upon the work, which took him to America, carried conviction
everywhere. It was, indeed, a sight to see this eloquent, sannyasin
preaching the religion of his fathers in regions, which send missionaries
to India to convert the Hindus into the Christian faith. The tide of
conversion seemed to have rolled back from the East to the West – the
tables were completely turned – and the Hindu mission in the West
was crowned with a greater and more glorious success than what has
ever been vouchsafed to Christian missions in the East.... It was
reserved for a native of Hindustan to sow in the East the seeds of the
religion, bequeathed to him as a priceless legacy by his noble ancestors,
whose benefit he wanted the entire world to share.... And all this has
been effected within the short space of three years. Where is the Hindu,
who cannot help a feeling of pride at this unique record, and who does
not long to clasp Vivekananda in a close and fervid embrace. He
deserves well of his brethren in the faith, for he has rendered yeoman's
service to the cause, which is so dear and near to their hearts... We
cannot yet understand the far-reaching consequences of the work, which
Vivekananda has achieved. The gift of the Seer has not been vouchsafed
to us, and the inspiration of prophecy is not yet one of our
acquirements. But if the present be the best prophet of the future, "if
coming events cast their shadows before," we may take it upon
ourselves to say that Vivekananda has forged the chain, which is to
bind the East and the West together – the golden chain of a common
sympathy, of a common humanity, and the common and universal
religion. Vedantism, as preached and inculcated by Swami Vivekananda,
is the bridge of love, which is to extend from the East right away to the
West, and make the two nations one in heart, one in spirit and one in
faith – a consummation so devoutly to be wished. Can humanity, then,
be ever too thankful to Vivekananda? Can his fellow countrymen be
ever too proud of him or be ever too grateful to him?"

1897 JAN. 23: Birth of **Subbash Chandra Bose** (d. 1945), Indian nationalist
leader, who organized and led the revolutionary Indian National Army in
the hope of emancipation of India from foreign domination.

As one of the foremost leaders of India's freedom struggle, Bose left
an indelible impress not merely on the history of modern India but on
the minds and hearts of the people of Asia.

1897 JAN. 26: The citizens of Pamban accorded **SWAMI VIVEKANANDA** a most cordial welcome, under a decorated *pandal.* The **Raja of Ramnad** added to this a brief personal welcome which was remarkable for its depth of feeling.

In his reply, the Swami pointed out that the backbone of Indian national life was neither politics nor military power, neither commercial supremacy nor mechanical genius, but religion and religion alone, and that the eyes of the whole world were now turned towards this land of India for spiritual food, and India must provide it for all the races. It was in India, he said, that the best ideal of mankind existed, and the Western savants were striving hard to understand this ideal enshrined in the Sanskrit literature and philosophy of India. A moral obligation therefore rested on the sons of this land to fully equip themselves for the work of enlightening the world on the problems of human existence. In conclusion Swamiji expressed his deep gratitude to His Highness, the Raja of Ramnad, who had first conceived the idea of going to Chicago, put it into his head and persistently urged him to accomplish it. Swamiji wanted at least half a dozen more such Rajas who would take real interest in their dear motherland and work for her amelioration in the spiritual line. The meeting over, the Swami was taken in a State-carriage drawn by the Raja himself along with other people in a big procession.

1897 JAN. 27: **SWAMI VIVEKANANDA** who paid a visit to the great temple of Rameswaram, delivered on request, a stirring address on the true significance of a *tirtha,* and of worship, charging the eager listeners and through them all his co-religionists to worship Shiva by seeing Him not in images alone, but in the poor, in the weak and in the diseased.

"This is the gist of all worship" pointed out the Swami, "to be pure and to do good to others. He who sees Shiva in the poor, in the weak and in the diseased, really worships Shiva: and if he sees Shiva only in the image, his worship is but preliminary. He who has served and helped one poor man, seeing Shiva in him, without thinking of his caste, or creed, or race, or anything, with him Shiva is more pleased than with the man who sees Him only in temples."

The Raja of Ramnad was beside himself with the great spirit of the occasion, and the very day fed and clothed thousands of poor people at Ramnad after the Swami arrived there. And in commemoration of this great occasion, the Raja erected a monument of victory, forty feet in height, bearing the following inscription: *"Satyameva Jayate.* The monument erected by Bhaskara Sethupathi, the Raja of Ramnad, marks the sacred spot, where His Holiness Swami Vivekananda's blessed feet first trod on Indian soil, together with the Swami's English disciples, on His Holiness' return from the Western hemisphere, where glorious and

unprecedented success attended His Holiness' philanthropic labours
to spread the religion of the Vedanta. January, 27, 1897"

1897 JAN. 29: In reply to the address of welcome presented by the **Raja
of Ramnad, SWAMI VIVEKANANDA** made a speech, which was
characterized by beauty of thought and inspiring eloquence; these, in
conjunction with the power of his personality roused the people to intense
enthusiasm for their religion and the ideal of their national life and their
duty to their motherland.

> The very opening sentence of his speech was captivating: "The long
> night seems to be passing away, the sorest trouble seems to be coming
> to an end at last, the seeming corpse appears to be awakening, and a
> voice is coming to us – away back where history and even tradition
> fails to peep into the gloom of the past, coming down from there,
> reflected as it were from peak to peak of the infinite Himalaya of
> knowledge, and of love, and of work, India, this motherland of ours – a
> voice is coming unto us, gentle, firm and yet unmistakable in its
> utterances and is gaining volume as days pass by, and behold, the
> sleeper is awakening: Like a breeze from the Himalayas, it is bringing
> life into the almost dead bones and muscles, the lethargy is passing
> away, and only the blind cannot see, or the perverted will not see, that
> she is awakening, this motherland of ours, from her deep long sleep.
> None can resist her any more; never is she going to sleep any more; no
> outward powers can hold her back any more; for the infinite giant is
> rising to her feet!"

> The Swami exhorted the audience in the following terms: "Let us all
> work hard, my brethren; this is no time for sleep. On our work depends
> the coming of the India of the future. She is only sleeping. Arise, and
> awake and see her seated here, on her eternal throne, rejuvenated more
> glorious than she ever was – this motherland of ours.'ʲ

This awakening led, within less than a decade, to political awakening
and the initiation of the people's struggle for political freedom. It started
with the *swadeshi* agitation in Bengal in 1905, passed through the
violent anarchist revolutionary movement thereafter and culminated in
the non-violent mass Gandhian *satyagraha* and 'Quit India' Movement
from 1920 to 1947 (*Swami Vivekananda–His Humanism,* p. 32).

1897 JAN. 30: The *Chicago Tribune* in reviewing **SWAMI
VIVEKANANDA'S** *Lectures on Raja Yoga* said as follows:

> "There is something delightfully refreshing in listening to the
> philosophy of the East. We have so long been accustomed to send out
> missionaries to convert the poor, ignorant Hindu that the idea of

reversing the situation and taking the Hindu as our teacher brings a mental shock which is most invigorating....

"Without any personal knowledge of the Swami, who was such a familiar figure in the Congress of Religions at the time of the World's Fair, without caring to inquire whether he came with due credentials from his home in the East, or whether he had a right to speak in the name of the great religion of the East, I can only say that a perusal of the modest volume lately published by him upon the philosophy of the *Raja Yoga* is calculated to open the eyes of pharisees and fanatics who set themselves upon a plane of thought far above that of the native of India. Indeed, there are thousands of those who profess and call themselves Christians who have never in their highest and best moments attained the level of universal tolerance which is the starting point of all Vivekananda's teaching. It would be impossible here to go into the details of the original *Raja Yoga*, nor would we find there the true essence of what its interpreter has to say. Vivekananda has attempted to apply the advanced ideas of Western philosophy to the old beliefs of the Brahmin religion, and although he might not admit it himself, he has read as much into the old forms as any commentator ever read into Shakespeare. But he has this in his favour; he is able to look upon Western thought and Western creeds from an outsider's point of view. He has criticized us fairly and truly, just as we may criticise Hinduism; only he has shown greater impartiality than any Christian would employ in judging the effete East. And this, perhaps, is one of the great advantages of brahminism, that it is universally tolerant. It has kept its hold upon millions of people of very diverse habitation and intelligence simply because it embraces everything that runs counter with it. Indeed it would embrace Christianity if we were only willing that it should be so.

"Life is wonderfully simple. One efficient energy or Spirit permeates all that exists. A few universal habits or laws characterise this energy in all phases of its infinitely varied manifestation. To feel this Spirit as a living reality within, to understand these simple laws and reduce life to wise obedience to them without, this it is to possess such peace, such happiness, and such power of doing good as the world in general knows not of. The entire secret could be told in a few words; that is so far as this great inner joy can be described by human speech. To cease the restless activity and pursuit which causes the unhappiness of finite life, and recognize that which is eternally with us, is in a word the method whereby the great secret may be learned." (*Brahmavadin*)

1897 FEB. 1: In the course of his reply to the address of welcome presented by the citizens of Paramakudi (near Ramad), **SWAMI VIVEKANANDA** pointed out in the clearest tones the dangers facing the West.

"The whole of Western Civilization", he predicted "will crumble to pieces in the next fifty years if there is no spiritual foundation. It is hopeless and perfectly useless to attempt to govern mankind with the sword. You will find that the very centre from which such ideas as 'Government by Force' sprang up are the very centres to degrade and degenerate and crumble to pieces. Europe, the centre of the manifestation of material energy, will crumble into dust within fifty years if she is not mindful to change her position, to shift her ground, and make spirituality the basis of her life. And what will save Europe is the religion of the Upanishads."

Since Swami Vivekananda uttered the warning the West has experienced two world wars the second more shattering than the first, with recurring political and economic crises in between. The end of the second world war found Europe disillusioned and at the end of its tether.

1897 FEB. 4: *The Madras Mail* reported about the arrival of **SWAMI VIVEKANANDA** to India:

"As soon as the vessel containing Sri Swami Vivekananda was sighted, the Sethupathi's joy knew no bounds. The Swami was received with every mark of respect by the Sethupathi (Rajah of Ramnad) who prostrated himself before him and placed him on a throne-like seat in a boat well decorated for the occasion.... The Sethupathi came flying from Ramnad to welcome the Swami thinking of nothing else but him. Putting sandals at the feet of the Swami, the Sethupathi expressd that he deemed it a highest honour and privilege to have been in a position to do this than to wear the richest diadem on his head. How noble and sublime this sentiment! In Pamban the carriage in which the Swami took his seat was drawn by the Sethupathi and his staff from the landing place to the Rajah's bungalow, a distance of nearly a mile."

1897 FEB. 6: **SWAMI VIVEKANANDA** was interviewed by the representative of *The Madras Mail*. He met the Swami in the train at Chenglepet Railway Station and travelled with him to Madras. The following is an extract from the report of the interview published in *The Madras Mail* of date:

"What was your first experience of America, Swamiji?"

"From first to last it was very good. With the exception of the Missionaries and 'Church Women', the Americans are most hospitable, kind hearted, generous and good natured."

"Who are these 'Church Women' that you speak, Swamiji?"

"When a woman tries her best to find a husband she goes to all the bathing places imaginable and tries all sorts of tricks to catch a man. When she fails in her attempts, she becomes what they call in America an 'old maid' and joins the Church. Some of them become very 'Churchy'. These 'Church Women' are awful fanatics. They are under the thumb of the priests there. Between them and the priests they make a hell of earth; and make a mess of religion. With the exception of these the Americans are very good people. They loved me so much: I love them a great deal. I felt as if I was one of them."

"What is your idea about the results of the Parliament of Religions?"

"The Parliament of Religions, as it seems to me, was intended for a 'heathen show' before the world; but it turned out that the heathens had the upper hand, and made it a 'Christian Show' all round; so the Parliament of Religions was a failure from the Christian standpoint. Seeing that, the Roman Catholics, who were the organizers of that Parliament, are, when there is a talk of another Parliament at Paris, now steadily opposing it. But the Chicago Parliament was a tremendous success for India and Indian thought. It helped on the tide of Vedanta which is flooding the world. The American people, of course, – minus. the fanatical priests and 'Church Women', – are only very glad of the results of the Parliament.

"What prospects have you, Swamiji, for the spread of your mission in England"

"There is every prospect. Before ten years elapse vast majority of the English people will be Vedantins. There is a greater prospect of this in England than there is in America. You see Americans make a fanfaronade of everything, which is not the case with Englishman. Even Christians cannot understand their New Testament without understanding the Vedanta. Vedanta is the rationale of all religions. Without the Vedanta every religion is superstition, with it everything becomes religion."

1897 FEB. 6 (A): *The Madras Times* reported:

"For the past few weeks, the Hindu public of Madras have been most eagerly expecting the arrival of **SWAMI VIVEKANANDA**, the great Hindu monk of world-wide fame. At the present moment his name is on everybody's lips. In the school, in the college, in the High Court, on the Marina and in the streets and bazars of Madras, hundreds of inquisitive spirits may be seen asking when the Swami will be coming. Large number of students from the mofussil, who have come up for the University Examinations are staying here, awaiting the Swami, and increasing their hostelry bills, despite the urgent calls of their parents to return home immediately. In a few days the Swami will be in our midst.

"It was Madras that first recognized the superior merits of the Swami and equipped him for Chicago. Madras will now have again the honour of welcoming the undoubtedly great man who has done so much to raise the prestige of his motherland. Four years ago, when the Swami arrived here, he was practically an obscure individual....

"The mission of Swami Vivekananda is essentially spiritual. He firmly believes that India, the motherland of spirituality, has a great future before her. He is sanguine that the West will more and more come to appreciate what he regards as the sublime truths of the Vedanta. His great motto is 'Help, and not Fight', 'Assimilation; and not Destruction', 'Harmony and peace, and not Dissension'. Whatever difference of opinion followers of other creeds may have with him, few will venture to deny that the Swami has done yeoman's service to his country in opening the eyes of the Western world to 'the good in the Hindu'. He will always be remembered as the first Hindu *sannyasin* who dared to cross the sea to carry to the West the message of what he believes in as a religious peace."

In the course of an interview Swami Vivekananda told the representative of *The Madras Times*:

"I have visited a good deal of Europe, including Germany and France, but England and America were the chief centres of my work. At first I found myself in a critical position, owing to the hostile attitude assumed against the people of this country by those who went there from India. I believe the Indian nation is by far the most moral and religious nation in the world and it would be a blasphemy to compare the Hindus with any other nation. At first, many fell foul of me, manufactured huge lies against me by saying that I was a fraud, that I had a harem of wives and half a regiment of children. But my experience of these missionaries opened my eyes as to what they are capable of doing in the name of religion. Missionaries were nowhere in England. None came to fight me. Mr. Lund went over to America to abuse me behind my back, but people would not listen to him. I was very popular with them. When I came back to England, I thought this missionary would be at me, but Truth silenced him. In England the social status is stricter than caste is in India. The English church people are all gentlemen born, which many of the missionaries are not...."

"A great number of people sympathised with me in America – much more than in England. Vituperation by the low-caste missionaries made my cause succeed better. I had no money, the people of India having given me my bare passage-money, which was spent in a very short time. I had to live just as here on the charity of individuals. The Americans are a very hospitable people. In America one-third of the people are Christians, but the rest have no religion, that is, they do not belong to any of the sects, but amongst them are to be found the most spiritual persons...." (*The Indian Mirror*)

1897 FEB. 6 (B): After his triumphant march through the West for four years, **SWAMI VIVEKANANDA** returned to India via Colombo etc. to Madras.

He arrived in Colombo on January 15, 1897. From there he went to Jaffna and set foot on the Indian soil at Pamban, where a delighted Raja of Ramnad gave him a rousing reception (see 1897 Jan. 26). He arrived in Madras after a victorious tour via Paramakudi, Madurai, Sivaganga and Kumbakonam. All through, jubilant crowds had given him rousing receptions and showed their pride and happiness and Madras was no exception.

On his arrival Swamiji was accorded a grand reception by the citizens of Madras. In the words of a devotee who had witnessed the reception: "Along with a friend of mine, I had gone to see the colourful procession in honour of the great Swami, starting from Egmore Railway Station and proceeding towards the Ice House at Triplicane beach. We climbed up a roadside tree, to have a glance at the Swami seated in a horse carriage, along with Swamis Niranjanananda, Saradananda, and Sri J. J. Goodwin – Swamiji's stenorgrapher. The carriage was being drawn manually in the place of horses. There was a unique charm in Swamiji's countenance. We were amazed to behold a halo of golden hue shining around Swami's divine face. This scene, I could never forget in my life. When the procession reached the destination viz. the 'Ice House', a huge public meeting in honour of Swamiji was held there in a specially erected pandal in front of the 'Ice House.' "

C. Rajagopalachari reminized: "I was a law student living in Castle Kernan on the Madras beach, when Swami Vivekananda arrived from Chicago in 1897, after becoming world famous by then. He stayed for nine days in Castle Kernan then, and I look back to those days with pride and joy. *Prabhudha Bharata* was started then and Madras was thrilled by Swamiji's lectures. Hinduism arose from the grave as Jesus did."

Indian Mirror published a report on 6. 2. 1897: "Castle Kernan, where Swami Vivekananda is lodged, presented a picturesque scene on Saturday evening. The castle itself is beautifully decorated and fitted up for the reception of the Swami and party. Two magnificent *pandals* have been put up, one at the entrance, which is purely ornamental, and another in the compound, which serves the purpose of the meeting hall, where the Swami patiently undergoes the severe cross examination to which he is subjected to on the technicalities and subtleties of Vedanta. A large number of gentlemen waited upon the Swami at the pandal that evening, when an acrostic poem in Sanskrit in honour of the Swami was read by Mr. R. Sivasankara Pandiaji. The Swami then offered to answer any questions that might be put to him."

A devotee reminisces: "Once he (Swamiji) was walking on the Marina Beach with my father and other friends and was challenged as a bachelor to wrestle with a *pahilwan*. Swamiji accepted the challenge and defeated him on the sands of the Triplicane Beach."

Swamiji loved to walk on the Marina beach in the evenings. It is said that once while he was in the beach, he saw a disembodied being drawing his attention to its miserable plight and sought his help to be free. Swamiji who took pity on it, sincerely prayed and as a result it got liberated and disappeared.

Swamiji stayed at the bungalow ('Ice House') on the beach near Triplicane in Madras for 9 days (Feb. 6 to 14). During his stay there, he delivered seven electrifying lectures revealing his plan of campaign to restore India to her pristine glory. (These lectures are now available in *"Lectures From Colombo to Almora"*. The bungalow where Swamiji stayed is now renamed as *"Vivekanandar Illam"*. Given on lease to the Ramakrishna Math, and thoroughly renovated, it was thrown open to the public as a Museum of Vivekananda thought and literature on 20th December,1999).

On the eve of his departure for Calcutta, the devotees of Madras requested Swami Vivekananda to open a permanent centre. Swamiji readily agreed and deputed his brother disciple Swami Ramakrishnananda to initiate the Ramakrishnan Order's activities in South India. [see 1897 Mar. 17 and 1897 Apr.].

1897 FEB. 14: SWAMI VIVEKANANDA who had just returned from the West, delivered the fourth and last public lecture at Madras, the subject being *The Future of India.*

Over 3000 people attended the lecture. The very opening words of the address went deep into the hearts of all in the vast audience, which listened spell-bound till the very end. As remarked by a professor who attended the lecture: "The Swami's oratory was at its best. He seemed like a lion, traversing the platform to and fro. The roar of his voice reverberated everywhere and with telling effect."

In the course of his lecture Swamji exhorted the audience: "For the next fifty years, let this alone be your key-note – this great Mother India. Let all other vain gods disappear for the time from our minds. This is the only God that is awake, our own race – everywhere His hands, everywhere His feet, everywhere His ears, He covers everything."

Exactly fifty years hence, i.e., in 1947, India attained independence from the British rule thanks to the great sacrifices made by innumerable Indian patriots who loved India very dearly as their 'Motherland'. The life and precepts of Swami Vivekananda and his triumphant tour in the United States, not only raised the prestige of India abroad but also exerted a potent influence on the Indians, thus quickening the sense of national pride and patriotism among them.

1897 FEB. 23: In a letter to the Editor of *The Indian Mirror,* a reader wrote:

"I would respectfully suggest to those Hindus, who sincerely wish that their religion should occupy the foremost place among the world's religions, to accord their fullest support to **SWAMI VIVEKANANDA,** who is unquestionably the greatest Hindu teacher this age has produced. He has evoked an enthusiasm, the like of which has not been witnessed for centuries, and it only requires support from the good and enlightened, even by a denial of their own superior abilities, to ensure a triumph of this great cause. Differences of opinion should not induce one to denounce his noble work, and impede it....

1897 FEB. 28: A public reception was given to **SWAMI VIVEKANANDA** by the citizens of Calcutta. The meeting was attended by about five thousand people including Rajas and scholars, illustrious citizens and hundreds of college students. The address of welcome was presented in a silver casket in an atmosphere of profound solemnity. The Swami was introduced by the President as the foremost national figure in the life of India.

Swamiji in reply gratefully acknowledged, the honour the citizens of Calcutta had shown to him on the occasion and expressed his heartfelt thanks for the recognition they had given to the humble services rendered by him to the humanity ar large. He made a specific mention of Sri Ramakrishna Paramahamsa – his teacher, master, hero, ideal and good in life, whose spirit was wholly responsible for his phenomenal success in the foreign lands. He spoke about the power that had come out of his Master's advent, which within ten years of his passing away had encircled the globe, and more wonderful manifestation of which would be seen before this generation passed away. He hit off the weakness of the modern Hindus and asked them to know their latent strength and become strong. We must conquer the world, he said, not by force of physical arms, but by spiritual forces, which are irresistible. Swamiji closed his address with a fervent appeal to the people of Bengal, specially the youth of the province. The inspired speech of Swamiji sent a thrill through the entire audience.

With the roll of years the explosive ideas articulated through this lecture began to electrify the young generation with a new hope and courage which eventually ushered in a New Order in the eventful annals of modern India.

1897 FEB. : *The Indian Social Reformer* wrote:

"Occultism, to our mind, has always appeared to be nothing but the deification of the underhand. And we quite agree with the learned Swami, in thinking that this hungering and thirsting after the underhand and the round-about, have had much to do with the deterioration of our vitality, morally and religiously as well as politically.... Without further preface we make room for **SWAMI VIVEKANANDA'S** letter (to the Editor of the *'East and the West'*), the trenchant indignation of which will no doubt be appreciated by our readers.

" I must frankly state," writes the Swami "that, in my lifelong experience in the work, I have always found 'occultism' injurious and weakening to humanity. What we want is strength. We, Indians, more than any other race, want strong and vigorous thought. We have enough of the superfine in all concerns. For centuries, we have been stuffed with the mysterious, the result is that our intellectual and spiritual digestion is almost hopelessly impaired and the race has been dragged down to the depths of hopeless imbecility never before or since experienced by any other civilized community. There must be freshness and vigour of thought behind, to make a virile race. More than enough to strengthen the whole world exist in the 'Upanishads'. The Advaita is the eternal mine of strength. But it requires to be 'applied'. It must first be cleared of the incrustation of scholasticism, and then in all its simplicity, beauty, and sublimity be taught over the length and breadth of the land as applied even to the minutest detail of daily life. 'This is a very large order' but we must work towards it nevertheless as it should be accomplished tomorrow. Of one thing I am sure that whoever wants to help his fellow-beings through genuine love and un-selfishness will work wonders."

1897 MAR. 8: *The Indian Nation* wrote:

"**SWAMI VIVEKANANDA** left India a pauper and returned a prince. We refer not to material resources but to popular esteem. He left his motherland a poor, unnoticed 'Calcutta boy'. He went to America, no one can say why. The Parliament of Religions was held in Chicago, nobody knows why. He was permitted to attend, nobody can say how. In that far-off town, however, he rose one morning and found himself famous. Destiny works through accidents, and in the present instance quite a number of them contributed to the distinction of the Swami and shaped his ends. The Shobhabazar meeting at which the address was presented to him was one of monstrous proportions.... The Swami delivered a lecture on Vedantism on Thursday at the Star Theatre. He is not able to deliver a series of discourses, however, for he stands in need of rest. He goes to Darjeeling at once, returns to Calcutta after a few days, delivers one more lecture, and then proceeds up-country before quitting the country for a fresh tour in the West."

1897 MAR. 17: Swami **Ramakrishnanada**, brother disciple of **SWAMI VIVEKANANDA**, arrived in Madras with **Swami Sadananda**.

After a short stay of a few day at the "Flora Cottage", a building on the Ice House Road (now Dr. Besant Road), shifted to "Ice House" and established a shrine for Sri Ramakrishna there. Thus, the first branch of the Ramakrishna Math was started in Madras.

1897 APR. 5: *The Madras Standard* wrote:

"**Swami Ramakrishnananda**, the brother disciple of Swami Vivekananda, having been deputed by the latter to carry on his mission in Madras, arrived there last week from Calcutta and is putting up in Ice House Road, Triplicane. It is said that he is to open three classes in different centres of the city, one at Triplicane, one at Mylapore and another at Black Town, for imparting regular instructions in *Gita, Upanishads* and *Brahmasutras*." (*The Indian Nation*).

1897 May 1: SWAMI VIVEKANANDA founded the **Ramakrishna Mission** in Calcutta with the help of the monastic and lay disciples of Sri Ramakrishna.

The aims and ideals of the mission propounded by the Swami were purely spiritual and humanitarian:

(a) to bring into existence a band of sannyasins devoted to a life of renunciation and practical spirituality, from among whom qualified teachers and workers could be sent out to spread universal message of Vedanta as illustrated in the life of Sri Ramakrishna;

(b) to carry on educational, philanthropic and social service work, in co-operation with lay members, looking upon all men, women and children, irrespective of caste, creed or colour, as veritable manifestation of the Divine.

1897 MAY 16: Referring to the noble work which **Swami Akhandananda**, a direct disciple of Sri Ramakrishna, has been doing for the relief of the famine stricken people in some places near Moorshidabad, Swami Nityananda, writes in a letter to the Editor of *The Brahmavadin*:

"Coming to help Swami Akhandananda on Friday, the heart-rending sights which I saw everywhere around me are simply beyond description. When the ragged men and women in every village come to us, and narrate their trouble, no man can remain unmoved to bear them. The husband of a certain woman, leaving his wife and children to their fate, has run away to save his own life from starvation. Another has hanged himself, being unable to see the extreme pains of his hungry wife and children. We are supplying the helpless wife and her children with rice. Two other men oppressed with hunger as well as disease, were going to commit suicide but timely help from us has prevented them from fulfilling their fatal intention. The majority of the people are simply living upon a little quantity of boiled pulse and pot-herb, but these too even are now becoming rare. Along with starvation diseases have also come to increase the distress of the people. No one who is not present on the scene, can ever realize the extreme distress to which they have been put for want of medicine. We are distributing rice as much as our means can allow. The people are almost naked. Clothes are required to cover their nakedness. The number of men and women suffering from privations is daily increasing." [see 1866-67, 1868-69, 1873 (b), 1874 (a), 1876-78, 1877 Jan. 1, 1878 (b), 1896-97, 1897 Jan.13, 1899-1900]

1897 JUNE. 23: *The Indian Mirror* wrote:

"The Christian Missionaries rage and fume over the success of **SWAMI VIVEKANANDA'S mission in America**. In its impotent fury, the *Missionary Review of the World* says that 'Swami Vivekananda is simply a specimen of the elation and inflation of a weak man over the adulations of some silly people. If America ever gives up Christ, it will be for the devil, not Buddha or Brahma or Confucius. It will be a lapse into utter apostasy, unbelief, and infidelity'. The writer, when penning these lines, was evidently under a fit of insanity brought on by the unlooked for spectacle of a Hindu preacher making disciples among American members of the Christian church...."

1897 JUN: Communal riots at Calcutta, due to the following reason:

Maharaja Sir Jatindra Mohan Tagore obtained by a decree of the court a plot of land at Talla, just outside the northern limits of the city of Calcutta. There was a small hut on the piece of land which the Mohammedans claimed to be a mosque. So when the Tagore's party went to take possession of the land, a large number of Mohammedans gathered with a view to resisting the demolition of the hut. Though they were dispersed by the Police, a group of them attacked the Calcutta water works pumping station in the neighbourhood. This was a signal for a number of riots in different parts of Calcutta by detached parties of Mohammedans during the nights of 30th June and 1st July in the course of which the Police opened fire on several occasions. (Bharatiya Vidya Bhavan's *History and Culture of the Indian People,* Vol. X, Part II, p. 334). [see 1874 Feb 13, 1877 Sept, 1885 (a), 1889 (m), 1891 (b), 1893 (c).]

1897 AUG. 22: *The Indian Mirror* wrote:

"Under the title *From Colombo to Almora,* the Vyjayanti Press, Egmore, Madras, has published a record of **SWAMI VIVEKANANDA'S return to India,** after his mission to the West, including reports of seventeen lectures, delivered by him in different parts of India. With regard to the publication, we fully endorse the remarks, made by Miss F. Henrietta Muller, who in the prefatory note, says, 'All Eastern students, and still more, perhaps, those of England and America will welcome this book, containing as it does, the latest utterances of their much loved teacher, for the lectures exhibit to the Hindu the fervid patriotism of the 'Calcutta boy', and to the American and the English that larger patriotism, which counts the world as its home, and all the people in it, as fellow-countrymen'. As the only authorized edition of the lectures, the book is one of immense value, but the 'record' gives quite an inadequate idea of the enthusiasm, with which the Swami was greeted during his progress through this country. Full descriptions of the reception, which were accorded to him in different parts of India, would, we venture to think, have given the volume a better air of completeness."

1897 SEP. 10: SWAMI VIVEKANANDA at Kashmir (Srinagar) on tour.

He was warmer in his praise of Kashmir in a letter to a devotee. Said he, "This Kashmir is a veritable paradise on earth. Nowhere else in the world is such a country as this...." A few days before he left Srinagar, 1st October 1897, he wrote to Miss Noble, "I shall not try to describe Kashmir to you. Suffice it to say, I never felt sorry to leave any country except this paradise on earth." In one of his letters to his disciple Swami Suddhananda dated 15 September 1897, he said "It is the one land fit for yogis, to my mind."

At this time Kashmir was virtually a Muslim land – about 85% of the population professing Islam – but to him it remained nevertheless a part of the Holy Land of *Aryavarta,* its culture essentially Hindu in spite of many elements having entered into it. He was confirmed in this view when a few days later he visited some Hindu temples, among them a great Marthanda Sun temple which stands on an open plain with dazzling of the Pir Punja range to watch over it through centuries (*A Comprehensive Biography of Swami Vivekananda,* Vol. II, p. 998).

1897 NOV. 5-15: SWAMI VIVEKANANDA in Punjab, on tour.

On his arrival at Lahore, the Swami was accorded a grand reception by the leaders, both of the Arya Samaj and of the Sanatana Dhartna Sabha. During his brief stay in Lahore, Swamiji delivered three lectures. In the very first lecture ('*The Common Bases of Hinduism*'), in words of matchless eloquence as well as deep sincerity and earnestness, he expressed himself thus: "This is the land which is held to be the holiest even in holy *Aryavarta;* this is the *Brahmavarta* of which our great Manu speaks. This is the land from whence arose the mighty aspiration after the spirit, aye, which in times to come, as history shows, is to deluge the world. This is the land where like its mighty rivers, spiritual aspirations have arisen and joined their strength till they travelled over the length and breadth of the world and declared themselves with a voice of thunder. This is the land which had first to bear the brunt of all inroads and invasions into India; this heroic land had first to bare its bosom to every onslaught of the outer barbarians into *Aryavarta*.... Wave after wave of barbarian conquest has rolled over this devoted land of ours. "*Allah Ho Akbar*" has rent the skies for hundreds of years, and no Hindu knew what moment would be his last. This is the most suffering and the most subjugated of all the historic lands of the world. Yet we still stand practically the same race, ready to face difficulties again and again, if necessary...."

Swami Vivekananda came to the Punjab with his heart full not only of admiration for the valour of its people but of reverence for its hoary past. He, however, was not unaware of the realities of the present times – the facts that of the population of Punjab about 51 per cent were Muslims, that the 'valiant Sikhs' were a small minority of about 12 percent only and that in the matter of education the Punjab was one of the most backward of the provinces of British India. But he thought that the Punjabis, – Hindus, Muslims, Sikhs and others – were all a common culture which was predominantly Hindu and as such, like Kashmiris, belonged to *Aryavarta*. At the time of Swamiji's visit, the Punjab was a land of sectarian quarrels of which the one that was very prominent was the controversy between the exponents of *Sanatana Dharma*, the old unreformed Hinduism, and the Arya Samaj, a reforming party who, taking their stand on the Vedas and Vedas alone, denounced some tenets and practices of Hindu religion and society. Swamiji deplored the lack of emotion in the Punjabis, remarking that the land of the five rivers was rather a dry place spiritually. But that was exactly the chief reason why he had come to the Punjab, said he: It was to find out points of agreement, not of difference and to understand on what ground all could meet and always remain as brothers, "upon what foundation the voice that has spoken from eternity may become stronger and stronger as it grows." His eye, above all, was on the future, "March ahead, children of the Aryans" he exhorted.

It has been claimed that Swamiji's visit to the city did have the desired effect of establishing, even if it was for the time being, some harmony and peace among its fighting sects. It certainly induced the leaders of the sects to have some thinking, or rethinking on their respective positions concerning some issues, even though it is quite likely that this did not have any appreciable or permanent results.

In the meantime, the Muslim proselytisers, who had been taking since decades, full advantage of the disunity and weaknesses prevailing in the Hindu society, were briskly engaged in Islamizing the land of five rivers. And by 1900 the Indus Valley – once the cradle of Vedic culture and civilization, turned into the cradle of Islamic India, consequent on ram- pant mass conversions effected over a period of about fifty years. According to the UNESCO *History of Mankind,* "By about 1900 all the 'low caste' inhabitants of Punjab had been converted to Islam...." Narrating the background and the modus operandi adopted by the muslim zealots for Islamization of Punjab, the UNESCO publication says: "All clear-sighted Muslims were aware that once the English left, the Muslim territories would be divided from the Hindu provinces. They must therefore make plans to establish reunification on religious principles beginning with the Indus Valley, the cradle of Islamic India. Here arose the problem of the Punjab, with its capital, Lahore, where Hindus and Sikhs had settled in the late eighteenth century, when the Mongol power began to decline. The ruler of Afghanistan, Ahmed (1747-73) had fought them and his successor, Taimur (1773-93) had taken Lahore and Multan from them; but the internecine warfare that broke out in Afghanistan after the death of Zeman (1793-1800) had left the field free for the Hindus and their friends. The Muslim population was obliged to put itself on a footing of self-defence (1826) and to make a spiritual conquest of the Pubjab by a puritan revival on the Wahabi model. In any case, the military occupation of Punjab by the British as a result of the Anglo-Sikh War (1894), left no possiblity of armed attack, so that ogranization of missions was the muslims' only remaining hope of eliminating the Hindu religion from the Punjab. The weak point of the Hindu system being the division of the community into castes, the Muslims proceeded to convert the 'low castes', the unfortunate proletariat of every organized Hindu community. They met with a remarkable success. By about 1900 all the 'low caste' inhabitants of the Punjab had joined Islam, which constituted a far more brilliant and decisive victory than any in tournaments held by the Afghan and Baluchi chivalry and recorded by poets in their epics." [*History of Mankind– Cultural and Scientific Development* – Vol. V, Part IV, p. 1078 and 1079]

1897 NOV. 5: In the course of his lecture *'The Common Bases of Hinduism'* at Lahore, **SWAMI VIVEKANANDA** proclaimed:

"....We are Hindus. I do not use the word Hindu in any bad sense at all, nor do I agree with those that think there is any bad meaning in it. In old times, it simply meant people who lived on the other side of the Indus; today a good many among those who hate us may have put a bad interpretation upon it, but names are nothing. Upon us depends whether the name Hindu will stand for everything that is glorious, everything that is spiritual, or whether it will remain a name of opprobrium, one designating the downtrodden, the worthless, the heathen. If at present the word Hindu means anything bad, never mind; by our action let us be ready to show that this is the highest word that any language can invent. It has been one of the principles of my life not to be ashamed of my own ancestors. I am one of the proudest men ever born, but let me tell you frankly, it is not for myself, but on account of my ancestry. The more I have studied the past, the more I have looked back, more and more has this pride come to me, and it has given me the strength and courage of conviction, raised me up from the dust of the earth, and set me working out that great plan laid out by those great ancestors of ours. Children of those ancient Aryans, through the grace of the Lord, may you have the same pride, may that faith in your ancestors come into your blood, may it become a part and parcel of your lives, may it work towards the salvation of the world!

"When a man has begun to be ashamed of his ancestors, the end has come. Here am I, one of the least of the Hindu race, yet proud of my race, proud of my ancestors. I am proud to call myself a Hindu, I am proud that I am one of your unworthy servants. I am proud that I am a countryman of yours, you the descendants of the sages, you, the descendants of the most glorious *rishis* the world ever saw. Therefore have faith in yourselves, be proud of your ancestors, instead of being ashamed of them.

"Let them talk of India's regeneration as they like. Let me tell you as one who has been working – at least trying to work – all his life, that there is no regeneration for India until you be spiritual. Not only so, but upon it depends the welfare of the whole world....

"If a Hindu is not spiritual I do not call him a Hindu. In other countries a man may be political first, and then he may have a little religion, but here in India the first and the foremost duty of our lives is to be spiritual and then, if there is time, let other things come. Bearing this in mind, we shall be in a better position to understand why, for our national welfare, we must first seek out at the present day all the spiritual forces of the race, as was done in days of yore and will be done in all times to come.

National union in India must be a gathering up of its scattered spiritual forces. A nation in India must be a union of those whose hearts beat to the same spiritual tune."

1897 NOV. 12: SWAMI VIVEKANANDA at Lahore on tour, delivered his third lecture, the subject being Vedanta. It was a triumphant success and lasted for over two hours. According to Mr. Goodwin who had attended many lectures that the Swami had delivered in India and abroad, it was a masterly exposition of the monistic philosophy and religion of India.

While at Lahore, Swami Vivekananda met **Sri Tirtha Ram Goswami**, then a professor of Mathematics in one of the Lahore Colleges. It was under his guidance that the students of the college took a leading part in arranging for public lectures which the Swami delivered there. The Professor was captivated by Swamiji's lectures. He was particularly struck by Swamiji's eloquence during the discourse on Vedanta. He wrote about the lecture as follows: "This lasted for full two and half hours. The listeners were so deeply engrossed and it created such an atmosphere that all ideas of time and space were lost. At times one reached the stage of realization of absolute 'abheda' between ourself and the cosmic 'Atman'. It struck at the roots of ego and pride in self. In short, it was such a grand success as you come by once in a way."

The relation between the Swami and Tirtha Ram grew so intimate and cordial that the latter presented the Swami with a gold watch on the eve of his departure from there. Swamiji took the watch very kindly but put it back in Tirtha Ram's pocket, saying "very well, friend, I shall wear it here in this pocket". The prophetic utterances of Swamiji did not take much time to fructify. For some time later, Prof. Tirtha Ram renounced the world, and became widely known as Swami Ram Tirtha, and subsequently preached Vedanta, both in India and America.

1897 NOV. 24: In a letter to a Western friend, SWAMI VIVEKANANDA wrote from Almora:

"....I feel my task is done – at most three or four years more of life are left. I have lost all wish for my salvation. I never wanted earthly enjoyments. I must see my machine in strong working order, and then knowing sure that I have put in a lever for the good of humanity, in India at least, which no power can drive back, I will sleep, without caring what will be next, and may I be born again and again, and suffer thousands of miseries so that I may worship the only God that exists, the only God I believe in, the sum total of all souls – and, above all, my God the wicked, my God the miserable, my God the poor of all races, of all species, is the special object of my worship.

'My time is short. I have got to unbreast whatever I have to say, without caring if it smarts some or irritates others. Therefore do not be frightened at whatever drops from my lips, for the power behind me is not Vivekananda but He the Lord, and He knows best. If I have to please the world, that will be injuring the world; the voice of the majority is wrong, seeing that they govern and the sad state of the world. Every new thought must create opposition – in the civilized a polite sneer, in the vulgar savage howls and filthy scandals."

1897 (A): The British in India were celebrating the **Diamond jubilee of Queen Victoria's rule.**

The plague epidemic, then raging in many parts of Maharashtra, claimed thousands of lives. Patriotic people strongly felt that these grand celebrations were an insult to the motherland at that juncture. There was protest all over and feelings ran high and the fearless Chapekar brothers shot dead two British plague inspectors at Poona, and the brave lads were summarily tried and hanged.

The assassination at Poona and the subsequent trial and imprisonment of B. G. Tilak, marked the rise of the extremist school of nationalism, in Maharashtra and Bengal.

1897 (B): **Half tones** were printed for the first time on a power press and on newsprint. The *New York Tribune* employed techniques developed by **Frederick E. Ives** and **Stephen Horgan.**

1897 (C): **J. J. Thompson** (1856-1940), British physicist, announced the **discovery of electron,** the first subatomic particle; he also determined experimentally the ratio of its mass to its charge.

Thompson's discovery was the result of his investigation of the cathode- rays. Working at the Cavendish Laboratory, Cambridge, Thompson showed that cathode rays were charged particles, with a mass only a small fraction of that of hydrogen, the lightest atom known. He eventually called the particles "electrons", using the word proposed in 1891 by the Irish physicist G. J. Stoney (1826-1911) for a hypothetical unit of electric current. Thompson showed that the electron is the basic unit of electricity and that all atoms contain electrons; he demonstrated that electrons were universal constituents of matter and thereby founded the field of sub-atomic physics.

Thompson thus helped revolutionize the knowledge of atomic structure by his discovery. His work led to a much greater understanding of electric currents as the current is made up of a flow of electrons.

1897 (D): A **cathode ray tube** (Braun tube) that pioneered development of television and other electronic communications was invented at Strassburg by German physicist, **Karl Ferdinand Braun,** 47, who improved the Marconi Wireless by increasing the energy of sending stations and arranging antennas to control the direction of effective radiation. [see 1884 (g), 1888 (c)]

The Braun tube was linked in 1907 to "electric vision" by Russian, physicist Boris Rosing.

1898 JAN. 15: **Bepin Chandra Pal**, a celebrated Indian publisher, wrote from London to the *Indian Mirror*:

"How deep and extensive **VIVEKANANDA'S work** has been in this country (England) will readily appear from the following incident.

"Yesterday evening I was going to visit a friend in the Southern part of London. I lost my way and was looking from the corner of a street thinking in which direction I should go, when a lady accompanied by a boy came to me, with the intention, it seemed, of showing me the way.... She said to me, 'Sir, perhaps you are looking to find your way. May I help you?....'" She showed me my way and said, 'From certain papers I learned that you are coming to London. At the very first sight of you I was telling my son, 'Look, there is Swami Vivekananda'. As I had to catch the train in a hurry, I had no time to tell her that I was not Vivekananda, and compelled to go off speedily. However, I was really surprised to see that the lady possessed such great veneration for Vivekananda even before she knew him personally. I felt highly gratified at the agreeable incident, and thanked my *gerua* turban which had given me so much honour. Besides the incident, I have seen here many educated English gentlemen, who have come to revere India and who listened eagerly to any religious or spiritual truths, if they belong to India." (*Indian Mirror,* February 15, 1898).

1898 JAN. 28: **Miss Margaret Elizabeth Noble** (b. 1867) who had first met **SWAMI VIVEKANANDA** in London (Nov. 1895) and regularly attended his classes, and imbibed the great Vedanta spirit, arrived at Calcutta, deciding to devote her life to the service of India and the Swami's work.

On March 25, 1898, Swamiji ordained her a *brahmacharini* (religious celibate). He also gave her the name of *'Nivedita'*, the 'Dedicated One', by which name she has ever since been cherished by the Indians with deep respect and affection. The ordaining ceremony performed in the chapel of the monastery, was in many respects a momentous event, as the Sister was the first Western woman novice received into any monastic Order in India.

1898 MAR. 5: In order to establish a permanent home for the Ramakrishna Order, **SWAMI VIVEKANANDA** purchased a plot of land (about seven acres in extent, altogether with a building, on the bank of the Ganges at Belur, five miles above Calcutta) for a sum of Rs. 39,000 which was donated by Swamiji's devoted English admirer Miss Henrietta F. Muller and his American follower Mrs. Ole Bull, and the work of construction was forthwith undertaken. [see 1895 (p)]

> The consecration of the newly purchased Math grounds was, celebrated in the same month. On this occasion, Swamiji himself carried on his shoulder the urn containing the hallowed remains of Sri Ramakrishna. All his brother disciples also accompanied him in a procession. When the procession reached the Math ground, the sacred urn was placed on a special seat and worshipped with solemn religious rites. Swamiji was now satisfied that a permanent place and sufficient means to build a temple for the Master with a monastery as the Headquarters of the Order had been found for the dissemination of the universal teachings of the Master. Swamiji said, "....Today I feel free from the weight of the responsibility which I have carried with me for twelve long years. And now the vision comes to my mind! This Math shall become a great centre of learning and *sadhana*...."

1898 MAR. 15: Death of **Sir Henry Bessemer** (b. 1813) English metallurgist and inventor of the Bessemer process for making steel which, by driving an air blast through molten pig iron (1856), greatly cheapened the cost of manufacture.

1898 APR: Plague broke out suddenly and in a virulent form in Calcutta.

SWAMI VIVEKANANDA who was then taking rest at Darjeeling, got the news and learnt about the widespread panic and confusion prevailing among the people. Though not in good health, he soon came to Calcutta (May 3), and made hurried preparations with the help of his *gurubhais* and disciples, including **Sister Nivedita**, to mitigate the sufferings of the afflicted and the terror-stricken. When one of his *gurubhais* told him about the dearth of funds to meet the situation, Swamiji emphatically declared: "Why? We shall sell the newly bought Math grounds, if necessary! We are *sannayasins*, we must be ready to sleep under the trees and live on daily *bhiksha* as we did before. What! Should we care for Math and possessions when by disposing of them we could relieve thousands suffering before our eyes!" Fortunately it was not necessary to take this extreme step, for very soon ample funds poured in for the purpose from other quarters. The relief rendered to the plague patients and measures adopted by the Swami and the heroic band of his selfless workers were very much appreciated both by the public and the Government, and made the infant organization extremely popular to the people at large.

In March 1899, plague reappeared in Calcutta, taking daily a heavy toll of lives, specially in the slums, and creating wild panic. Swami Vivekananda who had been long apprehensive of the possible reappearance of plague in Calcutta, promptly put into operation, measures which had already been contemplated in advance. On March 31, 1899, the **Ramakrishna Mission Plague Service** was finally initiated. Swamiji himself came to live in a poor locality to inspire courage in the people and cheer up the workers. The whole management was put in the hands of Sister Nivedita whose efforts were directed more to adopting measures to prevent and check the spread of the epidemic.

1898 MAY. 19: Death of **William E. Gladstone** (b. 1809), the greatest British statesman of the 19th century.

He led the Liberal Party and served as Prime Minister of England four times during the period from 1868-1894. His strong religious sense was an integral part of his political and social policies.

1898 JUN. 2: Death of J. J. Goodwin, an English stenographer, who rendered yeoman service to **SWAMI VIVEKANANDA** with unswerving spirit of devotion.

He was able to take down the Swamiji's lectures almost verbatim, with their prophetic and inspirational quality unimpaired.

An emigrant to the United States from England, Mr. Goodwin was engaged at New York, in December 1895, by the American disciples of Swamiji who were eager to have their Master's extempore lectures recorded. Goodwin transcribed exactly and accurately all the utterances of Swamiji. He worked day and night over the Swamiji's lectures, taking them down stenographically and then typewriting them, all the same day, in order to hand over the manuscript for publication. Swamiji's American lectures were thus fully and accurately recorded. Goodwin was also responsible for the reports of all those inspiring Indian lectures of the Swami which are now available in the famous book, *Lectures From Colombo To Almora.*

Mr. Goodwin accompanied Swamiji wherever he went, visiting Detroit and Boston, when the Swami went to those places in the spring of 1896, and later accompanying him to England and to India, where he died. At the news of Goodwin's premature death, the following touching tribute to his memory was sent by Swami Vivekananda to the papers:

"With infinite sorrow I learn the sad news of Goodwin's departure from this life, the more so as it was terribly sudden and therefore prevented all possibilities of my being at his side at the time of death. The debt of gratitude, I owe him, can never be repaid, and those who think they have been helped by any thought of mine, ought to know that almost every word of it, was published through the untiring and most unselfish exertions of Mr. Goodwin. In him I have lost a friend true as steel, a disciple of never failing devotion, a worker who knew not what tiring was, and the world is less rich by one of those few who are born, as it were, to live only for others."

1898 JUN: *The Brahmavadin* reported about the renowned *yogi* **Pavahari Baba** of Ghazipur who made a sacrifice of his body:

"The *yoga-siddha* familiarly known as Pavahari Baba who resided at the village of Kuta in the District of Ghazipur, for about thirty years, and has been the great source of spiritual influence to all grades of the Hindu community, put an end to his earthly career in rather a curious way. He owned nothing very important in the way of property except a small image of Rama his favourite Deity, the photos of Sri Ramakrishna Paramahamsa and a few others supposed to be presents from Keshab Chandra Sen, and a few utensils used in daily worship.... On the day previous to his end, it seems he hinted to his brother that the weight of the *Kaliyuga* was becoming too oppressive and that it was time that his spirit quitted this mortal body. His brother seems to have suspected nothing but learnt the grave significance of these words, the next day. The morning of June 10th, of the seventh day of the dark half of the lunar month, *Jyeshtha,* was the last time when the pious pedestrians on the fields of Kuta heard the familiar ringing of the *puja* bell of their beloved *yogin.* For it was on that day the venerable *sadhu,* after his customary ablutions, gathering of flowers and worship, is said to have smeared his body with clarified butter and sprinkled it over with incense and then set fire to the four corners of his room; and when the flames had taken hold on all sides, it is said, he deliberately went and sat in the sacrificial pit making his body an oblation...."

".... Our readers will better appreciate the glory of this saint from the eloquedt words of **SWAMI VIVEKANANDA**: 'There is a sage in India, a great yogi, one of the most wonderful men I have ever seen in my life. He is a peculiar man; he will not teach anyone; if you ask him a question he will not answer. It is too much for him to take up a position of a teacher; he will not do it. If you ask a question, and if you wait for some days in the course of conversation he will bring the subject out himself, and wonderful light will be then thrown on it. He told me once the secret of perfect work, and what he said was: 'Let the end and the means be joined into one, and that is the secret of work.' Again in another place Swamiji says: 'The great men in the world have passed away unknown. The Buddhas and the Christs that we know are but second-rate heroes in comparison with the greatest men of whom the world knows nothing. Hundreds of these unknown heroes have lived in every country working silently. Silently they live and silently they pass away; and in time their thoughts find expression in Buddhas or Christs, and it is those latter that become known to us. The highest men do not seek to get any name or fame from their knowledge. They leave their ideas to the world; they put forth no claim for themselves and establish no schools or systems in their name. Their whole nature shrinks from such a thing. They are the pure *sattvikas* who can never make any stir, but only melt down in love. I have seen one such *yogin* who lives in a cave in India. He is one of the most wonderful men I have ever seen. He has so altogether lost the sense of his own individuality that we may say that the man in him is completely gone, leaving behind only the all-comprehending sense of the divine. If an animal bites one of his arms, he is ready to give it his other arm also, and say that it is the Lord's will. Everything that comes to him is from the Lord. He does not show himself to men and yet he is a Magazine of love and of true and sweet ideas.' "

1898 JUL. 4: SWAMI VIVEKANANDA who was on a tour, arranged, personally the observance of the memorable date – the anniversary of the American Declaration of independence.

On this day he was travelling with several American disciples in remote Kashmir. As a surprise to his companions that day Swamiji composed and read to them a poem named: *To the Fourth of July.*

Vivekananda's utterances frequently revealed the deep impression he had absorbed in his association with the people of America. He felt a powerful affinity which their spirit of liberty had, with his own drive for universal tolerance and spiritual harmony. Significantly, the day of Swamiji's exit from the world happened to be a 4th July.

1898 JUL. 29: Birth of **Isidor Rabi**, American physicist, who pioneered in the development of precision atomic and nuclear-beam measurements.

1898 JUL. 30: Death of **Bismarck** (b. 1815), founder and first Chancellor of the German Empire (1871).

A leading diplomat of the late 19th century, Bismarck was known as the 'Iron Chancellor'.

1898 AUG. 2: SWAMI VIVEKANANDA on a tour to Kashmir, undertook a pilgrimage to the icy-cave-temple of Amarnath.

Accompanied by **Sister Nivedita,** and observing meticulously every little practice demanded by custom, the Swami entered the cave-temple, trembling with emotion. A great mystic experience came over him, of which he never spoke, beyond saying that Lord Shiva himself appeared before him.

1898 SEP. 30: *The Amrit Bazar Patrika* wrote in its editorial:

"It must be intolerable to a Christian to see a pagan preaching religion in Christian countries, at the cost of the blessed Christians themselves. The privilege of preaching religion to others than Christians is enjoyed by the Christian missionaries alone. Any non-Christian, therefore, who takes to preaching religion to others, especially in a Christian country, is an interloper....

"....The most natural thing in the world, according to the Christian missionaries, is that Christians should subscribe handsomely for the spread of Christianity and send batch after batch of missionaries to heathen countries. The most unnatural thing in the world, according to the same authority, is for the heathens to penetrate into the country of these Christians and preach religion, and that at the cost of the Christians themselves! Naturally, the sight of **Swami Abhedananda** (a brother disciple of **SWAMI VIVEKANANDA**) being honoured, feted and fed in the United States of America, is hateful to the sight of the missionaries.

"Viewing the thing from an impartial standpoint of view, we think that Abhedananda committed no wrong, and that the missionaries do commit a wrong in coming to this country....

"....Everything in the conduct of this Swami is straightforward and honourable. But that cannot be said of many of the missionaries.

"There is no doubt of it that one of the ways of raising money for missionary purposes in India is to blacken the character of the Hindus, by exhorting pious Christians to save the black pagans of India 'who ate their babies alive, burnt their women, offered human sacrifices and worshipped hideous idols!'

"The real fact is that the Hindus do not need that looking after as the Christians themselves do. As fighting men, as men of energy, the Christians are immensely superior to the Hindus, but in morality the Hindus are probably better than the Christians. And in proof of this we can show that the Hindus do not touch liquor. Charity must begin at home, and the duties of Christian missionaries and pious Christians is first to put their own house into order before saving strangers. A drunken Christian saved is likely to be a more pleasing sight to Christ than a sober heathen rescued. For, a drunken Christian disgraces his name and religion.

"We presume there is much to do nearer home, in Christian countries, than even in a heathen country like India. Besides, a Christian reclaimed, is a solid piece of work. The Christianized heathen in India is a farce, – he gains very little, as a rule, by his conversion. We have seen a good many converts who have only learnt to give air and nothing of any value. Our humble idea is that pious Christians should, first of all, try to improve the moral tone of their own community; and that will do more to spread Christianity than mere precepts.

"But we have no need to thrust our advice upon the Christians, though we have some to offer to our own countrymen. It is that, as Hindus, they have a duty to their fellows, namely the humanization of their fellow-beings. By Buddhism they humanized Asia, and by Vaishnavism they should humanize Europe and America. Is not the Czar trying to reduce the number of fighting men? What a reflection this against Christ and his teachings! What a piece of criticism this against the religion, which taught the brotherhood of man and fatherhood of God, and which further taught man to turn the right cheek when the left is hurt! Let Hindus send batch after batch of missionaries to all parts of the world, carrying the flag of Lord Gauranga – preaching love as the highest blessing of God to men."

1898 NOV. 8: While working with the cathode ray ultra-vacuum tube invented by English physicist Sir William Crookes, German physicist, **Wilhelm Konrad Roentgen** (1845-1925), discovered a new type of radiation, which he called **X-rays** and their use for obtaining picture of the interior structure of animate and inanimate bodies. He announced his discovery to the Wurzburg physical-Medical Society in December 28, in his paper.

The first X-ray picture taken by Roentgen in 1898 clearly showed the bone structure of his wife's hand. The technique soon revolutionized medical diagnosis. This discovery of X-ray also led to others of significance, e.g., that of radio-activity by Becquerel, which transformed physical science. Roentgen's epoch-making discovery earned him the Nobel Prize in Physics, of which he was the first recipient, in 1901.

1898 NOV. 13: SWAMI VIVEKANANDA attended the opening ceremony of Nivedita School at Calcutta. **The Holy Mother**, Sri Ramakrishna's consort, performed the opening ceremony of the school. At the end she prayed that the blessings of the Divine Mother might be upon the school and that the girls it trained be ideal women.

Nivedita who witnessed the ceremony with the Swamis of the Ramakrishna Order said: "I cannot imagine a grander omen than her blessings spoken over the educated Hindu womanhood of the future." The dedication of the school was the beginning of Nivedita's work in India.

1898 NOV. : **Max Muller** brought out his book entitled *Ramakrishna –
His Life and Sayings.*

The book had a rapid sale, the third edition coming out the following
May. In this context, Mrs. Georgina Max Muller wrote: "This Indian
saint (**SRI RAMAKRISHNA**), who died in 1886, had many devoted
followers and from them and various journals Max Muller collected his
sayings and materials for his life, feeling that attention ought to be drawn
in this country (England) to the utterances of men like Ramakrishna who
gather multitudes round them, and who exercise a powerful influence
not only on philosophy but on large masses of people. 'A country
permeated by thoughts as were uttered by Ramakrishna cannot possibly
be looked upon as a country of ignorant idolators, to be converted by
the same methods which are applicable to the races of Central
Africa' " *(The Life and Letters of Max Muller,* Vol. II, p. 399).

1898 DEC. 9: **Belur Math** (monastery at Belur, a small town on the West
bank of the Ganga, about five miles from Calcutta) was formally consecrated
by **SWAMI VIVEKANANDA**, with the installation of Sri Ramakrishna's
image in chapel.

On January 22, 1899, the Ramakrishna Math was finally removed to this
new monastery – it was occupied by the members of the Ramakrishna
Order. After establishing the Math in 1899 Swami Vivekananda turned
it over to a Board of Trustees drawn from the monastic members of the
Ramakrishna Order.

While Ramakrishna Math is a registered religious trust dedicated to the
nursing of the inner spiritual life of the monastic members of the
Ramakrishna movement, the Ramakrishna Mission is a charitable Society
registered under the Societies Registration Act of 1860 and dedicated
to the expression of the inner spiritual life in outward collective action
in the service of man. Though legally two distinct entities with separate
funds, the Ramakrishna Math and the Ramakrishna Mission are virtually
a single body; the members of the Math form the principal workers of
the Mission; the Trustees of the Math form the Governing Body of the
Mission, and the Belur Math is the headquarters of both. Both Math
and Mission now have branches all over India.

1898 (A): Research into the radioactivity of pitchblend, an ore of Uraniurn,
led **Marie** (1867-1934) and **Pierre Curie** (1859-1906), French physicists, to
discover the radioactive elements **Polonium** and **Radium.**

The Curies and Antoine Henri Becquerel (1852-1908) shared the 1903
Nobel Prize for physics for their discovery of radioactivity which laid
the foundation of later research in nuclear physics and chemistry.

1898 (B): Bubonic plague killed an estimated 3 million people in **China** and **India,** in the following decade.

1898 (C): Sir Pherozeshah Mehta (1845-1915), one of the founders of the Indian National Congress, and an outstanding leader of the Bombay Municipality, was named to the **Imperial Legislative Council,** and served with distinction until poor health forced his resignation.

1898 (D): Prarthana Samaj of Bombay started **Depressed Class Mission.**

1898 (E): The **Telegraphone** patented by Danish electrical engineer **Valdemer Paulsen** (1869-1942), was the world's first magnetic wire-recording device.

1898 (F): Sir Ronald Ross (1857-1932), British bacteriologist, successfully investigated the theory of a mosquito vector in the transmission of malaria.

His discovery of the **malarial parasite** in the gastro-intestinal tract of the Anopheles mosquito led to the realization that malaria was transmitted by Anopheles and laid the foundation for combating the disease.

He received the Nobel Prize in 1902 for discovery of how malaria enters an organism.

Ross's discovery led to the draining of swamps where mosquitoes breed, to expanded use of window screens and mosquito netting and – eventually – to widespread use of insecticides.

1898 (G): M. J. Owens (1859-1923) invented **automatic bottle-making machine.**

1898 (H): John Philip Holland (1840-1914), Irish American inventor, succeeded in designing and developing a **sub-marine vessel,** 'Holland', which is considered the principal forerunner of the modern submarines.

1898 (I): The **Graflex Camera** patented by U. S. inventor **Williarn F. Folmer,** 36, was the world's first high-speed multiple-split focal plane camera. In the same year photographs taken with artificial light were produced for the first time.

1898 (J): *The School and Society* by University of Chicago philosopher-psychologist **John Dewey,** 39, pioneered progressive education by challenging traditional teaching methods based on lectures, memorization, and mechanical drill. Dewey suggested that education was a process of accumulation and assimilation of experience whereby a child developed into a balanced personality with wide awareness.

1898 (K): **Alberto Santos Dumont** (1873-1932), Brazilian aviation pioneer, built a **model airplane** with an internal combustion engine.

Shortly after the successful flight by the Wright Brothers in 1903, Santos Dumont turned his attention to heavier-than-air machine. In 1909, he produced his famous monoplane, the forerunner of the modern flight plane.

1898 (L): **Spanish-American War** that lasted for 112 days, was initiated by America and fought ostensibly to end Civil War in Cuba and free the island from Spanish rule. But it also manifested America's desire to consolidate their strategic position and extend their economic penetration to the Carribean area.

The war was precipitated by a February 15 explosion that destroyed the U. S. battleship 'Maine' in Havana Harbour, killing 258 sailors and two officers. The Battle of Manila Bay began on May 1, in the morning. By the time a cease fire was ordered in the afternoon, all 10 ships in the Spanish squadron had been destroyed with a loss of 381 men, while 8 Americans had been slightly wounded and none killed. Admiral Dewy's victory at Manila Bay established the United States as a Pacific power in a brief war with Spain. Spain was forced to give up the Philippines, Guam and Puerto Rico. Cuba became independent, but was held closely under U. S. political and economic influence.

1898 (M): **'Gideons International'** had its beginning at Boscobel, Wis., where two travelling salesmen, John H. Nicholson and Sam Hill, shared a room at the Central Hotel and decided to form an Association of Christian businessmen and professional men to "put the word of God into the hands of the unconverted."

The Association raised money for their work, it placed 25 Bibles in Montana Hotel in 1908, and by 1976 the Gideons had placed 16.5 million Bibles per year in hotels, hospitals, prisons, schools, colleges and other locations.

1899 JAN. : **Swami Trigunatitananda**, a brother disciple of **SWAMI VIVEKANANDA**, in his capacity as the Manager, published the first number of the Bengali Magazine *Udbodhan* (The Awakener).

Swami Vivekananda selected the name for the magazine, and gave Swami Trigunatitananda his hearty blessings for its success. Swami Trigunatitananda would beg his food from householders of a devotional nature, or sometimes go without food, and would march ten miles on foot, on business relating to the Press and the magazine. There was no means at that time of employing a clerk and Swami Vivekananda had given strict orders not to spend a farthing out of the magazine fund for any other purpose than the interests of the magazine itself. And Swami Trigunatitananda carried out the orders to the letter, maintaining himself from *bhiksha* at the houses of *baktas* or by other means.

Swami Vivekananda wrote out the introduction to the magazine, and it was proposed that only the *sannyasin* and householder disciples of Sri Ramakrishna would write in this paper. Swamiji also warned the authorities against obscene advertisements being published in it. The members of the Ramakrishna Association, then an organized body, were called upon by Swamiji to contribute articles to the magazine and spread the religious views of Sri Ramakrishna through this paper among the general public.

1899 MAR. 19: **Advaita Ashram** was founded at Mayavati, Himalayas In the words of **SWAMI VIVEKANANDA**, "To give this One Truth (*Advaita*) a freer and fuller scope in elevating the lives of individuals and leavening the mass of mankind, we start this Advaita Ashram on the Himalayan heights....."

Ever since the visit to the Alps at Switzerland, Swami Vivekananda had been cherishing the desire to establish a monastery in the solitude of the Himalayas where non-dualism would be taught and practised in its pure form, and where the people from the East and the West could live together in spiritual comradeship and practise the Vedanta philosophy and get their outlook on life greatly widened by a mutual exchange of their highest cultural and spiritual ideas. In the course of his itinerary, he had searched in vain for a suitable site for such an Ashram in the hills. Eventually Mr. and Mrs. Sevier accompanied by Swami Swarupananda, travelled far into the interior of the District of Almora and after a diligent search, selected for the Ashram the estate of Mayavati lying at a distance of 50 miles from Almora at an altitude of 6800 ft. and commanding a magnificent view of the eternal snow ranges of the Himalayas. With the approval of the Swami, the spot was immediately purchased and the monastery under the name of the "Advaita Ashram" came into existence with his heartfelt blessings. In order that devotees hailing from different parts of the world and belonging to various faiths might carry on their spiritual practices without let or hindrance, it was enjoined by the Swami as a special rule that in that Ashram there would be no worship of images, pictures or symbols of God, nor any religious ceremony or ritual, not even the worship of Sri Ramakrishna. [see 1901 Jan. 7]

1899 MAR. 19: (a): *The Mahratta* wrote in its Editorial:

"In an interview with a representative of *The Madras Mail,* **Swami Abhayananda** is reported to have said the following: 'Missionary reports are spread in America that in India children are thrown in the Ganges and under the wheel of the car of Jagannath, and people in America are induced to believe these. I myself have been constantly asked how such things are possible in the land of the beautiful Vedanta Philosophy.'Asked as to whether she seriously suggested that such stories were told in America as descriptive of the present state of affairs in India, and whether the people there really believed such stories Swami Abhayananda reasserted her previous answer with emphasis and said, 'I am pained to say, yes. I shall be able after personal observation here to contradict many of these false stories when I return to America'.

"....The tenacity of the American missionaries in propagating in their land something that is not true about India, is not a new thing to the Indian public; but it more pointedly than ever thrusts upon our attention the consideration whether it is not high time that we did take some steps to dispel the impressions about us made on the misinformed American mind, whose good opinion and sympathy we cannot afford to lose. The venerable **SWAMI VIVEKANANDA** has shown us the right way to the attainment of our object and it would therefore be a pity if we do not send at least a couple of Hindu preachers, disciples of the Swami along with Swami Abhayananda to America." [see 1894 Nov. 7]

1899 APR. 11: Death of **Sir Monier-Williams** (b. 1819), English-Sanskrit scholar, who was largely responsible for the establishment at Oxford of the Indian Institute.

A prolific writer on Sanskrit, Hindustani and Indian religions, Monier-Williams' *Enghsh-Sanskrit Dictionary* (1851) and *Sanskrit-English Dictionary* (1872) are standard reference works. His *Indian Wisdom* (1875) is a source book representing mostly every field of classical Indian studies.

A staunch orientalist and admirer of Hindu faith, Sir Monier-Williams wrote: "And yet it is a remarkable characteristic of Hinduism that it neither requires nor attempts to make converts.... nor is it being driven out of the field by two such proselytizing religions as Mohammedanism and Christianity. On the contrary, it is at present rapidly increasing. And far more remarkable than this is that it is all receptive, all-embracing and all-comprehensive....

"It cares not to oppose the progress of Christianity nor of any other religion. For it has no difficulty in including all other religions with its all-embracing arms and ever-widening fold. And in real fact, Hinduism has something to offer which is suited to all minds. Its very strength lies in its infinite adaptability to the infinite diversity of human characters and human tendencies. It has its highly spiritual and abstract side suited to the philosophical higher classes. Its practical and concrete side suited to the man of affairs and the man of the world. Its aesthetic and ceremonial side suited to the man of poetic feeling and imagination. Its quiescent and contemplative side is suited to the man of peace and lover of seclusion.

"Indeed, Hindus were Spinozists 2000 years before the birth of Spinoza, Darwinians centuries before the birth of Darwin, and evolutionists centuries before the doctrine of evolution had been accepted by the Huxleys of our times, and before any word like evolution existed, in any language of the world. [see 1872 (c)]

1899 APR. 30: *The Mahratta* reported:

"The movement initiated by Ramakrishna Mission with the object of securing the voluntary services of natives in cleaning the insanitary districts and adopting plague preventive measures resulted on Saturday evening in a large representative meeting of the University professors and students.

"The Chairman, **SWAMI VIVEKANANDA,** in opening the proceedings, impressed upon the students the necessity of immediate and decisive action. There had been any amount of talk and theorising, but no practical work had been done by the Bengalis themselves tending towards checking the plague. He remarked that the Bengalis were getting crazy because of the severe criticism lately passed on them by an English newspaper correspondent, but unless they threw aside their lethargy and proved themselves to be men by actual practical action, and not mere puppets shut up in a glass case for show, they would not be able to dissipate the aspersions cast on them, nor wipe out the disgrace attaching to the country. Miss Noble also gave an address.

"At the close of the meeting a large number of students came up and enrolled themselves as volunteers for the proposed work.

"There were 74 deaths reported in Calcutta on Saturday against an average of 75. The plague cases reported numbered 21 and the deaths 13. The suspected plague cases were 6 and the deaths from suspected plague 5."

1899 APR. : The following is an interview which a representative of the *Prabuddha Bharata* had with **SWAMI VIVEKANANDA** on the bounds of Hinduism – about his views on reconversion to Hindusim:

Having been directed by the Editor, (writes the representative of *The Prabuddha Bharata*), to interview Swami Vivekananda on the question of converts to Hinduism, I found an opportunity one evening on the roof of a Ganges houseboat. It was after nightfall, and we had stopped at the embankment of the Ramakrishna Math, and there the Swami came down to speak with me.

Time and place were alike delightful. Overhead the stars, and around the rolling Ganges; and on one side stood the dimly lighted building, with its background of palms and lofty shady trees.

"I want to see you, Swami," I began, "on this matter of receiving back into Hinduism those who have been perverted from it. Is it your opinion that they should be received?"

"Certainly", said the Swami, "they can and ought to be taken."

He sat gravely for a moment, thinking, and then resumed. "Besides", he said, "we shall otherwise decrease in numbers. When the Mohammedans first came, we are said – I think on the authority of Ferishta, the oldest Mohammedan historian – to have been six hundred millions of Hindus. Now we are about two hundred millions. And then every man going out of the Hindu pale is not only a man less, but an enemy the more.

"Again, the vast majority of Hindu perverts to Islam and Christianity are perverts by the sword, or the descendants of these. It would be obviously unfair to subject these to disabilities of any kind. As to the case of born aliens, did you say? Why, born aliens have been converted in the past by crowds, and the process is still going on."

"In my own opinion, this statement not only applies to aboriginal tribes, to outlying nations, and to almost all our conquerors before the Mohammedan conquest, but also to all those castes who find a special origin in the Puranas. I hold that they have been aliens thus adopted."

"Ceremonies of expiation are no doubt suitable in the case of willing converts returning to their Mother-Church, as it were; but on those who were alienated by conquest – as in Kashmir and Nepal – or on strangers wishing to join us, no penance should be imposed."

"But of what caste would these people be, Swamiji?" I ventured to ask. "They must have some, or they can never be assimilated into the great body of Hindus. Where shall we look for their rightful place?"

"Returning converts", said the Swami quietly, "will gain their own castes, of course. And new people will make theirs. You will remember", he added, "that this has already been done in the case of Vaishnavism. Converts from different castes and aliens were all able to combine under that flag and form a caste by themselves, – and a very respectful one too. From Ramanuja down to Chaitanya of Bengal, all great Vaishnava teachers have done the same."

"And where should these new people expect to marry?" I asked.

"Amongst themselves as they do now", said the Swami quietly.

"Then as to names", I enquired, "I suppose aliens and perverts who have adopted non-Hindu names should be named newly. Would you give them caste-names, or what?"

"Certainly", said the Swami, thoughtfully, "there is a great deal in a name" and on this question he would say no more.

But my next enquiry drew blood. "Would you leave these newcomers, Swamiji, to choose their own forms of religious belief out of many-visaged Hinduism, or would you chalk out a religion for them?"

"Can you ask that?" he said. "They will choose for themselves. For unless a man chooses for himself, the very spirit of Hinduism is destroyed. The essence of our Faith consists simply in this freedom of the *Istha*."

I thought the utterance is weighty one, for the man before me has spent more years than any one else living, I fancy, in studying the common bases of Hinduism in a scientific and sympathetic spirit – and the freedom of the *Istha* is obviously a principle big enough to accommodate the world.

But the talk passed to other matters, and then with a cordial good night this great teacher of religion lifted his lantern and went back into the monastery, while I, by the pathless path of the Ganges, in and out amongst her crafts of many sizes, made the best of my way back to my Calcutta home. [see 1899 May, 1899 June 25]

1899 MAY 24: Birth of **Kazi Nazrul Islam,** the revolutionary poet of Bengal.

One of his poems: "Of equality I sing: where all barriers and differences between man and man has vanished, where Hindus, Muslims, Buddhists and Christians have mingled together. Of equality I sing".

1899 MAY. : *The Indian Social Reformer* wrote about Vivekananda's views on reconversion to Hinduism:

"SWAMI VIVEKANANDA said to an interviewer that 'every man going out of the Hindu pale is not only a man the less, but an enemy the more'. Therefore in his opinion converts to Christianity and Mohammedanism ought to be received back into Hinduism. Not only so, even born aliens should be received into the Hindu fold. As to their position in Hindu society he said that 'returning converts will gain their own castes, of course. And new people will make theirs. This has already been done in case of Vaishnavism. Converts from different castes and aliens were all able to combine under that flag and form a caste by themselves – and a very respectable one too. From Ramanuja to Chaitanya of Bengal, all great Vaishnava teachers have done the same.

As to the form of belief to be adopted by them, 'they will choose for themselves. The essence of our Faith consists simply in this freedom of *Istham.*' When the Hindu castes – at least – the higher ones – take back converts to Christianity and Mohammadanism the difficulty as to what caste they should form will very probably not exist at all." [see 1899 Apr., 1899 June 25]

1899 JUN. 2: The Bengal correspondent of *The Hindu* wrote:

"SWAMI VIVEKANANDA has not yet been able to completely shake off his ailment. Yet he has decided to leave for Europe and will probably embark early in June. The Swami, we believe, has a double object in view, viz., to benefit his health by the voyage, and to resume his work in England and America after complete recovery. We heartily wish the Swami a pleasant voyage, speedy restoration to his normal health and vigour and an active career to a preacher of the Higher Hinduism in the West." (*The Indian Mirror*)

1899 JUN. 20: Accompanied by **Sister Nivedita** and **Swami Turiyananda,** one of his brother monks, **SWAMI VIVEKANANDA** left for the West on his mission for the second time.

After consolidating his newly started activities in India, Swamiji had strongly felt an urge to take a trip to the West to personally inspect how far the work founded in the foreign lands had progressed during his absence. Besides, the doctors, apprehending a sudden physical break- down of the Swami due to the overstraining of his nerves in the midst of his whirlwind activities in India, had advised him to go on a sea-voyage to recoup his fast deteriorating health. So he boarded the S. S. Golconda in the Hoogli river at Calcutta and began his second and last voyage to the Western world.

1899 JUN. 25: *The Mahratta* wrote in its editorial about **SWAMI VIVEKANANDA'S views** on reconversion to Hinduism:

"A representative of *The Prabuddha Bharata* lately interviewed Swami Vivekananda, and drew him out on a most important question of social and religious reform. The Swami is of opinion that those persons who have been perverted from Hinduism can, and certainly ought to be taken back. Since the days of Ferista, the oldest Mohammedan historian, the Hindus have, the Swami calculates, been reduced in number from six to two hundred millions. And besides every man going out of the Hindu pale is 'not only a man less, but an enemy the more'. The vast majority of Hindu perverts to Islam and Christianity are perverts by the sword or descendants of these, and it would be obviously unfair to subject these to disabilities of any kind. Born aliens too could be received within the pale of Hinduism just as much as perverts and their descendants. The question of *prayaschitta* or penance is only a subordinate one. Reason would demand the enforcement of the *prayaschitta* in a case of those persons only who have been voluntary perverts and wish to be reconverted in their own life. The demand would evidently be not so imperative in the case of those upon whom excommunication has visited as a vicarious punishment, i.e., punishment for the sins of their parents or ancestors, or in the case of those who originally belonged to a different religion but are willing, by honest conviction, to change it in favour of Hinduism. As for the accommodation and adjustment in Society of converts to Hinduism the Swami is of opinion that while returning converts will gain their own castes, aliens will form a caste of their own. 'This has already been done', says the Swami, in the case of Vaishnavism. 'Converts from different castes and aliens were all able to combine under that flag and form a caste by themselves, and a very respectable one too. From Ramanuja to Chaitanya of Bengal all great Vaishnava teachers have done the same'. As for the form of religious belief the convert will of course choose his own. 'For unless a man chooses for himself the very essence of Hinduism is destroyed. The essence of our faith consists simply in this freedom of the *Istham.'* The above views are convincing proofs of the breadth and liberalism of the new Gospel which Swami Vivekananda has been preaching in India and the Western countries." [see 1899 April, 1899 May]

1899 JUL. 9: *The Mahratta* in its editorial:

"**SWAMI VIVEKANANDA** once more sailed for England with two of his disciples from Calcutta. On his way he was to have landed for some time at Madras. But the quarantine regulations in force at Madras Harbour, disappointed him as well as his Madras friends, who had made some preparations for receiving him. The object of the present visit of the Swami to England is, of course, to continue his mission of Hindu Evangelism. It appears from the letter which Mr. Alfred Webb recently wrote to India, that the missionaries have once more started a fresh crusade of calumny against the Hindu religion; and if that be so the Swami's visit to England may be regarded as quite opportune. Evidently the Swami's labours have begun to bear fruit in that land of materialism; and the awakened jealousy and spitefulness of the missionaries is a sure proof of it. We wish bon voyage to the Swami, and are confident that his present tour will prove as fruitful as the last. The grand exhibition at Paris is to come off next year and religion in one form or another is sure to be one of the exhibits at it. In fact we shall not be surprised to hear that the World's Parliament of Religions meets at Paris as it met on a similar occasion at Chicago. Such an opportunity must be very welcome to the Swami, and we may surely expect to hear of Swami's success as we did three years ago."

1899 JUL. 21: Death of **Robert Ingersoll** (b. 1833), American lawyer and orator, who popularized the higher criticism of the Bible, a humanistic philosophy, and a scientific rationalism; a champion of free thought, he became known as "The Great Agnostic". Nationally known as a lecturer, he was in great demand and received as much as $ 3,500 for a single evening's performance in which, with brilliant oratory and wit, he sought to expose the orthodox superstitions of the times.

While in America, **SWAMI VIVEKANANDA** met Ingersoll with whom the Swami on several occasions discussed religious and philosophical subjects. During the course of these conversations the great agnostic cautioned the Swami not to be too bold and outspoken, to be careful in his preaching of new doctrines and his criticisms of the way of life and thought of the people. When asked the reason why, Mr. Ingersoll replied: "Fifty years ago you would have been hanged if you had come to preach in this country or would have been burned alive. You would have been stoned out of the villages, if you had come even much later." The Swami was surprised; he could not believe that there was such a great amount of **fanaticism and bigotry in the American nation**, and he told Mr. Ingersoll as such.

"Ingersoll once said to me," said the Swami, in the course of a class talk, "I believe in making the most out of this world, in squeezing the orange dry, because this world is all we are sure of." I replied, "I know a better way to squeeze the orange of this world than you do; and I get more out of it. I know I cannot die, so I am not in a hurry. I know that there is no fear, so I enjoy the squeezing. I have no duty, no bondage of wife and children and property; and so I can love all men and women. Every one is God to me. Think of the joy of loving man as God! Squeeze your orange this way and get ten thousand fold more out of it. Get every single drop!"

1899 AUG. 17: *The Indian Mirror* comments on the *book, "Swami Vivekananda and His Guru With Letters From Prominent Americans on The Alleged Programme of Vedantism in United States"*, published by the Christian Literature Society for India, London and Madras, 1897:

"The object of the first part of this book is to show that, on account of his *shudra* birth and for his want of knowledge as well as on the part of his guru, Vivekananda is not qualified for teaching the Vedanta; that he, in consequence of his doings, is not entitled to be called a 'Swami', that Schopenhauer, the admirer of the Upanishads, was a bad man, and that Professor Max Muller (in connection with his opinion of Vedantic books) is a 'man having two voices'. The second part immediately concerns *The Indian Mirror.* It may be remembered that, on the 21 st

January, 1897, an article appeared in the paper, headed 'SWAMI VIVEKANANDA' in which it was stated that 'hundreds of men and women have enlisted themselves under the standard, which he unfolded in America, and some of them have even taken to the bowl and the yellow robes.' This statement proved too much for the serenity of the Rev. Dr. W. W. White, Secretary to the College Young Men's Christian Association of Calcutta and he forthwith set out to verify this statement by writing to a number of ladies and gentlemen of America, mostly belonging to missions and educational institutions, to whom copies of *The Mirror* were sent, and asking them if there was any 'likelihood of America abandoning Christianity and adopting either Hinduism or Mohammedanism, in its stead.' The replies received are inserted in the second part of the book, and they are of course, to the effect that neither Hinduism nor Mohammedanism has a chance of obtaining a foothold in America. Some of the writers say that Swami made no impression on the people, while some others assert that the Swami may have made a few converts, but such converts were vacillators and seekers of novelty. All of them consoled the enquirers with the assurance that Christianity has made a firm footing in America, and there is no fear of its being supplanted by any other religion.' [see 1895 May 19, 1895 May 31]

1899 SEP. 27: In a letter to the Editor of *The Indian Mirror* **Sri Sarat Chandra Chakravarthi,** a disciple of **SWAMI VIVEKANANDA,** wrote:

"....The Christian Missionaries of America, who lately have so terribly suffered from their pecuniary support being stopped by many enlightened millionaires of the United States who have heard Swami Vivekananda, give circulation to many unfounded stories against the Swamiji on many occasions.... the false report comes from a quarter where the Swamiji's work has been the most successful one in India, and where the Missionaries have been most terribly opposed in furtherance of their work of evangelization. Although it is better to ignore the calumnies of backbiters, yet we cannot help contradicting it, as it seems to have created a stir both in the European and Indian circles.

1899 OCT. 28: Death of **Ottmer Mergenthler** (b. 1854), German American inventor of the **Linotype,** who revolutionized the printing industry with his remarkable type-setting-type-casting machine.

1899 OCT. 30: In a letter of date, written from Ridgely Manor, U. S. A., **SWAMI VIVEKANANDA** confided to Mary Hale his views on British Rule in India – views which he could express publicly in India, or even in America, only at a great risk.

"Suppose you simply publish this letter", he told Mary, "The law just passed in India will allow the English Government in India to drag me from here and kill me without trial." He conceded that British rule in India had one redeeming feature; it had brought her out once more on the stage of the world. If this had been done with an eye to the good of the people, it would have as circumstances had favoured Japan with, produced more wonderful results, said he. "No good can be done when the main idea is blood-sucking", added he. In spite of massacres (as after the rising of 1857) and recurring famines "that take off millions" the population of India had increased, said he, but it had not yet come up to what it was before Muslim rule. (He quoted the Muslim historian Ferishta, circa 1570 to 1611 A. D.; as saying that in the 12th century the Hindus numbered 600 million whereas, said he, it was now less than 200 million). India can well support five times the present population, he said.

He spoke about the strangling of the press, the bit of self-government that was given to India being quickly taken off, the poor prospects of educational expansion, and Indians having been (of course) disarmed long ago.

"For writing a few words of innocent criticism men are being hurried to transportation for life, others imprisoned without any trial; and nobody knows when his head will be off .... there has been a reign of terror in India for some years. English soldiers are killing our men and outraging our women – only to be sent home with passage and pension at our expense. We are in a terrible gloom – where is the Lord? Mary, you can afford to be optimistic – can I?" *(A Comprehensive Biography of Swami Vivekananda*, Part I, p. 542 and 543).

1899 OCT. : In a long letter to **Pratap Chandra Mazumdar** (1840-1905), the disciple of Keshab Chandra Sen, and the leader of the more liberal portion of the Brahma Samaj, **Max Muller** suggested that his followers should call themselves Christians.

"Tell me some of your chief difficulties", wrote Max Muller, "that prevent you and your countrymen from openly following Christ. I shall do my best to explain how I and many who agree with me have met them and solved them.... From my point of view, India, at least the best part of it, is already converted to Christianity. You want no persuasion to become a follower of Christ. Then make up your mind to act for yourselves. Unite your flocks and put up a few folds to hold them together, and to prevent them from straying. The bridge has been built for you and those who came before you. Step boldly forward, it will not break under you, and you will find many friends to welcome you on the other shore, and among them none more delighted than your old friend and fellow labourer, F. Max Muller."

This letter remained unanswered for sometime, though, Mazumdar published it, with a rejoinder from himself, in some of the Indian papers. ... Max Muller's suggestion that the followers of Mazumdar should call themselves Christian, led to attacks from many different parties (*The Life and Letters of Max Muller,* Vol. II, p. 415 and 416).

1899 (A): First Hague Peace Conference (a tentative move towards internationalization at a time of rising European tension) was held at the suggestion of Russia, who could not afford to compete in the arms race.

1899 (B): The evolutionist or reformist current in social democracy was established by **Edward Bernstein** (1850-1932), German politician, in his writings, wherein he queried Marx's predictions and advocated evolutionary as distinguished from revolutionary socialism.

1899 (C): A. L. Debierne (1874-1949), French chemist, discovered the radioactive element '**actinium**'.

1899 (D): Aspirin (acetylsalicylic acid) was perfected by German researchers **Felix Hoffman** and **Hermann Dresser,** who had developed the powdered analgesic (pain-killer) and fever reducer from coal tar.

1899 (E): Lenin (1870-1924), Russian Communist leader, brought out his major works: *The Development of Capitalism in Russia.*

Analysing the first war of the Indian Independence, Lenin wrote elsewhere: "Only the Hindu society can free India from English colonial rule. Unfortunately, the Hindu society today is scattered and disunited. The Hindus must unite."

1899-1900: Severe famine in North India killed 2 million people.

The famine was due to complete failure of the South-West monsoon and drought, which as Sir John Elliot, the Government meteorologist, after- wards estimated, was "the greatest in extent and intensity" which India had experienced during the last 200 years. The famine affected parts covering an area extending over 400,000 square miles with a population of 25 million in British India and 35 million in the Native States. The area included the greater part of the Bombay Presidency, the whole of the Central Province, Berar, and much of the Punjab, Rajputana, the Nizam's territories, Baroda and the Central Indian principalities. Relief measures were undertaken on a wide and liberal scale.

In the wake of agonies of famine accompanied by devastations, pestilence, and deaths, the government of India appointed a **Famine Commission**, to examine the administration of relief in all its branches, the cost of operations and the extent of mortality etc.

Between 1866 and 1900 there were four major famines in India. In all,

over nine million people died of starvation. Hardly any part of India
was free from this curse. The Punjab, the Ganges valley, Orissa, Madras,
the Central Provinces and parts of Bombay were all affected at different
times. [see 1866-67, 1868-69, 1873 (b), 1874 (a), 1876-78, 1877 Jan. 1, 1878
(b), 1896-97, 1897 Jan. 13, 1897 May. 16]

1899-1902: **The South African War (Boer War)** – a struggle between
Britain and the Boer States of the Transval and the Orange Free State for
supremacy in South Africa.

It was the result of protracted dispute between British and Boers (the
descendants of Dutch settlers in South Africa) over British territorial
ambition. 450,000 British soldiers fought against 60,000 Boers, the total
casualties being 21,142 and. 26,000 respectively. It was one of the
longest and bloodiest wars fought south of Sahara in modern times and
lasted for over two and half years. The war ended with a victory for the
British and absorption of the Transval and Orange Free State into the
British Empire. When the two ex-republics were granted self-government
(1906-7), Africans living in them were not given political rights. The real
losers of the war were thus the African inhabitants of South Africa.

1899-1905. : **Lord Curzon** (1859-1925), the Viceroy of India.

At the height of one of the most severe famines in Indian history, he
wrote of "the extraordinary apathy and indifference of representative
natives. They leave the whole burden of the battle to be borne by the
European Officers. They do not visit the poor-houses.... they decline
to come forward with subscriptions; they illustrate irresponsibility and
indifference in every possible way. It is a curious thing that the Hindu,
who is so merciful and tender hearted in a lot of stupid ways, such as
saving the lives of pigeons, and peacocks, and monkeys, is almost
completely callous as regards the sufferings of his fellow-creatures."

1900 JAN. 1: **Swami Ram Tirtha** (1873-1906) predicted:

"Whether working through many souls or alone, I seriously promise to
infuse true life and dispel darkness and weakness from India within ten
years and within the first half of the twentieth century, India will be
restored to more than its original glory. Let these words be recorded."

1900 JAN. 20: Death of **John Ruskin** (b. 1819), British art critic and writer
on social problems.

Unto the Last (1860) was the most influential of his books, affecting
not only socialistic thought, but the attitude of the ordinary people to
art and taste. His writings combine enormous sensitivity and human
compassion with a burning zeal for moral values.

1900 FEB. 1: Referring to the *Gita*, in the course of his lecture on the *Mahabharata* delivered at Pasadena, California **SWAMI VIVEKANANDA** said:

> "I would advise those of you who have not read that book, to read it. If you only knew how much it has influencd your own country even! If you want to know the source of Emerson's inspiration, it is this book, the *Gita*. He went to see Carlyle and Carlyle made him a present of the *Gita*, and that little book is responsible for the Concord Movement. All the broad movements in America in one way or another, are indebted to the Concord party...." [see 1882 Apr. 27]

The *Gita* was first translated into English by Charles Wilkin in 1785.. Warren Hastings wrote a preface to it. In 1786, he "recommended" a translation of the *Gita* to the President of the East India Company, and wrote in the preface, "The writers of the Indian philosophies will survive when the British domain in India shall long have ceased to exist, and when the sources which it wielded of wealth and power are lost to remembrance." This work was well-known in its original English edition in New England circles and was reprinted in New York in 1867.

1900 FEB. 21: In a letter (written from California) to his brother disciple Swami Akhandananda, **SWAMI VIVEKANANDA** wrote:

> "In these days of dire famine, flood, disease and pestilence, tell me where your Congressmen are. Will it do to merely to say, 'Hand over the Government of the country to us'. And who is there to listen to them? If a man does work, has he to open his mouth to ask for anything? If there be two thousand people like you working in several districts, won't it be the turn of the English themselves to consult you in matters of political moment?"

Swami Vivekananda disliked politics, or at any rate thought that his own path was different and was out of the sympathy with the policy of mendicancy that the Indian National Congress was pursuing, in his opinion. His views on Congress policies did not make him popular with the leaders of the Congress with the exception perhaps of some who belonged to its extremist sections such as Mr. Tilak. (*A Comprehensive Biography of Swami Vivekananda.* Vol. II, p. 1396).

1900 FEB-MAY: During **SWAMI VIVEKANANDA'S stay** in California he received a gift of 160 acres of land through the generosity of Miss Minnie Boock, one of his devoted students. The place with its picturesque surroundings was ideally situated on the eastern slope of Mount Hamilton in Santa Clara country of California at an elevation of about 2500 ft. away from the din and bustle of town life.

Appropriately named **'Shanti Ashram'**, or Peace Retreat, it was first visited by **Swami Turiyananda** (a *gurubhai* of Swami Vivekananda) on 2nd August 1900. He was then accompanied by a party of twelve students whom he trained regularly in meditation, living with them the most austere life as in India. Gradually the silent but intensely spiritual life which Swami Turiyananda lived in the company of his students in that lonely Ashram exercised a great influence not only upon the select group of his young students but also upon all who, attracted by his luminous personality, came to the monastery for spiritual guidance. Thus the ideas spread far and wide and the work prospered under the able leadership of Swami Turiyananda.

1900 APR. 25: Birth of **Wolfgang Pauli** (d. 1958), Austrian theoretical physicist, who was awarded Nobel Prize for physics for his discovery of the exclusion principle, known as Pauli Principle.

Pauli became one of the most brilliant of the mid-20th century school of physicists. While still a student he wrote a masterly exposition of the theory of relativity. The work for which he received the Nobel Prize relates to the quantum theory and played an important part in the wave theory of the atom.

1900 JUN. 10: **SWAMI VIVEKANANDA** who came to New York from California, and stayed there in the Vedanta Society with Swami Turiyananda and Swami Abhedananda, lectured on the subject of *Vedanta Philosophy.* The rooms were filled to their utmost capacity with students and old friends of the Swami. **Sister Nivedita** who had come to New York in early June also attended the lecture. About this she wrote:

"I went early and took the seat at the left end of the second row....

"And then he came; his very entrance and his silence as he stood and waited to begin were like great hymn. A whole worship in themselves.

"At last he spoke – his face broke into fun, and he asked what was to be his subject. Someone suggested the Vedanta philosophy and he began....

"....The splendid sentences rolled on and on, and we, filled into the Eternities, thought of our common selves as of babies stretching out their hands for the moon, or the sun – thinking them as baby's toys. The wonderful voice went on.

"And for me I had found the infinitely deep things that life holds for us. To sit there and listen was all that it had ever been. Yet there was no struggle of intellectual unrest now – no tremor of novelty.

"This man who stood there held my life in the hollow of his hand – and as he once in a while looked my way, I read in his glance what I too felt

in my own heart, complete faith and abiding comprehension of purpose
– better than any feeling...."

1900 JUN. 24: *The Mahratta* wrote in its editorial:

"It is well-known, we presume, that **SWAMI VIVEKANANDA** is at
present in the United States of America, where he is doing good work
in connection with the Advaitic propaganda. After spending some
months in Los Angeles and the neighbourhood and giving numerous
public lectures and conventional addresses, he went at the end of
February last to San Francisco where he is now lecturing and teaching.
He is in excellent health and his friends feel that some of the best and
greatest work of his useful life is yet before him. *The Unity* of February
last gives an impressing account of his work in Los Angeles. This is
what *The Unity* says:

" 'Hindu missionaries are not among us to convert us to a better religion
than Christ gave us, but rather in the name of religion itself, to show us
that there is in reality but one Religion, and that we can do no better
than to put into practice what we profess to believe. We had lectures at
the Home by the Swami Vivekananda and all were intensely interesting....
There is combined in the Swami Vivekananda the learning of a University
President, the dignity of an archbishop, with grace and winsomeness
of a free and natural child. Getting upon the platform without a moment's
preparation, he would soon be in the midst of his subject, sometimes
becoming almost tragic as his mind would wander from deep
metaphysics to the prevailing condition in Christian countries today,
who go and seek to reform the Fillipinos with sword in one hand and
the Bible in the other, or in South Africa allow children of the same
Father to cut each other to pieces. In contrast to this condition of things
he described what took place during the last great famine in India where
men would die of starvation beside their cattle rather than stretch forth
a hand to kill.' "

1900 JUL. 8: *The Mahratta* wrote in its Editorial:

"We learn from *The Amrit Bazar Patrika* that the State Secretary for
India has, at the request of the Government of India, sanctioned the
deputation of **Prof. J. C. Bose** to attend the International Congress of
Physicists to be held in Paris and also the meeting of the British
Association, to enable him to lay before the scientific public in Europe
certain remarkable discoveries made by him. The Lieutenant Governor
of Bengal, Sir John Woodburn, is said to have taken the initiative in the
matter; and His Honour deserves the thanks of the Indian public for
thus showing an active appreciation of the merits of the great Indian
scientist. Besides Prof. J. C. Bose, another illustrious Indian to be present

at the function in connection with the Paris Exhibition is **SWAMI VIVEKANANDA** who, we learn, is going to Paris from America. The mission of the Swami will be to represent Hinduism at what will be like a Congress of the World's Religions in connection with the great Exhibition. Both the Swami and the Professor are personalities who, we are sure, will attract a good deal of attention." [1880 (b), 1894 (a), 1900 Aug-Oct, 1902 Jul. 9]

1900 AUG. 18: Birth of **Smt. Vijayalakshmi Pandit,** Indian nationalist, politician and diplomatist and a sister of Jawaharlal Nehru.

She was active in Indian freedom movement and held high national and international position.

1900 AUG. 25: Death of **Friedrich Nietzsche** (b. 1844), German philosopher, classical scholar, renowned for his provocative and highly original works of cultural criticism.

He had a powerful influence on continental philosophy and literature. His doctrine of the 'Superman', exerted tremendous influence in the early 20th century. [see 1884 (a)]

1900 AUG: A Conference of leading Muslims from all over North India was held at Lucknow.

It was attended by 400 delegates from the Punjab, Bombay, Central Provinces, U. P. and elsewhere. The Mullahs, landlords, merchants, lawyers, journalists and others who had flocked to the Conference called upon the "Muslim masses" to defend their "religion and culture" with all their might. Mohsin-ul-Mulk, Secretary of the Aligarh College, thundered: "Although we have not the might of pen....our hands are still strong enough to wield the might of the sword."

1900 AUG. - OCT. : SWAMI VIVEKANANDA in Paris, in connection with his participation in the Congress of History of Religions held on the occasion of the Universal Exposition.

The Paris Exposition was in commemoration of 'the end of a century of prodigious, scientific and economic effort'. It was also designed to further commercial and industrial interests. The 549-acre-wide site was filled mostly with artistically constructed stalls containing about 9 million exhibits and the total cost was £ 4,660,000. 39 million people visited this Exposition. [see 1867 (f-1), 1878 (d)]

In connection with the Exposition, besides the Congress of the History of Religions, a number of scientific meetings were held. In one of them viz, the International Congress of Physicists, the Indian scientist, Dr. Jagadish Chandra Bose, read a paper and thrilled the western scientists with his wonderful scientific discoveries. **SWAMI VIVEKANANDA** met this distinguished countryman. He had so much admiration for Dr. Bose that he would frequently point out to his numerous friends the shining genius of this Indian savant whom he called "the pride and glory of Bengal." [see 1880 (b), 1894 (a), 1900 Jul. 8, 1902 Jul. 9]

Swami Vivekananda had been invited by the Foreign Delegates' Committee of the Congress of History of Religions, to deliver lectures before the distinguished Assembly. Though Swamiji attended several sittings of the Congress, his health did not permit him to speak before the distinguished gathering more than twice. But his lectures were highly appreciated by the Western Orientalists. During this period of his stay in Paris, Swamiji got an opportunity to make a critical study of the French culture and also to come into contact with many celebrities.

The Congress of the History of Religions was held, though the original idea of holding a Parliament of Religions, Chicago-fashion, had been abandoned due to the opposition of the Roman Catholics, the pre-dominating influence in France. The latter feared that, as had been the case in Chicago, Oriental ideas might jeopardize the safety of Christianity.

1900 SEP. : **Wilbur** (1867-1912) and **Orville** (1871-1948) **Wright,** who were first to accomplish manned, powered flight in a heavier-than-air machine, set up a camp near the small town of Kitty Hawk, N. C., U. S. A. for their **gliding experiments.**

Their work culminated 3 years later in success. On Dec. 17, 1903, they executed the historic airplane flight at Kitty Hawk. [see 1893 (l)]

1900 OCT. 28: Death of **Max Muller** (b. 1823) orientalist and philologist.

He was a naturalized Englishman, whose life-work was the translating and editing of the *Rig-Veda.* From 1875 he edited *The Sacred Books of the East,* translated by various scholars and published in 51 volumes. His work stimulated widespread interest in the study of linguistics, mythology and religion. About Max Muller's great venture, **SWAMI VIVEKANANDA** once told one of his disciples: "Did you hear that the East India Company paid nine lakhs of rupees, in cash to have *Rig-Veda* published? Even this money was not enough. Hundreds of Vedic pandits had to be employed in this country on monthly stipends. Has anybody seen in this age here in this country such profound yearning for knowledge, such prodigious investment of money for the sake of light and learning? Max Muller himself had written in his preface that for twenty five years he prepared only the manuscripts. Then the printing took 25 years." [see 1867 Feb. 26, 1867 Dec. 9, 1868 Dec. 16, 1870 Mar., 1873 Dec. 3, 1874 Oct., 1874 Nov. (a), 1874 Dec., 1875 Dec 13, 1875 (b), 1882 May, 1894 Mar., 1894 Aug. 15, 1894 Aug. 15 (a), 1896 Mar. 28, 1896 May. 28, 1898 Nov., 1899 Aug. 17, 1899 Oct.]

1900 DEC. 9: After his second visit to the West, **SWAMI VIVEKANANDA** arrived at the Belur Math late at night.

> The monks had sat for dinner when *mali* (gardener) came running and out of breath to say that a *saheb* (European gentleman) had come. He was immediately sent back to the front gate with the key, while they kept on speculating who the *saheb* might be and why he had called at the Math at that late hour. Suddenly, in front of them they found the *saheb* standing and, Oh, he was Swamiji himself! (dressed in European clothes). The joy and excitement of the inmates of the Math knew no bounds when they discovered that the *saheb* was none other than their beloved leader who had come back so unostentatiously and so suddenly in their midst. They all at once got up, shouting excitedly, 'Oh, Swamiji has come, Swamiji has come!' He explained, a broad smile lighting up his face, that he had heard the gong announce the dinner and lest they finished everything before he was admitted in, had scaled the compound wall and so was now before them. Immediately an *asana* was spread for him and he sat down in the midst of the monks and the *brahmacharins* their hearts overflowing with joy. A large quantity of *khichuri* that had been cooked that night was served to him and he enjoyed it, his favourite dish, specially because he had not tasted it for a long time.

1900 DEC. 14: At a meeting of the **German Physical Society** in Berlin, **Max Planck** (1858-1947) German physicist, announced his sensational theoretical research into thermal radiation, and his discovery of quantum of action which provided the key concept for the development of **quantum theory**. According to Planck, bodies that radiated energy did not emit the energy constantly but rather in discrete parcels which he called 'quantums'. Max Plank observed: "As a physicist, i.e., as a man who has devoted his life to the most matter-of-fact branch of science, namely the investigation of matter, I am surely free from any suspicion of fanaticism. And so after my research into the atoms I say this you: there is no such thing as matter per se! All matter originated from and consists of force which sets the atomic particles in oscillation and concentrates them into minute solar systems of the atom. But as there is neither intelligence nor an internal force in the universe we must assume a conscious intelligent spirit behid the force. **This spirit is the basic principle of the matter**....".

> From that time on, a predominant role has been played in ever-increasing number of fields by quantum of action, introduced into physics by Planck, and it has proved to be of vital importance to the theory of structure of atomic dimensions. The quantum theory has, in fact, brought about fundamental changes in physics.

Because of its deviation from the fundamental principles of classical physics, the quantum theory was at first rejected by many physicists. It was only with the triumph of Niels Bohr (1885-1962), a Danish physicist, who in 1913, calculated for the first time the position of the special lines of the spectrum with the aid of the quantum theory that the theory became a spectacular success. In 1918 Max Planck was awarded the Nobel Prize for physics for his work. He took little part in the further rapid development of the quantum theory that reached a pinnacle in the 1920s by the efforts of the physicists Werner Karl Heisenberg (1901-1976), lrwin Schrodinger (1887-1961), Paul Adrien Maurice Dirac (1902) and others in formulating quantum mechanics.

1900 (A): In his *Memoirs of European Travel* written in the form of letters to one of his brother monks (Swami Trigunatitananda) who was the editor of the monthly *Udbodhan,* Calcutta, **SWAMI VIVEKANANDA** paid a touching tribute to the 'ever-trampled labouring classes of India':

"Those uncared-for lower classes of India – the peasants and weavers and the rest who have been conquered by foreigners and are looked down upon by their own people – it is they who, from the time immemorial, have been working silently, without even getting the remuneration of their labours. But what great changes are taking place slowly all over the world, in pursuance of nature's laws! Countries, civilizations and supremacy undergoing revolutions.

"Ye labouring classes of India, as a result of your silent, constant labours, Babylon, Persia, Alexandria, Greece, Rome, Venice, Genoa, Baghdad, Samarkand, Spain, Portugal, France, Denmark, Holland and England have successively attained supremacy and eminence! And you? – Well, who cares to think of you! My dear Swami, your ancestors wrote a few philosophical works, penned a dozen or so epics, or built a number of temples – that is all and you rend the skies with triumphant shouts, while those whose heart's blood has contributed to all the progress that has been made in the world – well, who cares to praise them?

"The world-conquering heroes of spirituality, war and piety, are in the eyes of all, and they have received the homage of mankind. But where nobody looks, no one gives a word of encouragement, where everybody hates – that, living amid such circumstances and displaying boundless patience, infinite love, in their homes day and night, without the slightest murmur – well, is there no heroism in this? Many turn out to be heroes, when they have got some great task to perform. Even a coward easily gives up his life and the most selfish man behaves disinterestedly, when there is a multitude to cheer them on; but blessed indeed is he who manifests the same unselfishness and devotion to duty in the smallest of acts, unnoticed by all – and it is you who are actually doing this, ye, the ever-trampled labouring classes of India! I bow to you."

1900 (B): 'Mitra Mela', a society was established at Nasik, by **V. D. Savarkar** (1883-1966), Indian revolutionary.

It was started in connection with the Ganapathy celebrations and in 1906 it was transformed into a revolutionary Association.

1900 (C): Genetic Laws revealed by Gregor Mendel in 1865 became generally known for the first time as Mandel's published work was discovered and Mendelian laws were made public by Dutch botanist **Hugo De Vries** (1848-1935) at the University of Amsterdam, by German Botanist **Karl Erich Correns,** 35 and by Austrian botanist **Erich Tschermak von Seysenegg,** 29, who worked independently of each other. [see 1865 (b), 1884 Jan. 6]

1900 (D): Bertrand Russell (1872-1970), British philosopher and mathematician, finished most of his major work, *The Principles of Mathematics.* "Intellectually", he later said "this was the highest point of my life."

A few years later, with A. N. Whitehead, he undertook the enormous project of trying to show that no underived concepts and non-proved assumptions need be introduced other than those of pure logic. The results were published as *Principia Mathematica* in three Volumes (1910-1913).

Russell's book, *Why I am not a Christian and other Essays on Religion and Related Subjects* is an invigorating challenge to set notions and a masterly presentation of a philosophical position. In it runs his reasoned opposition to any system of dogma which he feels may shackle man's mind. The book is in fact the most graceful and moving presentation of the free thinkers' position.

1900 (E): *The Interpretations of Dreams* by **Sigmund Freud** was based on psycho-analytic techniques that lean heavily on dream analysis.

1900 (F): Ferdinand Zeppelin (1838-1917), German army officer and inventor, built **the first rigid frame motor-driven airship** and launched it.

It caught the imagination of the German people, but failed to prove its worth in the First World War, since it was easily shot down.

1900 (G): The first modern submarine was purchased by the U. S. Navy. Invented by Irish-American engineer **John Phillip Holland,** 60, the submarine 'Holland' used electric motors under water and internal combustion engines on the surface, employing water ballast to submerge.

1900 (H): The first British gasoline-powered motor buses went into service in January, as single-deck buses began operating in Norfolk.

The first international championship motor car race was held on June 14 from Paris to Lyons.

The first U. S. National Automobile show opened on November 10, at New York's Madison Square Garden, with 31 exhibitors.

Contestants competed in starting and braking, and exhibitors demonstrated hill-climbing ability on a specially built ramp.

1900 (I): A **mercury-vapour electric lamp** was invented by U. S. electrical engineer **Peter Cooper Hewitt,** 40, whose father Abraham Stevens Hewitt produced the first American made steel in 1870.

1901 JAN. 7: SWAMI VIVEKANANDA (who was at the **Advaita Ashram at Mayavati**) was painfully surprised to see that a shrine room containing the image of Sri Ramakrishna had been established at the Ashrama and that regular *puja* was conducted in the shrine with ritualistic paraphernalia in contravention of the rules and regulations which he himself had formulated at the time of establishment of the monastery for its guidance. He said nothing at the time, but that evening when all were gathered about the fireplace, he spoke vehemently, disapproving of ceremonial worship in an Advaita Ashram and encouraging private meditation, individual and collective study of the scriptures, and the teaching of the highest spiritual monism. Returning to Belur Math, he alluded to the above occurrence and said, "I thought that there should be at least one centre where the external worship of Sri Ramakrishna should not find place but going there I found that the Old Man had already established himself even there! Well, Well!" [see 1899 Mar. 19]

Later, Swami Vimalananda who along with Swami Virajananda was among the inmates of the Mayavati Ashram who had been responsible for the setting up of a shrine-room there, wrote to the Holy Mother Sri Sarada Devi (the consort of Sri Ramakrishna) asking for her views on the subject. Her reply (from Jayarambati) dated 30 August 1902, was as follows: "Sri Ramakrishna was all Advaita and preached Advaita. Why should you not also follow Advaita? All his disciples are Advaitins". That settled the point once for all. In 1903 while executing a Trust Deed for the Mayavati Ashrama, it was distinctly stipulated that no ritual except the *viraja homa* – the ceremony for the vow of renunciation of the world – should be performed in the Mayavati Estate. (A *Comprehensive Biography of Swami Vivekananda,* Part III, p. 1334).

1901 JAN. 22: Death of **Queen Victoria** (b. 1819), at the age of 82, after a reign of nearly 64 years. (She became the Queen at the age of 18). The queen's 59 year old son, the Prince of Wales (1841-1910) succeeded to the throne as Edward VII.

The Victorian era had seen the peak of British Imperialism and industrial advance; a quarter of a globe had come under the British Flag.

1901 May 10: **Sir Jagadish Chandra Bose** (1858-1937), Indian physicist and plant physiologist, presented at the Royal Institute, a paper entitled: *"The Response of Inorganic Matter to Stimulus"*. His admirable series of experiments established, on a definite basis of physical facts, the **universality of life**.

He proved that the so-called "Inorganic matter" is responsive to stimulus, and that the response is identical from metals, vegetables, animals and man.

He arranged apparatus to measure the stimulus applied, and to show in curves, traced on revolving cylinder, the response from the body receiving the stimulus. He thus compared the curves obtained in tin and in other metals with those obtained from muscles, and found that the curves from tin were identical with those from muscle, and that other metals gave curves of like nature but varies in the period of recovery.

A stimulant will increase response, and as large and small doses of a drug have been found to kill and stimulate respectively, so have they been found to act on metals. "Among such phenomena", asks Jagadish Chandra Bose, "how can we draw a line of demarcation and say: 'Here the physical process ends, and there the physiological begins?' No such barriers exist".

Mr. Bose caried on a similar series of experiments on plants, and obtained similar results. A fresh piece of cabbage stalk, a fresh leaf, or other vegtable body, can be stimulated and will show similar curves; it can be fatigued, excited, depressed, poisoned. There is something rather pathetic in seeing the way in which the tiny spot of light, which records the pulses in the plant, travels, in ever weaker and weaker curves, when the plant is under the influence of poison, falls into a final despairing straight line, and stops. The plant is dead. One feels as though a murder had been committed – as indeed it has (vide *"Response in Living and Non-Living"*, by J. C. Bose).

These admirable series of experiments have established, on a definite basis of physical facts, the universality of life. [see 1880 (b), 1894 (a), 1900 Jul. 8, 1900 Aug-Oct., 1902 Jul. 9.]

1901 MAY: SWAMI VIVEKANANDA, though incapacitated by his illness to do any hard outdoor work, utilized his ample leisure for the study of the newly published edition of the *Encyclopaedia Britannica*.

When told by his disciple **Sarat Chandra Chakravarthy**, that it was a Herculcan task to go through all those twenty-five large volumes and to remember the contents thereof, the Swami who had already finished ten volumes and taken up the eleventh, replied with a mild surprise, "What do you mean? Ask me whatever you like from these ten volumes and I can tell you about it." The curiosity of the disciple was so much roused at the Master's words that he could not resist the temptation of asking him many difficult questions from different volumes, and his astonishment and admiration knew no bounds when the Swami did not only answer the question with all technical details and exactitude, but, in some cases, quoted the very language of the books! The Swami told the bewildered disciple that there was nothing miraculous about it. This kind of prodigious retentive power could be attained if one only observed the strictest *brahmacharya* (continence). He further added, "For the lack of this *brahmacharya,* we as a nation are becoming poorer and poorer in strength and intellect, and are losing our manhood."

1901 JUL. 4: Death of **John Fiske** (b. 1842), U. S. philosopher and historian, and the first important American exponent of the evolutionary theories of Herbert Spencer and Charles Darwin.

Fiske attempted to reconcile the then shocking Darwinian theory of evolution with Christian tradition. It was largely through his lectures and books that liberal Christians came to accept Darwin's theories.

1901 JUL. 6: Birth of **Shyama Prasad Mukherjee** (d. 1953), Indian nationalist, Parliamentarian and the founder of the Jan Sangh (1951).

1901 SEP. 6: The 25th U. S. President **Mckinley** was shot at point-blank range by Polish-American architect **Leon Czelgsoz,** during the President's visit to the pan-American Exposition at Buffalo, New York. The assassin, an avowed anarchist, defended the murder, claiming, "I don't believe we should have any ruler." As the wounds were not properly dressed, Mckinley died of gangrene (Sep. 14) at the age of 58.

He was succeeded in office by the Vice-President, Theodore Roosevelt (1858-1919), who became the youngest President in the history of the country.

1901 OCT. 8: **M. K. Gandhi** left Natal for India with his family.

On the eve of his departure, the Indian community at Natal offered him costly gifts which he returned and recommended a trust thereof for beneficial objects.

1901 NOV. : Two learned Buddhists from Japan, **Mr. Okakura** and **Rev. Oda** met **SWAMI VIVEKANANDA** at the Belur Math.

Mr. Oda told Swamiji that he had come to India with a special objective of inviting him to visit Japan so that he might attend a Congress of

Religions that was contemplated to be held there in the near future. "If such a distinguished person as you take part in the Congress," said Rev. Oda, "It will ensure its success. Japan stands in need of a religious awakening and we do not know of any one who can bring about this much desired consummation." Swamiji was deeply moved by Rev. Oda's appeal and though feeling that there was little chance of his being well enough again to be able to begin a mission in Japan, as he had done in the West in 1893, however much that was necessary, agreed to co-operate in the great task in which Rev. Oda and other seemed to be engaged.

1901 DEC. 5: Birth of **Werner Karl Heisenberg** (d.1976), German physicist, who was one of the most important scientists of the 20th century, chiefly because of his contribution to the development of quantum mechanics.

He is best known for his enunciation of the uncertainty principle, which states that there are fundamental limits on man's knowledge of nature at the atomic level. In 1932, he was awarded the Nobel prize in physics for his pioneer work in quantum mechanics. In his book *The Physical Principles of the Quantum Theory,* Heisenberg has given an exposition of the theoretical interpretation, experimental meaning and mathematical apparatus of quantum mechanics for professional physicists.

1901 DEC. 12: Using an aerial hung from a kite, **Guglielmo Marconi** (1874-1937), Italian electrical engineer, and his two assistants listened at St. Johns, Newfoundland, to the **wireless signals, sent across the Atlantic** from a station in Poldhu, Cornwall, nearly 2000 miles away. This successful transmission of wireless signals, for the first time, across the Atlantic ocean, created a world wide sensation.

Marconi built a station at Glace Bay, Nova Scotia, the following year, and he sent the **first readable message across the Atlantic** to begin regular transatlantic wireless service.

1901 DEC. 22: Rabindranath Tagore (1861-1941), poet and educationist, established a school at **'Shantiniketan',** [see 1886 (a)] 93 miles from Calcutta, where he sought to link up learning and living in an atmosphere of freedom in the midst of nature, in a community where teachers would be *gurus* and pupils disciples.

According to Tagore, "Firstly, true education should be a life of discipline in the home of a teacher, away from predetermined influence of a particular home and particular society under the soothing quietness of an environment congenial to the budding of a human personality. This is the period of vigorous discipline."

The school founded by Tagore developed into an international institution called 'Vishwabharati'. Now it is one of the Union Government Universities.

1901 DEC. 28 - 31: The seventeenth session of the Indian National Congress was held at Calcutta, in Beadon Square (now renamed Rabindra Kanon), with great eclat.

Mr. Dinshaw Wacha, was in the chair and delegates came from all the provinces of India for attending the session. **M. K. Gandhi** who had come to Calcutta, attended the Congress session for the first time. He made a speech while moving a resolution on the status of Indians in South Africa. He came to Congress as he said, as "a petitioner for 100,000 British Indians in South Africa", for whose recognition as citizens possessing equal rights with the white settlers he had been carrying on a heroic nonviolent struggle for many years. His request was granted by the Congress and he was permitted to move a resolution in support to his movement, which was carried out unanimously.

After the Congress session was over, M. K. Gandhi stayed in the house of **G. K. Gokhale** for whom he had the highest admiration. During his stay at Calcutta, M. K. Gandhi met and talked with some of the national leaders. He also visited the Kali Temple, and was shocked to see the rows of beggars and cripples pestering the visitors for arms.

1901 DEC. (last week): **B. G. Tilak** (1856-1920) Indian nationalist politician, met **SWAMI VIVEKANANDA.** [see 1892 Jun]

About this meeting, B. G. Tilak wrote later on in his reminiscences of Swami Vivekananda: "During one of the Congress sessions at Calcutta, I had gone with some friends to see the Belur Math of the Ramakrishna Mission. There Swami Vivekananda received us very cordially. We took tea. In the course of the conversation, Swamiji happened to remark somewhat in a jocular spirit that it would be better if I renounced the world and took up his work in Bengal, while he would go and continue the same in Maharashtra. "One does not carry," he said, "the same influence in one's own province as in a distant one."

1901 (A): Towards the latter part of the year some **Santal labourers** were employed in digging the ground in the campus of the Belur Math. **SWAMI VIVEKANANDA** who had profound love and sympathy for these poor Santals, served one day a hearty meal to them. The Swami himself supervised the arrangement and the serving of food to his guests watching whether each of them got what he relished and has his fill of it and conversing merrily with them while they ate on. The menu included *luchis,* curries, sweets, curds and a number of delicacies, things which the poor men had never tasted in life. "O Swami Baba," they exclaimed from time to time, "from where have you got such things? We have never tasted such in life."

After the feast, Swamiji told them, "You are Narayanas! Today I have entertained the Lord Himself by feeding you!" Thereafter turning to the *sannyasins* and *brahmacharins* of the Math, he said, "see how simple-hearted these poor illiterate people are! Can you mitigate their misery a little? If not, of what use is your wearing the *gerua* robe? Sacrifice everything for the good of others – this is true *sannyasa*.... What should we care for homes, we who have made trees our shelter? Alas! How can we have the heart to put a morsel to our mouths, when our countrymen have not enough wherewith to feed or clothe themselves! .... Alas! nobody in our country thinks of the low, the poor and the miserable! These are the backbone of the nation, whose labour produces our food. Where is the man in our country who sympathizes with them, who shares in their joys and sorrows.... Just see, for want of sympathy from the Hindus, thousands of *pariahs* in Madras are turning Christians. Don't think this is due simply to pinch of hunger; it is because they do not get any sympathy from us. We are day and night calling out to them, 'Don't touch us, Don't touch us'.... Unless they are raised, this motherland of ours will never awake!.... Let us open our eyes – I see as clear as day light that the same *Brahman*, the same *Shakti* that is in me is in them as well; only there is a difference in the degree of manifestation – that is all. In the whole history of the world, have you ever seen a country rise without a free circulation of national blood throughout its entire body? If one limb is paralysed, then even with the other limbs whole, not much can be done with the body – know this for certain. Your duty is to serve the poor and the distressed, without distinction of caste and creed.... Your duty is to go on working and everything will follow of itself.... Let this body go in the service of others – and then I shall know that your coming to me has not been in vain.... After so much *tapasya,* I have understood this as the highest Truth: 'God is present in every being. There is no other God besides that. He who serves all beings serves God indeed!"

1901 (B): The nationalists of Bengal organized **"Shivaji Utsav"** in Calcutta.

The idea was to get acquainted with the patriotic heroes of each province. But nobody dared to become the President of the public function. They were mortally afraid of the lynx-eyed watch of the Government. At last, Suresh Chandra Samajpati, the grandson of Pandit Ishwar Chandra Vidyasagar and a literateur sent his younger brother Jyotish to Belur Math to talk with **SWAMI VIVEKANANDA** about the difficulty and to request him to accept the presidentship of the *utsav* function. Swamiji hearing everything began to weep and said, "*beti* demands sacrifice. Go to Narendranath Sen, the Editor of the *Indian Mirror* and request him in my name to accept the Presidentship. If nobody accepts it, then I myself will be the President of the function."

Here the allusion is that the goddess *Shakti* wants sacrifice of life in her worship, and *"beti"* means daughter, a term of endearment applied to mother or to a younger woman. (*Swami Vivekananda – Patriot-Prophet,* by Bhupendranath Datta).

1901 (C): According to **the third All-India Census** taken in March this year, the total population of the Indian Empire was 294,361,066 of whom 207,147,026 (70.37 per cent) were Hindus, Muslims 21.22 per cent, Christians (534,940,000) and followers of Confucius (300,000,000). [see 1872 (b), 1881 (a), 1891 (a)]

If the estimates of H. Zeller be accepted, Hinduism thus stands numerically third among the religions of the world, being exceeded only by Christians (534,940,000) and followers of Confucius (300,000,000).

The distribution of Hindus throughout the Indian Empire is as follows: Orissa (in Bengal) 94.7 per cent; Mysore 92 per cent, Madras 89.1 per cent, Bombay (excluding Sind and Gujarat) 88.9 per cent; Hyderabad (the Dominions of the Nizam) 86.6 per cent, the United Provinces of Agra and Oudh 85.4 per cent, the Central Provinces 82.7 per cent; Central India 80.9 per cent, Baroda 79.2 per cent, Bombay (the whole Presidency) 76. 5 per cent, Travancore 68.9 per cent, Bengal (the whole Presidency) 63.3 per cent.

The least Hindu portions of the Empire are the N.W. Frontier Province with Punjab 35.6 per cent, Sind 23.4 per cent and Burma 4.3 per cent; in the first two Hinduism having given way to Islam, in the third to Buddhism. In Eastern Bengal the percentage of Hindus has been reduced by the notable extension of Mohammedanism, and in Travancore of Christianity.

During the twenty years preceding the census of 1901, the recorded proportion of Hindus to the total population fell from 74.32 to 70.37 per cent in the Empire as a whole; from 72.08 to 68.6 in the British provinces, from 82.99 to 77.56 in the Native States. On the other hand in the whole empire the percentage of Mohammedans has in the same period risen from 19.74 to 21.22 per cent; that of Christians from 0.73 to 0.99 per cent. The result is thus unfavourable to Hinduism.

The results of the three famines within the last ten years (1891-1901) and the increasing poverty of the Indian people, are shown in the census taken this year. There is a decrease in the population by some millions in Bombay, the Central Provinces, and the Native States affected by recent famines. In other words, the population of India today is less by some thirty millions than it would have been if the national increase of one per cent per annum had taken place during these ten years (vide *Indian Famines,* by R. C. Dutta, p. 2)

The reports of the **Indian Famine Commission** of 1880 and 1898 show that between 1860 and 1900, that is, within forty years, there were ten widespread famines in India. In 1860 a famine broke out in Northern India and the loss of life was estimated at two lakhs, but was probably much larger; in 1866 a famine in Orissa carried off one-third of the population, or about a million people; in 1869 there was another famine in Northern India, during which at least 1,200,000 people died; in 1874 Bengal was visited by famine, but land-tax in this province is light and is perrnanently settled; the people are therefore comparatively prosperous and resourceful, and there was no loss of life from this famine. The land-tax of Madras, on the contrary, is heavy and is enhanced from time to time, and the people are poor and resourceless; when, therefore, a famine broke out there in 1877 five millions perished. A third famine in Northern India in 1878 cost the lives of 1,250,000 people; and during the famine of 1889 in Madras and Orissa the loss of life was very severe, but no official figures are available. In 1892, there was a famine in Madras, Bengal, Burma and Rajputana, causing a heavy loss of life in Madras but none in Bengal. In 1897 famine swept all over northern India, Bengal, Burma, Madras, and Bombay. The number of people on relief works alone rose to three millions in the worst months. Deaths were prevented in Bengal and elsewhere, but in the Central Provinces the death rate rose from an average of thirty-three per mile to sixty-nine per mile during the year. The famine of 1900 in the Punjab, Rajputana, the Central Provinces, and Bombay was the most widespread ever known in India. The number of persons relieved rose to six millions in the worst months. In Bombay, in the famine camps, so Sir A. P. Macdonnell, President of the Famine Commission, reported, the people "died like flies."

1901 (D): **Europe's population** reached above 400 million, up from 188 million in 1800, with 56.4 million in Germany, 39.1 million in France, 34 in Austria, 33.2 in Italy; China had an estimated 373 million, India 294, Japan 44, Russia 117, Great Britain and Ireland 41.4, the United States more than 76.

1901 (E): **The Pan-American Exposition** was held at Buffalo.

The site of the exposition covered 350 acres; more than 8 million people visited the exhibition to view 3,500 exhibits costing £ 9,447,702 .

An exposition was also held at Glasgow. More than 11 million people visited the exposition to view exhibits costing £ 350,600.

1901 (F): **Adrenaline** (epinephrine) was isolated by Japanese-American chemist **Jokiche Takanine,** 47, a consultant to Parke, Davis and Company, and by Armour and Company scientist working with John Hopkins Medical

School Chemist-Pharmacologist, **John Jacob Abel,** 44. Secreted by the medullary portion of the adrenal glands, *levo-methylaminoethanolcatchetol* ($C_9 H_{13} ON_3$) was the first ductless gland secretion to be isolated by man. It was used in medicine as a heart stimulant to constrict the blood vessels, and to relax the bronchi in asthma.

1901 (G): Nobel Prizes were awarded for the first time from a fund (initially $ 9.2 million) established by **Alfred B. Nobel** (1833-1896), Swedish Chemist, engineer and the inventor of dynamite and other high explosives, who had added to his fortune by investments in Russia's Baku Oil Fields. [see 1866 (e), 1838 (g), 1896 Dec.10]

> "Inherited wealth is a misfortune which merely serves to dull man's faculties" said Nobel in 1895, and he had willed that his fortune be invested in safe securities.... that interest accruing from which shall be annually awarded in prizes."

> **The first Nobel Prizes** were awarded to the German Physicist, **W. C. Roentgen** (1845-1923), in physics for discovery of X-ray; to the Dutch physical chemist, **J. H. Van't Hoff** (1852-1911), in chemistry for discovery of laws of chemical dynamics and cosmotic pressure; to the German bacteriologist, **E. A. Von Behring** (1854-1917), in medicine for work on serum therapy; to the French poet and philosophical and critical writer **R. F. A. Sully Prudhomme** (1839-1907), in literature; to the Swiss humanitarian and founder of the Red Cross Society, **J. H. Dunant** (1828-1910) and French economist, **Frederic Passy** (1822-1912) jointly for peace. Since then the five prizes are awarded annually to the persons adjudged by Swedish learned societies to have done the most significant work during the year in physics, chemistry, medicine and literature and to the person who is adjudged by the Norwegian Parliament to have rendered the greatest service to the cause of peace.

1901 (H): **Leo Tolstoy** (1828-1910), Russian novelist and thinker, was **excommunicated** by the Synod of the Russian Church for his anti-orthodox writings.

> In his search for an answer to the meaning of life, Tolstoy turned to the orthodox Christianity in 1876. But soon he renounced the Church, as it could not satisfy his reason. He also rejected the authority of the Church. Incessant probing into the purpose of life, drove him to a state of spiritual crisis. Following this crisis, he devoted much of his time after 1880 to write a series of books and pamphlets in which he expounded the various aspects of his new religious and ethical teachings which can be summed up as rationalized Christianity, the foundation of which is non-violence. He thus came into open conflict with the established Church and this led to his excommunication by the Russian Synod.

According to Tolstoy, God is not personal, and there is no personal immortality. Jesus was a great man whose teaching is true but not because he was the Son of God, but because it coincides with the light of the human conscience. The Buddha or other men were as great and Jesus holds no monopoly of the truth. God and the Kingdom of God are "inside us". The aim of life is to achieve eternal happiness, which can be done only by doing right, loving all men, and by freeing oneself from the appetites of greed, lust and anger. The social order can become better only when all men have learned to love each other.

1901 (I): The first practical **electric vacuum cleaner** was invented by British bridge-builder and wheel-designer, **Hubert Booth.** His vacuum Cleaner Co. Ltd. sent vans round to houses and used the Booth machine to suck dust out of houses via tubes.

1901 (J): Sir F. G. Hopkins (1861-1947), English biochemist, discovered the **amino acids tryptophane,** isolated it from protein, and eventually (1906-1907) showed that it and certain amino-acids (known as essential amino acids) cannot be manufactured by certain animals from other nutrients and must be supported in the diet.

He received the 1929 Nobel Prize for physiology/medicine for discovery of essential nutrient factors – known as vitamins needed in animal diet to maintain health.

1901 (K): Trans-Siberian Railway was officially opened.

A decade ago (in 1891) work had begun on this Railway which was to link European Russia with Pacific coast. The longest continuous stretch of railway in the world (9,300 km), it made possible the large scale industrial development of Siberia.

1901 (L): William James (1842-1910), American philosopher and psychologist, delivered extraordinary lectures at Edinburgh under the title: *The Varieties of Religious Experience.*

This is regarded by many as the first great insightful application of psychology to the study of the religous life. The impact of these lectures was very great. The following year they were brought out in the form of a book. [see 1902 (b)]

Religious study absorbed lames from 1893-1903. **SWAMI VIVEKANANDA'S** *Raja Yoga* exerted a potent influence on him.

James' extraordinary treatise, *Principles of Psychology,* brought him world wide response and has continued everywhere to be regarded as one of the few great comprehensive treatises that modern psychology has produced.

1901 (M): **Andrew Carnegie** (1835-1919), U. S. steel magnate, gave the **New York Public Library** $ 5.2 million to open its first branches. In the following year, he gifted $ 10 million to establish the **Carnegic Institute of Washington** devoted to scientific research. [see 1889 (n)]

1901 (N): **John D. Rockefeller** (1838-1937), U. S. industrialist and philanthropist, endowed **Rockefeller Institute for Medical Research** (Now Rockefeller University).

Unlike European laboratories which are built around individuals such as the Pasteur Institute founded in 1888, the Rockefeller Institute offered facilities to groups of collaborating investigations and established a new pattern that others followed.

In 1891, Rockefeller had helped to establish Chicago University. He also endowed the General Education Board (1902), and the Rockefeller Foundation (1913) 'to promote the well-being of mankind'. From the late 1890s he was primarily concerned with the distribution of much of his vast wealth in charitable and philanthropic ventures. [see 1870 Jan. 10, 1876 (e), 1882 (c), 1889 (n), 1891 (j), 1894 Mar.-Apr.]

1901 (O): **The First four majour blood groups** A, O, B, and AB were discovered by Austrian-born U. S. pathologist **Karl Landsteiner**. M and N groups wre discovered in 1927.

1902 (A): **Swami Shraddhananda** (1856-1926), Arya Samajist, founded the **Gurukula Vishwavidyalaya** at Haridwar. It laid emphasis on the study of Indian culture.

1902 (B): Publication of *The Varieties of Religious Experience* by Harvard philosopher-psychologist **William James,** 60, whose Gifford Lectures at the University of Edinburgh comprise a classic reconciliation of science and religion. [scc 1901 (l)]

1902 (C): **Arthur Dehon Little** (1863-1935), American chemical engineer patented **rayon,** the first cellulose fibre, and also artificial silk.

1902 (D): *Mendel's Principles of Heredity – a Defence* by English biologist **William Bateson**, 41, supported the work by Hugo De Vries and others published 2 years ago. Bateson had explored the fauna of Salt Lakes in Western Central Asia, and in Northern Europe and introduced the term 'genetics'.

1902 (E): *Elementary Principles of Statistical Mechanics*, by Yale physicist **Jesiah Willard Gibbs,** 63, helped establish the basic theory for physical chemistry.

1902 (F): **Modern air-conditioning** was pioneered in a Brooklyn (New York) printing plant by U. S. engineer, **Willis Haviland Carrier,** 26. He designed a humidity control process to accompany a new air-cooling system for the plant.

1902 (G): The **hormone secretion** manufactured by glands on the walls of the small intestine was discovered by English physiologist **William Maddock Bayliss,** 42, and **Ernest Henry Starling,** 36, who introduced the word "hormone' in 1904. Working at London's University College, Bayliss and Starling found that secretion acts on the liver to increase the flow of pancreatic juice when the acid contents of the stomach enter the duodenum.

1902 (H): Death of **Cecil Rhodes** (b. 1853), British entrepreneur and states-man, who amassed a fortune in diamonds and gold in South Africa, during late 19th century.

He left £ 6 million, most of which went to Oxford University to establish the Rhodes Scholarships to provide places at Oxford for students from the United States, the British Colonies and Germany.

1902 (I): **Mont Pelee** of the French Caribbean Island, of Martinique, erupted inundating the capital and commercial centre St. Pierre with molten lava and ashes that destroyed the City's harbour and killed between 30,000 and 50,000. The 4,430 feet volcano had given premonitory signals but the people of St. Pierre had been preoccupied with an imminent local political contest; they had ignored the warnings.

1902 JAN. 19: **M. K. Gandhi** addressed a public meeting at Calcutta, on the question of Indians in South Africa. His second speech on 27th January dealt with the work done by the Indian Ambulance Corps in Boer War.

1902 JAN. 27: **Lord Curzon,** who sought to reorganize the educational institutions in India, appointed a **Universities Commission** "to inquire into the conditions and prospects of the Indian Universities, to report upon proposals which might improve their constitution and working, and to recommend such measures as might tend to elevate the standard of University teaching and to promote the advancement of learning."

The commission recommended introduction of post-graduate studies and residential system. The official element in the University Senates was to be strengthened and the Vice-Chancellors were to be appointed by the Government. Greater Government control over the affiliated colleges was to be established. These were sweeping reforms and were looked upon by the educated middle class as interference with their autonomous institutions particularly in the internal affairs of the affiliated colleges, and raised a storm of protests against the Universities

Act of 1904. The agitation against the Universities Act was but a prelude to the massive *swadeshi* movement which followed another administrative measure of Curzon viz., the Partition of Bengal (1905).

1902 JAN: Sri Brahmabandhav Upadhyay, Swami Vivekananda's friend in youth, reminisced: " .... I came across **VIVEKANANDA** by the side of the Hedua Park in Calcutta. I said to him, 'Brother, why are you keeping slient? Come, raise a stir of Vedanta in Calcutta. I will make all arrangements. You just come and appear before the public' Vivekananda's voice grew heavy with pathos. He said, 'Brother, Bhavani, **I will not live long. I am busy now with the construction of my Math, and making arrangements for its proper upkeep. I have no leisure now'.** At the pathetic earnestness of his words I understood that day that his heart was tormented with a passion and pain. Passion for whom? Pain for whom? Passion for the country, pain for the country.... I think of that pain and passion in Vivekananda, and ask, who is Vivekananda? Is it ever possible that passion for the Motherland becomes embodied? If it is, then only one can understand Vivekananda." [see 1902 Jul. 5 (a)]

1902 FEB. : During his stay in Calcutta with **Gokhale, Gandhiji** went to Belur Math one day with a keen desire to meet **SWAMI VIVEKANANDA.**

About this visit Gandhiji recorded later on, in his autobiography, as follows: "Having seen enough of Brahma Samaj, it was impossible to be satisfied without seeing Swami Vivekananda. So with great enthusiasm I went to Belur Math, mostly, or may be all the way, on foot. I loved the sequestered site of the Math. I was disappointed and sorry to be told that the Swami was at his Calcutta house, lying ill, and could not be seen."

Though unable to meet and talk with Swamiji, Gandhiji was deeply influenced by him. On the occasion of his visit he paid to Belur Math on 6th February 1921 and being requested to say something on Swamiji, he quietly walked to the upper veranda of the monastery (Belur Math) over-looking the Ganga and addressed the public on the lawn. He said, in substance, as follows: "I have come here to pay my homage and respect to the revered memory of Swami Vivekananda, whose birthday is being celebrated today. I have gone through his works very thoroughly and after having gone through them, the love that I had for my country became a thousandfold."

1902 MAR. 22: *The Indian Mirror* reported:

"The news of the very serious illness of **SWAMI VIVEKANANDA** will bring great grief to the Hindu community, and specially to the members of the Ramakrishna Mission. The Swami is suffering from a number of complications, and his medical advisers are rather gloomy over the case. We may, however, hope for the best."

1902 MAR. 28: There was a sport tournament at the Belur Math. Sister Nivedita was distributing the prizes. Miss. Macleod was standing at the window of Swamiji's bedroom, watching the event. Suddenly, **SWAMI VIVEKANANDA** said to her: "**I shall never see forty.**" This shocked her. He was running his fortieth year. She said to him, "But, Swami! Buddha did not do his great work until between the age of 40 and 80." "I have delivered my message and I must go", he said softly. "But why go?" She asked. He said, "The shadow of a big tree will not allow smaller trees to grow. I must go to make room."

1902 MAY 15: **SWAMI VIVEKANANDA** at Belur Math – premonition of his departure from this life:

"A great idea of quiet has come upon me. I am going to retire for good – no more work for me."

"I had a message from India to the West, and boldly I gave it to the American and English people."

"I have worked my best. If there is any seed of truth in it, it will come to life. I am satisfied in my conscience that I did not remain an idle Swami."

"I have roused a good many of our people; that was all I wanted. Let things have their course...."

"Oh, the grief! If I could get two or three like me, I could have left the world – convulsed."

"It may be that I shall find it good to get outside of my body – to cast it off like a worn out garment. But, I shall not cease to work! I shall inspire men everywhere."

"Let me die a true *sannyasin*, as my Master did, heedless of money, or women, and of fame!"

"Do you think that there will be no more Vivekanandas after I die!.... There will be no lack of Vivekanandas, if the world needs them.... Know for certain that the work done by me is not the work of Vivekananda, it is His work – Lord's own work! If one Governor-General retires, another is sure to be sent in his place by the Emperor."

"I have attained my aim. I have found the pearl for which I dived into the ocean of life, I have been rewarded. I am pleased...."

"I am more calm and quiet now than I ever was. My boat is nearing the calm harbour from which it is never more to be driven out."

"I have bundled my things and am waiting for the great deliverer."

"I am only the boy who used to listen with rapt wonderment to the wonderful words of Ramakrishna under the Banyan tree at

Dakshineswar. That is my true nature. Works and activities, doing good and so forth are all superimpositions. Now I again hear his voice; the same old voice thrilling my soul. Bonds are breaking – love dying, work becoming tasteless – the glamour is off life. Now the voice of the Master calling: 'I come, Lord, I come.' – 'Let the dead bury the dead, follow thou me.' – 'I come, my beloved, I come.' "

"Yes, *Nirvana* is before me. I leave none bound, I take no bonds."

"I feel freedom is near at hand."

"My dreams are breaking. *Om Tat Sat!*"

"I am attaining peace that passeth understanding, which is neither joy nor sorrow, but something above them both.... Now I am nearing that peace, the eternal silence. I preached the theory (of Vedanta) so long but Oh joy! I am realizing it now. Yes, I am. 'I am free.' 'Alone, alone, I am the one without a second.' " (*Swami Vivekananda on Himself,* pp. 310-317)

1902 JUN. 29: SWAMI VIVEKANANDA told Sister Nivedita: "Well, well, Margaret! Perhaps you are right. Only I feel I am drawing near to death, I cannot bend my mind to these worldly things now." And before parting from her, he took her head twice between his hands and blessed her.

1902 JUL. 2 (Wednesday): Sister Nivedita, on a sudden impulse, came to see SWAMI VIVEKANANDA and asked his advice about a particular subject to be taught in her school. The Master said, "Perhaps you are right, but my mind is given to other things. I am preparing for death." He also said: "**A great austerity and meditation are coming upon me. I am making ready for death.**" And, after the meals, he poured water over her hands and dried them with a towel. "It is I who should do these things for you, Swamiji!" protested Nivedita. "Not you, for me!" "Jesus washed the feet of his disciples," said Swamiji. "But that was only the last time, Swamiji" – she was about to say. But she checked herself: the words were inauspicious.

1902 JUL. 4 (Friday): Sister Nivedita, who had left Swamiji to go somewhere out of the city, had a dream. She saw Sri Ramakrishna Paramahamsa was dying again.

On this day SWAMI VIVEKANANDA got up early and, at 8. 30 a. m., went to the temple and meditated.

At 9.30 a. m., Swami Premananda came to the chapel for *puja.* Swami Vivekananda asked him to close all doors and windows. Closeted inside all alone for 1 1/2 hours Swamiji was in deep meditation and communion.

At 11 a. m., he came down singing a hymn to Mother Kali, Swami Premananda overheard Vivekananda whispering to himself, "If there were another Vivekananda, he would understand what Vivekananda has done. And yet – how many Vivekanandas shall be born in time!" Premananda was stunned.

Swamiji took his meals, and gave Sanskrit tuition to the *brahmacharins*. At 4 p. m., he went out for an evening walk with Premananda for about a mile. They both returned to the Math at 5. 30 p. m.

At 7 p. m., Swami Vivekananda went upstairs to his room, and asked for a rosary to be sent to him. He asked a *brahmacharin* to wait outside. Swamiji remained inside, meditating.

At 7. 45 p. m., he called in the *brahmacharin* and asked him to open the doors and windows of the room. He then lay down on the bed. He asked the disciple to fan him a little. Swamiji then told him to massage his feet.

At about 9 p. m., Swamiji's hands shook a little. He uttered a cry, breathed a deep breath, his head rolled down from his pillow. Another long breath and his eyes became "fixed in the centre of his eyebrows and his face assuming a divine expression, and all was over", Swami Sadananda said later. The scared disciple ran down and called in Swami Advaitananda. The latter came, then some more came. They saw that the pulse had stopped, the hands and feet were cold "Thinking that Swamiji was in *samadhi,* they whispered in his ear the name of Sri Ramakrishna; but Swamiji's body was immobile, immediately a doctor was called in who found "life suspended". Artificial respiration was given, but the man who had rejuvenated the people could not be rejuvenated by artificial respiration. **SWAMI VIVEKANANDA had attained** *mahasmadhi* (Final Ilumination). He was thirty-nine years, five months and-twenty-four days old, thus fulfilling the prophecy he had made that he would not live beyond forty.

1902 JUL. 5 (Saturday): In the morning **Sister Nivedita** was in high spirits. Three days ago, on July 2, **SWAMI VIVEKANANDA** had blessed her. There was now a knock on the door. She opened it. A monk came in with a sad face. "Swamiji died last night" said the messenger. She was shocked, stunned, paralysed. She left for the Math immediately.

She sat by her master's dead body, took it into her lap, stared at him with fixed eyes, fanned him, and recounted in her mind those loving, endearing moments when the Master resurrected her from the soil of Europe to give her a new life in the soil of India.

The body was brought down, covered with ochre robe, decorated with flowers, perfume and incense; with lights burning, conch-shells blowing, bells chiming.

The news had already spread that the maker and moulder of millions, Narendra, literally lion amongst men, had died. A large crowd had collected. Unable to steel her heart, Sister Nivedita, the anointed spiritual daughter of Swami Vivekananda, wept. Tears. More tears. Still more tears. A torrent of tears. She wept and wept like a child. Nobody could console her. Everybody was mourning. Suddenly she saw a cloth of Swami Vivekananda and asked Swami Sadananda: "Is this also going to be burnt? It is the last thing I ever saw him wear. Can I take it?" "Surely," said Sadananda. "You can take it." But she hesitated. It looked unbecoming. She wanted to give it to Josephine Macleod as a memento of Swamiji's last relic, last remembrance. She did not take it. Suddenly she felt something. She bent down and saw. Wonder of Wonders! A small piece of the same cloth, which she had wanted to take, came out of the burning and blackness of the charred body of Swami Vivekananda, blowing to her feet. She stared at the piece of cloth. Did she hear Swamiji saying, "Take it, my daughter! My last gift to you?" She picked up the sacred relic from the burning pyre with great reverence. It was a piece of ochre robe from the burning pyre that came to her feet with the breeze. It was a benediction and she sent it to Josephine, who preserved it.

Three days before Swamiji died he had even pointed out the particular spot near the Ganga where he was to be cremated.

"Go to Belur Math, and you will find that place where he was cremated. You will also find the room on the first floor where Swamiji had died – his bed, his tanpura, his chappal, his table – you will find them intact. The room is kept spotlessly clean even now. Swamiji's Spirit still pervades the room."

"You can visit that room today; it is still kept exactly as Vivekananda left it. But it does not seem museum-like or even unoccupied.... In the life of the Belur Math, Vivekananda still lives and is as much a participant in its daily activities as any of its monks"

Sister Nivedita records that during the final days and especially on the last, the Swamiji emanated great joy and radiance. There was nothing sad or grave about him:

"During the last days one was conscious all the while of a luminous presence about him.... None was prepared least of all on that happy Friday July the 4th, on which he appeared so much stronger and better than he had been years to see the end so soon. He had spent hours of that day in formal meditation. Then he had given a long Sanskrit lesson. Finally, he had taken a walk from the monastery gates to the distant high road. On his return from this walk, the bell was ringing for even song, and he went to his own room, and sat down facing towards the Ganges to meditate. It was the last time. The moment was come that had been foretold by his Master from the beginning. Half an hour went by and then on the wings of that meditation, his spirit soared whence there could be no return, and the body was left like a folded vesture, on the earth."

1902 JUL. 5 (A): **Sri Brahmabandhav Upadhyay**, Swami Vivekananda's friend in youth, reminisced: "For a few days I went on a trip to Bolpur. On my return as I stepped down at the Howrah Station, someone said, 'SWAMI VIVEKANANDA passed away yesterday.' At once an acute pain, sharp like a razor – not the least exaggerated – thrust into my heart. When the intensity of pain subsided, I wondered, 'How will Vivekananda's work go on ? He has, of course, well-trained and educated brother-disciples. Why, they will do his work!"

"Swamiji! I was your friend in youth. How much of merry-making I have enjoyed with you! With you I went on picnics and spent hours in talks and conversations. But then I never knew that there was a lion's strength in your soul, a volcanic pain and passion for India in your heart. Today with all my humble strength I have come to follow your way.... In the midst of this fierce struggle, whenever I get torn and tossed, whenever despondency comes and overwhelmes my heart, I look up to the great ideal you set forth, I recollect your leonine strength, meditate on the profound depths of your agony – then all at once my weariness withers away. A divine light and a divine strength comes from somewhere and fulfils my mind and heart." [see 1902 Jan].

OBITUARIES AND HOMAGES
[Jul. 6, 1902, to Feb. 1903]
(Excerpts)

1902 JUL. 6: *The Indian Mirror* in its Editorial:

"We deeply regret to announce the death of **SWAMI VIVEKANANDA**, the head of the Ramakrishna Mission. This melancholy event took place on Friday last at 10 p. m., at the Belur Math. He died at the rather early age of a little over 39 years. In him a star of great magnitude has disappeared from the Indian firmament. His work in America was of inestimable value both to that country and to this. It extended over a period of nearly three-and-a-half years. He proceeded to America sometime in 1893, and returned to India in February, 1897. Ever since his arrival in this country, he had been far from well. Lately, the area of the Ramakrishna Mission work in America had widened so much that Swami Vivekananda was called upon by his colleagues in that country to send ten more Hindu preachers there to supplement the labours of Swami Abhedananda and Swami Turiyananda? The Ramakrishna Mission has been doing good work in India quietly and unostentatiously for some years, chiefly in Madras, Mayavati near Almora, Murshidabad, Kishengarh in Rajputana, and Kankhal near Hardwar; its headquarters being at Belur near Howrah."

1902 JUL. 6 (A): *The Bengalee* in its Editorial:

"It is with the deepest regret we learn that **SWAMI VIVEKANANDA** is no more. The orange monk of Chicago fame, the loving and loved disciple of Ramakrishna, the great apostle of neo-Hinduism, has finished his earthly labours and been gathered by the side of the Lord, whose glory and love he had proclaimed on a hundred platforms, and whose banner he had unfurled even in foreign lands. His was a striking personality and his service to the cause of the national religion were immense.... If Hinduism today counts among its votaries many European and American ladies and gentlemen, if the ancient religion of India has risen in the estimation of Europeans and Americans, the late lamented Swami Vivekananda must mainly have the credit for the happy and much desired consummation. The Swami's death was truly saintly. For, on Friday last, he had his usual evening walk and on returning to the Mutt at Belur, gathered his followers by his bedside and after telling them that he was going to leave this mundane world, thrice drew heavy breaths and passed off quietly. With his countrymen, we regret his death and desire to console his disconsolate friends and followers with the well-known saying 'the good die first.' "

1902 JUL. 6 (B): *The Statesman* and *Friend of India* wrote:

"**SWAMI VIVEKANANDA** who, a few years ago, made a great stir in America by his lectures on rajayoga philosophy died at the Belur Math, Howrah, on Friday night. He was a robust, youngish looking man of striking appearance, and after his tour in Europe and United States he travelled round the country lecturing on his experiences in the Western hemisphere.... The Swami who was highly esteemed by a number of his own countrymen seems to have died rather suddenly. It appears that on returning to the Math after a short walk he felt unwell and lay down on his charpoy, where he expired within a few minutes"

1902 JUL. 7: *The Times of India* wrote:

"A very remarkable religious reformer (**SWAMI VIVEKANANDA**) passed away at Howrah on Friday evening.... His eloquence combined with a strong personal magnetism attracted enormous crowds to the public lectures he   delivered. ....The philosophy he preached was in many respects so attractive that he was able to make converts not only among his own people, but among Europeans. He visited America as the recognized representative of the Hindu community and his eloquence not only ensured him a hearing, but won him some very fervent disciples.... He was big and burly in appearance, very different from the ordinary conception of an Eastern Philosopher, and his movements and actions recalled rather the warrior than the priest."

1902 JUL. 7(A): *The Indian Nation* wrote:

"As we go to press we receive the distressing news that **SWAMI VIVEKANANDA** is no more. He passed into spirit life on Friday last at Belur in the Math of the Ramakrishna Mission. His soul shook off the flesh easily. He passed away in full consciousness, without a pang. After returning from a walk he laid himself down, informed his friends and disciples that his end was come, drew three long breaths and expired. Unfortunately the best men do not always make the easiest exit; in this case, however, the ideal was realized. ....Vivekananda more quicky assimilated and was more deeply inspired by the teachings of the seer (Sri Ramakrishna) whom he accepted as master and exemplar.... He gave formal and systematic expression to that teaching in Bengali and English and propagated it far and wide. His work was done. Loved of the gods he died early, but his was a crowded hour of glorious life. Released from the turmoil of this world, let him rest in the blessed company of his master and inspire the fellow-workers he leaves behind."

1902 JULY. 9: On hearing about the passing away of **SWAMI VIVEKANANDA, Dr. J. C. Bose** wrote from London:

"What a void this makes. What great things were accomplished in these few years. How one man could have done it all. And how all is stilled. And yet, when one is tired and weary, it is best that he should rest. I seem to see him just as I saw him in Paris two years ago – the strong man with the large hope, everything large about him.

"I cannot tell you what a great sadness has come. I wish we could see beyond it. Our thoughts are in India with those who are suffering" [see 1880 (b), 1894 (a), 1900 Jul. 8, 1900 Aug.-Oct.]

1902 JUL. 9 (A): *Native Opinion* wrote:

"We are extremely sorry to announce the death of **SWAMI VIVEKANANDA,** the most enthusiastic and earnest champion of Vedanta. The labours of Swami Vivekananda in the field of Hindu religious reforms are certainly admirable and his death will be mourned by all. His childlike simplicity, suavity of manners, willingness to confess his own faults and mistakes, – all these virtues have endeared him to many sons of India whether orthodox or reformer. The European missionaries had solely misrepresented Hindu religion in Europe and America, and the Swami's refutations were admitted to be sound and logical. It need hardly be said that the arguments of the Christian missionaries never stand the test of sound reasoning, and when they are likely to be defeated they malign advocates of other religions, and by that method attempt to convince the world that Christianity stands uppermost in every respect. Swami Vivekananda had to confront such persons and encounter difficulties of a complicated nature in carrying conviction to sensible men that Hinduism was the purest of all religions. The Swami explained the Hindu yoga philosophy to the American public and earned an everlasting name as a fair critic and a profound philosopher. That asceticism is essential for the study of yoga was the conviction of many, but he assured them that for rajayoga asceticism was not necessary. He was held in high estimation in every part of the country for pioneering a noble and a true cause. He was much deified in Bengal in spite of the efforts of some mischief mongers to throw cold water over his admirable exertions. May his soul rest in peace!"

1902 JUL. 10: *The Tribune* from Lahore wrote:

"On Friday last was gathered to shades of the *gurus* the English educated young Indian monk and preacher of philosophic Hinduism, who by sheer force of individuality rose by one leap from obscurity to renown and whose genius secured to the much maligned faith of his fathers a high place in the estimation of thoughtful people in the West.... SWAMI VIVEKANANDA was a truly remarkable man, a man of wonderful powers of persuasion and strength of will, who, with a larger experience of life and a deeper initiation into the realm of spirituality, might have worked wonders in the way of rousing his countrymen from their comatose condition in matters religious and social if his life had been spared. It is indeed a case of most promising career cut short, of the spark of life burning out before it reached its fulfilment. What the Swami, however, achieved during his short term of public life was no small thing. He it was who more than any other scholar or preacher contributed to establish the claim of philosophic Hinduism to respectful attention and careful study among the people of the West by standing forth in their midst as a concrete and brilliant example of the culture produced by it. His genius has brought into being a movement of practical benevolence. The Ramakrishna Mission is now a well-organized institution in the country whose members are seen working quietly in famine tracts or plague-infested areas, bringing relief to the needy and succour to the distressed according to the humble means. The monasteries established by the Swami, at Belur, Mayavati, and other places are centres for the cultivation, by educated men who have renounced the world, of the practical religion, preached by the Master, of service of humanity and devotion to the Lord. It was Vivekananda's genius that gave shape to this new and unique movement of a new school of monks in modern times.

"Vivekananda was great in action and organizing capacity. And as men of action have to come into contact and friction with the world, Vivekananda has his critics and detractors.... Not his severest critic would deny that Vivekananda was a remarkable personality and a heroic character the best of whose aspirations and energies were devoted not to the aggrandizement of self, but to the uplifting of his fallen countrymen."

1902 JUL. 10 (A): *The New India* wrote:

"The news of the sudden death of **SWAMI VIVEKANANDA**, on Friday last, at the early age of 39, has been received with profound regret, by the Indian public, and will cause considerable grief among the large circle of his acquaintances and admirers in England and America. Endowed with large powers, and a supremely magnetic personality, Vivekananda excited the wonder and admiration of large multitudes wherever he went. ....The great inspiration of his life came from Ramakrishna Paramahamsa, and in his intimate association with the life and teachings of the great Hindu Saint, lay the real secret of Vivekananda's unique popularity with his own countrymen. This popularity, however, would not have been one hundredth part as great and wide as it was, if Vivekananda had not produced the sensation he did in America, where, however, he did also solid pioneering work, in creating interest in Indian life and thought, among large numbers of people, who had been brought up to look down upon both, as little removed from primitive culture. As a teacher, Vivekananda's strength lay in his personal magnetism, more than in the depth of his insight, or the breadth of his grasp. ....He possessed the power of transmitting enthusiasm to the multitude, in an uncommon degree.... He had the making of a capable man of affairs in him, and the organization of which he was, until his death, the head and main prop bears testimony to his large capacities as a leader of men.... His memory will be held in honour as of one who sought to raise them in the estimation of civilized humanity, and thus awakened to some extent that national self-consciousness in them without which no people can realize its God-given destiny."

1902 JUL. 10 (B): *The Indian Mirror* in its Editorial:

"There is yet another aspect of the surpassing usefulness of the late Swamiji's closing years which has not been noticed in the obituary testimonials in the Press; or if noticed at all, in a brief line or two. When the Swami ceased to be a public speaker, it was, perhaps, he was not any longer wanted on the public platform, but, a great deal more, because he was absorbed in the work of silent but practical philanthropy. In that work, if his own countrymen or co-religionists would not take share, his American believers and admirers did take a very considerable and very practical share. Disease and pain and discouragement not withstanding, **SWAMI VIVEKANANDA** with the help of the faith which he had in himself, and with the help of the faith which his friends had in him, established Mutts and Ashrams in different localities in Bengal and Punjab. He created asylum for Hindu orphans – the waifs and strays left to the world's charity by two successive famines. These institutions still exist and flourish, and as to their excellence and self-sustaining power, every one who knows anything about them has borne eloquent and repeated testimony. The Swami also found, or helped to found,. two religio-philosophical Magazines – one in Madras and the other in Mayavati in Almora. These literary ventures have proved successful, and stimulated much research in the field of Vedantic religious thought among the Hindus. Swami Vivekananda made many friends in the West, and acquired some few disciples, and among the latter there is none more learned and loyal, and eloquent and self-sacrificing than that charming English lady, Miss Margaret Noble, who has become a *sannyasini* and prefers to be known by the name of Sister Nivedita. With this Sister's help, Swami Vivekananda achieved remarkable success in the work of social reform among the Bengali-Hindu community in Calcutta. They at no time claimed infallibility of perfection for their speech, or thought, or methods of work. They did not strive for effect. They lived in a poor locality in a poor house, facing disease and death itself in their local surroundings, but ever stimulating by life, voice, and example, earnest effort in others to alleviate the social misery which all around them was only too much in evidence. To refer to only one thing among many, Swami Vivekananda saw and wept for the abundant plague misery of Calcutta. We are all familiar with the late Laureate's lyric, which begins with the verse – "Tears, idle tears. I know not what they mean". The followers of Swami Vivekananda "wept tears bitter as blood", at the sight of the plague-devastation and destruction. But those were no "idle tears". From those tears flowed the streams of Rescue and Charity. We remember with admiration and gratitude, the work of rescue and succour, undertaken and accomplished by the members of the Ramakrishna Mission – we remember how they penetrated into the filthiest *bustis*, full of moral and material filth, how they consoled the plague-stricken population; how they helped to cleanse the moral and material plague-spots, and how they won love and gratitude everywhere. This altruistic work has a permanent record in the city's annals."

1902 JUL. 11: *The Behar Times* wrote:

"By the death of **SWAMI VIVEKANANDA** a remarkable personage has passed away.... He joined the Chicago Parliament of Religions as an Indian representative, where by his striking personality and stirring eloquence he impressed the soundness of Hindu Philosophy.... To his credit, it may be said, that the existing influence of Hinduism in foreign countries is due to his unaided exertions. All along he led a life of 'plain living and high thinking'. He died a saintly life at Howrah on Friday amidst his numerous followers and disciples assembled round him to bid their last farewell to him, he having foretold them of his approaching end."

1902 JUL. 13: *The Hindu* in its Editorial:

"The news that **SWAMI VIVEKANANDA** breathed his last in Calcutta on Friday, the 4th instant, has come upon us with a shock. Although it was known for a year or two that the heavy and tireless work he did in America and the Western world as an expounder of the ancient Hindu thought had considerably shattered his constitution, still it was believed recently that his health was improving and that he would soon be able to resume his work with his usual energy and enthusiasm. But the will of divine providence seems to have ordained otherwise, and now that he is no more, the least that we can do is to appraise justly the value of the work he did in his life, and to learn for ourselves, as well as to arrange to transmit to the posterity, all those lessons of nobility, self-sacrifice and enthusiastic patriotism which have so largely abounded in his career as a cosmopolitan Hindu *sannyasin*.

"What flowed from him was simply the old stream of Vedantic light and illumination: only the stream in its flow was more all-embracing than it ever seems to have been in the past in practice. And the great lesson that he wanted apparently to impress upon the mind of humanity was the lesson of the harmony of religions. How very largely the world stands today in need of learning that lesson can be well enough made out by all those who are able to perceive the clash and the turmoil that is even now noticeable in the creeds and religions.

"Swami Vivekananda's great work in life has been to endeavour to make the world realize this three-fold character of the teachings contained in the ancient Vedanta of India, to fight against the war of creeds and religions and to make all men and particularly his own countrymen realize that the soul of man is fundamentally divine in character, and that the divinity which is so found within each man and woman requires that the life which is lived by him or her should be divine in character and divine in all its motives.

"Swami Vivekananda was a *sannyasin,* and the serenely calm death that has come to him, at the conclusion of a life of such usefulness and divinely human service, is an event in relation to which nobody has any right to complain. He has done in a most admirable manner the work in life for which he prepared himself and paid his debt to nature. Today we feel proud that India produced him and that her title to honour in the pages of history has been considerably enhanced by him whose memory deserves to be cherished with reverence and love along with that of some of the greatest men known to the annals of humanity."

1902 JUL. 13 (A): *The Indian Social Reformer* wrote:

"We have received with much regret the news of the death of the **SWAMI VIVEKANANDA**, at the early age of thirty-nine, at the headquarters of the Ramakrishna Mission near Calcutta. We were among the small company which gathered at the Triplicane Literary Society ten years ago to meet Swami Vivekananda, then an obscure and unknown wanderer in South India. The incidents of the memorable evening will be found recorded in the pages of the *Reformer.* Sometime after that the late Swami was enabled to go to Chicago .... he became the hero of the hour, and his return was a royal procession from Ramnad to Madras....

"....The philanthropic work of the Ramakrishna Mission which he founded and controlled till his death, marks it out as a unique organization in the history of modern India. That alone is enough to raise him high among those who have laboured to infuse new life into the Indian people. It is a matter of melancholy satisfaction to us, who differed so much and so strenuously from the deceased Swami at one period of his remarkable life, to bear testimony, at his death which we sincerely deplore, to the greatness of his ideal, the magnetism of his personality, and the depth of his patriotism. India is poorer for the loss of Swami Vivekananda."

1902 JUL. 13 (B): *The Mahratta* in its Editorial :

"....The Swamiji's choice of the ideal of a spiritual as opposed to a material life, his successful attempt to wear Ramakrishna's mantle and to deserve it, and his great renunciation are the three key-notes of his short and sweet life. There is perhaps one more idea which has been carried out by **SWAMI VIVEKANANDA**, though it does not appear to have formed the subject of any of his guru's sayings; and it is that a sage should use patriotism as a fulcrum for the operation of his spiritual power and *tapas.* It is this last, perhaps, which made the difference between the practical aspects of the life of the great sage and his illustrious disciple, for whereas Sri Ramakrishna personally realized supreme bliss in a spiritual trance, Swami Vivekananda realized in superinducing something like a trance of enchantment upon his fellow-countrymen, by the magic of eloquent preaching with a view to rouse them in patriotic action.

"In Swami Vivekananda, therefore, we lose a patriot-sage who deserves the foremost rank among the national workers of the present age....

"It is now well-known how successful was the Swami's performance on the platform of the Parliament of the World's Religons at Chicago. His appearance there was the bursting of the Vedantic bombshell among the mob of Christian sects and the charm of his personal magnetism proved so patent, that even his opponents could not help liking him. *The New York Critic* certified: 'The most impressive figure of the Parliament was Swami Vivekananda. No one expressed so well the spirit of the Parliament as did the Hindu Monk. He is an orator by divine right.' *The Iowa State Register* had the following: 'During his stay in the city, which was happily prolonged, Vivekananda met many of the best people, in the city who found their time, well spent in discussing religious and metaphysical questions with him. But woe to the man who undertook to combat the monk on his own ground, and that was where they all tried it who tried it at all. His replies came like flashes of lightning and the venturesome questioner was sure to be impaled on the Indian's shining intellectual lance. The working of his mind, so subtle and so brilliant, so well-stored and so well-trained, some times dazzled his hearers; but it was always a most interesting study. Vivekananda and his cause found a place in the hearts of all true Christians.'

"It is due to Swami Vivekananda that the seeds of Vedanta have been sown in the American soil and the name of India is being respected in that distant land.

"....Can the death of such a man be regarded as anything less than a national calamity? We really doubt whether the last century produced another man within whom such true patriotism was combined with such religious fervour.... the Swami possessed that dash and that intense love for Hinduism, which both Ram Mohan Roy and Keshab Chander Sen lacked. ....Though they won admiration from Europeans, they could not make Hinduism as much respected as it is today owing to the efforts of Swami Vivekananda.

"The Swami's career has been brief and like a meteor of the first magnitude, he lighted up the face of his country and went down the horizon – all within ten short years. It is men like him that our country needs most at the present time; and though he is gone, the glory of his example will, we trust, remain long behind him."

1902 JUL. 13 (C): *The Native States* from Madras wrote:

"A strong and sublime personality closed his earthly career on the 4th night when **SWAMI VIVEKANANDA** after returning from a walk passed to eternal rest. The Swami was born a little over 39 years ago, and built for himself a world-wide reputation when he was about thirty as a masterly exponent of the Vedanta in the Parliament of Religions of 1893. Since his return in 1897 to India he was engaged, in spite of indifferent health, in a strenuous effort to found the Ramakrishna Mission on an enduring basis. But his friends were always deeply concerned in the failing health of the apparently strong stalwart-looking beloved leader of theirs. And now that the dreaded event has come to pass, to mourn and suffer seems to be the lot of India.

"Her choicest sons are snatched away before her expectations are realized. Her greatest men too early become mere names, – a thing of memory. Is it wrong then to hope? No; disappointments and sorrows are the steps that lead us to our goal. It is thus that we must receive the news of the death of Swami Vivekananda. He is dead. He has joined the ranks of those who live to us only in their works. It is too early now to form any idea as to the extent of the Swami's influence over the present generation, and through this generation on the future. The grandest and most enduring work that he did according to our view is the teaching of the gospel of strength and love. His lectures, although a noble commentary and exposition of the great Vedanta Philosophy, insisted with splendid force and reiteration on its practical side. From being an abstract speculation to many, it has through the Swami's teaching become an intensely practical guide in our life....

"Every man, great or small, high or low, is a centre of infinite power, infinite purity, infinite bliss, infinite existence. Only shake off the influence of the body, the power of the flesh, you will come to know the Atman, the pure, the eternal, the ever-present. You will then feel your power and strength. Thus the essence of all Swami's work is the gospel of strength and love.... The lips that sounded the bugle call and uttered these inspiring words of strength, of love and of hope are now silent for ever, and all that remains of him now is dearer to the country....

"Such was the man whose premature death has cast a gloom on India and left it poorer by one strong and sterling patriot who braced himself for a life of sacrifice and duty by drinking deep of the ancient founts of inspiration."

1902 JUL. 14: *Mysore Herald* wrote:

"**SWAMI VIVEKANANDA**, the foremost of the spiritual sons of India...., was a great master of Hindu religion and philosophy. He contributed more than anybody else to shed a spiritual lustre around the Vedanta Philosophy of India among the Westerners. By his death the philosophy and religion of India have sustained a loss which it is difficult to make good. We have many masters of Hindu Religion and Philosophy equal and even superior to Swami Vivekananda but we have yet to find one who has combined such mastery of the English language with such attainments in Hindu philosophy. It is however a consolation that in so short a time he has done so much to raise the name and fame of his motherland in the Western World."

1902 JUL. 16: *The Hindu Organ* from Jaffna wrote:

"....We need hardly say that a genuine feeling of very deep regret pervades the Hindu community here at the death of the Swami. It is but five years ago the Swami paid a visit to Jaffna and was accorded a most hearty and enthusiastic reception by the Hindu public. He then thrilled audiences composed not only of Hindus but also of Christians, by his unmatched eloquence and religious fervour; and this visit of the Swami is, and will always be, remembered by the Hindus of Jaffna as an important event connected with the revival of Hinduism here.

"The Swami was undoubtedly the greatest Hindu Missionary of modern times. All other great Hindu sages and reformers confined their action within the limits of India. But it was **SWAMI VIVEKANANDA** who preached Hinduism in America and Europe, convinced a large number of people in those continents of the truths of this ancient Religion, and made several converts to his faith. Although he has trained others to carry on the work which he had commenced in the West, yet his death is an irreparable loss to the cause of Hinduism and it would be long before his place can be filled."

1902 JUL. 20: *The Gujarati* in its Editorial:

"**SWAMI VIVEKANANDA** is no more. Like a meteor he suddenly appeared on the horizon full of brilliance and glory and in a short time vanished into infinite space.... His luminous exposition, his irresistible eloquence, the sublimity and grandeur of the philosophy he propounded with so much knowledge and skill, his simplicity and complete renunciation of the world – all these made a profound impression upon the learned expositors of the various creeds and religions of the world that had gathered there (at the Parliament of Religions at Chicago) and upon the mind of the vast audience that had come to hear them .... His remarkable eloquence and fascinating power of exposition constrained our contemporary of *The Hindu* to say that never within the memory of the oldest inhabitant had an orator of his brilliance been heard in Madras .... Let us hope the spirit of his teachings will continue to animate his sorrowing pupils. To India he has done invaluable service by showing to the Western nation what she is capable of achieving in the higher spheres of religion and philosophy. He rose like a resplendent star and has set with all his effulgence. His death is a heavy loss to the country, to the Indian community, and will be deeply mourned even in America where he was so widely known."

1902 JUL. 25: In a letter to the Editor of *The Indian Mirror* a reader wrote:

"**SWAMI VIVEKANANDA**, that powerful instrument in the hand of God, is no more.... The reason why the Swami's lectures were readily appreciated by the West is not far to seek. The West had reached the acme of material civilization. The time has now come for the people in the West to become introspective. If a number of young men like the Swami undertake the same mission, they will do lasting good to the country....

"The noble Swami's death was as calm as his mission was sublime. He was in the best of health on the day of his departure.... He taught his disciples that day a few chapters of *Yajur Veda*. He took a walk; returning he took a little rest. He, then, cried for sometime like a child, as he was accustomed to do when his communion with God was deepest. He was in a state of *samadhi*. The doctors could not say whether he was dead or alive. Not a muscle was strained, nor a feature was rigid. The face had not lost, but gained fulness from the touch of death...."

1902 JUL. 25 (A): A public meeting of the citizens of Madras was held at Pachiappa's college to give expression to the deep sense of the great loss which India has sustained in the death of **SWAMI VIVEKANANDA** and to take steps to perpetuate his memory in a suitable form. The meeting was largely attended and the proceedings were characterized by the great enthusiasm. The principal speakers were some of the lawyers of the High court. The Swami's work in America and his exposition of the Hindu religion and philosophy were the themes of appreciation. As there was the Swami's idea that in order to continue and complete the work he had begun there should be trained a band of earnest workers whose only work in life should be to spread the teachings of the Hindu Religion, it was the general view of the audience that any memorial that was to be found for him should embody that idea of his and aim at producing a stream of earnest workers to carry out his wishes.

It was unanimously resolved in the meeting to perpetuate the memory and continue the work of the late Swami Vivekananda by establishing an institution in the city for the study and propagation of Hindu religion and philosophy.

The meeting concluded with an earnest appeal from **Swami Ramakrishnananda**, who said:

"Now that Swami Vivekananda has entered the *mahasamadhi*, I as a fellow disciple of his under the great Paramahamsa Ramakrishna, approach you with the request that you should be pleased to render such help as is in your power to embody the great life-work of Swami Vivekananda in a local religious and educational institution, in accordance with his desire and the desire of many who have appreciated and admired the great Swami's personality and teachings. For the last five years I have myself been doing in my own humble way, under the late Swami's guidance and our common Master's inspiration, the work of expounding the higher truths of Hinduism to young and earnest students in more than one part of this city of Madras. It is here, by the intelligent and earnest citizens of this city of Madras, that Swami Vivekananda's great intellectual and moral worth was first recognized openly, and it is from here that he derived the support which sent him on to America to the Parliament of Reigions held at Chicago. Again it is here that he received the grandest public ovation on his return from America, after doing there the most signal and ever memorable service in behalf of the ancient philosophic religion of our ancient and holy country. There are reasons to believe that the loss sustained by the country in consequence of his departure from this life is very keenly felt in almost every part of India; and to you, the people of Madras, who loved him so well and honoured and appreciated him so much, it surely must be a source of great pleasure and satisfaction to render help in respect of the organization which will, in your midst, carry on the great Vedantic missionary work, which he started and for which he so heroically and successfully laboured during nearly the last ten years. What shape the contemplated institution may take is dependent upon the nature of the response to my appeal for help. It is a great cause – the cause of spreading and propagating the spiritual wisdom of India and her famous religious teachers. The world outside needs the light of their wisdom quite as much as we do in India, and I am hence anxious to see an 'Ananda-mandir' rise somewhere in a conspicuous part of Madras, from where that light might be made to radiate in an ever increasing proportion to all near as well as distant regions, so as to take away the overshadowing darkness of ignorance which is indeed responsible for all the weaknesses and miseries of man. I need not tell you that God always blessed those who bless His creatures by helpful service rendered unto them. Any contribution that you may make will be received with gratitude, will be treated as a sacred trust, and will be fully utilized in commemorating the great Swami Vivekananda so as to continue his life-work in Madras."

1902 JUL. (A): *The Advocate* from Lucknow wrote:

"It is with great regret that we announce the death of SWAMI VIVEKANANDA. The news everywhere will be received with feeling of deep regret and sorrow. In him we have lost not only one of the most popular Vedantists, but a patriot whose heart was full of love for mother India. Earnest and sincere, always trying to live the life of a practical Vedantist, full of noble emotions and thoughts, for the regeneration of the mother country, his life has been cut short in the very prime of manhood amidst the great sorrow of the community at large."

1902 JUL. (B): *Prabuddha Bharata* wrote:

"Our beloved SWAMIJI entered *mahasamadhi* on Friday night, the 4th of July, at the Math, Belur. On that morning, he meditated for more than two hours. During the day, he held a class on *Panini Grammar* for about three hours, and remarked how much better he was feeling. In the afternoon he took a short walk. In the evening, he went to his own room; a *brahmacharin* was in attendance. He took his beads and did *japam* and directed the *brahmacharin* to sit outside and do likewise. About 45 minutes later he called the *brahmacharin* in, asked him to fan his head and then went to sleep. At about nine, he gave a sudden start and then drew two long breaths. The *brahmacharin*, unable to understand what the matter was, immediately called an aged *sannyasin*, who, on coming, felt for his pulse but found it stopped.

"At first, it was taken to be a *samadhi* and a brother repeated the name of the Master in his ear. Seeing no sign of return of life, however, a doctor was called in who tried to induce breath artificially, but without success. The next day, Swamiji's body was cremated under a Bel tree on the Ganges, in the Math grounds."

1902 JUL. (C): *East and West* wrote:

"SWAMI VIVEKANANDA – the eloquent representative of Hinduism who took the Parliament of Religons at Chicago by storm is no more. His open, prepossessing countenance, his majestic bearing, and his orange coloured robe might have contributed in some measure to heighten the effect of his eloquence, but what struck his hearers most was the universality of his creed, the absence from it of that theological exclusiveness which is generally associated with the religions which seek to assert their superiority over others. The Hindu regards all religions with equal reverence, proclaimed the apostle of the Vedanta, and what higher goal could a Parliament of Religons attain?...."

1902 JUL. (D): Babu Romesh Chandra Dutt, Retd. I. C. S., wrote:

"I have heard the sad news of **SWAMI VIVEKANANDA'S death.** I never saw the Swami, I never closely followed his teachings, but you know how sincerely I appreciated and admired his high patriotism, his genuine belief in the greatness of his country, his manly faith in the future of his countrymen if they are true to themselves. That spirit of self-reliance, that determination to work out our own salvation, – that faith in our country and ourselves, – that conviction that our future rests in our own hands, – are the noblest lessons that we learn from the life of him whose loss we all lament today. India is poorer today for the untimely loss of an earnest worker who had faith in himself; to us in Bengal the loss is more of a personal nature; to you the bereavement is one which will cast a shadow over all your life. Only the thought of his earnestness and greatness, only the imperishable lessons which his life teaches, – may afford some consolation to those who have lost in him a friend, a helper in life, a teacher of great truths."

1902 JUL. (E): *The Journal of the Maha Bodhi Society* wrote:

"A veritable prince among men has passed away. **SWAMI VIVEKANANDA,** the foremost Hindu Missionary of the modern times, the most popular representative at the Parliament of Religions, the favourite 'Orange Monk of Chicago', breathed his last on Friday evening at the Belur Math. It is hard to enumerate his services today. Suffice it to say that he will be ever remembered by his countrymen as a foremost patriot capable in every way of the work of raising India in the estimation of Europe and America. His powerful exposition of Hindu religion has marked an epoch in the history of the religious movement of modern India. His writings and utterances, almost inspired, breathed a true catholic spirit and gave a new turn to the religious thought of India, and they will ever remain as a storehouse of spiritual truths. The great disciple of a great master, he showed in his person what an Indian was capable of. Possessed of a noble and feeling heart, he silently worked towards the amelioration of the condition of the poor and the distressed. In him, India has lost one of her gifted sons and ablest expositors of her ancient religion."

1902 JUL. (F): *The Kayastha Samachar* from Allahabad wrote:

"The loss of such a sincere and genuine patriot at the present juncture in our history is a truly irreparable loss, which we can hardly bear with equanimity. Though a worker in a different sphere of activity, no less heavy has been the loss to the country in the death of the young Bengali preacher – he was only 39 – who bore the name Narendranath Dutta, but was better known, all over the world, as the **SWAMI VIVEKANANDA....**

"Vivekananda's appearance on the Chicago platform, draped in the orange-coloured robe of a Hindu *sannyasin*, his lucid and learned exposition of the Vedanta philosophy, his command over the genius and the resources of the English language and his remarkable facility as a public speaker, all combined to create quite a stir in the New World and produced a deep sensation, even in that land of nine day's wonders....

"Short as his life was and few as the number of years were during which he worked for public welfare, the moral influence exercised by him and brought to bear upon his countrymen, has been large out of all proportion to the shortness of the period of his activities.... the death of the Swami Vivekananda has removed from our midst a towering and a unique personality, which we could ill afford to spare, just at present."

1902 JUL. (G): *The Indian Review* wrote:

"The glorious light is extinguished and a terrible gloom has been cast over the land. The brightest star for ten years and more proclaimed in all its splendour and grandeur the glory of God and the divinity of man, has vanished from mortal view. He that came of the Lord has gone unto the Lord. The noble soul that early in life cast off all that mortal man holds near and dear, donned the simple yellow robe of the ascetic, took the beggar's bowl in hand and wandered from one corner of the country to another, aye! crossed the distant seas to proclaim the glory of the Vedanta, is no more. We shall no longer see his majestic figure, nor hear his magnetic eloquence that kept under a spell all that came under its influence. On the fourth this month, **SWAMI VIVEKANANDA** who had been out for a walk in the evening, feeling ill, returned to the Mutt at Howrah, assembled all his brother *sannyasins*, announced that his master's call had come and in a few minutes passed in peace. It is impossible to adequately give expression to the feelings of genuine and profound sorrow which the news of the premature demise of this great *sannyasin* has caused throughout the land and the sorrow with which the sad tidings will be received in America, the land where he built his world-wide fame. It is equally impossible within the short space of a note written hastily under the influence of great sorrow even to describe in brief the glory of his mission and the greatness of his achievements .... The secret of his success lay in his sincere but enlightened love for the land of his birth and the religion of his *rishis*. His religion knew no caste, no creed, no colour; his philosophy knew no systems and sophistries; his sympathy was boundless, and he recognised a brother and sister in every man and woman he met.... He despised no religion, no form of worship.

"If often he laid stress on the glory of the Vedanta, it was because he felt indeed it proclaimed the great lesson which he incessantly voiced forth – the lesson of the harmony of all religions....

"The death of such a man leaves a void that will long remain unfulfilled. This is the great misfortune of India at present. Worthy and capable leaders are few and far between, and when they go, they leave no successors to carry on their work. Swami Vivekananda, however, was a teacher of a rare personal charm and power. May we hope that his blessed mantle has descended on some worthy pupil of his?"

1902 JUL. (H): *The Brahmacharin* wrote:

"**SWAMI VIVEKANANDA** was the greatest Hindu of modern India. He loved India, as no other Indian did, and made her name respected throughout the world. His countrymen can never forget the services he did to the cause of their religion and philosophy at the Chicago Parliament of Religions. Young in years, he was old in wisdom. His piety and self-sacrifice would serve as bright examples to his countrymen No one that has not come into contact with him, can form any idea of his strong personality, before which even crowned heads would not hesitate to bow down. He was truly a prince amongst men.

"....Swami Vivekananda revived the *sannyasa* of Buddha and Sankara, who considered their individual salvation as of no importance whatever compared with the good of humanity. If Swami Vivekananda gave up the world and all its good things, it was not for retiring into the forest and living a life of meditation only, but for doing active good to his fellowmen, free as he was from the trammels of a family life.

"If renunciation is the test of greatness, Swami Vivekananda was a truly great man. His ideal was ancient India of the *rishis*, who made India the teacher of all nations.... He has sown the seed, and we have no doubt it will germinate and grow into a goodly tree, if the workers he has left behind him, make the best use of their opportunities, and work as unselfishly for the cause of the country, as he himself did. The function of a *sannyasin*, a teacher, is man-making, and Swami Vivekananda was eminently successful in drawing his disciples from the various races of India, who, as well as his European and American disciples, are as devoted to the cause of India's religion and philosophy as was their master, and who will no doubt carry on the work, which he had begun but could not finish. Vivekananda though young worked hard for the country, and he deserved rest, and rest he has got. The mission of his life has been fulfilled, and the prophecy of his *guru* Sri Ramakrishna verified.

"Swami Vivekananda was a Vedantist, but his Vedantism was of a practical sort. He did not like his countrymen to be dreamy philosophers, but strong practical men, with love for God and man...."

1902 JUL. (I): *The Brahmavidin* wrote:

"It is with feelings of profound sorrow that we announce the passing away of **SWAMI VIVEKANANDA** on the evening of the 4th July, 1902, at the Belur Math on the banks of the sacred Bhagirathi near Calcutta. His immortal soul departed in solemn peacefulness to its divine abode of eternal freedom and enduring bliss. The zeal, which he displayed while here on earth in behalf of the spiritual elevation of humanity, so as to make men in general and his own countrymen in particular realize the glory and the power of the divinity dwelling within them, cannot but be a guarantee to all those, who have had the privilege of feeling the warmth and the glowing intensity of the zeal, that his soul, from its divine abode, will continue to watch with care and help on, in ways that frail man here, may not see, the progress of the work of human ennoblement for which he laboured so hard both in the East and in the West. Still the loss sustained by us and, as we may well say, by the world at large in the disappearance of this great personality from the earthly scene of his holy activity is immeasurably great, and appears to us to be almost irreparable. We have been too much within the brilliant halo of his magnetic influence to estimate justly either the great value of the work that he did in our midst or how that work will grow and prosper in the coming years so as to make the march of human civilization towards its God-appointed goal quicker and surer.

"....There is only one way of worthily honouring the memory of a great man that has been a great worker, and that one way consists in labouring steadily and strenuously towards the fulfilment of his high aims and aspirations. May God bless the departed Swami's soul with divine blessings, and may He also bestow on us the strength to bear up his loss and to carry on his mission of human elevation and ennoblement in India and elsewhere."

1902 JUL (J): *The South Indian Times* wrote:

"Another distinguished son of india is gone. And it is with deep sorrow that we record the death on Friday the fourth instant of **SWAMI VIVEKANANDA** the great scholar and preacher of the Hindu Vedantic philosophy....

"....It is with infinite credit to himself that he mastered the doctrines of other religions so well as to be able to meet their respective missionaries in their own fields and to even successfully maintain the truth, the dignity and the divinity of his own religion, Hinduism. Nothing is so difficult and even impossible as to expect a missionary of one religion to acknowledge some merit in another religion. This however, Swami Vivekananda has achieved in his remarkable career in Chicago during the famous Exhibition there. His addresses before the great Parliament of Religions held in Chicago in 1893 were received by foreign religionists with discriminating admiration, if we are to believe what the American newpapers wrote about the Swami at the time. The representatives of all creeds and denominations respected his views and even those that disagreed loved him as a man and a preacher – so winningly affable and so unoffending in his expressions and manners. Those who had the privilege of hearing his inspiring and spirited lectures in foreign lands – and he had visited many of them – and those who like us in Kumbhakonam have listened to his able exposition in his country will readily credit him with extraordinary powers of eloquence, deep wide knowledge and his philanthropic heart. Here do we recall a few random extracts from the comments of the American Press:

" 'The polished Hindu feared not to meet single-handed and alone, the combined attacks of all Christians of America. He had thus much confidence in his religion. Yet he did not seek to proselytize. Although his knife cuts deep sometimes, it is like that of the surgeon, in that it cuts only to be kind.'

" 'The most impressive figure of the Parliament was Swami Vivekananda. He is an orator by divine right and his strong, intelligent face in its picturesque setting of yellow and orange – was hardly less interesting than his earnest words and the rich, rythmical utterance he gave them.' *(New York Critic,* Nov. 7, 1893)

" 'Those who heard him once were so impressed by the magnetism of his fine presence, the charm and power of his eloquence, his perfect command of the English language and the deep interest in what he had to say, that they desired all the more to hear him again.' (Dr. H. W. Thomas of Chicago)

"That the ancient Hinduism is a whole and elevating religion has been acknowledged by its friends and enemies. Any time spent on its earnest study will result in personal happiness and beatitude. We but echo the unmixed sorrow of the Indian people at this calamitous news and we hope that the impressions left in them by his varied discourses will be lasting enough to ennoble their souls. We quote below most appreciatingly these few thoughts of the Hindu Sage whose demise we are mourning...."

1902 JUL. (K): In a communication addressed to the president of the Ramakrishna Mission, **Sri Norendronath Sen** wrote:

"As President of the Gita Society (Calcutta), I crave leave to lay before you the following message with reference to the melancholy death of **SWAMI VIVEKANANDA**. The resolution, I have the honour to submit, was carried with becoming solemnity at a special meeting of the society, held under my presidency on Sunday, the 6th July, the vast assembly standing up in utter grief to do honour to the sacred memory of the illustrious departed.

"Resolved that this Meeting desires to place on record its sense of deep sorrow at the sad and untimely death of Swami Vivekananda, who devoted the best years of his life with unflagging zeal and enthusiasm to the propagation of Vedantism and of Hindu Philosophy and theology generally in the West. By his death the Hindu community has suffered an irreparable loss, which is keenly felt throughout the length and breadth of the country.

"On behalf of the members of the Gita Society, I desire to offer you together with your brethren of the Ramakrishna Mission our sincerest and heartfelt condolence for the sad and untimely death of Swami Vivekananda. We mourn over his death because we are painfully conscious that a tower of strength for the Hindu community, that valiantly swept away the stronghold of prejudices against Hindu life and thought has suddenly disappeared, which might under God's providence have achieved incalculable good to the general cause of Indian reform. We venture to join our tears with those of his Mission and offer them our heartfelt condolence because we have the firm faith and abiding conviction that 'sorrow shared is sorrow soothed', and I am desired to submit that none shares your poignant grief with greater sympathy than the members of the Gita Society.

"We all pray to the Almighty, who is the giver of all good, that the immortal soul of the late lamented Swami Vivekananda, which has flown to Him may rest in peace for ever and ever. *Requiescat* in peace!"

Thankfully acknowledging the above letter from the Gita Society, **Swami Brahmananda**, the President of the Ramakrishna Order, wrote:

"Irreparable as the loss has been to ourselves, it gives us joy even at this time to think that the unselfish labours of our dear Swami on behalf of his motherland, are being appreciated in the midst of his own people, however slightly. Time alone will show the extent of his labours, and how much he has raised Mother India, in the estimation of the great nations of the West.

"The Sower has sown the seed and gone to his rest, but shall we be able to hold our own and carry on the great work, which he has so nobly begun? Let us hope so, in the meantime let us rally round the sacred memory of the great life that has been just taken away from among us, for united effort, for the regeneration of our own land and people." (*The Brahmavadin*)

1902 JUL (L): An obituary by 'A Western Disciple' appeared in *The Prabuddha Bharata*:

"By the death of **SWAMI VIVEKANANDA**, we have lost a dear friend, and suffered an irreparable loss. He is best remembered by us, as having been 'the greatest figure in the Parliament of Religions' held at Chicago in 1893, where he addressed crowded audiences, the quality of his teaching and his unaffected eloquence winning a most sympathetic hearing. He had a vivid, eager personality, singularly magnetic, persuasive and enthusiastic. He was no mere visionary anchorite of the Himalayas, giving out the truths of Indian philosophy. On the contrary, he was a man born with perfectly developed spiritual sense, discerning spiritual truths without effort; calm and steadfast, giving forth power from the spiritual centre within, and living for the advancement of his race; a true lover of his fellow-men, devoting his energies in trying to rouse them to their true selves, content to use up his gifts and talents for their benefit. Clad in his habit of red or ochre, did this Indian *sannyasin* standing upon all sorts of platforms, in all manner of places with a strong beautiful voice expound the philosophy of Vedanta. Again and again in his lectures did he recur to the central idea of Advaita, the One in everything, the potential divinity in all. Gifted with an original outlook upon life, he displayed that fervour and vigour that one associates with monks, who have for centuries held to their spirituality with a power and staunchness unrivalled with worldly affairs.

"He was widely travelled; he preached Vedanta from New York to Chicago; from Boston to California. Flitting through London, Paris and other cities, he passed through the vain show, as if unconscious of it, except, occasionally to hurl at his listeners a vehement denunciation of the frivolity, and lack of spirituality of the times. Speaking of India to Western people, his voice would drop, a wonderful smile would overspread his countenance, as he lovingly related the manners, customs, and characteristics of his beloved countrymen and women. What charming Indian legends and tales he could tell, delighting and enthralling the hearts of his hearers, betraying the sympathy and yearning he felt for his countrymen, feeling the pulsation of their hidden life, touching so tenderly on their little idiosyncrasies of temperament and custom.

"He has gone from amongst us, he who was instinct with so much inspiration, and who had in him so much of the seer of these latter days. His teachings have become an abiding possession with us, and a strength for ever-more."

1902 AUG. (A): *The Theosophist* wrote:

"On the Fourth of July last, **SWAMI VIVEKANANDA**, the distinguished pupil and disciple of the late Ramakrishna Paramahamsa departed this life, at Howrah, a suburb of Calcutta, in the 40th year of his age. His brief but brilliant career dates back from 1893, when he astonished all America by the eloquent orations in which he defended the Hindu religion and expounded the doctrine of the Vedanta. The scene at the platform in the great hall of the Parliament of Religions at Chicago, when the meeting broke up as described in the local newspapers of the day was most striking .... This quaintly garbed man with the brown skin and deep, penetrating eyes, whose platform oratory challenged comparison with that of the best American public speakers, came flashing before them like a brilliant meteor. Their first impressions were deepened by his subsequent public lectures; he was invited to all parts of the States, and remained in the country until 1897.... A Vedanta Society was formed, several of his fellow pupils of the Paramahamsa went to the States and are still working there, and a demand for ten more helpers was, it is said, recently sent to him.

"....The Swami has left behind him several works of a religious character, but it is as an orator and public teacher that he will be longest remembered. He had a strong personal magnetism and was naturally. combative.... He was an intense Hindu and a most able expounder of the school of philosophy to which he belonged."

1902 AUG. (B): *Malbar Mail* wrote:

"**SWAMI VIVEKANANDA** is dead. The prop of Hinduism is fallen in his quiet hermitage at Howrah, on the 4th of last month, that great leader of Hindu thought and ornament of the religion of the *rishis*, bade the last adieu to his country. God's will be done. To this ancient land, the heir of the most glorious past that the world has ever known, and to more than two hundred millions of grateful inhabitants, the great Swami whose premature demise we record today, was for the last ten years and more 'Like yon orb in Heaven without whom all were darkness.' The Hindus were taught by him both precept and example; their thoughts were shaped and their actions guided by his mighty intellect. The people of India know, why for the matter of that, the whole civilized world knew, first to admire and respect and then to love him like a master and adore him as a God. The world is certainly much poorer by the death of the Swami and the loss that the Hindus have been doomed to sustain today, in the untimely demise of the great Bengali Saint is one the like of which has not happened to them at any time in the near past, and will not, because it cannot, happen to them at any time in the near future. 'Whom the Gods love die Young.' So, in their despair cried the old philosophers of Greece. The Gods indeed have loved him but too well and deprived a weeping and woe-begone world of its lovely light and leader. The heart-rending news must have been received throughout the length and breadth of this empire, from Kashmir to Comorin and from Karachi to Kachar, as one of the heaviest national calamities that have befallen the Hindus. When we only remember, that even in distant continents like America and Europe and in the remotest corners of the world, the death of the great Hindu sannyasin will be looked upon as a direct, distinct and positive loss to the world, which nothing on earth can profess to replace, we must be in a position to realize the worth and magnitude of the work that the Swami was doing in his life. And now that our revered Saint is no more, what alone, we Hindus, who follow the religion that Swami Vivekananda preached, can hope to do, is to study his life and learn from it the many noble lessons of purity and self-sacrifice, which will last like beacon-lights to the end of the time for the guidance and correction of erring humanity.

"....The lectures that he delivered in that connection are some of the masterpieces of the world's religious literature and, many American Christians who had come to scoff at him, remained in the end to pray with him. Not only Chicago, the scene of the Swami's brilliant discourses, but the whole Republic of the United States was galvanized by his thrilling speeches and the great orator and thinker commanded, at times, the largest audience, that could ever be had for lectures on religion. It is due to the Swami's speeches and the classes he held in different parts of America that Hinduism has become an established religion at least in the Vedanta form, with thousands of men and women in that country....

"....God has taken away this person from us. But his spirit is still with us, and will guide and control us. Hindus are proud to cherish the memory of such a man, and Hindus will love and revere him, as long as they live. Swami Vivekananda was born in a country, which produced the authors of the *Bhagavad Gita* and the *Vedanta Sutras,* and he will be unhesitatingly ranked with them by the future historians of India. We who live today to record this, feel proud, that one from among us lived to attain that honour.

"Lord! Who hast snatched him from our midst, show us the way and make us live like him."

1902 OCT. 17: *The Indian Nation* published a tribute to the memory of **SWAMI VIVEKANANDA** from the San Francisco Class of Vedanta Philosophy:

"The sad news has just reached us by way of New York of the sudden taking off of the most worshipful Master Swami Vivekananda who peacefully passed into the arms of the Infinite Mother on July the Fourth.... As he loved and revered his Master, so we will love and cherish his sacred memory. He was one of the greatest souls that has visited the earth for many centuries. An incarnation of his Master, of Krishna, Buddha, Christ and all other great souls, he came fitted to fill the needs of the times as they are now. He was a twin soul to that of his Master who represented the whole philosophy of all religions, be they ancient or modern. Vivekananda has shaken the whole world with his sublime thoughts and they will echo down through the halls of time until time shall be no more. To him all people and all creeds were one. He had the patience of Christ and the generosity of the sun that shines and the air of heaven. To him a child could talk, a beggar, a prince, a slave or harlot. He said: 'They are all of one family. I can see myself in all of them and they in me. The world is one family, and its parent an infinite Ocean of Reality, *Brahman*'.

"Nature had given him a physique beautiful to look upon with features of an Apollo. But nature had not woven the warp and woof of his mortal form so that it might withstand the wear and tear of a tremendous will within and the urgent calls from without. For he gave himself to a waiting world. Coming to this country as he did, a young man, a stranger in a foreign land and meeting with the modern world's choicest divines and holding more great and critical audiences of the World's Congress of Religions in reverential awe, with his high spiritual philosophy and sublime oratory, was an unusual strain for one so young. No other person stood out with such magnificent individuality, no creed or dogma could so stand. No other one had a message of such magnitude. Professors of our great Universities listened with profound respect. 'Compared to whose gigantic intellect these were as mere children'. 'This great Hindu cyclone has shaken the world', this was said after he passed through Detroit, Mich. No tongue was foreign to him, no people and no clime were strange. The whole world was his field of labour. His reward is now a season of rest in the infinite Mother's arms, then to return to a waiting world. When he comes again then may we appreciate the fullness of his great spirit. And may we who know him latest be in the flesh at that time.

"While on a visit to this far Pacific coast, many of us had unusual opportunities of knowing him. The sad news of his untimely death comes to us with all the profound mystery of mortal death, intensified to a profound degree. He is to us what Jesus Christ is to many devout Christians. Although no more with us in flesh yet he is with us than before. We consider that we were exceedingly fortunate to have known him in the flesh, to have communed with him in person and to have felt the sweet influence of his divine presence.

"In the death of the Swamiji our cause at large has suffered the loss of a great and beloved leader, whose gentle smile, pleasant words and affable address made his presence ever welcome. His was a pronounced personality with the noblest of attributes, both human and divine; he gave himself to the world. He lived up to the highest standard of spirituality so that his name, character and memory are an inspiration and benediction to his followers.

"....We may not perfectly understand why our great leader has been so suddenly called from our midst, we reverently bow to the will of the Supreme Mother who is too wise to err and too good to be unkind.

"....Although we cannot satisfactorily philosophize over the death of our honoured Master, our confidence remains unshaken in the infinite spirit, and we firmly believe that his companion *sannyasins* will be sweetly and adequately comforted and receive the consolation of the Divine Spirit according to the measures of their need.

"....This expression of our love and affections for our dear departed Master be spread upon the records of the class, and that copies thereof be forwarded to his fellow *sannyasins* at the Math in India and elsewhere."

1902 OCT. 26: A memorial service in honour of late **SWAMI VIVEKANANDA** was held by the **Vedanta Society of New York**. Not only did the regular members come in large numbers, but also many outside friends, who, in loving devotion to their former Master, travelled, some of them, long distances to do honour to his memory.

The service opened with prayers, meditation, and an address by the Swami Abhedananda, during which were read extracts from the letters of brother Swamis in India describing the wonderful passing out of the great Soul. Although his emotion was so intense as at times well-nigh to master him, Swami Abbedananda was nonetheless able to bring home forcefully to his listeners all that they owed to the Swami Vivekananda as the daring pioneer who had first proclaimed the lofty truths of Vedanta to America.

Dr. Parker, the president of the Society, next dwelt with earnest reverence upon what it had meant to us and to the world to have known so profound a thinker and so great a spiritual leader, and how irretrievable must be his loss to all concerned in the uplifting of the human race. In conclusion he offered in the name of the Society a resolution 'expressing the great and irreparable loss felt by the members of the Vedanta Society and the students of the Vedanta Philosophy in the untimely passing away of the Blessed Swami Vivekananda, the founder, Master, and Spiritual Director of the Vedanta Society of New York.

The Society expressed 'deep sorrow and sent heartfelt sympathy to his brother *sannyasins*, disciples, followers, and co-workers residing in the monastery at Belur, in Madras and other parts of India, in Europe and America'.

Dr. Parker also expressed 'the desire of the Society to hold Memorial Services in a public hall in honour of Swami Vivekananda, and to raise funds to perpetuate his memory as the founder of the Vedanta Society'.

After Dr. Parker, Mr. Goodyear, the Society's treasurer and a warm personal friend of Swami Vivekananda in his turn paid glowing tribute to him, as did another disciple, Dr. Street, Miss Mcleod, who had been with the Swami not only in America but in India, told how dear India was to his heart; while Miss Sarah Farmer, the Founder of the Summer School for the comparative study of Religion at Greenacre, who could not be present, sent the following note which was read out during the memorial service:

"....My spirit will be with you all as you bear witness to the spiritual uplift which, under God, you all received from this dear brother. To know him was a renewed consecration; to have him under one's roof was to feel empowered to go forth to the children of men and to help them all to a realization of their birthright as Sons of God.

"What Greenacre owes to him cannot be put into words. A little band of people had started to prove the providing care of God for those who rely upon Him in utter faith and love. This great soul came into our midst and did more than any other to give to the work its true tone, for he lived everyday the truths which his lips proclaimed, and was to us the living evidence of the power manifested ninteen hundred years ago in that he went about his Father's business in perfect joyousness and childlike trust, without 'purse or script' and found all promises fulfilled, all needs met. Forever after, as he grew in knowledge and in power, his influence increased among us and helped to strengthen our faith, and today his powers for good is even greater and will continue to be, if we are true to Him who worketh in us 'to will and to do His good pleasure.'

"When the news of the transition of this beloved servant of God reached us, we assembled in the grove consecrated by him and his brothers and under 'the Prophet's Pine' gave thanks to God for what he had been to us, for what he is now and ever will be. It was a blessed hour, and I pray that tomorrow the Spirit of God may move mightily among you all, leading each to know the Unity of God, and find that in Him we are all one, visibly and invisibly, clothed upon with Him who is our Sun and Shield.

"May this transition give renewed impetus to his work here and in the far east. I shall always give thanks that I was permitted to work at his side when the first precious seeds were planted in New York. God bless you all."

Mrs. Ole Bull, who arrived from Europe just in time to attend the service and who like Miss Farmer, had witnessed the incalculable good accomplished by Swami Vivekananda at Greenacre as well as in other parts of the United States and in India among his own people, made an eloquent appeal for earnest workers, who in return for the priceless spiritual teaching which India had sent to them would go out to aid her in the reconstruction of her social fabric, not by offering her new ideals, but by helping her men and women to value and apply those given to them ages ago by their own Great Teachers.

So impressive and convincing were her words that few could have heard them without feeling the desire to share in the noble work already begun by Ramakrishna's disciples; and when at the close, Swami Abhedananda in ringing tones recited Swami Vivekananda's *Song of the Sannyasin* every heart must have felt renunciation a privilege, and the voice which had first uttered that loud call to freedom worth following wherever it might lead. (Reported in *The Brahmavadin,.* Jan. 1903)

1902 DEC. 16: An obituary from *The Illustrated Buffalo Express* (U. S. A.) reproduced in *The Bengali:*

"The recent death in India of **SWAMI VIVEKANANDA** results to recall to mind the brilliant figure of the young Hindu monk who was one of the chief attractions at the Parliament of Religions in Chicago in 1893. This Swami had the distinction of being the first accredited Hindu teacher ever to cross the sea on a religious mission from his own land to the people of the West, and so great was the impression he made on that occasion by his exposition of Vedanta Philosophy, the ancient religion of the Hindus, that people became much interested, and Vedanta Societies were formed in several cities where the Swami was invited to lecture after finishing his work at Chicago.

"He appeared before many learned bodies, talked at Harvard University and elsewhere, always creating a profound impression on account of his eloquence, and great learning.

"If it is true, as has been said, that some of the promoters of the Parliament of Religions wished merely to make of that gathering a sort of heathen show, reserving all the honour for Christendom, great must have been their disappointment when this young oriental delegate stepped forward and by the sheer force of his eloquence and superior logic took the palm for India. Not only was Vivekananda the most impressive speaker among the delegates at the Chicago Conference, but the magnetism of his fine presence, and his wonderful intellectual and spiritual power had made him one of the foremost religious teachers of his time.

"Swami Vivekananda was thus an excellent representative of Hinduism, exemplifying in his wonderful personality many of the ideas involved in his teachings.

"His success at Chicago was the more remarkable as it is said he made there his first appearance upon a public platform, having had no special preparation for the work; except a thorough knowledge of his subject.

"The Swami, besides being a gifted orator, was a scholar and poet, and possessed high scientific attainments. Though foreign born and bred, he was a master of English prose-style. Indeed, an English critic has said of him that his published writings enrich the language. Those works consist, for the most part, of lectures given here (in U. S. A.) and in England and several volumes on the Indian systems of philosophy."

1903 FEB. : An obituary by **S. E. Waldo** published in *The Anubis* and reproduced in *The Brahmavadin*:

"There recently passed away at Calcutta, India, one of the most remarkable men that the nineteenth century produced.

"....On the 4th of July last **SWAMI VIVEKANANDA** gave up the body passed beyond mortal men. It was a sublime death, a fitting close to the life that had preceded it and one in harmony with the grand philosophy of the Vedanta that he loved so well and taught so faithfully.

"Swami Vivekananda was a man who will be widely missed, and to India his loss will be incalculable. The extent of his work there, is far wider than is generally known, and friends and admirers in all classes of Hindu society will deplore the closing of a life that meant so much.

"Not only in India, but in nearly all quarters of the globe are to be found groups of men and women whose lives have been broadened and whose inspirations have been elevated through the ministrations of the noble soul whose departure from the tenement of flesh is a source of deep sorrow to the many who loved him. A great man has left the earth and all the world is the poorer in consequence. He lived a noble life and left behind him many mourning hearts."

1903 FEB (A): A loving tribute to **SWAMI VIVEKANANDA** from **Dr. John C. Wyman**, published in *The Brahmavadin*:

> A pure, grand soul hath left us journeying here
> While he, a victor crowned, hath sped to heav'nlier sphere:
> We mourn our loss, and sadly gaze, with grief untold,
> Along that shining way on which spirit bold,
> Yet calm and wise hath gone. Alas, no more
> Shall we his gentle presence know. This we deplore.
> "To live in hearts we leave behind is not to die",
> A poet sang. So lives he in our hearts for aye.
> The magic spell of his surpassing eloquence
> Oft filled our souls with longings deep, intense
> And prayerful, as the splendour of his thought,
> And glowing with a light from heaven caught,
> Moved us to wonder, rapture, smiles and tears,–
> Sweet memories to linger through th'eternal years.
> Farewell, Dear Brother. Thou wert one of "God's own kin",
> Thy home of peace and rest thou now hast entered in.

PART THREE

VIVEKANANDA – A VOICE FROM ACROSS THE CENTURY

"When will that blessed day dawn
when my life will be a sacrifice
at the altar of humanity?"

"I have given humanity enough
for the next fifteen hundred years.
....What is India or England or America to us?
We are the servants of that God
who by the ignorant is called man."

"He burst into the world like a bomb not to lick it into destruction with tongues of fire, but to rouse men from their spiritual stupor by the boom of his powerful voice. His words seem to gain greater force as they role down the years. He has transcended the limitations of human personality: he has become concretized into an impersonal institution which the world will not willingly let die: he is a system of thought: an attitude to men and things: an approach to life: a tradition which has woven itself inextricably into the world. His spirit is more alive today than his body was decades ago. It permeates a network of organizations spread over the whole world: it has expressed itself in diverse activities which have become institutionalized. It is this spirit which we should understand and catch if we want to make our lives fruitful. His message of spirituality can alone give solace and strength to the war-weary world."

PART THREE

CONTENTS:

VIVEKANANDA
A VOICE FROM ACROSS THE CENTURY

Vivekananda as a Divine Messenger to America
– M. V. Kamath

"Columbus had discovered the soil of America, but Vivekananda her soul"
– Bankim Chandra Chatterjee

"I have given humanity enough for the next fifteen hundred years."

"What is India or England or America to us? We are the servants of that God who by the ignorant is called man."

– Swami Vivekananda

No other country in Asia – or, for that matter, elsewhere in the world – has offered the United States alternative religious experience as India has, over the last one hundred years at least. America has been fascinated by the Indian spiritual experience with a consistency that has drawn to it good men and true as well as fakes and charlatans.

This has been primarily because religion in India is not organized but is a highly individual affair and permits of various interpretations. But leaders of acknowledged greatness have been received with the respect and the admiration due to them and they have invariably commanded a solid folowing.

Easily the first to make a very direct and personal impact was a young – and then unknown – monk from Calcutta – Swami Vivekananda. A disciple of the great Indian saint Sri Ramakrishna Paramahamsa, he had been persuaded to attend a Parliament of Religions that was to be held in 1893 in conjunction with the World's Columbian Exposition in Chicago. Vivekananda was keen to attend it and his own disciples and friends in India raised the money for his passage.

The Parliament of Religions proved to be a turning point in Vivekananda's own life. He was then a ridiculously young man – he was hardly thirty, born as he was on January 12, 1863. The other delegates to the Parliament were older, more prominent men, admirably representative of their respective faith. Vivekananda represented no established church or body.

Here was a man from the Mysterious East who was not *talking down* to them, but talking to them, as one searcher of Truth to another. Vivekananda's first speech was short and not one of his best. But as an introduction, it was most effective. From that moment onwards, he was one of the Parliament's outstanding personalities, summoned to speak when audience enthusiasm perceptibly lacked. The newspapers took him up.

Well-known periodicals quoted his talks in full. *The Review of Reviews* described his address as "noble and subline". *The Critic* called him "an orator by Divine Right". The Hon. Merwin-Marie Snell, writing about Vivekananda said people thronged about him wherever he went and hung with eagerness on his every word. The most orthodox Christians said of him: "He is indeed a prince among men!"

Dr. Annie Besant giving her impression of Vivekananda in that Parliament quoted a man as saying: "That man a heathen? And we send missionaries to his people? It would be more fitting that they should send missionaries to us!"

The point to Vivekananda's many speeches delivered both to the Parliament and elsewhere is that he never apologized about Hinduism nor felt it neccessary to paint Christanity in a flattering light.

The important thing is that he was not misunderstood "and his rebukes were accepted by a large majority of the audience in the same spirit of brotherhood in which he gave them" writes his biographer.

However, the climate was not all that propitious for a religous leader from India. He had often to face the rough and tumble of indiscreet publicity, well-meant but merciless curiosity and reckless slander. A whole generation had grown since the Transcendental Movement that was neither aware of the wisdom of the East nor of the men and women who lived in what was an alien culture. If there was a genuine thirst to know more about Hinduism, there was and equal measure of scorn for what the newcomer preached. But Vivekananda was outspoken, quick at repartee, dynamic, witty and courageous. Few men, before or since have stood between East and West impartially admiring the virtues and condemning the defects of both.

To Americans he was a new and fresh experience. "After hearing him" wrote the *New York Herald*, "we feel how foolish it is to send missionaries to this learned nation".

But Vivekananda had his detractors and his critics and they dogged his footsteps.

On March 25, 1896, Vivekananda was invited to lecture before the Graduate Philosophical Society of Harvard and after the lecture he was offered the Chair of Eastern Philosophy, 'an honour,' according to his biographer Marie Louise Burke, 'which, being a monk, he declined'. Vivekananda had other things on his mind. He returned to India and established the Ramakrishna Mission which today runs its own hospitals, dispensaries, high schools, industrial and agricultural schools and publishing houses and has done oustanding work in famine relief. In fact, the Ramakrishna Mission is synonymous today with humanitarian work of all kinds.

Vivekananda also founded the first American Vedanta Society in New York City. Subsequently centres have been established in other U. S. cities as well where Vedantic philosophy is available for those who wish to study it.

Although Vivekananda came to America as a messanger from India, as it were, to teach and to be a spokesman, he was also a student of the strange country he entered. His utterances frequently revealed the deep impression he had absorbed in his association with the people of America. He felt the powerful affinity which their spirit of liberty had with his own drive for universal tolerance and spiritual harmony. It is perhaps from this close bond that, on July 4, 1898, while travelling with several American desciples in remote Kasmir, the Swami was inspired to arrange an observance of the anniversary of the American Declaration of Independence. As a surprise for his companions that day, Vivekananda composed and read to them a poem he named *"To The Fourth of July."*

Vivekananda's Contribution to America Culture
– M. V. Kamath

It is now a hundred years since Vivekananda took the message of Vedanta to the United States during which time it has taken roots in the country. One of the first things that Vivekananda did after this visit to America was to send four other direct disciples of Sri Ramakrishna Paramahamsa to the West to spread the Vedantic message. One of them was Swami Turiyananda who founded the Shanti Ashram in a 200 acre piece of land in the San Antonio Valley of north California. Another was Swami Trigunatitananda who reached San Francisco in 1903 and was responsible for building a Hindu temple in the city – the first of its kind in America. Tragically, Trigunatitananda was to die in January 1915 of injuries caused by a bomb which was thrown during one of his lectures by a mentally unbalanced student. He was succeeded by Swami Prakashananda who took over the centre and stayed on until his passing away in 1927.

By the time the last direct disciple of Sri Ramakrishna left America in 1921, the New York, Boston, and San Francisco centres had become firmly established, with pockets of interest growing throughout the country. By January 1930 centres had been opened in Portland (1925), Providence (1928), Hollywood (1929) and Chicago (1930). By January 1940 another New York centre was founded (1933) along with Seattle (1939) centres.

In the late 1930s and forties the Vedanta work was still small enough for the swamis to devote their time to writing. Their books, often edited by an impressive circle of American intellectuals and published by respectable firms, sometimes as mass market editions, appeared in college syllabuses and on the shelves of libraries.

In January 1988 the Vedanta literary movement was augmented by the *Voice of India* journal. In the mid 1990s the Seattle Centre was to start a quarterly magazine called *Global Vedantist.*

One reason why the Vedanta movement gathered intellectuals around it was the high intellectual ratings of the swamijis themselves. Thus Swami

Prabhavananda drew men like Gerald Heard, Christopher Isherwood and Aldous Huxley to him. There were others like Dr. Joseph Kaplan, one-time chairman of the Geophysical Year who gave credence to Vedanta. The Ramakrishna-Vivekananda Centre at New York attracted scholars of the eminence of Joseph Campbell (Indologist), J. D. Salinger (author), Chester Carlson (inventor of Xerox), Mrs. Max Beckmann, Margaret Woodrow Wilson and Malvina Hoffman (sculptress). In an era of overt racial prejudice – especially in the deep south – Swami Satprakashananda could not have founded the St. Louis Centre in 1938 without the help of Dr. Huston Smith – celebrated religious historian and former president of the St. Louis Vedanta Society – who purchased the centre in his own name, to then turn it over to the Vedanta Society.

For the Vedanta Society monks life was not always easy. Sometimes they were close to starvation. But help came from well-meaning Americans and of such the instances are too many to recount.

Presently in America there exist seventeen official Vedanta Centres (including branch centres) and they contribute to a monastic body of approximately 110 members – about 45 of whom are nuns in the Vedanta Societies of southern and northern California. Membership in the Vedanta Societies totals approximately 2,200 with a collective mailing list that ranges from 7,975 and 8,525. Vedanta's non-sectarian appeal is widespread. Though many Vedanta Societies house a chapel and lecture hall, nine public templles have also been raised, three Indian-style, of which the first Hindu Temple in San Francisco and the Santa Barbara Temple elicit occasional magazine and newspaper write-ups.

"Vedanta's idea of karma yoga – serving God in every human being and bringing the concentration and calmness of meditation to the American workplace – has drawn the attention of the Christian clergy and other religious leaders. Today the growing inter-faith movement has requested Vedanta Societies, along with other religious organizations, to participate in social services such as Hospice; Transition House for the homeless; correspondence, book gifts and counselling to prisoners; charitable support to soup kitchens, the Salvation Army, Rescue Mission and Shelter for Battered Women; certified volunteer support to 'Reach to Recovery' for cancer patients, among others. In working side-by-side with volunteers from other faiths, Vedantists have elicited feelings of cooperation, reliance and respect from their communities and has further gained Vedanta's acceptance as a tangible contributor to American society".

America in Search of Spiritual Values
– M. V. Kamath

To many it has seemed paradoxical that Swami Vivekananda's visits and lectures in the United States in the final decade of the last century aroused such extraordinary interest – partly entusiastic, partly antagonistic. The paradox, it has been explained, arose from the very common image of nineteenth century America as a materialistic wasteland, ruled by robber barons and devoted exclusively in the building and acquisition of tangible things. What was forgotten was that there were other counter forces at work in American life such as an idealistic revulsion against certain evil effects of industrialisation, as exemplified in Edward Bellamy's famous novel *Looking Backward*. Even as industrialization marched triumphantly, there was a simultaneous search for spiritual values and a dramatic confrontation of orthodox 'fundamentalist' Christianity with a liberal and more tolerant kind of religion, which had been sprouting since the days of Ram Mohan Roy's influence in New England.

This was to lead to a greater desire to learn about other religions and make a comparative study of them. Books quickly came to be published such as *Ten Great Religions* by James Freeman Clarke, written from a liberal point of view and free from bigotry. This work included substantial chapters on Hinduism and Buddhism. Originally published in 1871, it went into twenty-two editions and found wide acceptance in American liberal circles. Clarke, born in 1810, a graduate of Harvard Divinity School, was a Unitarian, a friend of Emerson and one of the original members of the Transcendentalist Club.

Part of Freeman's chapter on Hinduism was included in Rev. Edward Hale's revised edition of *The Age of Fable* (1881) by Thomas Bulfinch. In his Introduction, Hale wrote: "During the last fifty years new attention has been paid to the systems of religion of the Eastern World. Even young readers will take an interest in such books as Clark's *Great Religions* and Johnson's *Oriental Religions*. The last reference is to Samuel Johnson's *Oriental Religions and their Relation to Universal Religion, India*".

Bulfinch's *The Age of Fable* was for decades a very popular family and school book in America and its material on Hindu mythology and Buddhism must have fascinated thousands of readers.

The American Oriental Society was founded in 1842, but the study of Sanskrit and the ancient texts written in it did not take root in American universities until some years later. The first American Sanskrit scholar of note was Edward Elbridge Salisbury who taught a few pupils at Yale between 1840 and 1850.

One of Salisbury's students at Yale was William Dwight Whitney, who was to become America's first great explorer of the Indian classics in their original languages.

Whitney taught scores of Yale students in Indian literature. His studies and editions of the *Atharva Veda* and *Sanskrit Grammer* are still considered standard.

Whitney's successor in the chair of Sanskrit Studies at Yale was Edward Washburn Hopkins (1857-1932). His book The *Religions of India* (1895) was for many years considered one of the principal authoritative guides to the subject available in America. A companion work *Ethics of India* (1924) won him critical praise, but it was his *Origin and Evolution of Religion* published in 1923 that appealed most to American popular interest and became a 'best-seller'.

Harvard University took some time to get into the study of Sanskrit, but when it finally did, in 1872 it gave birth to some great Sanskritists like Charles Rockwell Lanman, a student of Whitney's who taught for forty years and wrote, among other works, *Beginnings of Hindu Pantheism* (1890). But his greatest contribution to Oriental scholarship in America was the planning and editing of the Harvard Oriental Series that has run into forty substantial volumes. Among his students were a number who later achieved literary fame including T. S. Eliot and Irving Babbitt.

Admittedly, these scholars of oriental religions and especially Hinduism constituted a minuscule fraction of the American population. Nor can their influence be described as wide and far-ranging. But among intellectuals and liberals their presence, especially on the eastern seaboard, was palpable and felt. That, in its own ways, created waves of its own.

The American intllectual soil was ready to receive the spiritual wisdom of India. A host of movements came into being: The Self-realization Fellowship founded by Paramahamsa Yogananda, the Hare Krishna Movement founded by Swami Srila Prabhupada, the 3HO Foundation of Yogi Bhajan, the Muktananda Ashram (S. Y. D. A), the Sivananda Ashram, the Vishnu Devenanda Ashram, the Auroville Association, the Yoga Society of San Francisco, the Blue Mountain Meditation Centre, the Divine Life Mission branches and the California Institute of Asian Studies set up by the late Dr. Haridas Chaudhury, each in its own gracious way, fulfilling the needs of young and old alike. To the extent that these movements provided the anchorage and security that so many needed and sought, their relevance to contemporary American Society seems unchallengeable.

Vivekananda goes to America
– Christopher Isherwood

"The going forth of Vivekananda marked out by the Master (meaning Sri Ramakrishna) as the heroic soul destined to take the world between his two hands and change it, was the fist sign to the world that India was awake not only to survive but also to conquer...."

– Sri Aurobindo

In 1893, a Parliament of Religions was to be held at the World's Columbian Exposition in Chicago. Vivekananda was anxious to attend it, and his disciples and friends raised the money for the passage. What followed was a typically Indian comedy of errors. He arrived much too early in the United States. His funds ran out. He lost the address of his Chicago hosts, did not know how to use the telephone or the directory, and spent the night sleeping in a box in the freight-yards. Next morning, after much walking, he found himself in a fashionable residential district, without a cent in his pocket. There seemed no point in going any further. He sat down on the sidewalk and resigned himself to the will of God. Presently, a door opened, and a well-dressed lady came out. "Sir," she asked, "are you a delegate to the Parliament of Religions?" A few minutes later, he was sitting down to breakfast, with all his difficulties solved.

The other delegates to the Parliament were prominent men, admirably representative of their respective creeds. Vivekananda, like his Master, was unknown. For this very reason, his magnificent presence created much speculation among the audience. When he rose to speak, his first words, "Sisters and Brothers of America," released one of those mysterious discharges of enthusiasm which seem to be due to an exactly right conjunction of subject, speaker and occasion. People rose from their seats and cheered for several minutes. Vivekananda's speech was short, and not one of his best; but, as an introduction, it was most effective. Henceforward, he was one of the Parliament's outstanding personalities. The newspapers took him up. Invitations to lecture began to come in from all over the country. It was clear that he would have to remain in the United States for some time.

In those days, a foreign lecturer touring America found himself in a position midway between that of a campaigning politician and a circus performer. He had to face the rough-and-tumble of indiscreet publicity, well-meant but merciless curiosity, reckless slander, crude hospitality, endless noise and hurry and fuss. Vivekananda was surprisingly well-equipped for all these trials. He was outspoken, quick at repartee, dynamic, witty and courageous. Above all, he was a true monk; and only a monk could have preserved his inner calm amidst such a tumult. On one occasion, a party of cowboys fired pistols around his head during a lecture, for a joke. Vivekananda went on imperturbably. He said what he had to say, whether the audience liked it or not. "In New York," he used to remark, "I have emptied entire halls."

His main theme was the universality of religious truth, a dangerous topic in communities which still clung to a rigid Christian fundamentalism. To such listeners, the doctrine of the *Atman* must have sounded like the most appalling blasphemy: "Look at the ocean and not at the wave; see no difference between ant and angel. Every worm is the brother of the Nazarene ....Obey the Scriptures until you are strong enough to do without them.... Every man in Christian countries has a huge cathedral on his head, and on top of that a book.... The range of idols is from wood and stone to Jesus and Buddha...." Vivekananda is pre-eminently the prophet of self-reliance, of courage, of individual enquiry and effort. His favourite story was of the lion who imagined himself to be a sheep, until another lion showed him his reflection in a pool. "You are lions, you are pure, infinite and perfect souls. The might of the universe is within you.... After long searches here and there, at last you come back, completing the circle from where you started, and find that He, for whom you have been weeping and praying in churches and temples, on whom you were looking as the mystery of all mysteries shrouded in the clouds, is nearest of the near, your own Self, the reality of your life."

Vivekananda realy loved America: that was part of his greatness. As few men, before or since, he stood between East and West impartially, admiring the virtues and condemning the defects of both. To Americans and Englishmen, he preached india's religious tolerance, her freedom of spiritual investigation, her ideal of total dedication to the search for God. To Indians, he spoke severely of their sloth, their timid conservatism in manners and customs, and held up for their imitation the efficiency of the American and the Englishman's energy and tenacity.

In 1897, after two visits to England, he returned to India, where he witnessed the founding of the Ramakrishna Order, with its headquarters in Calcutta, and the establishment of several other monasteries. His progress through the country was triumphal; and his achievements in the West, real as they were, were wildly exaggerated by the enthusiasm of his Indian disciples. Yet, amidst all this adulation, Vivekananda never lost his emotional balance. Again and again, he paid homage to Brahmananda, whose spirituality was the inner strength of the movement and the inspiration of its growth. The relation between these two men, the ardent missionary and the calm, taciturn mystic remained deep and beautiful throughout their lives.

In 1899, Vivekananda returned to America. His second visit was less spectacular than his first; it was concerned chiefly with the development of small groups and the training of devotees in different parts of the country. But it made great demands upon his already failing strength. He came back to India by way of England and Europe at the end of 1900 sick and exhausted. His mood, too, had changed. He was weary of talk, of letter-writing, of the endless problems of organization. He was weary of activity. He longed for the Himalayas, and the peace of meditation. Through much struggle, he had learned resignation and acceptance. He was happier, perhaps, than at any other period of his life.

His departure from this life, on July 4th, 1902, had all the marks of a premeditated act. For some months, he had been quietly releasing himself from his various responsibilities and making final arrangements. His health gave no particular cause for alarm. He had been ill, and now seemed better. He ate his midday meal with relish, talked philosophy with his brother Swamis, and went for a walk. In the evening, he sat down to meditate, giving instructions that he was not to be disturbed. Presenty, he passed into *samadhi,* and the heart stopped beating. It all happened so quietly that nobody could believe this was the end. For hours, they tried to rouse him. But his Mother's work was done. And Ramakrishna had set him free at last.

I have already suggested that Vivekananda had two messages to deliver; one to the East, the other to the West. In the United States and in England, he preached the universality of religious truth, attacked materialism, and advocated spiritual experiment, as againgst dogma and tradition. In India, on the other hand, we find that he preferred to stress the ideal of social service. To each, he tried to give what was most lacking.

II

Vivekananda championed the cause of Hinduism in the Parliament of Religions held at Chicago (U. S. A) in 1893 in connection with the celebration of the 400th anniversary of the discovery of America by Columbus. There, in the presence of the representatives of all the religions from almost all the countries in the world, the young monk from India expounded the principles of Vedanta and the greatness of Hinduism with such persuasive eloquence that from the very first he captivated the hearts of vast audience. It would be hardly an exaggeration to say that Swami Vivekananda made a place for Hinduism in the cultural map of the modern world. The civilized nations of the West had hitherto looked down upon Hinduism as a bundle of superstitions, evil institutions, and immoral customs, unworthy of serious consideration in the progressive world of today. Now, for the first time, they not only greeted, with hearty approval, the lofty principles of Hinduism as expounded by Vivekananda, but accorded a very high place to it in the cultures and civilizations of the world. The repercussion of this on the vast Hindu community can be easily imagined. The Hindu intelligentsia were always very sensitive to the criticism of the Westerners, particularly the missionaries, regarding the many evils and shortcomings of the Hindu society and religion, as with their rational outlook they could not but admit the force of much of this criticism. They had always to be on the defensive and their attitude was mostly apologetic, whenever there was a comparative estimate of the values of the Hindu and Western culture. They had almost taken for granted the inferiority of their culture vis-a-vis that of the West which was so confidently asserted by the Western scholars. Now, all on a sudden, the table was turned and the representatives of the West joined in a chorus of applause at the hidden virtues of Hinduism which were hitherto unsuspected either by friends or foes. It not only restored the self-confidence of the Hindus in their own culture and civilization, but quickened their sense of national pride and patriotism. This sentiment was echoed and re-echoed in the numerous public addresses which were presented to Swami Vivekananda on his home-coming by the Hindus all over India, almost literally from Cape Comorin to the Himalayas. It was a great contribution to the growing Hindu nationalism.

On his return to India, Swami Vivekananda preached the spiritual basis of Hindu civilization and pointed out in his writings and speeches that the spirituality of India was not less valuable, nor less important for the welfare of humanity, than the much vaunted material greatness of the West which has dazzled our eyes. He was never tired of asking the Indians to turn their eyes, dazed by the splendour of the West, to their own ideals and institutions. By a comparative estimate of the real values of the Hindu ideals and institutions and those of the West he maintained the superiority of the former and asked his countrymen never to exchange gold for tinsels....

But Vivekananda was not prejudiced against the West nor insensible to the value of her achievements. He frankly admitted that Indian culture was neither spotless nor perfect. It has to learn many things from the West, but without sacrificing its true character.

– Dr. R. C. Majumdar

Vivekananda – His Bharata Parikrama and Participation in the World's Parliament of Religions, in Retrospect
– Dr. Shankar Dayal Sharma

"We are privileged to be living at the time of the centennial of Swami Vivekananda's visit to America in 1893. This centennial is a once in a hundred year opportunity to spread his message."

"Our effort should be to put Swami Vivekananda's message of Practical Vedanta in our own life and share his message with those who are eager to have new vision and new hope for mankind."

In this Centenary year (1992-93) of Swamiji's *Bharata Parikrama* and his brilliant participation in the World's Parliament of Religions, we do well to recall his teachings and his life's work in the service of humanity. Just as the *parikrama* helped to weave the threads of our cultural unity into a harmonizing pattern and became an important link in the re-awakening of our national consciousness, so also, in Chicago, Swamiji gave a new perspective of Religion and introduced India to the West, indeed to Indians themselves.

The spirit of Sri Ramakrishna and Swami Vivekananda is one of universal religion, embodying the principles of a truly spiritual life. In fulfilment of a divine, mission passed on to him by Sri Ramakrishna, Swami Vivekananda undertook the *Bharata Parikrama* and travelled extensively abroad.

Swamiji travelled to Varanasi and the *"tirthas"* in the Himalayas and to Dwaraka, holy with the memories and legends of Sri Krishna. At Pune, he was the guest of a towering hero of our freedom struggle, Lokamanya Tilak. "He had the wonderful faculty of answering many men and many questions at the same time. It might be a talk on Spenser or some thought of Shakespeare and Kalidasa, Darwin's theory of evolution, Jewish history, the growth of Aryan civilization, the *Vedas*, Islam or Christianity – whatever the question, the Swami was ready with an appropriate answer", stated a report on his stay in Kerala at that time. From Trivandrum, he went on to Rameshwarm and to Kanyakumari, the southernmost tip of the sub-continent, thus completing his great pilgrimage. And it was there, while reflecting and meditating on his beloved motherland that he received the enlightenment which gave him his mission in the service of humanity and his place in the history of mankind.

At the Chicago Parliament of Religions, Swamiji explained how Hinduism was itself a Parliament of Religions and held in equal esteem different paths to God. In the United States, the leading newspapers wrote eloquently about him, the *"New York Herald"* commenting, "He is undoubtedly the greatest figure in the Parliament of Religions.... It was now to be his mission to help all men rise to their heights by spiritual education and strive to alleviate the sufferings and remove the ignorance of his own countrymen.

Dr. Annie Besant has thus described her meeting with Swami Vivekananda at the Parliament of Religions: "A striking figure, clad in yellow and orange, shining like the sun of India in the midst of the heavy atmosphere of Chicago, a lion-head, piercing eyes, mobile lips, movements swift and abrupt – such was my first impression of Swami Vivekananda, as I met him in one of the rooms set apart for the use of the delegates in the Parliament of Religions.... Purposeful, virile, strong, he stood out, man among men, able to hold his own."

The news of Swamiji's thundering success at the Parliament was slow in reaching India but once it became known, it created an outburst of joy and national pride. Many recalled the old prophecy of Sri Ramakrishna: "Naren will shake the world to its foundations."

Both in India and abroad, Swamiji upheld the validity of all religions and their right to independent existence. He once concluded a discussion on the universality of religion with the following words: "Our watchword will be acceptance and not exclusion. Not only toleration but acceptance. Toleration means that I think that you are wrong and I am just allowing

you to live. I believe in acceptance. I accept all religions that were in the
past and worship them all. I worship God with every one of them, in
whatever form they worship Him... Salutations to all prophets of the past,
to all great men of the present and to all that are to come in the future."

Swami Vivekananda was steeped in the lore and learning of India. He
knew of the ancient basis of our approach to life and of our achievements
and he explained these to the people in a language which they understood
easily. But he did not limit himself to India and it was because of this that
his voice was listened to with great attention in other countries as well. He
said: "We should give positive ideas. Negative thoughts only weaken
men.... If you can give them positive ideas, people will grow up to be men
and learn to stand on their own legs. In language and literature, in poetry
and arts, in everything we must point out not the mistake that people are
making in their thoughts and actions, but the way in which they will be
able to do these things better."

What greater satisfaction can an admirer of Swami Vivekananda derive,
than recalling his monumental work for the uplift of human society through
sustained inculcation of moral and ethical values.

But it is not enough to only revere the person Vivekananda, his message
is to be understood, acted and implemented. Only then would we have truly
paid homage to Swamiji's hallowed memory and done justice to his legacy.

Vivekananda – His Historic Chicago Address
– K. Suryanarayana Rao

*"But then his speech was like a tongue of flame. Among the grey wastes of
cold dissertation it fired the souls of the listening throng. Hardly had he
pronounced the very simple opening words – 'Sisters and brothers of
America' – than hundreds rose in their seats and applauded. He wondered
if it could really be him they were applauding. He was certainly the first to
cast off the formalism of the Congress and to speak to the masses in the
language for which they were waiting. Silence fell again. He greeted the
youngest of the nations in the name of the most ancient monastic Order in
the world – in Vedic Order of Sannyasins. He presented Hinduism as the
mother of religions, who had taught them the double precept: Accept and
understand one another. He quoted two beautiful passages from the sacred
books: 'Whoever comes to me, through whatsoever form, I reach him.'
'All men are struggling through paths which in the end lead to Me.' "*

– Romain Rolland

It was exactly 100 years ago (1893) that Swami Vivekananda made his
celebrated speech at the World's Parliament of Religions at Chicago that
opened the eyes of the Westerners. It was a brief but intense speech which
Swamiji delivered in the afternoon session. Its spirit of universality,

earnestness and breadth of outlook completely captured the whole assembly. He cast off the formalism of the Parliament and spoke to nearly 7000 people assembled, in the language of the heart:

Sisters and Brothers of America,

It fills my heart with joy unspeakable to rise in response to the warm and cordial welcome which you have given us. I thank you in the name of the most ancient Order of monks in the world; I thank you in the name of the mother of religions; and I thank you in the name of millions and millions of Hindu people of all classes and sects.

My thanks, also, to some of the speakers on the platform who, referring to the delegates from the Orient, have told you that these men from far-off nations may well claim the honour of bearing to different lands the idea of toleration.

I am proud to belong to a religion which has taught the world both tolerance and universal acceptance. We believe not only in universal toleration, but we accept all religions as true. I am proud to belong to a nation which has sheltered the persecuted and the refugees of all religions and all nations of the earth.

I am proud to tell you that we have gathered in our bosom the purest remnant of the Israelites, who came to Southern India and took refuge with us in the very year in which their holy temple was shattered to pieces by Roman tyranny. I am proud to belong to the religion which has sheltered and is still fostering the remnant of the grand Zoroastrian nation.

I will quote to you, brethren, a few lines from a hymn which I remember to have repeated from my earliest boyhood, which is every day repeated by millions of human beings: "As the different streams having their sources in different places all mingle their water in the sea, so O Lord, the different paths which men take through different tendencies, various though they appear, crooked or straight, all lead to Thee."

The present convention, which is one of the most august assemblies ever held, is in itself a vindication, a declaration to the world of the wonderful doctrine preached in the *Gita*: "Whosoever comes to Me, through whatsoever form, I reach him; all men are struggling through paths which in the end lead to me." Sectarianism, bigotry, and its horrible descendant fanaticism, have long possessed this beautiful earth. They have filled the earth with violence, drenched it often and often with human blood, destroyed civilization and sent whole nations to despair.

Had it not been for these horrible demons, human society would be far more advanced than it is now. But their time is come; and I fervently hope that the bell that tolled this morning in honour of this convention may be the death-knell of all fanaticism, of all persecutions with the sword or with the pen, and of all uncharitable feelings between persons wending their way to the same goal.

On the 11th September 1893, history was made. Swami Vivekananda, a young sannyasin from Bharat, barely 30, burst upon the world with his message of universal all-embracing Hinduism. It was the opening day of the World's Parliament of Religions, held at Chicago.

The Western intelligentsia had organized the great Columbian Exposition to demonstrate to the world the achievements of the Industrial Revolution. It was a unique exhibition of scientific and technological developments accomplished by them. It was the desire of some to hold a World's Parliament of Religions also at the same time and venue. Some prominent clergymen opposed the move, on the plea that this would give recognition to and acceptance of other so-called religions, whereas actually there was no religion other than Christianity. Some of his young admirers, wanted Swamiji to attend the Parliament and expound the greatness of Hinduism.

Swami Vivekananda arrived at Chicago in July 1893. The Parliament was to be held in September, and none could be a delegate without having registered his name and without proper credentials.

One day Professor J. H. Wright of Harvard University, came to meet Vivekananda. The Professor was highly impressed. He said: "Swamiji, your ideas are not to be confined within the four walls of a room. You should give a talk and make the world know about your wonderful ideas."

Swamiji explained his predicament. Professor Wright remarked, "Swami, to ask you for credentials is like questioning the everbright Sun his right to shine!" He gave a letter of introduction to Rev. Barrows, the Chairman of the Parliament of Religions, in which he wrote about Swami Vivekananda: "Here is a man who is more learned than all the Professors of America put together."

At the beginning of the evening session, Rev. Barrows announced, "Swami Vivekananda, the Hindu monk from India, will speak now." Swamiji himself has recalled later his experience at that moment. With fear in his heart he got up and prayed to Saraswati, the goddess of learning, and at once there was a tremendous flow of strength. He stepped forward and uttered his first sentence. There was unprecedented clapping, thumping and a thunderous applause. It was all in response to the two words "Sisters and Brothers" with which he addressed the gathering.

These words conveyed the full message of Vedanta – unity of existence, universality of outlook and universal brotherhood, which he was to deliver. It was for the first time, the Western audience had heard this idea in such simple words. In fact those words not only conveyed but convinced them that the whole of humanity was one family and all were brothers and sisters.

While all the delegates had spoken about their religion as the only true religion, Swami Vivekananda expounded the Hindu idea of all-inclusive universal religion, vast as the sky and deep as the ocean. He quoted profusely from our scriptures: "As the different streams having their sources in different places all mingle their water in the sea, so, O Lord, the different paths which men take through their different tendencies, – various though they appear, crooked or straight, all lead to Thee", and said, this is repeated by millions of Hindus every day in Bharat. He also explained the wonderful doctrine preached in the *Gita*: "Whosoever comes to me, in whatever form, I reach him. All men are struggling through the path which in the end leads to Me."

The first speech was very short but it was so effective and universal in its appeal that the next day all the newspapers described him as "undoubtedly the greatest figure in the World's Parliament of Religions." The papers wrote: 'We are fools to send religious preachers to that great country from where the Swami hails. It is like carrying coal to Newcastle.'

Swami Vivekananda gave a few more lectures, one of which was his momentous paper on Hinduism. In the course of these talks he very ably propounded the all-embraching universal approach of the Hindu mind. Once he said: "Unity in variety is the plan of nature, and the Hindu has recognized it. Every other religion lays down certain fixed dogmas and tries to force the society to adopt them. It places before society one coat which must fit Jack, John and Henry, all alike. Hindus have discovered one coat for each according to his size!"

"Every one sits in his own little well and thinks the whole world is his well. I have to thank you of America for the great attempt you are making to break the barriers of this little world of ours."

In all his speeches he strained every nerve to explain to the world, the broad and   all-inclusive philosophy of the Hindus. He quoted from the *Rig Veda*: "*ekam sat viprah bahudha vadanti*" (Truth is one, the learned call it in many ways). He laboured hard to make the West understand the message of Vedanta as the universal principle basic to all religions.

Swamiji once declared: "Ye, the children of immortal Bliss, Divinities on earth, sinners? It is the greatest sin to call a human being a sinner!" The appeal of Swami, simple but straightforward words, his great personality, his bright countenance and his orange robes were so enchanting that the audience started moving in and out of the hall with him. After hearing him, they found the other speeches very insipid.

Swamiji was very much pained to find the atrocious methods that the Christian missionaries were adopting to invoke pity in the Western world to collect funds for their proselytizing activities. In the course of a forthright admonition he warned: "You Christians who are so fond of sending out missionaries to save the soul of the heathen, why do you not try to save their bodies from starvation? In India during the horrible famines, thousands died from hunger, yet you Christians did nothing! You erect churches all through India, but the crying need of the East is not religion. They have religion enough; but it is bread that the suffering millions of burning India cry out for with parched throats. They ask for bread but you give them stones. It is an insult to a starving people to offer them religion."

Though he was at the peak of his popularity in the affluent America, Swamiji was thinking of his poor brethren. He wrote to his *gurubhai* in Bharat: "Who cares for name and fame and all that. I have come here only with one idea: to fetch something to change the miserable life of the suffering millions of my country." Swamiji did not stop at appealing to the youth of India to devote themselves for the service of the poor and the downtrodden; he himself was an embodiment of service and sacrifice. After his return from the West he was busy establishing monasteries as centres of training and preaching, and organizing centres of service for the relief of famine and other kinds of distress and suffering.

His final testament was: "It may be that I shall find it good to get outside my body to cast it off like a worn-out garment. But I shall not cease to work. I shall inspire men everywhere until the world shall know that it is one with God." And "may I be born again and again, and suffer thousands of miseries so that I may worship the only God that exists, the only God I believe in, the sum total of all souls. And above all, my God the wicked, my God the miserable, my God the poor of all races, of all species, is the special object of my worship."

Vivekananda as the Education for the Whole World
– Swami Ranganathananda

More than ever, today, we need a philosophy that can deal with all aspects of human life in an integrated way ensuring all-round happiness, harmony, unity, mutual love and respect and welfare. The spark of divinity in each one of us has to be divined.

Most religions convey dogmas or creeds that cannot and should not be questioned. They have to be accepted, they have to be believed, they have to be followed blindly. Their validity is not allowed to be tested or experimented with. India also has a religious philosophy, developed scientifically and systematically, that provides for investigation, that welcomes and allows detailed inquiry into the 'Truth'.

India's scientific approach to religion stressed spiritual experience and spiritual growth in place of mere belief in creed or dogma or conformity. Much of religion today bereft of this stress on spiritual growth, has become, in the words of Vivekananda, 'lifeless mockery; what we want is character'. Ramakrishna came to stimulate that message throughout the world.

Vivekananda saw in the West that faith in religion was always accompanied by intolerance, fanaticism, violence, and war. This is the opposite of what has become the characteristic feature of Indian culture for thousands of years, due to her scientific approach to the subject of religion. Religion in India, accordingly, tolerated not only other religions but even the atheists and agnostics as well. The people of India have been deeply religious, and out of the depth of their religious faith (till Christianity and Islam came to India as conquerors with their semetic exclusive-mindedness and intolerance) the people of India respected all religions, lived in greater harmony. This harmony inspired also various political states, big or small, that history threw up from time to time. These states often patronized more than one religion and received with respect and understanding all religions that came to India from outside during the last two thousand years.

The only way to worship an infinite God is not to take a copyright on Him after your experience of Him through your religion, but to accept and respect the spiritual experiences of other religions also, in the knowledge that the infinite is inexhaustible. That attitude alone can make you not only tolerate other religions but also to accept them with reverence. This is mature Indian wisdom which alone can help to transform religions from mutually weakening, colliding units into working for betterment and peace.

Vedanta has no dogma to convey, only the 'Truth' realized by rational investigation or deep enquiry. You are allowed to test and experiment with it until you are convinced of its validity, until you are ready to accept it on conviction so that you can 'realize' the 'Truth' ultimately. Such a unique approach is not to be found elsewhere except in Vedanta – the Hindu philosophy of life. The Vedantic Truths enable you to realize that there is nothing alien, nothing foreign, – there exists only Humanity, the Oneness of everything, the 'Truth' – 'one for all, all for one.'

The Vedantic philosophy not merely deals with human uniqueness, they deal with something more – man's own true nature and how he can discover it for himself. It urges him to go deeper within himself, come in touch with his inner self and, thereby, unfold for himself the purer, vaster and more powerfully profound creative energy resources that lie dormant within. Its main message is "Manifest the divine dimension that is within you."

Vedanta issues a clarion call to all children of the earth thus: "O Ye children of immortal bliss all over the world! I have realized the Truth – the infinite man behind the finite man. Search and realize this Truth yourself and you would have gained the *summum bonum* of human existence."

The world is bound to change for the better if we put into practice the Vedantic concepts of strength, harmony, unity and human dignity enunciated by our seers hundreds and hundreds of years ago, which are more relevant today than ever.

A big change is coming over in the world of religion, which in spite of occasional set-backs, is moving in the direction of inter-religious harmony, as preached by the sages of India, ancient and modern. Religion which is so profound an experience of man, should not become poisoned at its very source through exclusiveness and intolerance. Then only will it be in a position to rescue modern man from the current evils of materialism, mad consumerism and 'slavery of the lower part of himself.' Here, Vivekananda stresses a character-excellence as an important constituent of total human excellence.

What must be the high level of character-excellence of the man in whom you have the all-enveloping universal attitude, sympathy and understanding! Sri Ramarkrishna himself was one such embodiment of this universality. To him went not only believing men and women of all sects, but also persons with agnostic and scientific attitudes. Sri Ramakrishna welcomed all of them with love and respect. In his life one may see one of the highest type of human excellence.

The second aspect of human excellence is the combination of strength and fearlessness, on the one side, and gentleness and peace, on the other. This is a very rare combination in one character. It is the fruit of very high spiritual development. The highest development in this line constitutes another manifestation of human excellence taught and exemplified by Vivekananda. Mahatma Gandhi belonged to this category.

These are wonderful ideas coming out of that 'personification of the harmony of all human energy' which Vivekananda was. The subject is fascinating from several points of view. The nine volumes of *The Complete Works of Swami Vivekananda* are available to everyone who wishes to read further. It is a literature of strength and fearlessness, love and compassion. There are also the six volumes on *Vivekananda in the West – New Discoveries.*

Vivekananda's works stress the need to educate modern man to combine productive efficiency in his outer life with spiritual efficiency in his inner life. It is education that lifts man from one-sidedness to all-sidedness in character; it is the combination of 'learning to be' with 'learning to do', as urged by the UNESCO Education Commission Report which itself has dealt with 'learning to be' only superficially.

Here is Vivekananda bringing to the modern West this Vedantic message of a profound and deep humanism based upon the divine spark in every human being, and presenting man's education and his life and work as the field to unfold that divine possibility. That is Vivekananda's message of human excellence for all children everywhere. It will take time for humanity to be influenced by these ideas; but they are bound to produce their effect, for they are rational and human. Today, thinkers like Romain Rolland have begun to recognize Vivekananda as the education for the whole world. This century may be considered, so far as this message is concerned, as seed-time, while the next century can be expected to be the harvest time.

It will be interesting to you to know about the impact of Vivekananda on India. He powerfully influenced India's Independence struggle and many progressive social reform movements, like the one for removal of untouchability, and others for the uplift of women and the weaker sections. His influence is deepening decade after decade. And something very significant has happened in a very humble way recently. The Government of India has presented Vivekananda before the youth of India, by its recent circular D.O. No. F. 6/1/84, dated 17th October, 1984: 'that the birthday of Swami Vivekananda is to be observed as National Youth Day every year from 1985 onwards as it was felt that the philosophy of Swamiji, and the ideals for which he lived and worked, could be a great source of inspiration for the Indian Youth.' It was a significant step towards educating youth in human excellence.

Swamiji sends out to everyone this inspiring message of the achieving total human excellence:

"Teach yourselves, teach everyone, his real nature; call upon the sleeping soul and see how it awakes, power will come, glory will come, goodness will come, purity will come, and everything that is excellent will come, when this sleeping soul is roused to self-conscious activity."

Vivekananda – His Vision and the Relevance of His Teachings to Contemporary India
– Dr. Shankar Dayal Sharma

"If you want to know India, study Vivekananda. In him everything is positive and nothing negative."

– Rabindranath Tagore

Swami Vivekananda ranks with the greatest religious seekers, spiritual teachers and social reformers of all times. A truly outstanding son of our country, Swamiji was a uniquely magnetic personality exuding vibrant energy and indomitable strength.

Swami Vivekananda's broad vision encompassed several fields and he packed into his short life a range of activities which would have taken others many decades to perform. He was a source of inspiration for those illustrious sons and daughters of India, old and young, whose sacrifices in the national cause led to political independence. Our great country has since made impressive strides in various sectors of economic development and all of us are engaged in the grand task of building a glorious India which Swami Vivekananda foresaw and dreamt of.

He set in motion a process of national rejuvenation and regeneration directed at ridding society of archaic and obscurantist practices and spreading the knowledge of Vedanta. He believed in building on the foundations of the past, shorn of its shortcomings and in the power of the spirit which alone can give the fuel for the successful operation of institutions and legislation and the strength and purity of individual character that alone can give life to the building up of a new society.

I have been attracted to Swami Vivekananda's personality and teachings since my own early days. I believe that today, more than ever before, our young men and women have to become more and more familiar with the teachings of Swami Vivekananda and draw inspiration from them. We have to read what he taught and wrote and learn from his teachings. And if we do so, I have no doubt that the different problems which face our country will become easier of solution.

The idea which he propounded were indeed revolutionary for the India of his day and age and had a tremendous impact on subsequent political thinking and action in the country.

His understanding of Vedanta made him an inveterate opponent of the terrible practice of untouchability which he strongly denounced. He stood for all such activity as would result in increase in production and the removal of poverty. To him, however, material development was only a transitional stage towards spiritual development and not a substitute for it. He was in favour of a limitation of material requirements. If he wanted material development, he did so especially for the masses so that they were able to meet their essential needs.

Swamiji's acute concern for the poor stood out when he said: "....Let each one of us pray day and night for the downtrodden millions of India who are held fast by poverty and tyranny, pray day and night for them. I came more to preach to them than to the high and the rich.... Him I call a mahatma who feels for the poor....

"Unfurl the banner of love", he told his disciples. "If you want to help others", he told them, "your little self must go.... In this age, as on the one hand people have to be immensely practical, so on the other hand they have to acquire deep spiritual knowledge."

Swami Vivekananda clearly saw the need to employ education as an instrument for social and economic progress. He was an ardent champion of women's education. He wanted women and the members of all classes to receive education and determine their status in the light of the enlightened perception of their own needs and requirements.

Swamiji realized that the foremost quality which a people require is strength and the lesson that he imparted, especially to the youth and the children of India, was the lesson of strength.

Let us, therefore, resolve anew to act upon Swami Vivekananda's inspiring message and endeavour to become strong of heart, strong of mind and have the strength never to submit to injustice and wrong-doing. It is my prayer and fervent hope that our countrymen of today and particularly our children and our youth, will try to emulate the shining example of Swami Vivekananda in successfully accomplishing the challenging tasks of national reconstruction and social change that lie ahead.

II

Though Swami Vivekananda lived and taught about a century back, his life and teachings have as much relevance today as they had a century ago. The reason for this is that he was ancient yet modern, one who combined in himself all the highest values for which our ancient civilization stood, together with all the aspirations which modern India has begun to cherish.

The highest value for which our country stood in the past is spirituality, a word which brings all sorts of curious and contradictory notions into the minds of people. The meaning that the Swami attached to it is acceptance and expression of the idea of the divinity of man. Man is not a mere body-mind as he feels himself to be in his natural state, but a spark of the divine, that Infinite Being of power and perfection, from whom the whole universe has come. To be established in the sense of this higher identity of man and to express the graces and excellences proceeding from this conviction in life in the world, is the essence of spirituality.

Swamiji held that, more than any other civilization of the world, Indian civilization had a hold on this view of life and that it continues to be so even today. He therefore held that India is the spiritual guru of mankind and that she should never give up this capacity in the midst of our efforts at what is called modernization.

– Swami Tapasyananda

III

While the teachings of Sri Ramakrishna exercised a profound influence upon Swami Vivekananda, it would be less than fair to look upon Swamiji as little more than a mere follower of his Master. We have only to focus our gaze momentarily upon a portrait of Swamiji to get a measure of the incisive intelligence, the restless energy and the spiritual vitality which shaped this personality.

Swami Vivekananda was, above all, a man of action, a doer of things, rather than a mere visionary or a fabricator of grand spiritual designs. Indeed he possessed qualities of both reflection and action which reside very rarely within a single person. This is the unique feature of Swami Vivekananda. He was not only great in himself but he was able to transmit something of that greatness because he was a man of action more than anything else.

Swamiji's belief that above everything else India needed a spiritual revolution stemmed from his conviction that lasting social dynamism could come to India only through the spiritual channel. His ultimate objective was social revolution and the channel through which he wanted to bring it about was the spiritual revolution. These two went side by side in his thinking.

The profound influence of Sri Ramakrishna upon Swami Vivekananda is sensitively reflected in Swamiji's formulation of the principles underlying the *Sanatana Dharma* of the Hindus and its relationship with other religious systems. Like his mentor, Swamiji looked upon Vedanta as the source of Hindu spirituality and the essential underpinning of the diverse moral systems located within Hindu society. As he put it, 'the word Vedanta must cover the whole ground of Indian religious life.'

While Swami Vivekananda was deeply influenced by the tolerance and catholicity of Sri Ramakrishna, his spiritual articulation was endowed with a life-force and a vital energy which was largely a reflection of his personal and spiritual and social dynamism. Indeed there is every reason to believe that Sri Ramakrishna chose him as his successor for these very qualities.

We get a vivid glimpse of the spiritual and social dynamism in Swami Vivekananda's polemic against those who ridiculed the so-called materialism of the West. Mind you, he was speaking these words in 1893, almost a hundred years ago. What he had said is this: "We talk foolishly against material civilization. The grapes are sour. Material civilization – nay, even luxury – is necessary to create work for the poor. I don't believe in a God who cannot give me my bread here, giving me eternal place in heaven." Now, can you imagine a more revolutionary approach, a more revolutionary statement, than this in 1893?

He was, in addition, totally in favour of borrowing liberally from the West to energize his country. "From the great dynamo of Europe", he said, "emerged the electric flow, that tremendous power vivifying the whole world. We want that energy, that love of Independence, that spirit of self-reliance, that immovable fortitude, that dexterity in action, that bond of unity of purpose, that thirst for improvement."

He saw all these qualities in the Western society as long back as a century ago (1893). He could choose the good while leaving out what was not so good. So he had that catholicity, he had that *samadrishti* as we call it, which is a great trait in any saint who becomes the leader of his people.

When Swami Vivekananda emerged as Sri Ramakrishna's principal disciple after his death in 1886, the social canvas on which he chose to work was wider than the one on which the saint of Dakshineshwar had inscribed his life's work. Since times immemorial the notion of a pilgrimage or a *Bharat Parikrama* across the country constituted an essential ingredient of the education of the spiritual men in India. In 1888 Swami Vivekananda undertook such a journey to interact with men of religion elsewhere within India and to gain an understanding of the social and spiritual climate of the country as a whole.

The *Bharat Parikrama* both widened and deepened his understanding of the spiritual unity of India, at the same time as it provided him with an assessment of the national work that needed to be done. Swamiji's spiritual wanderings finally brought him to Kanyakumari, the southern tip of the peninsula. While he was in Kanyakumari, he spent a full night awake reflecting what he had seen and heard during the course of his *parikrama*. In the course of these reflections, in the still of the night there emerged before him an inspired vision of India. Also, in the course of these reflections, Swamiji saw the role which could be played by dedicated *sannyasis* in improving the lot of the common-folk

The last stages of Swami Vivekananda's *Bharat Parikrama* were witnesses to a decision which affected his spiritual career in a most remarkable fashion. A World Conference of Religions was scheduled in

Chicago in 1893 and for that some time before Swamiji had toyed with the idea of placing before this assembly his understanding of the *Sanatana Dharma*. The experience of the *parikrama* encouraged Swamiji to decide in favour of attending the World Conference. To gain a full appreciation of Swamiji's spiritual achievement at the World Conference of Religions in Chicago in September 1893, it is necessary to dwell briefly on how the West perceived Hinduism in the last quarter of the 19th century.

India lay prostrate before British Imperialism at this juncture and she was known to humanity as a country burdened with poverty, ritual and superstition. She was, so the world believed, also bereft of any larger moral vision. An eminent Englishman described the religion of the Hindus as 'idolatory with all rabble of impure deities, its monsters of wood and stone, its false principles and corrupt practices and its lying legends and fraudulent impositions.' Now, you can imagine from that state of affairs where Swami Vivekananda brought India in the eyes of the Western people, of the whole world and that is a real measure of his greatness, of the service which he rendered to his motherland.

The words of Swami Vivekananda in Chicago took the assembly and indeed the entire Western world by storm. At a stroke Vivekananda had dramatically transformed the Western image of the *Sanatana Dharma* of the Hindus. As a delegate to the Conference observed, Vivekananda was beyond question the most popular and influential man in the gathering. An important newspaper in Chicago described him as an individual of towering stature and one who was the master of his situation.

I feel that the message of tolerance and openness of fellow-feeling and friendliness for all religions and of the essential unity of all spiritual experience which Swami Vivekananda delivered before the world a hundred years ago is as relevant for Hindus, Muslims, Christians, Sikhs and all the religions today as it was relevant for them when it was originally voiced. In fact, it is much more relevant today.

Swamiji captured in his inspired utterances the true spirit of the *Sanatana Dharma* as he saw it in the closing decade of the last century and as it indeed stands in our times today. Perhaps, the *rashtra-chetana* which we are seeking to arouse in our country can draw profitably upon the notion of what was noble and perennial in our *dharma* to fashion our nation into a harmonious polity where citizens can lead a life of moral dignity and material plenty. Such a consummation would be our best homage to Swami Vivekananda.

– P. V. Narasimha Rao

IV

When we try to comprehend the legacy of Swami Vivekananda against the background of our present-day national scenerio, we are sure to exclaim "Oh, never was Swamiji's message more relevant than it is today!" Indeed, there can be no two opinions about it – the urgent need for us to heed the thundering warnings of that leonine *sannyasi*.

As days are passing, the profound significance of the insights of Swami Vivekananda in shedding light on our present-day problem is becoming ever more pronounced, especially, when we observe how by our rejection of the same the nation's ship is dangerously floundering. And how if only we had stuck to Swamiji's guidelines, we as a nation could well have reached to our full heights as a world teacher of cultural and spiritual values, instead of going about knocking at everybody's door with a begging bowl in every single sphere of life.

Now let us begin from the beginning: that is, ourselves. Unless we know who we are, what our identity as a nation is, there can hardly be any hope of our nation's progress. A nation can march forward only when its direction, its goal of life reflecting its identity, is well etched on its mind. Otherwise, it will be only drifting, being tossed about by every single pull and push by interested forces inside and outside the country.

– H.V. Seshadri

The Man Who Manifested Vivekandanda's Secret of Action in Life
– S. J.

"My boy, when death is inevitable, is it not better to die like heroes than as stocks and stones? And what is the use of living a day or two more in this transitory world? It is better to wear out than to rust out."

"Let the body, since perish it must, wear out in action and not rust in inaction."

"When will that blessed day dawn when my life will be a sacrifice at the altar of humanity."

– Swami Vivekananda

Eknath Ranade, a dedicated soul, believed and acted on the dicta of Swami Vivekananda: Better wear out than rust out. Death is a must. Let the body fall in serving a noble cause.

The noble cause was the inspiring memorial which stands proudly in Kanyakumari and the 'Vivekananda Kendra' which Ranade established and nurtured with great devotion. The body, worn out with incessant work, sought rest on 22 August, 1982. Eknath's master would have approved the fact that it never gathered rust.

Devoid of any self-interest, dedicated in the execution of his life-mission, Ranade died in harness as a *karmayogin*. He reminds us of the incense stick that burns itself out without a trace, but leaves a sweet fragrance all around.

All that remain of Ranade to bear witness to his greatness are the twin monuments which he successfully erected, within the shortest period possible, in the hallowed memory of Swami Vivekananda. One, a 'physical monument', the historic Vivekananda Rock Memorial at Kanyakumari, and the other, a 'living monument' in the form of a service mission, 'Vivekananda Kendra' set up to create a band of dedicated young men and women who will give shape to Swamiji's dreams.

Wearing the layman's simple white robe, Ranade was a true *sanyasin* all the same, a rare phenomenon in todays murky atmosphere.

The idea of erecting a memorial on the sea-girt rock at Kanyakumarai, (whereon, immersed in deep meditation, Swami Vivekananda glimpsed the mission of his life prior to his sailing to America to participate in the World's Parliament of Religions in 1893) was mooted by the local Vivekananda Rock Memorial Committee (VRMC) in commemoration of the Swami's Birth Centenary (1963). It was as though Providence had got Ranade ready for the key role he was to play at Kanyakumari. Joining the VRMC as its Organizing Secretary, Ranade wholeheartedly addressed himself to the task. The local VRMC was turned into an all-India one, thanks to the organizing acumen and dynamic leadership which he provided to the all-India VRMC. An unassuming Ranade would never attribute the great achievement to himself. He would say that the rock memorial project grew, thanks to those who had opposed it. The more the opposition, the greater became the project: "We should really be thankful to those who opposed us in our noble venture and created impediments in our way. In fact, the opposition and hurdles were blessings in disguise. Only on account of them could we put to test our strength, both physical and intellectual and bring forth the best in us."

In the teeth of vehement opposition and even hostility, Ranade laboured with diligence and tenacity. He went on a whirlwind tour all over India and mobilized a strong public opinion in support of the cause. He even met the people's representatives in Delhi and sought their help. More than 300 MPs signed a memorandum urging the Government of India and the state government of Madras to help solve the problem at Kanyakumari. It was a unique venture in which the masses as well as the governments participated in a manner that cut across all barriers of distinction.

The campaign organized by Ranade fetched more than a crore of rupees from all over India. This amount was utilized for the first phase of the Vivekananda Memorial plan consisting of four items. The major portion of the funds, viz. about 80 lakhs of rupees, came from the masses who contributed in small sums according to their mite as their offering of love to the cause of Swami Vivekananda. The rest of the amount was gathered by way of contributions both from the state governments and the Government of India, besides those of industrialists and philanthropists.

Apart from the edifice, 'Vivekananda Mandapam', erected on the rock, the other items of the first phase were: (a) a campus of about one hundred acres, named 'Vivekanandapuram', at the entrance of the Kanyakumari township, catering to the needs of the pilgrims at Kanyakumari who visit the rock memorial as well as the ancient temple of the virgin goddess on the mainland; (b) a Pictorial Exhibition at Vivekanandapuram, depicting the life and mission of Swami Vivekananda and (c) free transport facilities for lodgers at Vivekandapuram, and other amenities for the pilgrims.

All these items of the first phase of the plan at Kanyakumari speak volumes for the organizing genius, as also the dedication of Eknath Ranade. Since its inauguration in 1970, the magnificent national monument has been attracting pilgrims in thousands from all over India and abroad. Millions have visited it and offered their homage to the hallowed memory of the great Patriot-Saint of modern India. The monument standing at a point where three seas mingle at Kanyakumari, has become the focal point of national and international integration.

Not being satisfied with the erection of a mere 'physical monument' to the memory of the mighty monk who was a great lover of the lowly and the downtrodden, Ranade brought into existence a 'Living Memorial' to Swami Vivekananda. This 'Living Memorial' is in the form of a spiritually oriented all-India Service Mission, the 'Vivekananda Kendra' with its headquarters at Vivekanandapuram, Kanyakumari, launched as the second phase of the overall plan with a significant programme of training a cadre of qualified and dedicated young men and women for social service all over India, spiritual regeneration and humanitarian work. The Vivekananda Kendra is a Lay Order of missionaries dedicated to life-long service of the motherland which was very dear to Swami Vivekananda. Since 1973, in its training centre at Vivekanandapuram, the Kendra has been training prospective life-workers drawn from all over India. The trained candidates have been sent to needy areas of the country, particularly backward and tribal areas, for social service, as also for gaining intensive field training.

The Kendra has set up several residential schools in the remote north-eastern region of our country and elsewhere which are all being administered by the trained life-workers of the Kendra. In some parts of the country, rural development activities have been undertaken. Yoga being the core of the Vivekananda Kendra Movement, training is also imparted in yoga in different centers sponsored by the Kendra. A yoga therapy and research centre is functioning under the supervision of qualified persons. Thus, the second phase initiated by Ranade is gradually gaining momentum.

Ranade had in mind a third phase as well, which envisaged the propagation of the message of Swami Vivekananda all over India and abroad (under the banner of 'Vivekananda Kendra International'). But before he could give it a concrete shape the curtain fell. Eknath Ranade had been incessantly working for the last few decades without any break. Rest was alien to his constitution. Continued hard labour naturally told upon his health, though physically he looked sturdy and bright. More than once, he was laid low by "heart trouble", but every time after a brief repose, he plunged into hectic activities, including touring all over India, in connection with his work. The 'ferry service problem' which dragged for years had sapped much of his precious energy and, in fact, dealt a mortal blow to his already delicate health.

In 1980, Ranade again suffered a stroke. He went into coma as a result, and his condition became very critical. But after a period of intensive care and medical treatment, he gradually recovered though not completely. After much persuasion by his physician and friends, he reluctantly subjected himself to a short period of rest. He was requested, time and again, by all who loved him that at least thereafter he should take complete rest. His forthright reply was, "This life is given for a cause. We have come here for work and not for any rest. Well, rest will come of itself in the end, once and for all." Thus, in spite of medical advice not to strain himself, he once again commenced a month-long tour and visited several places and persons in connection with the organizational work, and when returned to Madras he had a cardiac arrest. The end came on 22 August, 1982.

Even during his final sojourn at Madras, Ranade was not idle. With all the strain of a long tour, he carefully perused and edited the manuscript of a publication ("Sadhana of Service") comprising scores of his lectures delivered at Kanyakumari during the tenure of his service in the cause of Swami Vivekananda. Only recently the latest edition of his popular compilation, "Rousing Call to Hindu Nation" had come out of the press. This book was the result of his detailed and reverential study of the Vivekananda literature, while in Calcutta, before he embarked on the Vivekananda Rock Memorial project at Kanyakumari two decades ago. He said once that he did such a meticulous study because he felt that one who intended to work for the cause of Swami Vivekananda must be conversant with the Swami's unique life and message.

In the course of this deep study, Ranade culled out significant passages and exhortations from the speeches and writings of Swamiji which appealed to him most and compiled them in a book form and got it published in Calcutta during the Birth Centenary of Swami Vivekananda (1963) as his homage to the patriot-saint. It was Ranade's fond hope that such a compilation would serve as a source of inspiration for one and all.

Eknath Ranade to whom example was better than precept, truly manifested Vivekananda's secret of action in life. He lived an intensely active and dedicated life all through. He wore himself but in serving a noble cause. His life was an oblation on the altar of Swami Vivekananda. His rare accomplishments will remain a monument to his own genius and dedication. In a significant utterance Eknath Ranade has summed up the philosophy of his life. He has revealed therein the secret of his monumental achievement at the Land's End of India. It is in fact the charter of his intensely active and utterly dedicated life. It is also an abiding impetus for us in achieving our cherished aims in life:

*"There is one thing to which you can always turn for unfailing support....
You can safely rely at all times on your own self for the fulfilment of your
mission. All other help may fail, but there is a power within you which will
never let you down. It is your own Self. Depend on it and march ahead with
unceasing prayer to God to give you strength to fulfil His Will"* (vide
"Sadhana of Service").

Vivekananda – His Impact on Tata and Rockefeller
– S. J.

Two renowned entrepreneurs – one an Indian and the other, an
American, had the rare good fortune of meeting the great patriot-saint of
modern India – Swami Vivekananda, and being influenced by his exalted
personality, as a result of which, even while remaining extremely industrious
and innovative, they also turned philanthropic and became the benefactors
of mankind. The abundant riches conferred upon them by Providence,
flowed, as it were, through them generously for the commonweal – for the
well-being of mankind. Their entrepreneurship and munificence have
immortalized them!

During this eventful year (1993) of the Centenary of Swami
Vivekananda's appearance in the World's Parliament of Religions at Chicago
(U. S. A.), it is only fitting and proper that we remember these significant
events which had a great bearing on the life and activities of Sir Jamsetji
N. Tata and John D. Rockefeller. While the former met Swami Vivekananda
during his voyage to America to participate in the Chicago Parliament of
Religions, the latter called on Swamiji at Chicago, after the Parliament.

Vivekananda – The Force Behind the Tatas

The large number of educational institutions, industrial houses and
workshops established by the Tatas all over India, over a period of eight
decades, bear testimony to their perseverance and munificence. Pulsating
with confidence, discipline and vision, their organizations stand out as an
archetype of modern management, vigour and productive growth. And the
motive force behind all their achievement in the field of industry is their
illustrious Founder – Sir Jamsetji Nusserwanji Tata (1839-1904). But very
few know that the real force behind Jamsetji's thoughts and activities was
an exalted spiritual personage – Swami Vivekananda, the patriot-saint of
modern India. And the Tatas have a special reason to rejoice during this
centenary year (1993) of Swami Vivekananda's appearance in the World's
Parliament of Religions at Chicago. For, it was exactly hundred years ago
(1893), when Swami Vivekananda was on his way to Chicago that he met
Jamsetji, and it proved a turning point in the life of the latter. In fact this
meeting opened a new vista for Jamsetji – the potential industrialist.

How Jamsetji, the first great captain of Indian Industry, came under the
inductive effect of Swami Vivekananda – then quite an unknown young

sannyasin of 30, – and how the basic concept of scientific research as an essential pre-requisite for sound industrial development was first generated in the country by Swamiji, is strangely not known even to the larger section of the educated and enlightened people. The interesting episode of Jamsetji meeting Swamiji, throws light on the latter's attitude towards scientific and technological education and industrialization of India.

Swami Vivekananda was on an itinerant life soon after the passing away of his guru, Sri Ramakrishna. He was seeking ways and means to fulfil his life's mission entrusted to him by his guru. During the several years of his itinerant life in India, Swamiji was greatly distressed by the poverty, squalor and the economic misery of the Indian masses. In quest of an economic solution to this chronic problem, he made up his mind to go to America. And the Parliament of Religions offered him a unique, Providential opportunity.

Jamsetji, already a renowned personality in India, was a fellow-traveller on Swamiji's voyage from Japan to Chicago. Swamiji was on his way to attend the Parliament of Religions as an unknown monk without any credentials. Swamiji enquired of Jamsetji why he exported matches from Japan for sale in India; for that meant a heavy drain on national wealth. Swamiji then pleaded with Jamsetji that if, instead, he set up a match factory in India, that would not only give him a handsome profit, but also employment for quite a number of men and prevent the national wealth from going out of the country.

The admonition of an anguished *sannyasin* did not miss that target, and the potential industrialist immediately realized that here was an uncommon *sannyasin* with a sure professional approach towards the economic ills of the society. Though a Vedantist to the core, his approach to life was never negative. He was very much concerned about the basic needs and tears of the lowly placed, oppressed humanity. He was always after doing something concrete for the betterment of the condition of the poor and the downtrodden.

At a time when the educational system introduced by the then British rulers in India was absolutely unrelated to the needs of life and in no way did it help the promotion of nation's prosperity, Jamsetji came forward with a promise of huge financial assistance for clearing the way to the introduction of a new system of education tailored to the needs of the nation. It was the dynamic inspiration of Swami Vivekananda that moved Jamsetji to come forward in 1898, with a significant announcement about his scheme for promotion of basic scientific research for industrial development and economic resurgence in India. Since he valued higher education as a preparation for industrial and commercial vocation, and visualized the establishment of a postgraduate research institute of science, he made a magnificent gift of Rs. 30 lakhs for the purpose. The whole of India greeted him in a chorus of commendation. The proposed institute was admirably calculated to hasten the dawn of that industrial revival in India, upon which depends the salvation of her teeming millions. When founded, the institute initially was called the Indian Institute of Science and is also popularly known as Tata Institute. Located about 5 Km. from Bangalore, this great institution is noted for its contribution for the advancements in knowledge both of pure and applied Science.

Jamsetji sought the spiritual wisdom of Swamiji for the smooth functioning of such an institution. Swamiji evinced keen interest in the Tata-scheme. His friends and disciples undertook to work behind the scene to secure fulfilment of his desire. In this project, however, the role of Sister Nivedita was the more important. Tata-scheme being the embodiment of a cherished desire of her Master, Swami Vivekananda, she devoted every ounce of her energy for its implementation.

Although Swamiji and Jamsetii did not live to see the scheme materialize, Sister Nivedita must have been happy when the institute started functioning from July 1911. Possibly she could see the radiance of her Master illuminating this vast ancient land of her adoption – that is, a new-born Bharat.

II

Coming under the inductive effect of Swami Vivekananda and thereby being blessed by him, Jamsetji became an enlightened industrialist. Known as the Father of modern iron and steel industry in India, he was a vigorous and dynamic personality, with untiring energy and indomitable will. He had a versatile mind with a wide range of interests. His broad vision and wider genius, made a mark in many and diverse activities. His life had embraced a truly exceptional range of accomplishments – which were the fruits of a rich imagination, an innovative mind and almost limitless range of interests. Each of his enterprises was an answer to the question that was for ever in his mind – what does India need now?

It was clear to him that for India to gain economic independence she required three things: power for her industries, trained scientists for her economic development and iron and steel on which to base her industry. To these major goals he devoted the final years of his life and much of his fortune.

Animated by a spirit of enterprise and adventure and inspired by patriotic fervour, he struggled against heavy odds and pioneered, planned and organized number of schemes, big and small, for the economic advancement of India. A man of keen intellect and penetrating vision, he realized the importance of science as the basis of industrial advancement and founded, as already mentioned, an institute to promote scientific education and research.

Among his many achievements, he had helped pioneer India's textile. industry, he had built Bombay's first modern hotel, and planned a hydroelectric scheme which was to make India among the first countries in the world to exploit its natural resources for this purpose, and conceived the then revolutionary idea of a modern iron and steel industry in India, he had set-up fruit-farms, experimented with horticulture and advanced the production of silk. But his greatest achievement was the luster he had brought to the family name of Tata and the honour and reputation he had earned for it.

Like all geniuses, Jamsetji left much of his work unfinished and many of his dreams unfulfilled. His visions were however translated into reality by his successors. The force of his examples and the memory of his achievement both as an industrialist and as a benefactor of education and arts, have always guided the destiny of his house and reinforced the abilities of his successors. The achievements of the House of Tata, both in his own time and today are all well-known.

Though Jamsetji was renowned for his charity, he did not seek any reward for his many generous benefactions. Wealth for him was but a means to an end. The end was the good of the nation, its economic advancement, its prosperity.

As aptly pointed out by the *Prabuddha Bharata* (1904) which openly supported the interest Swami Vivekananda evinced in the Tata-scheme, "The making of a prosperous Indian nation depends on the qualities of head and heart like those possessed by Mr. Tata. A few more Tatas would change the face of India. Let our wealthy countrymen imitate the Parsi patriot, the direction and munificence of his charity."

How Vivekananda influenced Rockefeller

John D. Rockefeller (1839-1937), American industrialist and world's richest man, was foremost among men who created the modern petroleum industry. His career is often regarded as a prime example of the American self-made man.

It was in 1894 (March/Apirl) that Rockefeller called on Swami Vivekananda who was then resting for a while at a house at Chicago, after going through his two strenuous and triumphant lecture programmes at Detroit and elsewhere in U. S. A.

Swamiji made Rockefeller understand that "he was only a channel and that his duty was to do good to the world – that God had given all his wealth in order that he might have an opportunity to help and do good to people." About a week later, when Rockefeller met Swamiji again the second time, he told Swamiji of his plan to donate an enormous sum of money towards the financing of a public institution. Three years hence (1897) Rockefeller devoted himself completely to philanthropy. He spoke his philosophy as follows: "There is more to life than the accumulation of money. Money is only a trust in one's hand. To use it improperly is a great sin. The best way to prepare for the end of life is to live for others. This is what I am trying to do." This seemed to echo Swamiji's own words: "They alone live who live for others; the rest are more dead than alive."

Philanthropy in large scale was Rockefeller's second career in which he became renowned. From the late 1890s he was primarily concerned with the distribution of much of his vast wealth in charitable and philanthropic ventures. In pioneering large-scale philanthropy, he started the forces that modernized American medical science. He devoted hundreds of millions of dollars to the improvement of American medical practice, education and research. He is believed to have given away some 550 million dollars in his lifetime, including major endowments to the University of Chicago (1892), the Rockefeller Institute for Medical Research (1901) – renamed Rockefeller University; and the General Education Board (1902). He also established the Rockefeller Foundation in 1913, "to promote the well-being of mankind" throughout the world. While the Rockefeller Foundation was the chief vehicle for his philanthropy, the General Education Board was devoted to improving the standard of education.

The University of Chicago was founded with a munificent donation of 30 million dollars from John D. Rockefeller. He gave it over 80 million dollars during his lifetime.

Rockefeller's benefactions during his lifetime totalled more than $ 500,000,000, while his and his son's totalled more than $ 2,500,000,000 by 1955.

As early as in 1863, Rockefeller built his first oil refinery, near Cleveland, and thereafter he devoted himself exclusively to the oil business. In 1870, he founded Standard Oil Company in Ohio, with a capital of one million dollars. His oil business absorbed many Cleveland refineries and expanded into Pennsylvania oil fields to become the world's largest refinery concern. The division of the operations into 18 companies – later to include more than 30 companies – under the umbrella of Standard Oil of New Jersey (1899) helped him to accumulate a personal fortune of over one billion dollars.

In 1882 Rockefeller created America's first great Trust. It had a capital of about 70 million dollars and was the world's largest and rich industrial organization.

After his retirement in 1911, Rockefeller expanded his efforts in philanthropy, which claimed about one half of his fortune. He firmly believed that he had a duty to transfer some of his huge fortune to humanitarian use rather than merely leave it to his heirs.

Vivekananda – A Dynamic Spiritual Force
to Shape the Future of Humanity
– Swami Budhananda

"Whether we regard Swami Vivekananda as a teacher, patriot or saint and whether we accept his teachings only partially or in their entirety, no one can deny that in his life there was made manifest a tremendous force for the moral and spiritual welfare and upliftment of humanity, irrespective of caste, creed, nationality or time."

"Vivekananda's name is a passport to the cultural centres of the West and his disciples and grand disciples are really cultural Ambassadors to the Western world."

The magnificence and munificence of Swami Vivekananda as a spiritual architect of humanity cannot be sufficiently measured unless we see in a single sweep his wonderful life-work. In his oceanic heart enlightened by the realization of the Supreme Spirit, Swami Vivekananda felt the agonies of entire humanity. Commissioned by Sri Ramakrishna to do the 'Mother's work,' he faced the magnitude of his task with the vision of the *rishi* that he was and planned and executed his work with the dexterity of an Apostle of Destiny. Realizing well that the world malady was in the ultimate analysis a spiritual problem though its expressions in the two hemispheres were different, and that the advent of Sri Ramakrishna was for the good of entire humanity, he felt deeply the urgency of spreading his message throughout the world. This was why he went to America in 1893 to represent Hinduism at the Parliament of Religions. In broadcasting the message of the Master he brooked no opposition and spared no exertion. He knew for certain that the Vedanta as lived and taught by Sri Ramakrishna when applied variously in varying situations could help all in progressively realizing the ultimate end of life.

Vivekananda came to the West in obedience to the directions of the Divine. Readers of his biography know this fact. It was the part of his mission of removing miseries of human beings and bringing them knowledge.

Vivekananda's going to the West and working in the midst of the Western people during the prime part of his ministry was, so to say, an actualization of divine intervention in the history of the Western man. As far as we know, no *Brahmajnani* of his type had walked on the soil between the Atlantic and the Pacific in America. Besides, he was the chosen messenger of the Lord manifest in the world.

These facts have gone into the history of the Western man with all their implications. If it is sure that tomorrow you are going to witness the rising sun, you may be equally sure that what Vivekananda did for the West is going to unfold itself in a most beneficent manner.

It is true that there has yet to be a full recognition of Vivekananda's services to the West by the Western leaders of thought. Notwithstanding that, his ministry has been all the time leavening in depth the essential religious thinking and also the spiritual life of those who have been seeking an inspiration which is unafraid of truth and can show the path to illumination.

Vivekananda, contrary to common notion, did not have an easy walk-over in America. After the initial success at the Parliament of Religions he had to march like a benign warrior through an organized and powerful opposition. He knew his mission, which was nothing less than regeneration of entire mankind and he could not permit human follies to claim much of his attention.

One more invaluable legacy of far-reaching historical import mankind has inherited as the outcome of Swamiji's work in the West, is the enduring bridge of understanding he built on the foundation of mutuality of regard between the East and the West. This work has released more creative forces of great significance in the human civilization, than have so far been perceptively read by the students of history.

One other momentous outcome of Swamiji's work in the West was the self-perpetuating stirring of the soul it caused in prostrate India of that time. Of even greater practical import was the fact that while deeply engaged in giving his message to the West, he simultaneously set in motion his future work in India through the power of his thoughts and words conveyed in his inspiring letters to his brother disciples and disciples in India.

II

A few broad channels of influence radiating from the personality, work and spiritual milieu of Swami Vivekananda can easily be traced. Foremost among them is Swamiji's contribution to our understanding of Vedanta, the philosophy of all mankind, teaching us that One divinity pervades all creation. It can be called by many names and that man is divine. Vedanta became the basis of his life and work.

Swami Vivekananda's interpretation of religion as Vedantic Unity in practice through service, based on equality and *tyaga* turned the traditional religious concepts upside down. He brought men, societies and religions nearer to God. Service as a pathway to God became Swami Vivekananda's great contribution to religion.

Swami Vivekananda's understanding and presentation of India as the living and loving embodiment of Vedanta, made him appreciate her role in the world at large. To Swami Vivekananda and to those inspired by him, regeneration of India became the first step in reconstructing the spiritual order of the world. The world itself has to be prepared to receive the time-tested Vedantic message of India, as and when Mother India became fit and ready to deliver it. Hence, Swami Vivekananda's visit to the West, opening the gates, hearts and intellects of the world, to India and the later day Indian spiritual ambassadors.

The world in general, and the West in particular, may not be able to soak in the nourishment of Vedantic truth hidden in the meat of Indian texts and rituals. Therefore, Swami Vivekananda had to speak the language of science.

Swami Vivekananda's influence on societies and individuals can be classified into: 1) His impact as a teacher of Vedanta, 2) His stress on the practice of religion of service, based on equality and *tyaga*, 3), His role as an awakener, builder and organizer of modern India with its patriotic, spiritual and service movements, 4) His contributions as a cultural and spiritual emissary of India to the West, 5) His work as an interpreter of Indian values in the universal language of science and, 6) His influence in taming and unifying science itself.

Add to these contributions, the personality of the man who was a living poem, his powerful and clear language of electrifying impact, and his utter humility when he traces all that is good in him to the grace of his Master Sri Ramakrishna, the task of one who sets out to assess the impact of Swami Vivekananda becomes unenviable indeed.

The Ramakrishna Movement is the outcome of the great Ramakrishna-Vivekananda phenomenon. One was the cause and the other the effect. One was lightning, the other was thunder. One was fire, the other was its glow. Humanity has not yet opened fully the gift it has received from Sri Ramakrishna, the gift of the advent and work of Swami Vivekananda. We can only envy the future world, which will be delighted and blessed with this gift, which it has been ready to receive but slow to uncover.

– Dr. M. Lakshmi Kumari

III

"Swami Vivekananda was a colossus whose foot-prints have left an indelible impression on the sands of Time. Many, many are those that were influenced by him; many are those that still carry the Swami's message in their heart, trying to give practical expression whenever possible; and many, not only in this country but also abroad, will continue to draw inspiration from his life and message."

One of the most competent persons to have deeply studied and ably commented on the spiritual signification of the Ramakrishna phenomenon in regard to human development was **Sri Aurabindo.** The Yogi of Pondicherry was undoubtedly inspired by the power that was released from Dakshineswar, and responded to it, in his own and singular way.

Tracing the history of the modern spiritual renaissance in India, he wrote about the significance of "the going forth of Vivekananda" in the history of mankind. What spiritual import this going forth of Vivekananda had for Sri Aurobindo's personal yoga has been narrated by Sri Anil Baran Roy, a faithful disciple: "....I asked Sri Aurobindo wherefrom he got this idea. He said when he was in Alipore Jail Vivekananda appeared before him and

told him about this. At that time Vivekananda was not in this world. I asked
whether it was a vision that he saw. He replied, 'No, if it had been a vision
I would not have believed it'. He had not the slightest doubt that it was
not an illusion but a reality. I said, 'Do you really think it to be possible?'
He replied enigmatically, 'It is both possible and impossible'.

This "possible and impossible" thing only indicates that in the regions
beyond the ken of common men's understanding the Ramakrishna
Movement has been having its dynamic sway, and that its institutional part
of manifestation is only the visible tip of the ice-berg. In the depth of human
consciousness, in the summits of superconsciousness its sun-glow
overspreads the expanding horizons of vast unreckoning. It is no poetry
but a conservative statement of fact.

Rabindranath Tagore knew Sri Ramakrishna and Swami Vivekananda
personally. And he lived long enough to view the gradual growth of the
Ramakrishna Movement from his watch-tower. He was perhaps never
emotionally involved with the Movement and hence could mingle marked
detachment with a poet's deep-seeing appraisal.

The poet touches one of the main notes of the grand music that is
Ramakrishna Movement when he says the Vivekananda's was "a call of
awakening to the totality of the manhood of man. Like the ever rolling waves
of the ocean the call goes on ceaselessly sounding and resounding all over
the world, bringing out a variety of responses and the resultant
regeneration."

There can be no doubt that Gandhiji's inner life was influenced by Sri
Ramakrishna, and he has also acknowledged how after reading the works
of Swami Vivekananda his patriotism increased manifold. What an increase
of the patriotism in the life of **Gandhiji,** meant to India and the world history,
is well-known. Gandhiji of course greatly differed from Swamiji in his political
views but he largely accepted Swamiji's programme of removal of
untouchability and constructive work for the uplift of the masses and
advancement of women.

Chakravarty Rajagopalachari, a man of great intellect, who lived a long
life of sacrificial action for the independence and uplift of India, summed
up in a few words what the Ramakrishna Movement, as embodied and
spearheaded by Swami Vivekananda really meant to the history of this land:
"Swami Vivekananda saved Hinduism and saved India. But for him we would
have lost our religion and would not have gained our freedom. We,
therefore, owe everything to Swami Vivekananda." These are the words of
a man of great learning and wisdom who himself has been the witness and
one of the makers of modern Indian history. If Swami Vivekananda saved
Hinduism this meant an invaluable abiding service to religion as such
against all the forces ranged against it, and if he has been instrumental in
gaining freedom for India, this meant setting in motion freedom movement
all over the world as a historic force.

Subhas Chandra Bose was one of those heroes of recent Indian history, who exemplified in his life what Rabindranath Tagore meant to be the response to Vivekananda's "call of awakening to the totality of our manhood". Subhas Chandra wrote: "Few Indeed could comprehend or fathom Vivekananda – even among those who had the privilege of becoming intimate with him. His personality was rich, profound and complex and it was this personality as distinct from his teachings and writings, which account for the wonderful influence he has exercised on his countrymen.... He was a rare personality in this world of ours."

Bearing testimony to the fact how the freedom movement in India received effective fillip from the Ramakrishna Movement as embodied by Swami Vivekananda, Pandit **Jawaharlal Nehru** said: "....He was no politician in the ordinary sense of the word and yet he was, I think, one of the great founders – if you like you may use any other word – of the national modern movement of India, and a great number of people who took more or less an active part in that movement in later date, drew their inspiration from Vivekananda. Directly or indirectly, he has powerfully influenced the India of today."

Striking a note of urgency, **Dr. Radhakrishnan** emphasizes the importance of working out in the life of the individual and in our corporate action, the implications of the inspiration that flows out of the Ramakrishna Movement. Though a powerful purveyor of mystical traditions which concern themselves chiefly with transcendentalism and the life of the spirit, Sri Ramakrishna lived very close to common man his illumined life. Hence, his life produced several social results.

Dr. Radhakrishnan writes: "....If you really believe in the divine spark in man, do not for a moment hesitate to accept the great tradition which has come to us, of which Swami Vivekananda was the greatest exponent."
"It is essential, therefore, that we should remember what this great soul stood for, and what he taught us. It is not merely a question of remembering it, but trying to understand what he wished us to do. We should assimilate his teachings, incorporate them in our being, and make us worthy to be the citizens of the country which produced Vivekananda."

From a historian's perspective which envisages the movements of events as purposive forces at work for the progress or regress of man, **Dr. R. C. Majumdar,** the celebrated historian writes: "....By an inscrutable dispensation of Providence the mantle of the old Hindu Missionaries fell upon Swami Vivekananda. When he left the Indian shores as a cultural ambassador of India to the West, he unlocked the door, barred for a thousand years, and placed the cultural heritage of India again at the service of the whole world." That was in a sense a foreign obligation that the Ramakrishna Movement was fulfilling through Swami Vivekananda.

Because the Ramakrishna Movement has issued forth from the very central radiance of the *Sanatana Dharma*, it has set in motion not only the present Hindu renaissance, but cast new sunshine of the spirit on distant skies in which great minds read the portents of a new age dawning.

Prof. F. Max Muller was advanced in age and wisdom when he sat with young Vivekananda across the table at his Oxford home and talked and listened about his Master. He was about the first among the Western savants, who discovered in Sri Ramakhshna, *A Real Mahatma*. This he did after his life-long critical and scholarly studies of Vedic literature.

After Max Muller, **Romain Rolland** was the most eminent Western savant who presented Ramakrishna-Vivekananda and their message to the people of the Western hemisphere with rare depth of empathy and understanding. One must read his two fascinating books *The Life of Ramakrishna* and *The Life of Vivekananda* for experiencing the elevating joy of going through two finest pieces of world's hagiography. Romain Rolland was the one European savant who became awakened and aware of the creative sweep of the beneficent implications of the lives of Vivekananda and his Master not only for India but for the entire human race though most of the world may not yet be aware of it. Romain Rolland's thoughts continue to be echoed by eminent Western academicians, savants, scholars and thinkers.

Prof. A. L. Basham wrote: "The last eighty years have seen the foundation of societies in Europe and America, looking for inspiration to the saintly 19th century Bengali mystic, Paramahamsa Ramakrishna, and his equally saintly disciple, Swami Vivekananda."

What Vivekananda personified and what he did through his spiritual ministry have all entered into the history of the Western people, more particularly that of the American people, with the divine dynamism. Working through all the opposing forces which resisted his ministry, Vivekananda went right into the heart of the spiritual need of Western civilization and fulfilled the mandate of his Master: "Narendra will teach."

Not many though, a few talented Americans, have discovered Vivekananda as a maker of history in America. Among them the most noteworthy is **Marie Louise Burke.** She had found the calling of her life in announcing to whoever would care to listen that the advent of Swamiji in America was more than common history. It was the prophet doing your gardening in the inner quarter of your being, and your not fully looking at his face and not enough knowing who he was. She wrote: "Almost a whole nation had barked after Swamiji, but he had strode unperturbed, chastising where it was necessary with one or two well-directed blows, awakening and quickening the minds of thousands, and bestowing his blessings upon friends and foes alike. Both America and Swamiji had changed from a year and a half's contact with each other.... Swamiji himself had developed and given form to many of his ideas, he had learned the need of the West for the philosophy of Vedanta and he had seen how that philosophy could be applied to every problem of modern man...."

"During his travel he was consciously or unconsciously, fulfilling the function of a divine prophet to America – scattering seeds of spirituality wherever he went and bestowing his blessings upon innumerable men and women."

Should it have to survive for any meaningful future, there is no alternative for the human race but to learn to live and grow into a single family. But who will inspire and guide the people of this world in this new adventure? **Dr. Arnold Toynbee** wrote: "....At this supremely dangerous moment in human history, the only way of salvation for mankind is an Indian way. The Emperor Ashoka's and Mahatma Gandhi's principle of non-violence and Sri Ramakrishna's testimony to the harmony of religions; here we have the attitude and the spirit that can make it possible for the human race to grow together into a single family and, in the Atomic Age, this is the only alternative to destroying ourselves."

One American academician, **Prof. Carl Thomas Jackson,** of the University of California, Los Angeles, has produced valuable thesis, after painstaking research on *The Swami in America: A History of the Ramakrishna Movement in the United States 1893-1960.* This thesis proves that the impact of Ramakrishna, and what has flowed out of his life and teaching, are no longer confined to "stranded lonely hearts", but have attracted disciplined and thorough-going studies by urban and "cold-hearted" academicians. Prof. Jackson's thesis is a significant undertaking in that he pursued this non-sentimental study from the historical perspective, and produced a thesis of the Ramakrishna Movement in America, so far unsurpassed in its thoroughness and wealth of details.

Dr. Claude Alan Stark, in his book *God is All* makes a deliberate attempt to introduce Sri Ramakrishna to the academicians. He prefaces his book with the words: "The objective of this work is to introduce Sri Ramakrishna's approach to the scholarship community; first to the Christian world since I am a Christian, and then to the broad fellowship of world religions.... It is submitted that his approach to the dilemma of religious plurality is a significant one in religious history and merits further study...."

More than even the growing Vedanta Movement in the West, the effect of Swamiji's spiritual ministry is discernible in what has been happening to Christianity as a religion.

The West today is in the throes of a great religious ferment. Pope John's Ecumenical Council; rejection by the new generation of Catholic priests some of the cherished dogmas like infallibility of the Pope, original sin, and 'pining for heaven'; honest-to-God religious thinking of the Anglican Church; avant-garde thinking in the Fourth World Council of Churches at Upsala and many other signs will indicate that the whole religion of Christianity is seeking a renewal from within in order to tide over the crisis of irrelevancy forced on it by the developing empirical sciences and find an adequacy of faith commensurate with the demands of an age of science.

Exactly seventy-five years after Swami Vivekananda's spiritual ministry to humanity through the Parliament of Religions in 1893 at Chicago a symposium was held on September 15, 1968, in commemoration of that historic event. From what **Father Campbell,** a Catholic Professor of Theology, DePaul University, Chicago, said, we can have some idea how deeply and in what a far-reaching manner Vivekananda's work and thought have been influencing the Western religious thinking. Referring to the aforesaid ferment in Western religious thinking, what he chose to call 'possibly the worst crisis in Christianity', Father Campbell said: "I know Swami Vivekananda, the great Swami who spoke here in Chicago seventy-five years ago at the first Parliament of the Religions would himself look with favour on most of the trends in the direction of humanistic Christianity, because one of his sayings was, 'Don't be concerned about doctrines or dogma or church or temples', and liberal Christians echo those sentiments one hundred percent. Also, Swami Vivekananda said that formerly in the old religions the atheist was the man who did not believe in God and he said that now in the new religion we call an atheist a man who does not believe in himself and in mankind, and, once again, this attitude would be echoed wholeheartedly by the humanistic, the modernistic, Christian approach. Although Swami Vivekananda would not endorse all the attitudes of the new humanistic Christianity, perhaps the moral code, he would not endorse one hundred percent, still I think he would be in favour of this trend. Especially because it seems to be making more likely the development of the oneness of religions for which he was hoping. Ecumenism, for example, flourishes among liberal Christians....

"For this reason, I think this trend in the direction of humanism would be applauded by Swami Vivekananda were he here today, because it does seem to be breaking down to a large extent, previous divisions between religions and leading conceivably to one world religion in the future."

Swami Vivekananda's ministry to the West is more than its effect as religious ferment would indicate. He dowered the West with the solvent of the problems that were yet to come to the reckoning of the people. That is how the "divine prophet of America" worked for the Western man.

The Western problems of living that have been exasperating the thinkers of the technologically advanced affluent countries of the world, issue from an imbalance. This imbalance originates from the fact that in the West man's control over outer nature has far superseded the control over the inner nature of man. Western civilization could have no creative and forward looking future unless this imbalance could be corrected. Vivekananda's preaching of Vedanta and Yoga in the West was directly addressed to this desideratum in depth of the Western civilization, about which thinkers have of late started becoming aware.

The greatest need was to hold the whole life-process in perspective and correlate every effort of living human beings to the movement towards ultimate freedom and order society accordingly. Therefore, Vivekananda taught that 'the goal was to be free'. If we become more and more bound to senses and matter through advancement, then our civilization has failed as far as we are concerned, and it calls for inner revolution for the sake of redemption of man.

Vivekananda's teachings set in motion those forces which could eventually bring in the Western civilization the needed qualitative changes. So he preached Vedanta and Yoga. Vedanta conceptualizes reality in terms acceptable to the scientifically minded West and Yoga provides the know-how of being free.

– Swami Budhananda

IV

Just in these troublous times when humanity is fast slipping into savagery, when the rumbling echoes of the explosion of bombs, the wreckage of ships, the crash of planes and the massacre of men are filling men's minds with agitation and anxiety, contemplation on the life of Swami Vivekananda has added appropriateness, special significance. His message of spirituality can alone give solace and strength to the war-weary world. He was indeed Narendra, monarch among mortals, who burst into the world like a bomb not to lick it into destruction with tongues of fire, but to rouse men from their spiritual stupor by the boom of his powerful voice. His words seem to gain greater force as they roll down the years.

Swami Vivekananda is no mere hero who was in the footlights of the world for sometime and cast a spell over his immediate contemporaries: even after several decades of his passing away, his name is no mere memory, labouriously sought to be kept green in men's minds. He has transcended the limitations of human personality: he has become concretized into an impersonal institution which the world will not willingly let die: he is a system of thought: an attitude to men and things: an approach to life: a tradition which has woven itself inextricably into the world. His spirit is more alive today than his body was decades ago. It permeates a network of organizations spread over the whole world: it has expressed itself in diverse activities which have become institutionalized. It is this spirit which we should understand and catch if we want to make our lives fruitful.

– Dr. S. Balakrishna Joshi

The Memorable Year 1893!
Some Significant Events, in Retrospect
– S. J.

The year 1893 was a unique one. It was the year in which Swami Vivekananda delivered his historic Chicago Address. In the same year there were also quite a few significant events connected with the important contemporary personalities like Sri Aurobindo, Sri M. K. Gandhi, Sri B. G.

Tilak and Mrs. Annie Besant. While two of them had met Swami Vivekananda and known him personally, the others were greatly inspired by him. All of them played a key role in the national regeneration in India. Paramahamsa Yogananda was born in the very same year. All these events have been woven into this write-up. From the time Swami Vivekananda sailed for America (on May 31) and till the final session of the Chicago Parliament, his movements in America and participation in the Parliament of Religions have also been depicted in the following pages. A graphic description of the World's Columbian Exposition opened (on May 1) can also be found. All these events highlighted here have been brought together from the Chronicle part of this book where they are found scattered. In the context of the Centenary of Swami Vivekananda's visit to America, these events, in retrospect, will enable the reader to appreciate Swamiji's unique role in the national and international regeneration and his spiritual ministry to mankind.

For other significant events, national and international, of the year, the reader may refer to the Chronicle, under 1893.

Birth of Paramahamsa Yogananda

Paramahamsa Yogananda was born on January 5, in Gorakhpur, U. P. An enlightened exponent of the science of yoga, he was the first Indian yogi to live in the West for a long period of over a quarter of a century initiating over a lakh of students in yoga – the scientific techniques for awakening the divine consciousness in man. "As a bright light shining in the midst of darkness, so was Yogananda's presence in this world. Such a great soul comes on earth only rarely, when there is a real need among men." His *Autobiography of a Yogi,* has remained a classic in its field since its publication in 1946. Through 'Yogoda Satsanga Society' (1917) and 'Self-Realization Fellowship' (1926) established in India and in America respectively, the wisdom of the Great Yogi is made available to seekers of Truth in all parts of the world.

When Swami Vivekananda was addressing the World's Parliament of Religions in September, 1893, in Chicago, he was approached, with gratitude, by a 17-year old lad, Dickinson, who was saved from drowning by Swami Vivekananda twelve years earlier in a miraculous way. Dickinson wanted to become his disciple. Swami Vivekananda read his thought. With his beautiful, piercing eyes he gazed at Dickinson and said "No, my son, I am not your guru." "Your teacher will come later. He will give you a silver cup." After a little pause, Swami Vivekananda added, smiling,"He will pour out to you more blessings than you are now able to hold." The prophecy of Swami Vivekananda came true after 33 years. The guru referred by Swami Vivekananda was Paramahamsa Yogananda.

Sri Aurobindo returns from England

On February 6, Sri Aurobindo (1872-1950) returned to India, completing his studies in England where he spent 12 years from the age of six. The moment he set foot an the Indian soil at Apollo Bunder, Bombay, he had the first notable spiritual experience of infinite calm. Vadodara (Baroda) was his immediate destination and abode from 1893 till 1906. He mastered the Vedas and the essential heritage of India incredibly fast while at Baroda. Coming down to Calcutta in 1906, he edited the revolutionary daily *"Bandemataram"*, giving a shake to the passive national politics of those days and making the Congress take a radical stance with freedom for its goal. He also spent a year in Alipore jail. From 1910 to 1950 he remained engrossed in his yoga and explored the mystic world for a clear visualization of what man is and what is his destiny.

Sri Aurobindo has clearly stated how he was inspired by Swami Vivekananda, long after the latter had left his mortal coil. During the jail period, for a short time, Sri Aurobindo used to hear the voice of Swami Vivekananda instructing him on a particular aspect of *sadhana*. "It is a fact" Sri Aurobindo wrote, "that I was hearing constantly the voice of Vivekananda speaking to me for a fortnight in the jail in my solitary meditation and felt his presence. The voice spoke on a very important field of spiritual experience." Years later Sri Aurobindo spoke categorically about Vivekananda having been to him the very first messenger to reveal the lore of the Supramental Truth. "It was the spirit of Vivekananda who first gave me a clue in the direction of the Supermind. This clue led me to see how the Truth-consciousness works in everything. He did not say, 'Supermind'. 'Supermind' is my own word. He just said to me, 'This is this, this is that' and so on. That was how he proceeded – by pointing and indicating. He visited me for fifteen days in Alipore jail, and until I could grasp the whole thing, he went on teaching me and impressed upon my mind the working of the Higher consciousness, the Truth-consciousness in general – which leads towards the Supermind. He would not leave until he had put it all into my head.... I had never expected him and yet he came to teach me and he was exact and precise even in the minutest details." Aurobindo had another direct experience of Vivekananda's presence when he was practising hathayoga. He felt this presence standing behind and watching over him!

M. K. Gandhi sails for Durban

In the month of April, M. K. Gandhi (1869-1948) sailed for Durban, readily grasping an opportunity of legal work there. During his stay in South Africa when the Natal Indians were deprived of franchise, consequent on the introduction of Disenfranchisement Act of 1896 by the British rulers, M. K. Gandhi became a vigorous champion of the rights of Indian settlers. By the time he returned to India, in January 1915, he had become known as "Mahatmaji", a title given to him by poet Rabindranath Tagore (1861-1941).

During his stay in Calcutta (February, 1902) with Gokhale, Gandhiji went to Belur Math one day with a keen desire to meet Swami Vivekananda. About this visit Gandhiji recorded later on, in his autobiography as follows:· "Having seen enough of Brahma Samaj, it was impossible to be satisfied without seing Swami Vivekananda. So with great enthusiasm I went to Belur Math, mostly, or may be all the way, on foot. I loved the sequestered site of the Math. I was disappointed and sorry to be told that the Swami was at his Calcutta house lying ill, and could not be seen." Though unable to meet and talk with Swamiji, Gandhiji was deeply influenced by him. On the occasion of his visit he paid to Belur Math on 6th February, 1921, and being requested to say something on Swamiji, he quietly walked to the upper veranda of the monastery (Belur Math) overlooking the Ganga and addressed the public on the lawn. He said, in substance, as follows: "I have come here to pay my homage and respect to the revered memory of Swami Vivekananda, whose birthday is being celebrated today. I have gone through his works very thoroughly and after having gone through them, the love that I had for my country became a thousand-fold."

Bal Gangadbar Tilak and Ganesh Puja Festival

This was the year in which Bal Gangadhar Tilak (1856-1920), Indian nationalist leader and a major force in the Indian nationalist movement (1890-1920), transformed the traditional worship of Ganapathy in Maharashtra, into an altogether new forum and inaugurated the Shivaji Festival (1896), with the sole motto of bringing people together to ensure their awakening and involvement in the freedom struggle, He used the 'national opportunity' that these festivals provided for the spread of national feeling among the Hindu masses. He sought to mobilize popular support and create a militant, nationalist ideology. His emphasis was on 'Hindutva' (Hinduness), the organic links between Hindus in all parts of India. Sharing Swami Vivekananda's view in respect of Religion and Religious appeal as a powerful lever to move and magnetize, awaken, integrate and energize the people, Tilak made full use of the Ganesh Puja Festival, leading to its celebrations widely and on a larger, more enthusiastic scale, unifying the people and awakening them to a sense of self-respect, dignity and pride in their past, as a people. He was disappointed with the Congress Party, and anxious either to reform it or to replace it with a more militant organization which would preserve rather than weaken the cultural basis of the Hindu Nation. Tilak made it the great object of his life to diffuse the spirit of patriotism and nationalism among masses.

The Ganesh Puja Festival celebrated with great gusto and fervour as was rightly envisaged by Tilak vindicates his wisdom and the view of Swami Vivekananda in the matter of religion being the keynote of India's heart as a nation, moving and moulding as no other force can. Gandhiji could sense and see this as Jawaharlal Nehru could not and did not. So he planned for a secular India, while Gandhiji was wiser and more in tune with the genius of the Indian people. Gandhiji was absolutely in tune with Swami Vivekananda in the matter of Religion occupying the centre stage in India. Science is now approaching and accepting the truths of Spirituality. Even a scientific historian like Toynbee regards revival of religion as the key to the crisis of civilization, today, vindicating what Vivekananda proclaimed and Gandhiji, in line with the sages of the East and the wise ones of the West.

As an itinerant monk when Swami Vivekananda visited Poona (1892, June), he was the guest for several days of Bal Gangadhar Tilak, with whom the Swami had many interesting conversations on various topics. The Swami avoided mixing with society and did not make any public speeches but once, when he accompanied Tilak to the Deccan Club, rose to reply to a speech made by one of the members on a philosophical subject. He then pointed out, in fluent English, the other aspect of the subject. As Tilak said, at home the Swami talked frequently about Advaita philosophy and Vedanta.

The Swami had remained anonymous during his stay at Tilak's house, for, when they first met in the railway carriage at Bombay, the Swami, being asked his name, had said that he was just a *sannyasin*, and courtesy forbade Tilak to put the question again to him, A couple of years later when Swami Vivekananda returned to India with world-wide fame owing to his grand success at the Parliament of Religions Tilak happened to see his likeness in some of the newspapers, and from a similarity of features thought that the Swami who had resided in his house must have been the same. He wrote to him accordingly enquiring if his inference was correct and requesting him to kindly pay a visit to Poona on his way to Calcutta. The Swami sent a "fervent reply", frankly admitting that he was the same *sannyasin* and expressing his regret that he was not able to visit Poona then. It was not till about four years later when Tilak came to Calcutta to attend a session of the Indian National Congress that another meeting between the two persons took place (in the last week of December, 1901). About this meeting Tilak wrote in his reminiscences of Swami Vivekananda: "During one of the Congress sessions at Calcutta, I had gone with some friends to see Belur Math of the Ramakrishna Mission. There Swami Vivekananda received us very cordiaiiy. We took tea. In the course of the conversation, Swamiji happened to remark somewhat in a jocular spirit that it would be better if I renounced the world and took up his work in Bengal, while he would go and continue the same in Maharashtra. "One does not carry", he said "the same influence in one's own province as in a distant one."

Swami Vivekananda disliked politics, or at any rate thought that his own path was different and was out of the sympathy with the policy of mendicancy that the Indian National Congress was pursuing, in his opinion.

His views on Congress policies did not make him popular with the leaders of the Congress with the exception of nationalists such as Tilak. In this connection, it is worth noting what Swami Vivekananda wrote in a letter (dated 21-2-1900) written from California to one of his brother disciples: "In these days of dire famine, flood, disease and pestilence, tell me where your Congressmen are. Will it do to merely say, 'handover the Government of the country to us'. And who is there to listen to them? If a man does work, has he to open his mouth to ask for anything? If there be two thousand people like you working in several districts, won't it be the turn of the English themselves to consult you in matters of political moment?"

Mrs. Annie Besant arrives at Madras

On November 16, Mrs. Annie Besant (1847-1933), the British social reformer and Theosophist, arrived at Madras to take charge of the growing Theosophical Movement. In 1907, she succeeded Colonel Olcott and became the President of the Theosophical Society.

Mrs. Besant believed that a revival and re-introduction of India's ancient ideals and institutions could solve most of her problems. With a view to providing Hindu religious instruction, she founded the Central Hindu School at Varanasi in 1898, and this developed later into the Banaras Hindu University. She rose to fame as the creator of Home Rule League in 1916, and the next year she was elected President of the Indian National Congress. Mrs. Besant was a leader among Europeans in receiving and disseminating of Hindu Religion and culture. As commented by *The Amrit Bazaar Patrika* (dated 15-8-1894) in its editorial: "That Hinduism is making its existence felt more and more all over the world, is a spectacle which is now too patent to be ignored. Prof. Max Muller has admitted, to the infinite wonder of learned Europe, that the Vedanta philosophy has realized the highest aspirations of humanity. The miracle of an intellectually great English lady like Mrs. Besant, with such pronounced free-thinking tendencies kneeling before the image of Sri Krishna, has produced no little wonder in the world."

Mrs. Besant who saw Swami Vivekananda in America, wrote about him thus: "A striking figure, clad in yellow and orange, shining like the sun of India in the midst of the heavy atmosphere of Chicago, a lion-head, piercing eyes, mobile lips, movement swift and fast – such was my first impression of Swami Vivekananda as I met him in one of the rooms set apart for the use of the delegates to the Parliament of Religions. Monk, they called him, not unwarrantably, but warrior-monk he was, and the first impression was the warrior rather than of the monk, for he was off the platform, and his figure was instinct with pride of country, pride of race – the representative of the oldest of living religions, surrounded by curious gazors of nearly the youngest, and by no means inclined to give step, as though the hoary faith he embodied was in aught inferior to the noblest there. India was not to be shamed before the hurrying arrogant West by this her envoy and her son. He brought her message, he spoke in her name, and the herald remembered the dignity of the royal land whence he came. Purposeful, virile, strong, he stood out, a man among men, able to hold his own.... Enraptured, the huge multitude hung upon his words; not a syllable must be lost, not a cadence, missed! 'That man a heathen!' said one, as he came out of the great Hall, and we send missionaries to his people! It would be more fitting that they should send missionaries to us."

World's Columbian Exposition openes in Chicago

On May 1, World's Columbian Exposition (World Fair) was officially opened in Chicago, U. S. A., by President Cleveland. It was an international Exposition to observe the 400th anniversary of discovery of America, by Christopher Columbus (1461-1506) in 1492. It was also a demonstration of the growth of America to world status as an economic power.

Magnificent ceremonies dedicated the Exposition in October, 1892. In pursuance of a public demand for some fitting commemoration of the discovery of America, the U. S. Congress had passed an Act (April 25. 1890) authorizing an "Exhibition of the arts, industries, manufactures and products of the soil, mine and sea." The American President, Harrison, had recommended a sum of "not less than 10 million dollars" be allotted for the Fair. The estimated expenditure was given as over 22 million dollars.

The site of the Exposition covered 200 acres and extended about 2 miles along the shores of Lake Michigan. More than 21 million people visited the fair to view some 60,000 exhibits costing about 30 million dollars. After a period of six months, the Exposition was formally closed on 30th October.

Built largely on reclaimed swamp land, the World's Columbian Exposition was a spectacular "White City" of classically designed plaster structures (One major building – 600,000 sq. ft. – of the Exposition, is now housing the Museum of Science and Industry, a great Public Educational Exhibition which has been called a permanent World Fair).

For the first time electric light was lavishly used. George Westinghouse (1846-1914), U. S. Engineer, displayed at the World's Columbian Exposition, for the first time, the alternating current generator, later to become the basis of lighting and electric power.

An interesting feature of the World's Columbian Exposition was the Congress held at the grounds under the auspices of the World's Congress Auxiliary. The Congress discussed the leading phases of professional, scientific, economic, educational and religious thought; the World's Parliament of Religion's (held from 11th to 27th September and attended by Swami Vivekananda) attracted the most general attention.

Swami Vivekananda sails for America

On May 31, Swami Vivekananda sailed for America to attend the World's Parliament of Religions. He was helped by a group of brilliant students of the Madras University, who energetically took steps to organize ways and means of his going to America to represent Hinduism at the proposed World's Parliament of Religions at Chicago. He was also aided by a few of the enlightened native princes. And armed with the blessings of Sarada Devi, the Holy Mother, he set sail for the United States, from Bombay. Passing Colombo, Penang, Singapore, Hongkong, Canton, Nagasaki, Kobe, Osaka, Kyoto, and Yokohama, he landed at Vancouver and thence reached Chicago by train on 28th July, 1893. From there on upto his first speech at the Parliament of Religions at Chicago on the 11th September, 1893, he had to face many hardships and sharp moments of despair.

Swami Vivekananda meets Prof. J. H. Wright of Harvard University

On August 5, Swami Vivekananda met Prof. John H. Wright of Harvard University, at Annisquam (Mass.). The Professor had invited the Swami to spend the week-end at his place. Swamiji promptly responded to this invitation from a reputed scholar. Prof. Wright was so deeply impressed with the profundity of scholarship and the versatility of genius of this young Hindu monk that he himself insisted that he should represent Hinduism in the Parliament of Religions. Swamiji explained the peculiar difficulties that stood in his way in the fulfilment of his objective, and said that he did not posses any credentials whereby to introduce himself to the organizers of the Parliament. Prof. Wright, who had already discovered the sparkling intelligence and the rare ability of the Swami, said, "To ask you, Swami, for your credentials is like asking the sun to state its right to shine." Prof. Wright, who was well-known to the life of the city of Chicago and also to many distinguished personages connected with the Parliament, wrote at once to his friend, the Chairman of the Committee on the selection of delegates, stating, "Here is a man who is more learned than all our learned Professors put together." Moreover, he gave letters of introduction to the Committee which had the responsibility of providing accommodation for Oriental delegates. Knowing that the Swami was short of funds, he himself purchased a ticket for him to enable him to go to Chicago.

The World's Parliament of Religions opens at Chicago

On September 11, the World's Parliament of Religions opened in the morning, in the great Hall of Columbus, Art Institute, Michigan Avenue, Chicago, U. S. A.

A notable event in mankind's long search for spiritual harmony, it emphasized the accord between "Unity in Diversity" and "Diversity in Unity" of outlook and urged a cultural fellowship and mutual understanding between Western and Eastern worlds. The stated objectives of the Parliament were, briefly:

"To bring together in conference, for the first time in history, leading representatives of the great historic religions of the world; to demonstrate in the most impressive way, what and how many important truths the various religions held and taught in common; to set forth, by those most competent to speak, what are deemed the important distinctive truths held and taught by such each religion and by the various branches of Christendom; to enquire into the mimesis of religions; to discover what light religion can shed on the great problems of the time especially temperance, labour, education, wealth and poverty; to bring the nations of the earth into more friendly fellowship in the hope of securing permanent international peace."

At 10 a.m., ten solemn strokes of the New Liberty bell on which was inserted, "A new commandment I give unto you, that ye love one another", proclaimed the opening of the Congress – each stroke representing one of the chief ten religions, listed by President Bonney as Judaism, Mohammedanism, Hinduism, Buddhism, Taoism, Confucianism, Shintoism, Zoroastrianism, Catholicism, the Greek Church and Protestantism. "The sight", says Houghton, "was most remarkable. There were strange robes, turbans and tunics, crosses and crescents, flowing hairs and tonsured heads." In the midst of this sat Swami Vivekananda conspicuous in his orange turban and robe or as Rev. Mr. Wente put it, for his "gorgeous red apparel, his bronze face surmounted with a turban of yellow." The auditorium was jam-packed with men and women, intellectuals of the day, both clerical and secular. "Such a scene", writes Houghton again, "was never witnessed before in the world's history." Of this scene and the moment Swamiji later wrote, "My heart was fluttering and my tongue nearly dried up."

Of what followed Marie Louise Burke says: "Suddenly the great organ of the gallery burst forth with the strains of the 'Doxology' and the entire assembly rose to sing, 'Praise God from whom all blessings flow; Praise Him, all creatures here below; Praise Him above ye heavenly hosts; Praise Father, Son and Holy Ghost'. At the end of the hymn, a deep silence was sustained by the uplifted hand of the Cardinal. Then into this impressive hush, he began the words of the Lord's prayer, 'Our Father who art in heaven' – and every voice in the hall joined his." "The supreme moment of the nineteenth century", says Houghton, "was reached."

Swami Vivekananda speaks at the World's Parliament of Religions

(On September 11) Swami Vivekanada spoke at the World's Parliament of Religions during the first day's afternoon session, after four delegates had read their prepared speeches.

The spacious hall at the Art Institute of Chicago was packed with nearly 7000 people, representing the best of culture of the country. On the platform every organized religion from all corners of the world had its representative. Conspicuous among them was Swami Vivekananda who, with his bright countenance, crimson robe, and yellow turban, easily attracted the attention of the assembled thousands. When he addressed the gathering as "Sisters and Brothers of America" the entire audience broke into prolonged applause and greeted him with unprecedented enthusiasm – not merely because he addressed them as "Sisters and Brothers", for they had already heard many speak on the themes of Universal Brotherhood, but because his words, completely free from platitudes, reflected spontaneous realization of the spiritual oneness of mankind.

In fact there was an electric effect on the audience when Swamiji spoke the first five words of his address. Both Barrows and Houghton comment on the fact that "when Mr. Vivekananda addressed the audience as 'Sisters and Brothers of America', there arose a peal of applause for several minutes" and Swamiji himself tells that "a deafening applause for several minutes followed...." Another reference to this incident comes from Mrs. S. K. Blodgett, who later became Swamiji's hostess in Los Angeles. "I was at the Parliament of Religions in Chicago in 1893", she once told. "When the young man got up and said, 'Sisters and Brothers of America', seven thousand people rose to their feet as a tribute to something they knew not what." In this way, in the words of *Chicago Inter Ocean,* Swamiji "with an eloquence and power not only won admiration for himself but consideration of his own teachings."

It was a brief but intense speech which the Swamiji delivered in the afternoon session. Its spirit of universality, earnestness, and breadth of outlook completely captured the whole assembly. He cast off the formalism of the Parliament and spoke to the people in the language of the heart. The Parliament gave him a tremendous ovation that afternoon, and the American nation, infused by the streamer headlines of the newspapers of his contribution at the Parliament, gave him its silent ovation the next day morning,

During the ensuing seventeen sessions of the Parliament, Swami Vivekananda, in the course of his illuminating address, laid particular stress on the requirements of the day in the domain of religion and culture.

Swami Vivekananda reads his celebrated paper on Hinduism

On September 19, Swami Vivekananda read his celebrated paper on Hinduism at the World's Parliament of Religions at Chicago.

Chicago Inter Ocean depicted a picture of the tremendous excitement that prevailed that day. It reported "great crowds of people most of whom were women, pressed around the doors leading to the Hall of Columbus, an hour before the time stated for opening the afternoon session, for it had been announced that Swami Vivekananda, the popular Hindu monk who looks so much like Macullough's Othello, was to speak."

As reported by the *Chicago Daily Tribune,* "Dr. Noble presided at the afternoon session of the Parliament of Religions in Chicago. The Hall of Columbus was badly crowded. Dr. Noble then presented Swami

Vivekananda, the Hindu monk, who was applauded loudly as he stepped forward to the centre of the platform. He wore an orange robe bound with a scarlet sash, and a pale yellow turban. The customary smile was on his handsome face and his eyes shone with animation.... When the applause had ceased, Swami Vivekananda went to read his paper on 'Hinduism.' "

It was a fairly long document, being a masterly summary of the philosophy, psychology, and general ideas and statements on Hinduism, in its all-inclusive aspects. On this day the Hall was crowded to its fullest capacity, women vastly out-numbering the men, and many had to be turned away.

Swami Vivekananda in the final session of the Parliament

On September 27, in the final session of the Parliament, Swami Vivekananda made a grand appeal for the harmony of religious faiths.

He said: "The Christian is not to become a Hindu or Buddhist, nor is a Buddhist or a Hindu to become a Christian. But each must assimilate the spirit of the others and yet preserve his individuality and grow according to his own law of growth. If the Parliament has shown anything to the world, it is this: It has proved to the world that holiness, purity and charity are not the exclusive possessions of any Church in the world and that every system has produced men and women of the most exalted character. In the face of this evidence, if anybody dreams of the exclusive survival of his own religion and the destruction of the others, I pity him from the bottom of my heart."

The mighty words which were addressed by the Swami to the entire humanity over the heads of the official representatives in the Parliament made a tremendous appeal to the conscience of the people at large. The *New York Herald,* one of the most popular and widely circulated newspapers, editorially remarked, "He is undoubtedly the greatest figure in the Parliament of Religions. After hearing him we feel how foolish it is to send missionaries to his learned nation."

Soon after the termination of the historic sessions of the Parliament of Religions, it became the main object of Swami Vivekananda to acquaint the peoples of the West with the ideals of the civilization and the religious consciousness of his own race, to learn the secret of the material greatness of the Occident and also to collect adequate funds wherewith to provide his countrymen with scientific methods for the improvement of their economic condition. With this dual purpose in view he visited the important cities of America and delivered a series of illuminating lectures on a variety of subjects which comprised not only the history of the Indian people, the religion of the Vedanta and his future plan of work in India, but also the cardinal teachings of the other leading faiths of the world and a comparative study of the cultures and civilization of the East and the West.

Vivekananda as an Ardent Student of History
– M. P. Pandit

It appears, once when lecturing in London, Swami Vivekananda was asked: "But why did not your *rishis* come to England to teach us?" Swamiji quipped: "Because there was no England to come to. Would they preach to the forests?"

Swamiji had keen interest not only in the history of India but the whole world. Even before the end of the last century he had felt and expressed the need for an Indian School of Historical Research to arrive at correct appraisal of the nation's past. He was more than a student of history; he was a prophet who correctly envisaged the unfolding of events in the twentieth century. Note his repeated insight into the rise of the working classes in Russia and China, the collapse of the European civilization under the weight of its unbalanced development and unjust exploitation of countries in Asia and Africa. "He traces the origin of nearly all civilizations in the world to the Aryan civilization which he categorizes under three types – The Roman type which represents organization, conquest and steadiness, but lacks in appreciation of beauty and higher emotions; the Greek type is essentially enthusiastic for the beautiful; the Hindu type is essentially metaphysical and religious but lacks in the elements of organization and work."

Swamiji does not accept the theory of the Aryan invasion of Dravidian India. To him the two are not distinct ethnic groups but two linguistic cultural groups. Swamiji observes "The Dravidians were a race of central Asia who preceded the Aryans and those of Southern India were the most civilized.... They subsequently divided, some going to Egypt, others to Babylonia and the rest remaining in India."

While lauding the intellectual achievements of the Greeks, Swamiji notes: "It never occurred to the Greeks to pry into the secrets after death. But here from the beginning was asked again and again 'what am I?' "

Swamiji's evinced deep interest in the movement of Buddhism which he summed up in three periods: "Five hundred years of Law, the Hinayana phase; five hundred years of images, the Mahayana phase; five hundred years of Tantras, the declining phase characterized by hideous rituals and other forms of corruption."

Regarding India itself, he took pains to point our that *varna* is not *jati*. The four distinct features of human temperament are to be observed in all societies in the world. Caste is an unfortunate deformation of a universal principle. Swamiji's account of the major contributions of the Indian people to the world is noteworthy: "The influence of Buddhism on Christianity is unmistakable.... She (India) gave ideas on medical sciences by discovering various chemicals which could be used as cures for various diseases. She has done much more in the field of mathematics in its different branches – algebra, geometry, astronomy etc. Her most valuable gift was the ten numerals which is the very cornerstone of all present-day civilization.... In philosophy, India is head and shoulders above any other nation. In music, India has given to the world the system of notation with the seven cardinal notes and the diatonic scale.... She has given to the world the games of chess and dice. With regard to manufacture, India was the first country to make cloth out of cotton, muslin and silk."

Swamiji notes that India has not been a political nation; its forte has been spirituality and that is the direction in which she is going to serve the world.

Swami Vivekananda's perceptions in world history are striking. To cite a few: Competitive examination for recruitment was first introduced in China. Political revolutions occur when the masses are not involved in the governing process. Feudalism was introduced into Europe by Mohammedans. And last: "If it is possible to form a state in which the knowledge of priest period, the culture of the military, the distributive spirit, of the commercial and the idea of equality of the last can all be kept intact *minus* their evils, it will be an ideal state. But is it possible?"

In appreciation of the personality and vision of Swami Vivekananda Sri Aurobindo said: "The going forth of Vivekananda marked out by the Master (meaning Sri Ramakrishna) as the heroic soul destined to take the world between his two hands and change it, was the first visible sign to the world that India was awake not only to survive but to conquer. Swami Vivekananda was a soul of puissance, if ever there was one, a very lion among men, but the definite work he has left behind is quite incommensurate with our impression of his creative might and energy. We perceive his influence still working gigantically, we know not well how, we know not well where, in something that is not yet formed, something leonine, grand, intuitive, upheaving, that has entered the soul of India, and we say, Behold! Vivekananda still lives in the soul of his Motherland, and in the soul of her children."

Vivekananda as a Bridge Between The East and the West
– Dr. V. Sukumaran Nair

Swami Vivekananda's mission had two major aspects; one world- moving and the other nation-making.

Towards the culmination of his wandering days at Kanyakumari in December 1892, he decided to go to the West for spreading his Master's message of universal brotherhood and love. In his famous speech at Chicago on September 11, 1893, he expounded briefly the cardinal virtues of *Sanatana Dharma*. Humanism and universalism were so curiously blended in his words that the West was deeply impressed by the moral and spiritual grandeur of Indian national culture. He earnestly wished that the bell that tolled at the Parliament of Religions must put an end to fanaticism, superstition and ignorance.

From September 11, 1893, till the later part of August 1895, Swamiji had hectic work, giving lectures to the American people about India and Vedanta. His stay in the West which lasted till 1896 was packed with intense activity. It is of great significance that Vivekananda spent nearly four years of his public life in the West. Also, of the nine volumes of his published works, nearly seven comprise the lectures he delivered in the West.

He presented before his Western audience a new religious programme emphasising the oneness of God, the freedom of man, the equality of man and laid solid foundation of Vedantic thought both in New York and London. Swamiji interpreted Vedanta as the truly perennial and universal gospel, a religion relevant to all mankind. His exposition about religion and human life are forceful, clear and profound and in conformity with the modern historical sense and scientific thought. He preached before mankind the spiritual content of Vedic revelations that "each soul is potentially divine". He viewed religion as the manifestation of divinity in man. To him the Hindu religion represented a synthesis of all the religions of the world. He converted the Vedantic philosophy from a jumble of logical disputation to meaningful technique of human development.

On return from the West, Swamiji continued his mission in India. Between the day of his arrival at Colombo in January 1897 and the day of his *mahasamadhi* in July 1902, he worked day-in and day-out organizing relief centres, monasteries etc. for the betterment of society. His contribution to the awakening of modern India is unique in its quality and variety. His second visit to America by August 1899 was for a very short period during which he was able to establish Vedanta Societies in the West.

Vivekananda convinced the West that he stood for the harmony and synthesis of the entire humanity. In his writings and discourses he propagated the importance of human conscience and its sanctity in social and political relations. Swamiji emphasized the need for constant probing to find out the truth in the internal realms of human nature. The human society is to be trained in analysing the higher aspects and values of life apart from the transient and fleeting gains in social life.

He wanted the evolution of a cosmopolitan humanist culture comprising the best elements of the Orient and Occident. He believed in the regeneration of the spirit of the masses all over the world. As a great educator, Vivekananda had given to the world the message of fearlessness and strength. His outstanding legacy was that he reconciled life and religion and said 'strength is life, weakness is death.'

According to Swamiji the Vedanta had been not merely a philosophy for ascetics, but a living factor in the process of modernization. Religion signified to him the eternal principles of moral and spiritual advancement throughout the ages. He emphasized that behind all the differences of caste, colour and sex there existed the real human spirit. He firmly believed that Indian thought had influenced great personalities like Socrates, Plato and

Pythagoras. He sincerely hoped that Vedanta would save the West from rank materialism.

Swamiji heroically championed the cause of spiritual equality and pleaded for a happy synthesis between Indian ideal of contemplation and the Western ideal of mastering the external nature. He upheld the glory of India's ancient heritage and pleaded for making spirituality the basis of all human endeavours. His concept of socialism was not based on economic factors but on man's cultural growth through self-respect and self-expression. He always pleaded for equilibrium and synthesis in social and political relations. The Western ideas of organized charity, industrialisation, education of women, etc. had their deep impact on him and so he took the best out of them to be planted in India.

Vivekananda regarded all religious faiths as revelations of divine truth. He wanted the West to learn the lessons of religious toleration from the East. The West should supply to East their science and technology. He sincerely felt the need for a world culture and world conscience. He pointed out that the common tenets of Eastern and Western thoughts could easily bring about a philosophical bridge between the two cultures. His discussions with great personalities like Max Muller, were highly useful in procuring a favourable public opinion in West on behalf of India. In his opinion, the Occident had rated its values on the utilitarian ethics. He insisted both on the moral purification of every individual and the necessity of social reconstruction.

What made Vivekananda irresistible to his learners of the East and the West was that he interpreted the fundamental principle of the Vedanta in consonance with the findings of modern science. The contribufing factor to the leadership of Vivekananda was that he championed the cause of unity in human relation.

The Relevance of Vivekananda to the West

Sri Ramakrishna, the prophet of harmony of religions, and Swami Vivekananda, India's spiritual ambassador to the West, can be treated as a composite personality, as the facets of the same thing. They together make the circuit of galvanic spirituality complete. The marvellous union of these two – the Great Master and his foremost disciple, has ushered into the world a flood of spirituality which was never before witnessed on earth.

Through Sri Ramakrishna's blessings, Swami Vivekananda got the highest spiritual realization in the very prime of youth, and succeeded in perfectly assimilating it before he attained the age of thirty. As soon as he was ripe to deliver his message of uplift to the world, there was field ready for him in the Parliament of Religions held in Chicago in 1893. To move the world a good fulcrum is needed and the Chicago Parliament served as that point to Swamiji.

The Chicago Parliament where Swamiji made a tremendous impact, is one of the turning points of human history. Swamiji's talks at that august and celebrated Parliament had revealed to an astounded American public the moral and spiritual grandeur of India's religious culture. The doors of the civilized world were thrown open to Swamiji. America and Europe listened with admiration to the words of this young scion of the ancient rishis of India. He boldly voiced forth the teachings of the Vedanta, clothing the wonderful truths of unity-in-variety with a forceful and intelligible language so that the modern man and woman might grasp them with ease. Quite literally he planted the seeds of spirituality deep in the hearts of innumerable human beings, changing the course of their lives for ever.

In Swamiji's comprehensive message, science and religion, reason and faith, the secular and the sacred, the modern and the ancient and the East and the West became unified and he himself was the personification of that union, nay, his life became a confluence where the Eastern and Western ideals and ideas could meet, resulting in a vast universal synthesis that would give birth to a new moral order for humanity. Indeed his life and message have given the necessary impetus for the ushering in of a new era in the history of the civilization of man.

Vivekananda had made a deep and comparative study of world history, modern western science, and the thought and culture of different countries of the East and the West in general and of India in particular. He had possessed a keen intelligent understanding of the various forces that operated and the needs of mankind in the East and the West. He had also acquired a deep insight into the significance of the Indian spiritual and philosophical thought in the light of his Great Master's life and realizations. Moreover, besides his giant intellect and the towering catholic spirituality, Vivekananda had an intensely feeling heart which loved mankind. And his compassion for humanity was of a higher order! It was based on actual spiritual kinship with all men and women. He saw the Divine in all beings, and service of man was for him worship of God. And this moved him to sacrifice his all for the removal of the sufferings of humanity and its spiritual upliftment. He expressed his wish in the following words: "When will that blessed day dawn when my life will be a sacrifice at the altar of humanity?" And time has proved the truth of the words he uttered before his death: "It may be that I shall find it good to get outside my body – to cast it off like a worn-out garment. But I shall not cease to work! I shall inspire men everywhere until the world shall know that it is one with God!"

Swamiji was a champion of freedom, justice and equality everywhere. He welcomed science and technology, because he recognized their potentiality to promote material growth. But he rejected the view that material prosperity was an end in itself. His message was that this should be matched by spirituality which alone makes for a complete man, endowed with the 'inner character efficiency' coupled with the 'external productive efficiency', thereby resulting in peace and happiness for one and all.

At a time when the spectacular achievements of science and technology, art and politics, had drawn heavily on the spiritual reserves of the world, and the material life and physical enjoyment had become the primary concern of the people, Swamiji had declared: "Today man requires one more adjustment on the spiritual plane; today when material ideas are at the height of their glory and power, today when man is likely to forget his divine nature, through his growing dependence on matter, and is likely to be reduced to a mere money-making machine, an adjustment is necessary. The voice has spoken, and the power is coming to drive away the clouds of gathering materialism. The power has been set in motion which, at no distant date, will bring unto mankind once more the memory of its real nature."

Swami Vivekananda defined religion as "the manifestation of the Divinity already in man". In his inimitable words he summed up what religion is: "Each soul is potentially divine. The goal is to manifest this Divinity within by controlling nature external and internal. Do this either by work or worship or psychic control or philosophy – by one or more or all of these – and be free. This is the whole of religion. Doctrines or dogmas or rituals or books or temples or forms are but secondary details."

Man is essentially divine and the main task of his life is to assert his potential divinity. Religion does not consist in attempt to believe certain dogma, but in realizing – not believing, but being and becoming. The future universal religion will be a religion which will have no place for persecution or intolerance in its polity, which will recognize divinity in every man and woman, and whose whole scope, whose whole force will be centred in aiding humanity to realize its own divine nature.

If we look into the present literary activities of India and abroad, into what is being given out from Press and Platform, do we not find everywhere an echo of peace, harmony and freedom, of brotherliness and love for which the Swamiji stood pledged and which he so eloquently proclaimed before all the world? Some acknowledge the indebtedness, others may not, but the careful reader never fails to understand where the wind is blowing from. And the spirit of Swamiji must be glad at the phenomenon.

Although Vivekananda's teachings are not to be found yet in the mainstream of Western thought and culture, the Christian Church in the West, both Protestent and Roman Catholic, are taking deep interest in Eastern thought. Without quite knowing the source, the Americans are influenced by Vivekananda in their 'search for a life within'.

Today a reversal is taking place in the West where the people cloyed with material surfeit are searching for the inner being. The 'spiritual jolt' which Vivekananda gave to the West early in the century is now proving its impact. The West horrified by the destructive powers of the nuclear forces, is really corroborating the teachings of Vivekananda that a "man with excess of knowledge and power without holiness is a devil."

The Western problems of living that have been exasperating the thinkers of the technologically advanced affluent countries of the world, issue from an imbalance. This imbalance originates from the fact that in the West man's control over outer nature has far superseded the control over the inner nature of man. Western civilization could have no creative and forward looking future unless this imbalance could be corrected. Vivekananda's preaching of Vedanta and yoga in the West was directly addressed to this desideratum in depth of the Western civilization, about which thinkers have of late started becoming aware.

The greatest need was to hold the whole life-process in perspective and correlate every effort of living human beings to the movement towards ultimate freedom and order society accordingly. Therefore, Vivekananda taught that 'the goal was to be free'. If we become more and more bound to senses and matter through advancement, then our civilization has failed as far as we are concerned and it calls for inner revolution for the sake of redemption of man.

Vivekananda's teachings set in motion those forces which could eventually bring in the Western civilization the needed qualitative changes. So he preached Vedanta and yoga. Vedanta conceptualizes reality in terms acceptable to the scientifically minded West and yoga provides the know-how of being free.

We are privileged to be living at the time of the centenary of Swami Vivekananda's visit to America and his historic appearance in the World's Parliament of Religions held in Chicago on Septernber 11, 1893. This centenary is a unique opportunity to spread his message which is sufficiently powerful to influence the whole mankind in bringing about a radical spiritual regeneration in the world.

The main concern of the world today is peace and harmony. The path that the world has until now traversed in pursuit of technological mastery has imperilled peace. If peace and harmony are to rise and reign in the hearts and minds of human beings all over the world, they should have an opportunity to be exposed to the revealing insights of spirituality which Swami Vivekananda has bequeathed to humanity. Hence an earnest and vigorous propagation of his spiritual teachings is the most important means of serving that divine mission. The more the life and teaching of the great Swamiji are made known, the more will the spiritual perspective of humanity be widened, thereby resulting in world peace which today everyone is hankering for.

Swami Vivekananda – 100 years later *
– Bansi Pandit

Glen Ellyn, IL. : "In a world that is in constant pursuit of material happiness, our young men and women are tending to become hedonistic, thereby losing the true perspective of life," says Swami Jyotirmayananda of Madras, India, who has arrived in Chicago to attend the forthcoming World's Parliament of Religions. In his recently published book *Vivekananda – A Comprehensive Study*, Jyotirmayananda clearly brings

* *Weekly Spotlight*, Chicago, August 27, 1993.

home the universal message of oneness Swami Vivekananda delivered to the World's Parliament of Religions, hundred years ago. This book carries Vivekananda's message of hope for an inner transformation, resulting in a spritually oriented 'character efficiency' to go hand-in-hand with the present-day technologically oriented 'external productive efficiency,' to pave the way for universal peace and harmony.

According to Swami Jotirmayananda, the path that the world has until now traversed in pursuit of technological mastery has imperilled peace and environment and failed to provide prosperity and equality for all people of the world. Hosts of problems are cropping up, bringing in its train a lot of tension, anxiety, worries and frustration. Beset with psychological, social, economic, ethnic, political and environmental problems, which defy solution, the people of today's world are becoming the beasts of burden. Can anybody help and rescue those who are constantly being buffeted by these and the other problems? Can they themselves solve their problems by dint of their self-effort? Or can their Governments or social organizations, or even the mighty world organization – the United Nations – find a permanent solution for today's human crisis? The answer is emphatically negative. At best they can find some temporary remedies which can act as just palliatives. In any case it is certain that none of them can create in all the people of the world a total awareness for higher and enduring values, the inculcation of which alone can regenerate human life and reform the character. No amount of state authority can bring an essential change in human nature. 'Neither science nor politics can give man perfect peace and happiness. The ills of life cannot be cured by political, social or other mechanical remedies which human beings are constantly attempting and which have always failed," says Jyotirmayananda.

Nevertheless, there is an abiding solution for all human problems. Swami Vivekananda, the prophet of spirituality, whose mission was to make human life sublline and fruitful, emphatically affirms the fact that the world will change when the human beings, who constitute it, change from within. The "inner man" is to be set right first and the externals will take care of themselves. So the solution of problems which Vivekananda offers is not by external means, though these also have to be used, but essentially by an inner change, a complete transformation of man's consciousness and nature. Unless the man's psyche changes, the society cannot by deeply and permanently changed. The various social, political, and economic problems of today's world are only the outward symptoms of an inner psychological malaise. So it is the spiritual awareness alone that generates the real peace and happiness, and love and unity in the world.

Swami Vivekananda, therefore, advocates self-culture and self-tansformation, and teaches the technique of change within. He loves to call this process as "Man-making". This is the panacea of all the maladies of today's world. Although modern technology and science has placed enormous power at the disposal of man, he cannot use this power for the peace and prosperity of the human race, until his own mind is cultured. Excess of knowledge and power, without holiness, can easily make human beings devils, warns Swami Vivekananda. "We must progress materially and spiritually, side by side. Material properity should not be at the expense of spiritual advancement. They must go hand-in-hand. Then only we can have integral evolution. Then and then alone we can expect to have a socially more useful and individually peaceful and spiritually enlightened life," says Swami Jyotirmayananda.

Hundred Years after
the Historic 'Chicago Address'
Vivekananda Centenary Celebrations in America, in Retrospect

In connection with the centenary of Swami Vivekananda's appearance at the World's Parliament of Religions at Chicago in 1893, I was in the U. S. A. (from 1st August, 1993) for nearly six months and returned on the 17th January, 1994, after a tour in the East coast. The following are a few excerpts from my notes on the trip. The focus here is mainly on the centenary celebrations in which I participated:

Major Programmes

The major programmes I attended were the Vivekananda Centenary Celebrations at Washington and Chicago. I also attended the Parliament of the World's Religions held at the Palmer House Hilton at Chicago.

Hiduism Today (North America Edition, October and November 1993 issues) published a faithful account of those programmes. Let me therefore begin with a few lines therefrom to highlight the significance and uniqueness of the historic occasion:

'Global Vision 2000' Conference

The Largest U. S. A. gathering of Swamis highlighted the three-day 'Global Vision 2000' conference at Washington D. C. (August 6-8) where 10,000 rallied to honour Swami Vivekananda and mark the 100th anniversary of his arrival in America. Speakers boldly proclaimed that the spiritual concepts propounded by Swami Vivekananda in the last century contain the solutions to the problems of the next. There were pressing appeals for spreading the ancient Hindu values, beginning with *vasudhaiva kutumbakam* – 'the world is one family' – the message that Swami Vivekananda dilated upon at the Parliament of Religions in Chicago in 1893.

As an event, 'Global Vision 2000' was more than a sucess – double the number of expected three-day participants (4000 in all) showed up, overwhelming the staff. Despite some very difficult logistics, including the feeding of unexpected large numbers of people, the conference fulfilled all its planned objectives: to bring together a large gathering of Hindus for spiritual celebration of Swami Vivekananda's arrival in the West; to involve the youths in substantial numbers; and to bring Eastern and Western philosophers together to examine the ideal of the oneness of all creation.

Parliament of the World's Religions

One hundred years ago (in 1893), while hosting the World's Columbian Exhibition, celebrating the 400th year of Columbus' discovery of the America, Chicago also become the home of the first-ever interfaith gathering. Roaring like a lion at that first assembly of all faiths, Swami Vivekananda overawed the audience with his knowledge, his love of Hinduism and its olympian tolerance. By his eloquent depiction of the Hindu faith, it saw in this thirty-year-old monk the highest expression of Hindu intuitive wisdom.

One hundred years later, at the second Parliament of the World's Religions held from August 28th to September 5th in Chicago, 600 world spiritual leaders and dignitaries, explored the hope of realizing interfaith harmony.

That single saffron robe of 1893 had turned to hundreds in 1993. A few Eastern souls had turned to thousands. There in the crowded hall, mingling with indigenous American Indians, jostling shoulder-to-shoulder with Christian and Jewish leaders, were the new-comers. The Jains were there, along with the Sikhs, the Buddhists and the Hindus. There were also a few Mohammedans.

The Parliament was a clinching proof of the emerging multiracial society in America. No one could ignore the Indian presence. It was a kind of Chicago *Kumbha Mela.*

There were the seminars, panels, lectures, inspirational readings and discourses on all spiritual traditions. Much was said of interfaith harmony and understanding. There was genuine sharing and a true tolerance that transcended the reluctant toleration of a century ago. In essence, the Parliament revolved around 600 world spiritual leaders and dignitaries gathered to share their faith with over 6,500 participants. Clearly it had a message of profound interest to the world at large. Besides heavy North American representation, participants also came from every continent, and carried the message when they went back home.

At the Art Institute of Chicago

About a thousand devotees participated in the 100th anniversary celebration (11th September, 1993) to commemorate Swami Vivekananda's famous 'Chicago Address'. The function, sponsored by the Vivekananda Vedanta Society of Chicago and the Consul General of India, was held at the Art Institute of Chicago – the very place where the Swamiji had made history

100 years ago. I had a rare privilege to pay a reverential homage to the great Swamiji on that day in the Art Institute (see *Appendix II*).

The Hindu Representative at the Parliament

It was the first day of the Parliament and the opening session was about to commence. The Grand Ball Room of the Palmer House Hilton was jam-packed with the delegates from all over the world. The representatives of the leading faiths were present on the platform. When the session started, the representatives of different faiths were called one by one, and they made their invocation speeches. The Hindu representative fared excellently well, as did Swami Vivekananda himself 100 years ago in the opening session of the Parliament. Sant Keshavadas made an extempore, inspiring speech, paying rich tributes to the hallowed memory of Swami Vivekananda who made history in the Parliament of Religions a century ago. The moment Sant Keshavadas reminded the audience about that great Hindu Monk of India and his historic 'Chicago Address' in 1893, there was a loud and prolonged applause from the audience at the Grand Ball Room. It appeared as if the scene of the first day of the 1893 Parliament at the Art Institute of Chicago was re-enacted at the Palmer House Hilton in 1993! Indeed Sant Keshavadas echoed in his own inimitable style the grand message of the *Sanatana Dharma* contained in the famous 'Chicago Address' of Swami Vivekananda.

Incidently, what did Swami Vivekananda proclaim 100 years ago in the World's Parliament of Religions at Chicago? Note his impassioned plea: "The Christian is not to become a Hindu or Buddhist, nor is a Buddhist or a Hindu to become a Christian. But each must assimilate the spirit of the others and yet preserve his individuality and grow according to his own law of growth. If the Parliament has shown anything to the world, it is this: It has proved to the world that holiness, purity and charity are not the exclusive possessions of any church in the world, and that every system has produced men and women of the most exalted character. In the face of this evidence, if anybody dreams of the exclusive survival of his own religion and the destruction of the others, I pity him from the bottom of my heart". In contrast to this statement of Swami Vivekananda, note the following report from *The New York Times* dated 30th August, 1993: "....But even within the religious world, there is disagreement about the Parliament's merits. The Southern Baptist Convention, for instance, is among groups that declined to send a representative. *Many evangelical and fundamentalist Christians believe that such gatherings are at best a disraction from spreading the Gospel and at worst a confusing compromise of their belief that Christianity is the only way to salvation.*"

'The Star of the 1893 Assembly'

Recalling the World's Parliament of Religions held at Chicago 100 years ago and the 'star of the 1893 assembly', Swami Vivekananda, and the impact of his dynamic spiritual message on contemporary America, *The New York Times* dated 30th August, 1993, stated:

"This meeting is the centennial of the 1893 World's Parliament of Religions, held on the site of what is now the Art Institute of Chicago, was a landmark in American religious history.... The star of the 1893 assembly was Swami Vivekananda, a thirty-year-old spokesman for Hinduism.

" 'Do not care for dogmas, or sects....' he preached. 'They count for little compared with the essence of existence in each man which is spirituality.' It was a message that struck chords in an America where school children encountered similar thoughts in the writings of Ralph Waldo Emerson and Thomas Jefferson.

"Swami Vivekananda demounced the sectarianism that 'has filled the earth with violence, drenched it often and often with human blood,' and he called for 'the death-knell of all fanaticism.' "

Evidently, Peter Steinfels, the reporter of *The New York Times* quoted above, realized the relevance and significance of Swami Vivekananda and his message to the West, nay, to mankind. All kudos to him!

A Holy Mother at the Parliament

On one of the days of the Parliament at Chicago, Mata Amritanandamayi, the renowned saint from Kerala, kept the audience spellbound for about an hour, with her spiritual discourse. She spoke in the Grand Ball Room of the Palmer House Hilton, where I was present among the audience. In consonance with the teachings of Swami Vivekananda, she emphasized spirituality and spiritual experience as the essence of religion. Said she, *inter alia*: "Religion leads us to know we are the all-powerful God. God is in us all. He is like the space. Space is everywhere. Suppose we build a house, space existed before the house came into being, and after the house is demolished the space is unchanged. God is like that, everywhere and unchanged. God is all-pervasive, and is the Light of Consciousness within us. Heaven and hell are created by the mind. Rising in love is religion." No sooner did she finish her discourse than the audience surged towads her. She received and blessed them affectionately.

I had visited her Ashram in Kerala, about a decade ago (in 1984, vide my book: Beloved Mother – Amritanandamayi). So it was a pleasant surprise to her when I met her at the Grand Ball Room of the Palmer House Hilton at Chicago and presented to her a copy of the International Edition of my book on Swami Vivekananda. In less than a decade, her divine mission has flourished phenomenally, both in India and abroad. She is today a great solace to the careworn and heavy-ladden humanity. The enlightened saints are verily the salt of the earth.

Pilgrimage in Swamiji's Footsteps: Chicago

In the context of the Vivekananda Centenary Celebrations, in the month of September, 1993, the Vivekananda Vedanta Society of Chicago arranged for the devotees a pilgrimage to various places connected with Swami Vivekananda at Chicago. I too joined the band of enthusiastic devotees and had the privilege of visiting the places intimately connected with Swamiji during his stay at Chicago, a century ago. This was a cherished wish of mine even before I left for the U. S. A. and now it was amply fulfilled.

Other than the Art Institute of Chicago (the venue of the Parliament of Religions a hundred years ago, where Swamiji delivered the historic 'Chicago Address'), the places connected with Swamiji we visited were: The Hale House, John B. Lyons House, Fine Arts Building, Lincoln Park near Dearborn Street, and the house at 1210 N. Astor Street.

It is opposite to the Hale House, across the street, that Swamiji sat down exhausted after his long walk from the Railway Station (September, 10, 1893), where Mrs. Hale welcomed him. At John B. Lyons house, the Lyons family hosted Swamiji throughout the Parliament and often afterwards at the then 262 Michigan Avenue. At the Fine Arts Building, Swamiji gave several classes in the studios of Florence Adams – a noted devotee and friend. At the entrance of Lincoln Park near Dearborn Street, Swamiji often used to sit, while staying with the Hales. One mother impressed by his imposing apperance asked if she could leave her six-years-old child in his charge while she was shopping; since he agreed, she did so several times. Later, that child – Agnes Ewing – became a student of Swami Akhilananda. From 1897, the house at 1210 N. Astor Street was the residence of the Hale family. Here Swamiji stayed during his last two Chicago visits.

The Programme I missed

The Ramakrishna-Vivekananda Centre of New York also organized a three-day Vivekananda Centennial Celebrations at New York (November, 5-7, 1993). One of the programmes was held at the United Nations Auditorium. It was presented in co-operation with the Permanent Mission of India to the United Nations, and more than a dozen distinguished participants paid rich tributes to the hallowed memory of the Swamiji. Unfortunately, I missed the entire programme.

Excellent Facilities for Students

My stay for a fortnight at the International House located in the Hyde Park by the campus of the University of Chicago was providential. I was staying at Bolingbrook which was far away from downtown Chicago where the Parliament of Religions was to be held at the Palmer House Hilton. Dr. Shyam L. Bhatia (a Ramakrishna-Vivekananda devotee residing in Hyde Park) whom I had met in the College of DuPage campus, Glen Ellyn, in the second week of August, was kind enough to introduce me to the International House to which I shifted, thus being able to attend the week-long Parliament punctually. The House is about fifteen minutes away from the downtown by commuter trains which stop one block away.

An autonomous department of the University of Chicago and a self-supporting educational residence for students from around the world, the International House was founded in 1932 through a munificent gift from John D. Rockefeller, Jr. – son of the renowned philanthropist, John D. Rockefeller (1839-1937) who had met Swami Vivekananda in Chicago, in 1894, and about which I have incorporated a write-up in my book on Swami Vivekananda – the International House is a great boon to the international students and scholars. They are provided with all amenities for a comfortable stay, besides facilities for their social and cultural development. Verily, the International House symbolizes Rockefeller's love for students and his patronage to the cause of higher education.

Need of the Hour: A Coming Together of the East and the West

In conclusion, some observations:

At the zenith of material prosperity and technological achievement, America seems to be at the crossroads on account of a lack of concern for spiritual values in life. A 'moral vacuum' can be palpably felt in their hectic life even as one finds a chronic 'material vacuum' (abject poverty and squalor) in India despite its lofty spiritual inheritance. This imbalance can go if only India and America join hands. America needs India as much as India needs America. Swami Vivekananda is the harbinger of such a commingling of the East and the West. His teachings set in motion those forces which could eventually bring to the Western civilization the needed qualitative changes. So he preached Vedanta and Yoga in the West, and at home emphasized the need for useful and dynamic activity, the education of the Indian masses and the service of the poor and the downtrodden without disturbing their faith and tradition.

We are privileged to be living at the time of the centenary of Swami Vivekananda's visit to America and his historic apperance at thee World's Parliament of Religions held in Chicago in 1893. This centenary is a unique opportunity to spread his message which is powerful enough to influence the whole mankind in bringing about a radical spiritual revolution in the world.

Widening the Spiritual Perspective of Humanity

The main concern of the world today is peace and harmony. The path that the world has until now traversed in pursuit of technological mastery, has imperilled peace. If peace and harmony are to rise and reign in the hearts and minds of human beings all over the world, they should have an opportunity to be exposed to the revealing insights of spirituality which Swami Vivekananda has bequeathed to humanity. Hence an earnest and vigorous propagation of his spiritual teachings through books is the most important means of serving that divine mission. The more the life and teachings of the great Swamiji are made known, the more will the spiritual perspective of humanity be widened, thereby paving the way for enduring world peace everyone is hankering for.

– S. J.

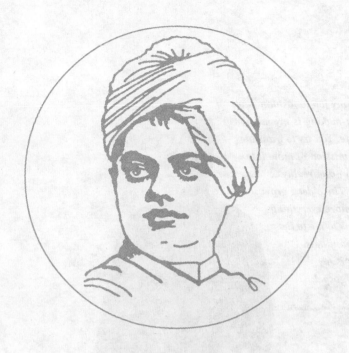

PART FOUR

VIVEKANANDA
IN PICTURES

This Part pesents a selection of about eighty photographs projecting tapestry-like a visual review of the evolution of Naren into Vivekananda the prophet of Prabudha Bharata, of man's awakening into his true self, and of the efflorescence of the Divine in everyday human life.

For the Vivekananda buff, the true admirer, there is a portfolio of eighty pictures. That comes as a bonus.

– M. V. Kamath

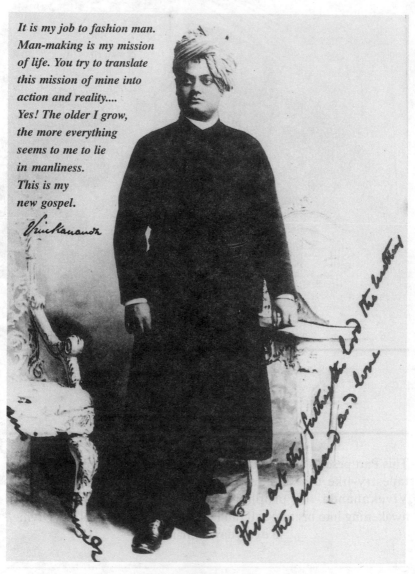

It is my job to fashion man. Man-making is my mission of life. You try to translate this mission of mine into action and reality.... Yes! The older I grow, the more everything seems to me to lie in manliness. This is my new gospel.

Vivekananda

One single man changed the current of thought of half the globe
– that was his work.

– Christina Albers

LIST OF PICTURES

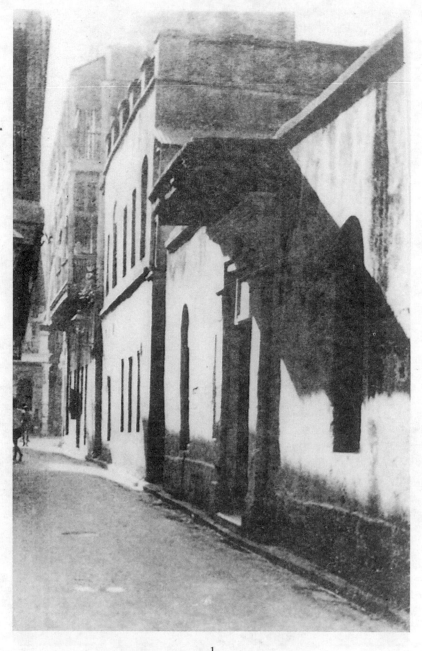

1
Where Narendra was born
(3, Gour Mohan Mukherjee Lane, Calcutta)

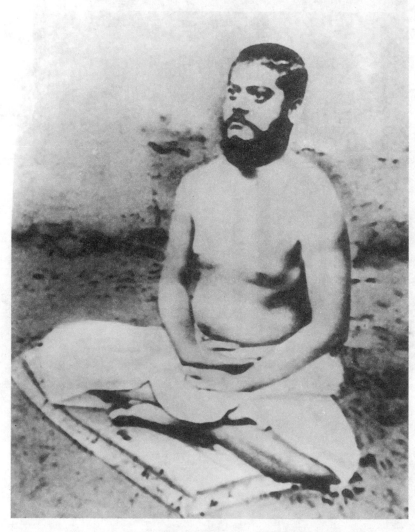

2
Narendra meditating at Cossipore Garden (1886)

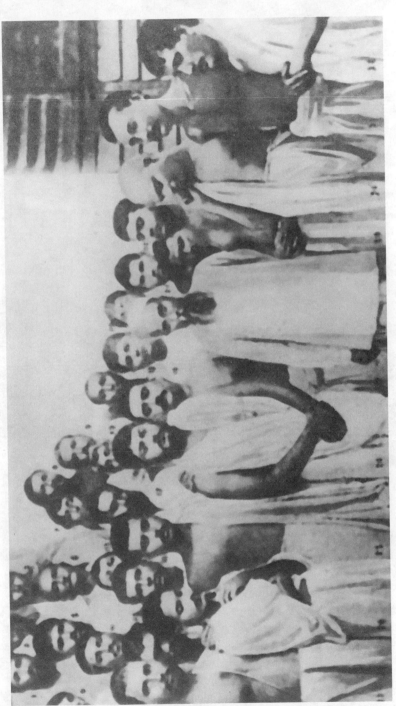

3

Narendra in a group of devotees immdiaely after
the passing away of the Master (August 16, 1886)

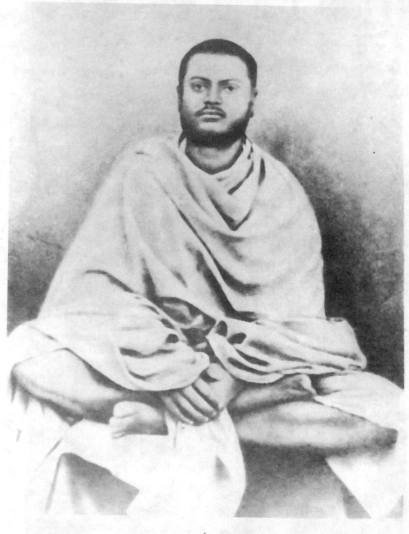

4
Swamiji in Calcutta (1886)

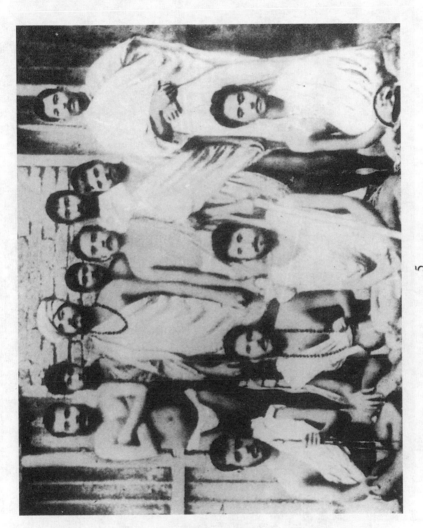

5

With *gurubhais* at the Baranagore Math (1887)

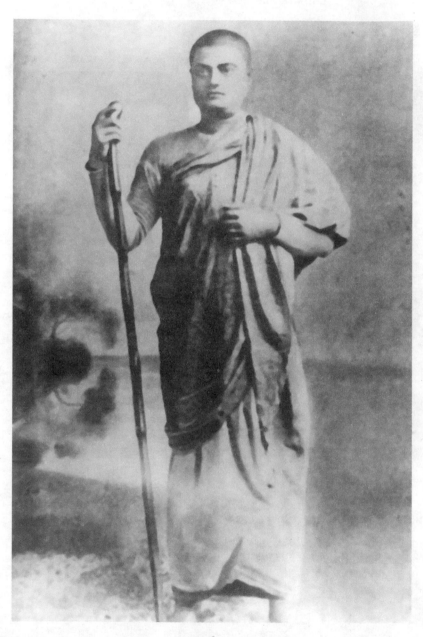

6
As *parivrajaka*

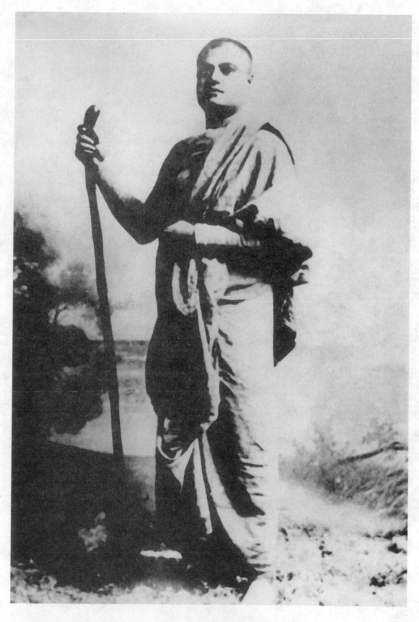

7
As parivrajaka

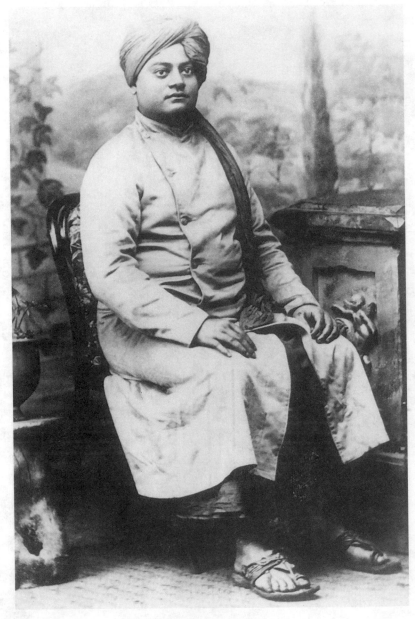

8
At Belgaum (October, 1892)

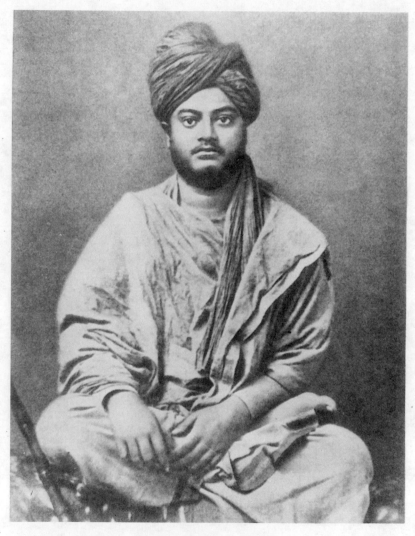

9
At Belgaum (October, 1892)

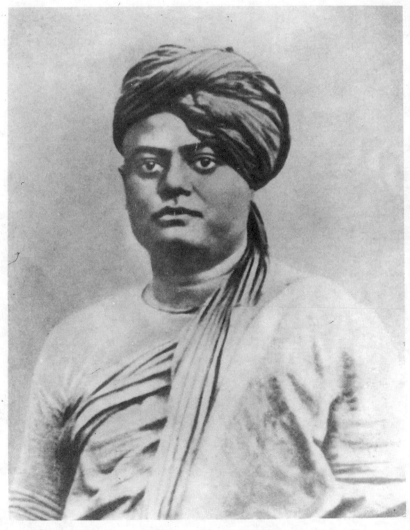

10
At Trivandrum (December, 1892)

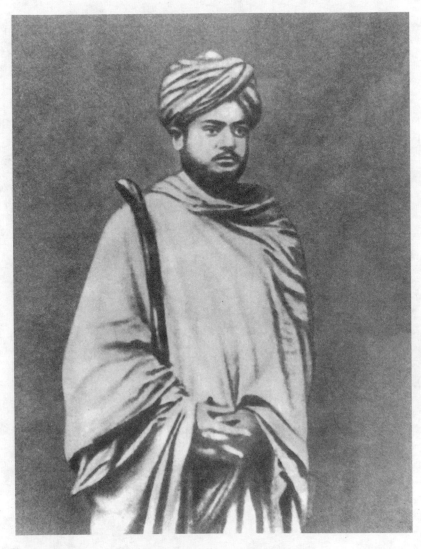

11
At Hyderabad (February, 1893)

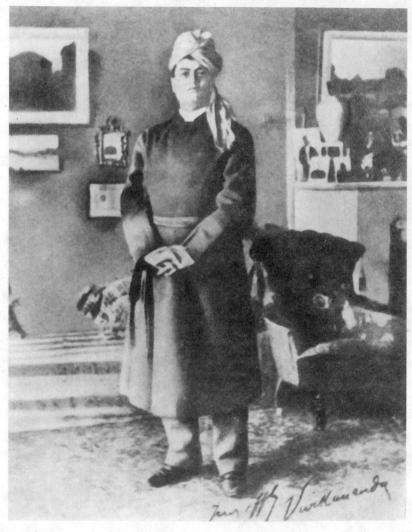

12
In America (1893)

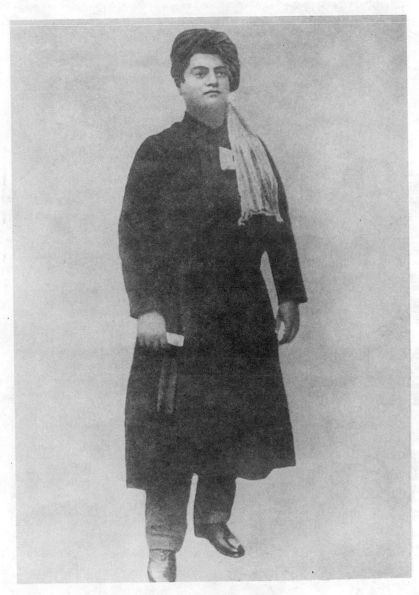

13
Entering the Parliament of Religions, Chicago (1893)

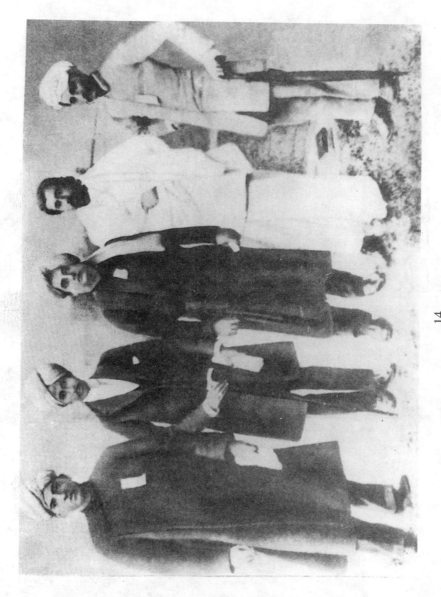

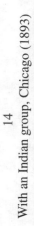

14

With an Indian group, Chicago (1893)

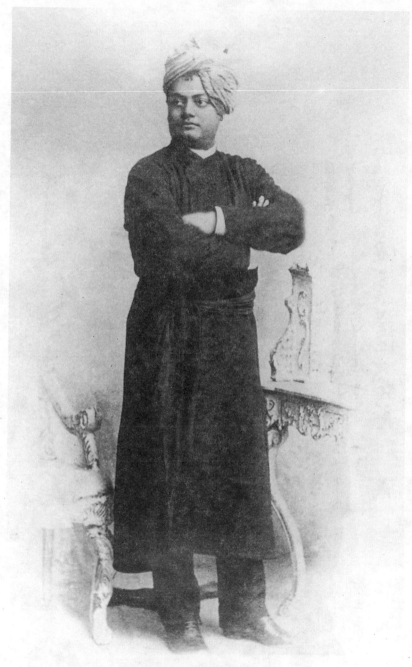

15
The Lion of Vedanta at the Parliament of Religions (1893)

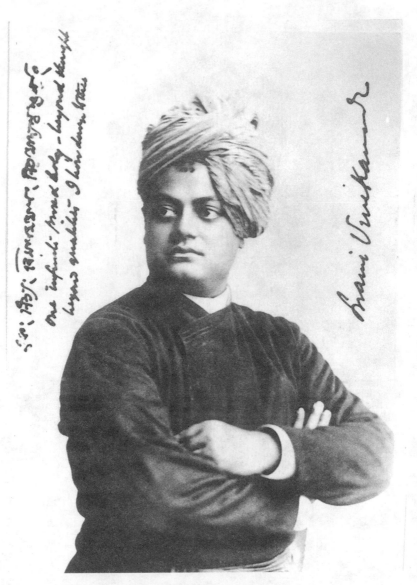

16
The Familiar Pose: Chicago (1893)

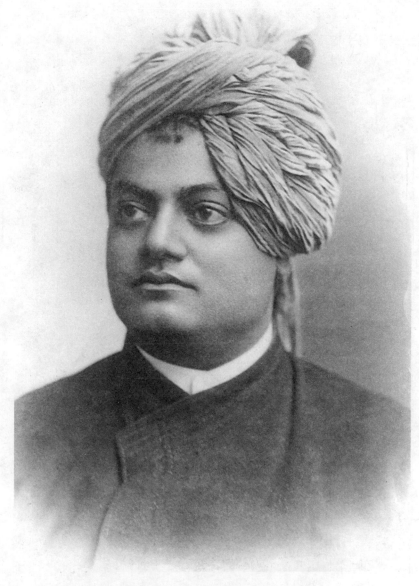

17
At the Parliament of Religions (1893)

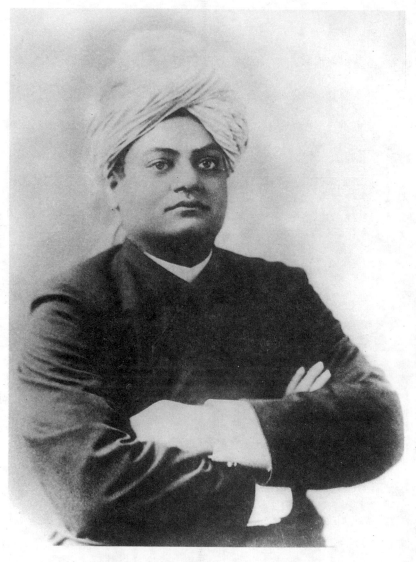

18
At the Parliament of Religions (1893)

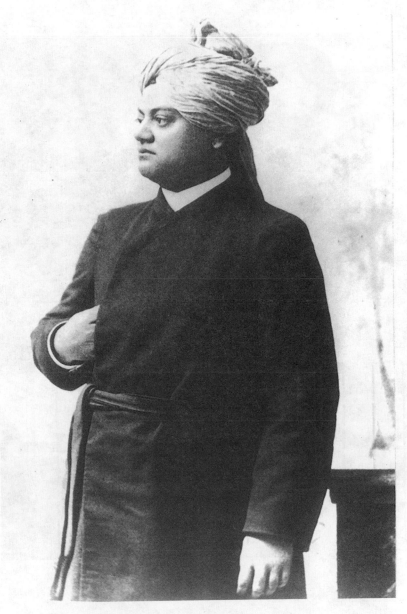

19
At the Parliament of Religions (1893)

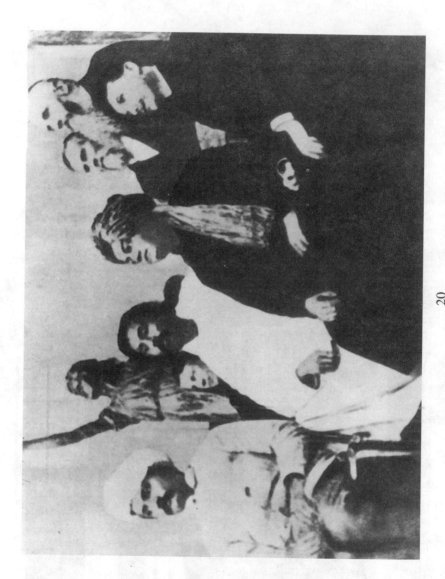

20

On the dais at the Parliament of Religions (1893)

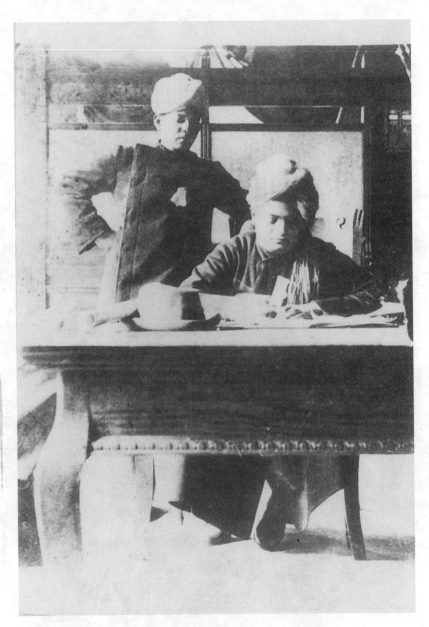

21
At the writing desk with Narasimhacharya

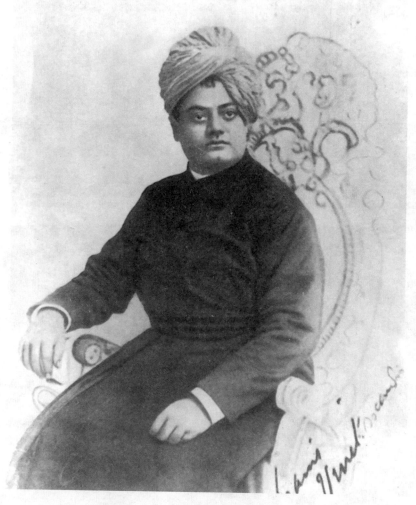

22
The Uncrowned King, Chicago (September, 1893)

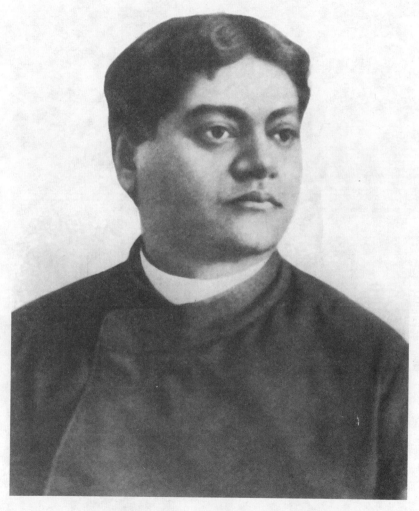

23
The Radiant Goodness, Chicago (1893)

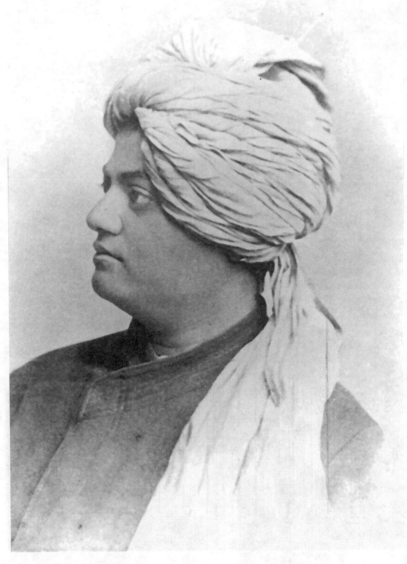

24
The Orator by Divine Right, Chicago (October, 1893)

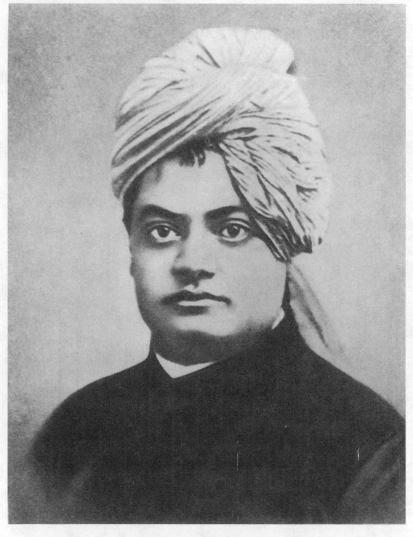

25
The arresting gaze, Chicago (October, 1893)

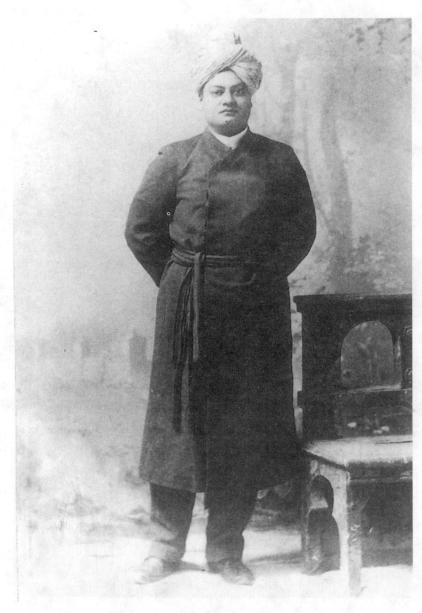

26
In America (1893)

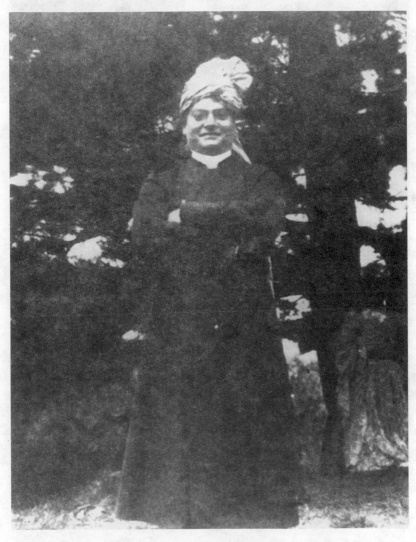

27
In tune with Nature at Greenacre (1894)

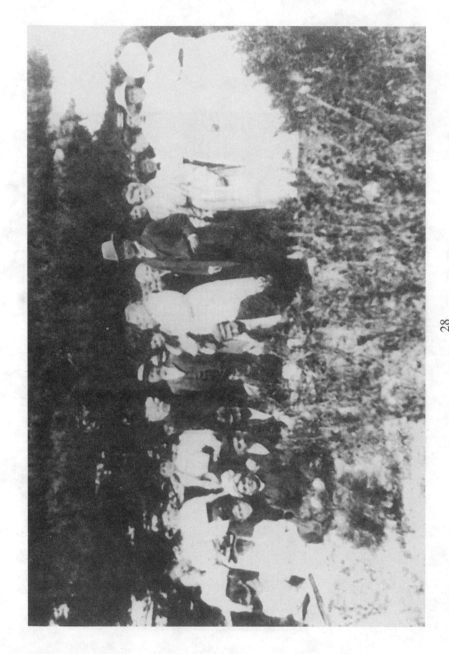

28
With friends at Greenacre (1894)

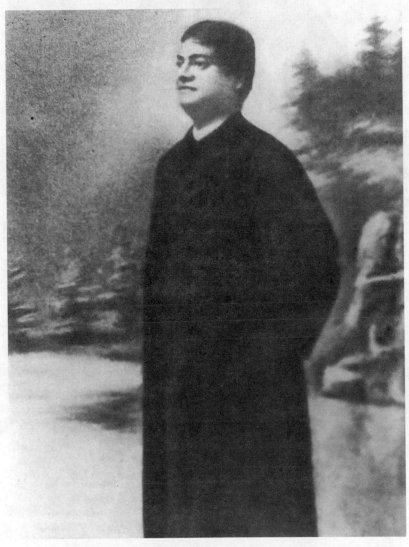

29
The Inspired Talker at the Thousand Island Park

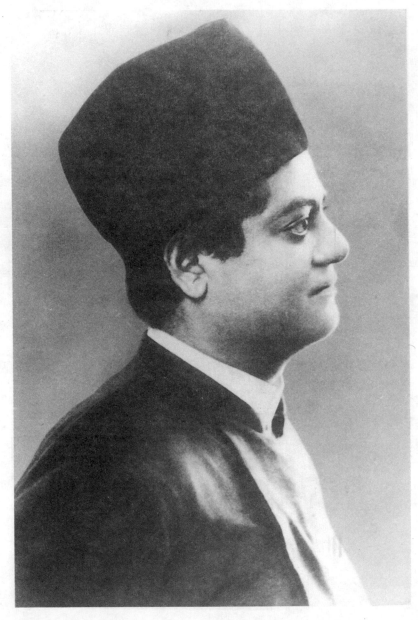

30
In London (October 1895)

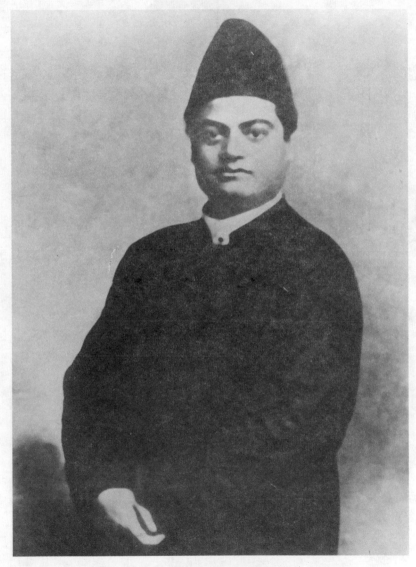

31
In London (October 1895)

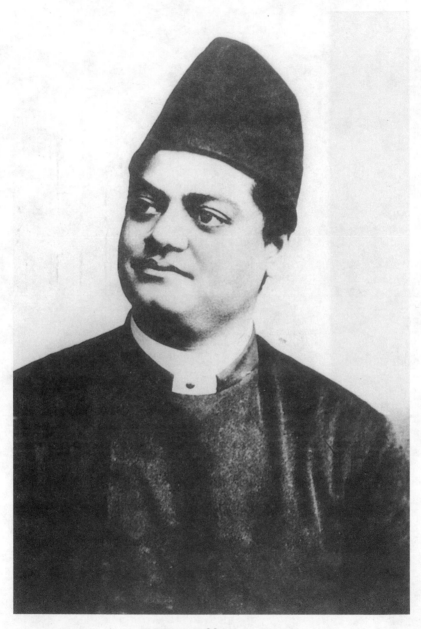

32
In London (October 1895)

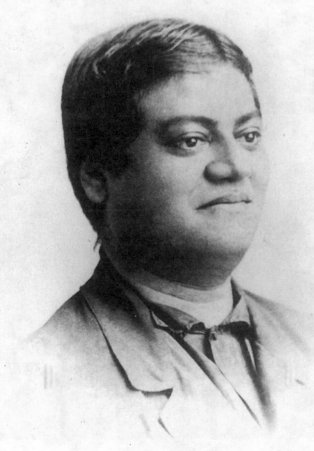

33
Prince Charming, London (May, 1896)

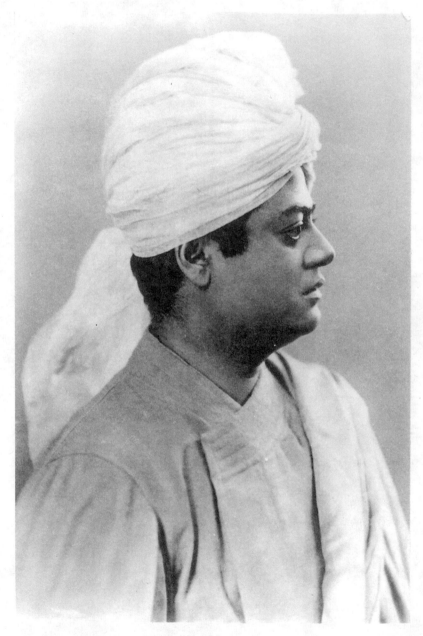

34
The symbol of Freedom, London (May, 1896)

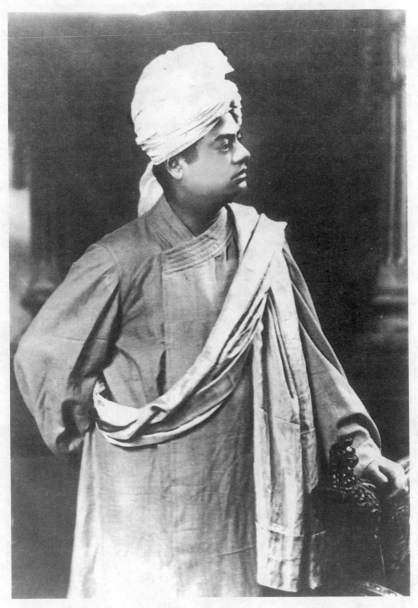

35
The Preacher of Strength, London (May, 1896)

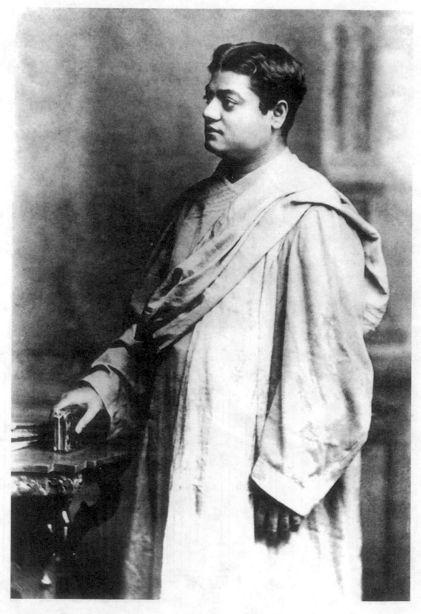

36
The Supreme Faith, London (May, 1896)

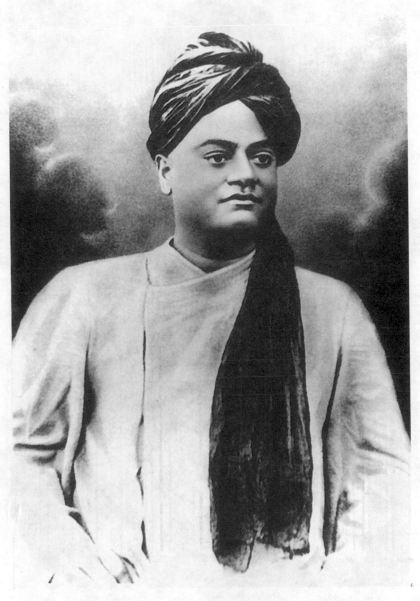

37
The Indian in London (May, 1896)

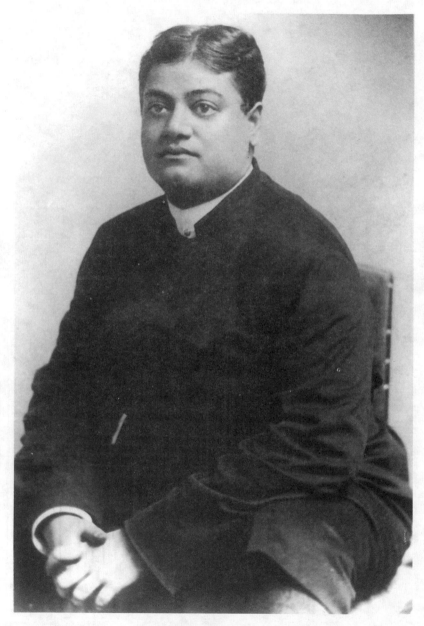

38
The exponent of *Advaita*, London (July, 1896)

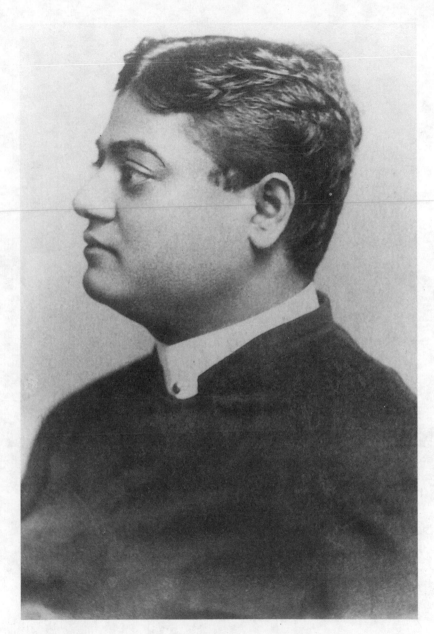

39
In London (1896)

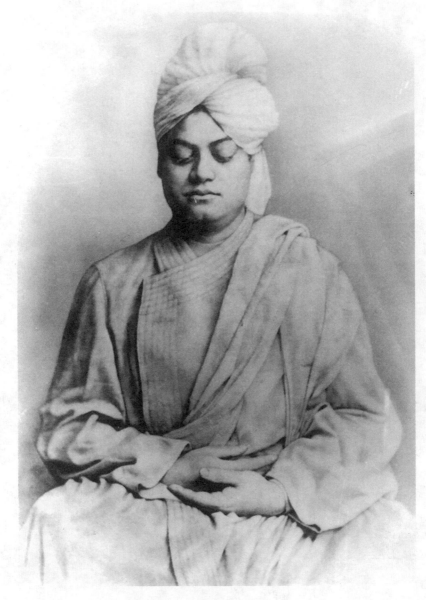

40
Meditation, London (1896)

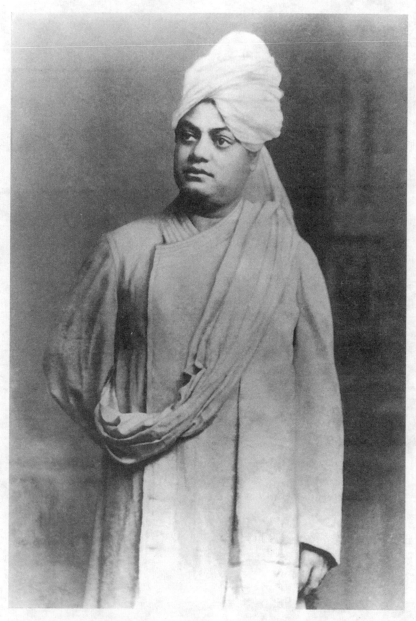

41
The call to action, London (December, 1896)

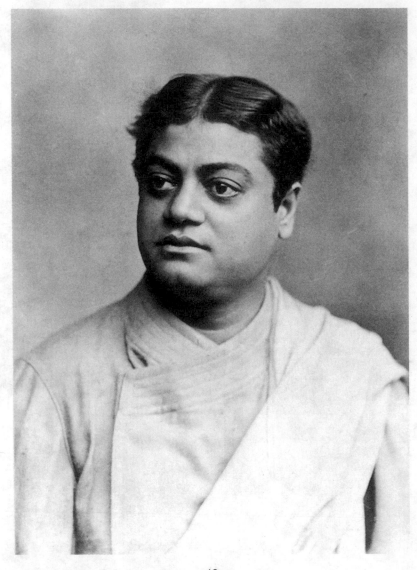

42
The Exponent of disciplined Freedom, London (1896)

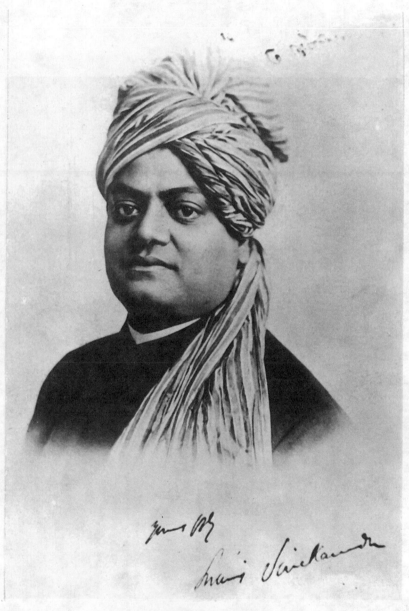

43
Adieu to London (1896)

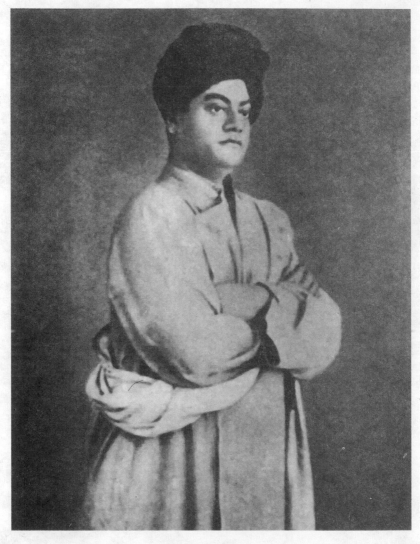

44
The Hero returns, Colombo (January, 1897)

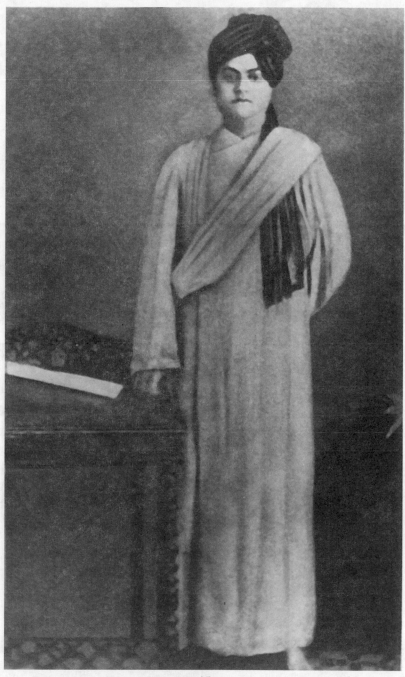

45
The First Talk to his Countrymen, Colombo (January, 1897)

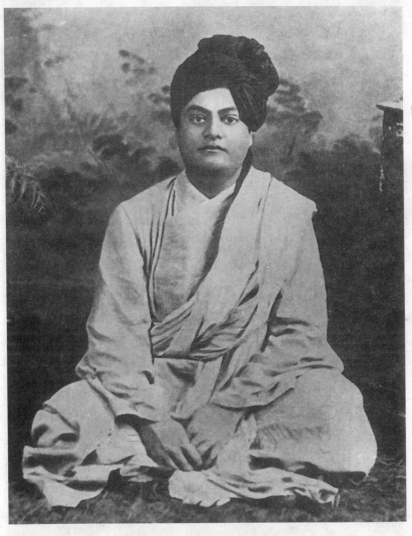

46
Discourse in Colombo (January, 1897)

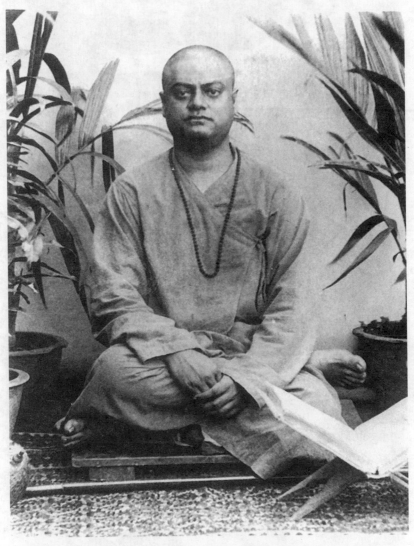

47
The Acharya, Madras (February, 1897)

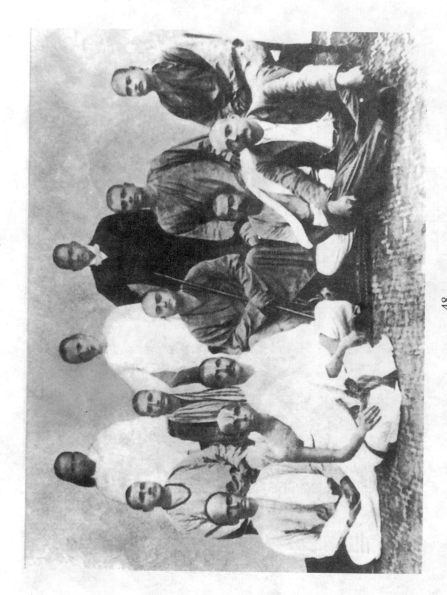

48

The Madras Circle (February, 1897)

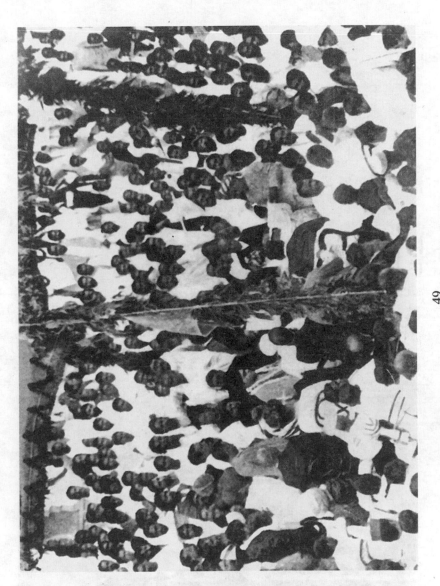
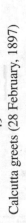

49
Calcutta greets (28 February, 1897)

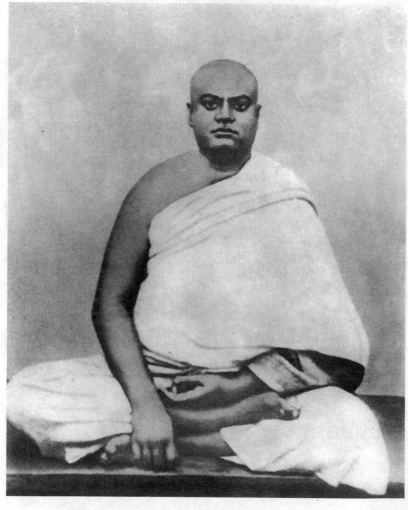

50
At home in Calcutta (February, 1897)

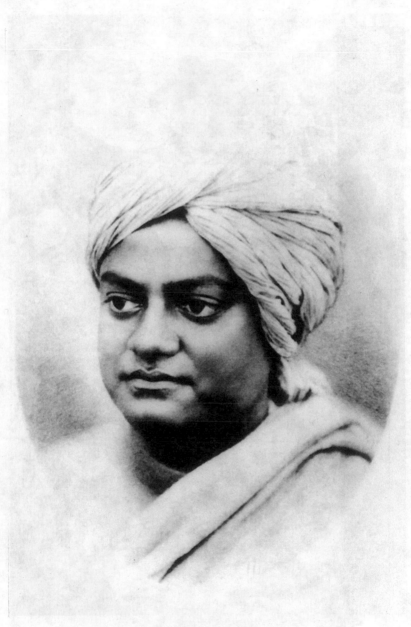

51
Planning the future, Calcutta (February, 1897)

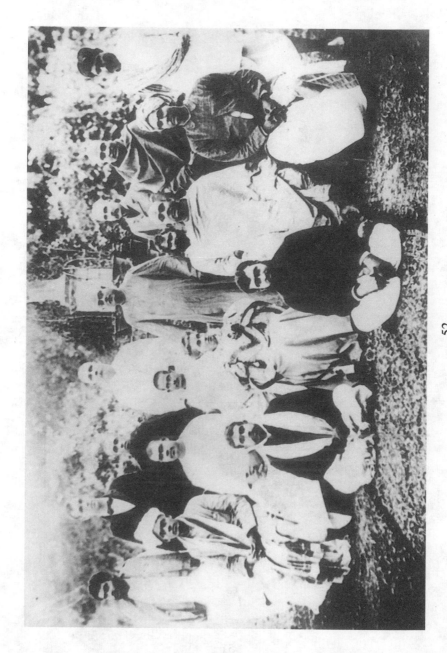

52
The Calcutta Circle

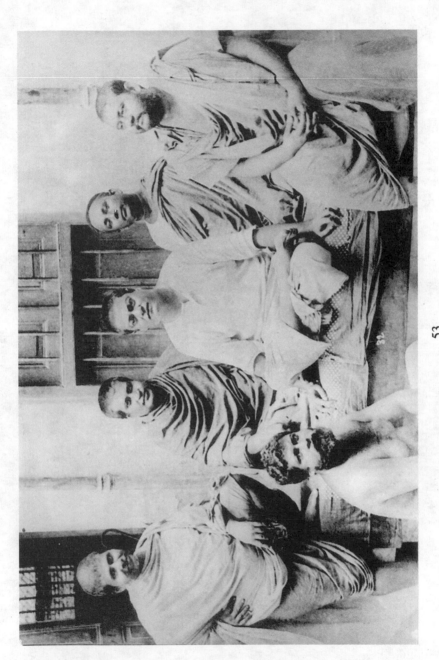

53
With *gurubhais*, Calcutta (1897)

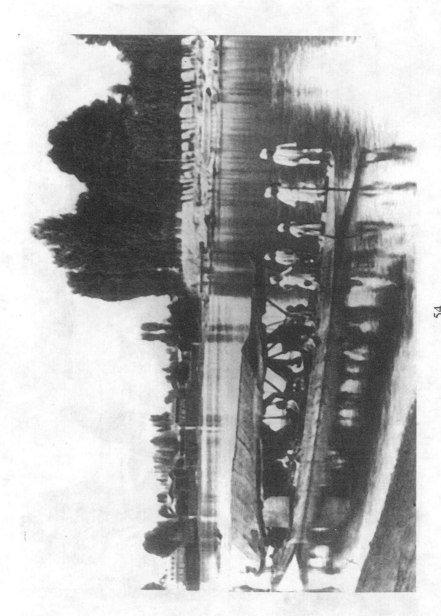

54

Afloat in Kashmir (1898)

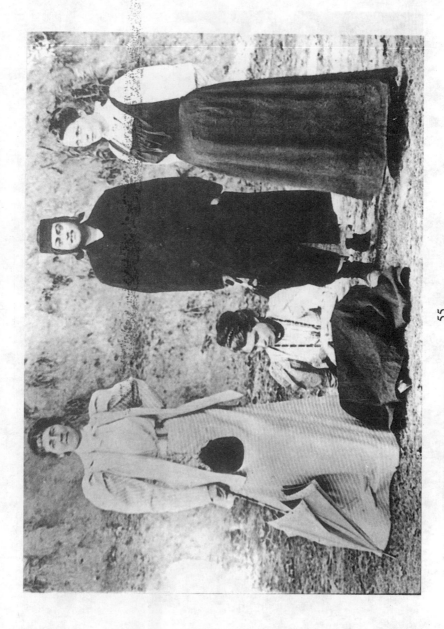

55

With Western Disciples in Kashmir

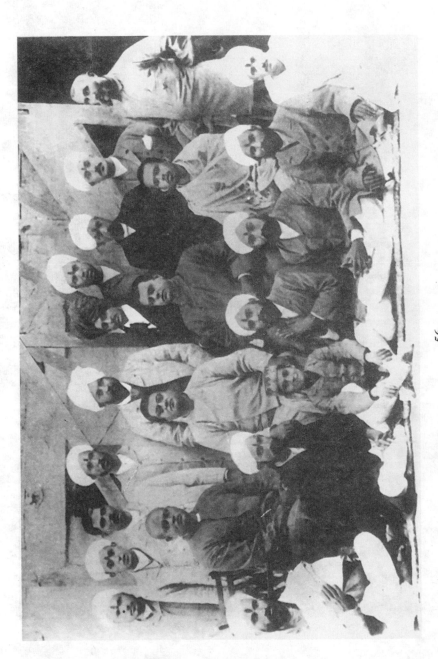

56

The Kashmir Circle

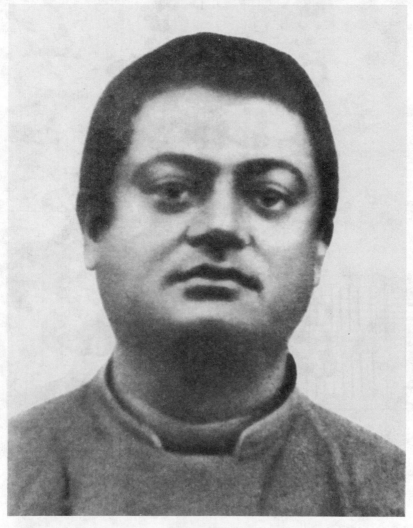

57
The calm of the sannyasin, Kashmir (July, 1898)

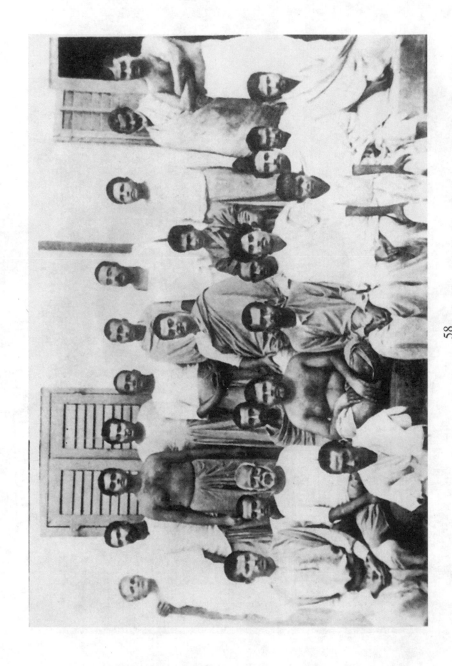

58
At Belur Math (1899)

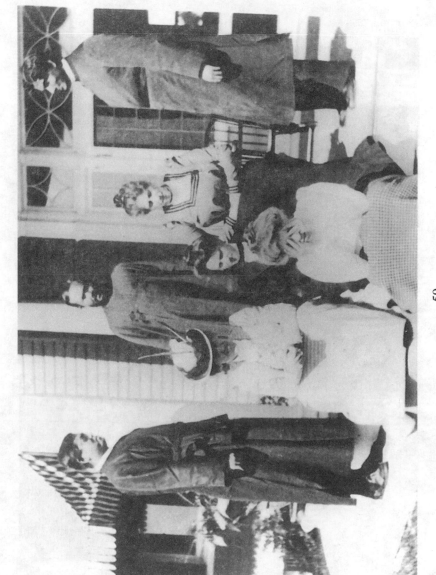

59
At Ridgely Manor (1899)

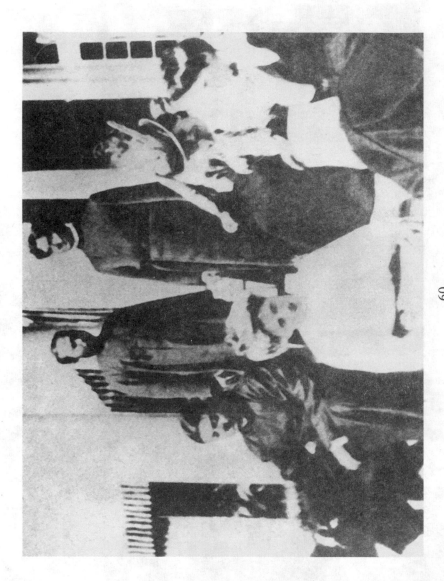

60

At Ridgely Manor (1899)

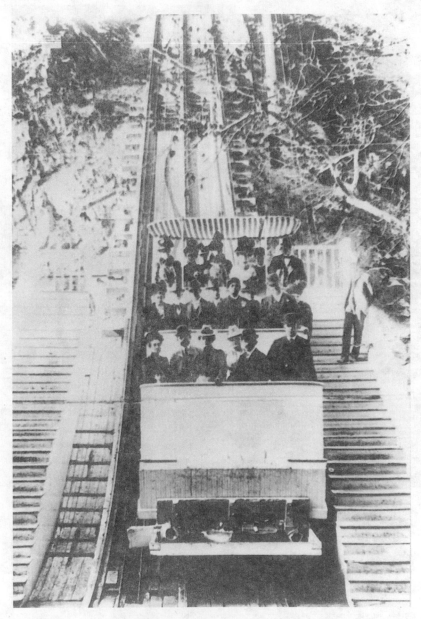

61
By cable up Mt. Lowe, Pasadena (January, 1900)

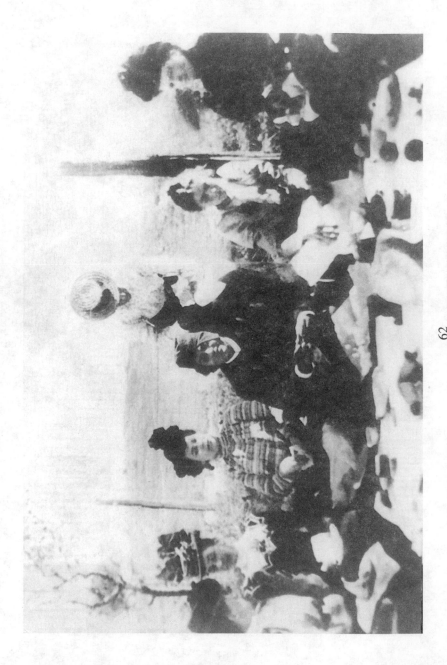

62

Picnic at Pasadena (1900)

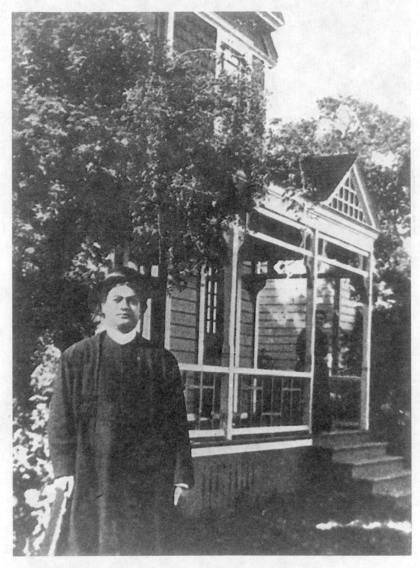

63
The Prophet at Pasadena (1900)

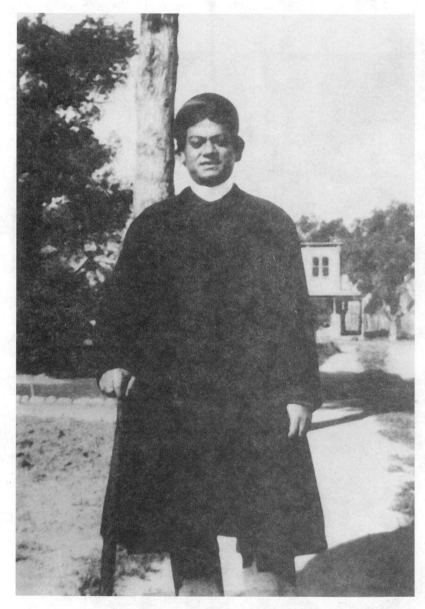

64
The Prophet at Pasadena (1900)

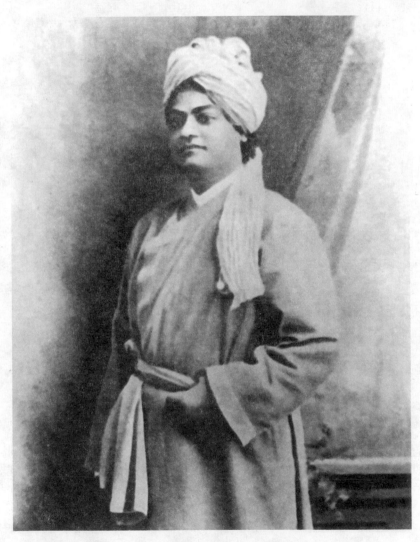

65
At San Francisco (February, 1900)

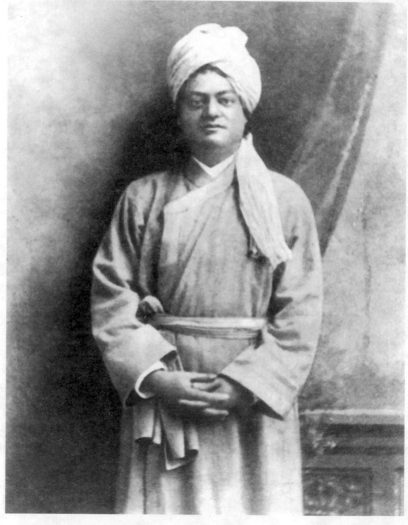

66
The Power of Renunciation, San Francisco (1900)

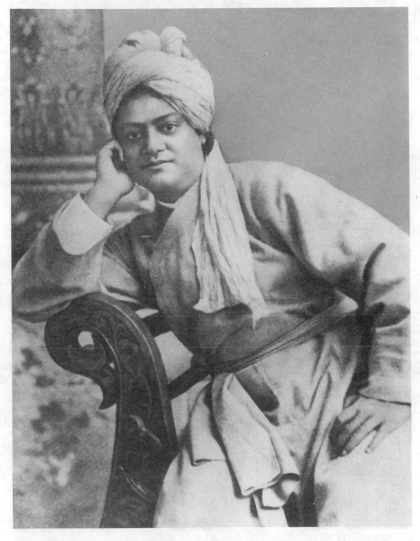

67
Pariprasna: Questions and Answers; San Francisco (1900)

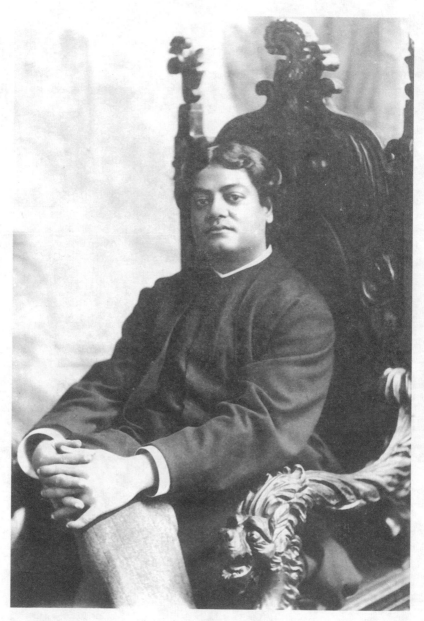

68
'Do you know?'; San Francisco (1900)

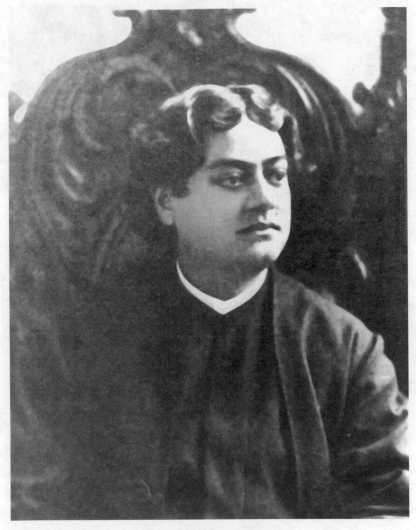

69
The heart that understands; San Francisco (1900)

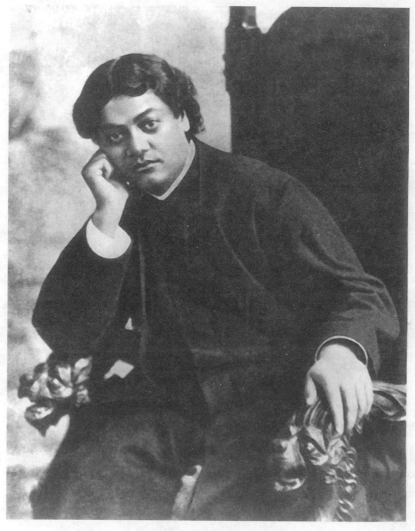

70
'What then?'; San Francisco (1900)

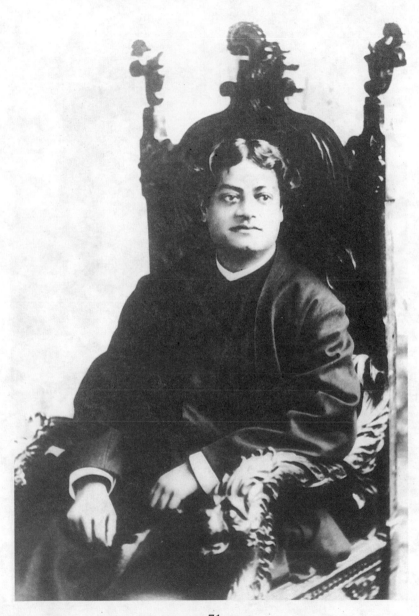

71
'To work we have the right, not to the fruits thereof';
San Francisco (1900)

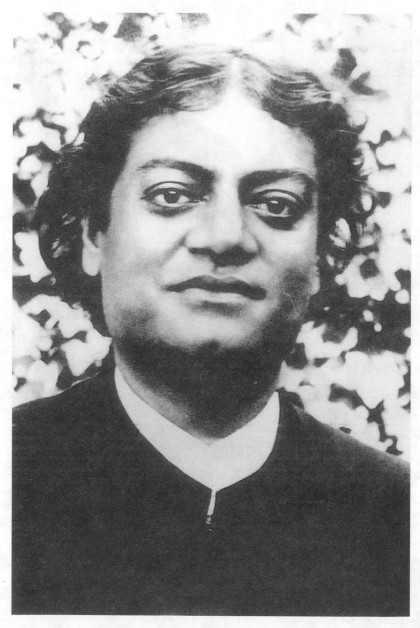

72
The Joy of Peace, Alameda (April, 1900)

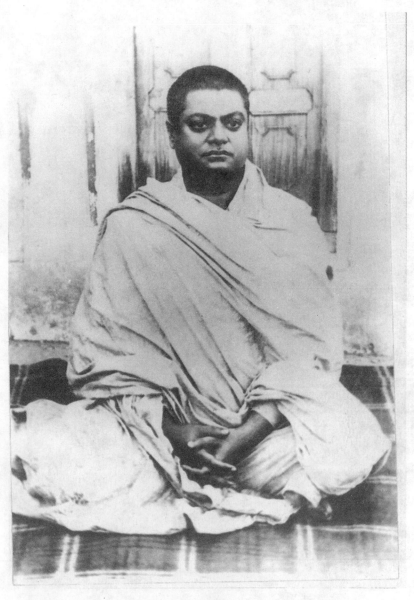

73
The Rishi, Calcutta (1901)

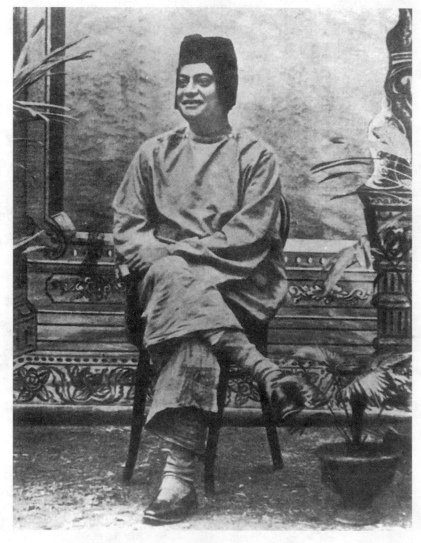

74
Retreat at Shillong (1901)

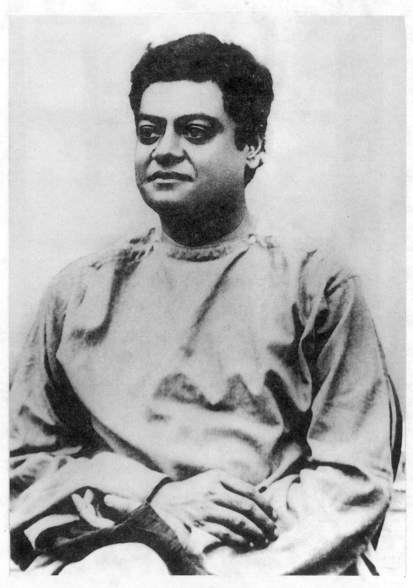

75
Relaxing at Shillong (1901)

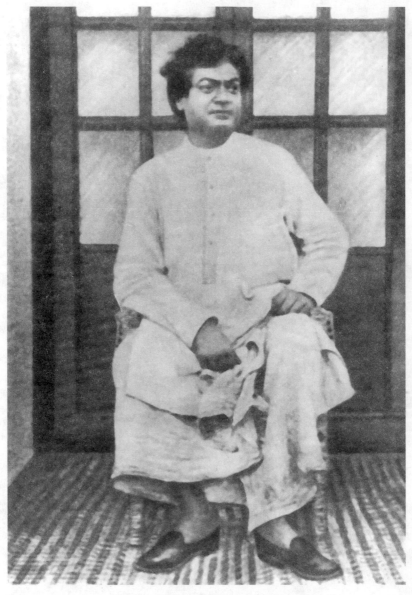

76
Not so well, Shillong (1901)

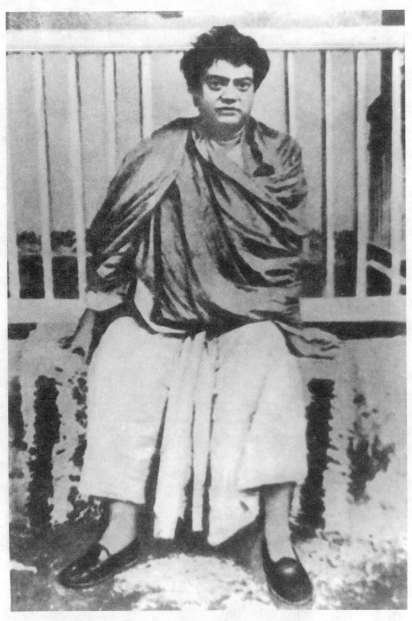

77
After an illness, Shillong (1901)

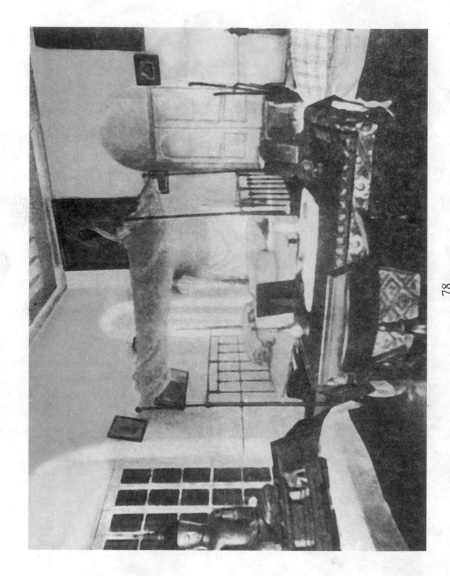

78
Mahasamadhi (4th July, 1902)

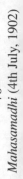

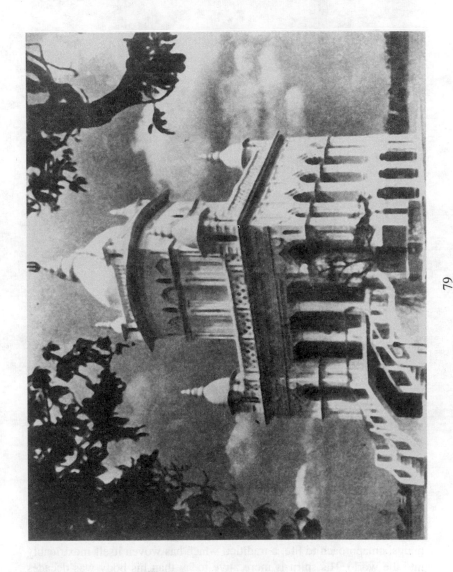

79

The Final Rest on the bank of the Ganges

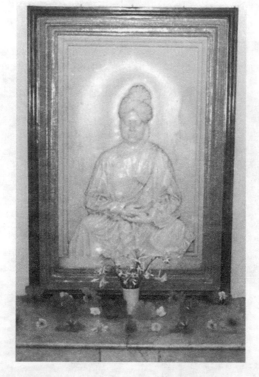

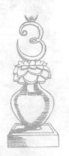

80

"I am a voice without a form".

(Vivekananda's bas-relief where his body was cremated)

Time has proved the truth of the words he uttered before his death:

> *"It may be that I shall find it good to get outside my body – to cast it off like a worn out garment. But I shall not cease to work. I shall inspire men everywhere until the world shall know that it is one with God"*

Vivekananda is today a voice without form. He has transcended the limitation of human personality. He has become concretized into an impersonal institution. He is a system of thought, an attitude of men and things, an approach to life, a tradition which has woven itself inextricably into the world. His spirit is more alive today than his body was decades ago. It permeates the re-awakening India. It revitalizes man. It infuses new life and strength. Acquaintance with him opens a new portal to life. Accepting his message and applying it in full makes one's life exalted.

VIVEKANANDA AND HIS NEW GOSPEL
– A RECAPITULATION

His multi-faceted life and work, and the invigorating message
for the spiritual regeneration of India and the world

"It is my job to fashion man. Man-making is my mission of life. You try to translate this mission of mine into action and reality.... Yes! The older I grow, the more everything seems to me to lie in manliness. This is my new gospel."

His rare personality

It is indeed seldom that such an eminent personage of light and leading as Swami Vivekananda appears amongst mankind. His was a multi-faceted personality whose emotions, words and deeds exhibited a profound harmony. Endowed with a sharp intellect, noble heart, and a powerful mind, his whole being was ever engaged in the amelioration of the suffering humanity. Immaculate purity, voluntary poverty, self-abnegation, deep devotion to his Master and disinterested love for humanity were the major characteristics of this great servant of God. He exemplified the ideal of the fourfold yogas. He was indeed the living example of Vedanta.

His source and support

Sri Ramakrishna Paramahamsa was undoubtedly the source and support of his intellectual and spiritual effulgence. It was Paramahamsa's divine touch that awakened all the latent powers in Swami Vivekananda and charged him with the mission of rediscovering for India its soul and quickening a mighty renaissance in every field of creative work. Swami Vivekananda was thus Sri Ramakrishna's gift not only to India but to the whole humanity.

His mission in the West

In fulfilment of his spiritual mission, Vivekananda attended the World's Parliament of Religions held at Chicago in 1893. He was indeed India's first spiritual ambassador to the West, where he delivered the message of Vedanta as lived and exemplified by his Great Master Sri Ramakrishna. It was the message of India's eternal wisdom, a message of harmony and goodwill, of strength and fearlessness, of unity of existence, of universal love and service. While Vivekananda delivered his message eloquently, forcefully and logically, he also carried out his mission with sincerity, statesmanship and with deep respect for other faiths. His message of Vedanta had a tonic effect on the materially affluent but spiritually impoverished life of the Occident.

His mission in India

Being successful in planting the seeds of India's spiritual wisdom in the very heart of the English speaking world – in New York and London,

Swami Vivekananda came home to be welcomed as a conquering hero by his proud and grateful countrymen. His achievements abroad created in the average Indian mind a pride in the past and a confidence in the future. It looked as though a miracle had happened and the country apperared to be waiting for his message. And the Swamiji set about his task with systematic thoroughness. He felt the pulse of India and found out what she wanted. Through his soul-stirring outpourings he roused the slumbering spirit of his countrymen and galvanized it into dyanamic activity. He sought to draw out the spiritual resources of the people. He endeavoured to enkindle the fire of manliness and vigour in them. He emphasized the greatness of the spiritual ideas enunciated in the Vedanta, the important role it was destined to play in elevating the whole of mankind. But, he said, this great mission of India would remain unfulfilled as long as India continued in her present state of abject poverty and squalor. The material greatness of India was, therefore, indissolubly bound up with the spiritual regeneration of India and mankind.

His dynamic and dedicated life in a short span

Swami Vivekananda's public life covered a period of about ten years from 1893, when he appeared at the Parliament of Religions in Chicago, to 1902, when he gave up his body. These were years of great physical and metal strain as a result of extensive travels, adaptations to new environments, opposition from detractors both in his native land and abroad, incessant public lectures and private instructions, a heavy correspondence and the organizing of the Ramakrishna Order in India. Hard work and ascetic practices undermined his health. Nevertheless he kept himself engaged in some work or the other. "When death is inevitable, let the body fall in serving a noble cause." "Let this body, since perish it must, wear out in action and not rust in inaction" – that was his firm resolve till the last. "Let this body which is here put to the use of others. The highest truth is this: There is no other God to seek. He alone serves God who serves all beings" – that was his sublime realization. "Have immense faith in yourself. That faith calls out the Divinity within" – these were his watchwords. Time and again he exhorted everyone to be strong, fearless, cheerful and charitable. He insisted on everyone living upto the teachings of Vedanta, as that was what the world needed. He regularly imparted his instruction in this regard and also set himself to mould the character of his followers, until the fourth of July, 1902, when he shed his body, as a true yogi and liberated himseldf from all bonds, by entering into the state of superconsciousness, from which he never returned, thus fulfilling the prediction of his Master, that when he would accomplish his divinely ordained mission on earth, he would get back at the time of giving up the body the treasure of spiritual realization.

He owed everthing to his Guru

Only one person was able to gauge the potential of the phenomenon known to the world as Swami Vivekananda and that person was his own

Master Sri Ramakrishna, to whom he was totally dedicated and in whose hands he became a humble instrument. His *Gurubhakti* was unique. Whatever he could achieve, in thought, word and deed, during his brief earthly sojourn, he offered it all at the holy feet of his Guru. He owed everthing to Him. In fact, Vivekananda considered himself as the most obedient servant of his Great Master. He said that he had not one word of his own to utter, not one infinitesimal thought of his own to unfold; everything, all that he was himself, all that he could be to others, all that he might be to the world came from that single source, Sri Ramakrishna. "All that I am, all that the world someday be, is owing to my Master, Ramakrishna. If there has been anything achieved by my thoughts or words, or if from my lips has ever fallen one word that has helped anyone in the world, I lay no claim to it; it was all His. All that has been weak has been mine, and all that has been life-giving, strengthening, pure and holy, has been His inspiration, His word – and He Himself. I am an instrument and He is the operator. Through this instrument He is rousing the religious instincts in thousands. 'He makes the dumb eloquent and makes the lame cross mountains'. I am amazed at His will – I am a voice without a form". "My supreme good fortune is that I am his servant through life after life.....If there has been a word of truth, a word of spirituality that I have spoken in this world, I owe it to my Master. Only the mistakes are mine."

He lives for ever!

In the words of Sister Nivedita: "The *Shastras*, the Guru and the Motherland – are the three notes that mingle themselves to form the music of the works of Vivekananda....These are the three lights burnings within that single lamp which India by his hands lighted and set up for the guidance of her own children and the world".

Swamiji said he would continue his work even after he left his body. This is his touching testament: "It may be that I shall find it good to get outside my body – to cast it off like a worn out garment. But I shall not cease to work. I shall inspire men everywhere until the world shall know that it is one with God.... And may I be born again and again and suffer thousands of miseries so that I may worship the only God that exists, the only God I believe in – the sum total of all souls. And above all, my God the wicked, my God the poor, of all races and species, shall be the special object of my worship".

II

A new gospel

"Man-making is my mission of life", declared Swami Vivekananda, "you try to translate this mission of mine into action and reality." He also said, "The older I grow the more everything seems to me to lie in manliness. This is my new gospel." And in consonance with his "new gospel" he wanted to make man his own master, to give him self-confidence and to show him how to draw forth, from within himself, by himself, the infinite power of spirit. Vivekananda therefore declared that his ideal was to rouse in all people the awareness of the ever present focus of human dignity and glory, namely the Atman, the Divine spark in all men and women, and to help them to manifest that glory in every movement of their life. He pointed out that enormous potential is within us, if only we would assiduously actualize it. When we realize the profundity of our spiritual life, our external life beomes smoother, tension-free and radiant. Vivekananda exhorted: "Awake from this hypnotism of weakness. None is really weak, the soul is infinite, ominipotent and omniscient. Stand up, assert yourself, proclaim the God within you.... Teach yourself, teach everyone his real nature, call upon the sleeping soul and see how it awakes. Power will come, glory will come, goodness will come, purity will come and everything that is excellent will come, when the sleeping soul is roused to self-conscious activity."

The greatest benefaction

The greatest of all nenefactions, according to Swami Vivekananda, is the act of rousing man to the glory of the divinity within. The awakened man solves for himself all his problems. Once the awareness of divinity inherent in man is awakened, his service to fellowmen becomes worship of God in them and that divine love can only encrown the humanity with prosperity and peace. The ideal is rather to make men serve efficiently in the already existing schools, colleges, and hospitals, than to go in for the establishment of the new ones.

Emergence of a new man

"The solution to all human problems is in man's becoming Man in all his dimensions, by manifesting his divinity. Problems are understandably many. But the solution is one – to become the new kind of man, who being simultaneously scientific, eventually becomes free. It is this new man, pure in heart, clear in mind, unselfish in motivation, who works in a blanced manner with his head, heart and hand, who has shed all his smallness and illusions, who has experienced unity of existence in his expanded consciousness – this selfless, spotless and fearless man of character, enlightenment and love, is the hope of the world. The more such men we have the greater the hope of the world. Hope is not in more machinery, wealth, politics of cleverness and power. The world is looking forward to the coming of this new man – who is aware of his own divinity and is always anxious to discover and worship the same divinity in all others – in ever increasing numbers." This, in short, is "Man-making" as envisaged by Swami Vivekananda.

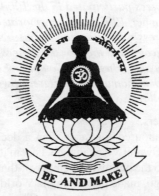

"First, let us be Gods, and then help others to be Gods.
'Be and make', let this be our motto."

Each soul is potentially Divine.
The goal is to manifest this Divinity within
by controlling nature, external and internal.
Do this either by work or worship or psychic control or philosophy
– by one or more or all of these – and be free.

Vivekananda

The monosyllable ॐ superimposed on the bosom of man symbolizes his intrinsic Divinity which is his real nature.

The prayer: "*tamaso maa jyotirgamaya*" – 'Lead me from darkness to Light' quoted in the inner orb, is indicative of man's spiritual quest – his aspiration to discover, realize and manifest the innate Divinity.

The meditative posture of man, the brilliant sun behind him, the lotus on which he is seated and the waves beneath it are symbolic of mystic communion, pursuit of knowledge, devotional absorption and selfless work, respectively.

The design thus depicts the gospel of Swami Vivekananda, according to which man can discover, realize and manifest the Divinity enshrined in him, by cultivating an integrated life, with due emphasis on pursuit of knolwdge, devotional absorption, mystic communion and selfless service.

"Be and Make" – is an epigram of Swamiji exhorting man to unfold his intrinsic divinity through the cultivation of an integrated life and also to help others march towards that end.

A HOMAGE TO SWAMI VIVEKANANDA
(on the 11th September, 1993, at the Art Institute of Chicago, U. S. A.)

About a thousand devotees participated in the 100th anniversary celebration (on the 11th September, 1993) to commemorate Swami Vivekananda's famous 'Chicago Address'. The function, sponsored by the Vivekananda Vedanta Society of Chicago and the Consul General of India, was held at the Art Institute of Chicago, where the Compiler-Editor of this book had an opportunity to render homage to the great Swami on that day. As a prelude he spoke as follows:

Dear Sisters and Brothers,

As one who has laboured for more than a decade, in preparing and bringing out a book on Swami Vivekananda, I deem it a rare privilege to pay a reverential homage to the hallowed memory of that great Hindu Monk of India who, a century ago, made history in the World's Parliament of Religions held in this very place, on this very day. The homage is in the form of a Sanskrit composition depicting Vivekananda – the Man and His Mission.

[*Before singing the Sanskrit poem, the English version of the same was read out to the audience. It is given herebelow along with the corresponding stanzas in transliteration*]:

> *vishwahitaishi mahaamanishi janaseva-taapasi*
> *jayatu Vivekananda Swami, jayatu veera sannyasi //*

Victory be unto Swami Vivekananda, the intrepid Hindu Monk of India, who was endowed with a poised mind and a scintillating intellect, who was keenly interested in the welfare of the entire mankind, and to whom the service of man was verily the *tapas* (spiritual practice) for God-realization.

> *nipeeya sakalam tattwajnaanam*
> *paanchabhautikam nava vijnaanam*
> *jagaditihaasa puraana darshanam*
> *parameshwara darshane manaswi*
> *yo nitaraam abhilaashi, jayatu veera sannyasi //*

Victory be unto that intrepid Hindu Monk of India, who was well-versed in all branches of philosophy including the metaphysics, and well-acquainted with the modern material science, World History, *Puranas* and *Darshanas*, and ever intensely aspired for God-realization.

> *sakaladharma patha parama saadhakam*
> *vividha dharma mata marma bodhakam*
> *bhogavaada naastikya rodhakam*
> *jagadgurum tam vilokya sahasaa*
> *jaato dradhataapasi, jayatu veera sannyasi //*

Victory be unto that intrepid Hindu Monk of India, who was instantly transformed and established in spiritual practice on account of his mere glance at
the World Teacher, Sri Ramakrishna, the practitioner supreme of all religious
paths, who preached the inner core of all religions, and who is a bulwark
against atheism and hedonism.

> *graame graame nagare nagare*
> *nadi nadaanaam teere teere*
> *guha gahware vipine ghore*
> *vilokya jana jivanam vipannam*
> *yo vivhala maanasi, jayatu veera sannyasi //*

Victory be unto that intrepid Hindu Montk of India who, as an itinerant
monk, travelled all over India – visiting villages, towns and cities, river
banks, caves and dense forests, and witnessing the deplorable living
conditions of the poor and the downtrodden, the distressed and the diseased
masses, was greatly pained at heart and felt intensely compassionate for
them, and was spurred on to find ways and means to mitigate their sufferings.

> *vishwadharma sammelana pithe*
> *vividha dharma guru garva garishte*
> *naanaa dharma dhwaja pratishte*
> *navayuga maanavadharma ghoshanaa*
> *jagarjayo saahasi, jayatu veera sannyasi //*

Victory be unto that intrepid Hindu Monk of India, who proclaimed with a
leonine roar, as it were, the *dharma* for the mankind of the New Age, from the
platform of the World's Parliament of Religions at Chicago, whereon had
assembled the religious leaders of all faiths of the world, with all their pride
and privilege, and with all their banners unfurled, to proudly proclaim and
establish the supremacy of their own creeds.

> *Mahaveera iva parama viraagi*
> *Krista-Buddhavat karuno tyaagi*
> *Shankara iva digvijayi yogi*
> *udaara charito vishwa kutumbi*
> *janagana hrdaya nivasi, jayatu veera sannyasi //*

Victory be unto that intrepid Hindu Monk of India, who is supremely
dispassionate like Mahavira, kind, compassionate and renunciate like the
Christ and the Buddha, a yogi par excellence like Adi Shankara who held
sway over his opponents in all the four quarters, who was extremely generous
and endowed with a noble character, to whom the whole world was one big
family, and who is ever residing in the hearts of hosts of people.

GLOSSARY *

abhaya – Fearlessness; an epithet of the Supreme Being (Brahman).

abheda – Non-difference.

abhih – Fearless.

abhyasa – Constant practice.

acharya(s) – Spiritual teacher.

adhar – Support.

Adi Brahmo Samaj – The first Brahmo Samaj. This is how the theistic organization founded by Raja Rammohan Roy (1774-1833) came to be known, after its renowned adherent, Keshab Chandra Sen (1838-1884), ceceded therefrom and formed a new organization called "The Brahmo Samaj of India", in 1866.

Advaita – Non-duality; a school of the Vedanta philosophy, declaring the oneness of God, soul, and universe.

Advaita sadhana – Sadhana according to Advaita.

Advaita siddhi – Siddhi attained through Advaita sadhana.

Advaita Vedanta – Non-dualistic system of Vedanta expounded by Sri Sankaracharya (A. D. 788-820).

Advaitic – Pertaining to Advaita.

Advaitin(s) – An adherent of Advaita.

Advaitism – An anglicized derivation from Advaita denoting the Advaita system of philosophy.

Advaitist(s) – Same as Advaitin(s).

ahamkara – Ego or "I-consciousness".

ahimsa – Non-injury in thought, word and deed, which is one of the five-fold preliminary disciplines, a sine qua non, for the practice of rajayoga.

akasha – Ether or space; the first of the five elements evolved from Brahman – the Supreme Reality. It is the subtlest form of matter, into which all the elements are ultimately resolved. The four other elements are *vayu* (air), *agni* (fire), *ap* (water) and *prthvi* (earth).

akhil Bharatiya – All-India.

Alwars – The twelve Vaishnavaite saints of Tamil Nadu who, in the medieval period, propagated Vaishnavism through Tamil devotional poems compiled under the title "*Naalaayira Divya Prabandham*".

Amarnath – (Lit., the Lord of Immorality) A holy place of pilgrimage in Kashmir, renowned for its icy-cave-temple dedicated to Lord Shiva.

amrtasya putrah – "Children of Immorality", as proclaimed by the Upanishadic rishis.

Ananda – Bliss.

Anandmath – The best-known novel of Bankim Chandra Chatterjee (1838-1894), Bengali novelist, containing the famous hymn '*Vande Mataram*'.

Antaryamin – The Inner Controller.

anubhava – Experience.

apara vidya – Secular knowledge.

Arjuna – A hero of the *Mahabharata* and the friend and disciple of Sri Krishna.

---

* 's' in bracket (s) at the end of certain Sanskrit words in the Glossary indicates the anglicized plural form of those words, but the meaning given is for the singular only.

Arsha Dharma – Dharma founded by the rishis of yore; Sanatana Dharma.

artha – Wealth, one of the four ends of human pursuits.

Arya(s) – (Lit., noble) In ancient times, an inhabitant of Aryavarta or Vedic India; in later times, a member of any of the first three castes of the Hindu society.

Arya Dharma – Dharma of the Aryas; Sanatana Dharma.

Arya Samaj – A powerful religious and social reformist movement (which played an important role in the awakening of Indian national consciousness), founded by Swami Dayananda Saraswati (1824-1883), a great scholar of the Vedas.

Aryan(s) – Same as Arya(s).

Aryan rishis – Rishis of the Vedic period.

Aryavarta – Vedic India – the land of Aryans.

asana – Seat; also a posture adopted by the yogi in the practice of yoga.

ashraddha – The spirit of levity; lack of respect.

Ashram(s) – A place of religious retreat, a hermitage.

Ashrama – Any of the four stages of life: the celibate student stage (brahmacharya), the married householder stage (grhastha), the stage of retirement and contemplation (vanaprastha), and the stage of religious mendicancy (sannyasa).

Ashvaghosha – The author of *Buddha Charita*.

asura – Demon.

asuric – Demonic.

Atharva Veda – One of the four Vedas, the most sacred and revered scriptures of the Hindus.

Atman – Self or soul; denotes also the Supreme Soul, which, according to Advaita Vedanta, is one with the individual soul.

Atmano mokshartham jagaddhitaya cha – For one's own liberation and welfare of the world.

Atmavai putranamasi – The son is only oneself by another name.

Atma-vidya – Science of the divine Self within.

Atma-vichara – Self-enquiry, 'Who am I ', as taught by Sri Ramana Maharshi (1879-1950), the sage of Arunachala at Tiruvannamalai.

Aurobindo – The celebrated yogi of Pondichery and one of the most dominant figures in the history of the Indian renaissance and Indian nationalism (1872-1950).

avatar(a) – Incarnation of God.

avidya – Ignorance.

Ayodhya – The capital of Sri Rama's kingdom in northern India; modern Oudh.

bahujana hitaya – For the commonweal of the society at large.

bahujana sukhaya – For the happiness of the society at large.

beti – (Lit., daughter) – a term of endearment applied to mother or to a young woman; also an epithet for goddess Shakti, the Divine Mother.

Bhavad Gita – An important and well-known scripture comprising eighteen chapters, embodying the teachings of Sri Krishna, and contained in the *Mahabharata*.

Bhagavan – (Lit., One endowed with six attributes, viz. infinite treasure, strength, glory, splendour, knowledge, renunciation) An epithet of godhead; also the personal God of the devotees.

Bhagavata – The well-known Hindu devotional scripture dealing mainly with the life and divine sports of Sri Krishna.

Bhagavata Dharma – Dharma according to the *Bhagavata*; the path of divine love; the virtuous actions performed in the spirit of divine worship.

Bhagavata saints – Saints following the Bhagavatadharma.

bhairavi – A nun of the Tantrick sect.

Bhairavi Brahmani – (Brahmani, lit., brahmin woman) The brahmin woman who taught Sri Ramakrishna (1836-1886) the Vaishnava and Tantra disciplines.

bhakta(s) – Devotee of God.

bhakti – Love of God; single-minded devotion to one's Chosen Ideal; divine love.

bhaktimarga – Path of devotion.

Bhakti Yoga – A book by Swami Vivekananda teaching man how to train emotions in order to attain his spiritual end. The aspirant is asked to practise pure love of God, through which he attains the highest knowledge and realizes the oneness of the lover, love and the beloved.

bhaktiyoga – The science of devotion followed by dualistic worshippers to realize God.

bhaktiyogi(s) – The adherent of bhaktiyoga.

Bharata – India, so named in honour of Bharata (the son of Rishbha), the celebrated hero and monarch of ancient India from whom a long line of kings decended.

Bharata Mata – Mother India.

Bharata Parikrama – A wayfarer's spiritual excursions across the length and breath of India. Since times immemorial the notion of a pilgrimage across the country constituted an essential ingredient of the education of the spiritual men of India. In 1888 Swami Vivekananda undertook such a journey to interact with men of religion elsewhere within India and gain an understanding of the social and spiritual climate of the country as a whole. The journey lasted for more than four years till he left for the U. S. A. in 1893, to participate in the Chicago Parliament of Religions.

Bharatavarsha – India, so called from Pauranic times.

Bharata-yatra – All-India tour.

Bharatiya samaj – Indian society.

bhiksha – alms.

Bhoodan – Land gift to the landless poor.

Bipin Chandra Pal – A celebrated Indian publisher, prominent freedom fighter and revolutionary Hindu leader of Bengal who was among the renowned trinity of Indian freedom struggle: Bal-Pal-Lal, the other two being Lala Lajpath Rai (1865-1928) and Bal Gangadhar Tilak (1856-1920).

Brahma – The Creator God; the First Person of the Hindu Trinity, the other two being Vishnu and Shiva.

brahmachari(s) – A religious student devoted to the practice of spiritual discipline; a celibate belonging to the first stage of life.

brahmacharin(s) – Same as brahmachari(s).

brahmacharini – An unmarried woman leading the life of brahmacharya.

brahmacharya – The first of the four stages of life: the life of an unmarried student; celibacy; continence.

Brahmajnani – A knower of Brahman.

Brahman – The Absolute; the Superme Reality of the Vedanta philosophy.

brahmana – Same as brahmin.

Brahma Sutras – An authoritative treatise on Vedanta philosophy ascribed to Vyasa.

Brahma-teja – Spiritual glory.

Brahmavarta – India, so called in ancient texts.

brahmin – The first of the four castes of the Hindu society; same as brahmana; refers also to a holyman.

Brahmo – Member of the Brahmo Samaj.

Brahmo Samaj – A theistic organization of India founded by Raja Rammohan Roy (1774-1833), the great Indian social and religious reformer, who believed in a formless God and deprecated the worship of idols.

Brahaspati – Preceptor of gods.

Buddha – (Lit., one who is enlightened) The founder of Buddhism who is considered by the Hindus to be an incarnation of God.

busti(s) – A slum; colony of labourers.

Chaitanya – Spiritual Consciousness; also the name of a prophet born in A. D. 1485, who lived at Navadvip, Bengal, and emphasized the path of divine love for the realization of God; he is also known as Gauranga.

chakra – Wheel; an emblem (Ashoka Chakra) adorning Indian national flag .

chandala(s) – an untouchable.

charya – Conduct; the process.

chela – disciple.

chinmudra – One of the yogic symbols in which the thumb and forefinger are brought together to represent Om.

Chit – Consciousness.

chitta – The mind-stuff.

chitta-vritti – Modifications of the mind-stuff.

Dakshin – South.

daridra devo bhava – Let the poor be your God.

Daridranarayana – God in the form of the poor and the needy.

Dasbodh – A didactic treatise in Marathi verses by Samarth Ramdas (1608-1682), the guru of Shivaji (1630-1680). A valuable treatise for spiritual aspirants, comprising twenty chapters, it poetically delineates the fundamentals of the Vedanta philosophy.

Dayananda Saraswati – The founder of Arya Samaj (1824-1883), and a great scholar of the Vedas.

deva(s) – (Lit., shining one) A god.

Deva Samaj – Society of the holy.

Devendranath Tagore – A religious leader of Sri Ramakrishna's time; father of Rabindranath Tagore.

devi(s) – Goddess.

dharma – Righteousness, duty; the law of being; the inner constitution of a thing which governs its growth; one of the four ends of human pursuits; generally translated as "religion", it signifies rather the inner principle of religion.

dharmabhoomi – Land of righteousness.

dharmachakra pravartana – The wheel of dharma in motion.

dharmik(a) – Religious, righteous, pious.

dhyana – Concentration; meditation; a constant, uninterrupted flow of mind towards a particular object or an idea symbolizing the Divine, to the exclusion of all other ideas and thoughts.

drshta – Seer.

durbar – A formal Stately Assembly.

Dvaita – The philosophy of Dualism propounded by Sri Madhvacharya.

ekam sat viprah bahudha vadanti – "Truth is one, but the learned call it in many ways", a well-known declaration in *Rig Veda*.

fakir – Beggar.

Gandhi, M. K. – Apostle of non-violence and Indian national leader (1869-1948), whose distinguished leadership won for India liberation from British domination.

Gargi – A woman seer mentioned in the Upanishads.

gerua – (Lit., ochre) The ochre cloth of a monk.

Gita – Same as *Bhagavad Gita.*

Gitacharya – (Lit., the teacher of the *Gita*) Sri Krishna.

Gokhale – The Indian nationalist leader, humanitarian and social reformer (1866-1915), and the founder of the 'Servants of India Society'.

grhastha – Householder.

Guhaka – An untouchable who was a friend of Sri Rama.

gurubhai(s) – Brother disciple of the same guru or spiritual teacher.

gurubhakti – Devotion to guru.

guru(deva) – Spiritual preceptor.

Guru Gobind Singh – The tenth Guru of the Sikhs who founded the Sikh Khalsa, a militant army wing of Sikhs constituted for the protection of Hindu Dharma from the onslaughts of Muhammadan rulers of Mughal period.

gurugrhavasa – Residing at the house of the preceptor during the prosecution of one's studies, as in the olden days in India.

gurukula(s) – Residential educational institution.

gurukulavasa – Residing at the gurukula.

Harijana – "The Men of God"

hathayoga – A school of yoga that aims chiefly at physical health and well-being as a preparation for the higher yogic practices.

Hinayana – A name given by the followers of Mahayana Buddhism to the more orthodox of early Buddhism, which survived in Sri Lanka as Thervada school.

Hindu Dharma – Hindu Religion, known from times immemorial as Sanatana Dharma.

Hindu shatras – Sacred scriptures of the Hindus.

Hindutva – Hinduness, Hindu identity; the organic links between Hindus in all parts of India.

hookah – An oriental tobacco pipe with a long flexible tube which draws the smoke through water in a bowl.

Ishta(m) – Same as Ishta(devata).
Ishta(devata) – The Chosen Ideal, Spiritual Ideal or Deity of the devotee.
Ishvara – The personal God.
Ishvarakoti(s) – A perfected soul born with a special spiritual message for humanity.
iti iti – (Lit., "this, this") The path of bhakti or the path positive.

jagadguru – The World Teacher.
jagriti – Awakening.
Janardhana – A name of Sri Krishna.
Janata – People; masses.
japa(m) – Constant repetition of a mantra which is a sacred formula, into which a disciple is traditionally initiated by a guru.
jai Ram – Victory to Ram.
jati – Caste.
jayakars – Expression of greetings and praises.
jihad(s) – A traditional war enjoined on and undertaken by Muhammadans against other religionists. It is in fact a Muhammadan struggle to firmly establish Muhammadanism on every bit of earth's surface, to the exclusion of all other religions, particularly Hindu religion which is referred to as religion of the Idolators, Pagans or Kafirs. Terrorism is an important component of this jihad. Every follower of Muhammadanism has to join the "Muhammadan jihad" at every stage of his life.
jiva – The embodied soul; a living being, an ordinary man; the individual soul which in essence is one with the Universal Soul.
jnana – Knowledge of Reality arrived at through reasoning and discrimination; also the process of reasoning by which the Ultimate Truth is attained. The word is generally used to denote the knowledge by which one is aware of one's identity with Brahman.
Jnanadeva – A renowned saint of Maharashtra during the Bhakti Movement and the renaissance period in India; a contempory of saint Tukaram.
jnanamarga – The path of knowledge.
jnanayoga – The science of knowledge, consisting of discrimination, renunciation and other disciplines, to realize God.
Jnana Yoga – A book by Swami Vivekananda based upon the teachings of the Upanishads, showing the way to realize the oneness of the individual soul and the Supreme Soul, through the discipline of discrimination between the real and the unreal. The contents of this book, originally delivered as lectures in America and England, deal with Swami's direct experience of Truth.
jnanayogi – The follower of jnanayoga.
Jnaneshvar – The well-known saint of Maharashtra, and the author of *Jnaneshvari*, a popular commentary in Marathi on the *Bhagavad Gita*.
jnani(n) – One who follows the path of knowledge; generally used to denote a non-dualist.

Jyeshtha – Seventh day of the dark half of the lunar month; one of the stars according to the Hindu calender; also means the elder brother or sister.

kabadi – A popular south Indian game.

Kabir – A medieval religious reformer, saint, and composer of devotional songs.

Kali – A name of the Divine Mother; the Primal Energy.

Kaliyuga – The worst of the four yugas or cycles. In the Kaliyuga there is a minimum of virtue and a great excess of vice. The world is said to be now passing through the Kaliyuga.

kalpa(s) – The period between the creation and the end of the world; a cycle; one aeon.

kama – Fulfilment of desire, one of the four ends of human pursuit.

Kamadeva – God of love; cupid.

kama-kanchana – 'Lust and gold', a term used to refer to an insatiable craving in man for the enjoyment of sense pleasures and a longing for material possessions.

Kamsa – Sri Krishna's uncle, the personification of evil, whom Sri Krishna ultimately killed.

karma – Action in general; duty; ritualistic worship.

karmabhoomi – Land of service.

karmayoga – (Lit., union with God through action) The path by which the aspirant seeks to realize God through work without attachment; also the ritualistic worship prescribed in the scriptures for realizing God.

Karma Yoga – The outstanding book among the works of Swami Vivekananda, showing the way to perfection for the active man of the world, who may be sceptical about the God of the theologians or the various untested dogmas of religion.

karmayogi(n) – The follower of karmayoga.

Kartabhaja – A minor Vaishnava sect which teaches that men and women should live together in relationship of love and gradually idealize their love by looking upon each other as the Divine.

Kerala Pratibha – The glory of Kerala.

kichuri – Rice and vegetables cooked together.

kirtan – Devotional music, often accompanied by dancing.

Krishna – An Incarnation of God as described in *Bhagavata*.

kshatra-virya – Manliness of a warrior.

kshatriya – The second or warrior caste in Hindu society.

Kshir-Bhavani – A sacred place of pilgrimage in Kashmir, renowned for the temple dedicated to the Divine Mother Bhavani who is offered *kheer* (thickened milk).

Kundalini – (Lit., the Serpent Power) – It is the spiritual energy lying dormant in all individuals. This 'Serpent Power' lies coiled at the base of the spine.

Kundaliniyoga – Yoga seeking to arouse the 'Serpent Power' latent at the sacral plexus which, when awakened, passes through the six dynamic centres in the human body and culminates in the topmost centre at the cereburm. This is the highest goal, and here the awakened spiritual energy manifests itself in its full glory and splendour.

loka-uddharak(a) – World-redeemer.
luchi(s) – A thin bread made of flour and fried in butter.

Mahabharata – A celebrated Hindu epic.
Maharaja – Emperor
maharshi – A great rishi or seer of truth.
mahasamadhi – The highest state of God-realization; the word also signifies the death of an illumined person.
mahat – The cosmic mind; a term used in the Sankhya philosophy, denoting the second category in the evolution of the universe.
mahatma – A high-souled person; a holy man; a sage.
Mahatmaji – A title by which M. K. Gandhi was popularly known.
Mahavirabhava – Intense absorption in and total identification with Hanuman, Sri Rama's devotee.
Mahayana – One of the two major traditions of Buddhism, practised especially in China, Tibet, Japan and Korea.
mahayogi – A great yogi.
Maitreyi – Wife of rishi Yajnavalkya who aspired to attain the Highest in life, which is Self-realization (or God-realization).
Makarasankranti – An auspicious time when the sun starts moving northward.
mali – Gardner; sweeper.
mamata – (Lit., mineness) Attachment, desire, longing.
manava – Man
mantra(m) – Holy Sanskrit text; also the sacred formula used in japam.
mantra(s) – Plural of mantra(m).
Manu – The great Hindu lawgiver.
margadarshak(a) – Pathfinder; one who shows the way.
Martanda Varma – The first Prince of Travancore State.
mata – Religion; also means opinion.
math(s) – Monastery.
maya – A term of Vedanta philosophy denoting ignorance obscuring the vision of Reality; the Cosmic Illusion on account of which One appears many, the Absolute as the Relative.
mayavadi(n) – A follower of the maya theory of the Vedanta philosophy, according to which the world of names and forms is illusory, like a dream.
mlechcha – A non-Hindu, a barbarian. This is a term of reproach applied by the orthodox Hindus to foreigners, who do not conform to the established usages of Hindu religion and society. The word corresponds to the "heathen" of the Christians and the "kafir" of the Muhammadans.
moksha – Liberation from the thraldom of wordly existence and release from the cycle of rebirth, culminating in the attainment of Eternal Happiness, which is the supreme goal of life and the end and aim of all spiritual practices.
mukta – The liberated one.
mukti – Same as moksha.
murkha devo bhava – Let the ignorant be your gods.
mutt(s) –Same as math(s).

Nagarjuna – A Buddhist monk and scholar who was in the Buddhist university at Kanchipuram and later carried Buddhism to Tibet and China.

Narada – A great sage, a propounder of the path of devotion, as delineated in his important work entitled, *"Narada Bhakti Sutras"*.

Narayana – A name of Vishnu; also refers to God.

Narayana Guru – The harbinger of peaceful revolution in the conditions of the depressed people in Kerala (1856-1928).

Nayanmars – Sixty-three Shaivaite saints who flourished during the Bhakti Movement period in Tamil Nadu and whose Tamil poetic works are incorporated in *"Panniru Thirumurai"* and *"Periya Puranam"*.

Nava Vidhan – 'New Dispensation' – a new creed proclaimed in 1881 by Keshab Chandra Sen (1838-1884), the celebrated Brahmo leader. It signified the harmony of religions, a presentation of the teachings of Sri Ramakrishna (1836-1886) as far as Keshab was able to understand them.

Neo-Vedanta – Also called 'Practical Vedanta' as propounded by Swami Vivekananda, it seeks to make the sublime but abstruse philosophy of the traditional Vedanta concrete and living in everyday life.

neti neti – (Lit., "not this, not this") Path of jnana or the path negative.

Nirvana – Final absorption in Brahman, or the all-pervading Reality, by the annihilation of the individual ego; a transcendent state without desires or sufferings, but with perfect and abiding Happiness.

nirvakalpa samadhi – The highest state of samadhi in which the aspirant realizes his total oneness with Brahman.

nishada – hunter.

nityasiddha – Eternally perfect and endowed with great spiritual power.

Nivedita – The 'Dedicated One', as Swami Vivekananda named his disciple, Margaret Elizabeth Noble (1867-1911), an irish teacher, who came to India and dedicated her life for the cause of Hinduism and India.

nivrtti – Renunciation.

nivrtti-marga – The path of detachment or renunciation (of desires).

Om – The most sacred word of the Vedas; also written as Aum. It is the symbol of God and of Brahman.

Om Tat Sat – Om (that) is the Truth.

ota-prota – Through and through.

padre(s) – Clergyman, Christian missionary.

pahilwan – Wrestler.

pandal – A temporary thatched roof.

Panini Grammar – A well-known Sanskrit grammar composed by Panini.

paramahamsa – One belonging to the highest order of sannyasins.

Paramahamsa – A name for Sri Ramakrishna (1836-1886).

paramartha – Goal Supreme.

parartha – For others' sake.

para vidya – Supreme knowledge; knowledge of the Self; spiritual knowledge.

pariah(s) – Untouchable. This term and the social restrictions accompanying it were declared illegal in the constitution of India in 1949. The official term today is 'Scheduled caste'.

parikrama – Going round the country as a wayfarer, visiting the holy places and pilgrimage centres.

parivrajaka – An itinerant monk.

Patanjali – A renowned yogi of yore who codified the *Yoga Sutras* extant during his time and formulated the yoga system, one of the six systems of orthodox Hindu philosophy, also known as the yoga philosophy or "*Patanjala*", named after the codifier.

Pauranic – Pertaining to Puranas.

Prabuddha Bharata – Awakened India.

Practical Vedanta – Same as Neo-Vedanta of Swami Vivekananda.

prana – The cosmic emergency latent in man which is responsible for all his psycho-physical functions; the vital breath that sustain life in a physical body.

Pranava – Om.

Prarthana Samaj – A religious body similar to Brahmo Samaj founded in Bombay, under the influence of Keshab Chandra Sen (1838-1884), the celebrated Brahmo leader, who paid a visit to Bombay in 1864. It was led by Dr. Atmaram Pandurang (1823-1898).

pratishtita prajna – Wisdom well-established.

pravartana – Movement; operation; action for national reconstruction; social development and the upliftment of the poor and downtrodden.

pravrtti – Involvment in activities.

pravrtti-marga – The path of activity characterized by desire.

Prayaga – A pilgrimage centre at the confluence of the sacred rivers, Ganga, Yamuna and Saraswati, which is also known as the Triveni Sangam, now part of Allahabad city near Benaras in Uttar Pradesh.

prayaschitta – Atonement.

preyas – The real gain in life; worldly prosperity.

puja – Ritualistic worship.

punarutthana – Re-awakening, revival, renaissance.

pundit – Erudite scholar.

punyabhoomi – Sacred land.

Purana(s) – Books of Hindu mythology.

Purusha – (Lit., a man) A term of the Sankhys philosophy, denoting the eternal Conscious Principle. The universe evolves from the union of Prakriti and Purusha. The word also denotes the soul and the Absolute.

Rabindranath Tagore – Great Indian poet and educationist of Nobel fame (1861-1941).

Rahula – Son of Buddha, the founder of Buddhism.

raja – King.

rajas – The principle of activity or restlessness and passion.

rajayoga – A system of yoga ascribed to Patanjali, dealing with concentration and its methods, control of the mind, samadhi and allied matters.

Raja Yoga – A book by Swami Vivekananda consisting of the yoga aphorisms of Patanjali with the Swami's masterly introduction and penetrating commentary, which is the most widely read of his books in Europe and America. It deals with various disciplines for the practice of self-control, concentration, and meditation, by means of which the truth of religion are directly experienced.

rajayogi – The follower of rajayoga.

Rama(chandra) – The hero of the *Ramayana*, regarded by the Hindus as a Divine Incarnation.

Ramamantra – The sacred formula incorporating the name of Sri Rama considered to be the most powerful mantra which is also known as the Taraka Mantra.

Ramanuja – A famous saint and philosopher of southern India, the founder of the school of Qualified Non-dualism or Vishistadavaita (A. D. 1017-1137).

Ramarajya – Kingdom of God; a welfare state.

Ramayana – A famous Hindu epic.

Rammohan Roy – The great Indian social and religious reformer (1774-1833), and the founder of Brahmo Samaj.

rashtra – Nation.

rashtra-chetana – National awakening.

rashtra-guru – National preceptor.

Rig Veda – One of the Vedas, the revered scriptures of the Hindus.

rishi(s) – A seer of Truth; the name is also applied to the pure souls to whom were revealed the words of the Vedas.

sadguru – True teacher.

sadhana(s) – Spiritual discipline.

sadhu(s) – Holy man, sage, ascetic; a term generally used with reference to a monk.

saheb – Europen gentleman.

sajeeva Bhagavan – Living God.

samadhi – Ecstasy, trance, a superconscious state; communion with God.

samadrshti – Equal vision.

samskara(s) – Subtle mental impressions; a tendency inherent in the mind.

samskrti-devata – Goddess of culture.

Sanatana Dharma – (Lit., eternal religion) Hindu religion (Hinduism) formulated by the Vedic rishis. "It is wholly free from the strange obsession of some faiths that the acceptance of a particular religious metaphysics, doctrine or dogma is necessary for salvation, and non-acceptance thereof is heinous sin meriting eternal punishment.... Heresy-hunting, the favourite game of many religions, is singularly absent from Hinduism.... It insists not on religious conformity but on a spiritual and ethical outlook in life. Wars of religion (crusades and jihads) which are the outcome of fanaticism that prompts and justifies the extermination of aliens of different faiths were practically unknown in Hindu India...."

Sankara – A name of Shiva; also short for Sankaracharya (A. D. 788-820).

Sankaracharya – One of the greatest philosophers of India, an exponent of Advaita Vedanta.

Sankhya philosophy – One of the six systems of the Hindu philosophy.

Sankhya system – Same as Sankhya philosophy.

sannyas(a) – The monastic life, the last of the four stages of life.

sannyasi(s) – A Hindu monk who has renounced the worldly attachments in order to realize God.

sannyasin(s) – Same as sannyasi(s).

sannyasini(s) – A Hindu nun.

sannyasinism – An anglicized derivation from sannyasin denoting monkhood or sannyas.

saptarishis – Seven sages.

Saraswati – The goddess of learning and music.

Sariputta – One of the prominent disciples of Buddha.

Sarvodaya – Welfare of all; commonweal.

Satchidananda – Same as Sat-Chit-Ananda.

Sat-Chit-Ananda – (Lit., Existence-Knowledge-Bliss) A term for Brahman, the Ultimate Reality.

sattva – The quality of tranquillity, purity, virtue and illumination; one of the three *gunas* (qualities or strands) constituting the Prakriti (Primordial Nature), in contrast with Purusha (the eternal Conscious Principle).

sattvikas – Those possessed of sattva.

satyagraha – A method of peaceful and non-violent agitation to establish one's rights and freedom, introduced by Mahatma Gandhi (1869-1948).

Satyameva Jayate – "Truth alone triumphs", a declaration in *Mundaka Upanishad*, accepted as the Indian national slogan.

sevak(s) – Servant.

Shakti – Power, generally the Creative Power of Brahman; the name of the Divine Mother.

shaktis – Special powers.

Shaktiyoga – Worship of God as the Divine Mother.

Shantih – Peace.

shastras – Scriptures; sacred books; code of laws.

shastric – pertaining to shastras.

Shiva – The Destroyer God; the Third Person of the Hindu Trinity, the other two being Brahma and Vishnu.

Shivaji – The king and emperor of Maharashtra (1630-1680) who, under the guidance of the renowned saint, Samarth Ramdas (1608-1682), founded the *"Hindu-pada-paadashaahi"* – the Hindu empire as a bulwark against the Mughal marauders.

Shivamatmani pasyanti – Seeing the Lord in one's own heart.

Shodashi – Of the age of sixteen; one of the names of Kali, the Divine Mother.

Shodashi Puja – Worship of the Divine Mother.

shraddha – Faith.

shreyas – The temporal gain in life.

shruti(s) – (Lit., what is heard) The Vedas, being the revelations of the eternal verities to the enlightened rishis of yore.

shudra(s) – The fourth caste in Hindu society.

shudra shakti – Power of the proletariat.

siddha – A perfected soul.

siddhi – The eight occult powers which the yogi acquires through the practice of yoga; perfection in spiritual life.

sishya – Disciple.

smriti(s) – The law books, subsidiary to the Vedas, guiding the daily life and conduct of the Hindus.

"Soham" – (Lit., "I am He") One of the sacred formulas of the Non-dualistic Vedantist.

stuti – Praise.

Subhas Chandra Bose – One of the greatest leaders of India's freedom struggle (1897-1945), who founded the Indian National Army which dealt the final blow to the British empire in India.

Suka(deva) – The narrator of the *Bhagavata* and the son of Vyasa, regarded as one of India's ideal monks.

sukta – A hymn.

suprabhata – Auspicious dawn.

sutras – Aphorisms.

swadeshi – Of one's own country.

Swadeshi Movement – A movement exhorting the citizens to use only the products made in their own country.

swadharma – One's duty.

swarajya – Self-rule.

swartha – Selfishness.

swatantra – Independent.

tamas – The principle of inertia and dullness.

tamasika – Pertaining to, or possessed of, tamas.

tamoguna – Same as tamas; also means unwisdom.

Tantra(s) – A system of religious philosophy in which the Divine Mother, or Power is the Ultimate Reality; also the scriptures dealling with this philosophy.

Tantra shastra – Treatise dealing with Tantra.

Tantrik(a) – A follower of Tantra; also, pertaining to Tantra.

Tantrika sadhana – Practices related to Tantra.

tapas – Spiritual austerity.

tapasya – Same as tapas.

Tattvajnana – The knowledge of Reality.

tat tvam asi – (Lit., "That thou art") A sacred formula of the Vedas denoting the identity of the individual self and the Supreme Self.

Thakur – Master.

Theosophical Society – The organization started by Madame Blavatsky (1831-1891) in 1875 to integrate the philosophies of the major world religions.

Tilak – One of the great patriots and leaders of the Congress Movement (1856-1920) who led the extremist group and declared, "Swaraj is my birthright", demanding absolute freedom from the British yoke.

tirtha(s) – Holy place.

Tukaram – The name of a saint of Maharashtra.

tyaga – Renunciation.

tyagabhoomi – Land of renunciation and self-sacrifice.

Upanishad(s) – The well-known Hindu scriptures containing the philosophy of the Vedas. They are one hundred in number, of which eleven are called major Upanishads.

Upanishadic – Pertaining to Upanishads.

utsav – Festival.

vairagya – Renunciation.

Vaishnavism – Philosophy of the Vaishnavas – the followers of Vishnu, a dualistic sect which emphasizes the path of devotion as a spiritual descipline. Vaishnavas are generally the followers of Sri Chaitanya in Bengal and of Ramanuja and Madhva in south India.

vaishya – The third or merchant caste in Hindu society.

vak – Speech.

Vali – A monkey chieftain mentioned in the *Ramayana* and killed by Sri Rama.

Valmiki – the author of the *Ramayana*.

'Vande Mataram' – 'Salutation to the Motherland', the famous hymn by the Bengali novelist Bankim Chandra Chatterjee (1838-1894), which inspired people to sacrifice all for their motherland.

varna – (Lit., colour) Now it is applied to the concept of caste.

vasana(s) – The subtle mental impressions; desire for possession.

Veda(s) – The most ancient and sacred scriptures of the Hindus, consisting of the *Rig Veda, Yajur Veda, Sama Veda* and *Atharva Veda*.

Vedanta – One of the six systems of orthodox Hindu philosophy, formulated by Vyasa.

Vedanta Kesari – The lion of Vedanta.

Vedanta Sutras – Same as *Brahma Sutras*.

Vedantic – Pertaining to Vedanta.

Vedantin – Same as Vedantist.

Vedantism – An anglicized derivation from Vedanta denoting the philosophy of Vedanta.

Vedantist(s) – A follower of Vedanta.

Vedic – Pertaining to Vedas.

veena – A stringed musical instrument.

veer sannyasi – Heroic monk.

Vidura – The name of a great devotee of Sri Krishna mentioned in the *Mahabharata*.

vidya – Knowledge leading to liberation, i.e. to the Ultimate Reality.

viraja homa – A Vedic preparatory to one's entering the life of sannyas, consisting of offering oblations into the sacred fire with the chanting of certain Vedic mantras indicating renunciation.

virat – The first progeny of Brahman in Hindu cosmology; the Spirit in the form of the universe; the all-prevading Spirit; also all those around, being the cosmic form of the Absolute.

Vishishtadvaita – The philosophy of Qualified Non-dualism as expounded by Sri Ramanujacharya.

Vishwamitra – The name of a sage in the *Ramayana*. He was a companion and counsellor of Sri Rama. Though born a kshatriya, by dint of his austerities he was raised to the status of a brahmin.

Vishwanatha – (Lit., Lord of the universe) Shiva who is the chief deity at Kashi, the most sacred pilgrimage centre of the Hindus.

viveka – Discrimination.

vrtti – Modifications, ripples or waves.

vyakarana – Grammar.

Vyasa(deva) – The compiler of the Vedas, reputed author of the *Brahma Sutras,* and father of Sukadeva.

Yajur Veda – One of the four Vedas, the revered scriptures of the Hindus.

yoga – Union of the individual soul and Universal soul; also the method to realize this union. The yoga system of philosophy, ascribed to Patanjali, is one of the six systems of orthodox Hindu philosophy, and deals with the realization of Truth through the control of mind.

yogas – Mainly four: Jnanayoga, Karmayoga, Bhaktiyoga and Rajayoga. Expounded by Swami Vivekananda, these four yogas serve a very useful purpose for the spiritual development of the four types of men – the intellectual, the active, the emotional, and the psychic or introspective. They also help the individual to integrate his diverse faculties and thus endow his actions with grace and meaning.

yoga-siddha – Adept in the practice of yoga.

Yoga Sutras – Aphorisms of yoga codified by sage Patanjali; an authentic and authoritative treatise on the yoga philosophy.

yogi(n) – a practitioner of yoga.

yogic – Pertaining to yoga.

yogism – An anglicized derivation from yoga denoting the philosophy of yoga.

Yogiswara – Lord of yoga.

yuga – A cyale of world period. According to Hindu mythology the duration of the world is divided into four yugas, namely, Satya, Treta, Dwapara, and Kali.

Yugavatara – Incarnation of the Age.

yuj – to unite, to join, to yoke.

BIBLIOGRAPHY
(Chronicle)

ASIMOV, ISSAC,
Biographical Encyclopedia of Science and Technology,
Pan Books Ltd., London, 1972.

BARKER, L. MARY,
Pears Encyclopedia,
Pelham Books Ltd., U.K., 1975.

CARRUTH, GORTON, AND ASSOCIATES (Editors),
The Encyclopedia of American Facts and Dates,
Thomas Y. Crowell Co., New York, 1970.

CAXTON PUBLICATION,
The New Caxton Encyclopedia,
The Caxton Publishing Co., London, 1977.

CHAUDHURY, NIRAD, C.,
Scholar Extraordinary (The Life of Prof., the Rt. Hon. Friedrich Max MullerP.C.)
Oxford University Press, Delhi, 1974.

CHANDRA NATH, RAKHAL,
The New Hindu Movement (1886-1911),
Minerva Associates, Pvt. Ltd., Calcutta, 1982.

DHAR, Prof. S. N.,
A Comprehensive Biography of Swami Vivekananda (in two Volumes),
Vivekananda Kendra, Madras.

HOPKINS, JOSEPH G. E.,
Concise Dictionary of American Biography,
Charles Scribner's Sons, New York, 1977.

HOWAT, C. M. D.,
Dictionary of World History,
Thomas Nelson and Sons, London, 1973.

LAMPLIGHT PUBLICATION,
Modern Illustrated Library – World History Science,
Lamplight Publishing.

LANCER, WILLIAM L. (Compiler and Editor),
An Encyclopedia of World History,
George C. Harrap and Co., London, 1972.

MACMILLAN PUBLICATION,
The Macmillan Family Encyclopedia,
Macmillan London Ltd., London, 1980.

MAJUMDAR, R. C. (Editor),
The History and Culture of the Indian People, Vol. X, Part. II,
Bharatiya Vidya Bhavan, Bombay, 1965.

MAXMULLER, Mrs. GEORGINA (Editor),
The Life and Lettors of the Rt. Hon. Friedrich Max Muller (in two Volumes),
Longman's, Green and Co., 1903.

MeGRAW-HILL PUBLICATION,
Encyclopedia of World Biography,
McGraw-Hill Book Co., New York, 1973.

MORRIS, RICHARD B.,
Encyclopedia of American History,
Universal Book Stall, Delhi, 1965.

PHILIPS, C.H.,
The Evolution of India and Pakistan (1858-1947) – Select Documents,
The English Language Book Society and Oxford University Press, London. 1965.

PURNELL PUBLICATION,
Knowledge (Vol. I–XVIII),
Purnell and Sons Ltd., London,1960.

PURNELL PUBLICATION,
365 Days to Remember,
Purnell Books, Berkshire, 1981.

READER'S DIGEST PUBLICATION,
Heritage of Britain, Reader's
Digest Association Ltd., London, 1975.

READER'S DIGEST PUBLICATION,
Family Encyclopedia of American History,
Reader's Digest Association Inc.,New York, 1975.

ROBERTS, J. M.,
History of the World,
Hutchinson and Co., London, 1976.

ROBERTSON, PATRICK,
The Shell Book of Firsts,
Ebury Press and Michael Joseph Ltd., London, 1974.

SABEL (LYNNE) AND STEEL (PHILLIP),
1000 Great Events.

SEN, S. P. (Editor),
Dictionary of National Biography (in four volumes),
Institute of Historical Studies, Calcutta, 1972.

SHARMA, JAGDISH SARAN,
*India since the advent of the British – A Descriptive Chronology from
1600 - October 2, 1969,*
S. Chand and Co., New Delhi, 1970.

SHARMA, JAGDISH SARAN,
Encyclopedia Indica,
S. Chand and Co., New Delhi, 1975.

SHARMA, IAGDISH SARAN,
Encyclopedia of Indian Struggle for Freedom,
S. Chand and Co., New Delhi, 1971.
STUTTMAN CO. PUBLICATION,
The Illustrated Science and Inventions Encyclopedia,
H. S. Stuttman Co., New York, 1977.
TRAGER, JAMES (Editor), *People's Chronology,*
William Heinemann Ltd.,London, 1980.
UNESCO PUBLICATION, *UNESCO History of Mankind – Cultural and*
Scientific Development – Vol. V,
George Allen and Unwin Ltd., London, 1976.
WEEKS, MARY ELVIRA, *Discovery of Elements,*
Paico Publishing House, Cochin, 1968.
WILLIAMS, NEVILLE, *Chronology of the Modern World (1763-1965),*
Barrie and Jenkins Ltd., London.

British Historicmal Facts (1830-1900)
European Political Facts (1848-1918).
Penguin's Dictionary of Modern History (1889-1945).
Indian Gazetteer (In two Volumes).
Encyclopedia Britinnica – Micropedia.
Encyclopedia Britinnica – Macropedia.

VIVEKANANDA LITERATURE
Books by and on Vivekananda

Swami Vivekananda's writings and speeches are collected in *The Complete Works of Swami Vivekananda* (in 9 volumes), and published by the Advaita Ashram, 5 Dehi Entally Road, Calcutta-700 014. They have also brought out many other books by and on Swami Vivekananda among which the reader may consult the following with profit:

Life of Swami Vivekananda (in two volumes),
  by HIS EASTERN AND WESTERN DISCIPLES.
Swami Vivekananda – A Biography
  by SWAMI NIKHILANANDA.
The Life of Vivekananda and the Universal Gospel
  by ROMAIN ROLLAND.
Vivekananda – A Biography in Pictures (Album containing 170 pictures).
Reminiscences of Swami Vivekananda
  by HIS EASTERN AND WESTERN ADMIRERS.
Swami Vivekananda in the West – New Discoveries (in six volumes)
  by MARIE LOUISE BURKE.
What Religion is (in the words of Swami Vivekananda)
  by SWAMI VIDYATMANANDA.
Swami Vivekananda: Vedanta – Voice of Freedom
  by SWAMI CHETANANANDA.
Swami Vivekananda's Four Yogas.
The Philosophical and Religious Lectures of Swami Vivekananda.
The Natonalisitc and Religious Lectures of Swami Vivekananda.
– Condensed and Retold.
  by SWAMI TAPASYANANDA.
Swami Vivekananda – A Historical Review,
  by R. C. MAJUMDAR
Living at the Source: Yoga Teachings of Vivekananda,
  Edited by ANN MYREN and DOROTHY MADISON.
"My Faithful Goodwin",
  by PRAVRAJIKA VRAJAPRANA.
Swamiji and His Message
  by SISTER NIVEDITA.
Lectures from Colombo to Almora.
Letters of Swami Vivekananda.
Teachings of Swami Vivekananda.
Talks with Swami Vivekananda.
Swami Vivekananda's Second Visit to West.
Swami Vivekananda's Contribution to the Present Age.
Swami Vivekananda: A Study of Religion.

Vivekananda – Great Spiritual Teacher.
Vivekananda – The Man and His Message.
Selections from the Complete Works of Swami Vivekananda.
Last Days of Swami Vivekananda.
A Short Life of Swami Vivekananda.
Salvation and Service: Swami Vivekananda.
Hail Independent India: Swami Vivekananda.
India: Vivekananda.
Jnana Yoga
Raja Yoga
Karma Yoga
Bhakti Yoga

Other Publications:

ABHEDANANDA, SWAMI
  Swami Vivekananda and His Work, Ramakrishna Vedanta Math, Calcutta.
AHLUWALIA, B. K., and SHASHI AHLUWALIA
  Vivekananda and Indian Renaissance, Associated Publishing Co.,
  New Delhi.
AMAL, BRAHMACHARI
  A Simple Life of Swami Vivekananda,
  Ramakrishna Mission Ashrama, Narendrapur.
ANANDA
  – A Vivekananda View of Mythology,
  Sri Ramakrishna Math, Belur Math, Howrah.
  – Statistics and Dynamics of Progress: *The Vivekananda Concept,*
  Ramakrishna Mission Seva Pratisthan, Calcutta.
ARORA, V. K
  The Social and Political Philosophy of Swami Vivekananda,
  Punthi-Pustak, Calcutta.
ASSOCIATED UNIVERSITY PRESS, London,
  Swami Vivekananda: A Reassessment.
ASYLUM, LAWRENCE, Madras,
  Swami Vivekananda, Disciple of Ramakrishna Paramahamsa at the
  Parliament of Religions.
ATHALYE, D.V.
  – Quintessence of Yoga Philosophy: *An Exposition of Swami*
    Vivekananda's Conception of Practical Vedantism.
  – An Exposition of Swami Vivekananda's Concept of Vedantism.
  Taraporevala, Bombay.
  – Swami Vivekananda: A Study,
  Ashish Publishing House, New Delhi.

AVINASHILINGAM, T. S.
— *The Educational Philosophy of Swami Vivekananda.*
— *Make Me a Man.*
— *National Seminar on the Relevance of Swami Vivekananda's Message   in the Context of National Education Policy.*
Ramakrishna Mission Vidyalaya, Coimbatore.
AVYAKTANANDA, SWAMI
— *The Teachings of Swami Vivekananda.*
— *Vivekananda: The Nation Builder.*
Ramakrishna Ashram, Patna.
BANHATTI, G. S.
Quintessence of Vivekananda,
Suvichar Prakashan Mandal, Nagpur.
BASU, PRAMATH NATH
Swami Vivekananda (4 volumes).
BASU, S. P. and S. B. GHOSH
Vivekananda in Indian Newspapers (1893-1902),
Basu Bhattacharya and Co., Calcutta.
BASU, SANKARI PRASAD, Ed.,
Swami Vivekananda in Contemporary Indian News (1898-1902), with Sri Ramakrishna and the Mission,
The Ramakrishna Mission Institute of Culture, Calcutta.
BHATTACHARYA, BEJOY CHANDRA
Karl Marx and Vivekananda, Author, Calcutta.
BHATTACHARYA, MANMATHA NATH
Vivekananda Centenary Souvenir, Dhiraj Basu, Calcutta.
BHISHMADEV, ACHARYA
A Call to Rising Generation: Foundation of True Education,
Bharatiya Vidya Bhavan, Bombay.
BISWAS, ARUN KUMAR
Swami Vivekananda and the Indian Quest for Socialism,
Firma KLM, Calcutta.
BOSE, MEMAI SADHAN,
Swami Vivekananda,
Sahitya Academy, New Delhi.
BROWN, Dr.
The White Umbrella (a chapter on Vivekananda).
BUDHANANDA, SWAMI
Ramakrishna's Naren, Naren's Ramakrishna,
Ramakrishna Mission, New Delhi.
BURDWAN, UNIVERSITY OF BURDWAN
Vivekananda Commemoration Volume.
BURKE, MERIE LOUISE
Swami Vivekananda: Prophet of the Modem Age,
The Ramakrishna Mission Institute of Culture, Calcutta.

CHAKRAVORTY, TARINI SANKAR
Patriot-saint Vivekananda,
Ramakrishna Mission Sevashrama, Allahabad.

CHAUDHURI, TAPAN ROY
Europe Reconsidered: Perceptions of the West in Ninteenth Century
Bengal,
Oxford University Press, Delhi.

CHATTERJEE, SIBRANJAN
Indian National Congress and Swami Vivekananda,
Ananda Gopal Mukherjee, Durgapur.

CHETANANDA, SWAMI
East Meets West: Vivekananda
Vetanta Society, St. Louis, U. S. A

CHOWDHURY, SANJIB
Vision of Vivekananda, Author, Calcutta.

CHUAN, HUANG XIN
Modern Indian Philosopher Vivekananda: A Study.

CHUNDER, DR. P. C.
Brother Vivekananda,
Lodge Anchor and Hope, Calcutta.

DAS GUPTA, R. K.
– *Revolutionary Ideas of Swami Vivekananda*
– *Swami Vivekananda on Indian Philosophy and Culture.*
– *Swami Vivekananda's Vedantic Socialism.*
The Ramakrishna Mission Institute of Culture, Calcutta.

DAS GUPTA, SANTWANA
Vivekananda: The Prophet of Human Emancipation, Calcutta.

DAS, PROF. TRILOCHAN
The Social Philosophy of Swami Vivekananda,
Co-operative Book Depot Calcutta.

DESAI, RAMPRASAD K.
Life of Swami Vivekananda, Baroda.

DEV, GOVINDA CHANDRA
The *Philosophy of Vivekananda and Future of Man,*
Ramakrishna Mission, Dacca.

DHAR, NIRANJAN
Vedanta and Bengal Renaissance, Minerva Associates, Calcutta.

DHAR, PROF. S. N.
A *Comprehensive Biography of Swami Vivekananda,*
Vivekananda Kendra, Madras.

DUTTA, BHUPENDRANATH
– *Swami Vivekananda, the Socialist,*
Swaraj Ashrama, Khulna.
– *Swami Vivekananda, Patriot-Prophet: A Study,*
Navabharat Publishing Co., Calcutta.

DUTTA, TAPASH SANKAR
  A Study of The Philosophy of Vivekananda,
  Sribhumi Publishing Co., Calcutta.
GANGULY, HEMANT KUMAR
  Radicalism in Advaita Vedanta: A Comprehensive Critique of the
  Theories of Vivarta, Drishtisrishti and Neo-Vedtanta of Swami Vivekananda,
  Indian Publicity Society, Calcutta.
GANGULY, MANOMOHAN
  Swami Vivekananda: A Study, Sarada Press, Calcutta.
GERMAN-INDIAN ASSOCIATION, Calcutta
  Swami Vivekananda in Germany.
GHANANANDA, SWAMI and GEOFFREY PARRINDER
  Swami Vivekananda in East and West,
  The Ramakrishna Vedanta Centre, London.
GHOSH, ANIL CHANDRA
  Swami Vivekananda: His Life and Message,
  Presidency Library, Calcutta.
GNANESWARANANDA, SWAMI
  Yoga for Beginners, Sri Ramakrishna Math, Madras.
GNATUK-DANIL' CHUCK, DR. A. P.
  Tolstoy and Vivekananda,
  The Ramakrishna Mission Institute of Culture, Calcutta.
GUPTA, HARISH C.
  Swami Vivekananda, Studies in Soviet Union (in Russia),
  The Ramakrishna Mission Institute of Culture, Calcutta.
GUPTA, NAGENDRANATH
  Ramakrishna-Vivekananda, Ramakrishna Math, Bombay.
HARSHANANDA, SWAMI
  – Sri Vivekananda Karma Yoga Sutra Satakam,
  Sri Ramakrishna Math, Bangalore.
  – Reconstruction of India According to Swami Vivekananda,
  Samskrita Sangha, Indian Institute of Science, Bangalore.
HOSSAIN, MUSARAF
  Swami Vivekananda's Philosophy of Education,
  Ratna Prakashan, Calcutta.
INDIRA PATEL
  Vivekananda's Approach to Social Work,
  Sri Ramakrishna Math, Madras.
JACKSON, PROF. CARL THOMAS
  The Swami in Amerca: A History of the Ramakrishna Movement in
  the United States (1893-1960), University of California, Los Angeles.
JAGADEESWARANANDA, SWAMI
  Swami Vivekananda and Modern India,
  Ramakrishna Vedanta Math, Calcutta.

JAGTIANI, G. M.
– *Swami Vivekananda: The Militant Hindu Monk.*
– *Swami Vivekananda: Redeemer of our Faith.*
– *The Fire and Flame of Swami Vivekananda.*
Author, Bombay

JITATMANANDA, SWAMI
– *Swami Vivekananda: Prophet and Pathfinder.*
Sri Ramakrishna Math, Madras.
– *Modern Physics and Vedanta.*
Bharatiya Vidya Bhavan, Bombay.

KAMATH, M. V.
The United States and India: 1776-1996: The Bridge Over The River Time.
Indian Council for Cultutal Relations, New Delhi.

KAPOOR, SATISH K.
Cultural Contact and Fusion: Swami Vivekananda in the West (1893-96),
ABS Publications, Jalandhar.

KARANDIKAR, DR. V. R
Ramakrishna and Vivekananda, Bharatiya Vidya Bhavan, Bombay.

KASTURI, N.
Swami Vivekananda, The Patriot Monk of Modern India,
Ramakrishna Ashram, Mysore.

KEENE, CAROLYN
Swamiji's Ring.
Armada Books, U. S. A.

LAHIRI, K. C.
Vivekananda: A Dialect of Power and a Dialect of Pain, Sushila,
Howrah.

LAKSHMI KUMARI, DR. M.
Swami Vivekananda: The Master Builder of Our Nation,
Vivekananda Kendra, Kanyakumari.

LINDA PRUGH
Josephine MacLeod and Vivekananda's Mission,
Ramakrishna Math, Chennai.

LOKESWARANANDA, SWAMI
– *World Thinkers on Ramakrishna-Vivekananda,*
The Ramakrishna Mission Institute of Culture, Calcutta.
– *The Perennial Vivekananda: A Selection,*
Sahitya Academy, New Delhi.

MAJUMDAR, AMIYA KUMAR
Understanding Vivekananda, Sanskrit Pustak Bhandar, Calcutta.

MAJUMDAR, AMIYA KUMAR, and FRED W. TREMBOUR
Swami Vivekananda and America,
United States Information Service, New Delhi

MAJUMDAR, B.
Vivekananda, The Informer of Max Muller,
Scientific Book Agency, Calcutta.
MAJUMDAR, DR. R. C.
– *Swami Vivekananda: A Historical Review,*
General Printers and Publishers, Calcutta.
– *Swami Vivekananda Centenary Memorial Volume,*
163, Lower Circular Road, Calcutta.
MALCOM-SMITH, E. F.
Vivekananda, V. Sundaram Iyer and Sons, Trichur.
MINISTRY OF INFORMATION AND BROADCASTING
(Govt. of India), Publication Division – *Vivekananda.*
MITRA, KAMAKHYANATH
*Swami Vivekananda, The Great World Teacher and Prophet of
New India,* Vedanta Society, Calcutta.
MITTAL, DR. S. S.
The Social and Political Ideas of Swami Vivekananda,
Metropolitan Book, New Delhi.
MOOKERJEE, NANDA
Vivekananda's Influence on Subhas, Jayasree Publication, Calcutta.
MUKHERJEE, HIREN
Swami Vivekananda and Indian Freedom,
The Ramakrishna Mission Institute of Culture, Calcutta.
MUKHERJEE, SANTILAL
*The Philosophy of Man-making: A Study in Social and Political Ideas
of Swami Vivekananda,* New Central Book Agency, Calcutta.
MUKHOPADHYAY, NABANIHARAN
– *Vivekananda – A Study.*
– *Swami Vivekananda and The World of Youth,*
Akhil Bharat Yuva Mahamandal, Calcutta.
MURDOCH, JOHN
*Swami Vivekananda on Hinduism: An Examination of His Address at
the Chicago Parliament of Religions,* Christian Literature Society, Madras.
MUTTUCUMARU, T.
Vivekananda: Prophet of the New Age of India and The World,
The Ramakrishna Mission, Colombo.
NAIR, V. SUKUMARAN
Swami Vivekananda: The Educator, Sterling Publishers, New Delhi.
NARAYANSWAMI, T. V.
Life of Swami Vivekananda, Central Chinmaya Mission Trust, Bombay.
NATESON AND CO., G. A., Madras,
– *Swami Vivekananda: A Sketch of His Life and Teachings.*
– *Chaitanya to Vivekananda.*

NATESON, M. S.
   Swami Vivekananda: A Sketch, Sri Vanivilas Press, Srirangam.
NATONAL LIBRARY, Calcutta,
   Swami Vivekananda Centenary Exhibition, 1964: A Bibliography and a Brief Chronology.
NEHRU, JAWAHARLAL
   Sri Ramakrishna and Swami Vivekananda, Advaita Ashrama, Almora.
NIKHILANANDA, SWAMI
   Vivekananda: The Yogas and Other Works,
   Ramakrishna-Vivekananda Centre, New York.
NIRVEDANANDA, SWAMI
   – *Swami Vivekananda and Spiritual Freedom,*
   Sri Ramakrishna Math, Belur Math, Howrah.
   – *Swami Vivekananda on India and Her Problems,*
   Advaita Ashram, Calcutta.
NIVEDITA, SISTER
   – *The Master as I saw Him.*
   . – *Notes of Some Wanderings with Swami Vivekananda.*
   Udbohan Office, Calcutta.
   – *Swamiji and His Message,*
   Sri Ramakrishna Math, Belur Math.
PARAMESWARAN, P.
   – *Beyond All Isms to Humanism: A Study of Swami Vivekananda's Relevance Today,*
   Sri Ramakrishna Math, Puranattukara, Trichur.
   – *Marx and Vivekananda: A Comparative Study.,*
   Sterling Publishers, New Delhi.
PHILLIPS, JAMES E.
   Vedanta Philosophy: An Examination of Vivekananda's Karma Yoga,
   Traders' Union Labour, London.
PILGRIM (P. M.)
   Emersion of Vivekananda From The Clouds of Hearsay and The Storms Eclat,
   Sailendra Krishna Chowdhury, Calcutta.
PILLAI, DR. P. K. NARAYANA
   Vishwabhanu: The Universal Light, Author, Trivandrum.
PRABHANANDA, SWAMI
   Swami Vivekananda's Vision of Rural Development.
PRABHAVANANDA, SWAMI
   Religion in Practice, George Allen and Unwin, London.
PRABUDDHA BHARATA
   Swami Vivekananda Centenary Volume,
   Prabuddha Bharata Office, Calcutta.

PRINTWELL PUBLISHERS, Jaipur,
   Speeches and Writings of Swami Vivekananda (in two volumes).
PUSALKAR, A. D.
   Swami Vivekananda: Patriot-saint of Modern India, Bombay.
RADICE W.
   Swami Vivekananda and the Modernzsation of Hinduism,
   Oxford University Press, London.
RAMABHADRAN, R. S.
   Swami Vivekananda: Divinity on Earth, Vivekananda Literature Society, Madras.
RAMAKRISHNA MATH, Chennai.
   – *Inspired Talks.*
   – *Facets of Vivekananda.*
   – *Swami Vivekananda: The Wisdom and Bliss.*
   – *Sarat Chandra Chakravarthy – A Disciple of Swami Vivekananda.*
RAMAKRISHNA MATH and RAMAKRISHNA MISSION.
   Belur Math, Horah, W. B.
   Swami Vivekananda: A Hundred Years Since Chicago – A
   Comprehensive Volume.
RAMAKRISHANA MISSION, Dacca,
   A Short Account of The Life and Teachings of Swami Vivekananda.
RAMAKRISHNA MISSION ASHRAMA, Patna,
   Swami Vivekananda Birth Centenary Souvenir.
RAMAKRISHNA MISSION ASHRAMA INSTITUTE OF SOCIAL
   EDUCATION AND RECREATION, Narendrapur, *Swami Vivekananda*
   Centenary Celebration and the Sixth Sri Ramakrihana Mela.
RAMAKRISHNA MISSION INSTITUTE OF CULTURE, Calcutta,
   – *Pearls of Wisdom.*
   – *Books on Vivekananda: A Bibliography.*
   – *Words of Inspiration.*
   – *A Concord to Swami Vivekananda – Vol. I (A to H).*
   – *Vivekananda : Prophet of Modern Age.*
   – *My India – The India Eternal.*
RAMAKRISHNA SEVA SAMITHI, SRI, Bapatla, (A. P.),
   Vivekananda on Organisation and Organised Work.
RAMAKRISHNA TAPOVANAM, Tirupparaithurai, Tamil Nadu,
   The Man-making Message of Swami Vivekananda.
RAMAKRISHNA VIVEKANANDA PRACHAR, Howrah,
   Swamiji and Social Ideals.
RAMAKRISHNAN. R.
   Swami Vivekananda: Patriot-saint of Modern India,
   Sri Ramakrishna Math, Madras.
RANADE, EKNATH
   Rousing Call to Hindu Nation,
   Vivekananda Kendra, Kanyakumari.

RANGANATHANANDA, SWAMI
- *The Meeting of East and West in Swami Vivekananda,*
- *Swami Vivekananda: His Life and Mission,*
- *Swami Vivekananda's Synthesis of Science and Religion,*
The Ramakhshna Mission Institute of Culture, Calcutta.
- *Swami Vivekananda's Vision of Free India.*
- *Swami Vivekananda on Universal Ethics and Moral Conduct.*
Bharatiya Vidya Bhavan, Bombay .
- *Swami Vivekananda: His Humanism.*
- *Swami Vivekananda and Human Excellence,*
Advaita Ashram, Calcutta.

RAO, K. VYASA
The Master and the Disciple, V. R. Sastralu, Madras.

RAO, T. N. VASUDEVA
Swami Vivekanada's Idea on History with Special Reference to Indian History and Culture,
R.. K. M. Vidyapith Institute of Vivekananda Studies, Madras.

RAO, V. K. R.V.
- *Swami Vivekananda: The Prophet of Vedantic Socialism,*
Publication Division, Government of India.
- *Vivekananda's Message to the Youth,*
Bharatiya Vidya Bhavan, Bombay.

REDDY, A.V. RATHNA
Political Philosophy of Swami Vivekananda,
Sterling Publishers, New Delhi.

ROLLAND, ROMAIN
- *The Godman Ramakrishna and Universal Gospel of Vivekananda,*
Rotapfet-Verlag, Zurich & Leipzig.
- *Prophets of the New India,*
Cassell, London.

ROY, BENOY K.
Socio-political Views of Vivekananda,
People's Publishing House, New Delhi.

ROY, BHUPENDRANATH
Vivekananda, Golmara High School, Purulia.

ROY, SANAT KUMAR
Swami Vivekananda: The Man and His Mission,
Scientific Book Agency, Calcutta.

SADASHIVANANDA, SWAMI
Swami Vivekananda, My Master, Author, New Delhi.

SAMBUDDHANANDA, SWAMI
- *Swami Vivekananda on Himself,*
163, Lower Circular Road, Calcutta.
- *Swami Vivekananda's Ideal of Renunciation.*

SARKAR, PROF. BENOY KUMAR
– The Might of Man in the Social Philosophy of Ramakrishna and
Vivekananda,
Sri Ramakrishna Math, Madras.
– Creative India From Mahenjodaro to The Age of Ramakrishna-
Vivekananda,
Motilal Banarasidas, New Delhi.
SATPRAKASHANANDA, SWAMI
Swami Vivekananda's Contribution to The Present Age,
Vedanta Society of St. Louis, Missouri, U. S. A.
SEAL, BROJENDRANATH
My Reminiscences of Vivekananda.
SEN, GAUTAM,
The Mind of Swami Vivekananda, Jaico Publishing House, Bombay.
SEN GUPTA, SUBODH CHANDRA
Swami Vivekananda and Indian Nationalism,
Shishu Sahithya Samsad, Calcutta.
SHARMA, ARAVIND
Ramakrishna and Vivekananda: New Perspective,
Sterling Publishers, New Delhi.
SHARMA BENISHANKAR
Swami Vivekananda: A Forgotten Chapter of His Life,
Oxford Book and Stationary Co., Calcutta.
SHARMA, D. S.
The Master and The Disciple, Sri Ramakrishna Math, Madras.
SHARMA, G. RANJIT
The Idelistic Philosophy of Swami Vivekananda,
Atlantic Publishers and Distributors, Delhi.
SHASTRI, K. S. RAMASWAMI
The Message of Swami Vivekananda to The Modern World,
Ramakrishna Math, Madras.
SHEAN, VINCENT
Lead Kindly Light (a chapter on Vivekananda and Ramakrishna).
SINGH, DR. KARAN
The Message of Swami Vivekananda, Vivekananda Kendra, Madras.
SINGH, DR. SHAIL KUMARI
Religious and Moral Philosophy of Swami Vivekananda,
Janaki Prakashan, Patna.
SOMESWARANANDA, SWAMI
Vivekananda's Concept of History, Samata Prakashan, Calcutta.
SOPER, DR.
The Inevitable Choice (the author finds in the Swami's harmonizing ideas a
great challenge to all 'special' revelations).

SRINIVAS IYENGAR, K. R.
Swami Vivekananda, Samata Books, Madras.
SUBRAHMANYAM, K.
Vibhooti Vivekananda, Ramana Publications,
Tiruvedakam West, Tamil Nadu – 624217.
SUDDHASATWANANDA, SWAMI and K. JAYARAMAN
Swami Vivekananda Birth Centenary (1863-1963)
Commemoration Souvenir,
Swami Vivekananda Centenary Committee, Madras.
SWAMI VIVEKANANDA CENTENARY COMMITTEE, *Calcutta,*
– *Swami Vivekananda Centenary: General Report of*
Celebrations in India and Abrod.
– *Parliament of Religions: 1963-64.*
TAPASYANANDA, SWAMI
Swami Vivekananda: His Life And Legacy,
Sri Ramakhshna Math, Madras.
TEJASANANDA, SWAMI
Swami Vivekananda And His Message,
Ramakrishna Mission Saradapith, Belur, Howrah.
THOMPSON, E. W.
The Teachings of Swami Vivekananda.
VASWANI, T. L.
The Voice of Vivekananda.
VEDANTA KESARI
Swami Vivekananda Centenary Volume,
Sri Ramakrishna Math, Madras.
VIVEKANANDA COLLEGE, Madras.
Viveka: The Vivekananda College Magazine Centenary Number (1964).
VIVEKANANDA KENDRA, Kanyakumari,
– *The Wandering Monk.*
– *Impact of Swami Vivekananda On Society And Individuals.*
VIVEKANANDA ROCK MEMORIAL COMMITTEE, *Madras,*
Vivekananda Commemoration Volume.
VIVEK SADHANA SANGHA, *Bangalore,*
Vivekavani: Swami Vivekananda Birth Centenary Number.
WILLIAM, GEORGE M.
The Quest For Meaning of Swami Vivekananda:
A Study of Religious Change,
New Horizon Press, California.

BRIEF INTRODUCTION TO THE AUTHORS

*(excerpts from whose writings have been incorporated in
Part One – Section II, and Part Three of this book)*

SWAMI ABHEDANANDA (1866-1939), one of the direct disciples of
Sri Ramakrishna and a spiritual brother of Swami Vivekananda. From 1897 to
1921 he was in the U. S. A. propagating the Message of Vedanta as taught
and lived by Sri Ramakrishna-Vivekananda.

SWAMI ADIDEVANANDA was the Head of the Ramakrishna
Math, Mangalore, till 1966, and later a trustee and the treasurer of the
Ramakrishna Order. A good Sanskristist, he is best known for his lucid
translation of the *Prasthanathraya* in Kannada.

SWAMI BHASHYANANDA was the spiritual Head of the Vivekananda
Vedanta Society, Chicago, U. S. A., for nearly three decades from 1965.
Known for his dynamism and dedication, his tenure was distinguished by
vigorous spiritual activity and expansion. A landmark was the establishment
(in 1971) of a Monastery and Retreat in Ganges Township, Fennville,
Michigan, in a farmland which now consists of 101 acres.

SWAMI BHAVYANANDA was the spiritual Head of the Ramakrishna
Vedanta Centre in Buckinghamshire, U. K., and the editor of *Vedanta for
East* and *West* published from his Centre.

SWAMI BUDHANANDA (1917-1983), a well-known scholar, who was
sometime the Editor of *The Vedanta Kesari and Prabuddha Bharata*. He
was later the President of the Advaita Ashram, Mayavati, and the Secretary
of the Ramakrishna Mission, New Delhi.

SWAMI GABHIRANANDA, a good Sanskritist, he is presently the Head
of the Ramakrishna Ashram, Vytila, Kerala.

SWAMI GNANESWARANANDA (1893-1937), a powerful speaker, he
was the Founder and Head of the Vivekananda Vedanta Society, Chicago,
U. S. A.

SWAMI HARSHANANDA , a Senior Monk of the Ramakrishna Order,
he is the President of the Ramakrishna Math, Bangalore. A good Sanskritist,
singer, speaker and writer, he has to his credit several works, including books
on yoga and temples etc.

SWAMI NIKHILANANDA was the Head of the Ramakrishna-
Vivekananda Centre, New York. A prolific writer, he is best known for his
English translation of *The Gospel of Sri Ramakrishna* from the original
Bengali by 'M'.

SWAMI PAVITRANANDA (1886-1977), an initiated disciple of Swami
Brahmananda, he was the Editor of *Prabuddha Bharata,* and later the Head
of the Vedanta Society of New York, from 1951 until his death in 1977.

SWAMI PRABHAVANANDA (1930-1976) was the Founder of the Vedanta Society of Southern California, Hollywood, U.S.A. A disciple of Sri Ramakrisna's disciple Swami Brahmananda, he preached the spiritual message of India in the West for more that half a century.

SWAMI RAMDAS (1884-1963), endearingly called by his devotees as *'Papa'*, he attained the Highest by chanting the Divine Name – *Ramnam,* incessantly, and with a yearning heart for spiritual illumination. Later, in 1930, founding the Anandashram, (at Kanhangad, Kerala) with the ideal of 'Universal Love and Service', he propagated the glory of the Divine Name in India and abroad. He authored several books including *"In Quest of God",* being his autobiography after he took to monastic life and till he attained spiritual illumination.

SWAMI RANGANATHANANDA (b. 1908) is the President of the Ramakrishna Order, Belur Math. Renowned for his oratory, he undertook extensive lecture tours from 1946 to 1972 covering 50 countries and spreading the Message of Vedanta as taught and lived by Sri Ramakrishna-Vivekananda. He has a versatile and facile pen, and has to his credit a number of publications.

SWAMI SIDDHINATHANANDA , a Senior Monk of the Ramakrishna Order, he was the Head of Ramakrishna Mission Sevashram Calicut, Kerala, till he retired recently. A prolific writer in both English and Malayalam, he has a number of philosophical works to his credit.

SWAMI SWAHANANDA (b 1921), a Senior Monk of the Ramakrishna Order, he is the spiritual Head of the Vedanta Society of Southern California, Hollywood, U.S.A. A former editor of *The Vedanta Kesari*, he has written several books including *Service and Spirituality*.

SWAMI TAPASYANANDA (1904-1991) was one of the Vice-Presidents of the Ramakrishna Order, Belur Math. A good Sankritist, he has several books to his credit, some of them being lucid translations of Sanskrit works like *Srimad Bhagavatam, Adhyatma Ramayanam, Saundarya Lahari* etc.

SWAMI VIDYATMANANDA , a Senior Monk of the Ramakrishna Order, a creative thinker and gifted writer, he was the editor of *Vedanta and the West*, and was based at the Centre Vedantique Ramakrichna, Gretz, France.

SWAMI VIJNANANDA was the Secretary of Ramakrishna Mission Ashram, Salem, Tamil Nadu. Earlier, he was the Head of the Ramakrishna Ashram, Mangalore, South Kanara, Karnataka.

SWAMI VIMALANANDA (1903-1985) a Senior Monk of the Ramakrishna Order, he lived a retired and inward life at a sequestered place near Trivandrum, Kerala. An erudite scholar in Sanskrit, he is best known for his prominent work – *Mahanarayanopanishad*, with introduction, translation, interpretation in Sanskrit, and critical and explanatory notes.

SWAMI VIRESWARANANDA (1892-1985), an initiated disciple of the Holy Mother Sarada Devi, he was the tenth President (1965-1985) of the Ramakrishna Order, Belur Math. He is known for his lucid translations of the *Gita*, Sankara's and Ramanuja's commentaries on *The Brahma Sutras*.

PROF. R. K. DASGUPTA Formerly Director, National Library, Calcutta, he is intimately associated with the Ramakrishna Mission Institute of Culture, Calcutta.

CHRISTOPHER ISHERWOOD a writer of world-repute, with an intimate knowledge of Vedanta and Hindu ways of life, has to his credit a number of books and articles on these subjects. He has collaborated with Swami Prabhavananda in translating many of the spiritual classics of India.

Dr. S. BALAKRISHNA JOSHI , a leading, educationist of Madras, he was the Head and Correspondent of the Hindu Theological School, Madras. He was an ardent devotee of Sri Ramakrishnan-Vivekananda.

R. N. HALDIPUR, the former Lt. Governor of Arunachal Pradesh and Pondicherry. Spiritually inclined , he is based at Bangalore and now leading a retired and inward life.

M. V. KAMATH, renowned author and journalist based in Mumbai, he currently writes for over a dozen newspapers and periodicals. He has authored over 40 books (on a wide range of subjects), including *The United States and India 1776-1996: The Bridge Over the River Time* which contains an illuminating chapter on Swami Vivekananda and his contribution to American culture.

DR. M. LAKSHMI KUMARI, former President of Vivekananda Rock Memorial and Vivekananda Kendra, she is a good speaker and writer as well. She is now the Founder-President of Vivekananda Vedic Vision Foundation, Kodungallur, Kerala.

DR. R. C. MAJUMDAR , a renowned historian, he was a Fellow of Royal Asiatic Society, the Vice-Chancellor of Dacca University and Visiting Professor of Universities of Chicago and Pennsylvania, U. S. A. He has edited and authored several books including *Vivekananda – A Historical Perspective*.

DR. H. NARASIMHIAH, formerly Vice-Chancellor of the Bangalore University, he is an ardent devotee of Sri Ramakrishna-Vivekananda. He is closely associated with the National College, Bangalore.

BANSI PANDIT, an engineer based at Glen Ellyn, near Chicago, Illinois, U. S. A., he is an author and speaker on religious and spiritual topics, and his works include, *The Hindu Mind* and *Hindu Dharma*. A dedicated worker for the Hindu causes, he is a veritable Hindu missionary working silently in association with the like-minded organizations in U. S. A

M. P. PANDIT, an authority on the philosophy of Sri Aurobindo, he was the Secretary of Sri Aurobindo Ashram, Pondicherry, for decades. Widely travelled abroad, he was a good speaker and writer and has scores of books to his credit.

PROF. S. S. RAGHAVACHAR was the Head of the Department of Philosophy, Mysore University. Intimately associated with the Ramakrishna Ashrams at Mysore and Mangalore, he was an ardent devotee of Sri Ramakrishna-Vivekananda. His works include *Naishkarmyasiddhi*.

PROF. C. S. RAMAKRISHNAN, is an ex-editor of *The Vedanta Kesari* and has a long association with the Ramakrishna Math, Chennai, and its activities.

EKNATH RANADE, a senior dedicated worker of the Rashtriya Swayamsevak Sangh, he was the Founder-President of the Vivekanmda Rock Memorial and Vivekananda Kendra, Kanyakumari. A silent and tenacious worker, endowed with the organizing genius, he successfully involved the entire country in the project for the erection of a magnificent Memorial for Vivekananda at the Land's End of India. His works include *Swami Vivekananda's Rousing Call to Hindu Nation,* and *The Story of the Vivekananda Rock Memorial.*

K. SURYANARAYANA RAO, a senior dedicated worker and one of the All India leaders of the Rashtriya Swayamsevak Sangh, he is a good speaker inspired by the life and teachings of Swami Vivekananda.

P. V. NARASIMHA RAO, former Prime Minister of India and a seasoned Parliamentarian. He is a good writer and his *Insider* is a modified Autobiography.

PROF. D. S. SARMA , a well-known educationist and teacher of English in the first half of the century, he was the first Principal of the Vivekananda College, Madras. An ardent devotee of Sri Ramakrishna-Vivekananda, he has written about them, and his works include The *Hindu Renaissance.* His *A Primer of Hinduism,* teaches the tenets of the Hindu religion to the younger generation in the form of questions and answers.

H. V. SESHADRI is a senior dedicated worker and the former General Secretary of the Rashtriya Swayamsevak Sangh. An inspiring speaker in Kannada, Hindi and English, he is also a prolific writer, and has several books to his credit, both in Kannada and English.

DR. SHANKAR DAY.AL SHARMA, the former President of India, he was a man of letters and a distinguished scholar in Hindi and Sanskrit. Unlike other politicians of his time, he was deeply imbued with and grounded in Hindu religion and spirituality.

S. J., the Compiler-Editor of this volume.

DR. JOHN W. SPELLMAN, formerly Head of the Asian Cultures Institute, Windsor University, Oratorio, Canada.

ARNOLD TOYNBE , English Historian best known for his comparative study of civilizations. His major work, *A Study of History* (1934-54) was published in ten volumes. He was an ardent student of Sri Ramakrishna-Vivekananda.

GENERAL INDEX
(For the Chronicle)

Instructions:

The General Index commencing in the next page enables easy and immediate location of any desired information contained in the Chronicle. Before consulting it please note the following:-

1. In the Index, page numbers have been substituted by the year, month and date in order to make it easier to locate the entry about the events, place, person or subject in the Chronicle.

2. Every entry in the Index is followed by year, month and date (e.g. 'Abolition of slavery in U. S. A., 1865 Dec. 18') indicating thereby that, for details, reference should be made to that particular year, month and date in the Chronicle.

3. Where the date of an event is not known, only the year and month are mentioned (e.g. 'Anti-sepsis, method of, 1877 Oct.'); where even the month is not known, only the year is mentioned.

4. Where the months and dates of more than one event transpiring in the same year could not be indicated, a letter of the alphabet (in brackets) has been appended to the year to enable identification and location, e.g. 'Alasinga, 1863 (c)'.

5. The General Index is followed by a Subject Index which provides, in a short compass, different particulars of kindred nature scattered in the Chronicle. But to locate the details thereof in the Chronicle, the General Index may be consulted (e.g. under the head 'Political Events', one of the entries is: 'All India National Congress'. On consulting the General Index it will be seen that reference thereto has been made against the entry under 1883 Dec. 28-30 in the Chronicle).

GENERAL INDEX

(see instructions)

Anti-sepsis, method of,1877 Oct. Antiseptic surgery, 1865 (c), 1895 Sep. 28

Anubis, The, 1903 Feb.

Appeal Avalanche, 1894 Jan. 16, 1894 Jan. 21

Appearance and Reality, 1893 (j)

Apollo Bunder, 1893 Feb. (a)

Arabs, 1894 Feb.' 16

Arc lamp, 1879 (i)

Arc-welding, 1886 (f)

Arctic region, 1863 (j)

Argon, 1894 (d)

Arrhenius, Svante Aug., 1887 (d)

Armat, Thomas, 1889 (h)

Armour and Co., 1901 (f)

Arnold, Matthew, 1888 Apr. 15

Arnold, Sir Edwin, 1879 (c), 1886 (o), 1894 Sep. 25, 1885 (j)

Art Institute, Chicago,1893 Sep. 11

Artificial silk, 1883 (f), 1902 (c)

Arya Dharma, 1894 Sep. 5

Arya Samaj:
1869 (a), 1873 (a), 1874 Jun. 12, 1875 Apr. 10, 1883 Oct. 30, 1897 Nov. 5-15

Aryan invasion of India, Theory of, 1866 Apr. 10

Aryans, 1866 Apr. 10

Aryavarta, 1897 Sep. 10, 1897 Nov. 5-15

Asceticism, 1902 Jul. 9 (a)

Ashrams, 1896 (m), 1899 Mar. 19, 1902 Jul. 10 (b)

Asia,
1869 Nov. 17, 1878 (c), 1888 (early part), 1894 Feb. 18 (a), 1895 Jul., 1897 Jan. 23, 1896 (f), 1898 Sep. 30

Asia's Message to Europe, 1883 (a)

Asiatist, ardent, 1882 Apr. 27

Aspirin, 1899 (d)

Association of Christian Businessmen, 1898 (m)

Asthma, 1901 (f)

Astronautics, works on, 1895 (g)

Astrophysics, theoretical, 1877 Sep.11, 1888 Dec. 28,

Atman, 1896 Mar. 28, 1896 Apr. 2, 1897 Nov. 12

Atma-vichara, 1879 Dec. 30

Atlantic, 1866 Jul. 27; cable across, 1867(e); Ocean, Wireless signals across, 1895 (a), 1901 Dec. 12

Atlee, Clement, 1883 Jan. 23

Atomic
bomb, 1879 Mar. 14; dimension, 1900 Dec. 14; physics, 1885 Oct. 7; structure, 1897 (c); structure and radiation, 1885 Oct. 7; theory, 1885 Oct.7

Atoms,
first artificial splitting, 1871 Aug. 30; nuclear, 1871 Aug. 30; theory of, 1885 Oct. 7

'Atonement by proxy', 1894 Mar. 18

Audion, 1873 Aug. 26

Augsburg-Nuremburg Machine Tools Factory, 1895 (e)

Aurobindo, Sri:
1872 Aug. 15, 1874 Jan. 30,1879 (d), 1893 Feb. (a)

Australian continent, telegraphic lines across, 1872 (k)

Autochrome process, 1895 Mar. 22

Automatic
filler and capper, 1892 (d); electric signalling, 1872 (e)

Automobile, 1885 (b); electric, 1892 Sep.; the first, 1883 (e); the world's first successful, 1885 (b)

Aviation, 1896 (l)

Awakened India, 1896 June 14, 1896 June 14 (a)

Awards, International, 1896 Dec.10

A Week on the Concord and Merrimack Rivers, 1882 Apr. 27

Azad, Abul Kalam, 1888 (d)

Duplicating machine, 1888 (h)
Durant,
    Albert, 1878 (j); Will, 1885 Nov. 5
Durbar, 1885 Mar. 4, 1881 (b)
Duryea,
    Charles and Franklin, 1892 Sep.;
    Motor Wagon Co., 1896 (k)
Dutt,
    Babu Romesh Chandra, 1902 Jul.
    (d); NARENDRANATH, 1894
    Aug. 8 (a) 1902 Jul. (f)
Dvaita, 1895 Jun. 18-Aug. 7
*Dynamic Theory ot Electromagnetic
    Field,* 1864 (f)
Dynamite, 1866 (e), 1888 (g), 1901 (g)
Dynamo,
    1867 Aug. 25; improved, 1879 (i);
    industrial, 1872 (g)
Dysprosium, 1879 (q)

East,
    African highlands, 1884 (c); India
    Co, 1877 Jan. 1; 1900 Feb. 1, 1900
    Oct. 28, London Revival Society,
    1865 (a); and the West, 1897 Feb.,
    1902 Jul. (c)
Eastman,
    George, 1868 (b), 1884 (e),1888(i),
    1892 (b), 1895 (d); Kodak Co., 1884
    (e), 1893 (i), 1892 (b)
Eberthella typhi,1880 (d)
Eberth, Karl Joseph, 1880 (d)
ECG, 1887 (h)
Economic Depression in U. S. A,
    1892 (c)
Economic History of India, 1866 - 67
Economics, 1889 (j)
Eddington, Arthur S, 1882 Dec. 28
Eddy, Mary Baker, 1879 (c), 1886 (o)
    1894 Sep. 25,
Edison,
    Thomas Alva,1864 (e),1867 (d),
    1877 Nov. 29, 1878 (h), 1882 (c),
    1883 (c), 1883 (d), 1889 (h), 1891

Dec. 29, 1893 (h), 1895 Mar. 22;
    Co., 1888 (f); Effect, 1883 (d)
Edourd, 1888 Oct. 31, 1893 (k)
Education
    Act, 1870 (b), 1886 Apr.. 6; Natio-
    nal system of, 1886 Apr. 6; Progre-
    ssive, 1898 (j); a process of accu-
    mulation and assimilation, 1898 (j);
    according to Tagore, 1901 Dec. 22;
    English, 1863 (b)
Educational Institutions in India,
    1902 Jan. 27
Edward VII, 1873 (h), 1901 Jan. 22
Eiffel,
    Alexandre Gustav, 1889 (l); Tower,
    1899 (l), 1889 (m)
Einhorn, N. O., 1896 (n)
Einstein, Albert, 1868 Mar. 28,
    1879 Mar. 14, 1896 Feb.(a)
Einthoven, Willem, 1887 (h)
Electric
    current, 1867 Aug. 25, 1878 (h),
    1897 (c); eyes, 1893 (d); fan, the
    world's first, 1882 (f); flat iron,
    1882 (f); generating system 1864
    (e); generator, Westinghouse, 1895
    Aug. 26; lamp, 1900 (i), 1864 (e);
    motor, 1867 Aug. 25, 1888 (f);
    power, the first commercial, 1895
    Aug. 26; signal, automatic, 1872 (e);
    signal, station, 1864 (e), 1867 (e);
    street car, 1874 (d); trolly, the
    world's first, 1885 (g), typewriter,
    1867 (d); vacuum cleaner, 1901 (i);
    vision, 1897 (e);
Electrical system, 1883 (c); waves, 1894
    (a)
Electricity
    drew machinery for the first time,
    1873 (c); used to draw locomotive
    for the first time, 1879 (a); and
    Magnetism, 1879 Nov. 5, 1867 Aug.
    25
Electric System, world's first public,
    1882 (e)

16, 1898 Jun., 1899 Jan., 1902 Jul.
6 (a), 1902 Jul. 10 (a), 1902 Jul. 13
(b), 1902 Jul. 25 (a), 1902 Jul. (h),
1902 Aug. (a); completed *Tantrika
sadhana*, 1863 (a); initiated into
sannyas by Totapuri, 1864 (a);
attained *nirvikalpa samadhi*, 1864
(a); in *advaita* plane for six months,
1866 (a); practised Islam, 1866 (b);
worshipped his wife as the Divine
Mother, 1872 May; met Swami
Dayananda, 1873 (a); his remarks
about Dayananda, 1873 (a);
practised Christianity, 1874 Nov.;
met Keshabchandra Sen, 1875 Mar.,
1884 Jan.; and Brahmo Samaj, 1878
(a); first publication of the Sayings
of, 1878 (a); and '*Nava Vidhan*',
1881 Jan. 25; NARENDRA heard
about, 1881; NARENDRA saw at
Calcutta, first time, 1881 Nov.; and
N A R E N D R A N A T H a t
Dakshineswar, 1881 Dec.; met
Ishwarchandra Vidyasagar, 1882
Aug. 5; his reaction on hearing
Keshab's death, 1884 Jan.; with
Bankim, 1884 Dec.; showered
grace on his disciples, his powerful
touch, 1886 Jan.1; rebuked
NARENDRANATH, 1886; 'locks'
NARENDRANATH'S spiritual
experience, 1886; 'NARENDRA
would pass away of his own will',
1886; undergoing treatment at
Cossipore Garden House, 1886
Apr.; initiated NARENDRA with
Ramamantra, 1886 Apr.; '*Avatar* of
Rama and Krishna',1886 Aug.;
transmitted spiritual powers to
NARENDRANATH ,1886Aug.;
entered *Mahasamadhi*, 1886
Aug.16; the power, 1886 Aug.16;
VIVEKANANDA had the vision
of, 1890 Feb.4; VIVEKANANDA

presented to his American stud-
ents for the first time a vivid picture
of, 1895 Jun. 18-Aug. 7;
VIVEKANANDA speaks to Max
Muller about, 1896 May 28; *A Real
Mahat-man,* 1896 May 28; The life
and Sayings of, 1896 May 28
RAMAKRISHNA MATH, 1898 Dec.
9, 1899 Apr., 1896 Jun. 27, 1896
Jul. 9; first branch at Madras, 1897
Mar. 17
RAMAKRISHNA MISSION
1892 Dec., 1897 May 1, 1898 Dec.
9, 1899 Apr. 30, 1901 Dec.; 1902
Mar. 22, 1902 Jul. 6, 1902 Jul. 7 (a),
1902 Jul. 10, 1902 Jul. 10 (b), 1902
Jul. 13 (a), 1902 Jul. (c), 1902 Jul.
(k); aims and ideals of, 1897 May1
RAMAKRISHNA MOVEMENT,
1898 Dec. 9.
RAMAKRISHNA ORDER, 1898 Dec.
9; president of, 1902 Jul. (k)
RAMAKRISHNA-VIVEKANANDA,
the prophets of New India, 1866
Jan. 29
RAMAKRISHNA'S DISCIPLES, 1902
Oct. 26
RAMAKRISHNANANDA, SWAMI,
1897 Feb. 6 (b), 1897 Mar. 17,
1897Apr. 5, 1902 Jul. 25 (a)
Ramalingam, Swami, 1874 Jan. 30
Ramamantra, 1886 Apr.
Ramana Maharshi, 1879 Dec. 30
Raman, C. V., 1888 Nov. 7
Raman Effect, 1888 Nov. 7
Ramanuja, 1895 Jun. 18-Aug. 7; 1896
Mar. 28, 1899 Apr., 1899 May,
1899 Jun. 25
Ramanujan, Srinivasa, 1887 Dec. 22
Ramatirtha, Swami, 1873 Oct. 22, 1897
Nov. 12, 1900 Jan. 1
Rameswaram, VIVEKANANDA at,
1897 Jan. 27
Ramlal, 1886 Jan. 1

SUBJECT INDEX

(Chronicle)

This Index provides, in a short compass, different particulars of kindred nature scattered in the Chronicle, such as: Political Events of the period (1863-1902); Social, Political, Religious and Cultural Organizations; Researches; Educational and Philanthropic Activities; Enterprises; Explorations and Expeditions; Transport and Communication; 'Firsts'; prominent Publications; Indian and Foreign Contemporaries; Inventors and Discoverers; Inventions and Discoveries etc. But to locate the details thereof in the Chronicle, the body of the 'GENERAL INDEX' may be consulted.

Political Events:

Abolition of slavery in U. S. A.
All India National Conference
American Civil War
Annexation of Tanganyika and
    Zanzibar by Germany
Annexation of Zululand by Britain.
Anglo-Burmese War
Assassination of U. S. President
    Garfield
Assassination of U. S. President
    McKinley
Assassination of Russian Czar
    Alexander II
Battle of Gettysburg
Battle of Manilla Bay
Battle of Solferino
Boer Struggle for Independence
Bombardment of Alexandria
Delhi Durbar
First session of Indian National
    Congress
Franco-Prussian War
Ganapathi festival
Hay Market massacre
Native Marriage Act
Paris under seige
Rendition of Mysore
Shivaji festival

Sino-Japanese War
South African War (Boer War)
Spanish-American War
Vernacular Press Act
War of Pacific
Zulu War

Organizations, Social and Political:

All-England Croquet Club
American Federation of Labour
Bernardo Homes
Central National Muslim Association
Fabian Society
First Socialist International
First Women's Suffrage Committee
Gideons International
Indian Association
Indian National Congress
Ku Klux Klan
Labour Party
League of Struggle
National Society
Red Cross
Salvation Army
Second Socialist International
Society for the Promotion of National
    Feeling among the Educated Natives
    of Bengal
United Patriotic Association
Upper India Muslim Defence Association

Railway between Punjab and Delhi

St. Gotthard Tunnel

Suez Canal

Telegraph line across Australia

Trans-continental Railway

Trans-Siberian Railway

'Firsts':

The first rigid frame motor-driven airship

The first automobile by Daimler

The first comprehensive work on Bacteriology

The first operation for the removal of a brain tumour

The first light-weight all metal bicycle

The first large scale manufacture of safety bicycle

The first recorded bicycle race

The first College for women

The first major conflict between two nations

The first solo circumnavigation of earth

The first simple, inexpensive camera

The first central power station

The first cellulose fibre

The first synchronous census in India

The first all-India Census (not synchronous)

The first Diptheria antitoxin

The first human application of the Diptheria vaccine

The first Employer's Liability Act

The first dynamo

The first demonstration of the existence of electromagnetic waves

The first flight of a mechanically propelled flying machine

The first manned, powered flight in a heavier-than-air machine

The first vacuum flask

The first gasoline engine

The first Governor General of India

The first incandescent lamp

The first session of the Indian National Congress

The first Library School in U. S. A

The first direct casting Linotype

The first newspaper to use Linotype

The first gasoline-engined motorcycle to appear publicly

The first motor car of Henry Ford

The first International championship for motor car race

The first electromagnetic motor

The first motor cycle

The first Hague Peace Conference

The first pearl farm

The first man-made plastic

The first production of the photograph taken with artificial light

Pneumatic tyres were first applied to vehicles

Electricity was used to draw railroad locomotive for the first time

The first photographic reproduction in newspaper

The first trichromatic half-tone process printing plates

The first motor car to be equipped with pneumatic tyres

The first laboratory devoted to entirely. experimental psychology

The first course in psychology in U. S. A

The first transmission of radio-signals across the Atlantic

The first of a series of racing cars

The first recording of human voice

The first submarine

The first administration of the anti-rabies vaccine

The first electric sewing machine

The first modern submarine

The first sun photography

The first complete steel frame structure,

The first public stage in Calcutta

The first Womens Suffrage Committee

Papers:

Contemporaries and Near-Contemporaries (Indian) :

Saints and Savants

Inventions and Discoveries:

Transport and Communication
Internal Combustion Petrol engine
Diesel engine
Highspeed engine
Gas Engine
Improved Carburettor
Flatfeed Carburettor
Automobile
Electric automobile
Electrie street Car
Electric Locomotive
Airbrake
Automatic airbrake
Automatic Electric signalling
    for railroads
Electric trolley
Motor trolley
Motor cycle
Safety Bicycle
Pneumatic Rubber tyre
Petrol tractor
Submarine
Torpedo
Steam turbine
Multistage steam turbine
Rigidframe airship
Model Airplane with an internal
    combustion engine
Radar
Telephone
Coin-operated telephone
Automatic system of telephone
Telephone transmitter
Multiple Switch board
Photophone
Telegraph
Automatic Telegraph repeater
Receiver for submarine Telegraph
Morse code
Wireless telegraph

Electrical
Electron
Fluorescent lamp
Incandescent electric lamp
Mercury-vapour electric lamp
Arc lamp
Induction motor
Electric Motor (A/C)
Central Power Station
A/C electric system
Single phase, high voltage A/C system
Tesla coil (Transformer)
Improved dynamo
Industrial dynamo
Copper Oxide battery
Electric Flat iron
Electric Fan
System of Arc Welding
Gas mantle
Escalator
Phenomenon of electromagnetic
    induction
Principle of rotary magnetic field
Principle of clectrir motor

Photography
Roll film
Kodak box camera
Brownie box camera
Graflex camera
Colour photograph
Bakelite
Celluloid
Velox

Audio-visual
Peepshow machine
Vitascope
Cinematograph
Cathode-ray tube
Rotating scanning disk
Audion
Phonograph